OXFORD MEDICAL PUBLICATIONS

Osteoarthritis

Dedication

This book is dedicated to our patients with osteoarthritis

Osteoarthritis

Edited by

KENNETH D. BRANDT

Professor of Medicine and Head,
Rheumatology Division,
Indiana University School of Medicine,
Indianapolis, USA

MICHAEL DOHERTY

Professor of Rheumatology,
University of Nottingham Medical School,
Nottingham, UK

and

L. STEFAN LOHMANDER

Professor in Orthopaedics,
University Hospital, Lund, Sweden

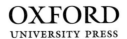

OXFORD

UNIVERSITY PRESS

OXFORD

UNIVERSITY PRESS

Great Clarendon Street, Oxford OX2 6DP

Oxford University Press is a department of the University of Oxford.
It furthers the University's objective of excellence in research, scholarship,
and education by publishing worldwide in

Oxford New York

Athens Auckland Bangkok Bogotá Buenos Aires Calcutta
Cape Town Chennai Dar es Salaam Delhi Florence Hong Kong Istanbul
Karachi Kuala Lumpur Madrid Melbourne Mexico City Mumbai
Nairobi Paris São Paulo Singapore Taipei Tokyo Toronto Warsaw

with associated companies in Berlin Ibadan

Oxford is a registered trade mark of Oxford University Press
in the UK and in certain other countries

Published in the United States
by Oxford University Press Inc., New York

A catalogue record for this book is available from the British Library

Library of Congress Cataloging in Publication Data
Osteoarthritis/edited by Kenneth D. Brandt, Michael Doherty, and
L. Stefan Lohmander.
(Oxford medical publications)
Includes bibliographical references and index.
1. Osteoarthritis.   I. Brandt, Kenneth D.   II. Doherty, M., M.D.
III. Lohmander, Stefan.   IV. Series.
[DNLM: 1. Osteoarthritis.   WE 348 08458 1998]
RC931.0670866   1998   616.7'223—dc21   97-11747
ISBN 0 19 262735 X

Printed in Great Britain
on acid-free paper by
The Bath Press, Bath

Contents

Acknowledgments

The efficient and highly competent secretarial support which the editors received from Joanna Ramowski in Nottingham and Anne Ekman in Lund is hugely appreciated; without their efforts this book would not have seen the light of day. Kathie Lane, in Indianapolis, has our gratitude for her initiative, energy, and professionalism in working with the editors, authors on both sides of the Atlantic, and representatives of Oxford University Press. Without her skill in tracking those chapters which seemed to be in limbo, we could not have met our deadlines.

Preface

A number of exciting new developments make it highly desirable, at this time, to summarize the large body of knowledge related to the etiopathogenesis and management of osteoarthritis. For years, many primary care physicians and, indeed, many rheumatologists have considered osteoarthritis to be a boring condition for which they had little to offer patients. Osteoarthritis has been viewed by physicians and surgeons, erroneously, as an inevitable consequence of aging or repetitive usage of a joint and a condition which, once it becomes symptomatic, progresses inexorably. Doctors and allied health professionals have conveyed these misconceptions and oversimplifications to millions of patients. Consider the nihilism, pessimism, and futility engendered in those patients by such remarks!

But things are changing — and changing rapidly. Our understanding of mechanisms underlying the breakdown of articular cartilage in osteoarthritis has grown greatly in the past several years — perhaps to an even greater extent than our awareness that osteoarthritis is not a disease simply of cartilage, but of an organ, the diarthrodial joint. Osteoarthritis represents failure of the joint. It may be due in some instances to a primary abnormality in the articular cartilage, but in other cases the initial problem resides in the underlying bone, the synovium, the supporting ligaments, or the neuromuscular system. The section of this book dealing with the pathogenesis of osteoarthritis is written from this perspective.

Exciting new evidence from studies of animal models has made it apparent that the development and progression of osteoarthritis may be prevented or retarded pharmacologically. Clinical trials of such therapy have already been initiated in humans. The next several years will surely witness further progress with regard to the development of disease-modifying drugs for osteoarthritis and methodologies for their evaluation. A significant component of this book is, therefore, devoted to a discussion of the pharmacologic modification of tissue damage in osteoarthritis and to the outcome measures available for assessment of this effect.

Meanwhile, as prospects increase for the development of drugs that may modify tissue damage in osteoarthritis, a sea change is occurring in treatment of the symptoms of this disease. Although, in overwhelming numbers, physicians prescribe nonsteroidal anti-inflammatory drugs for patients with osteoarthritis, recognition is growing that, in many patients, comparable symptomatic relief may be achieved with analgesics that have no effect on inflammatory processes — or, indeed, with non-pharmacologic measures, such as physical therapy and psychosocial interventions.

It is being recognized increasingly that optimal management of osteoarthritis requires a comprehensive program involving drugs and non-medicinal components and, in some cases, surgery. Sections on both non-surgical and surgical therapy are contained within Chapter 9, 'Management of Osteoarthritis'. The decision to organize the material in this fashion reflects, in part, an attempt to avoid perpetuation of the notion that medical management is 'conservative', while surgery is 'radical' therapy. Indeed, the opposite is often true — that is, to withhold surgery from the patient with advanced disease who suffers daily from joint pain and becomes increasingly deconditioned may, in fact, be the 'radical' approach; it may be much more conservative to operate. Rather, for each patient, the full range of treatments — physical, pharmacologic, surgical, supportive — must be considered and the right blend chosen by the skilled physician working with the patient. Maintenance of sharp boundaries between various therapeutic modalities merely perpetuates our narrow-minded biases.

It is important to acknowledge that significant differences often exist between the perception of the patient and that of the physician with regard to what is important in treating the osteoarthritis in that individual, and to recognize that this dichotomy represents a barrier to optimal care. And, given the sharper focus on the treatment of disease processes as well as of symptoms in this disease, it is obvious that valid, simple, reliable, and inexpensive outcome measures are needed for optimal evaluation of both. Accordingly, sections of the text deal specifically with outcome measures related to joint pain and function, on the one hand, and to changes in joint pathology on the other. Furthermore, the Appendices provide a compilation of commonly employed instruments for assessment of such outcomes.

This book is written principally for the clinical rheumatologist, although primary care physicians, orthopedic surgeons, allied health professionals, basic researchers, members of the pharmaceutical industry who are involved in drug research and development, and regulatory agency staff also should find it useful. The high prevalence of osteoarthritis — which will become even greater in the next several years because of the increasing 'greying' of the population — assures that primary care physicians and specialists in musculoskeletal disease, in every developed country, will continue to see large numbers of patients with osteoarthritis. A review of the current understanding of the management of this disorder and of the basic mechanisms involved in its etiopathogenesis provides the rationale for publication of this book, whose contributing authors include experts on osteoarthritis from both shores of the Atlantic.

Indianapolis, USA   K.D.B.
Nottingham, UK   M.D.
Lund, Sweden   L.S.L.
September 1997

List of contributors

Altman, Roy D; Department of Medicine, University of Miami and Miami Veterans Affairs, Miami, FL, USA

Ayral, Xavier; Clinique de Rhumatologie, Hopital Cochin, Université René Descartes, Paris, France

Barton, Rebecca; Graduate Programs in Occupational Therapy, University of Indianapolis, Indianapolis, IN, USA

Bayliss, Michael; Department of Veterinary Basic Sciences, The Royal Veterinary College, London, UK

Bellamy, Nicholas; Department of Medicine, Epidemiology, and Biostatistics, University of Western Ontario, London, Ontario, Canada

Billingham, Michael EJ; Rheumatology Unit, University of Bristol, Bristol, UK

Bradley, John D; Department of Medicine, Indiana University School of Medicine, Indianapolis, IN, USA

Brandt, Kenneth D; Division of Rheumatology, Indiana University School of Medicine, Indianapolis, IN, USA

Buckland-Wright, J Christopher; Division of Anatomy and Cell Biology, UMDS of Guy's & St Thomas's Hospitals, London, UK

Buckwalter, Joseph; Department of Orthopaedic Surgery, The University of Iowa, Iowa City, IA, USA

Burr, David; Departments of Anatomy and Orthopaedic Surgery, Indiana University School of Medicine, Indianapolis, IN, USA

Buschmann, Michael D; Biomedical Engineering Institute, Ecole Polytechnique, Canada

Caldwell, David S; Division of Rheumatology and Immunology, Department of Medicine, Duke University Medical Center, Durham, NC, USA

Cooper, Cyrus; MRC Epidemiology Unit, Southampton General Hospital, University of Southampton, Southampton, UK

Cushnaghan, Janet; Rheumatology Department, Hereford County Hospital, Hereford, UK

Dennison, Elaine; MRC Environmental Epidemiology Unit, Southampton General Hospital, University of Southampton, Southampton, UK

Dexter, Phyllis A; Indiana University School of Nursing, Center for Research, Indianapolis, IN, USA

Doherty, Michael; Rheumatology Unit, Nottingham City Hospital, Nottingham, UK

Doherty, Niall S; Central Research Division, Pfizer Inc, Groton, CT, USA

Edwards, Jo; Department of Rheumatology, Arthur Stanley House, London, UK

Feinburg, Judy; Department of Orthopaedic Surgery, Indiana Unviersity School of Medicine, Indianapolis, IN, USA

Felson, David; Boston University Arthritis Center and the Department of Medicine at Boston City and Boston University Medical Center Hospital, Boston, MA, USA

Flores, Raymond; Department of Medicine, University of Maryland School of Medicine, Baltimore, MD, USA

Forster, Susan; Rheumatology Department, Hereford County Hospital, Hereford, UK

Garcia, A Minerva; Departments of Electrical and Mechanical Engineering, MIT, Cambridge, MA, USA

Griffin, Marie R; Departments of Preventive Medicine & Medicine, Vanderbilt University School of Medicine, Nashville, TN, USA

Griffiths, RJ; Central Research Division, Pfizer Inc, Groton, CT, USA

Grodzinsky, Alan J; Departments of Electrical and Mechanical Engineering, Massachusetts Institute of Technology, Cambridge, MA, USA

Hadler, Nortin M; Department of Medicine, University of North Carolina at Chapel Hill School of Medicine, Chapel Hill, NC, USA

Hart, Deborah J; Department of Rheumatology, St Thomas' Hospital, London, UK

Hayes, John R; Delivery System, St. Vincent Hospitals and Health Services, Indianapolis, IN, USA

Heinegård, Dick; Department of Cell and Molecular Biology, University of Lund, Lund, Sweden

Hochberg, Marc; Departments of Medicine and Epidemiology and Preventive Medicine, University of Maryland School of Medicine, Baltimore, MD, USA

Howell, David S; Geriatric Research, Education and Clinical Center, Miami Veterans Affairs Medical Center, Miami, FL, USA

Hunziker, Ernst B; ME Müller Institute for Biomechanics, University of Bern, Switzerland

Ike, Robert W; Department of Internal Medicine, University of Michigan Medical Center, Ann Arbor, MI, USA

Jewell, Frank M; Department of Clinical Radiology, Gloucestershire Royal Hospital, Gloucester, UK

Jimenez, Sergio A; Departments of Medicine, Biochemistry and Molecular Biology, and Radiology, Jefferson Medical College, Thomas Jefferson University, Philadelphia, PA, USA

Jones Adrian C; Rheumatology Unit, Nottingham City Hospital, Nottingham, UK

Karasick, David; Departments of Medicine, Biochemistry and Molecular Biology, and Radiology, Jefferson Medical College, Thomas Jefferson University, Philadelphia, PA, USA

Kashikar-Zuck, Susmita; Pain Management Program, Department of Psychiatry and Behavioral Sciences, Duke University Medical Center, Durham, NC, USA

Keefe, Francis J; Pain Management Program, Duke University Medical Center, Durham, NC, USA

Kim, Young-Jo; Department of Orthopaedic Surgery, Harvard Medical School, Boston, USA

Knutson, Kaj; Department of Orthopaedics, University Hospital, Lund, Sweden

Lark, Michael W; Department of Immunology and Inflammation Research, Merck Research Laboratories, Rahway, NJ, USA

Liang, H Matthew; Department of Medicine, Harvard Medical School, Brigham & Women's Hospital, Boston, MA, USA

Lidgren, Lars; Department of Orthopaedics, University Hospital, Lund, Sweden

Lohmander, L Stefan; Department of Orthopedics, University Hospital, Lund, Sweden

Lorenzo, Pilar; Department of Cell and Molecular Biology, Lund University, Lund, Sweden

Lorig, Kate; Stanford University, Palo Alto, CA, USA

Mazzuca, Steven A; Rheumatology Division, Indiana University School of Medicine, Indianapolis, IN, USA

Mow, Van C; Department of Orthopaedic Surgery, Columbia University, New York, NY, USA

Myers, Stephen; Rheumatology Division, Indiana University School of Medicine, Indianapolis, IN, USA

O'Reilly, Sheila; Rheumatology Unit, Nottingham City Hospital, Nottingham, UK

Peterfy, Charles; Musculoskeletal Radiology, University of California, San Francisco, CA, USA

Pettifer, ER; Central Research Division, Pfizer Inc, Groton, CT, USA

Pritzker, Kenneth PH; Department of Pathology and Laboratory Medicine, Mount Sinai Hospital, Toronto, Ontario, Canada

Quinn, Thomas M; ME Mueller Institute for Biomechanics, University of Bern, Switzerland

Ray, Wayne A; Vanderbilt Unviersity of School of Medicine, Nashville, TN, USA

Rivest, Charles (deceased); University of Montreal, Notre Dame Hospital, Montreal, Canada

Rogers, Juliet; Bristol Royal Infirmary, Bristol, UK

Sandy, John; Shriners Hospital, Tampa, FL, USA

Schauwecker, Donald; Department of Radiology and Nuclear Medicine, Indiana University School of Medicine and Wishard Memorial Hospital, Indianapolis, IN, USA

Schumacher, Ralph H Jr; Arthritis & Immunology Center, Philadelphia, PA, USA

Setton, Lori A; Department of Biomedical Engineering, Duke University, Durham, NC, USA

Spector, Tim D; Department of Rheumatology, St Thomas' Hospital, London, UK

Tyler, Jenny; Strangeways Research Laboratory, Cambridge, UK

van Beuningen, Henk M; Department of Rheumatology, University Hospital, Nijmegen, The Netherlands

van den Berg, Wim; Department of Rheumatology, University Hospital, Nijmegen, The Netherlands

van der Kraan, Peter M; Department of Rheumatology, University Hospital, Nijmegen, The Netherlands

Vilensky, Joel A; Indiana University School of Medicine, Fort Wayne, IN, USA

Watt, Iain; Department of Clinical Radiology, Bristol Royal Infirmary, Bristol, UK

Weinberger, Morris; Roudebusch VA MC, Indianapolis, IN, USA

Williams, Charlene J; Departments of Medicine, Biochemistry and Molecular Biology, and Radiology, Jefferson Medical College, Thomas Jefferson University, Philadelphia, PA, USA

Yelin, Edward; Arthritis Research Group, University of California, San Francisco, CA, USA

1 | Definition and classification of osteoarthritis

Raymond H. Flores and Marc C. Hochberg

Osteoarthritis (OA), formerly referred to as osteo-arthrosis and degenerative joint disease, is the most common form of arthritis[1,2]. Prior to 1986, no standard definition of OA existed; most authors described OA as a disorder of unknown etiology in which articular cartilage and subchondral bone were primarily affected — in contrast to rheumatoid arthritis, which primarily affects the synovial membrane. In 1986, the Subcommittee on Osteoarthritis of the American College of Rheumatology Diagnostic and Therapeutic Criteria Committee, proposed the following definition of OA: 'A heterogeneous group of conditions that lead to joint symptoms and signs which are associated with defective integrity of articular cartilage, in addition to related changes in the underlying bone at the joint margins.'[3].

A more comprehensive definition of OA was developed at a conference on the Etiopathogenesis of Osteoarthritis sponsored by the National Institute of Arthritis, Diabetes, Digestive and Kidney Diseases, the National Institute on Aging, the American Academy of Orthopedic Surgeons, the National Arthritis Advisory Board, and the Arthritis Foundation[4]. This definition summarizes the clinical, pathophysiologic, biochemical, and biomechanical changes that characterize OA:

Clinically, the disease is characterized by joint pain, tenderness, limitation of movement, crepitus, occasional effusion, and variable degrees of local inflammation, but without systemic effects. Pathologically, the disease is characterized by irregularly distributed loss of cartilage more frequently in areas of increased load, sclerosis of subchondral bone, subchondral cysts, marginal osteophytes, increased metaphyseal blood flow, and variable synovial inflammation. Histologically, the disease is characterized early by fragmentation of the cartilage surface, cloning of chondrocytes, vertical clefts in the cartilage, variable crystal deposition, remodeling, and eventual violation of the tidemark by blood vessels. It is also characterized by evidence of repair, particularly in osteophytes, and later by total loss of cartilage, sclerosis, and focal osteonecrosis of the subchondral bone. Biomechanically, the disease is characterized by alteration of the tensile, compressive, and shear properties and hydraulic permeability of the

cartilage, increased water, and excessive swelling. These cartilage changes are accompanied by increased stiffness of the subchondral bone. Biochemically, the disease is characterized by reduction in the proteoglycan concentration, possible alterations in the size and aggregation of proteoglycans, alteration in collagen fibril size and weave, and increased synthesis and degradation of matrix macromolecules.

A more recent definition was developed in 1994 at a workshop entitled 'New Horizons in Osteoarthritis' sponsored by the American Academy of Orthopedic Surgeons, the National Institute of Arthritis, Musculoskeletal and Skin Diseases, the National Institute on Aging, the Arthritis Foundation, and the Orthopaedic Research and Education Foundation[5]. This definition underscores the concept that OA may not represent a single disease entity:

Osteoarthritis is a group of overlapping distinct diseases, which may have different etiologies but with similar biologic, morphologic, and clinical outcomes. The disease processes not only affect the articular cartilage, but involve the entire joint, including the subchondral bone, ligaments, capsule, synovial membrane, and periarticular muscles. Ultimately, the articular cartilage degenerates with fibrillation, fissures, ulceration, and full thickness loss of the joint surface.

Classification of osteoarthritis

OA, as noted above, is a disorder of diverse etiologies which affects both small and large joints, either singly or in combination. A classification schema for OA developed at the 'Workshop on Etiopathogenesis of Osteoarthritis' is shown in Table 1.1[4]. Idiopathic OA is divided into two forms: localized or generalized; the latter represents the form of OA described by Kellgren and Moore involving three or more joint groups[6]. Hence, patients with OA localized to the hands but involving three joint groups, that is distal and proximal interphalangeal joints and the thumb base, would be classified as having idiopathic generalized OA.

Table 1.1 Classification of osteoarthritis[*]

I   Idiopathic
   A   Localized
       1   Hands: e.g. Heberden's and Bouchard's nodes (nodal), erosive interphalangeal arthritis (non-nodal), carpal-1st
           metacarpal
       2   Feet: e.g. hallux valgus, hallux rigidus, contracted toes (hammer/cockup toes), talonavicular
       3   Knee: (a) medial compartment; (b) lateral compartment; (c) patello-femoral compartment
       4   Hip: (a) eccentric (superior); (b) concentric (axial, medial); (c) diffuse (coxae senilis)
       5   Spine: (a) apophyseal joints; (b) intervertebral joints (discs); (c) spondylosis (osteophytes); (d) ligamentous
           (hyperostosis, Forestier's disease, DISH)
       6   Other single sites: e.g. glenohumeral, acromioclavicular, tibiotalar, sacroiliac, temporomandibular
   B   Generalized (GOA) includes three or more areas above (6)
II Secondary
   A   Trauma
       1   Acute
       2   Chronic (occupational, sports)
   B   Congenital or developmental diseases
       1   Localized diseases: e.g. Legg–Calve–Perthes, congenital hip dislocation, slipped epiphysis
       2   Mechanical factors: e.g. unequal lower extremity length, valgus/varus deformity, hypermobility syndromes
       3   Bone dysplasias: e.g. epiphyseal dysplasia, spondyloapophyseal dysplasia, osteonychondystrophy
   C   Metabolic diseases
       1   Ochronosis (alkaptonuria)
       2   Hemochromatosis
       3   Wilson's disease
       4   Gaucher's disease
   D   Endocrine diseases
       1   Acromegaly
       2   Hyperparathyroidism
       3   Diabetes mellitus
       4   Obesity
       5   Hypothyroidism
   E   Calcium deposition diseases
       1   Calcium pyrophosphate dihydrate deposition disease
       2   Apatite arthropathy
   F   Other bone and joint diseases
       1   Localized: e.g. fracture, avascular necrosis, infection, gout
       2   Diffuse: rheumatoid (inflammatory) arthritis, Paget's disease, osteopetrosis, osteochondritis
   G   Neuropathic (Charcot) arthropathy
   H   Endemic disorders
       1   Kashin–Beck
       2   Mseleni
   I   Miscellaneous conditions
       1   Frostbite
       2   Caisson's disease
       3   Hemoglobinopathies

[*] Reproduced from reference 4 with permission

Furthermore, generalized OA may occur with or without Heberden's and Bouchard's nodes, that is nodal and non-nodal forms.

Patients with an underlying disease which appears to have caused their OA are classified as having secondary OA. Some risk factors for idiopathic OA, for example chronic joint trauma from leisure and/or occupational activities, may be considered, alternatively, as causes of secondary OA (see Chapter 2). A detailed discussion of secondary OA can be found elsewhere[7].

Diagnostic criteria for osteoarthritis

Radiographic criteria

Classically, the diagnosis of OA in epidemiologic studies has relied on the characteristic radiographic changes described by Kellgren and Lawrence in 1957[8] and illustrated in the *Atlas of standard radiographs*[9]. These features include: (1) formation of osteophytes on the joint margins or in ligamentous attachments, as on the tibial spines; (2) periarticular ossicles, chiefly in relation to distal and proximal interphalangeal joints; (3) narrowing of the joint space associated with sclerosis of subchondral bone; (4) cystic areas with sclerotic walls situated in the subchondral bone; and (5) altered shape of the bone ends, particularly the head of the femur. Combinations of these changes considered together led to the development of an ordinal grading scheme for severity of radiographic features of OA: 0 = normal; 1 = doubtful; 2 = minimal; 3 = moderate; and 4 = severe. Different joints were graded using different characteristics; for the small joints of the hands, knees and hips these differences are summarized

in Tables 1.2–1.4 and illustrated in Fig 1.1–1.5 respectively.

Recently, potential limitations of the use of the Kellgren–Lawrence grading scale, as illustrated in the *Atlas on standard radiographs*, have been noted[10,11]. In an attempt to address the limitations of a global grading scale, several groups have developed radiographic grading schema which focus on individual radiographic features of OA at specific joint groups; reliable grading scales have now been published for the hand[12], hip[13,14], knee[15,16] and for all three of these peripheral joint groups[17].

Rating methods used in these scales for grading individual features are outlined in Tables 1.5–1.8 respect-

Table 1.2 Grades of severity of osteoarthritis in the small joints of the hands[*]

Distal interphalangeal joints:
Grade 1	Normal joint except for one minimal osteophyte.
Grade 2	Definite osteophytes at two points with minimal subchondral sclerosis and doubtful subchondral cysts, but good joint space and no deformity.
Grade 3	Moderate osteophytes, some deformity of bone ends and narrowing of joint space.
Grade 4	Large osteophytes and deformity of bone ends with loss of joint space, sclerosis and cysts.

Proximal interphalangeal joints:
Grade 1	Minimal osteophytosis at one point and possible cyst.
Grade 2	Definite osteophytes at two points and possible narrowing of joint space at one point.
Grade 3	Moderate osteophytes at many points, deformity of bone ends.
Grade 4	Large osteophytes, marked narrowing of joint space, subchondral sclerosis and slight deformity.

First carpometacarpal joint:
Grade 1	Minimal osteophytosis and possible cyst formation.
Grade 2	Definite osteophytes and possible cysts.
Grade 3	Moderate osteophytes, narrowing of joint space and subchondral sclerosis and deformity of bone ends.
Grade 4	Large osteophytes, severe sclerosis and narrowing of joint space.

[*] Modified from reference 9. Reproduced from Silman, A.J. and Hochberg, M.C. (1993). *Epidemiology of the rheumatic diseases*. Oxford University Press, Oxford.

Table 1.3 Grades of severity of osteoarthritis of the knee[*]

Grade 1	Doubtful narrowing of joint space and possible osteophytic lipping.
Grade 2	Definite osteophytes and possible narrowing of joint space.
Grade 3	Moderate multiple osteophytes, definite narrowing of joint space and some sclerosis and possible deformity of bone ends.
Grade 4	Large osteophytes, marked narrowing of joint space, severe sclerosis and definite deformity of bone ends.

[*] From reference 9. Reproduced from Silman, A.J. and Hochberg, M.C. (1993). *Epidemiology of the rheumatic diseases*. Oxford University Press, Oxford.

Table 1.4 Grades of severity of osteoarthritis of the hip[*]

Grade 1	Possible narrowing of joint space medially and possible osteophytes around femoral head.
Grade 2	Definite narrowing of joint space inferiorly, definite osteophytes and slight sclerosis.
Grade 3	Marked narrowing of joint space, slight osteophytes, some sclerosis and cyst formation and deformity of femoral head and acetabulum.
Grade 4	Gross loss of joint space with sclerosis and cysts, marked deformity of femoral head and acetabulum and large osteophytes.

[*] From reference 9. Reproduced from Silman, A.J. and Hochberg, M.C. (1993). *Epidemiology of the rheumatic diseases*. Oxford University Press, Oxford.

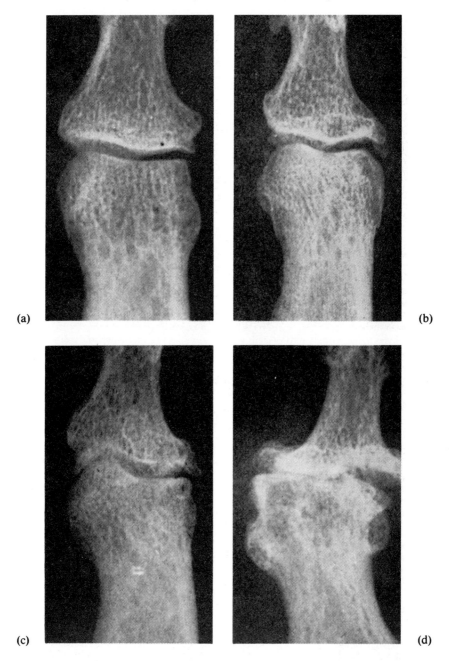

(a)

(b)

(c)

(d)

Fig. 1.1 Grades of severity of osteoarthritis of the distal interphalangeal joints. (a = Grade 1, b = Grade 2, c = Grade 3, d = Grade 4). Reproduced from Silman, A.J. and Hochberg, M.C. (1993). *Epidemiology of the rheumatic diseases*. Oxford University Press, Oxford.

ively. Using published atlases, trained readers have been shown to have excellent intra-reader and very good-to-excellent inter-reader reliability in measuring the presence and severity of OA of the hand, hip and knee; results of reproducibility studies have been reviewed recently by Hart and Spector[18] and Lane and Kremer[19].

The validity of using individual radiographic features and a revised composite grading scale has been demonstrated in several studies. Croft *et al.* examined the

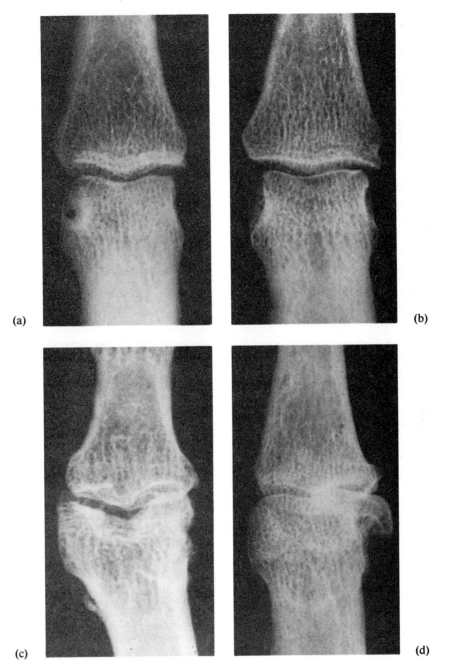

Fig. 1.2   Grades of severity of osteoarthritis of the proximal interphalangeal joints. (a = Grade 1, b = Grade 2, c = Grade 3, d = Grade 4). Reproduced from Silman, A.J. and Hochberg, M.C. (1993). *Epidemiology of the rheumatic diseases*. Oxford University Press, Oxford.

association of individual radiographic features of OA of the hip with reported hip pain in 759 men, 60–75 years of age, who had undergone intravenous urograms[13]. The radiographic feature most strongly asso-ciated with reported hip pain was joint space, at the narrowest point, measured in millimeters; in addition, an overall qualitative grade of 3 or higher (see Table 1.7) was strongly associated with reported hip pain.

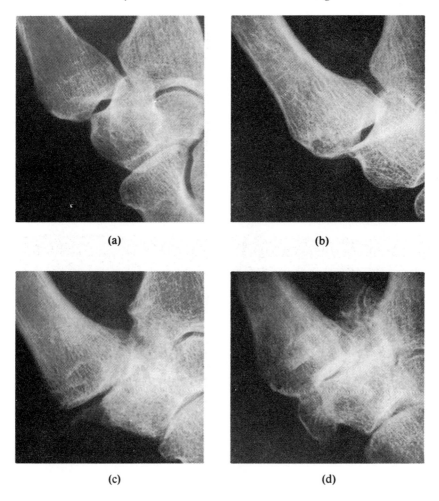

Fig. 1.3 Grades of severity of osteoarthritis of the first carpo-metacarpal joint. (a = Grade 1, b = Grade 2, c = Grade 3, d = Grade 4). Reproduced from Silman, A.J. and Hochberg, M.C. (1993). *Epidemiology of the rheumatic diseases*. Oxford University Press, Oxford.

These findings were subsequently confirmed by Scott *et al.* in an analysis of data from women age 65 and older, who had pelvic radiographs obtained at entry into the Study of Osteoporotic Fractures, a longitudinal epidemiologic study of risk factors for osteoporotic fractures[20]. Based on the validity of the association of individual radiographic features with hip pain, and the greater reliability of scoring individual features, as compared to the global Kellgren–Lawrence score[13,14], future population-based epidemiologic studies of OA of the hip should rely on the presence of individual radiographic features and modified global scales, rather than on the Kellgren–Lawrence grading scale, for classifying cases of OA of the hip.

Spector *et al.* examined the association of individual radiographic features of knee OA with reported knee pain in 977 women aged 45–64 years who were participants in the Chingford Study, a longitudinal study of musculoskeletal disease in women recruited from a single general practice in Chingford, East London, England[21]. They noted that, among the individual radiographic features of OA, a definite osteophyte in the medial compartment was most strongly associated with reported knee pain. The odds ratio for the association of grade 1–3 osteophytes with knee pain and the proportion of subjects with grade 1–3 osteophytes who had knee pain were both similar to those for Kellgren–Lawrence grade 2–4 changes.

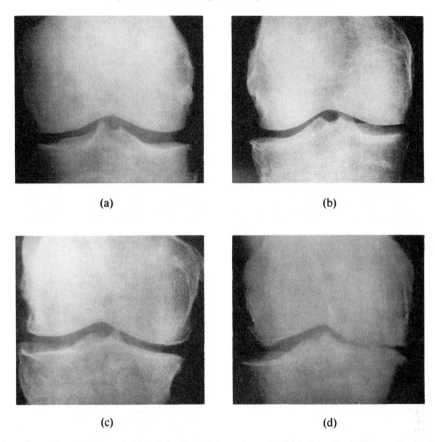

Fig. 1.4 Grades of severity of osteoarthritis of the knee joints. (a = Grade 1, b = Grade 2, c = Grade 3, d = Grade 4). Reproduced from Silman, Hochberg, M.C. (1993). *Epidemiology of the rheumatic diseases*. Oxford University Press, Oxford.

Table 1.5 Baltimore Longitudinal Study of Aging grading scale for osteoarthritis of the hand[*]

Feature	Grade	Definition
Osteophytes	0	None
	1	Small (definite) osteophyte
	2	Moderate osteophyte
	3	Large osteophyte
Joint space narrowing	0	None
	1	Mild definite narrowing
	2	Moderate-to-severe narrowing
	3	Bone-on-bone at > 1 point
Subchondral sclerosis	0	Absent
	1	Present
Subchondral cysts	0	Absent
	1	Present
Lateral deformity	0	Absent
	1	Present
Collapse	0	Absent
	1	Present

[*] Modified from reference 12.

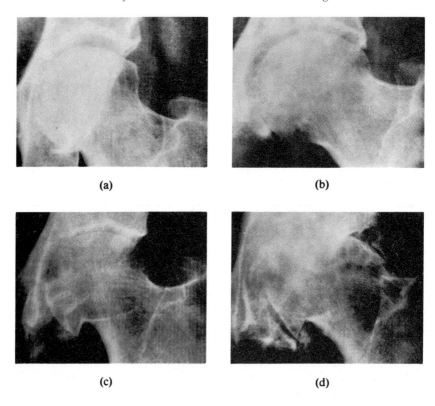

(a)   **(b)**

(c)   **(d)**

Fig. 1.5 Grades of severity of osteoarthritis of the hip joints. (a = Grade 1, b = Grade 2, c = Grade 3, d = Grade 4). Reproduced from Silman, A.J. and Hochberg, M.C. (1993). *Epidemiology of the rheumatic diseases*. Oxford University Press, Oxford.

Table 1.6 Baltimore Longitudinal Study of Aging grading scale for osteoarthritis of the knee[*]

Feature	Grade	Definition
Osteophytes	0	None
	1	Small (definite) osteophyte
	2	Moderate osteophyte
	3	Large osteophyte
Joint space narrowing	0	None
	1	Mild definite narrowing
	2	Moderate narrowing
	3	Severe narrowing
Subchondral sclerosis	0	Absent
	1	Present
Sharpening of tibial spine	0	Absent
	1	Present
Chondrocalcinosis	0	Absent
	1	Present

[*] Modified from reference 16.

In an analysis of data from the Baltimore Longitudinal Study on Aging, Lethbridge-Cejku *et al.* examined the association of individual radiographic features and the global Kellgren–Lawrence grade with reported knee pain among 452 men and 223 women, age 18 and older[22]. In support of the findings of Spector *et al.*[21], they found that the strength of the association of definite grade 1–3 osteophytes with

Table 1.7 Croft's overall qualitative grade of osteoarthritis of the hip*

Grade	Definition
0	No changes of osteoarthritis
1	Osteophytosis only
2	Joint space narrowing only
3	Two of osteophytosis, joint space narrowing, subchondral sclerosis, and cyst formation
4	Three of osteophytosis, joint space narrowing, subchondral sclerosis, and cyst formation
5	As in grade 4, but with deformity of femoral head

* Modified from reference 13.

Table 1.8 Study of Osteoporotic Fractures grading scale for osteoarthritis of the hip*

Grade	Definition
0	Normal film
1	Mild (grade 1) osteophyte and/or mild (grade 1) narrowing
2	Moderate (grade 2) narrowing and/or moderate-to-severe (grade 2–3) osteophyte
3	Severe (grade 3) narrowing and mild-severe (grade 1–3) osteophytes

* Modified from reference 14.

current knee pain was similar to that for grade 2 or higher OA, using the Kellgren–Lawrence scale; the odds ratios were 4.4 (95 per cent confidence intervals: 2.6, 7.5) and 4.8 (2.5, 8.5), respectively. This relationship was stronger, and remained consistent, among the more severe grades of OA: grade 2–3 osteophytes were associated with current knee pain with an odds ratio of 17.1 (7.5, 38.7), while a Kellgren–Lawrence grade of 3–4 was associated with current knee pain with an odds ratio of 20.8 (8.6, 50.4). Based on the validity of the association of individual radiographic features with knee pain, and the comparable reliability of scoring individual features and of grading OA severity by the global Kellgren–Lawrence scale, future population-based epidemiologic studies of OA of the knee could rely on either approach to classify cases.

Clinical criteria

As noted above, there are potential limitations to the use of only radiographic criteria for case definition, especially in clinical studies of OA. In particular, although a statistical association exists between radiographic changes of OA and reported pain at both the hip and knee, in the individual patient there is often a poor correlation between the severity of radiographic changes and clinical symptomatology.

At the Third International Symposium on Population Studies of the Rheumatic Diseases in 1966, the Subcommittee on Diagnostic Criteria for Osteoarthrosis recommended that population-based studies should

investigate the validity of certain historical, physical and laboratory findings in predicting the typical radiographic features of OA on a joint-by-joint basis[23]. Such historical features include pain on motion, pain at rest, nocturnal joint pain, and morning stiffness. Features present on physical examination include bony enlargement and expansion, limitation of motion, and crepitus. Laboratory features include the erythrocyte sedimentation rate, tests for rheumatoid factor, serum uric acid concentration and appropriate analyses of synovial fluid.

In 1981, the Subcommittee on Osteoarthritis of the American College of Rheumatology Diagnostic and Therapeutic Criteria Committee was established to develop clinical criteria for the classification of OA[24]. Over the last decade, the Subcommittee has developed and published sets of classification criteria for OA of the knee[3], hand[25] and hip[26]. Altman has amplified the criteria sets into algorithms, facilitating their use in clinical research and population-based studies[27]. Because the major inclusion parameter is joint pain on most days of the prior month, these criteria sets identify patients with clinically important OA. This contrasts with the identification of cases of OA based on radiographic features alone, insofar as many, if not most, subjects with radiographic evidence of OA do not report joint pain[28]. Therefore, estimates of the prevalence of OA will be lower when based on the American College of Rheumatology criteria as compared to traditional radiographic criteria[29]: readers need to be aware of this difference when reviewing published studies.

The algorithms for classification of OA of the knee (Table 1.9), hand (Table 1.10) and hip (Table 1.11), were all developed using patients with site-specific joint pain due to other types of arthritis or musculoskeletal diseases as the comparison groups. For OA of the knee, data on 85 historical, physical, laboratory and radiographic features were collected from 130 patients with symptomatic OA of the knee and 105 control patients with knee pain due to other etiologies; 55 of the controls had rheumatoid arthritis[3].

McAlindon and Dieppe reviewed both the process of development of, and the final published American College of Rheumatology criteria for OA of the knee[30]. They noted several potential limitations, including lack

Table 1.9 Algorithm for classification of osteoarthritis of the knee, Subcommittee on Osteoarthritis, American College of Rheumatology Diagnostic and Therapeutic Criteria Committee[*]

Clinical
  1 Knee pain for most days of prior month
  2 Crepitus on active joint motion
  3 Morning stiffness < 30 minutes in duration
  4 Age > 38 years
  5 Bony enlargement of the knee on examination

Osteoarthritis present if items 1, 2, 3, 4 *or* items 1, 2, 5 *or* items 1, 5, are present. Sensitivity is 89% and specificity is 88%.

Clinical, Laboratory and Radiographic
  1 Knee pain for most days of prior month
  2 Osteophytes at joint margins (X–ray spurs)
  3 Synovial fluid typical of osteoarthritis (laboratory)
  4 Age > 40 years
  5 Morning stiffness < 30 minutes
  6 Crepitus on active joint motion
Osteoarthritis present if items 1, 2 *or* items 1, 3, 5, 6 *or* items 1, 4, 5, 6 are present. Sensitivity is 94% and specificity is 88%.

[*] Modified from references 3 and 27. Reproduced from Silman, A.J. and Hochberg, M.C. (1993). *Epidemiology of the rheumatic diseases.* Oxford University Press, Oxford.

Table 1.10 Algorithm for classification of osteoarthritis of the hand, Subcommittee on Osteoarthritis, American College of Rheumatology Diagnostic and Therapeutic Criteria Committee[*]

Clinical
  1 Hand pain, aching, or stiffness for most days of prior month.
  2 Hard tissue enlargement of ≥ 2 of 10 selected hand joints[#]
  3 Fewer than 3 swollen MCP joints.
  4 Hard tissue enlargement of 2 or more DIP joints.
  5 Deformity of 2 or more of 10 selected hand joints.

Osteoarthritis present if items 1, 2, 3, 4 *or* items 1, 2, 3, 5 are present. Sensitivity is 92% and specificity is 98%.

Abbreviations: DIP = distal interphalangeal; PIP = proximal interphalangeal; MCP metacarpophalangeal; CMC = carpo-metacarpal
[*] Modified from reference 25 and 27. Reproduced from Silman, A.J. and Hochberg, M.C. (1993). *Epidemiology of the rheumatic diseases.* Oxford University Press, Oxford.
[#] 10 selected hand joints include bilateral 2nd and 3rd DIP joints, 2nd and 3rd PIP joints and 1st CMC joints.

Table 1.11 Algorithm for classification of osteoarthritis of the hip, Subcommittee on Osteoarthritis, American College of Rheumatology Diagnostic and Therapeutic Criteria Committee*

Clinical, Laboratory and Radiographic
  1 Hip pain for most days of the prior month
  2 Femoral and/or acetabular osteophytes on radiograph
  3 Erythrocyte sedimentation rate < 20 mm/hr
  4 Axial joint space narrowing on radiograph
Osteoarthritis present if items 1, 2 *or* items 1, 3, 4 are present. Sensitivity is 91% and specificity is 89%.

* Modified from references 26 and 27. Reproduced from Silman, A.J. and Hochberg, M.C. (1993). *Epidemiology of the rheumatic diseases.* Oxford University Press, Oxford.

of age-matched and gender-matched controls, inclusion of controls with rheumatoid arthritis, use of criterion items which were largely subjective and not validated, and the absence of a definition or test for OA. Their comments were subsequently addressed by Altman *et al.* who noted that the methodology used to construct the criteria adjusted for differences between cases and controls, and that the final items included in the criteria sets could be reliably and objectively measured[31].

For OA of the hand, the Subcommittee collected data on 51 historical, physical, laboratory and radiographic features from 100 patients with symptomatic hand OA and 99 control patients with hand pain of other etiologies: 74 had rheumatoid arthritis[25]. For OA of the hip, data on 76 historical, physical, laboratory and radiographic features were collected from 114 patients with symptomatic OA of the hip and 87 control patients with hip pain of other etiologies: 37 had rheumatoid arthritis[26]. At all joint sites, the sensitivity, specificity, and accuracy of these algorithms approached or exceeded 90 per cent. Misclassification bias, therefore, would not likely be a major problem in clinical research studies which employed these criteria. However, in population-based studies, misclassification, particularly of false-negative cases, may be considerable because of the high proportion of subjects with radiographic evidence of OA who do not have joint pain.

In summary, OA is a complex disorder which may result from many potential etiologies. Definitions of OA developed at multidisciplinary conferences, with international representation of experts, reflect this complexity. It is difficult, however, to apply these definitions to case definition and diagnosis in the community or clinic setting.

In the community setting, criteria for case definition have traditionally relied on the presence of radiographic features of OA, codified using the Kellgren–Lawrence grading schema as illustrated in the *Atlas of standard radiographs*. Recently, however, the use of reliable atlases for grading the severity of individual radiographic features of OA and of modified global scales has received enthusiastic attention among rheumatic disease epidemiologists. In the clinic setting, however, classification criteria based on radiographic features alone have limitations. For purposes of clinical research, including therapeutic trials, classification schema have been developed which utilize combinations of symptoms, physical findings, laboratory data, and radiographic features, and have high levels of sensitivity and specificity.

References

1. Kelsey, J.L. and Hochberg, M.C. (1988). Epidemiology of chronic musculoskeletal disorders. *Annual Review of Public Health*, 9, 379–401.
2. Scott, J.C. and Hochberg, M.C. (1993). Arthritis and other musculoskeletal diseases. In *Chronic disease epidemiology and control* (ed. R.C. Brownson, P.L. Remington, and J.R. Davis), pp. 285–305. American Public Health Association, Washington, DC.
3. Altman, R., Asch, E., Bloch, D., Bole, G., Borenstein, D., Brandt, K., *et al.* (1986). Development of criteria for the classification and reporting of osteoarthritis: classification of osteoarthritis of the knee. *Arthritis and Rheumatism*, 29, 1039–49.
4. Brandt, K.D., Mankin, H.J., and Shulman, L.E. (1986). Workshop on etiopathogenesis of osteoarthritis. *The Journal of Rheumatology*, 13, 1126–60.
5. Keuttner, K. and Goldberg, V.M. (ed.) (1995). *Osteoarthritic disorders*, pp. xxi–v. American Academy of Orthopedic Surgeons, Rosemont.
6. Kellgren, J.H. and Moore, R. (1952). Generalised osteoarthritis and Heberden's nodes. *British Medical Journal*, 1, 181–7.
7. Schumacher, H.R. Jr (1993). Secondary osteoarthritis. In *Osteoarthritis: diagnosis and surgical management*, (2nd edn) (ed. R.W. Moskowitz, D.S. Howell, V.M. Goldberg, and H.J. Mankin), pp. 367–98, W.B. Saunders Company, Philadelphia.
8. Kellgren, J.H. and Lawrence, J.S. (1957). Radiologic assessment of osteoarthrosis. *Annals of the Rheumatic Diseases*, 16, 494–501.
9. The Department of Rheumatology and Medical Illustration, University of Manchester (1973). *The epidemiology of chronic rheumatism, Vol. 2, Atlas of standard radiographs of Arthritis*, pp. 1–15, F.A. Davis Company, Philadelphia.
10. Spector, T.D. and Cooper, C. (1993). Radiographic assessment of osteoarthritis in population studies: whither Kellgren and Lawrence? *Osteoarthritis and Cartilage*, 1, 203–6.
11. Spector, T.D. and Hochberg, M.C. (1994). Methodological problems in the epidemiological study of osteoarthritis. *Annals of the Rheumatic Diseases*, 53, 143–6.
12. Kallman, D.A., Wigley, F.M., Scott, W.W. Jr, Hochberg, M.C., and Tobin, J.D. (1989). New radiographic grading scales for osteoarthritis of the hand. *Arthritis and Rheumatism*, 32, 1548–91.
13. Croft, P., Cooper, C., Wickham, C., and Coggon, D. (1990). Defining osteoarthritis of the hip for epidemiologic studies. *American Journal of Epidemiology*, 132, 514–22.
14. Lane, N.E., Nevitt, M.C., Genant, H.K., and Hochberg, M.C. (1993). Reliability of new indices of radiographic osteoarthritis of the hand and hip and lumbar disc degeneration. *The Journal of Rheumatology*, 20, 1911–18.
15. Spector, T.D., Cooper, C., Cushnaghan, J., Hart, D.J. and Dieppe, P.A. (1992). *A radiographic atlas of knee osteoarthritis*. Springer-Verlag, London.

16. Scott, W.W. Jr, Lethbridge-Cejku, M., Reichle, R., Wigley, F.M., Tobin, J.D., and Hochberg, M.C. (1993). Reliability of grading scales for individual radiographic features of osteoarthritis of the knee: the Baltimore Longitudinal Study of Aging atlas of knee osteoarthritis. *Investigative radiology*, **28**, 497–501.

17. Altman, R.D., Hochberg, M.C., Murphy, W.A. Jr, Wolfe, F., and Lequesne, M. (1995). Atlas of individual radiographic features in osteoarthritis. *Osteoarthritis and Cartilage*, **3**, (Suppl A), 3–70.

18. Hart, D.J. and Spector, T.D. (1995). The classification and assessment of osteoarthritis. *Bailliere's Clinical Rheumatology*, **9**, 407–32.

19. Lane, N.E. and Kremer, L.B. (1995). Radiographic indices for osteoarthritis. *Rheumatic Disease Clinics of North America*, **21**, 379–94.

20. Scott, J.C., Nevitt, M.C., Lane, N.E., Genant, H.K., and Hochberg, M.C. (1992). Association of individual radiographic features of hip osteoarthritis with pain. *Arthritis and Rheumatism*, **35**(**Suppl 9**), S81.

21. Spector, T.D., Hart, D.J., Byrne, J., Harris, P.A., Dacre, J.E., and Doyle, D.V. (1993). Defining the presence of osteoarthritis of the knee in epidemiologic studies. *Annals of the Rheumatic Diseases*, **52**, 790–4.

22. Lethbridge-Cejku, M., Scott, W.W. Jr, Reichle, R., Ettinger, W.H., Zonderman, A., Costa, P., *et al.* (1995). Association of radiographic features of osteoarthritis of the knee with knee pain: Data from the Baltimore Longitudinal Study of Aging. *Arthritis Care and Research*, **9**, 182–8.

23. Bennett, P.H. and Wood, P.H.N. (ed.) (1968). *Population studies of the rheumatic diseases. International Congress Series No. 148*, pp. 417–19. Excerpta Medica Foundation, Amsterdam.

24. Altman, R.D., Meenan, R.F., Hochberg, M.C., Bole, G.G. Jr, Brandt, K., Cooke, T.D.V., *et al.* (1983). An approach to developing criteria for the clinical diagnosis and classification of osteoarthritis: a status report of the American Rheumatism Association Diagnostic Subcommittee on Osteoarthritis. *The Journal of Rheumatology*, **10**, 180–3.

25. Altman, R., Alarcon, G., Appelrough, D., Bloch, D., Borenstein, D., Brandt, K., *et al.* (1990). The American College of Rheumatology criteria for the classification and reporting of osteoarthritis of the hand. *Arthritis and Rheumatism*, **33**, 1601–10.

26. Altman, R., Alarcon, G., Appelrough, D., Bloch, D., Borenstein, D., Brandt, K., *et al.* (1991). The American College of Rheumatology criteria for the classification and reporting of osteoarthritis of the hip. *Arthritis and Rheumatism*, **34**, 505–14.

27. Altman, R. (1991). Classification of disease: osteoarthritis. *Seminars in Arthritis and Rheumatism*, **20**(6,**Suppl 2**), 40–7.

28. Lawrence, J.S., Bremner, J.M., and Bier, F. (1966). Osteoarthritis: prevalence in the population and relationship between symptoms and X-ray changes. *Annals of the Rheumatic Diseases*, **25**, 1–25.

29. Hart, D.J., Leedham-Green, M., and Spector, T.D. (1991). The prevalence of knee osteoarthritis in the general population using different clinical criteria: the Chingford Study. *British Journal of Rheumatology*, **30**(Suppl 2), 72.

30. McAlindon, T., and Dieppe, P. (1989). Osteoarthritis: definitions and criteria. *Annals of the Rheumatic Diseases*, **48**, 531–2.

31. Altman, R.D., Bloch, D.A., Brandt, K.D., Cooke, D.V., Greenwald, R.A., Hochberg, M.C., *et al.* (1990). Osteoarthritis: definitions and criteria. *Annals of the Rheumatic Diseases*, **49**, 201.

2 | *Epidemiology of osteoarthritis*

David T. Felson

Osteoarthritis (OA) is the most common form of arthritis. Its high prevalence, especially in the elderly, and the frequency of OA-related physical disability make OA one of the leading causes of disability in the elderly, especially with respect to weight-bearing functional tasks[1]. Conservative estimates indicate that patients with OA in the United States account for 46 million physician visits, 3.7 million hospital admissions (20–30 times more admissions than for rheumatoid arthritis), 185 million bed days, 68 million work days lost per year[2], and for one of every eight days of restricted activity among the elderly[3]. As noted in a recent report on the prevalence of arthritis: 'By 2020 the estimated number of persons with arthritis is projected to increase by 57% and activity limitations associated with arthritis by 66%. These projected increases are largely attributable to the high prevalence of OA among older persons and the increasing average age of the US population[4].'

Epidemiology is the study of disease in populations and its association with characteristics of people and their environments. Epidemiologic studies document the burden of disease in society and evaluate risk factors for disease that, if modified, might lead to disease prevention and a lessening of the burden of disability associated with disease. Identifying modifiable risk factors for OA is the first step to prevent this disease and lowering its formidable burden in our society.

Prevalence and incidence

OA is an extremely common joint disorder in all populations. It often affects certain joints, yet spares others. For example, in the hands, the distal interphalangeal (DIP), proximal interphalangeal (PIP) joints and the carpometacarpal (CMC) joint of the thumb are frequently involved. Other joints commonly affected include the cervical spine, lumbosacral spine, hip, knee, and first metatarsophalangeal (MTP) joint. Notably,

the ankle, wrist, elbow and shoulder are usually spared. Disease predilection is for lower extremity weightbearing joints and hand joints which are involved in pincer grip. Our joints were designed and shaped, in an evolutionary sense, when humans were brachiating apes. Only later in evolution did humans develop pincer grip capability[5] and full weightbearing on their legs. These evolutionary differences in joint function and, possibly, differences in the composition of articular cartilage among different joints, predispose some joints to cartilage breakdown, leading to OA.

Whereas structural (radiographic) evidence of OA is most common in hands and feet, hand OA is less frequent and less severely symptomatic than OA in other joints. While the lumbar spine is also frequently affected, the correlation between radiographic OA and symptoms in the lumbar spine is poor. This correlation is better for hips and knees, in which symptoms are often disabling.

According to the United States National Arthritis Data Work Group[6], radiographic OA of the hand occurs in approximately 32.5 per cent of adults. The frequency of radiographic OA of hips and knees has been difficult to quantify because of systematic underreading of radiographs[7] in the large nationwide study of this disease, the National Health and Nutrition Examination Survey (NHANES I)[8]. The Framingham Study suggests radiographic knee OA occurs in 33 per cent of people aged 63 years and over[9].

The prevalence of symptomatic OA has been assessed in population-based studies in England, in the Framingham Study and in NHANES I. The latter provides the lowest estimates. Symptomatic knee OA may occur in 1.6[8] to 9.4 per cent[10] of adults; the Framingham Study estimated its prevalence in elders to be 9.5 per cent[9]. Symptomatic hip OA occurs in 0.7 per cent to 4.4 per cent of adults and symptomatic hand OA, based on British data from the 1960s[10], in approximately 2.6 per cent of adults.

The prevalence of OA in all joints is strikingly correlated with age. Regardless of how OA is defined, it is uncommon in adults under age 40 and becomes extremely prevalent above age 60. Radiographic hand OA, for example, was present in only about 5 per cent of adults under age 35, but was seen in over 70 per cent of those who were age 65 or older[11].

OA has a higher prevalence, and more often exhibits a generalized distribution, in women than in men. Before the age of 50 years, men have a higher prevalence of this disease than women, but after age 50 women have a higher prevalence and this sex difference in prevalence then increases with age[9,12]. These gender and age-related prevalence patterns are consistent with a role of post-menopausal hormone deficiency in increasing the risk of OA (see p. 00).

Cross-national and cross-racial studies can often produce insights about disease etiology. With respect to OA, black women have been reported to have higher rates of knee OA than white women[13,14], even after adjustment for age and weight. Results in black men have been inconsistent. However, studies suggest very low rates of hip OA among black populations in Jamaica, South Africa, Nigeria and Liberia (1–4 per cent for radiographic OA), in comparison with European populations (7–25 per cent).

Rates of hip OA may also be much lower in Asians than in Caucasians. Hoaglund[15] found that only 1 per cent of Hong Kong residents age 55 and older had hip OA, although hand OA was as prevalent among Chinese as Europeans. The rate of hip arthroplasty for OA in people of Asian extraction is lower than that in caucasians in the United States[16]. Although it was initially felt that these racial differences in prevalence might be attributed to an absence of developmental hip abnormalities in Asians and, possibly, blacks, recent studies of Chinese in Hong Kong[15,18] fail to confirm a lower prevalence of developmental hip abnormalities, so that the explanation for these racial differences in prevalence is unclear. In Blackfeet and Pima native Americans, rates of hip OA are intermediate between those for blacks and whites[19], even though the Pimas weigh more, on average, than caucasians.

Because the risk of mortality may be increased in those with OA[20,21], prevalence estimates may give erroneous estimates of actual disease incidence, that is the new occurrence of disease. The most accurate way of quantifying the occurrence of OA, evaluating its occurrence by age and sex, is to study the incidence of the disease. A recent large-scale study from a Massachusetts health maintenance organization[22] reported that the age- and sex-standardized incidence rate for symptomatic hand OA was 100 per 100 000 person years. For hip OA the rate was 88 per 100 000 person years and for knee OA 240 per 100 000 person years. The incidence of hand, knee and hip OA all increased with age (Fig. 2.1) and for each joint was higher in women than in men after age 50. These findings confirm those of the prevalence studies. At age

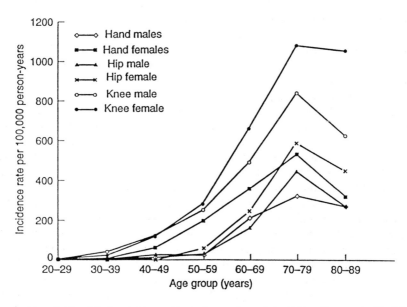

Fig. 2.1   Incidence of osteoarthritis of the hand, hip, and knee, in members of the Fallon Community Health Plan, 1991–1992, by age and sex. (From Oliveria *et al.* 1995.[22])

70 to 89, knee OA rates among women reached a maximum incidence of 1 per cent per year. Interestingly, a leveling off or decline in the incidence of symptomatic OA occurred in both sexes around age 80. In another study, in which serial knee radiographs were obtained[23], female Framingham elders had a rate of incident symptomatic OA of 1 per cent per year, identical to that in the health maintenance organization mentioned above. Radiographic OA of the knee (often asymptomatic) was more frequent in these elders, and occurred at a rate of 2 per cent per year.

Modifiable risk factors for OA

Weight and OA

Risk factors for OA probably depend on the joint affected. Knee injuries, as sustained in football, predispose to knee OA but, obviously, not to hand OA. Some risk factors may have purely local effects, whereas others have systemic effects. For body weight, local and systemic effects may both be relevant.

Population-based studies consistently show that overweight persons are at higher risk of having knee OA than non-overweight controls. Estimates of risk vary from population to population and depend, to some degree, on the criteria for overweight and the definition of OA. In NHANES I, which was conducted throughout the United States from 1971–1975[13], the risk of radiographic OA in obese women [body mass index (BMI) greater than 30 but less than 35] was almost four times that in women whose BMI was lower than 25. For men in the same overweight category the risk was 4.8 times greater than that for men of normal weight. Approximately there to six times body weight is exerted across the knee during single leg stance in walking[24]. Therefore, any increase in weight may be multiplied by this factor to reveal the excess force across the knee of an overweight person during walking. In addition to increasing the risk of tibiofemoral OA, which was the focus of most studies, the preponderance of recent evidence[25,26] suggests that those who are overweight also are at increased risk for patellofemoral OA.

While studies such as the above have shown a cross-sectional association of obesity and OA, the possibility exists that persons become overweight after developing OA because of their knee pain and sedentary level of activity. Recent studies[27,28], however, have disproved this notion and show that obesity *precedes* development of knee OA.

Overweight persons also appear to have an increased risk of hip OA, although the association of weight with hip OA is not as strong or as consistent across studies as for knee OA. This difference between hip and knee OA could possibly be due to different multiplier effects of body weight across the two joint sites or differences in distribution of load across the hip and knee during weightbearing[29].

Surprisingly, people who are overweight also appear to be at higher risk of hand OA[30]. Because the force across hand joints is not necessarily greater in overweight persons than in those who are not overweight, the relationship between overweight and OA remains enigmatic.

Weight could act to cause OA via two mechanisms: first, and most logically, because it increases the amount of load across a joint, obesity could induce cartilage breakdown simply on the basis of excess load, leading to OA. This could account for the apparent causal relationship between weight and knee and hip OA. Indeed, the association of obesity and knee OA is so strong that it is not likely to be explained by confounding factors. The load theory, however, does not explain the relationship between overweight and hand OA, which suggests involvement of a systemic factor. Following this line of reasoning, it has been speculated that a circulating factor that acts to accelerate cartilage breakdown may be present in overweight persons, serving as a second mechanism leading to OA.

In addition, bone mineral density is increased in overweight persons and this (or the absence of osteoporosis) may be a risk factor for OA[31]. Additional evidence in favor of a systemic factor is the possibility that the relationship between overweight and OA is stronger in women than men[32].

Does losing weight lower the risk of OA? For Framingham women whose baseline BMI values were greater than 25, that is, greater than the median, weight loss significantly lowered the rate of incident symptomatic knee OA[33]. The adjusted odds ratio per two units of BMI (approximately 5 kg for a woman of normal height) was 0.41, a reduction of more than 50 per cent in the risk of developing knee OA. Weight gain was associated with a slightly increased rate of subsequent knee OA (odds ratio 1.28 for a two-unit weight gain). For women whose baseline weight was lower than the median, neither weight gain nor weight loss significantly affected their risk of later disease.

Using data from the Framingham OA Study (unpublished observations), we estimated that substantial weight loss (dropping from obese to overweight, or from overweight to normal weight range) would prevent about 21 per cent of knee OA in men; in women (in whom the association of obesity and knee OA is stronger), 33 per cent of knee OA would be prevented. For women, weight accounts for more OA than any other known factor; for men, overweight is second to knee injury as a preventable cause of knee OA.

Not only does being overweight increase the risk for OA but, for those with established knee OA, it increases the odds of disease progression[33,34,35]. Furthermore, those with OA in one knee are at high risk of developing OA in the other knee if they are overweight[36]. The effect of obesity on OA progression in joints other than the knee has not been studied.

In those who already have OA, weight change is likely to affect symptoms. McGoey *et al.*[37] studied morbidly obese women at the time of their gastric stapling operation and one year later, at which time their mean weight loss was approximately 45 kg. The proportion with knee symptoms dropped from 57 per cent to 14 per cent during this interval and the prevalence of other regional symptoms, for example, hip pain and back pain, fell commensurately. Unfortunately, the authors did not definitively ascertain whether these subjects had OA.

In another study, 30 obese women (48.7 per cent above ideal weight) with knee or hip OA were randomized to phentermine, an appetite suppressant, or placebo, with all subjects instructed to eat a low energy diet[38]. Six months later, among 22 patients who remained in the trial, those taking phentermine had lost 6.3 kg and those in the placebo group 4.5 kg (p = NS). The amount of weight loss correlated significantly with improvement in a clinical score, which combined symptoms and physical findings. For knee OA, the correlation between weight loss and improvement was especially strong (r = 0.66, p < 0.01).

Joint injury and OA

In theory, joint cartilage could be damaged either by a sudden injury or by repeated stereotyped activity that exceeds the ability of periarticular muscle to withstand such use, transmitting force to cartilage. Sudden knee injuries, such as fractures and ligamentous tears, best parallel the model of acute joint injury; long-distance running, or jobs which require repetitive stereotyped use of a joint, are excellent examples of repeated impact loading of joints.

Acute major knee injuries, including cruciate ligament and meniscal tears, are common causes of knee OA, especially among men[39]. Those with a history of major knee injury are at high risk of later, usually ipsilateral, knee OA. In the Framingham study[40], men with a history of major knee injuries had a relative risk of 3.46 for subsequent knee OA; for women the relative risk was 2.18 (both p < 0.05). Major joint injury may account for a large proportion of all cases of OA at sites in which the disease is generally uncommon, for example, tibiotalar and glenohumeral joints.

With respect to repeated joint use, studies have focused on occupational and athletic activities. Farmers are at high risk for hip OA. Standing, bending, walking long distances over rough ground, lifting, moving heavy objects, and tractor driving all appear to pose high risks for hip OA, while climbing was not implicated as a risk factor[41].

Jackhammer operators have a high rate of OA in upper extremity joints that are otherwise rarely affected by OA. Jackhammers impart tremendous impact loads across joints that are ill-designed to sustain them. Vibratory tools may subvert the effectiveness of joint shock absorbers, such as muscles, leading to transmission of excess stress across the joint.

Miners have high rates of OA in knee and spine[42], while shipyard and dockyard workers have a higher prevalence of OA in knees and fingers than office workers. Lawrence[43] found a higher rate of Heberden's nodes and hand OA in cotton mill workers than in age-matched control women, but the prevalence of spinal OA was not increased.

Which specific job-related activities predispose to OA? Studying three occupational groups in a Virginia textile mill, Hadler[44] found that women whose jobs required fine pincer grip (increasing the stress across DIP joints) had significantly more DIP joint OA than those whose jobs required repeated power grip, a motion which does not stress the DIP joints. Workers whose jobs require regular knee bending[13,26] and lifting or carrying heavy loads[13,45,46] have a higher rate of knee OA than workers whose jobs do not entail these activities.

The risk of OA is increased also among other occupational groups. The rate appears to be highest in men and women who work as laborers. In a recent Swedish study[47], farmers, firefighters, millworkers, butchers, dockers and, to a lesser degree, unskilled manual workers, fishermen, and miners all had a higher than expected risk of hip OA. Increased rates of knee OA were observed in firefighters, farmers, construction workers and, to a lesser extent, unskilled manual workers and truck and crane operators.

With respect to prevention of OA, the relationship of the disease to occupational activities may be extremely important. In a study of older workers, the proportion of OA potentially attributable to occupational knee bending was higher (32 per cent) than that attributable to obesity (24 per cent)[13].

If specific job-related tasks which are associated with an increased risk of OA were changed or avoided, it is possible that many cases of OA would be prevented. Unfortunately, occupation-related OA is not an easy target for disease prevention. Jobs contain complex ergonomic activities; isolating the injurious ones will be difficult. Also, workers often change jobs or rotate to other tasks. Lastly, because OA takes years to develop, analyses of other (concomitant) risk factors must be incorporated into any study of occupational tasks and OA. Elimination of all jobs involving substantial physical labor is not realistic, but minor alterations in ergonomic activities might lower job-related OA risk if specific tasks could be shown to be linked to a high rate of OA.

The association of OA with jogging and other habitual leisure time sports activities is of special interest. Most studies evaluating the link between athletic activities and OA have, unfortunately, not included information about major joint injury. For example, former American football players have high rates of knee OA[48], but most subjects with OA in these groups had sustained previous major injuries and many had undergone knee surgery.

Much of the increased risk of knee OA in soccer players[46] can be explained by known injuries, such as cruciate ligament tears and meniscectomy. The risk for hip OA may also be increased among former soccer players[49] and track and field athletes[50].

Data on the risk of knee OA in runners is conflicting (Table 2.1); recent studies[51] suggest that radiographic changes of OA are more common in this group than expected. The changes, such as osteophytes, however, are not necessarily associated with an increased risk of knee symptoms.

With respect to hip OA, although a controlled study of marathon runners 20 years after they had ceased long-distance running[52] detected no increase in the proportion with hip OA, two other controlled studies[53,54] have found an increased risk of hip OA in long-distance runners.

Studies of this issue have been flawed, however, by failure to study those who stopped running because they developed knee or hip problems, by failure to incorporate a long-term follow-up, and by failure to adjust for potential confounders, such as a history of major knee injury.

Generalized disease Hereditary factors

Generalized OA involves hand joints, including DIP, PIP and the first carpometacarpal joints; cervical spine; lumbosacral spine and knees; and may include hips. There are two types of generalized OA: nodal OA (Heberden's nodes) and non-nodal OA[55]. There is little question that this entity exists; OA in one joint is associated with the presence of OA in other joints, even after adjusting for age and sex. Generalized OA is most

Table 2.1   Studies on running and osteoarthritis

Author (year)	Joint	No. of subjects	Time elapsed since running (years)	Controls	Results
Sohn and Micheli (1985)	Knee	504	25	Yes	No increase in knee complaints over controls (swimmers)
McDermott and Freyne (1983)	Knee	20	0	No	6/20 had X-ray OA
Lane *et al.* (1993)	Knee	33	5	Yes	No increase in OA
Panush (1994)	Knee	12	8	Yes	No increase in OA
Harris *et al.* (1994)[51]	Knee	73	0–40	Yes	Increase in osteophytes in runners
Kujala *et al.* (1995)[26]	Knee	28	35	Yes	Non-significant increase (OR = 4.8) of knee OA in runners vs. shooters
Puranen (1975)[52]	Hip	60	20	Yes	No increase in OA
Marti *et al.* (1989)[53]	Hip	27	15	Yes	Runners had more OA than controls
Vingard *et al.* (1993)[54]	Hip	233	20–50	Yes	Runners had more OA (RR = 2.1, p = NS)
Kujala *et al.* (1994)	Knee, hip and ankle	100	30	Yes	Runners had more hospitalizations for knee and hip OA (RR = 1.8; 95% CI 0.9–3.6)

common in older women and may be inherited in a polygenic pattern[56].

The tendency of some patients to deposit calcium crystals in degenerated cartilage may be a potential cause of generalized OA. Crystals of calcium pyrophosphate dihydrate (CPPD) are found in 18–60 per cent of synovial fluids of patients with OA who have knee effusions[57]. Furthermore, 21 per cent of patients with generalized OA have radiographic evidence of cartilage calcification, suggesting CPPD deposition.

However, CPPD may not be a major cause of generalized OA. Radiographic features of CPPD disease are substantially different from those of primary OA. CPPD affects joints which are not usually affected by OA, such as the elbow, wrist, and MCPs, and produces a different spectrum of pathologic and radiographic changes. CPPD deposits may be prevalent in subjects with OA because the prevalence of both OA and CPPD increases with age. However, chondrocalcinosis and OA are associated even after adjusting for age, although the association may not be strong[58].

Crystals of basic calcium phosphate (hydroxyapatite) have been found in 44 per cent of synovial fluid samples from patients with OA and are present universally in cartilage specimens from patients with severe OA[59]. Like CPPD, they may be common in joints of aged individuals and are not confined to joints with OA. However, both apatite and CPPD crystals are common in joints with severe OA, suggesting that crystals may promote acceleration of the disease process or may merely be an epiphenomenon of severe disease. The role of these crystals in inducing joint damage is unclear.

Genetic defects which produce generalized OA are currently under investigation. A study[60] of two families with a predisposition to develop generalized OA at an early age showed a clustering of OA among family members with an abnormality in the type II procollagen gene on chromosome 12. Other genetic defects predisposing to early and widespread OA have also been discovered (see Chapter 4), although many of these defects produce a disease that is phenotypically different from idiopathic OA, including epiphysial dysplasia or facial developmental abnormalities.

Osteoporosis and OA

Radin[61] has suggested that subchondral bone deformation during impact loading of the joint protects the articular cartilage from damage. Those with more deformable bone may be less susceptible to OA. Patients with osteopetrosis and, presumably, stiff subchondral bone have high rates of OA; while those with osteoporosis exhibit a lower than expected rate of OA[62]. Bone density is greater in patients with OA than in age-matched controls, even at sites distant from the OA joint[63,64]. Much of the increase in bone mass may be explained by the association of OA with obesity, which protects against osteoporosis. Some[64] argue, however, that obesity causes OA by producing stiff non-deformable bones. It is possible that osteophyte formation, but not cartilage loss, is linked to high bone mass[65]. This would suggest the presence of a circulating bone growth factor in those with osteophytes.

Congenital and developmental deformities and hip OA

Three uncommon developmental abnormalities, congenital dislocation, Legg–Perthes disease, and slipped femoral capital epiphysis, lead invariably to hip OA in later life. Milder developmental abnormalities, including subclinical variants of these developmental diseases may also presage hip OA, although the evidence for this is far from clear[17].

Circumstantial evidence for this link includes the unusual predominance of hip OA in men[66], the striking racial disparities in the prevalence of hip OA (see p. 00), and the weak association with hip OA of such traditional risk factors as obesity, suggesting the importance of other risk factors. Acetabular dysplasia, a mild variant of congenital dislocation in which the acetabulum is shallow, may account for a substantial proportion of hip OA in women, although probably not in men[67]. More evidence that mild structural abnormalities predispose to hip OA is needed.

Estrogen and OA

In addition to the high incidence of OA in women after age 50 — the approximate age of menopause — some women develop 'menopausal arthritis', (rapidly progressive hand OA) at the time of menopause[55]. These gender and age-related prevalence patterns are consistent with a role for post-menopausal hormone deficiency in increasing the risk of OA. In coronary artery disease, gout, and osteoporosis — diseases for which the risk in women rises dramatically after menopause as it does in OA — estrogen loss has been strongly implicated as a risk factor.

Recent epidemiologic studies[68–71] provide evidence that estrogen replacement therapy (ERT) is associated with a reduction in the risk of knee and hip OA (Table 2.2). All four studies evaluated prevalent disease, and two examined primarily the presence of radiographic disease. All showed an inverse association between ERT and the prevalence of OA, although in one study the odds ratio was close to unity (0.9). Additional corroborative evidence of a protective effect is that both the Study of Osteoporotic Fractures (SOF)[68] and the Framingham Study[69] have reported a stronger inverse association of ERT with OA among those reporting long-term use of ERT, than among non-users or among women who used ERT for shorter periods; (OR for more than 10 years of ERT use, for both SOF and the Framingham Study = 0.6). In both studies the inverse association was stronger when analysis was restricted to more severe OA or to bilateral radiographic OA.

Other risk factors

Recent investigations have focused on other risk factors for OA. This area of inquiry may provide insights into the etiology of generalized disease and clues to the development of new therapies.

Evidence of an association between diabetes and OA is inconsistent[27,72]. The discrepant findings may be explained by the association between diabetes and diffuse idiopathic skeletal hyperostosis (DISH), which may be mistaken for OA. While early studies suggested an association between OA and a high serum urate concentration, recent studies have failed to confirm this. Two studies have suggested an association of knee OA with hypertension[72,73], even after adjusting for obesity. Evidence is conflicting on a negative correlation of smoking with OA[72,74,75]; a biologic rationale is lacking. Other factors which have inconsistently been reported to be linked with OA are hysterectomy[76], hyperglycemia[72] and hypercholesterolemia[71]. The relation between NSAID use and OA development or progression is unknown. Risk factors for knee OA and hip OA are summarized in Tables 2.3 and 2.4, respectively.

Risk factors for symptoms of OA

Factors differentiating symptomatic OA from asymptomatic radiographic disease are unknown. This issue is important because such factors might cause symptoms in susceptible patients. Subjects with severe radiographic OA more often have symptoms than those with milder radiographic abnormalities. Also, females with knee OA are more likely to have symptoms than males, even after adjusting for disease severity.

Lawrence et al.[10] found that obese subjects with knee OA were more likely to have symptoms than non-obese subjects, but this has not been confirmed in recent studies[77,78].

Table 2.2   Epidemiologic studies of estrogen replacement therapy (ERT) and OA

Author (year)	No.	Design	Joint(s)	Definition of OA	Results*
Nevitt et al. (1994)[68]	4366	Cohort Cross-sectional	Hip	X-ray OA, Symptomatic OA	8.9% of ERT users with X-ray OA vs. 12.9% non-users; adjusted OR = 0.7 (0.5, 0.9).
Hannan et al. (1990)[69]	831	Cohort Cross-sectional	Knee	X-ray OA	For > 2 exams of ERT use, adjusted OR of X-ray OA = 0.7 (0.4, 1.2).
Wolfe et al. (1994)[70]	1329	Case-control Cross-sectional	Hip and knee	Symptomatic OA	For ever use of ERT adjusted OR = 0.9 (0.7, 1.2). ERT users with milder X-ray OA than non-users.
Samanta et al. (1993)[71]	690	Case-control Cross-sectional	Large joint (knee, hip) and hand	Symptomatic OA	For use of ERT at any time, crude OR of large joint OA = 0.3 (0.1, 1.4); of hand OA = 0.6 (0.2, 1.9).

* OR adjusted for at least age and BMI (or weight). All OR reported with 95% confidence intervals.

Table 2.3 Risk factors for knee osteoarthritis*

Definite	Probable	Possible/reported	Disproved

Age (+)
Female (after age 50)(+)
Obesity (+)
Major knee injury (+)
Part of generalized
   diathesis, inherited
   (?) crystal-related (+)
Prior inflammatory
   joint disease (+)
	Occupational knee
	bending/lifting (+)
		Running (+)
		Smoking (–)
		Early hysterectomy (+)
		Osteoporosis (–)
		Estrogen therapy (–)
		Black race (women) (+)
		Hypercholesterolemia (+)
		Hypertension (+)
		Hyperglycaemia (+)
		IGF 1 (–)
			Hyperuricemia

* (+) increases OA risk; (–) decreases OA risk.

Table 2.4 Risk factors for hip osteoarthritis*

Definite	Probable	Possible/reported

Age (+)
Diagnosed developmental
   abnormality (+)
Part of generalized
   diathesis, inherited (+)
Farming (+)
	Running (+)
	Obesity (+)
	Caucasian race (+)
	Undiagnosed developmental
	   abnormality (+)
	Occupations with
	   physical labour (+)
		Osteoporosis (–)
		Male sex (+)
		Estrogen therapy (–)

* (+) increases OA risk; (–) decreases OA risk.

References

1. Guccione, A.A., Felson, D.T., Anderson, J.J. Anthony, J.M., Zhang, Y., Wilson, P.W.F., *et al.* (1994). The effects of specific medical conditions on the functional limitations of elders in the Framingham Study. *American Journal of Public Health*, **84**, 351–8.
2. Kramer, J.S., Yelin, E.H. and Epstein, W.V. (1983). Social and economic impacts — four muscularskeletal conditions: A study using national community-based data. *Arthritis and Rheumatism*, **26**, 901–7.
3. Kosorok, M.R., Omenn, G.S., Diehr, P., Koepsell, D.D. and Patrick, D.L. (1992). Restricted activity days among older adults. *American Journal of Public Health*, **82**(9), 1263–7.
4. US Department of Health and Human Services. (1995). CDC: Prevalence and impact of arthritis among women — United States, 1989–1991. *MMWR*, **44**, 329–334.
5. Hutton, C.W. (1987). Hypothesis. Generalised osteoarthritis: an evolutionary problem? *The Lancet*, **1**, 1463–5.
6. Felson, D.T. (for National Arthritis Data Work Group). Osteoarthritis. *Arthritis and Rheumatism*, in press.
7. Helmick, C.G. and Pollard R.A. (1994). Evidence for underreading of radiographic osteoarthritis of the hips and knees in the First National Health and Nutrition Examination Survey (NHANES I). *Arthritis and Rheumatism*, **37** (Supplement), S301.
8. Maurer, K. (1979). Basic data on arthritis of knee, hip, and sacroiliac joints in adults ages 25–74 years, United States, 1971–1975. Rockville MD: National Center for Health Statistics, (**Series 11, no. 213, PHS publication no. 79–1661**).
9. Felson, D.T., Naimark, A., Anderson, J., Kazis, L., Castelli, W. and Meenan, R.F. (1987). The prevalence of knee osteoarthritis in the elderly. *Arthritis and Rheumatism*, **30**(8), 914–18.
10. Lawrence, J.S. and Bremner, J.M. (1966). Osteoarthrosis prevalence in the population and relationship between symptoms and X-ray changes. *Annals of the Rheumatic Diseases*, **25**, 1–24.
11. Engel, A. (1968). Osteoarthritis and body measurements. Rockville MD: National Center for Health Statistics, (Series 11, no. 29, PHS publication no. 1999).
12. Van Saase, J.L.C.M., Van Romunde, L.K.J., Cats, A., Vandenbroucke, J.P. and Valkenburg, H.A. (1989). Epidemiology of osteoarthritis: Zoetermeer survey. Comparison of radiological osteoarthritis in a Dutch population with that in 10 other populations. *Annals of the Rheumatic Diseases*, **48**, 271–80.
13. Anderson, J. and Felson, D.T. (1988). Factors associated with osteoarthritis of the knee in the First National Health and Nutrition Examination Survey (NHANES I). *American Journal of Epidemiology*, **128**, 179–89.
14. Bremner, J.M., Lawrence, J.S. and Miall, W.E. (1968). Degenerative joint disease in a Jamaican rural population. *Annals of the Rheumatic Diseases*, **27**, 326–32.
15. Hoaglund, F.T., Yau, A.C.M.C. and Wong, W.I. (1973). Osteoarthritis of the hip and other joints in Southern Chinese in Hong Kong. *Journal of Bone and Joint Surgery*, **55-A**, 545–57.

16. Hoaglund, F.T., Oishi, C.S. and Gialamas, G.G. (1995). Extreme variations in racial rates of total hip arthroplasty for primary coxarthrosis: A population-based study in San Francisco. *Annals of the Rheumatic Diseases*, **54**, 107–10.

17. Croft, P., Cooper, C., Wickham, C. and Coggon, D. (1991). Osteoarthritis of the hip and acetabular dysplasia. *Annals of the Rheumatic Diseases*, **50**, 308–10.

18. Lau, E. and Lin, F. (1994). Low prevalence of osteoarthritis of the hip in Chinese men. *Arthritis and Rheumatism*, **37** (**Supplement**), S239.

19. Lawrence, J.S. and Sebo, M. (1980). The geography of osteoarthritis. In *The aetiopathogenesis of osteoarthritis*, pp. 155–83.

20. Cerhan, J.R., Wallace, R.B., El-Khoury, G.Y., Moore, T.E. and Long, C.R. (1995). Decreased survival with increasing prevalence of full-body, radiographically defined osteoarthritis in women. *American Journal of Epidemiology*, **141**, 225–34.

21. Monson, R.R. and Hall, A.P. (1976). Mortality among arthritics. *Journal of Chronic Diseases*, **29**, 359–467.

22. Oliveria, S.A., Felson, D.T., Reed, J.I., Cirillo, P.A. and Walker, A.M. (1995). Incidence of symptomatic hand, hip, and knee osteoarthritis among patients in a health maintenance organization. *Arthritis and Rheumatism*, **38**, 1134–41.

23. Felson, D.T., Zhang, Y., Hannan, M.T., Naimark, A., Weissman, B., Aliabadi, P., *et al.* (1995). The Incidence and natural history of knee osteoarthritis in the elderly: The Framingham Osteoarthritis Study. *Arthritis and Rheumatism*, **38**, 1500–5.

24. Maquet, P. (1976). *Biomechanics of the knee*. Springer Verlag, New York.

25. McAlindon, T., Zhang, Y., Hannan, M., Felson, D., Naimark, A., Weissman, B., *et al*. Are risk factors for patellofemoral and tibiofemoral knee osteoarthritis different? *Journal of Rheumatology*, in press.

26. Kujala, U.M., Kettunen, J., Paananen, H., Aalto, T., Battie, M.C., Impivaara, O., *et al.* (1995). Knee osteoarthritis in former runners, soccer players, weight lifters and shooters. *Arthritis and Rheumatism*, **38**, 539–46.

27. Felson, D.T., Anderson, J.J., Naimark, A., Walker, A.M. and Meenan, R.F. (1988). Obesity and knee osteoarthritis. *Annals of International Medicine*, **109**, 18–24.

28. Schouten, J. (1991). A 12-year follow-up study of osteoarthritis of the knee in the general population. Thesis, Erasmus University, pp. 149–64.

29. Heliovaara, M., Mkel, M. and Impivaara, O. *et al.* (1993). Association of overweight, trauma and workload with coxarthrosis: a health survey of 7,217 persons. *Acta Orthopedica Scandinauica*, **64**, 513–18.

30. Carman, W.J., Sowers, M.F., Hawthorne, V.M. and Weissfeld, L.A. (1994). Obesity as a risk factor for osteoarthritis of the hand and wrist: a prospective study. **139**, 119–29.

31. Hannan, M.T., Anderson, J.J., Zhang, Y., Levy, D. and Felson, D.T. (1993). Bone mineral density and knee osteoarthritis in elderly men and women: the Framingham Study. *Arthritis and Rheumatism*, **36**, 1671–80.

32. Felson, D.T., Zhang, Y., Anthony, J.M., Naimark, A. and Anderson, J.J. (1992). Weight loss reduces the risk for symptomatic knee osteoarthritis in women. *Annals of International Medicine* **116**, 535–9.

33. Schouten, J.S.A.G., van den Ouweland, and Valkenburg, H.A. (1992). A 12-year follow-up study in the general population on prognostic factors of cartilage loss in osteoarthritis of the knee. *Annals of the Rheumatic Diseases*, **51**, 932–7.

34. Dougados, M., Gueguen, A., Nguyen, M., Thiesce, A., Listrat, V., Jacob, L., *et al.* (1992). Longitudinal radiologic evaluation of osteoarthritis of the knee. *Journal of Rheumatology*, **19**, 378–83.

35. Altman, Rd., Fried, J.F., Bloch, D.A., Carstens, J., Cooke, T.D., Genant, H., *et al.* (1987). Radiographic assessment of progression in osteoarthritis. *Arthritis and Rheumatism*, **30**, 1214–25.

36. Spector, T.D., Hart, D.J., Doyle, D.V., (1994). Incidence and progression of osteoarthritis in women with unilateral knee disease in the general population: the effect of obesity. *Annals of the Rheumatic Diseases*, **53**, 565–8.

37. McGoey, B.V., Deitel, M., Saplys, R.J.F. and Kliman, M.E. (1990). Effect of weight loss on musculoskeletal pain in the morbidly obese. *Journal of Bone and Joint Surgery*, **72B**, 322–3.

38. Williams, R.A. and Foulsham, B.M. (1981). Weight reduction in osteoarthritis using phentermine. *The Practitioner*, **225**, 231–2.

39. Jacobsen, K. (1977). Osteoarthrosis following insufficiency of the cruciate ligaments in man. *Acta Orthopedica Scandinauica*, **48**, 520–6.

40. Felson, D.T. (1990). The epidemiology of knee osteoarthritis: results from the Framingham osteoarthritis study. *Seminarsin Arthritis and Rheumatism*, **20**, 42–50.

41. Croft, P., Coggon, D., Cruddas, M. and Cooper, C. (1992). Osteoarthritis of the hip: an occupational disease in farmers. *British Medical Journal*, **304**, 1269–72.

42. Kellgren, J.H. and Lawrence, J.S. (1952). Rheumatism in miners. II: X-ray study. *British Journal of Industrial Medicine*, **9**, 197–207.

43. Lawrence, J.S. (1961). Rheumatism in cotton operatives. *British Journal of Industrial Medicine*, **18**, 270–6.

44. Hadler, N.M., Gillings, D.B., Imbus, R. *et al.* (1978). Hand structure and function in an industrial setting. *Arthritis and Rheumatism*, **21**, 210–20.

45. Felson, D.T. Hannan, M.T., Naimark, A., Berkeley, J., Gordon, G., Wilson, P.W.F., *et al.* (1991). Occupational physical demands, knee bending, and knee osteoarthritis: results from the Framingham Study. *Journal of Rheumatology*, **18**, 1587–92.

46. Cooper, C., McAlindon, T., Coggon, D., Egger, P. and Dieppe, P. (1994). Occupational activity and osteoarthritis of the knee. *Annals of the Rheumatic Diseases* **53**, 90–3.

47. Vingard, E., Alfredsson, L., Goldie, I. and Hogstedt, C. (1991). Occupation and osteoarthrosis of the hip and knee: A register-based cohort study. *International Journal of Epidemiology*, **20**, 1025–31.

48. Rall, K.L., McElroy, G.L. and Keats, T.E. (1964). A study of long-term effects of football injury to the knee. Mo Med **61**, 435–8.

49. Roos, H., Lindberg, H., Gärdsell, P., et al. The prevalence of gonarthrosis in former soccer players and its relation to meniscectomy. *American Journal of Sports Medicine* in press.

50. Lindberg, H., Roos, H. and Gädsell, P. (1993). Prevalence of coxarthrosis in former soccer players: 286 players compared with matched controls. *Acta Orthopedica Scandinauica* **64**(2), 165–7.

51. Harris, P.A., Hart, D.J., Jawad, S., Woman, R., Doyle, D.V. and Spector, T.D. (1994). Risk of osteoarthritis associated with running: a radiological survey of ex-athletes. *Arthritis and Rheumatism*, **37 Supplement**, S369.

52. Puranen, J., Ala-Ketola, L., Peltokallio, P., et al. (1975). Running and primary osteoarthritis of the hip. *British Medical Journal*, **1**, 424–5.

53. Marti, B., Knobloch, M., Tschopp, A., Armin, J. and Howald, H. (1989). Is excessive running predictive of degenerative hip disease? Controlled study of former elite athletes. *British Medical Journal*, **299**, 91–3.

54. Vingard, E., Alfredsson, L., Goldie, I. and Hogstedt, C. (1993). Sports and osteoarthrosis of the hip. An epidemiologic study. *American Journal of Sports Medicine* **21**, 195–200.

55. Kellgren, J.H. and Moore, R. (1952). Generalized osteoarthritis and Heberden's nodes. *British Medical Journal*, **1**, 181–7.

56. Lawrence, J.S. (1977). Osteoarthrosis. In *Rheumatism in populations*, (ed. J.S. Lawrence). Heinemann Medical Books Ltd., London.

57. Schumacher, H.R., Gordon, G., Hernando, P., et al. (1981). Osteoarthritis, crystal deposition, and inflammation. *Seminars in Arthritis and Rheumatism*, **10** (**supplement 1**), 116–19.

58. Felson, D.T., Anderson, J.J., Naimark, A., Kannel, W. and Meenan, R.F. (1989). The prevalence of chondrocalcinosis in the elderly and its association with knee osteoarthritis: the Framingham Study. *Journal of Rheumatology*, **16**, 1241–5.

59. Ali, S.Y. and Griffiths, S. (1983). Formation of calcium phosphate crystals in normal and osteoarthritic cartilage. *Annals of the Rheumatic Diseases*, **42** (**supplement**), 45.

60. Palotie, A., Ott, J., Elima, K., Cheah, K., Peltonen, L., et al. (1989). Predisposition to familial osteoarthrosis linked to type II collagen gene. *The Lancet*, **1**, 924–7.

61. Radin, E.L. (1976). Mechanical aspects of osteoarthritis. *Bull Rheum Dis*, **26**, 862–5.

62. Hart, D.J., Mootoosamy, I., Doyle, D.V. and Spector, T.D. (1994). The relationship between osteoarthritis and osteoporosis in the general population: the Chingford Study. *Annals of the Rheumatic Diseases*, **53**, 158–62.

63. Gevers, G., Dequeker, J., Martens, M., et al. (1989). Biomechanical characteristics of iliac crest bone in elderly women according to osteoarthritis grade at the hand joints. *Journal of Rheumatology*, **16**, 660–3.

64. Dequeker, J., Goris, P. and Utterhoeven, R. (1983). Osteoporosis and osteoarthritis (osteoarthrosis): anthropometric distinctions. *Journal of the American Medical Association*, **249**, 1448–51.

65. Hannan, M.T., Anderson, J.J., Zhang, Y., Levy, D. and Felson, D.T. (1993). Bone mineral density and knee osteoarthritis in elderly men and women. *Arthritis and Rheumatism* **36**, 1671–80.

66. Kellgren, J.H. (1961). Osteoarthritis in patients and populations. *British Medical Journal*, **243**, 1–6

67. Solomon, L. (1976). Patterns of osteoarthritis of the hip. *Journal of Bone and Joint Surgery*, **58-B**, 176–83.

68. Nevitt, M.C., Cummings, S.R., Lane, N.E., Genant, H.K. and Pressman, A.R. (1994). Current use of oral estrogen is associated with a decreased prevalence of radiographic hip OA in elderly white women. *Arthritis and Rheumatism*, **37 supplement**, S212.

69. Hannan, M.T., Felson, D.T., Anderson, J.J., Naimark, A. and Kannel, W.B. (1990). Estrogen use and radiographic osteoarthritis of the knee in women. *Arthritis and Rheumatism*, **33**, 525–32.

70. Wolfe, F., Altman, R., Hochberg, M., Lane, N., Luggan, M. and Sharp, J. (1994). Postmenopausal estrogen therapy is associated with improved radiographic scores in OA and RA. *Arthritis and Rheumatism*, **37 supplement**, S231.

71. Samanta, A., Jones, A., Regan, M., Wilson, S. and Doherty, M. (1993). Is osteoarthritis in women affected by hormonal changes or smoking? *British Journal of Rheumatology*, **32**, 366–70.

72. Hart, D.J., Doyle, D.V. and Spector, T.D. (1995). Association between metabolic factors and knee osteoarthritis in women: the Chingford Study. *Journal of Rheumatology*, **22**, 1118–23.

73. Lawrence, J.S. (1975). Hypertension in relation to musculoskeletal disorders. *Annals of the Rheumatic Diseases*, **34**, 451–6.

74. Felson, D.T., Anderson, J.J., Naimark, A., Hannan, M.T., Kannel, W.B. and Meenan, R.F., (1989). Does smoking protect against osteoarthritis? *Arthritis and Rheumatism*, **32**(2), 166–72.

75. Kraus, J.F., D'Ambrosia, R.D., Smith, E.G., van Meter, J., Borhani, N.O., Franti, C.E., et al. (1978). An epidemiological study of severe osteoarthritis. *Orthopedics*, **1**, 37–42.

76. Spector, T.D., Brown, G.C. and Silman, A.J. (1988). Increased rates of previous hysterectomy and gynaecological operations in women with osteoarthritis. *British Medical Journal*, **297**, 899–900.

77. Hartz, A.J., Fischer, M.E., Brill, G., et al. (1986). The association of obesity with joint pain and osteoarthritis in the HANES data. *Journal of Chronic Diseases*, **39**, 311–19.

78. Hochberg, M.C., Lawrence, R.C., Everett, D.F. and Cornoni-Huntley, J. (1989). Epidemiologic associations of pain in osteoarthritis of the knee: Data from the National Health and Nutrition Examination Survey and the National Health and Nutrition Examination-I epidemiologic follow-up survey. *Seminars in Arthritis and Rheumatism*, **18**, 4–9.

3 | *The economics of osteoarthritis*

Edward Yelin

Introduction

Demographers and economists traditionally divide chronic diseases into two groups: those of high prevalence and low average impact, for example, chronic sinusitis; and those of low prevalence and high average impact, for example, systemic lupus erythematosus[1]. Osteoarthritis (OA) sits astride these two major classifications: it is clearly a high prevalence condition, but it also must be classified as one with at least a moderate, if not a high level of impact. More importantly, because OA is associated with age[2], the aging of the population puts a higher proportion of the population at risk for OA. Moreover, once the onset of OA occurs, the aging of the population puts a higher proportion of persons in the ages of greatest severity. This combination of high and growing prevalence, and moderate to severe impact, makes OA an important condition in health policy concerns.

Interestingly, the condition has received relatively scant attention in the cost-of-illness literature. Instead, health services researchers from the rheumatology community have focussed on the cost of rheumatoid arthritis (RA) in clinical samples, probably because it is a more prominent condition in the practices of rheumatologists[3–6]. On the other hand, in their own studies, the demographers and economists tend to focus on the more encompassing rubrics of musculoskeletal disease or all forms of arthritis, probably because the data sets they analyze do not include discrete diagnoses, such as OA. However, persons with OA constitute a large fraction of all persons with musculoskeletal conditions and, therefore, of the costs of these diseases.

This chapter reviews the studies of the economic impact of musculoskeletal disease and all forms of arthritis, conducted on random samples of the population; summarizes the small literature on the cost of OA, using clinical samples; compares the results from the clinical studies of OA and RA; and then uses the 1979–1981 National Health Interview Survey to make preliminary estimates of the absolute national cost of arthritis and of the increment in costs experienced by persons with arthritis compared to those of similar age, sex, and race without arthritis. The pharmacoeconomics of the treatment of OA are discussed specifically in Chapter 8.

Cost of illness methods

The costs of illness are divided into two distinct spheres, those due to direct expenditures for medical care services and those due to the indirect impact of illness on function, principally measured by lost wages due to reduced work effort or total cessation of work activities[7]. Indirect costs also include the implied losses when homemakers are no longer able to function as well as before the onset of illness and the family substitutes for the homemaker's activities, and the explicit cost incurred when the family hires someone to replace those lost functions[8]. Finally, indirect costs also include the value of activity losses in non-work domains, such as leisure, although such losses are difficult to price in monetary terms[9,10]. As a practical matter, most cost-of-illness studies limit the estimate of indirect costs to lost wages and the proxy value of lost function among homemakers.

National studies of the cost of musculoskeletal diseases

Four studies of the cost of musculoskeletal diseases in the US have been published, the most recent of which presented the costs of arthritis separately. In addition, a study of the economic impact of musculoskeletal disease on Canada has recently been completed. Table 3.1 summarizes the results of these studies. In any one year, the estimate of the direct and indirect costs of illness is a function of the prevalence and impact of the disease in question, as well as of the relative prices of medical care and wages. In the first systematic study of the cost of illness, Rice[7] reported that

Table 3.1   Cost of musculoskeletal diseases in current US and Canadian dollars and as a % of Gross National Product (GNP)

Year	Direct ($ billion)	Indirect ($ billion)	Total ($ billion)	% of GNP
1963	2	2	4	0.7
1972	4	5	9	0.7
1980	13	8	21	0.8
1988	60	64	124	2.5
1988 (includes arthritis only)	13	42	55	1.2
		Canada		
1986	2	6	8	1.7

Source: US data: Refs 10–13 Canadian data: Ref. 15.

in the United States in 1963, musculoskeletal conditions accounted for $4 billion in total costs, half from the direct costs of medical care and half from wage losses and the imputed value of homemaker losses. This sum was equivalent to 0.7 per cent of that year's gross national product (GNP). By way of comparison, economists state that we are in a recession when the economy contracts by one per cent or more.

The relative magnitude of the total costs of musculoskeletal disease in the US remained fairly stable through 1980, though the proportion due to medical care and wage losses changed substantially[11,12]. In the 1960s, real wages were rising rapidly, while medical care inflation had not yet become a significant problem. Accordingly, the proportion of total costs due to wage losses rose between the 1963 and 1972 studies. In contrast, after the oil shock of the early 1970s, real wages stagnated while medical care prices rose quickly. By 1980, direct costs of musculoskeletal disease accounted for more than 60 per cent of the total costs of this group of illnesses.

The most recent national study of the costs of musculoskeletal conditions concerned 1988[13]. In that year, the total costs of these illnesses amounted to $124 billion, or more than 2.5 per cent of GNP. Slightly less than half of the total was due to direct costs of medical care and the balance was due to wage losses. In this same study, the costs of arthritis alone was estimated to be $55 billion, with three-quarters due to lost wages. In a paper published by the National Arthritis Data Work Group, we estimated that approximately half of the increase in the cost of musculoskeletal conditions between 1980 and 1988 was due to increases in the prevalence and severity of the conditions, and the remainder was an artifact of such methodological improvements as more accurate coding of medical conditions and more thorough allocation of costs to musculoskeletal disease[14].

The relative magnitude of the costs of musculoskeletal conditions would appear to be similar in Canada and the United States. Thus, in 1986 the total costs of musculoskeletal conditions in Canada was approximately 1.7 per cent of GNP, or about halfway between the estimates for the United States for 1988 of the costs of all forms of arthritis alone and all forms of musculoskeletal disease[15]. The exact conditions subsumed in the musculoskeletal rubric and the exact methods of study notwithstanding, these conditions have an impact on the economy equivalent to a severe recession, roughly comparable to the recession in the United States and Canada experienced at the beginning of the 1980s. Moreover, while recessions are temporary, the impact of arthritis on the economy is felt year after year.

Costs of osteoarthritis from studies using clinical samples

There have only been three studies of the costs of osteoarthritis derived from clinical samples and in only one of these was indirect costs due to lost wages assessed. Table 3.2 summarizes the result of these studies, expressing all costs in 1994 terms. The study by Liang *et al.*[16] derives from a random sample of those who had ever attended a tertiary care facility. They reported that physician visits accounted for a small portion of direct costs of medical care; the majority of direct costs were due to a handful of hospital admissions and to the category 'other', which includes prescription and non-prescription drugs and medical devices. Indirect costs of OA dwarfed medical costs, averaging $10,705 in 1994 terms among all persons with OA.

The study by Holman *et al.*[17] was limited to costs of physician visits and hospital admissions. It was con-

Table 3.2 Costs of osteoarthritis in 1994 dollars from three studies using clinical samples

| Study | Direct costs ($ billion) | | | | Indirect costs ($ billion) | Total ($ billion) |
	Physician	Hospital	Other	Total		
Liang *et al.* 1984	163	559	852	1574	10 705	12 279
Gabriel *et al.* 1995				2159		
Holman *et al.* 1988	1151	753		1919		

Notes: All costs expressed in 1994 by terms by inflating study year costs by the change in the Consumer Price Index ([22], p. 482). In the study by Liang *et al.*[16], indirect costs were estimated jointly for persons with OA and RA; this amount was applied here for the persons with OA. The study by Gabriel *et al.*[18] Reported the frequency of changes in employment, but not the associated indirect costs. In the study by Holman *et al.*[17], neither 'other' costs nor indirect costs were reported.

ducted in Northern California and included respondents receiving care in the fee-for-service sector, in a pre-paid group practice, and in an experimental center designed to lower utilization rates. The authors reported that the magnitude of the costs of hospitalization in their study was similar to the study by Liang *et al.* but they also reported much higher costs due to physician visits, and overall direct medical care costs more than 20 per cent higher, even though the costs of drugs and devices were not estimated. Interestingly, costs were lower in the experimental setting than in the pre-paid group practice, and lower in the pre-paid group practice than in fee-for-service. This suggests that medical care costs of OA are subject to reduction through both financial incentives facing providers and the persons with OA, and through non-monetary incentives of a practice designed to reduce utilization through a more interactive relationship among patients and physicians.

In the final study using clinical samples, Gabriel *et al.*[18] assembled a database of all persons with a diagnosis of OA among residents of Olmstead County, Minnesota. This sample comes closest to a true population-based study, with the caveat that those who have OA but have not received a diagnosis would not appear in the database. In this study, the authors did not report direct medical costs by category. Moreover, they only accounted for costs that generate medical bills. Even so, their estimate of overall annual direct medical care costs for OA — $2159 per person exceeds the estimates from the two previous studies. Although Gabriel *et al.* did not estimate the wage losses associated with OA, they did report that about 11 per cent of persons with OA reduced their hours of work, 9 per cent reported being unable to get a job, and 14 per cent retired early due to this condition.

Comparison of the costs of OA and RA

Table 3.3 compares the per case costs of OA and RA by averaging values from each of the studies using clinical samples. Not surprisingly, the per case costs of RA exceed the costs of OA in every category, with the costs of hospital admissions accounting for the largest relative difference. Overall, the per case cost of RA is 1.71 times as great as the per case cost of OA. Nevertheless, because the prevalence of OA is so great, it has a far

Table 3.3 Costs of rheumatoid arthritis and osteoarthritis from averages of clinical studies in 1994 dollars

| Study | Direct costs ($ billion) | | | | Indirect costs ($ billion) | Total ($ billion) |
	Physician	Hospital	Other	Total		
OA	657	656	852	2165	10 705	12 870
RA	963	2990	1243	5201	16 821	22 026

Notes: All costs expressed in 1994 terms by inflating study year costs by the change in the Consumer Price Index ([22], p. 482). The costs of OA were estimated by averaging the studies summarized in Table 3.2, or, where only one study provided as estimate, using that one value. The costs of RA were estimated in a similar fashion, using the studies of Meenan *et al.*[3] and Lubeck *et al.*[4].

greater overall impact on the economy than RA. Assuming a liberal estimate of the prevalence of RA of 1.0 per cent of the population and a conservative estimate of the prevalence of OA of 4.2 per cent of males and 9.0 per cent of females 20 years of age or over[2], there are 2.52 million persons with RA and 12.06 million with OA in the nation. Accordingly, the total costs of OA, at $15.52 billion, are about 2.8 times as large as the total costs of RA, at $5.56 billion. Even using the highest published estimates for the prevalence of RA — 2 per cent[2], the national costs of OA would still exceed the national costs of RA by about 50 per cent.

National, community-based estimates of the impact of arthritis

In studies using clinical samples, researchers are able to customize data collection to ensure relatively complete enumeration of the impacts of illness. However, the sample of persons with the illness is biased, either because those who receive a diagnosis may have inherently better access to care, or because they may have more severe illness, than those who do not.

In part, to avoid the bias from sampling in clinical environments, the federal government instituted an annual community-based survey of the health of the population — the National Health Interview (HIS)[19]. In the HIS, individuals self-report their symptoms and, unless a physician has told the individual a specific diagnosis associated with the symptoms, a general diagnostic code, such as arthritis is given. The analysis reported below provides estimates of the impact of all forms of self-reported arthritis for the years 1989 through 1991 (using three years reduces the sampling variability associated with any one year's data). Osteoarthritis accounts for most of those in this diagnostic classification[20].

Over the period 1989 through 1991, an average of 30.8 million individuals self-reported symptoms consistent with arthritis, for an overall prevalence rate of 12.3 per cent, roughly twice the rate from epidemiologic studies of OA based on physician examination[2]. Table 3.4 summarizes the average and total health care utilization of these individuals self-reporting arthritis. Overall, they made a mean of 7.34 visits to physicians in the year prior to interview, or 226.3 million visits overall. In addition, they experienced an average of 0.22 hospital admissions per person, amounting to 6.9 million admissions in the nation as a whole. These hospital admissions totalled 48.8 million days, for an average length of stay of 7.07 days per admission.

Table 3.5 provides estimates of the economic impact of this medical care use utilization and of the wage losses associated with arthritis. These estimates were made by multiplying the number of units of physician visits used by $75, the approximate average of the costs of physician visits in the nation, and the number of hospital admissions by $6136, the average cost of all hospital stays in the US. Using these unit prices, all persons self-reporting arthritis incurred $16.97 billion in costs due to physician visits and $42.33 billion in costs due to hospital admissions in the years 1989 through 1991. Because many of the hospital admissions for arthritis include surgical procedures, including total joint replacement surgery, and surgical admissions are more expensive than this average, the 'true' cost of the admissions probably exceeds the $42.33 billion estimate. Even without adjusting the unit price of hospital admissions to take surgery into account, the annual cost of medical care for arthritis is at least $59.30 billion. Including the costs of drugs and devices, not enumerated in the HIS, would increase the total substantially.

In addition, 14.1 per cent fewer of those with arthritis are in the labor force than persons without arthritis. Thus, 2.34 million persons with arthritis were not working who would have been if they had the same

Table 3.4 Per capita and total utilization of persons reporting arthritis, US, 1989–1991

Type of utilization	Mean	Total (million)
Visits to physicians	7.34	226.3
Hospital admissions	0.22	6.9
Hospital days	1.58	48.8
Length of admissions (in days)	7.07	

Source and note: Author's analysis of 1989 through 1991 National Health Interview Surveys. Estimates based on averaging across the three surveys.

Table 3.5 Estimates of the absolute national costs of arthritis in 1994 dollars, US, 1989–1991

Direct costs					Indirect costs			Total costs
Physician visits			Hospital admissions					
Number	Unit price	Total	Number	Unit price*	Total	Total	Number leaving work†	Unit price‡	Total	
226.3 mil.	$75	$16.97 bil.	6.9 mil.	$6136	$42.33 bil.	$59.30 bil.	2.34 mil.	$24 076	$56.34 bil.	$115.64 bil.

Source and notes: Author's analysis of 1989 through 1991 National Health Interview Surveys.

* Unit price of hospital admission based on average cost of patient stay in US short-term hospitals in 1992 ([22], p. 127), with the value inflated to 1994 terms using the Medical Care Component of the Consumer Price Index.

† Number of persons who left work based on difference in age, sex, and race matched labor force participation rates of persons without arthritis and actual labor force participation rate of persons with arthritis (14.1%).

‡ Unit price of cessation of work based on US median weekly wage times 52 weeks ([22], p. 429).

labor force participation rates as persons without arthritis. Applying a unit price for wage losses based on average earnings among all US workers, the indirect costs of arthritis totals at least $56.34 billion. This figure omits all losses due to a reduction in hours or the lesser degree of career advancement experienced by persons with arthritis in comparison with those without arthritis.

Even though the estimate of the direct costs omits common expenses for arthritis, and the estimate of indirect costs omits partial work disability, the estimate of the total cost of arthritis – $115.64 billion — represents 2.1 per cent of average GNP for the years 1989 through 1991.

Table 3.5 provides estimates of the total costs incurred by persons with arthritis. Table 3.6, in contrast, shows the increment in costs experienced by persons with arthritis relative to the remainder of the population and assuming persons with arthritis had the same age, race, and sex distribution as those without arthritis. Persons with arthritis make slightly less than one extra visit a year to the physician than similar persons without arthritis. Accordingly, the incremental costs of their physician visits are relatively small, $2.28 billion. The incremental cost of their hospital admissions is much larger. Based on an excess of 0.06 admissions per capita and a unit cost of $6136 per admission, the increment in the costs of the hospital admissions of persons with arthritis is $11.41 billion. Thus, of the total incremental medical care costs of $13.69 billion incurred by persons with arthritis, more than 80 per cent is due to excess hospital admissions.

However, the incremental costs of wage losses dwarf even those due to hospitalization. In the period 1989 through 1991, an extra 1.0 million persons with arthritis were out of work, relative to the expected labor force participation rate of persons with their age, sex, and race characteristics but without arthritis. After multiplying this number by the average wages among US workers, the increment in wage losses totals $24.08 billion. All told, the increment in wage losses of persons with arthritis relative to those without is far larger than the increment in direct medical care costs.

Policymakers concerned about the medical care costs of arthritis would do well to focus on reducing hospital admissions, since excess admissions are responsible for the bulk of the increment in medical care costs. Although one cannot easily attribute surgical procedures to particular conditions in the National Health Interview Survey, from other sources of data we know that surgical admissions account for a large proportion of the increment in costs attributable to hospitalization[21]. In a similar fashion, policymakers would do well to emphasize the impact of arthritis on work, since wage losses account for almost two-thirds of the incremental cost of arthritis.

Summary and conclusions

In contrast to RA, the cost of OA has been the subject of few studies. Accordingly, it is necessary to piece together evidence from several kinds of sources to provide an indication of the economic impact of OA. These sources include studies of the national impact of all forms of musculoskeletal disease, the few studies of the costs of OA using clinical samples, and new estimates using information from the 1989 through 1991 National Health Interview Survey concerning the impact of all forms of arthritis.

From these sources, the annual cost of OA would appear to approach $13 000 per case, with most of the costs due to wage losses. Though lower than RA, because of the much larger prevalence of OA, the overall economic impact of OA is much greater. However, it is very difficult to provide a good estimate of the exact magnitude of the economic cost of OA for the nation. In self-report studies, such as the National Health Interview Survey, the prevalence of OA is under-reported; most OA is classified under the more encompassing rubric of 'all forms of arthritis'. Indeed, a diagnosis of OA occurs relatively infrequently in the clinical environment, since physicians often do not differentiate among musculoskeletal complaints in their treatment plans. As shown above, it can be estimated that the economic impact of this more encompassing rubric is $115.64 billion, and that people with arthritis incur incremental costs of about $37.77 billion, mostly due to wage losses. Both the estimate of the per cost and the estimate of the national impact must be viewed as preliminary, in the former case because the clinical studies are few and not as systematic as the studies of the cost of RA, in the latter case because of our inability to separate OA from other forms of musculoskeletal disease.

However, to a certain extent these shortcomings in the literature reflect a shortcoming of concern about OA itself. Even these preliminary findings should indicate to policymakers that the combination of high prevalence, and moderate to high impact, combine to make OA a costly illness. It is time to conduct more systematic studies on the economic impact of OA, so

Table 3.6 Estimates of the incremental national costs of arthritis in 1994 dollars, US, 1989–1991

Direct costs							Indirect costs			Total costs
Physician visits			Hospital admissions			Total				
Incremental number*	Unit price	Total	Incremental number*	Unit price#	Total		Incremental number leaving work†	Unit price‡	Total	
0.98 mil.	$75	$2.28 bil.	0.06 mil.	$6136	$11.41 bil.	$13.69 bil.	1.0 mil.	$24 076	$24.08 bil.	$37.77 bil.

Source and notes: Author's analysis of 1989 through 1991 National Health Interview Surveys.

* Incremental number of physician visits and hospital admissions per person based on regressions estimating the utilization among persons with OA assuming the age, sex, and race distribution in the remainder of the population.

Unit price of hospital admission based on average cost of patient stay in US short-term hospitals in 1992 ([22], p. 127), with this value inflated to 1994 terms using the Medical Care Component of the Consumer Price Index.

† Number of persons who left work based on difference in labor force participation of persons without arthritis, and the estimated labor force participation rate of persons with arthritis and the same distribution of age, sex, and race as persons without arthritis (6.0%).

‡Unit price of cessation of work based on US median weekly wage times 52 weeks ([22], p. 429).

that we can plan adequately for the pandemic of OA we face with the aging of the population.

References

1. Verbrugge, L. and Patrick, D. (1995). Seven chronic conditions: their impact on US adults' activity levels and use of medical services. *American Journal of Public Health*, **85**, 173–82.
2. Silman, A. and Hochberg, M. (1993). *Epidemiology of the rheumatic diseases*, pp. 257–88. Oxford University Press, Oxford.
3. Meenan, R., Yelin, E., Henke, C., Curtis, D. and Epstein, W. (1978). The costs of rheumatoid arthritis. *Arthritis and Rheumatism*, **21**, 827–33.
4. Lubeck, D., Spitz, P., Fries, J., Wolfe, F., Mitchell, D. and Roth, S. (1986). A multicenter study of annual health services utilization and costs in rheumatoid arthritis. *Arthritis and Rheumatism*, **29**, 488–93.
5. Thompson, M., Read, J. and Liang, M. (1984). Feasibility of willingness-to-pay measurements in chronic arthritis. *Medical Decision Making*, **4**, 195–212.
6. Stone, C. (1984). The lifetime costs of rheumatoid arthritis. *Journal of Rheumatology*, **11**, 819–27.
7. Rice, D. (1966). Estimating the cost of illness. *Health Economics Series*, No. 6. (National Center for Health Statistics.)
8. Walker, K. and Gauger, W. (1970, revised 1980). The dollar value of household work. *Information Bulletin No. 60*. (New York State College of Human Ecology,) Ithaca, New York.
9. Lubeck, D. and Yelin, E. (1988). A question of value: measuring the impact of chronic disease. *Milbank Quarterly*, **66**, 445–64.
10. Reisine, S., Goodenow, C. and Grady, K. (1987). The impact of rheumatoid arthritis on the Homemaker. *Social Science and Medicine*, **25**, 89–95.
11. Cooper, B. and Rice, D. (1976). The economic cost of illness revisited. *Social Security Bulletin*, **39**, 21–35.
12. Rice, D., Hodgson, T. and Kopstein, A. (1985). The economic costs of illness: a replication and update. *Health Care Finance Review*, **7**, 61–80.
13. Rice, D. (1992). Cost of muscloskeletal conditions. In *Musculoskeletal conditions in the US*, pp. 143–70. (ed. A. Pramer, S., Furner and D. Rice), American Academy of Orthopedics, Chicago.
14. Yelin. E. and Callahan L. (in press). The economic cost and social and psychological impact of musculoskeletal conditions. *Arthritis and Rheumatism*.
15. Badley, E. (1995). The economic burden of muscu-loskeletal disorders in canada is similar to that for cancer, and may be higher. *Journal of Rheumatology*, **22**, 204–6.
16. Liang, M., Larson, M., Thompson, M., Eaton, H., McNamera, E., Katz, R., *et al.* (1984). Costs and out-comes in rheumatoid and osteoarthritis. *Arthritis and Rheumatism*, **27**, 522–9.
17. Holman, H., Lubeck, D., Dutton, D. and Brown, B. (1988). Improving health service performance by modi-fying medical practices. *Transactions of the Association American Physicians*, **101**, 173–9.
18. Gabriel, S., Crowson, C. and O'Fallon, W. (1995). Costs of osteoarthritis: estimates from a geographically defined population. *Journal of Rheumatology*, **22 (Supplement 43)**, 23–5.
19. Kovar, M. and Poe, G. (1985). National Health Interview Survey design, 1973–1984 and procedures, 1975–1983. *Vital and Health Statistics*, **Series. 1, No. 18**.
20. LaPlante, M. (1988). *Data on disability from the National Health Interview Survey*. National Institute on Disability and Rehabilitation Research, Washington, DC.
21. Felts, W. and Yelin, E. (1989). The economic impact of the rheumatic diseases in the United States. *Journal of Rheumatology*, **16**, 867–84.
22. USGPO. (1993). *Statistical Abstract of the US, 1993*, pp. 127, 429, 482.

4 | *Hereditary osteoarthritis*

Sergio A. Jimenez, Charlene J. Williams, and David Karasick

Introduction

Human osteoarthritis (OA) is a heterogeneous and multi-factorial disease with multiple pathogenetic mechanisms implicated in its development and progression. Despite its complex pathogenesis, it is clear that certain subsets of OA exhibit a hereditary pattern[1–7]. The concept of hereditary OA has evolved since the original description by Heberden of 'little hard knots, about the size of a small pea' in the dorsal aspect of the distal interphalangeal joints of the hands — that allowed him to distinguish OA from other forms of arthritis such as gout[8]. Subsequently, Haygarth expanded the clinical description of Heberden's nodes to include their association with simultaneous involvement of multiple joints[9]. Similar bony enlargements of the proximal interphalangeal joints of the hands were described by Bouchard[10]. These lesions, now known as 'Heberden's and 'Bouchard's nodes', were considered of diagnostic value to separate 'hypertrophic arthritis' from 'arthritis deformans' by Osler[11]. The familial occurrence of Heberden's nodes was first documented by Stecher and Hersh, who concluded that these lesions were inherited as a single autosomal dominant gene with strong female preponderance[1]. Subsequent studies provided additional evidence for the familial occurrence of Heberden's and Bouchard's nodes, and of degenerative arthritis involving multiple joints[2–7,12,13], although other studies suggested a polygenic inheritance rather than a single gene defect[14,15].

Clinical spectrum of hereditary OA

The spectrum of hereditary OA is quite varied encompassing mild disorders, which do not become clinically apparent until late adult life, to very severe forms that manifest clinically during childhood. Although many of these disorders have been previously classified as secondary OA[16], they all have the common characteristic of being caused by mutations in the genes encoding macromolecules expressed exclusively or predominantly in cartilaginous tissues. The genes that may be responsible for these diseases include: those encoding cartilage-specific collagens (Types II, IX, X, and XI); proteoglycan core protein and link proteins; non-collagenous components of the cartilage matrix; growth factors involved in the process of cartilage differentiation or in the regulation of chondrocyte proliferation and specific gene expression; and genes encoding enzymes involved in various cartilage-specific metabolic pathways. Thus, these disorders represent a truly distinct sub-group of OA that must be separated from secondary OA. Diseases that can be classified within the spectrum of hereditary OA are as follows:

- primary generalized osteoarthritis
- familial calcium pyrophosphate deposition disease
- familial hydroxyapatite deposition disease
- chondrodysplasias

    — spondylo-epiphyseal dysplasias
    — hereditary arthroophthalmopathy (Stickler syndrome)
    — Kniest dysplasia

- multiple epiphyseal dysplasias
- osteochondrodysplasias.

Genes that have been demonstrated to contain mutations that cause these disorders or are considered likely candidates implicated in their etiology are as follows:

- cartilage – specific collagens

    — type II collagen
    — type IX collagen
    — type X collagen
    — type XI collagen

- proteoglycan (aggrecan) core protein
- proteoglycan link proteins
- cartilage oligomeric matrix protein (COMP)
- other non-collagenous cartilage proteins
- growth factors (fibroblast growth factor, others)

- growth factor receptors
- other regulatory factors
- enzymes involved in cartilage-specific functions.

The distinction between hereditary OA and secondary OA is not an artificial one since it is based on clear-cut differences in their etiology and pathogenesis, as well as in their course of evolution and prognosis. Furthermore, there are also clear differences in the therapeutic approaches for these two forms of OA *see* Table 4.1. Whereas in secondary OA treatment must be directed toward the primary disease, in hereditary OA the ideal treatment would be the correction of the causative gene mutation. Although at the present time this approach is not feasible, the rapid advances in genetics and molecular biology in the recent past have made the prospects for gene therapy plausible in the future[17,18].

This chapter will review the most important clinical and radiographic features of various forms of hereditary OA and will describe the gene defects that have been identified or have been suspected as the cause of these diseases.

Primary generalized OA (PGOA)

This most common form of hereditary OA, was first recognized as a discrete clinical entity by Kellgren and Moore[2]. PGOA is characterized by the familial development of Heberden's and Bouchard's nodes and the premature degeneration of the articular cartilage of multiple joints[6,13]. Typically, the clinical and radiographic features have a precocious onset and an accelerated progression. It is generally accepted that the loss of articular cartilage in PGOA is usually concentric or uniform, particularly in the knees and hips[3,19,20]. This pattern of cartilage loss is not constant and the radiographic appearance of affected joints is indistinguishable from that of non-hereditary OA, except for their premature occurrence, their increased severity, and their rapid progression. In the hand, the pattern of distribution favors the distal and proximal interphalangeal joints, with prominent bone reaction resulting

in formation of Heberden's and Bouchard's nodes, and with frequent involvement of the first carpometacarpal joint. Degenerative changes of the hip typically develop early in adult life. The femoral heads tend to become flattened as the disease progresses. Sclerosis, pseudocysts, and femoral head deformity are seen with advanced disease and usually occur more rapidly than in sporadic OA.

Although there is controversy regarding the etiopathogenesis of PGOA, multiple studies have shown that a genetic predisposition plays an important role in its development and progression[3,5–7,21]. One study found that Heberden's and Bouchard's nodes were present in 36 per cent of the relatives of male individuals with OA and in 49 per cent of relatives of women with PGOA, in comparison to expected frequencies in the general population of 17 per cent and 26 per cent, respectively[6]. The frequency of nodal generalized OA increased to 45 per cent if only first degree female relatives of individuals with nodal OA were studied. The familial pattern of PGOA is also supported by studies that examined the inheritance of various genetic markers in affected individuals with PGOA and in their non-affected relatives. For example, a genetic predisposition to the disease was suggested by the demonstration of an increased frequency of the HLA A1 B8 haplotype[15,22], and of the MZ isoform of α_1 antitrypsin[22]. More recently, the relative contribution of genetic and environmental factors to OA affecting the hands and knees was investigated employing a classic twin study[23]. In this study, 130 identical and 120 non-identical female twins were examined radiographically for the presence of OA changes in hands and knees. The results demonstrated a clear genetic influence on the development of PGOA, with a calculated score for heritability influence ranging from 40 to 70 per cent, independently of known environmental or demographic confounders. The concordance of radiographic changes of OA at all sites examined was consistently two-fold higher in identical twins than non-identical, providing conclusive evidence for the hereditary nature of the disease.

Table 4.1 Differences between hereditary osteoarthritis and secondary osteoarthritis

	Hereditary OA	Secondary OA
Etiology	Mutations in genes expressed in articular cartilage	Various hereditary or acquired diseases
Pathogenesis	Alterations in structural or functional components of articular cartilage	Secondary effects to diseases not exclusively affecting articular cartilage
Therapy	Gene therapy to correct gene defect	Treatment of primary disease

Familial calcium pyrophosphate deposition (CPPD) disease

A second type of hereditary OA is that associated with familial CPPD disease, also known as familial chondrocalcinosis. Following the initial description of the disease in five Czech families[24,25], multiple ethnic series have been reported from throughout the world[26–39]. Most cases appear to be inherited in an autosomal dominant manner with precocious onset and severe clinical expression. The radiographic features include chondrocalcinosis most frequently seen in the knee, symphysis pubis, and triangular fibrocartilage of the wrist. These changes may precede frank OA changes of the affected joints. The arthropathy of CPPD radiographically resembles non-hereditary, sporadic OA but its distribution is distinctive; it occurs in sites less commonly involved in the usual form of OA such as the metacarpophalangeal, radioscaphoid, and patellofemoral articulations[40]. Subchondral cysts are more common, frequently being numerous and large. On occasion, the abnormalities can resemble neuropathic arthropathy with considerable bone debris and joint disorganization.

The mechanisms responsible for the tissue deposition of the crystals are not known, although some studies indicate that structural changes in articular cartilage matrix might promote crystal formation[41–44]. In support of this suggestion are results of a study of articular cartilage from a Swedish patient with familial CPPD disease, showing decreased collagen content in the middle zone of the cartilage matrix with some fragmentation of the collagen fibers[41,42]. Since these changes were in crystal-free areas of the matrix, it was postulated that a matrix abnormality may predispose the tissue to CPPD and to its degeneration. Other matrix abnormalities have also been reported in sporadic cases of CPPD[43,44]. However, to date no specific defect in the components of articular cartilage has been conclusively identified in familial CPPD disease.

Familial hydroxyapatite deposition disease (HADD)

Another form of inherited crystal deposition disease is due to the deposition of hydroxyapatite crystals in articular cartilage[45–53]. The mode of inheritance is that of an autosomal dominant pattern with full penetrance. This disorder results in periarticular disease in the form of tendinitis or bursitis and, less frequently, true articular disease. Calcium hydroxyapatite deposits in bursae and tendon sheaths are radiographically visible either as poorly defined linear densities or dense, homogeneous, well-delineated masses. The most common locations of HADD are the shoulders, hips, and wrists. In the shoulder, calcifications are visible in the rotator cuff and adjacent bursae. Calcification of the supraspinatus tendon is common and occurs in close proximity to the greater tuberosity of the humerus. Additional sites include gluteal insertions on the greater trochanter and surrounding bursa. Triceps tendon calcification at its insertion on the olecranon is occasionally observed. In the wrist, both flexor and extensor tendon calcifications can be seen. Calcific tendinitis may also occur in the neck, within the longus colli muscle tendon; it is visualized below the anterior arch of C_1 and is accompanied by retropharyngeal soft tissue swelling.

The clinical features and pathologic manifestations of HADD joint involvement have been recognized and characterized more recently than those of calcific bursitis and tendinitis[48,54,55]. Generally, these are essentially identical to those of CPPD disease except for the nature of the crystalline material that is deposited in the tissues. These features were examined in detail in a long-term prospective study of a large family with HADD[56]. This study showed the occurrence of premature OA in many affected members, with a high frequency of typical OA changes in the hands and large joints. These changes were associated with the occurrence of spinal and epiphyseal alterations in the majority of affected individuals. Although the presence of hydroxyapatite crystals in the synovium and articular cartilage was demonstrated, it is not clear whether the OA changes in affected members of this family are related to the spondylo-epiphyseal dysplasia or to the deposition of hydroxyapatite crystals. The effects of hydroxyapatite crystal deposition on the structural integrity of articular cartilage have not been defined to date. One study examined the formation of hydroxyapatite crystals in normal and OA articular cartilage[57], and another study described the ultrastructural alterations in articular cartilage matrix in HADD[58]. The results indicated the occurrence of severe structural alterations in the extracellular matrix in areas of crystal deposits, but there was no indication of ultrastructural abnormalities in collagen fibers or matrix in crystal-free regions.

The chondrodysplasias (CD)

The CD are a group of clinically heterogeneous hereditary disorders characterized by abnormalities in the growth and development of articular and growth plate cartilages. Various classification schemes have been proposed for this large group of disorders. However, most of these schemes are based on the clinical and radiographic features of affected individuals. As the gene mutations responsible for these diseases are identified it will be possible to establish a classification based on the nature of the genetic defect. Among the CD, several distinct entities are more likely to result in premature OA. These include spondylo-epiphyseal dysplasias, Stickler syndrome, and Kniest dysplasia. These disorders will be briefly reviewed here. Detailed descriptions of these diseases and of other CD can be found in several extensive publications[59-63]. Indeed, the term 'chondrodysplastic rheumatism' has been coined to refer to this form of OA[64].

Spondylo-epiphyseal dysplasias (SED)

The SED comprise a heterogeneous group of autosomal dominant disorders characterized by abnormal development of the axial skeleton and severe alterations of the epiphyses of long bones, often resulting in dwarfism with marked shortening of the trunk and, to a lesser extent, of the extremities[59-63]. The phenotype of the SED is quite varied, ranging from very severe forms that are clinically apparent at birth (SED congenita), to milder forms that manifest in childhood or early adolescence (late onset SED or SED tarda).

In the congenital form, ossification is generally delayed or absent in the pubic bones, distal femoral, and proximal tibial epiphyses, calcaneus, and talus. Platyspondyly is seen with a trapezoidal configuration of the vertebral centra due to a shortening of the pedicles and posterior portion of the vertebral bodies. The iliac bones are broad at the base giving them a rounded shape. The acetabular roofs are horizontal with deep fossae and there is severe varus deformity of the femoral necks. The thorax is bell-shaped and the anterior rib ends are flared. During the first year of life, the pubic bones remain under-ossified and the femoral heads do not ossify. Knee ossification centers are irregular and appear late. During childhood, the platyspondyly persists and a dorsolumbar lordosis progresses. Ossification of the capital femoral epiphyses is delayed and it may occur in multiple foci, producing a mottled appearance, resulting in irregular and flattened epiphyses. Metaphyseal abnormalities may also occur. The metaphyseal ossification may be slightly or grossly irregular with spur formation and metaphyseal splay-

ing. In adults, platyspondyly is severe and disc space narrowing produces marked short trunk dwarfism, often accompanied by severe scoliosis and progressively increasing lumbar lordosis. The severe coxa vara persists, and the femoral capital epiphyses remain small and irregular and possibly unfused. The long bones are short and display metaphyseal flaring. Genu valgus and patellar dislocations are also very common (Fig. 4.1).

In the late-onset form, SED becomes clinically apparent during prepuberty and manifests a peculiar 'hump-like' deformity of the lumbar spine with a deep, narrow pelvic configuration. Radiographically, there is disc space narrowing, platyspondyly, and mild kyphoscoliosis (Fig 4.2). Early degenerative changes are seen in multiple joints. Hip OA may develop in adolescence, worsening in early adulthood, and is characterized by marked joint narrowing, cystic changes, spur formation, and production of new bone. Resultant deformities of the femoral head and neck are commonly seen. There may be mild epiphyseal abnormality in the peripheral joints including the metacarpophalangeal joints. The most constant features of peripheral joint involvement include flattening of the articular surface of the ankles and the knees, and shallowness of the femoral intercondylar notches. In milder cases, the features of SED are not clinically obvious and these patients present with severe OA affecting multiple joints. In such cases, a careful and detailed family history and an extensive radiographic evaluation of hands, hips, knees, and spine are needed to uncover subtle epiphyseal alterations and, therefore, to establish the diagnosis of SED.

Stickler syndrome

This familial form of OA is characterized by prominent ocular involvement associated with severe premature degenerative arthritis. This syndrome, known as hereditary arthroophthalmopathy, or Stickler syndrome[65], is a relatively common autosomal dominant condition (1 case in 10 000 births). The disease is characterized by vitreous degeneration, retinal detachment, and premature degenerative joint disease which often develops in the second or third decade[66]. Associated clinical symptoms include myopia, progressive sensorineural hearing loss, cleft palate and mandibular hypoplasia (Pierre–Robin anomaly), and epiphyseal dysplasia. Although the ocular features of the syndrome are a hallmark of the disease, some of its clinical features often overlap with a number of other heritable dis-

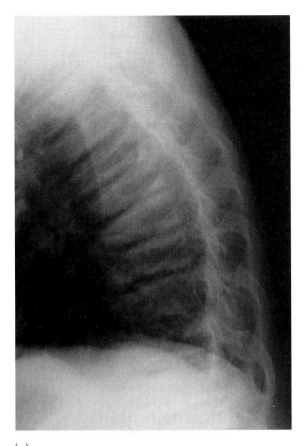

(a)

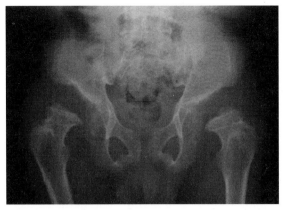

(b)

(c)

Fig. 4.1 SED congenita. (a) Lateral radiograph of the thoracic spine of a 13-year-old male showing severe platyspondly with kyphosis, marked disc space narrowing, and vertebral end-plate irregularities. (b) Radiograph of the hips and pelvis of a 16-year-old male showing deformities of the iliac bones, flattened acetabular roofs with deep fossae, and severe epiphyseal dysplasia of the femoral heads. (c) Radiograph of the knees of the patient shown in (b). Note flattened and irregular epiphyses, metaphyseal flaring and spurs of both tibiae, and severe valgus deformity of both knees.

eases, including the occurrence of marfanoid features and joint hypermobility in some kindreds[67–69]. The clinical spectrum is varied and several distinct subsets have been described, including the Wagner syndrome which is characterized by predominant ocular involvement and mild osteoarticular alterations. Radiographic studies of affected joints from patients with Stickler syndrome in the neonatal period show enlarged epiphyses, particularly of the proximal femur and distal tibia. With growth, epiphyseal dysplasia develops with irreg-

ular ossification of the epiphyses and subsequent progressive degenerative changes. In the spine, there is mild irregular platyspondyly, occasionally with end-plate irregularity and anterior wedging (Fig. 4.3). Although there is substantial overlap in the clinical phenotype of Stickler syndrome with that of late-onset SED, the more severe spinal and epiphyseal involvement, the presence of delayed ossification and striking dwarfism, and the lack of ocular manifestations in SED usually allow their differentiation.

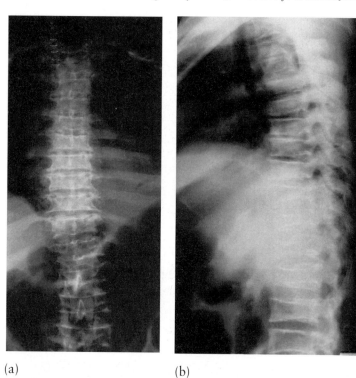

(a)   (b)

Fig. 4.2 SED tarda. (a) Anterior-posterior radiograph of the thoracic and lumbar spine of a 57-year-old male showing platyspondyly with severe degenerative arthritis, osteophytes, and disc degeneration at multiple levels. Mild thoracolumbar scoliosis is also noted. (b) Lateral radiograph of the spine of the same patient further illustrates the platyspondyly and the disc degeneration.

Kniest dysplasia

Kniest dysplasia is a disorder characterized by an autosomal dominant pattern of inheritance displaying shortening of the trunk and limbs, flattening of the face and the nose bridge, protuberance of eye globes, and severe joint abnormalities[70,71]. The joints are usually very large at birth and continue to enlarge during childhood and early adolescence. Myopia, hearing loss, cleft palate, and clubfoot are common, and the majority of affected individuals develop severe, premature degenerative joint disease which is most prominent in the knees and hips. Radiographically, flat, markedly elongated and irregular vertebral bodies with supero-inferior defects in the mid portion are seen during infancy and early childhood. Dumb-bell-shaped long bones are seen, with marked delay in epiphyseal ossification, and irregularity and expansion of the metaphyses with cloud-like defects on both sides of the epiphyseal plate. Flattened and squared epiphyses of the joints in the hands are seen with joint space narrowing. The findings in the spine include irregular platyspondyly with anterior wedging. The radiographic appearance of affected joints is shown in Fig. 4.4. The characteristic evolution of changes in the ends of the long tubular bones differentiates Kniest dysplasia from SED con-

genita. The articular cartilage is soft and has decreased resiliency, and histologically shows large cystic lesions giving a typical appearance that has been compared to that of Swiss cheese. Large inclusions have been found in dilated rough endoplasmic reticulum within chondrocytes. These inclusions have been shown to contain the carboxyl-propeptide of type II procollagen and it has been suggested that the disease results from abnormalities in the processing of type II procollagen[72].

Multiple epiphyseal dysplasias (MED)

The MED are a heterogeneous group of disorders characterized by alterations in epiphyseal growth that subsequently cause irregularity and fragmentation of the epiphyses of multiple long bones. Characteristically, spinal alterations are minimal or absent. The epiphyseal abnormalities often result in precocious, crippling OA of both weight-bearing and non-weight-bearing joints. MED is inherited in an autosomal dominant manner with a high degree of penetrance. These diseases include various phenotypes such as those described by Fairbanks[73] and Ribbing[74]. The common manifestations of affected individuals are a reflection of abnormalities in the development of the epiphyseal

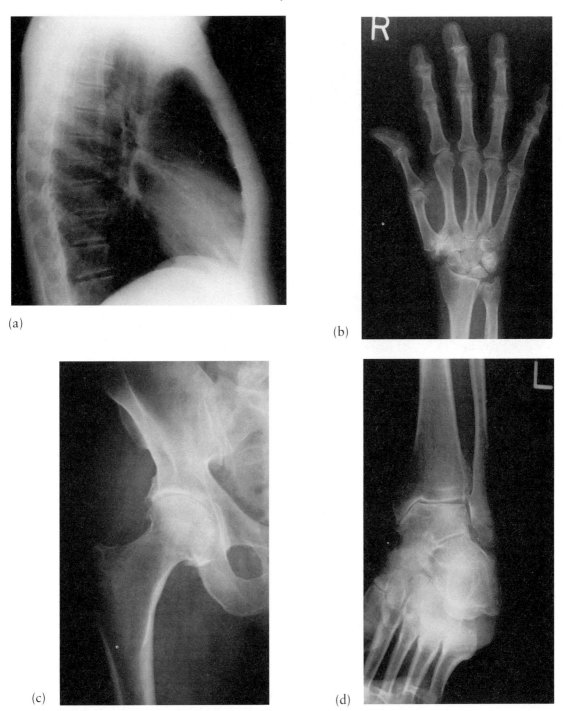

Fig. 4.3 Stickler Syndrome. (a) Lateral radiograph of the thoracic spine of a 67-year-old male showing mild vertebral end-plate abnormalities with only minimal flattening of the vertebral bodies. (b) Radiograph of the hand from the same patient. Note flattened metacarpal and proximal phalangeal heads, reflecting mild dysplasia, and severe degenerative arthritis in the proximal and distal interphalangeal joints. (c) Radiograph of the hip from the same patient. Note the mild flattening and small size of the femoral head, with associated degenerative arthritis manifest by uniform narrowing of the articular space and marginal osteophyte formation. (d) Radiograph of the ankle from the same patient. Note dysplastic epiphyses resulting in squared talar dome and tibial plafond. Degenerative changes, with joint space narrowing and subchondral sclerosis, are also present.

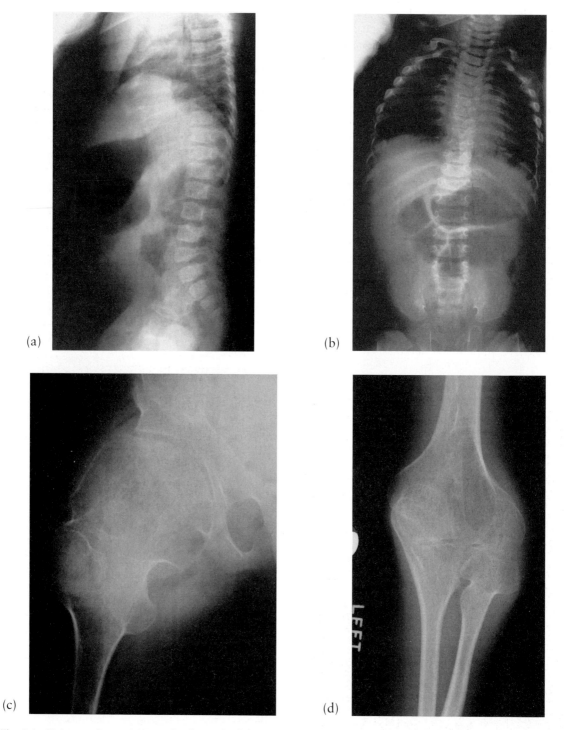

(a)

(b)

(c)

(d)

Fig. 4.4 Kniest syndrome. (a) Lateral radiograph of the spine of a one-year-old child showing mildly flattened and elongated vertebral bodies with anterior wedging noticeable in the thoracic spine. (b) Radiograph of the chest and pelvis of the same child illustrating flattening of vertebral bodies, dysplastic and unformed acetabular roofs, and delayed capital femoral epiphyseal ossifications. (c) Radiograph of the hip of a 16-year-old male showing marked enlargement of the femoral head (megaepiphysis) with clouding of its architecture. (d) Radiograph of the elbow of the same patient. Note the marked enlargement of epiphyses and flaring of the metaphyseal ends.

growth plates of long bones. These abnormalities are usually multiple and symmetric, particularly involving the knees, hips, hands, wrists, and shoulders. Most of the affected individuals develop symptoms early in childhood with pain and stiffness of multiple joints, and abnormal gait. These symptoms become progressively more severe and joint alterations evolve relentlessly into severe degenerative arthritis. Although there is no severe dwarfism, affected individuals are usually shorter than their unaffected siblings, and have characteristic short and stubby fingers. Patients with MED do not have ocular or retinal abnormalities, and spinal alterations are limited to the occurrence of irregular end-plates with varying degrees of flattening of vertebral bodies particularly in the lower dorsal spine. The most characteristic radiographic features are marked irregularity of multiple epiphyses predominantly at the hips, knees, and shoulders. The joints are nearly always symmetrically involved. Centers of ossification are late in appearing, frequently being fragmented and irregular. The capital femoral epiphyses are nearly always involved and the femoral heads become subsequently flattened (Fig. 4.5). In the more severe cases, mild

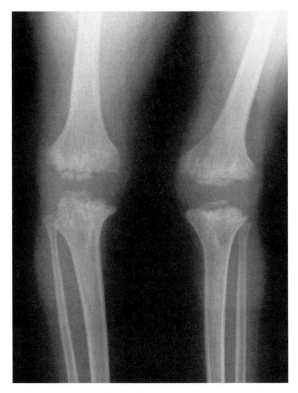

Fig. 4.5 Multiple epiphyseal dysplasia. Radiograph of the knees of a 10-year-old boy showing symmetrically flattened epiphyses with fragmentation of ossification centers.

tubular bone shortening, and cone-shaped deformation of the epiphyses in the hands can be found.

Metaphyseal chondrodysplasias

Another family of related heritable cartilage disorders that may present with precocious OA are the metaphyseal chondrodysplasias[75-77]. These disorders comprise a heterogeneous group of intrinsic alterations of metaphyseal bone. The clinical features of the affected individuals include short stature with short limbs, bowed legs, and a waddling gait. As a group, the metaphyseal chondrodysplasias are fairly common and over 150 different types have been described[75-77]. Three of the most well characterized syndromes within this group are the Jansen, Schmidt, and McKusick types. The skeletal abnormalities are similar in the three groups but differ in their degree of severity, being most severe in the Jansen type and mildest in the Schmidt type. Also, there are often manifestations reflecting alterations in other organ systems such as the immune and digestive systems, and the integument. A common characteristic of the metaphyseal chondrodysplasias is the presence of pronounced alterations in the organization and structure of growth plate cartilage, which displays clusters of proliferating and hypertrophic chondrocytes surrounded by thickened septa and disorganized matrix, with unmineralized cartilage extending into the subchondral bone. One of the most common metaphyseal chondrodysplasias is the Schmidt type[77]. This syndrome, like most other CD, is an autosomal dominant disorder. The radiographic features include coxa vara, shortening and bowing of tubular bones, and cupping and fraying of the metaphyses with more pronounced proximal than distal femoral metaphyseal involvement (Fig. 4.6). The most prominent alterations occur in the growth plates of long bones which are irregular, disorganized, and markedly widened, especially at the knees.

Gene mutations in hereditary OA

Following the initial descriptions of genetic linkage between the phenotype of precocious OA and the type II procollagen gene (COL2A1)[78,79], a large number of mutations in the genes encoding structural and functional components of articular cartilage have been identified in various hereditary diseases affecting this tissue. Several recent reviews on this subject have listed the numerous mutations responsible for these

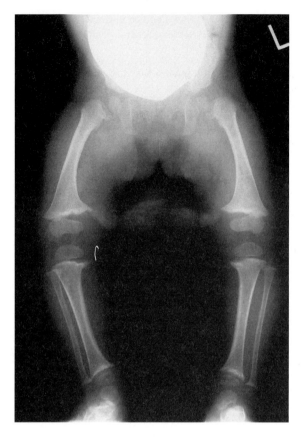

Fig. 4.6 Metaphyseal dysplasia, Schmid type. Radiograph of the knees of a 2-year-old child showing marked shortening and bowing of the long bones, with pronounced femoral and tibial metaphyseal cupping and flaring in association with growth plate irregularity.

diseases[80-82]. Progress on the elucidation of gene mutations in hereditary OA has been most substantial for COL2A1, the gene encoding the most abundant collagen present in articular cartilage, and the term 'type II collagenopathies' has been used to describe hereditary

cartilage diseases in which the primary defects are mutations in COL2A1[83]. Fig. 4.7 illustrates a recent list of documented COL2A1 mutations in various heritable diseases of cartilage[82], and Table 4.2 shows the approximate frequency of COL2A1 mutations in these diseases.

Mutations in COL2A1 have been identified in affected members of several families with a phenotype of generalized OA, with premature onset, and rapid progression. However, all these families display evidence of a mild SED besides precocious OA. The first report of a COL2A1 mutation in a PGOA / mild SED kindred was an $Arg^{519} \rightarrow Cys$ base substitution[84]. The pedigree and radiographic features of this family are shown in Fig. 4.8. Three additional families with an identical mutation have now been identified[85,86]. A second Arg $\rightarrow$ Cys base substitution, at position 75 of the type II collagen triple helix, has been identified in another kindred with precocious OA and mild SED[87], although the SED phenotype is not identical to that seen in the original $Arg^{519} \rightarrow Cys$ kindred. Like the $Arg^{519} \rightarrow Cys$ mutation, the $Arg^{75} \rightarrow Cys$ base substitution has recently been shown to occur in an additional, presumably unrelated, family[88]. Thus, it has been suggested that these COL2A1 regions may be highly prone to the occurrence of mutations[86,89]. Another COL2A1 mutation has been identified in a kindred with PGOA / mild chondrodysplasia $(Gly^{976} \rightarrow Ser)^{90}$ and a different Gly $\rightarrow$ Ser change $(Gly^{493} \rightarrow Ser)$, which results in a similar clinical and radiographic phenotype, has been described[91]. Interestingly, several other point mutations very near to this position have been identified in COL2A1 that resulted in the more severe phenotypes of SED congenita $(Gly^{997} \rightarrow Ser)^{92}$; and achondrogenesis II / hypochondrogenesis $(Gly^{988} \rightarrow Arg)^{93}$, $(Gly^{604} \rightarrow Ala)^{94}$, $(Gly^{769} \rightarrow Ser)^{95}$, $(Gly^{691} \rightarrow Arg)^{96}$, $(Gly^{310} \rightarrow Asp; Gly^{805} \rightarrow Ser)^{97}$. These observations demonstrate that amino acid substitutions in neighboring regions of

Table 4.2   Approximate frequency of COL2A1 mutations in selected heritable cartilage diseases

Syndrome	% of families with COL2A1 mutations
Hypochondrogenesis / achondrogenesis II	90–100
SED congenita / tarda	50
PGOA	10–20
Kniest dysplasia	40–50
Stickler / Wagner syndromes	25–50
MED	0
Calcium pyrophosphate / hydroxyapatite deposition disease	0

SED: spondyloepiphyseal dysplasia
PGOA: primary generalized osteoarthritis
MED: multiple epiphyseal dysplasia

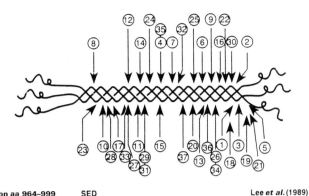

1	Deletion aa 964–999 (exon 48)	SED	Lee *et al.* (1989)
2	Gly^{943} → Ser (Exon 46)	Achondrogenesis II/Hypochondrogenesis	Vissing *et al.* (1989)
3	Duplication aa 970–984 (exon 48)	SED	Tiller *et al.* (1990)
4	Arg^{519} → Cys (Exon 31)	OA with mild chondrodysplasia	Ala-Kokko *et al.* (1990) Moskowitz *et al.* (1992) Williams *et al.* (1995)
5	Gly^{997} → Ser (Exon 48)	SED	Chan & Cole (1991)
6	Arg^{732} → Stop (Exon 40)	Stickler syndrome	Ahmad *et al.* (1991)
7	Gly^{574} → Ser (Exon 33)	Hypochondrogenesis	Horton *et al.* (1992)
8	Arg^{9} → Stop (Exon 7)	Stickler syndrome	Ahmad *et al.* (1993)
9	Arg^{789} → Cys (Exon 41)	SED	Chan *et al.* (1993)
10	Arg^{75} → Cys (Exon 11)	SED	Williams *et al.* (1993)
11	Gly^{247} → Ser (Exon 19)	SED	Ritvaniemi *et al.* (1994)
12	Gly^{154} → Arg (Exon 15)	SEMD	Vikkula *et al.* (1993)
13	Frame Shift (Exon 40)	Stickler syndrome	Brown *et al.* (1992)
14	G + 5IVS20	SED	Tiller *et al.* (1992)
15	Gly^{493} → Ser (Exon 30)	SED	Katzenstein *et al.* (1992)
16	Gly^{853} → Glu (Exon 43)	Hypochondrogenesis	Bogaert *et al.* (1992)
17	Deletion IVS12	Kniest/Stickler Syndrome	Winterpacht (1993)
18	Gly^{976} → Ser (Exon 48)	OA with mild SED	Williams *et al.* (1993)
19	Gly^{988} → Arg (Exon 48)	Hypochondrogenesis	Ganguly *et al.* (1993)
20	Gly^{691} → Arg (Exon 38)	Achondrogenesis II/Hypochondrogenesis	Williams *et al.* (1995)
21	Frame Shift (Exon 48)	Stickler syndrome	Brown *et al.* (1993)
22	Frame Shift (Exon 43)	Stickler syndrome	Ritvaniemi *et al.* (1993)
23	Gly^{67} → Asp (Exon 10)	Wagner syndrome	Körko *et al.* (1993)
24	G → A + 5IVS24	Kniest dysplasia	Wilkin *et al.* (1993)
25	Gly^{709} → Cys (Exon 39)	SEMD	Tiller *et al.* (1993)
26	Gly^{817} → Val (Exon 42)	Achondrogenesis II	Cohn *et al.* (1993)
27	A → G-2 IVS17	Stickler syndrome	Williams *et al.* (1994)
28	Δ 21 bp (Exon 12)	Kniest dysplasia	Wilkin *et al.* (1994)
29	Gly^{304} → Cys (Exon 21)	SEMD (Strudwick)	Tiller *et al.* (1994)
30	Δ 9 bp (Exon 44)	Kniest dysplasia	Winterpacht *et al.* (1994)
31	Δ Exon 21 (In-frame)	Kniest dysplasia	Winterpacht *et al.* (1994)
32	Δ 19 bp (Exon 34)	Kniest dysplasia	Winterpacht *et al.* (1994)
33	Gly^{171} → Arg (Exon 15)	SED	Winterpacht *et al.* (1994)
34	Duplication 9 bp (Exon 42)	SED	Winterpacht *et al.* (1994)
35	Gly → Ile (Exon 31)	Achondrogenesis II	Winterpacht *et al.* (1994)
36	Gly^{769} → Ser (Exon 41)	Achondrogenesis II	Chan *et al.* (1994)
37	Gly^{604} → Ala (Exon 35)	Hypochondrogenesis	Freisinger *et al.* (1994)

Fig. 4.7   Mutations in COL2A1 which have been reported for heritable cartilage diseases as of September, 1995. SED: spondyloepiphyseal dysplasia; SEMD: spondyloepimetaphyseal dysplasia; ED: epiphyseal dysplasia; POA: precocious osteoarthritis; Δ: deletion.

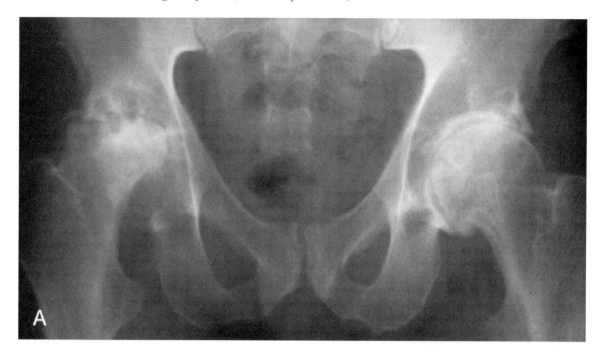

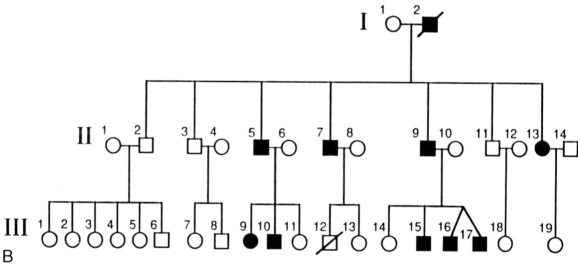

Fig. 4.8   (a) Radiograph of the hips of one affected individual from a family with PGOA associated with mild epiphyseal dysplasia. Note severe bilateral hip OA with mild dysplastic changes in the femoral heads. (b) Pedigree of the family with PGOA / mild epiphyseal dysplasia. (Reproduced with permission, Ref. 79.)

the type II collagen triple helix can result in a broad spectrum of clinical phenotypes.

Although the studies described above have provided conclusive evidence that mutations in COL2A1 are present in affected individuals from some families displaying the phenotype of PGOA / mild SED, multiallelic polymorphism analysis and genetic analysis of

sibling pairs of families with PGOA have shown that COL2A1 is not the disease locus in families which exhibit the clinical and radiographic features of PGOA in the absence of SED changes[98,99]. A recent study analyzing COL2A1 for mutations in affected individuals from 47 families with the phenotype of early onset familial OA without an SED phenotype, did not identify any mutations in the gene and a possible COL2A1 mutation was detected in only one case[100].

The COL2A1 gene has also been considered as a candidate gene for mutations responsible for CPPD. A recent study with a large family from Maine excluded linkage of the precocious OA and CPPD phenotype to the COL2A1 locus. However, genetic linkage was demonstrated between the disease phenotype and a genomic region in chromosome 8q[101]. Linkage of CPPD disease and COL2A1 was also excluded in multiple, large families from the Chiloe Islands[102]. However, an Arg[75] → Cys COL2A1 mutation was identified in one of the families in which affected individuals displayed severe SED with associated CPPD in multiple joints and fibrocartilages[102]. A recent study, conducted with a British family with a phenotype of CPPD and associated changes of mild SED[38], demonstrated genetic linkage to the genomic region 5p[103]. The results of these studies indicate that familial CPPD is a heterogeneous disease at the genetic level and that mutations in at least two different genes may eventually lead to the expression of the CPPD phenotype. Additional studies with other kindreds should determine whether there are differences in the phenotypes resulting from mutations in the genes residing in either of these two chromosomal regions.

Genetic linkage analyses in families with HADD have been more limited. A recent genetic linkage study of a large Argentinean family with HADD associated with SED, excluded several candidate genes including types II and X collagens[56]. However, no linkage to a chromosomal location has been described to date in this or in other HADD families.

Linkage analysis of several Stickler syndrome kindreds have shown that the disease is linked to COL2A1 in a high proportion of affected families[104,105], but not in others[106]. In one of these latter families, linkage to one of the type XI collagen genes on chromosome 6[107] and a mutation in the gene encoding the α2 XI collagen chain was demonstrated[108]. In this mutation, a splice donor site change resulted in an 'in frame' exon skipping. Mutations in COL2A1 have been identified and characterized in several families[109-113]. All described mutations in Stickler syndrome kindreds have shown the generation of a stop codon in the coding region of COL2A1 resulting from point mutations, or from frame shifts caused by insertions or deletions. The COL2A1 mutation in the original kindred described by Stickler in 1965 was shown to result from a base substitution in the 3′ splice acceptor site of intron 17 and the utilization of a cryptic splice acceptor site in exon 18, giving rise to the deletion of 16 bp of exon 18. The resultant frame shift eventually generates a stop codon[113].

Many laboratories have examined a variety of CD in attempts to link their phenotype to a deleterious genetic locus. The results of these studies indicate that there is a considerable degree of genetic heterogeneity among these diseases. Linkage to COL2A1 has been demonstrated in some cases and excluded in others[114-117]. COL2A1 mutations have been identified in many achondrogenesis / hypochondrogenesis and SED families (Fig. 4.7). These have included point mutations, a splicing mutation, an exon deletion, and a duplication of an exon[87-95,118-129]. Also, numerous mutations in COL2A1 have been identified in Kniest syndrome kindreds[130-135].

As abnormalities in the epiphyseal growth plate are the hallmark of MED, it has been suspected that a defect in one of the genes encoding growth plate cartilage macromolecules may be responsible for the disease. Linkage analyses of MED, and of the clinically related pseudoachondroplasia syndrome, excluded the genes for collagen types II and VI, chondroitin sulfate proteoglycan core protein, and cartilage link protein[136,137]. However, close linkage of these two disease to the pericentromeric region of chromosome 19 was found more recently[138,139]. Subsequent studies identified mutations in the gene encoding the cartilage oligomeric protein (COMP) in three patients affected with MED/pseudoachondroplasia[140]. Because the three mutations occurred in a region of the gene encoding the calcium binding domain in COMP, it is likely that the calcium binding function of the protein is essential for the normal development of growth plate cartilage. However, genetic heterogeneity of MED has recently been demonstrated, as affected members of one family with the Fairbanks type MED did not show linkage of the disease phenotype to the chromosomal region harboring COMP[141], and another family showed linkage to a region of chromosome 1 containing one of the genes for type IX collagen[142].

Several recent studies have examined the genetic mutations responsible for Schmid metaphyseal chondrodysplasia. Because the most prominent alterations in this disease occur in growth plate cartilage, the genes expressed specifically in this tissue have been considered highly likely candidates. Type X collagen is expressed almost exclusively in hypertrophic growth plate chondrocytes. Thus, the gene encoding this collagen (COL10A1) has been examined extensively for mutations in various osteochondrodysplasias. Indeed, recent studies have documented numerous distinct COL10A1 mutations in affected members of families with Schmid osteochondrodysplasia[143-149]. All the mutations identified to date have been localized to the gene region corresponding to the carboxy-terminal domain of the protein. These mutations would be expected to result in the synthesis of type X collagen polypeptides that are unable to assemble properly into a mature, fully functional protein and thereby would be expected to cause severe abnormalities in the structural organization of the growth plate. This is discussed in greater detail in a recent review[150].

Conclusion

The studies reviewed in this chapter provide conclusive demonstration that certain inherited forms of OA are caused by mutations in genes expressed in cartilage, including those encoding the cartilage specific types II, IX, X, and XI collagens, and COMP. Further study of other forms of familial OA, with the innovative techniques of molecular biology now available or being developed, will allow definition of the exact molecular cause of those diseases in which a gene defect has not been identified to date. Eventually, these studies may lead to a classification of these disorders based on the exact causative gene defect, rather than on their vastly variable clinical and radiographic phenotype. Also, these studies will lead to the development of simple DNA tests that will permit definitive diagnosis of molecular defects in individual patients in whom it may be possible to initiate preventive therapy. Furthermore, these studies will open the way (in the future) for the application of gene therapy for the correction of the causative gene defects.

References

1. Stecher, R.M. and Hersh, A.H. (1994). Heberden's nodes: the mechanisms of inheritance in hypertrophic arthritis of the fingers. *Journal of Clinical Investigation*, 23, 699–704.
2. Kellgren, J.H. and Moore, R. (1952). Generalized osteoarthritis and Heberden's nodes. *British Medical Journal*, 1, 181–7.
3. Stecher, R.M., Hersh, A.H., and Hauser, H. (1953). Heberden's nodes: the family history and radiographic appearance of a large family. *American Journal of Human Genetics*, 5, 46–69.
4. Stecher, R.M. (1955). Heberden's nodes: a clinical description of osteoarthritis of the finger joints. *Annals of the Rheumatic Diseases*, 14, 1–10.
5. Allison, A.C. and Blumberg, B.S. (1958). Familial osteoarthropathy of the fingers. *Journal of Bone and Joint Surgery*, 40B, 538–40.
6. Kellgren, J.H., Lawrence, J.S., and Bier, F. (1963). Genetic factors in generalized osteoarthritis. *Annals of the Rheumatic Diseases*, 22, 237–55.
7. Nuki, G. (1983). Osteoarthritis: some genetic approaches. *Journal of Rheumatology*, supplement 9, 29–31.
8. Heberden, W. (1803). *Commentaries on the history and cure of diseases*, (2nd edn). T. Payne, London.
9. Haygarth, J. (1805). *A clinical history of diseases*, pp. 147–68. Cadell and Davies, London.
10. Bouchard, C.J. cited in Benedek, T.G., and Rodnan, G.P. (1982). A brief history of the rheumatic diseases. *Bulletin of the Rheumatic Diseases*, 32, 59–68.
11. Osler, W. (1909). *The principles and practice of medicine*, (7th edn). D. Appleton and Co., New York.
12. Crain, D.C. (1961). Interphalangeal osteoarthritis characterized by painful inflammatory episodes resulting in deformity of the proximal and distal articulations. *Journal of the American Medical Association*, 175, 1049–51.
13. Buchanan, W.W. and Park, W.M. (1983). Primary generalized osteoarthritis: definition and uniformity. *Journal of Rheumatology*, Supplement 9, 4–6.
14. Lawrence, J.S. (1977). *Rheumatism in populations*. Heinemann Medical Books, London.
15. Lawrence, J.S., Gelsthorpe, K., and Morell, G. (1983). Heberden's nodes and HLA markers in generalized osteoarthritis. *Journal of Rheumatology*, supplement 9, 32–3.
16. Schumacher, Jr., H.R. (1992). Secondary osteoarthritis. In *Osteoarthritis: diagnosis and medical/surgical management* (ed. R.W. Moskowitz, D.S. Howell, V.M. Goldberg, and H.J. Mankin), pp. 367–98. W.B. Saunders, Philadelphia.
17. Mulligan, R.C. (1993). The basic science of gene therapy. *Science*, 260, 926–32.
18. Crystal, R.G. (1995). Transfer of genes to humans: early lessons and obstacles to success. *Science*, 270, 404–10.
19. Kellgren, J.H. and Lawrence, J.S. (1957). Radiologic assessment of osteoarthritis. *Annals of the Rheumatic Diseases*, 16, 494–502.
20. Marks, J.S., Stewart, I.M., and Hardinge, K. (1979). Primary osteoarthritis of the hip and Heberden's nodes. *Annals of the Rheumatic Diseases*, 38, 107–11.
21. Harper, P. and Nuki, G. (1980). Genetic factors in osteoarthritis. In *The aetiopathogenesis of osteoarthritis*, (ed. G. Nuki), pp. 184–201. Pitman, Tunbridge Wells, England.
22. Pattrick, M., Manhire, A., Ward, A.M., and Doherty, M. (1989). HLA-AB antigens and α1-antitrypsin phenotypes in nodal generalized osteoarthritis and erosive arthritis. *Annals of the Rheumatic Diseases*, 48, 470–5.
23. Spector, T.D., Cicuttini, F., Baker, J., Loughlin, J.A., and Hart, D.J. (1996). Genetic influences on

osteoarthritis in females: a twin study. *British Medical Journal*, **312**, 940–3.

24. Zitnan, D. and Sitaj, S. (1960). Chondrocalcinosis polyarticularis (familiaris). *Radiologia Diagnostica*, **1**, 498.

25. Zitnan, D. and Sitaj, S. (1963). Chondrocalcinosis articularis. Section I: clinical and radiologic study. *Annals of the Rheumatic Diseases*, **22**, 142–69.

26. Moskowitz, R.W. and Katz, D. (1964). Chondrocalcinosis (pseudogout syndrome). A family study. *Journal of the American Medical Association*, **188**, 867–71.

27. Louyot, P., Peterschmitt, J., and Barthelme, P. (1964). Chondrocalcinose articulaire diffuse familiale. *Revue du Rhumatisme* **31**, 659–63.

28. van de Korst, J.K., Geerards, J., and Driessens, F.C.M. (1974). A hereditary type of idiopathic articular chondrocalcinosis. *American Journal of Medicine*, **56**, 307–14.

29. Reginato, A.J., Hollander, J.L., Martinez, V., Valenzuela, F., Schiapachasse, V., Covarrubias, E., *et al.* (1975). Familial chondrocalcinosis in the Chiloe Islands, Chile. *Annals of the Rheumatic Diseases*, **34**, 260–8.

30. Gaucher, A., Faure, G., Netter, P., Pourel, J., Raffoux, C., Streiff, F., *et al.* (1977). Hereditary diffuse articular chondrocalcinosis. Dominant manifestation without close linkage with the HLA system in a large pedigree. *Scandinavian Journal of Rheumatology*, **6**, 217–21.

31. Gaudreau, A., Camerlain, M., Piborot, M.L., Beauregard. G., Lebiun, A., and Petitclerc, C. (1981). Familial articular chondrocalcinosis in Quebec. *Arthritis and Rheumatism*, **24**, 611–15.

32. Bjelle, A.O. (1982). Pyrophosphate arthropathy in two Swedish families. *Arthritis and Rheumatism*, **25**, 66–74.

33. Sakaguchi, M., Ishikawa, K., Mizuta, H., and Kitagawa, T. (1982). Familial pseudogout with destructive arthropathy. *Ryumachi*, **22**, 4–13.

34. Richardson, B.C., Chafetz, N.I., Ferrell, L.D., Zulman, J.I., and Genant, H.K. (1983). Hereditary chondrocalcinosis in a Mexican–American family. *Arthritis and Rheumatism*, **26**, 1387–96.

35. Rodriguez-Valverde, V., Zuñiga, M., Casanueva, B., Sanchez, S., and Merino, J. (1988). Hereditary articular chondrocalcinosis. Clinical and genetic features in 13 pedigrees. *American Journal of Medicine*, **84**, 101–6.

36. Balsa, A., Martin-Mola, E., Gonzalez, T., Cruz, A., Ojeda, S., and Gijon-Baños, J. (1990). Familial articular chondrocalcinosis in Spain. *Annals of the Rheumatic Diseases*, **49**, 531–5.

37. Eshel, G., Gulik, A., Halperin, N., Avrahami, E., Schumacher, Jr., H.R., McCarty, D.J., *et al.* (1990). Hereditary chondrocalcinosis in an Ashkenazi Jewish family. *Annals of the Rheumatic Diseases*, **49**, 528–30.

38. Doherty, M., Hamilton, E., Henderson, J., Misra, H., and Dixey, J. (1991). Familial chondrocalcinosis due to calcium pyrophosphate dihydrate crystal deposition in English families. *British Journal of Rheumatology*, **30**, 10–15.

39. Hamza, M., Meddeb, N., and Bardin, T. (1992). Hereditary chondrocalcinosis in a Tunisian family. *Clinical and Experimental Rheumatology*, **10**, 43–9.

40. Riestra, J.L., Sanchez, A., Rodriguez-Valverde, V., Alonso, J.L., de la Hera. M., and Merino, J. (1988). Radiographic features of hereditary articular chondrocalcinosis. A comparative study with the sporadic type. *Clinical and Experimental Rheumatology*, **6**, 369–72.

41. Bjelle, A.O. (1972). Morphological study of articular cartilage in pyrophosphate arthropathy (chondrocalcinosis articularis or calcium pyrophosphate dihydrate crystal deposition disease). *Annals of the Rheumatic Diseases*, **31**, 449–56.

42. Bjelle, A. (1981). Cartilage matrix in hereditary pyrophosphate arthropathy. *Journal of Rheumatology*, **8**, 959–64.

43. Ishikawa, K., Masuda, I., Ohira, T., Kumamoto-Shi, Yokoyama, M., and Kitakyushu-Shi. (1989). A histological study of calcium pyrophosphate dihydrate crystal deposition disease. *Journal of Bone and Joint Surgery (America)*, **71**, 875–86.

44. Masuda, I., Ishikawa, I., and Usuku, G. (1991). A histologic and immunohistochemical study of calcium pyrophosphate dihydrate crystal deposition disease. *Clinical Orthopedics*, **263**, 272–87.

45. Sharp, J. (1954). Heredo-familial vascular and articular calcifications. *Annals of the Rheumatic Diseases*, **13**, 15–16.

46. Zaphiropoulos, G. and Graham, R. (1973). Recurrent calcific periarthritis involving multiple sites. *Proceedings of the Royal Society of Medicine*, **66**, 351–2.

47. Cannon, R.B. and Schmid, F.R. (1973). Calcific periarthritis involving multiple sites in identical twins. *Arthritis and Rheumatism*, **16**, 393–5.

48. Dieppe, P.A., Huskisson, E.C., Crocker, P., and Willoughby, D.A. (1976). Apatite deposition disease: a new arthropathy. *Lancet*, **1**, 266–9.

49. Marcos, J.C., De Benyacar, M.A., Garcia-Morteo, O., Arturi, A.S., Maldonado-Cocco, J.R., Morales, V.H., *et al.* (1981). Idiopathic familial chondrocalcinosis due to apatite crystal deposition. *American Journal of Medicine*, **71**, 557–64.

50. Hajiroussou, V.J. and Webley, M. (1986). Familial calcific periarthritis. *Annals of the Rheumatic Diseases*, **42**, 469–70.

51. Caspi, D., Rosembach, T.O., Yaron, M., McCarty, D.J., and Graff, E. (1988). Periarthritis associated with basic calcium phosphate crystal deposition and low level of alkaline phosphatase. Report of three cases from one family. *Journal of Rheumatology*, **15**, 823–7.

52. Fernandez-Dapica, M.P., Gomez-Reino, J., and Reginato, A.J. (1993). Familial periarticular calcification in a Spanish kindred. *Revista Española de Rheumatologia*, **20**, 403. (Abstract)

53. Ferri, S., Zanardim M., Barozzi, L., Williams, C., and Reginato, A.J. (1994). Familial apatite deposition disease (FADD) in a Northern–Italian kindred. *Arthritis and Rheumatism*, **37**, S413. (Abstract)

54. Schumacher, Jr., H.R., Smolyo, A.P., Maurer, J., Tse, R., and Maurer, K. (1977). Arthritis associated with apatite crystals. *Annals of Internal Medicine*, **87**, 411–16.

55. Halverson, P.B. (1992). Arthropathies associated with basic calcium phosphate crystals. *Scanning Microscopy*, 6, 791–7.

56. Marcos, J.C., Arturi, A.S., Babini, C., Jimenez, S.A., Knowlton, R., and Reginato, A.J. (1995). Familial hydroxyapatite chondrocalcinosis with spondyloepiphyseal dysplasia: clinical course and absence of genetic linkage to the type II procollagen gene. *Journal of Clinical Rheumatology*, 1, 171–8.

57. Ali, S.Y. and Griffiths, S. (1983). Formation of calcium phosphate crystals in normal and osteoarthritic cartilage. *Annals of the Rheumatic Diseases*, supplement 42, 45–58.

58. Ohira, T. and Ishikawa, K. (1987). Hydroxyapatite deposition in osteoarthritic articular cartilage of the proximal femoral head. *Arthritis and Rheumatism*, 30, 651–60.

59. Spranger, J. (1976). The epiphyseal dysplasias. *Clinical Orthopaedics and Related Research*, 114, 46–59.

60. Rimoin, D.L. and Lachman, R.S. The chondrodysplasias. (1990). In *Principles and practice of medical genetics* (ed. A.E.H. Emery and D.L. Rimoin), pp. 895–907. Churchill Livingstone, New York.

61. Horton, W.A. and Hecht, J.T. (1993). The chondrodysplasias. In *Connective tissue and its heritable disorders* (ed. P.M. Royce and B. Steinman), pp. 641–675. Wyley–Liss, New York.

62. Pyeritz, R.E. (1993). Heritable and developmental disorders of connective tissue and bone. In *Arthritis and allied conditions*, (12th edn) (ed. D.J. McCarty and W.J. Koopman), pp. 1483–509. Lea and Febiger, Philadelphia.

63. Byers, P.H. (1994). Molecular genetics of chondrodysplasias, including clues to development, structure, and function. *Current Opinion in Rheumalogy*, 6, 345–50.

64. Kahan, M.F., Jurman, S.H., and Bourgeois, P. (1977). Le rhumatisme chondrodysplasique. A propos de 50 cas. *Annales de Medecine Interne* (Paris), 128, 857–60.

65. Stickler, G.B., Belau, P.G., Farrell, F.J., Jones, J.D., Pugh, D.G., Steinberg, A.G., et al. (1965). Hereditary progressive arthro-ophthalmopathy. *Mayo Clinic Proceedings*, 40, 433–55.

66. Rai, A., Wordsworth, P., Coppock, J.S., Zaphiropoulos, G.C., and Stuthrers, G.C. Hereditary arthro-ophthalmopathy (Stickler syndrome): a diagnosis to consider in familial premature osteoarthritis. *British Journal of Rheumatology*, 33, 1175–80.

67. Herrmann, J., France, T.D., Spranger, J.W., Opitz, J.M., and Wiffler, C. (1975). The Stickler syndrome (hereditary arthro-ophthalmopathy). *Birth Defects*, 11, 76–103.

68. Liberfarb, R.M., Hirose, T., and Holmes, L.B. (1981). The Wagner–Stickler syndrome: a study of 22 families. *Journal of Paediatrics*, 99, 394–9.

69. Niffenegger, J.H., Topping, T.M., and Mukai, S. (1993). Stickler syndrome. *International Ophthalmology Clinics*, 33, 271–80.

70. Kniest, W. and Leiber, B. (1977). Kniest syndrom. *Monatsschrift Kinderheilkunde* 125, 970–3.

71. Maroteaux, P. and Spranger, J. (1973). La maladie de Kniest. *Archives Francaises de Pediatrie* 30, 735–50.

72. Poole, A.R., Pidoux, I., Reiner, A., Rosenberg, L., Hollister, D., Murray, L., et al. (1988). Kniest dysplasia is characterized by an apparent abnormal processing of the C-propeptide of type II cartilage collagen resulting in imperfect fibril assembly. *Journal of Clinical Investigation*, 81, 579–89.

73. Fairbanks, T. (1947). Dysplasia epiphysialis multiplex. *British Journal of Surgery*, 34, 224–32.

74. Ribbing, S. (1937). Studien über hereditäre multiple epiphysenustörungen. *Acta Radiologica*, supplement 34.

75. Sutcliffe, J. and Stanley, P. (1973). Metaphyseal chondrodysplasias. *Progress in Pediatric Radiology*, 4, 250–69.

76. Kozlowski, K. (1976). Metaphyseal and spondylometaphyseal chondrodysplasias. *Clinical Orthopedics*, 114, 83–93.

77. Lachman, R.S., Rimoin, D.L., and Spranger, J. (1988). Metaphyseal chondrodysplasia, Schmid type. Clinical and radiographic delineation with a review of the literature. *Pediatric Radiology*, 18, 93–102.

78. Palotie, A., Vaisanen, P., Ott, J., Ryhanen, L., Elima, K., Vikkula, M., et al. (1989). Predisposition to familial osteoarthritis linked to type II collagen gene. *Lancet*, 1, 924–7.

79. Knowlton, R.G., Katzenstein, P.L. Moskowitz, R.W., Weaver, E.J., Malemud, C.J., Pathria, M.N., et al. (1990). Genetic linkage of a polymorphism in the type II collagen gene (COL2A1) to primary osteoarthritis associated with a mild chondrodysplasia. *New England Journal of Medicine*, 322, 526–30.

80. Williams, C.J. and Jimenez, S. (1993). Heredity, genes and osteoarthritis. *Rheumatic Disease Clinics of North America*, 19, 523–43.

81. Vikkula, M., Metsaranta, M., and Ala-Kokko, L. (1994). Type II collagen mutations in rare and common cartilage diseases. *Annals of Medicine*, 26, 107–14.

82. Williams, C.J. and Jimenez, S.A. (1995). Heritable diseases of cartilage caused by mutations in collagen genes. *Journal of Rheumatology*, Supplement 43, 28–33.

83. Spranger, J., Winterpacht, A., and Zabel, B. (1994). The type II collagenopathies: a spectrum of chondrodysplasias. *European Journal of Pediatrics*, 153, 56–65.

84. Ala-Kokko, L., Baldwin, C.T., Moskowitz, R.W., and Prockop, D.J. (1990). Single base mutation in the type II procollagen gene (COL2A1) as a cause of primary osteoarthritis associated with a mild chondrodysplasia. *Proceedings of the National Academy of Sciences, USA*, 87, 6565–8.

85. Williams, C.J., Rock, M. Considine, E., McCarron, S., Gow, P., Ladda, R., et al. (1995). Three new point mutations in type II procollagen (COL2A1) and identification of a fourth family with the COL2A1 Arg[519]→Cys base substitution using conformation sensitive gel electrophoresis. *Human Molecular Genetics*, 4, 309–12.

86. Pun, Y.L., Moskowitz, R.W., Lie, S., Sundstrom, W.R., Block, S.R., McEwen, C., et al. (1994). Clinical correlations of osteoarthritis associated with a single base mutation (Arginine[519]→Cysteine) in type II procollagen gene: a newly defined etiopathogenesis. *Arthritis and Rheumatism*, 37, 264–9.

87. Williams, C.J., Considine, E.L., Knowlton, R.G., Reginato, A., Neumann, G., Harrison, D., et al. (1993). Spondyloepiphyseal dysplasia and precocious

osteoarthritis in a family with an Arg[75]→Cys mutation in the procollagen type II gene (COL2A1). *Human Genetics*, **92**, 499–505.

88. Bleasel, J.F., Bisagni-Faure, A., Holderbaum, D., Vacher-LaVenu, M.C., Haqqi, T.M., Moskowitz, R.W., *et al.* (1995). Type II procollagen gene (COL2A1) mutation in exon 11 associated with spondyloepiphyseal dysplasia, tall stature and precocious osteoarthritis. *Journal of Rheumatology*, **22**, 255–61.

89. Bleasel, J.F., Holderbaum, D., Haqqi, T.M., and Moskowitz, R.W. (1995). Clinical correlations of osteoarthritis associated with single base mutations in the type II procollagen gene. *Journal of Rheumatology*, **Supplement 43**, 34–6.

90. Williams, C.J., McCarron, S., and Considine, E. (1993). A point mutation in one allele of the type II procollagen gene produces a Gly[976]→Ser substitution of the gene in a family with severe degenerative arthropathy of the hip associated with probable epiphyseal dysplasia. *American Journal of Human Genetics*, **53**, A1252. (Abstract)

91. Katzenstein, P.L., Campbell, D.F., Machado, M.A., Horton, W.A., Lee, B., and Ramirez, F. (1992). A type II collagen defect in a new family with SED tarda and early-onset osteoarthritis (OA). *Arthritis and Rheumatism*, **35**, S41. (Abstract)

92. Chan, D. and Cole, W.G. (1991). Low basal transcription of genes for tissue-specific collagens by fibroblasts and lymphoblastoid cells: application to the characterization of a glycine 997 to serine substitution in α1 (II) collagen chains of a patient with spondyloepiphyseal dysplasia. *Journal of Biological Chemistry*, **266**, 12487–94.

93. Ganguly, A., Rock, M., and Considine, E. (1993). Conformation sensitive gel electrophoresis of polymerase chain products of the type II procollagen gene reveals a heterozygous Gly[988]→Val mutation in a baby with hypochondrogenesis. *American Journal of Human Genetics*, **53**, A1159. (Abstract)

94. Freisinger, P., Ala-Kokko, L., LeGuellec, D., Franc, S., Bouvier, R., Ritvaniemi, P. *et al.* (1994). A mutation in the COL2A1 gene in a patient with hypochondrogenesis. Expression of the mutated COL2A1 gene is accompanied by expression of the genes for type I procollagen in chondrocytes. *Journal of Biological Chemistry*, **269**, 13663–9.

95. Chan, D., Cole, W.G., Chow, C.W., Mundlos, S., and Bateman, J.F. (1994). A COL2A1 mutation in achondrogenesis type II results in the replacement of type II collagen by type I and III collagens in cartilage. *Journal of Biological Chemistry*, **270**, 1747–53.

96. Mortier, G.R., Wilkin, D.J., Wilcox, W.R., Rimoin, D.L., Lachman, R.S., Eyre, D.R., *et al.* (1995). A radiographic, morphologic, biochemical and molecular analysis of a case of achondrogenesis type II resulting from substitution for a glycine residue (Gly[619]→Arg) in the type II collagen trimer. *Human Molecular Genetics*, **4**, 285–8.

97. Bonaventure, J., Cohen-Solal, L., Ritvaniemi, P., Van Malderge, L., Kadham, N., Delezoide, A.L., *et al.* (1995). Substitution of aspartic acid for glycine at position 310 in type II collagen produces achondrogenesis

II, and substitution of serine at position 805 produces hypochondrogenesis: analysis of genotype-phenotype relationships. *Biochemical Journal*, **307**, 823–30.

98. Vikkula, M., Nissila, M., Hirvensalo, E., Nuotio, P., Pallotie, A., Aho, K., *et al.* (1993). Multiallelic polymorphism of the cartilage collagen gene: no association with osteoarthrosis. *Annals of the Rheumatic Diseases*, **52**, 762–4.

99. Loughlin, J., Irven, C., Fergusson, C., and Sykes, B. (1994). Sibling pair analysis shows no linkage of generalized osteoarthritis to the loci encoding type II collagen, cartilage link protein or cartilage matrix protein. *British Journal of Rheumatology*, **33**, 1103–6.

100. Ritvaniemi, P., Korkko, J., Bonaventure, J., Vikkula, M., Hyland, J., Paassilta, P., *et al.* (1995). Identification of COL2A1 mutations in patients with chondrodysplasias and familial osteoarthritis. *Arthritis and Rheumatism*, **38**, 999–1004.

101. Baldwin, C.T., Farrar, L.A., Dharmavaram, R., Jimenez, S.A., and Anderson, L. (1995). Linkage of early-onset osteoarthritis and chondrocalcinosis to human chromosome 8q. *American Journal of Human Genetics*, **56**, 692–7.

102. Reginato, A.J., Passano, G.M., Neumann, G., Falasca, G.F., Diaz-Valdez, M., Jimenez, S.A., *et al.* (1994). Familial spondyloepiphyseal dysplasia tarda, and precocious osteoarthritis associated with an Arginine[75]→Cysteine mutation in the procollagen type II gene in a kindred of Chiloe Islanders. I: clinical, radiographic, and pathologic findings. *Arthritis and Rheumatism*, **37**, 1078–86.

103. Hughes, A.E., McGibbon, D., Woodward, E., Dixey, J., and Doherty, M. (1995). Localisation of a gene for chondrocalcinosis to chromosome 5p. *Human Molecular Genetics*, **4**, 1225–8.

104. Francomano, C.A., Liberfarb, R.M., Hirose, T., Maumenee, I.H., Streeten, E.A., Myers, D.A., *et al.* (1987). The Stickler syndrome: evidence for close linkage to the structural gene for type II collagen. *Genomics*, **1**, 293–6.

105. Knowlton, R.G., Weaver, E.J., and Struyk, A.F. (1989). Genetic linkage analysis of hereditary arthroopthalmopathy (Stickler syndrome) and the type II procollagen gene. *American Journal of Human Genetics*, **45**, 681–8.

106. Bonaventure, J., Philippe, C., Plessis, G., Vigneron, J., Lasselin, C., Maroteaux, P., *et al.* (1992). Linkage study in a large pedigree with Stickler syndrome: exclusion of COL2A1 as the mutant gene. *Human Genetics*, **90**, 164–8.

107. Brunner, H.G., von Beersum, S.E., Warman, M.L., Olsen, B.R., Ropers, H.H., and Mariman, E.C. (1994). A Stickler syndrome gene is linked to chromosome 6 near the COL11A2 gene. *Human Molecular Genetics*, **3**, 1561–4.

108. Vikkula, M., Mariman, E.C.M., Lui, V.C.H., Zhidkova, N.I., Tiller, G.E., Goldring, M.B., *et al.* (1995). Autosomal dominant and recessive osteochondrodysplasias associated with the COL11A2 locus. *Cell*, **80**, 431–7.

109. Ahmad, N.N., Ala-Kokko, L., Knowlton, R.G., Jimenez, S.A., Weaver, E.J., Maguire, J.I., *et al.* (1991).

Stop codon in the procollagen gene (COL2A1) in a family with the Stickler syndrome (arthro-ophthalmopathy). *Proceedings of the National Academy of Sciences, USA*, **88**, 6624–7.

110. Ritvaniemi, P., Hyland, J., Ignatius, J., Kivirikko, K.I., Prockop, D.J., and Ala-Kokko, L. (1993). A fourth example suggests that premature termination codons in the COL2A1 gene are a common cause of the Stickler syndrome: analysis of the COL2A1 gene by denaturing gradient gel electrophoresis. *Genomics*, **17**, 218–21.

111. Korkko, J., Ritvaniemi, P., Haataja, L., Kaariainen, H., Kivirikko, K., Prockop, D.J., *et al.* (1993). Mutation in type II procollagen (COL2A1) that substitutes aspartate for glycine α1–67 and that causes cataracts and retinal detachment. Evidence for molecular heterogeneity in the Wagner syndrome and the Stickler syndrome (arthro-ophthalmopathy). *American Journal of Human Genetics*, **53**, 55–61.

112. Brown, D.M., Vandenburgh, K., Kimura, A.E., Weingeist, T.A., Sheffield, V.C., Stone, E.M., *et al.* (1995). Genetic mutations in the procollagen II gene (COL2A1) associated with Stickler syndrome (hereditary arthro-ophthalmopathy). *Human Molecular Genetics*, **4**, 141–2.

113. Williams, C.J., Ganguly, A., McCarron, S., Considine, E., Michels, V., and Prockop, D.J. (1996). An A^{-2}→G transition at the 3′ acceptor splice site of IVS17 characterizes the COL2A1 gene mutation in the original Stickler kindred. *American Journal of Medical Genetics*, **63**, 461–7.

114. Peltonen, L., Palotie, A., Vaisanen, P., Vuorio, E., and Ott, J. (1988). Linkage analysis of type II collagen in the inherited and acquired collagen disorders. *Collagen Related Research*, **8**, 509–10.

115. Wordsworth, P., Ogilvie, P., Priestley, L., Smith, R., Wynne-Davies, R., and Sykes, B. (1988). Structural and segregation analysis of the type II collagen gene (COL2A1) in some heritable chondrodysplasias. *Journal Medical Genetics*, **25**, 521–7.

116. Priestley, L., Fergusson, C., Ogilvie, D., Wordsworth, P., Smith, R., Pattrick, M., *et al.* (1991). A limited association of generalized osteoarthritis with alleles at the type II collagen locus: COL2A1. *British Journal of Rheumatology*, **30**, 272–5.

117. Anderson, I.J., Goldberg, R.B., Marion, R.W., Upholt, W.B., and Tsipouras, P. (1990). Spondyloepiphyseal dysplasia congenita: genetic linkage to type II collagen (COL2A1). *American Journal of Human Genetics*, **46**, 896–901.

118. Vissing, H., D'Alessio, M., Lee, B., Ramirez, F., Godfrey, M., and Hollister, D.W. (1989). Glycine to serine substitution in the triple helical domain of proα1(II) collagen results in a lethal perinatal form of short-limbed dwarfism. *Journal of Biological Chemistry*, **264**, 18265–7.

119. Lee, B., Vissing, H., Ramirez, F., Rogers, D., and Rimoin, D. (1989). Identification of the molecular defect in a family with spondyloepiphyseal dysplasia. *Science*, **244**, 978–80.

120. Tiller, G.E., Rimoin, D.L., Murray, L.W., and Cohn, D.H. (1990). Tandem duplication within a type II collagen gene (COL2A1) exon in an individual with spondy-

loepiphyseal dysplasia. *Proceedings of the National Academy of Sciences, USA*, **87**, 3889–93.

121. Horton, W.A., Machado, M.A., Ellard, J., Campbell, D., Barley, J., Ramirez, F., *et al.* (1992). Characterization of a type I collagen gene (COL1A1) mutation identified in cultured chondrocytes from human hypochondrogenesis. *Proceedings of the National Academy of Sciences, USA*, **89**, 4583–7.

122. Bogaert, R., Tiller, G.E., Weis, M.A., Gruber, H.E., Rimoin, D.L., Cohn, D.H., *et al.* (1992). An amino acid substitution (Gly^{853}→Glu) in the collagen α1(II) chain produces hypochondrogenesis. *Journal of Biological Chemistry*, **267**, 22522–6.

123. Tiller, G.E., Weiss, M.A., Polumbo, P.A., Gruber, H.E., Rimoin, D.L., Cohn, D.H., *et al.* (1995). An RNA-splicing mutation (G+5IVS20) in the type II collagen gene (COL2A1) in a family with spondyloepiphyseal dysplasia congenita. *American Journal of Medical Genetics*, **56**, 388–95.

124. Chan, D., Taylor, T.K.F., and Cole, W.G. (1993). Characterization of an Arg^{789}→Cys substitution in α1(II) collagen chains of a patient with spondyloepiphyseal dysplasia. *Journal of Biological Chemistry*, **268**, 15238–45.

125. Vikkula, M., Ritvaniemi, P., Vuorio, A.F., Kaitila, I., Ala-Kokko, L., and Peltonen, L. (1993). A mutation in the amino-terminal end of the triple helix of type II collagen causing severe osteochondrodysplasia. *Genomics*, **16**, 282–5.

126. Tiller, G.E., Weis, M.A., Lachman, R.S., Cohn, D.H., Rimoin, D.L., and Eyre, D.R. (1993). A dominant mutation in the type II collagen gene (COL2A1) produces spondyloepimetaphyseal dysplasia (SEMD), Strudwick type. *American Journal of Human Genetics*, **53**, A209. (Abstract)

127. Cohn, D.H., Solsky, M.A., Polumbo, P.A., Rimoin, D.L., and Tiller, G.E. (1993). A Gly^{817}→Val substitution in α1(II) collagen produces achondrogenesis type II. *American Journal of Human Genetics*, **53**, A208. (Abstract)

128. Ritvaniemi, P., Sokolov, B.P., Williams, C.J., Considine, E., Yurgenev, L., Meerson, E.M., *et al.* (1994). A single-base mutation in the type II procollagen gene (COL2A1) that converts glycine α1-247 to serine in a family with late onset spondyloepiphyseal dysplasia. *Human Mutation*, **3**, 261–7.

129. Winterpacht, A., Schwarze, U., Menger, H., Mundlos, S., Spranger, J., and Zabel, B. (1994). Specific skeletal dysplasias due to type II procollagen gene (COL2A1) defects. *Matrix Biology*, **14**, 392. (Abstract)

130. Wilkin, D.J., Weis, M.A., Gruber, H.E., Rimoin, D.L., Eyre, D.R., and Cohn, D.H. (1993). An exon-skipping mutation in the type II collagen gene (COL2A1) produces Kniest dysplasia. *American Journal of Genetics*, **53**, A210. (Abstract)

131. Winterpacht, A., Hilbert, M., Schwarze, U., Mundlos, S., Spranger, J., and Zabel, B.U. (1993). Kniest and Stickler dysplasia phenotypes caused by collagen type II gene (COL2A1) defects. *Nature Genetics*, **3**, 323–6.

132. Wilkin, D.J., Bogaert, R., Wilcox, W.R., Rimoin, D.L., Eyre, D.R., and Cohn, D.H. (1994). Identification of a mutation hotspot in the type II collagen gene

(COL2A1): a common point mutation in two unrelated individuals with Kniest dysplasia. *Matrix Biology*, **14**, 390. (Abstract)

133. Spranger, J., Menger, H., Mundlos, S., Winterpacht, A, and Zabel, B.U. (1994). Kniest dysplasia is caused by dominant collagen II (COL2A1) mutations: parental somatic mosaicism manifesting as Stickler phenotype and mild spondyloepiphyseal dysplasia. *Pediatric Radiology*, **24**, 431–5.

134. Wilkin, D.J., Bogaert, R., Lachman, R.S., Rimoin, D.L., Eyre, D.R., and Cohn, D.H. (1994). A single-amino-acid substitution (G103D) in the type II collagen triple helix produces Kniest dysplasia. *Human Molecular Genetics*, **3**, 1999–2003.

135. Bogaert, R., Wilkin, D.J., Wilcox W.R., Lachman, R., Rimoin, D., Cohn, D.H., *et al.* (1994). Expression, in cartilage, of a 7-amino-acid deletion in type II collagen from two unrelated individuals with Kniest dysplasia. *American Journal of Human Genetics*, **55**, 1128–36.

136. Weaver, E.J., Summerville, G.P., Yeh, G., Hervada-Page, M., Oehlman, R., Rothman, R., *et al.* (1993). Exclusion of type II and type VI procollagen gene mutations in a five-generation family with multiple epiphyseal dysplasia. *American Journal of Human Genetics*, **45**, 345–52.

137. Hecht, J.T., Blanton, S.H., Wang, Y., Daigier, S.P., Horton, W.A., Rhodes, C., *et al.* (1992). Exclusion of human proteoglycan link protein (CRTL1) and type II collagen (COL2A1) genes in pseudoachondroplasia. *American Journal of Human Genetics*, **44**, 420–4.

138. Hecht, J.T., Francomano, C.A., Briggs, M.D., Deere, M., Conner, B., Horton, W.A., *et al.* (1993). Linkage of typical pseudoachondroplasia to chromosome 19. *Genomics*, **18**, 661–6.

139. Oehlmann, R., Summerville, G.P., Yeh, G., Weaver, E.J., Jimenez, S.A., and Knowlton, R.G. (1994). Genetic linkage mapping of multiple epiphyseal dysplasia to the pericentromeric region of chromosome 19. *American Journal of Human Genetics*, **54**, 3–10.

140. Briggs, M.D., Hoffman, S.M.G., King, L.M., Olsen, A.M., Mohrenweiser, H., Leroy, J.G., *et al.* (1995). Pseudoachondroplasia and multiple epiphyseal dysplasia due to mutations in the cartilage oligomeric matrix protein gene. *Nature Genetics*, **10**, 330–6.

141. Deere, M., Halloran-Blanton, S., Scott, C.I., Langer, L.O., Pauli, R.M., and Hecht, J.T. (1995). Genetic het-

erogenity in multiple epiphyseal dysplasia. *American Journal of Human Genetics*, **56**, 698–704.

142. Briggs, M.D., Choi, H., Warman, M.L., Laughlin, J.A., Wordsworth, P., Sykes, B.C., *et al.* (1994). Genetic mapping of a locus for multiple epiphyseal dysplasia (EDM2) to a region of chromosome 1 containing a type IX collagen gene. *American Journal of Human Genetics*, **55**, 678–84.

143. Warman, M.L., Abbott, M., Apte, S.S., Hefferon, T.W., McIntosh, I., Cohn, D.H., *et al.* (1993). A type X collagen mutation causes Schmid metaphyseal chondrodysplasia. *Nature Genetics*, **5**, 79–82.

144. McIntosh, I., Abbott, M.H., Warman, M.L., Olsen, B.R., and Francomano, C.A. (1994). Additional mutations in type X collagen confirm COL10A1 as the Schmid metaphyseal chondrodysplasia locus. *Human Molecular Genetics*, **3**, 303–7.

145. Dharmavaram, R.M., Elberson, M.A., Peng, M., Kirson, L.A., Kelley, T.E., and Jimenez, S.A. (1994). Identification of a mutation in type X collagen in a family with Schmid metaphyseal chondrodysplasia. *Human Molecular Genetics*, **3**, 507–9.

146. Wallis, G.A., Rash, B., Sweetman, W.A., Thomas, J.T., Super, M., Evans, G., *et al.* (1994) Amino acid substitutions of conserved residues in the carboxyl-terminal domain of the $\alpha 1(X)$ chain of type X collagen occur in two unrelated families with metaphyseal chondrodysplasia type Schmid. *American Journal of Human Genetics*, **54**, 169–78.

147. McIntosh, I., Abbott, M.H., and Francomano, C.A. (1995). Concentration of mutations causing Schmid metaphyseal chondrodysplasia in the C-terminal non-collagenous domain of type X collagen. *Human Mutation*, **5**, 121–5.

148. Bonaventure, J., Chaminade, F., and Maroteaux, P. (1995). Mutations in three subdomains of the carboxyl-terminal region of collagen type X account for most of the Schmid metaphyseal dysplasias. *Human Genetics*, **96**, 58–64.

149. Chan, D., Cole, W.G., Rogers, J.B., and Bateman, J.F., (1995). Type X collagen multimer assembly *in vitro* is prevented by a Gly^{619}→Val mutation in the $\alpha 1(X)$ NC1 domain resulting in Schmid metaphyseal chondrodysplasia. *Journal of Biological Chemistry*, **270**, 4558–62.

150. Jacenko, O., Olsen, B.R., and Warman, M.L. (1994). Of mice and men: heritable skeletal disorders. *American Journal of Human Genetics*, **54**, 163–8.

5 | *Pathology of osteoarthritis*

Kenneth P.H. Pritzker

Osteoarthritis (OA) can be considered as a group of joint diseases characterized by degenerative, regenerative, and reparative structural changes in all joint tissues including cartilage, bone, synovium, capsule, and periarticular soft tissues[1–5]. These architectural and compositional changes may progress to functional joint failure. These changes are driven by both local and systemic biologic mechanisms which vary in relative influence with the etiology, anatomical site, and stage of the disease process. As defined above, OA is distinct from the generalized tissue atrophy[6,7], amyloid deposition[8], and lipid pigment accumulation[9] associated with joint aging. OA occurs under three general conditions. First, OA can develop as a polyarticular joint disease from the reaction of joint tissues to as yet unknown systemic stimuli. Second, osteoarthritic changes can develop following known local or general disorders which promote deleterious changes in joint structures. Mechanical injury is a common example of a local stimulus[2–4]; acromegaly is an example of systemic disease[10]. Third, OA can supervene in advanced inflammatory arthritis of various etiologies. Post-inflammatory OA is distinct because inflammation inhibits regenerative and reparative changes in connective tissues. Under these conditions, osteoarthritic changes usually occur secondarily to structural degradation induced by inflammation, only after the inflammatory process becomes quiescent.

In this chapter, our discussion will be restricted to the reactions to injury of joint tissues in primary OA. Nonetheless, stimulated by similar pathogenic mechanisms, many OA morphologic features can be present in the other conditions noted above. Further, our discussion will focus on structural changes in the earlier phases of OA, rather than secondary changes and end-stage disease.

As OA is a dynamic structural disorder, the morphology of joint tissues reflects both the activity and progression of the disease within each particular joint at the time of sampling[5,11–14]. Because the joint tissues are affected by common pathogenic mechanisms, it might be expected that at each stage the various tissues within a joint will show common morphologic features. Moreover, because systemic factors may drive the morphologic changes, similar morphologic features may be seen in multiple joints at the same stage of disease. The countervailing reality is that within each joint, and between joints of different sizes at various anatomical sites, the specific architectural structure has been pre-adapted to different mechanical forces. Within each joint, this results in lesions with heterogeneous morphologic patterns. In active disease, typically this involves a mixture of tissue domains in which the force-bearing domains may exhibit predominantly degenerative changes, whereas the adjacent or lightly-loaded domains show more prominent regeneration[15]. Therefore, as the disease progresses, structural heterogeneity within the joint also progresses: a process which can further destabilize the structural and functional integrity of the articular tissues. Adaptation to mechanical forces affects the morphologic pattern of structural failure differently, in different joints. For example, in the phalangeal joints where articular cartilage is thin, the most prominent OA feature is osseous proliferation in marginal osteophytes. In contrast, within the knee joint, articular cartilage and synovial tissue changes are dominant.

There are two special features about each tissue within joints. First, each major tissue — cartilage, fibrocartilage, and bone — is characterized by a cell population that is phenotypically monomorphic, such as chondrocytes or osteocytes. Although these cell populations are stable, with appropriate stimuli they can replicate and remodel the composition of their extracellular environment. These changes occur focally within each tissue, resulting in functional differentiation of the cells and heterogeneity of the extracellular matrix. Second, joint function is dependent on both the architectural and compositional properties of an extracellular matrix, characterized by well-defined organization of the fibrillar (principally collagen) and amorphous (proteoglycans, non-collagenous protein) solute components. This matrix is produced and actively regulated by the cell population. As the cells regulate a matrix environment 15–30 times the volume of each cell, the matrix composition at locations further from the cell is less closely regulated than those adjacent to the cell. Particularly in cartilage, this means that matrix degradation products at a distance from the cell are cleared more slowly, and may accumulate. Therefore, OA pathology can be understood by observing how the extracellular matrix architecture and composition, changes in response to physical, chemical, and biochemical stimuli directly both on matrix components and on the participating connective tissue cells.

Formerly, OA was thought to be a disease of 'wear and tear', that is, a disorder in which mechanical forces physically degraded the joint material, independent of biologic response. While some direct physical effects on joint tissues as a material can be seen in OA, the pathologic features of OA are predominantly a result of inadequate or inappropriate response to injury of the affected tissues. As in other tissues, this reaction to injury has a defined sequence involving extracellular edema, matrix degradation by ambient enzymes, cell apoptosis, cell necrosis, followed by resorption of extracellular matrix and cell debris. Subsequently, repair and regeneration take place, with cell replication and restoration of the extracellular matrix organization by the endogenous cells. Within each tissue domain, the reaction to injury follows the same sequence. The intensity and the extent of the reaction depends both on the severity of the stimulus and the structural substrate, shaped by preceding reactions. In OA, the reaction to injury has features which are special to the histologic organization of the articular tissues. First,

under some conditions, the reaction to injury may be induced endogenously by stimulation of the connective tissue cells within the joints, rather than by exogenous injury. Second, the reaction may be sufficiently mild to be reversible without permanent structural change. These reversible changes are indicators of OA activity. Third, the reaction to injury initially centers on force-bearing avascular tissue such as cartilage. Consequently, the vascular reaction of OA is seen adjacent to the site of injury, namely in synovium, capsule, ligaments, and subchondral bone. Further, this reaction is subdued compared to inflammatory arthritis.

In summary, OA is a degenerative disease process involving reaction to injury which although similar in sequence, varies topographically in amplitude and duration from joint to joint, and within each joint. The reaction to injury is characterized by destruction and resorption of tissues, followed by proliferation of the participating cells. This results in hyperplasia, particularly of articular chondrocytes, as well as remodeling of articular tissue matrix. This remodeling process results in hypertrophy and architectural distortion of the joint (Table 5.1).

Cartilage

Synovial joint articular surfaces are lined by hyaline articular cartilage, which consists of a firm isotropic matrix containing as major components, Type II collagen fibers, aggrecan type proteoglycans, and

Table 5.1 Pathologic features of osteoarthritis

Tissue	Activity	Progression	
		Early	**Advanced**
Cartilage	• Matrix edema • Prominent chondrons with pericellular proteoglycan • Chondrocyte apoptosis and necrosis	• Superficial fibrillation • Chondrocyte proliferation • Reduplication of tidemark	• Deep fibrillation • Matrix delamination • Matrix erosion • Perichondronal fibrosis • Reparative fibrocartilage • Disruption of articular plate
Bone	• Osteoblast / osteoclast activity • Subchondral bone plate thickness	• Subchondral bone thickening • Capillary blood vessel penetration through the articular plate	• Articular plate fractures • Osteophyte formation • Osteonecrosis
Synovium	• Edema • Vascular congestion • Occasional lymphocytes and plasma cells	• Synovial lining cell hyperplasia • Lymphoid follicles	• Subintimal and perivascular fibrosis

water[1,12]. Articular cartilage appears on gross examination as a white firm homogeneous tissue and, on conventional histology, as amorphous extracellular substance interspersed by ovoid chondrocytes. However, with special techniques, articular cartilage is characterized by matrix domains organized in layers parallel to the joint surface, extending from the joint space to the subchondral bone[1,13-16]. These layers vary in thickness depending on the modality used for visualization. For example, magnetic resonance imaging of articular cartilage demonstrates a thicker superficial layer than does histology[14-16]. The most superficial layer is relatively rich in collagen fibers. These collagen fibers are organized horizontally as a mesh, containing elongated, flattened chondrocytes oriented parallel to the articular surface[17,18]. The intermediate and deeper layers consist of an interterritorial matrix containing vertically oriented collagen fibers, separating chondrons; structures that contain vertical aligned ovoid chondrocytes and their associated matrix[17,19]. In the deepest layers, the matrix surrounding the chondrocytes shows orderly calcium apatite calcification[20-24]. There is a thin distinct layer of enhanced calcification parallel to the articular surface, between the uncalcified and calcified cartilage matrix. This zone is commonly called the 'tidemark'. In all uncalcified layers of cartilage, water is the dominant component. The amount and distribution of water is closely regulated by the arrangement and concentration of the protein and proteoglycan matrix components, which in turn is regulated by the chondrocytes.

The first recognizable change in OA is edema of extracellular matrix, principally affecting the intermediate layer[25]. The cartilage becomes softer and more susceptible to injury. In conditions such as chondromalacia patellae, edema can become the dominant feature[26] and can be sufficiently prominent to form a mucinous cyst within the cartilage. Cartilage edema appears to result from the focal proteolytic and proteoglycan degradation activities of the chondrocytes. With the establishment of edema, the chondrocytes may produce proteoglycans in excess, with a cycle that permits the cartilage to absorb more water and to hypertrophy, as a tissue. Direct physical forces on the softened cartilage can produce matrix fibrillation and delamination of matrix fragments, features traditionally considered typical pathologic characteristics of OA[27,28] (Figs 5.1 and 5.2). Initially, the fibrillation is parallel to the articular surface, reflecting the arrangement of superficial collagen fibers and shear forces. Vertical propagation of the clefts is a feature of OA

progression. Frequently, at the base of the fibrillation clefts, the adjacent chondrocytes show necrosis[29] and apoptosis[30]. The selective cell death of chondrocytes in OA appears to result not from direct mechanical trauma, but rather from chemical signals derived from matrix degradation products or adjacent cells[30,31]. Adjacent to these areas of necrosis, clustering of chondrocytes and chondrocyte proliferation is observed[29,32,33]. Characteristics of OA progression include: regenerative changes, such as chondrocyte proliferation (hyperplasia) as well as chondrocyte enlargement (hypertrophy), and elaboration of cytoplasmic proteolytic enzymes such as Cathepsin B[33-43]; degenerative changes, such as cartilage matrix erosion, collagen condensation around chondrons, and amianthoid thickening of collagen fibers; and reparative changes, such as fibronectin deposition in superficial cartilage and proteoglycan accumulation within the chondrons.

Further, the cartilaginous matrix can exhibit biochemical features similar to growth plate cartilage. Biomarkers of these latter changes include elaboration of alkaline phosphatase on the chondrocyte cell membranes[44] and the presence of Type X collagen within the cartilage matrix[45]. Recently, magnetic resonance imaging studies have confirmed the progressive heterogeneity of cartilage matrix as OA advances[14,15]. These studies have also confirmed that cartilage tissue thickens (hypertrophies) as OA proceeds[15,16].

The complex regulation of the repair process has been observed in experimental OA, where there is discordance of the Type II collagen:aggrecan mRNA ratios, from those of normal cartilage[46]. In this model, disproportionate mRNA of Type II collagen is seen. These observations illustrate that while cartilage matrix maintenance and repair are temporally and spatially similar, individual sequences of the repair process may differ considerably in amplitude. With disease progression in force-bearing areas, particularly, there is erosion of the cartilage, often to the subchondral bone which is thicker than normal. In the deep cartilage, there is a tidemark layer of increased calcification separating the calcified from the uncalcified cartilage. Reduplication of this tidemark is a common feature, reflecting discrete events which have altered mechanical forces and have enlarged the domains of calcified cartilage[20-24]. As well, with OA there is penetration of capillary blood vessels into, and through, the calcified cartilage layer[20]. These vessels contribute to the increased remodeling of cartilage, by providing a direct route for penetration of systemic hormones and paracrine factors into the deepest cartilage layers.

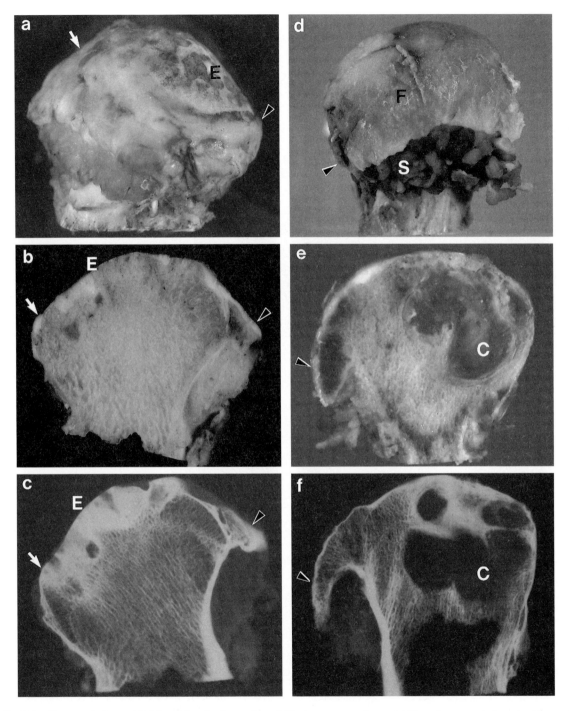

Fig. 5.1 Gross pathology of OA involving the femoral head. To demonstrate the variability of gross pathology, two femoral heads surgically removed for OA are illustrated. Both specimens show extensive remodeling. Figs (a), (b), and (c) show a femoral head with extensive eburnation of the surface and articular plate bone sclerosis: (a) surface; (b) cut surface; (c) specimen X-ray of (b). Prominent OA features include: cartilage erosion (➔); bone eburnation (E), osteophyte formation (➤). (Figs (d), (e), and (f) show a femoral head with relative preservation of cartilage, extreme subchondral bone cyst formation, and extreme osteophyte formation: (d) surface; (e) cut surface; (f) specimen X-ray of (e). Prominent OA features include: cartilage fibrillation (F); synovial hypertrophy (S); osteophyte formation (➤); cyst formation (C).

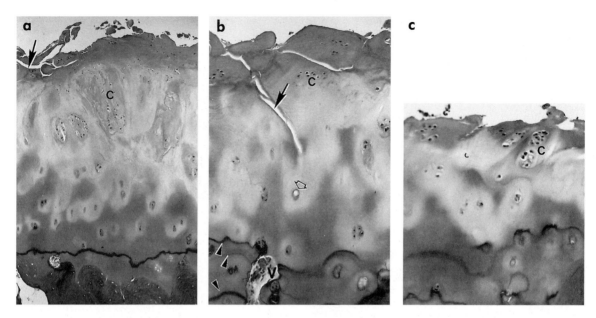

Fig. 5.2 Microscopic pathology of osteoarthritic articular cartilage. Note photomicrographs are taken from different areas of the same specimen. (a) Early OA. Horizontal fibrillation (→), chondrocyte clusters (C). (b) Moderate OA. Vertical cleft (→), chondrocyte death (⊅), tidemark duplication (➤), vascular penetration into cartilage (V), chondrocyte clusters (C). (c) Advanced OA. Shows cartilage erosion, cartilage matrix disorganization, and chondrocyte clusters (C). (Hematoxylin and eosin stain, magnification ×40)

Mechanically, blood vessel penetration through the subchondral bone and calcified cartilage provides sites for microfractures extending into the cartilage[47]. At these sites, there is ingrowth of fibrocytes. These cells undergo cartilaginous metaplasia[48] and elaborate a fibrous matrix containing Type I collagen. Fibrocartilage is also elaborated, in and above, microfractures within the articular bone plate that is present on articular surface denuded of cartilage. Compared to hyaline cartilage which contains Type II collagen in an isotropic arrangement, reparative fibrocartilage contains the less hydrated Type I collagen[49], usually organized with thicker fibers oriented perpendicularly to the surface[48]. Although fibrocartilage provides a less adequate articular covering, the reparative fibrocartilage in OA can provide an acceptable articular surface. With passive or active motion, this fibrocartilage can assume many characteristics similar to hyaline cartilage[50]. Indeed, following femoral osteotomy, clinical improvement occurs coincident with the extension of reparative fibrocartilage to cover the entire femoral head surface[51]. Delaminated articular cartilage fragments can persist within the joint space, as loose bodies. These structures are *in vivo* cartilage explants, which can enlarge by chondrocyte proliferation and elaboration of concentric layers of cartilaginous matrix[52].

Fibrocartilage

The knee, wrist, and temporomandibular joints contain meniscal structures composed of fibrochondrocytes embedded in a matrix with highly oriented Type I collagen fibers[53]. Except at the margins, these structures are avascular. Injury involves vertical disruption of collagen fiber bundles, with the cleft formation usually parallel to their alignment. With progression, complete tears and disruption of the meniscus, with formation of loose bodies, can occur. Meniscal tears can result from trauma and can persist without degenerative changes in the adjacent cartilage[54,55]. Meniscal tears associated with OA are usually connected with regenerative changes in the adjacent tissue[56–59]. The response to injury consists of focal proliferation and enlargement of fibrochondrocytes adjacent to the clefts, followed by elaboration of proteoglycans and production of reparative Type I and Type III collagen fibers[53–58]. This repair capacity is variable and is usually observed adjacent to clefts or complete tears[55,57,58]. When the reparative process is arrested at the proteoglycan production phase, a mucin-filled cyst can develop[60,61]. Meniscal structures are usually resistant to vascularization but, with advanced OA, it can occur at the meniscal margins.

Crystals and osteoarthritis

The relationship of crystal deposition to OA is controversial[62]. In gout, where monosodium urate crystals are deposited on the cartilage surfaces, osteoarthritic changes proceed either coincidentally, or secondarily, as a consequence of repeated episodes of acute gout. In pseudogout, or calcium pyrophosphate dihydrate (CPPD) crystal arthropathy, crystals form within hyaline and fibrocartilage matrix[63]. It is now known that the kinetic and biological conditions in which these crystals form are at variance with the conditions present in cartilage matrix, in active OA[64]. Therefore, when OA and CPPD crystal arthropathy are present together, it is likely that either the OA preceded the crystal deposition or, as in gout, OA has followed as a secondary consequence of matrix damage related to crystal deposition. The role of calcium apatite crystals in OA is also in dispute[65]. Apatite crystals may be present in osteoarthritic synovial fluids but these crystals may be derived from necrotic bone, or calcified cartilage at the articular surfaces, or from nodules of calcified cartilage usually within reparative cartilaginous tissues. In general, the presence of crystal agglomerates within the synovial space, or in cartilaginous structures, will alter biomechanics and may provide the stimulus for activation of the joint remodeling process.

Bone

In OA, the subchondral bone participates in the reaction to injury in a similar manner to the cartilage of the articular plate[66-68]. Initially, activation of the osteoclast–osteoblast system results in bone resorption and formation, which is preferentially restricted to subchondral bone within and adjacent to the articular plate. Subjacent to domains of greatest force, bone formation predominates and bone thickness increases within the articular plate (Fig. 5.3). However, this remodeled bone matrix is more hydrated, less dense, and less stiff than bone more remote from the joint[67]. As part of the bone resorption process, capillary blood vessels penetrate through the subchondral bone to the

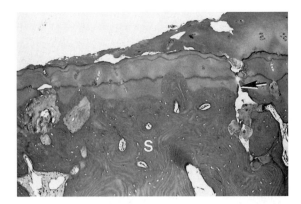

Fig. 5.3 Photomicrograph of the articular plate in advanced OA: cartilage is eroded; subchondral bone (S) is thickened; a fracture is present through the subchondral bone and calcified cartilage (→). (Hematoxylin and eosin stain, magnification ×20)

calcified articular cartilage. In zones where the cartilage has been eroded completely from bone, the bone surfaces become smooth and burnished, or shining, often with ridges aligned parallel to the joint movement. In advanced OA, this eburnated surface indicates that osseous surfaces can adapt to functions formerly performed by articular cartilage. At the joint margins, the cartilage bone interface is usually thin and, therefore, very susceptible to the remodling that occurs in OA. In this zone, there is an outgrowth of fibroblasts which elaborate collagenous fibrous tissue. This tissue undergoes metaplasia to bone, forming an osteophyte. Subsequent remodeling of this tissue results in a structure containing cortical bone, cancellous bone, and bone marrow. With further remodeling, this marrow becomes contiguous with the bone marrow in the interior of the bone. At sites where the osteophytes impinge on the joint surface, the fibrous tissue undergoes metaplasia to fibrocartilage, which often becomes an extension of the articular surface (Fig. 5.4). While under some conditions, osteophyte formation may have a function of stabilizing the joint, osteophytes can develop in size and shape disproportionate to any known structural function. This indicates that bone growth and remodeling are part of the general joint growth and remodelling characteristic of OA.

Osteonecrosis and OA

The role of osteonecrosis in the development of OA is also controversial[69]. In osteonecrosis which results

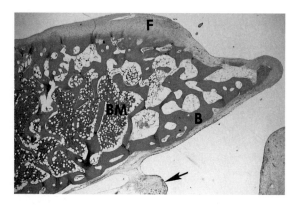

Fig. 5.4 Photomicrograph of an osteophyte at the articular margin: fibrocartilage (F); bone (B); hematopoietic bone marrow (BM), synovium (→). (Hematoxylin and eosin stain, magnification ×30)

from disruption of subchondral bone blood supply, the articular cartilage remains intact, with repair beginning by regrowth of blood vessels and resorption of bone. Resorption of subchondral necrotic bone leads to failure of the articular surface, disrupting the articular cartilage and distorting the joint architecture. In such cases, OA is a secondary event. However, in advanced primary OA, microfracture of the articular plate can lead to osteonecrosis and reparative new bone formation. Compared to primary osteonecrosis, the osteonecrosis which occurs late in OA is more limited in extent and in depth from the articular surface. Microfracture, though an intact articular plate, can occur also in patients with osteoporosis or joint laxity without prior OA[70]. In such cases, osteonecrosis is limited to the articular plate. In these patients, failure of adequate repair can lead to OA which is often more severe on the opposite articular surface[70].

Bone cysts and OA

The articular plate remodeling associated with OA, alters the forces on the joint and results in adaptation by the subjacent bone. In areas of increased force, this can result in osteosclerosis; in areas of decreased force, bone resorption can lead to domains of osteoporosis. Bone cysts are often misnamed 'geodes' by radiologists[71]. These cysts develop beneath joint surfaces which are both denuded of cartilage and remodeled such that the tissues are subject to lesser forces than their usual anatomical position would indicate[71]. Geode is a misnomer as, unlike geological structures of

the same name, the cysts in OA do not contain crystals. These cysts arise from microfractures from the joint surface to subjacent osteoporotic domains, with insudation of synovial fluid and the resultant encapsulation by surrounding new bone. These cysts initially contain loose connective tissue or even tissue resembling synovium. With repair, the connective tissue within the cyst becomes more fibrous and less vascular.

Synovium

In humans, the synovium consists of a single discontinuous intimal layer of cells, with no barrier to diffusion between the synovial space and the adjacent connective tissue. The early phases of OA are characterized by edema within the synovium. As it resorbs, edema is followed by proteoglycan secretion, microvascular congestion, and a slight inflammatory reaction. With the onset of OA, the synovial lining becomes more continuous as intimal cells proliferate, and as macrophages migrate and adhere to the synovial lining[72-75]. Although not proven, it is useful to consider that the stimulus for the synovial cell proliferation in OA is similar to that for chondrocytes. The synovial lining cells elaborate hyaluronate and proteolytic enzymes. Hyaluronate facilitates the presence of the synovial effusion and the retention of macrophages within the joint. In OA, the proteolytic enzymes secreted by synovium act principally to digest cartilage matrix that has been sheared mechanically from the joint surface. The established synovial inflammatory reaction consists of synovial lining cell hyperplasia with synovial frond formation; scattered lymphocytes and perivascular lymphoid aggregates are observed. In the subintimal synovium, this reaction, which is not as intense as that seen in rheumatoid arthritis, is followed by elaboration of collagen fibers parallel to the synovial surface and circumferential to small blood vessels (Fig. 5.5). In contrast to rheumatoid arthritis, there is insufficient activity of the synovial lining cells to erode articular cartilage at the joint margin, or to disrupt the cartilage surface. A characteristic feature of the synovitis in established OA is the presence of perivascular lymphoid follicles containing T cells, B cells, and macrophages. Quantitatively, the synovial lining cell proliferation may approximate to that of rheumatoid arthritis but, in OA, the synovial cells show a more prominent cytoskeleton[75] and nuclear lamina[76]. Again, in contrast to inflammatory arthritis, the synovium in OA shows relatively few neutrophils and fewer plasma

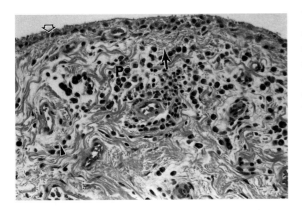

Fig. 5.5 Osteoarthritic synovium: synovial lining cells (⇨); subintimal fibrosis (→); perivascular fibrosis (➤); plasma cell and lymphocyte inflammatory infiltrate (P). (Hematoxylin and eosin stain, magnification ×40)

cells, with less immunoglobulin synthesis activity[73,74,77,78]. In advanced OA, circumferential perivascular fibrosis, a hallmark of previous perivascular inflammation, is seen in addition to the lamellar collagen fiber formation in the subintimal synovium.

With cartilage erosion, fragments of cartilage matrix and necrotic bone may become incorporated into the synovial membrane and surrounded by macrophages, including foreign body giant cells. Whilst modest amounts of cartilage and bone fragments can be found particularly in synovium from the recesses of the joints, when this material is prominent, a rapidly destructive arthritis with a neurogenic component must be considered.

Clinically, patients with OA may have an acute inflammatory episode superimposed on the chronic disease[79-80]. Most frequently, these episodes occur at the onset of interphalangeal OA. This inflammation may produce clinically tender synovial cysts over the dorsal aspect of the distal phalangeal joints. These cysts contain mucin and a few inflammatory cells. Inflammatory OA affecting other joints may show a neutrophil-rich exudate in the synovial fluid. Usually, this reaction is secondary to release of crystals or matrix products, the latter possibly related to microfracture of the articular plate.

Capsule, intra articular ligaments, and bursae

Joint capsules and intra-articular ligaments share structural features of highly oriented Type I collagen fiber bundles arranged between elongated fibrocytes. Small capillary blood vessels are present in this tissue. In joint capsules, the reaction to injury in OA is similar to that of synovium[81]. This reaction is characterized by edema and proteoglycan elaboration, followed by additional collagen fiber formation both parallel to the plane of the synovial intima and also in a perivascular pattern. During OA, vascular dilatation and congestion can be prominent. In ligaments, these changes are observed but to a lesser extent. In joint capsules and synovial membranes, perineurial and endoneurial fibrosis is frequently seen in OA. With these post-inflammatory changes, these neural structures may be a morphologic substrate of the chronic pain found in the joints of OA patients[82].

In advanced OA, the persistence of synovial effusions tends to expand the joint space and distort the architecture of the joint capsule. The ensuing fibrous reaction alters the physiology of the capsule, making the joint space less compliant, as well as creating a relative barrier to fluid diffusion. The expansion of the synovial space and the persistence of effusions expand the bursal structures communicating with the joint space. With advanced OA, these structures may participate in mild chronic synovitis. With deformation of the joint, movement of soft tissues about osteophyte structures can create additional bursae, which also can communicate with the joint and participate in the synovial reaction.

Collagenase, and other proteolytic enzymes elaborated by the synovium and inflammatory cells reacting to matrix fragments, can induce edema and proliferative responses in the ligament and capsular tissue in close proximity to synovium. In OA joints in which there is increased laxity, the intra-articular ligaments are more susceptible to mechanical injury, which in turn alters adversely the forces bearing on the articular cartilage, thereby facilitating incremental joint injury.

Extra-articular connective tissues and muscle

The arrangement and physiology of the extrinsic connective tissue in muscles contribute greatly to the range of joint movement and joint stability. Depending on the circumstances, OA joints can be either relatively stiff or relatively lax. In joints where there is continuing limitation of movement because of pain, the range of movement may ultimately become limited by muscular adaption, and fibrosis of capsular and extrinsic connective tissue structures. Joint laxity develops partly by adaption of the extrinsic structures to repeated effusions. As well, the systemic hyperplastic stimuli that activate cartilage and bone cells to remodel their matrix, also affect tendon and ligament insertions (entheses) in a similar manner. Joint laxity leads to mechanical instability which can suddenly alter the forces bearing on the articular surfaces, thus provoking additional joint injury.

OA: *diagnostic pathology*

Practical tissue diagnosis of OA has three major limitations. First, the opportunity to sample affected tissues is usually restricted to larger joints and then, only at the time of synovial fluid aspiration, synovial biopsy, arthroscopy, or joint replacement. Second, OA has a heterogeneous pattern of disease within each joint and this heterogeneity is observed both spatially and temporally. Third, as osteoarthritic structural changes can supervene secondarily in other forms of arthritis, the contribution of other types of arthritis, particularly crystal associated arthropathy or inflammatory arthropathies, must be determined in assessment of OA joint tissues.

The positive tissue diagnosis of OA is dependent on identifying characteristic degenerative and regenerative features in articular tissues (Table 5.1). Examination of synovial fluid, after centrifugation, may show particulates of cartilage matrix in which features such as fibrillation and chondrocyte clusters can be observed[83]. Frequently, these particles are trapped in a thick mucin which also contains a macrophage cell population. This cytologic pattern differs substantially from the pattern of thin mucin, degraded collagen fragments, fibrin and abundant neutrophils which characterize the synovial inflammatory exudate seen in rheumatoid arthritis. With arthroscopy, in addition to mechanical tears, cartilage fibrillation and cartilage hypertrophy can be seen. In OA, the synovium is focally involved and is usually most severely affected in the synovium adjacent to the articular cartilage[82]. Therefore, synovial biopsy is most likely to yield diagnostic tissue when the site is visualized through the arthroscope[84,85]. The examination of surgical specimens obtained at arthroplasty, provides a major opportunity to determine the presence of OA, its extent, and its coexistence with other disease processes. With examination of these tissues, it is important to orient fragmented gross specimens, to

describe the articular surface and deep portions of the articular plate, and to note the locations of cartilage erosion and the presence of osteophytes. It is also advisable to X-ray and section every specimen, to determine such features as the presence of crystals or osteonecrosis. In addition to cartilage, bone, synovium and capsular tissues should be sampled. Examination of the joint tissue in the manner described above permits confirmation that the disease is indeed OA. Further, with the above approach, the activity of the OA can be assessed and the question whether the OA is primary or secondary in nature may be resolved.

As disease-modifying drugs become more available for OA, it is highly desirable to have structural biomarkers that can be identified and quantified against the potential benefit of therapy. The development of such markers awaits not only cost-effective and less invasive methods of sampling joint tissue, but also, a more precise understanding of how cartilage, bone, and synovial cell populations change, and how the composition of the articular extracellular matrices evolve with OA progression.

References

1. Gardner, D.L. (1992). *Pathological basis of the connective tissue diseases*, pp. 842–943. Lea and Febiger, Philadelphia.
2. Moskowitz, R.W., Howell, D.S., Goldberg, V.M., and Mankin, H.J. (ed.) (1992). *Osteoarthritis. Diagnosis and medical/surgical management*, (2nd edn), pp. 1–761. W.B. Saunders, Philadelphia.
3. McCarty, D.J. and Koopman, W.J. (ed.) (1993). *Arthritis and allied conditions. A textbook of Rheumatology*, (12th edn), pp. 1699–1772 Lea and Febiger, Philadelphia.
4. Schumacher, H.R. Jr (ed.), Klippel, J.H., and Robinson, D.R. (Assoc. ed.) (1988). *Primer on the rheumatic diseases*, (9th edn), pp. 171–7. The Arthritis Foundation, Atlanta.
5. Pritzker, K.P.H. (1994). Animal models for osteoarthritis: processes, problems and prospects. *Annals of the Rheumatic Diseases*, 53, 406–20.
6. Karvonen, R.L., Negendank, W.G., Teitge, R.A., Reed, A.H., Miller, P.R., and Fernandez-Madrid, F. (1994). Factors affecting articular cartilage thickness in osteoarthritis and aging. *Journal of Rheumatology*, 21, 1310–8.
7. Goffin, Y. and De Doncker, E. (1980). Altérations histologique et histochimique de la capsule articulaire dans l'arthrose et chez les sujets séniles. *Revue du Rhumatisme*, 47(1), 15–20.
8. Egan, M.S., Goldenberg, D.L., Cohen, A.S., and Sega, D. (1982). The association of amyloid deposits and osteoarthritis. *Arthritis and Rheumatism*, 25(2), 204–8.

9. van der Korst, J.K., Sokoloff, L., and Miller, E.J. (1968). Senescent pigmentation of cartilage and degenerative joint disease. *Archives of Pathology*, **86**, 40–7.

10. Bluestone, R., Bywaters, E., Haratog, M., Holt, P.J.L., and Hyde, S. (1971). Acromegalic arthropathy. *Annals of the Rheumatic Diseases*, **30**, 243–58.

11. Macys, J.R., Bullough, P.G., and Wilson, P.D. Jr. (1980). Coxarthrosis: a study of the natural history based on a correlation of clinical, radiographic, and pathologic findings. *Seminars in Arthritis and Rheumatism*, **10(1)**, 66–80.

12. Pritzker, K.P.H. (1992). Cartilage histopathology in human and rhesus macaque osteoarthritis. *Articular cartilage and osteoarthritis*, (ed. K. Kuettner *et al.*), pp. 473–85. Raven Press Ltd., New York.

13. Benninghof, A. (1925). Form unn bau der gelenkknorpel in ihren Beziehungen zur function. II. Der aufbau nes gelenkknorpels in seinen Beziehungen zur function. *Zeitschrift für Zellforschung und mikroskopische Anatomie*, **2**, 783–862.

14. Gahunia, H.K., Babyn, P., Lemaire, C., Kessler, M.J., and Pritzker, K.P.H. (1995). Osteoarthritis staging: comparison between magnetic resonance imaging, gross pathology and histopathology in the rhesus macaque. *Osteoarthritis and Cartilage*, **3**, 169–80.

15. Gahunia, H.K., Lemaire, C., Babyn, P., Cross, A.R., Kessler, M.J., and Pritzker, K.P.H. (1995). Osteoarthritis in Rhesus Macaque knee joint: quantitative magnetic resonance imaging tissue characterization of articular cartilage. *Journal of Rheumatology*, **22**, 1747–56.

16. Modl, J.M., Sether, L.A., Haughton, V.M., and Kneeland, J.B. (1991). Articular cartilage: correlation of histologic zones with signal intensity at MR imaging. *Radiology*, **181**, 853–5.

17. Hwang, W.S., Li, B., Jin, L.H., Ngo, K., Schachar, N.S., and Hughes, G.N.F. (1992). Collagen fibril structure of normal, aging, and osteoarthritic cartilage. *Journal of Pathology*, **167**, 425–33.

18. Teshima, R., Otsuka, T., Takasu, N., Yamagata, N., and Yamamoto, K. (1995). Structure of the most superficial layer of articular cartilage. *Journal of Bone and Joint Surgery*, **77-B**, 460–4.

19. Poole, C.A., Flint, M.H., and Beaumont, B.W. (1987). Chondrons in cartilage: ultrastructure analysis of the pericellular microenvironment in adult human articular cartilage. *Journal of Orthopaedic Research*, **5**, 509–22.

20. Lane, L.B. and Bullough, P.G. (1980). Age-related changes in the thickness of the calcified zone and the number of tidemarks in adult human articular cartilage. *Journal of Bone and Joint Surgery*, **62-B(3)**, 372–5.

21. Green, W.T., Jr, Martin, G.N., Eanes, E.D., and Sokoloff, L. (1970). Microradiographic study of the calcified layer of articular cartilage. *Archives of Pathology*, **90**, 151–8.

22. Redler, I., Mow, V.C., Zimny, M.L., and Mansell, J. (1975). The ultrastructure and biochemical significance of the tidemark of articular cartilage. *Clinical Orthopaedics*, **112**, 357–62.

23. Bullough, P.G. and Jagannath, A. (1983). The morphology of the calcification front in articular cartilage: its significance in joint function. *Journal of Bone and Joint Surgery*, **65-B**, 72–8.

24. Revell, P.A., Pirie, C., Amir, G., Rashad, S., and Walker, F. (1990). Metabolic activity in the calcified zone of cartilage: observations on tetracycline labelled articular cartilage in human osteoarthritic hips. *Rheumatology International*, **10**, 143–7.

25. Venn, M. and Maroudas, A. (1977). Chemical composition and swelling of normal and osteoarthritic femoral head cartilage. *Annals of the Rheumatic Diseases*, **36**, 121–9.

26. Ohno, O., Naito, J., Iguchi, T., Ishikawa, H., Hirohata, K., and Cooke, D.V. (1988). An electron microscopic study of early pathology in chondromalacia of the patella. *Journal of Bone and Joint Surgery*, **70-A(6)**, 883–99.

27. Bartel, D.L., Bicknell, V.L., Ithaca, M.S., and Wright, T.M. (1986). The effect of conformity. Thickness and material on stresses in ultra-high molecular weight components for total joint replacement. *Journal of Bone and Joint Surgery*, **68A**, 1041–51.

28. Meachim, G. and Fergie, I.A. (1975). Morphological patterns of articular cartilage fibrillation. *Journal of Pathology*, **115**, 231–40.

29. Meachim, G. (1972). Articular cartilage lesions in osteoarthritis of the femoral head. *Journal of Pathology*, **107**, 199–210.

30. Erlacher, L., Maier, R., Ullrich, R., Kiener, H., Aringer, M., Menschik, M., *et al.* (1995). Differential expression of the proto-oncogene bcl-2 in normal and osteoarthritic human articular cartilage. *Journal of Rheumatology*, **22**, 926–31.

31. Sokoloff, L. (1990). Acquired chondronecrosis. *Annals of the Rheumatic Diseases*, **49(4)**, 262–4.

32. Poole, C.A., Matsuoka, A., and Schofield, J.R. (1991). Chondrons from articular cartilage. III. Morphologic changes in the cellular microenvironment of chondrons isolated from osteoarthritic cartilage. *Arthritis and Rheumatism*, **34**, 22–35.

33. Rothwell, A.G. and Bentley, G. (1973). Chondrocyte multiplication in osteoarthritic articular cartilage. *Journal of Bone and Joint Surgery*, **55B(3)**, 588–94.

34. Hirotani, H. and Ito, T. (1975). Chondrocyte mitosis in the articular cartilage of femoral heads with various diseases. *Acta Orthopedica*, **46**, 979–86.

35. Jones, K.L., Brown, M., Ali, S.Y., and Brown, R.A. (1987). An immunohistochemical study of fibronectin in human osteoarthritic and disease-free articular cartilage. *Annals of the Rheumatic Diseases*, **46**, 809–15.

36. Mitchell, N. and Shepard, N. (1981). Percellular proteoglycan concentrations in early degenerative arthritis. *Arthritis and Rheumatism*, **24(7)**, 958–64.

37. Baici, A., Hörler, D., Lang, A., Merlin, C., and Kissling, R. (1995). Cathepsin B in osteoarthritis: zonal variation of enzyme activity in human femoral head cartilage. *Annals of the Rheumatic Diseases*, **54**, 281–8.

38. Baici, A., Lang, A., Hörler, D., Kissling, R., and Merlin, C. (1995). Cathepsin B in osteoarthritis: cytochemical and histochemical analysis of human femoral head cartilage. *Annals of the Rheumatic Diseases*, **54**, 289–97.

39. Fassbender, H.G. (1987). Role of chondrocytes in the development of osteoarthritis. *American Journal of Medicine*, **83(supplement 5A)**, 17–24.

40. Mankin, H.J. and Lippiello, L. (1970). Biochemical and metabolic abnormalities in articular cartilage from osteoarthritic human hips. *Journal of Bone and Joint Surgery*, **52-A(3)**, 424–34.

41. Mankin, H.J., Dorfman, H., Lippiello, L., and Zarins, A. (1971). Biochemical and metabolic abnormalities in articular cartilage from osteoarthritis human hips. *Journal of Bone and Joint Surgery*, **53-A(3)**, 523–37.

42. Weiss, C. and Mirow, S. (1972). An ultrastructural study of osteoarthritic changes in the articular cartilage of human knees. *Journal of Bone and Joint Surgery*, **54-A(5)**, 954–72.

43. Ghadially, F.N., Lalonde, J-M.A., and Yong, N.K. (1979). Ultrastructure of amianthoid fibers in osteoarthrotic cartilage. *Virchows Archives of Cell Pathology*, **31**, 81–6.

44. Rees, V.A. and Ali, S.Y. (1988). Ultrastructural localization of alkaline phosphatase activity in osteoarthritic human articular cartilage. *Annals of the Rheumatic Diseases*, **47**, 947–53.

45. von der Mark, K., Kirsch, T., Nerlich, A., Kuss, A., Weseloh, G., Glückert, K. *et al.* (1992). Type X collagen synthesis in human osteoarthritic cartilage. Indication of chondrocyte hypertrophy. *Arthritis and Rheumatism*, **35(7)**, 806–11.

46. Matyas, J.R., Adams, M.E., Huang, D., and Sandell, L.J. (1995). Discoordinate gene expression of aggrecan and type II collagen in experimental osteoarthritis. *Arthritis and Rheumatism*, **38**, 420–5.

47. Sokoloff, L. (1993). Microcracks in the calcified layer of articular cartilage. *Archives of Pathology and Laboratory Medicine*, **117**, 191–5.

48. Meachim, G. and Osborne, G.V. (1970). Repair at the femoral articular surface in osteoarthritis of the hip. *Journal of Pathology*, **102(1)**, 1–8.

49. Grynpas, M.D., Eyre, D.R., and Kirschner, D.A. (1980). Collagen type II: native molecular packing differs from type I. *Biochemica et Biophysica Acta*, **626**, 346–55.

50. Kim, H.K.M., Moran, M.E., and Salter, R.B. (1991). The potential for regeneration of articular cartilage in defects created by chondral shaving and subchondral abrasion. An experimental investigation in rabbits. *Journal of Bone and Joint Surgery*, **73**, 1301–15.

51. Byers, P.D. (1974). The effect of high femoral osteotomy on osteoarthritis of the hip. *Journal of Bone and Joint Surgery*, **56B(2)**, 279–90.

52. Barrie, H.J. (1978). Intra-articular loose bodies regarded as organ cultures *in vivo*. *Journal of Pathology*, **125(2)**, 163–9.

53. McDevitt, C.A. and Webber, R.J. (1990). The ultrastructure and biochemistry of meniscal cartilage. *Clinical Orthopaedics and Related Research*, **252**, 8–18.

54. Noble, J. and Hamblen, D.L. (1975). The pathology of the degenerate meniscus lesion. *Journal of Bone and Joint Surgery*, **57-B(2)**, 180–6.

55. Fahmy, N.R.M., Williams, Ea., and Noble, J. (1983). Meniscal pathology and osteoarthritis of the knee. *Journal of Bone and Joint Surgery*, **65-B(1)**, 24–8.

56. Hough, A.J. and Webber, R.J. (1980). Pathology of the meniscus. *Clinical Orthopaedics*, **252**, 32–40.

57. Meachim, G. (1976). The state of knee meniscal fibrocartilage in Liverpool necropsies. *Journal of Pathology*, **119**, 167–73.

58. Merkel, K.H.H. (1980). The surface of human menisci and its aging alterations during age. A combined scanning and transmission electron microscopic examination (SEM, TEM). *Archives of Orthopedic Trauma Surgery*, **97**, 185–91.

59. Ferrer-Roca, O. and Vilalta, C. (1980). Lesions of the meniscus. Part I: macroscopic and histologic findings. *Clinical Orthopaedics and Related Research*, **146**, 289–300.

60. Ferrer-Roca, O. and Vilalta, C. (1980). Lesions of the meniscus. Part II: horizontal cleavages and lateral cysts. *Clinical Orthopaedics and Related Research*, **146**, 301–7.

61. Barrie, H.J. (1979). The pathogenesis and significance of menisceal cysts. *Journal of Bone and Joint Surgery*, **61-B(2)**, 184–9.

62. Dieppe, P. and Watt, I. (1985). Crystal deposition in osteoarthritis: an opportunitistic event? *Clinics in Rheumatic Diseases*, **11(2)**, 367–92.

63. Pritzker, K.P.H., Cheng, P-T., and Renlund, R.C. (1988). Calcium pyrophosphate crystal deposition in hyaline cartilage: ultrastructural analysis and implications for pathogenesis. *Journal of Rheumatology*, **15**, 828–35.

64. Cheng, P-T. and Pritzker, K.P.H. (1983). Pyrophosphate, phosphate ion interactions: effects on calcium pyrophosphate and hydroxyapatite crystal formation in aqueous solutions. *Journal of Rheumatology*, **10(5)**, 769–77.

65. Dieppe, P.A. (1991). Inflammation in osteoarthritis and the role of microcrystals. *Arthritis and Rheumatism*, **11**, 121–2.

66. Oettmeier, R. and Abendroth, K. (1989). Osteoarthritis and bone: osteologic types of osteoarthritis of the hip. *Skeletal Radiology*, **18**, 165–74.

67. Grynpas, M.D., Alpert, B., Katz, I., Leiberman, I., and Pritzker, K.P.H. (1991). Subchondral bone in osteoarthritis *Calcified Tissue International*, **49**, 20–6.

68. Grynpas, M.D., Huckell, C.B., Reichs, K.J., Derousseau, C.J., Greenwood, C., and Kessler, M.J. (1993). Effect of age and osteoarthritis on bone mineral in rhesus monkey vertebrae. *Journal of Bone and Mineral Research*, **8**, 909–17.

69. Ilardi, C.F. and Sokoloff, L. (1984). Secondary osteonecrosis in osteoarthritis of the femoral head. *Human Pathology*, **15**, 79–83.

70. Houpt, J.B., Pritzker, K.P.H., Alpert, B., Greyson, M.D., and Gross, A.E. (1983). Osteonecrosis of the knee – a review. *Seminars in Arthritis and Rheumatism*, **13**, 212–27.

71. Bullough, P.G. and Bansal, M. (1988). The differential diagnosis of geodes. *Radiologic Clinics of North America*, **26(6)**, 1165–84.

72. Arnoldi, C.C., Reimann, I., and Bretlau, P. (1980). The synovial membrane in human coxarthrosis: light and electron microscopic studies. *Clinical Orthopaedics and Related Research*, **148**, 213–20.

73. Soren, A., Cooper, N.S., and Waugh, Th.R. (1988). The nature and designation of osteoarthritis determined by its histopathology. *Clinical and Experimental Rheumatology*, **6**, 41–6.

74. Revell, P.A., Mayston, V., Lalor, P., and Mapp, P. (1988). The synovial membrane in osteoarthritis: a his-

tological study including the characterisation of the cellular infiltrate present in inflammatory osteoarthritis using monoclonal antibodies. *Annals of the Rheumatic Diseases*, **47**, 300–7.

75. Meek, W.D., Raber, B.T., McClain, O.M., McCosh, J.K., and Baker, B.B. (1991). Fine structure of the human synovial lining cell in osteoarthritis: its prominent cytoskeleton. *The Anatomical Record*, **231**, 145–55.

76. Ghadially, F.N., Oryschak, A.F., and Mitchell, D.M. (1974). Nuclear fibrous lamina in pathological human synovial membrane. *Virchows Arch. Abt. B Zellpathologie Cell Pathology*, **15**, 223–8.

77. Huth, F., Soren, A., Rosenbauer, K.A., and Klein, W. (1973). Fine strucutral changes of the synovial membrane in arthrosis deformans. *Virchows Arch. Abt. A Pathologische Anatomie Pathology*, **359**, 201–11.

78. Fritz, P., Mischlinski, A., Grau, A., Tuczek, H.V., Wegner, G., Müller, J., *et al.* (1986). *In situ* evaluation of immunoglobulin synthesis of synovial plasma cells in rheumatoid arthritis and osteoarthritis by plug photometry. *Pathology Research and Practice*, **181**, 243–8.

79. Utsinger, P.D., Resnick, D., Shapiro, R.F., and Wiesner, K.B. (1978). Roentgenologic, immunologic, and therapeutic study of erosive (inflammatory) osteoarthritis. *Archives of Internal Medicine*, **138**, 693–7.

80. Altman, R.D. and Gray, R. (1985). Inflammation in osteoarthritis. *Clinics in Rheumatic Diseases*, **11**, 353–65.

81. Dettmer, N. and Barz, B. (1977). Morhologische veränderungen der synovialen gelenkkapselznteile bei arthrosis deformans. *Archiv für orthopädische und Unfall-Chirurgie*, **89**, 61–79.

82. Rabinowicz, T. and Jacqueline, F. (1990). Pathology of the capsular and synovial hip nerves in chronic hip diseases. *Pathology Research and Practice*, **186**, 283–92.

83. Freemont, A.J., Denton, J., Chuck, A., Holt, P.J.L., and Davies, M. (1991). Diagnostic value of synovial fluid microscopy: a reassessment and rationalisation. *Annals of the Rheumatic Diseases*, **50**, 101–7.

84. Lindblad, S. and Hedfors, E. (1987). Arthroscopic and immunohistologic characterization of knee joint synovitis in osteoarthritis. *Arthritis and Rheumatism*, **30**(10), 1081–8.

85. Revell, P.A. (1987). The synovial biopsy. *Recent Advances in Histopathology*, **No. 6**, 79–93.

6 | Paleopathology of osteoarthritis

Juliet Rogers

Paleopathology is a term that was first defined by Sir Marc Armand Ruffer[1] at the beginning of the twentieth century as 'the study of disease in the past'. Ruffer was a pathologist in Cairo, his interest being aroused by the study of the extensive collection of mummies and other human remains which were being discovered with great frequency at this period. Paleopathological evidence is, of course, not restricted to the study of mummified human remains although, because of soft tissue preservation, they are ideal. Paintings, drawings, sculpture, literature, and early medical texts can all be used as evidence for the presence and identification of early disease. The most widespread, common, and direct type of evidence, however, is that derived from the study of human skeletal remains from archeological sites. Apart from the interest in the occurrence of particular disease at different time periods, paleopathology can provide invaluable evidence for the frequency, distribution, and variation of expression of individual pathologies through time[2].

From the earliest organized studies of human skeletal remains, it has been evident that joint disease is the most frequent type of postcranial pathology to be seen. Despite diagnostic confusion and variation in terminology, what is now recognized as osteoarthritis (OA) is, by far, the most common form of these joint diseases: it is reported in hominid fossils[3], from Neolithic sites[4], and from Egyptian mummies[5]. The presence of OA is ubiquitous in all other skeletal sites from earliest times to the postmedieval period[6], in the UK, Europe[7], the United States[8], and other areas of the world[9].

Recognition of OA

OA is customarily recognized in skeletal material by a combination of morphological changes. As in other paleopathological conditions, these are generally very easy to see, although postmortem damage may mask some changes. As in the clinical situation, OA may be noted at any of the synovial joints. The advantage of skeletal material over clinical observations, is the opportunity for direct viewing of every joint in the body thus allowing recording of OA in unreported or underreported situations. Conversely, there is the disadvantage that all joints may not be present in every skeleton, reducing the quantity and completeness of information for analysis.

The most frequent change is the presence of a rim of osteophyte at the margin of the joint surfaces. Osteophytes are also frequently observed along the upper or lower margins of the vertebral bodies. Around the articular margins, the osteophyte may take the form of a thin sharp rim, a flat ribbon, or a large florid and irregular fringe of bone (Fig. 6.1). They may circle the entire joint margin, or only a part. The joint surface itself may exhibit several different abnormalities, alone or in combination. There may be small areas of new bone formation, one to two centimetres in diameter, in the form of 'buttons' or 'pancakes' of osteophyte on the articular surface itself (Fig. 6.2). There are frequently areas of pitting, with the openings occasionally visibly connecting with subchondral cysts (Fig. 6.3). The pits can also be very small in diameter, and they

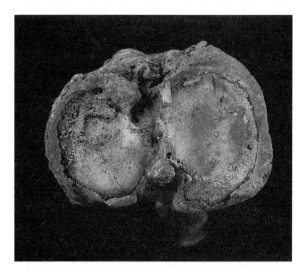

Fig. 6.1 The tibial plateau of a knee joint with prolific osteophyte around the entire joint margin.

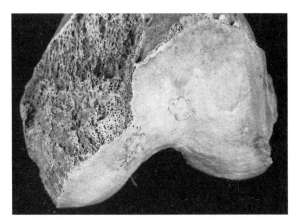

Fig. 6.2 The anterior surface of a distal femoral condyle. There is extensive postmortem damage to the medial condyle but it is still possible to see surface osteophyte both on the medial condyle and the patello-femoral joint.

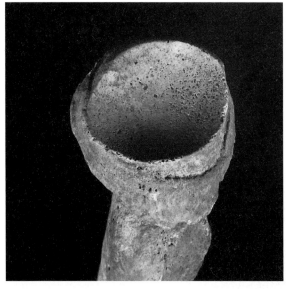

Fig. 6.4 Proximal radial joint with marked bony contour change and eburnation.

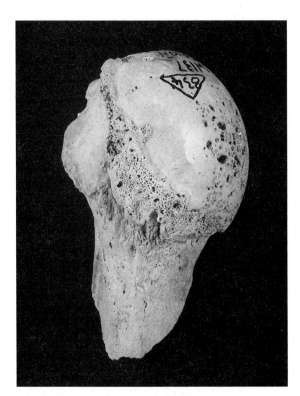

Fig. 6.3 Humeral head with marginal osteophyte, eburnation and pitting of the articular surface. In this example the pits are restricted to the eburnated area.

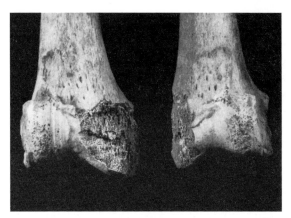

Fig. 6.5 Patello-femoral joints in medieval knees, from the site at Barton-on-Humber. Despite postmortem damage, grooves can clearly be seen on the eburnated lateral facet of the PF joint.

grooved or scored[10] (Fig. 6.5). This polishing is caused by the total degradation of cartilage, and the friction of the two opposing bone surfaces rubbing together is an unequivocal marker of the presence of OA. One other change in OA joints is alteration of bony contour.

may be widely spaced or crowded together. The most striking abnormalities, however, are clearly delineated areas of eburnation or polishing of the joint surface (Fig. 6.4). On some joints, the eburnated areas are

Disease definition and assessment

The relationship between these morphological changes has always been assumed to be linear, as in the radiological stages developed by Kellgren and Lawrence[11]. In this model, osteophyte on its own is scored as being the mildest and earliest sign of OA, developing to the most severe and latest stage marked by the presence of eburnation with grooves. However, osteophytes are an extremely common phenomenon and are very easily seen by direct observation of joints. If, therefore, a positive score for OA is recorded whenever osteophyte is present on its own, this may help to explain why OA has been reported to have an unexpectedly high frequency in some joints — the shoulder, for example. It is still the case that in many reports considering OA in skeletal populations, it is not always clear which diagnostic criteria have been used to score OA as present or absent. A study on the interobserver variation in coding OA in skeletal material[12] found that there was frequently incomplete agreement as to whether particular pathological changes were present, and only half the observers agreed on the severity of the changes. It is the case that many different scoring systems can and have been used[13]. These often bear no relationship to clinical scoring systems, which can add to the confusion and may impair the comparison of skeletal data both between archeological populations and with clinical data.

Examination of the relationship between visual, radiographic, and pathological changes can be used, however, to standardize the diagnostic criteria for OA in a paleopathological context. Inspection of a series of cadaveric knees with OA demonstrates that the region of cartilage degradation has a sharply delineated margin enclosing an area of eburnation. Because of this exact correlation of eburnation with the phenomenon of cartilage degradation, the presence of eburnation is taken as a pathognomic sign of the presence of OA. Osteophyte is more problematic, however; there is a strong association with aging[14] and a likelihood of osteophyte being formed more readily in some subsets of the population than others[15]. For this reason, the presence of osteophyte on its own is not regarded as a marker for OA. In paleopathology, the relationship of pitting and bony contour change to the soft tissue pathology, and how this relates in dry bone to the X-ray changes is also unclear; so again, the presence of pitting or contour change on their own will not be used as a marker for OA. Only if two of the group (pitting of joint surface, osteophyte, bony contour change) are present together[16] will OA be counted as occurring.

There are, of course, many other changes that can be recognized on joints, such as erosion, septic reaction, or trauma, which in the main are due to other forms of arthropathy, but which may give rise to secondary OA change.

In only one skeleton, a female recovered from a site in London, has a diagnosis of erosive OA (EOA) been suggested[17]. The distribution of the erosions on the articular surfaces of the interphalangeal joints and in the carpal bones, with proliferative new bone around the joint margins, is characteristic of EOA (Fig. 6.6). The radiological appearance confirmed the main involvement of the proximal and distal interphalangeal joints. The predominant abnormality was ill-defined bone destruction at the articular surfaces, producing in some fingers a 'gull wing' abnormality. One proximal interphalangeal joint was ankylosed.

The aim of most research into the occurrence of OA in the past is to compare the frequency of the disease both as a whole and in different joints, as between one population and another, and how this might differ from the present. Another aim will be to examine the distribution of OA within joints and, again, to compare any variation between ancient and current populations, and to interpret and explore the implications that any variation may have had for the population under investigation. For this one needs agreed and comparable data, and recent work has begun to address this problem[18,19,13]. Even with agreed operational definitions for OA in paleopathological material, as discussed above, there may still be some drawbacks. In order that data collected from ancient skeletal populations can be compared to modern information, it must be comparable. Clinical data are frequently obtained from radiological sources[11,20]. The visual inspection of skeletal material enables morphological alterations to be observed very easily, but it is not always clear that the visual and radiographic assessment of an osteoarthritic joint are comparable. A study by Rogers *et al.*[21] demonstrated a frequency of OA in a series of 24 skeletal knees ranging from 21 per cent by visual assessment to 8 per cent in the same knees radiologically assessed (Table 6.1). There is also considerable variation between authors in the way that individual joints are classified. The shoulder joint, for instance, may be defined as the glenohumeral joint or as the glenohumeral joint and acromioclavicular joint[6,8]. Clearly, differences in the definition of what constitutes a particular joint can also produce widely varying values. The knee is another joint that can suffer from confusion over definition between different researchers, some collecting data on the joint as a whole, and others recording compartmental changes as separate joints.

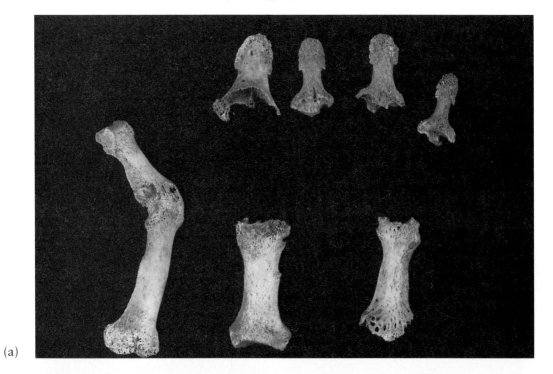

(a)

(b)

Fig. 6.6 (a) Selected medial and distal phalanges of skeleton showing areas of erosion and fusion of one proximal and medial phalanx. (b) X-ray of hand bones from same skeleton: a possible diagnosis of erosive OA was made for this specimen.

Table 6.1 Frequency of OA in a series of 24 skeletal knees[21]

	Visual appearance		Radiological appearance
Normal	Osteophyte only	OA (eburnation)	OA
8 knees (33.3%)	11 knees (41%)	5 knees (21%)	2 knees (8%)

Reported prevalence and distribution of OA

Despite the above constraints and potential problems much valuable information on the overall prevalence of OA in different populations has been obtained.

Most authors reporting on many different skeletal groups from a wide and varying time span agree that OA is the most commonly reported pathological change and the most frequently occurring joint disease[22]. In a group of Roman British skeletons from Cirencester, for example, Wells[23] reported that 44.8 per cent of the adult population had OA somewhere in the skeleton. When these figures were examined by sex, 51.5 per cent of males and 32.9 per cent of females were affected. In a medieval site in York[24], at Fishergate, 46.9 per cent of adults had OA in at least one joint — 48 per cent of males and 43.8 per cent of females. Rogers[25] found that only 15 per cent of adult Roman British skeletons had OA — but there were only 15 Roman British skeletons recovered from the site (St Oswald's Priory, Gloucestershire). Larger numbers were recovered for the periods dating respectively 900–1120, 1120–1230, and 1600–1850. For the first of these periods, 22 per cent of adults were reported as having OA — 28.5 per cent of males and 26.6 per cent of females. The second, later medieval period had 24 per cent of adults with OA — 37.5 per cent of males and 25 per cent of females; and, in the postmedieval period dating 1600–1850, the frequency of OA in all adults was 34 per cent — 33.3 per cent of males and 39.4 per cent of females. Another site which yielded contemporary skeletal material to support the findings of the last phase of St Oswalds Priory was Christ Church, Spitalfields, in London. Three hundred and eighty-seven named skeletons were recovered from among a larger assemblage from the crypt of this church. Waldron[26] reported a prevalence of 30.9 per cent of adults with OA, with 34.5 per cent of males and 24.3 per cent of females showing signs of OA change.

Site-specific prevalence

Many reports do not present an overall prevalence of OA for their skeletons but concentrate on the frequency of occurrence at particular joints. The majority of authors agree that OA most commonly affected the spinal facet joints, although Waldron[6] and Bridges[8] found the shoulder the most frequently affected joint. However, this discrepancy is due to the definition of the shoulder by these two authors as comprising both the acromio-calvicular and the glenohumeral components (see above). As the acromioclavicular joint is the second most affected joint, with OA in 36.5 per cent of Saxon skeletons from Trowbridge[27], for example, this elevation of frequency of 'shoulder' OA is not surprising.

The prominence of spinal OA is a reasonably constant finding. When more detailed analysis of the peak level of affected vertebrae is undertaken, there is also uniformity. Waldron[26] reports that the Spitalfields skeletons have peak occurrence at Cervical 4/5, Thoracic 4/5, and Lumbar 5. Jurmain and Kilgore[28] find an almost identical picture in a medieval Nubian sample. Merbs[30], in a detailed and extensive study of Innuit skeletons, found a very similar distribution with peaks of OA frequency at Cervical 2/4, Thoracic 4/5, and Lumbar 5. As well as facet joint involvement of the cervical spine, OA of the odontoid component of atlanto axial joints is also frequently observed (Fig. 6.7).

The frequency of OA at peripheral joints varies more widely between populations with Jurmain and Kilgore[28], for instance, stating that shoulder and hip are less involved than knee or elbow, whereas Waldron[6] found the converse. Table 6.2 displays the frequency of OA at different joint sites reported by seven authors for seven different skeletal assemblages. It will be seen that there is a wide variation, some of which can be explained by inclusion of the acromio-clavicular joint within the scoring of the shoulder (Waldron[6] and Bridges[8]). Other variations are likely to be due to inclusion of too wide a range of bony change within the definition of OA[7,24,8]. The variations seen from the skeletons from the other sites are likely to be

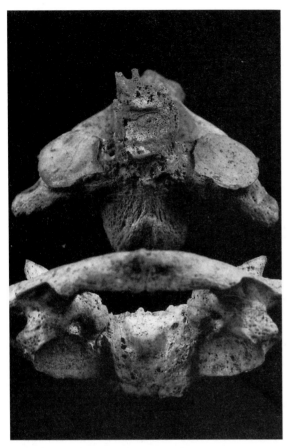

Fig. 6.7 OA of the odontoid articulation of first and second cervical vertebra, with osteophyte and eburnation.

real, as the data was collected using the same operational definition of OA.

It can be seen from Table 6.2 that the ankle is very rarely involved in OA, which is similar to the pattern seen today. However, other differences are apparent. The findings[6,7,24] (Table 6.2) confirm those reported by Rogers and Dieppe[29] that in the earlier historical period, hip OA was more frequent than knee OA, but that this ratio changed in the postmedieval period with knee OA becoming more frequent than hip OA. This differs from the pattern most frequently seen in archeological skeletons in the USA[8,28], where hip OA is less common than knee OA. Not many skeletal reports have covered the precise distribution of knee OA into its component subjoints of patellofemoral and tibiofemoral compartments. In the same study of over 785 skeletons[29], despite the changing frequency of knee OA, the majority of affected compartments were patellofemoral. This finding has been confirmed by Waldron[6]; but again skeletal populations from the USA seem to differ. Merbs[30] reported that the lateral compartment was more frequently involved than the other compartments. In some US populations the medial and patellofemoral compartments are equally involved. Further investigation is needed to find the true prevalence of different joint involvement in different groups. Further work with larger samples should also compare age-specific prevalences of OA at different joint sites for modern and ancient populations. However, the aging methods[19] used by biological anthropologists are generally imprecise, only allowing for aging within a decade after skeletal maturation has been achieved, and with no differentiation after the age of 50, in most cases.

It is very rare for an individual skeleton to be aged precisely, except in exceptional circumstances when

Table 6.2 OA of different joints in various skeletal populations

Archeological Site	Joints (% skeletons affected)						
	Spine	Shoulder	Elbow	Wrist	Hip	Knee	Ankle
SE USA[8]	–	35.0	40.0	15.0	3.0	27.0	8.0
Fishergate, York[24]	–	12.5	17.0	15.0	18.2	15.2	4.0
Dordrecht, Holland[7]	36.8	14.3	5.6	–	12.0	5.2	–
Trowbridge, Wilts.[27]	–	2.9	1.9	1.4	3.4	1.4	0.4
Castledyke, N. Lincs.[37]	–	7.6	1.8	5.2	2.3	3.8	0.0
England							
premedieval	31.9	31.9	2.1	8.5	12.8	2.1	0.0
medieval	31.7	33.5	2.1	3.6	5.7	5.0	0.0
postmedieval	24.0	27.7	2.6	1.9	2.9	4.4	0.0
St Oswald's Priory, Glos.[25]							
early medieval	18.6	0.0	0.9	5.7	1.9	0.0	0.0
medieval	22.5	0.9	0.0	2.7	4.6	0.9	0.0
post medieval	25.9	0.0	4.6	8.0	3.4	5.7	0.0

graves or coffins can be identified, as happened at Spitalfields[26]. However, in most populations the correct rank order can be achieved.

In most osteoarcheological and paleopathological investigations there is perhaps more interest in the precise pattern and distribution of OA in different populations. This is because the perception of the pathogenesis is of OA resulting from biomechanical stress and that, thus, the pattern of involvement is an imprint of the activity or occupations of the early populations under investigation. A quotation by Calvin Wells[23] perhaps best exemplifies this approach: '*It is the most useful of all diseases for reconstructing the lifestyle of early populations. Its anatomical localisation reflects very closely their occupation and activities...*'

This concept has helped the widespread dissemination of a preconceived idea of OA as only being caused by activities and occupation. For instance in a report[33] on the examination of over a thousand skeletons from the Romano–British site at Poundbury, the discussion of OA and other joint disease is placed in a chapter entitled 'Lifestyle and occupation'.

But this approach has also led to some extremely thorough and detailed examinations of the patterns and distributions of the series of bony changes seen in OA, and some of the variations of distribution are, in fact, very likely to be influenced by biomechanical and activity related changes. However, this somewhat simplistic approach of equating a particular pattern with a particular activity is now being questioned[32]. It is very difficult, if not impossible, to test the connection between activity and OA pattern and distribution in an archeological sample, as it is not usually known how representative of the whole historic population the excavated skeletons are, and there is rarely, if ever, documentation to link skeletons with particular activities.

The excavation of the 387 named skeletons from Christ Church, Spitalfields, provided a unique opportunity to investigate this further, as there was evidence for the occupation actually followed by these populations. Many of them had been weavers. Waldron and Cox[33], in a case control study, found no relationship between occupation and OA of the hands or any other joint site.

Comparative animal data

Investigation of the variance of distribution between human populations and primate skeletons is also proving a useful area of investigation, providing more insight into the potential contribution of mechanical factors in the pathogenesis of OA at particular joint sites. Jurmain and Kilgore[28], and Lim *et al.*[34] have shown that there is a similar distribution of OA of the interphalangeal joints between an age-matched group of macaque and human skeletons, but that there was a much lower frequency of thumb-base OA in the macaque group. Investigation of knee OA in the same group of subjects also showed differences, with the humans having a high prevalence of patellofemoral OA; the converse being true for the macaques[35].

Conclusion

It is clear from the brief discussion of the paleopathology of OA that there are many limitations both in the material, and in the methodology and interpretation of findings. Nevertheless, it is also clear that the investigation of the nature and epidemiology of a disease such as OA in earlier populations can provide a valuable type of information to enhance and complement the current research into OA[30,36]. Furthermore, the access to skeletal material provides a unique resource for the investigation of specific questions such as the relationship between the visual, radiological, and pathological appearance of particular pathological changes. Skeletal material can also provide a source of information about the relationship of changes[37,38] throughout the entire skeleton, rather than being restricted to a few symptomatic joints, thus enhancing the possibility of learning something about a systemic bony response.

References

1. Ruffer, M.A. (1913). Studies in palaeopathology in Egypt. *Journal of Pathology and Bacteriology*, **18**, 149–62.
2. Rogers, J. and Dieppe, P. (1990). Skeletal Palaeopathology of the rheumatic diseases. Where are we now? *Annals of the Rheumatic Diseases*, **49**, 885–6.
3. Strauss, W.L. and Cave, A.J. (1957). Pathology and posture of Neanderthal man. *Quarterly Reviews of Biology*, **32**, 348–63.
4. Rogers, J.M. (1990). The skeletal remains. In *Hazelton long barrow*, (ed. A. Saville), English Heritage, London, pp. 182–97.
5. Ruffer, M.A. (1918). Arthritis deformans and spondylitis in ancient Egypt. *Journal of Pathology and Bacteriology*, **22**, 152–96.

6. Waldron, T. (1995). Changes in the distribution of OA over historical time. *International Journal of Osteoarchaeology*, 5, 385–9.

7. Maat, G., Mastwijk, R.W., and van der Velde, E.A. (1995). Skeletal distribution of degenerative changes in vertebral osteophytosis, vertebral OA and DISH. *International Journal of Osteoarchaeology*, 5:3, 289–98.

8. Bridges, P. (1991). Degenerative joint disease in hunter gatherers and agriculturalists from the South Eastern United States. *American Journal of Physical Anthropology*, 85, 379–91.

9. Kricum, M.E. (1994). Paleoradiology of the prehistoric Australian aboriginies. *American Journal of Roentgentology*, 163, 241–7.

10. Rogers, J. and Dieppe, P. (1993). Ridges and grooves on the bony surfaces of osteoarthritic joints. *Osteoarthritis and Cartilage*, 1, 167–70.

11. Kellgren, J.H. and Lawrence, J.S. (1957). Radiological assessment of OA. *Annals of the Rheumatic Diseases*, 16, 494–501.

12. Waldron, T. and Rogers, J. (1991). Inter-observer variation in coding OA in human skeletal remains. *International Journal of Osteoarchaeology*, 1, 49–56.

13. Bridges, P. (1993). The effect of variation in methodology on the outcome of osteoarthritic studies. *International Journal of Osteoarchaeology*, 3, 289–95.

14. Hernborg, J. and Nilsson, B.E. (1973). The relationship between osteophytes in the knee joint, OA and ageing. *Acta Orthopedica Scandinavica*, 44, 69.

15. Rogers, J., Young, P., and Dieppe, P. (1993). Bone formers. Positive correlation between osteophytes and enthesophyte formation. *British Journal of Rheumatology*, 32, supplement 2, 51.

16. Rogers, J. and Waldron, T. (1995). A field guide to joint disease in archaeology. John Wiley, London, pp. 32–46.

17. Rogers, J., Waldron, T., and Watt, I. (1991). Erosive osteoarthritis in a mediaeval skeleton. *International Journal of Osteoarchaeology*, 1, 151–3.

18. Rogers, J. Waldron, T., Dieppe, P., and Watt, I. (1987). Arthropathies in palaeopathology: the basis of classification according to most probably cause. *Journal of Archaeology and Science*, 16, 611–25.

19. Buikstra, J.E. and Ubelaker, D.H. (1994). Standards for data collection from human skeletal remains. *Arkansas Arch Survey Research Series*, No. 44.

20. van Saase, J., van Romande, I.K., Cars, A., Vandenbrouke, J., and Valkenberg, H. (1989). Epidemiology of OA: the Zoctermeer survey. Comparison of radiological arthritis in a Dutch population with that in 10 other populations. *Annals of the Rheumatic Diseases*, 48, 271–80.

21. Rogers, J., Watt, I., and Dieppe, P. (1990). Comparison of visual and radiographic detection of bony changes at the knee joint. *British Medical Journal*, 300, 367–8.

22. Ortner, D.J. and Putschar, W. (1985). Identification of pathological conditions in human skeletal remains. *Smithsonian Contributions to Anthropology*, No. 28, p. 419

23. Wells, C. (1982). *The human burials in Romano–British cemeteries at Cirencester* (ed. A. McWhirr, L. Viner, and C. Wells), p. 152. Cirencester Excavation Committee.

24. Stroud, G. (1993). *The human bones in cemeteries of St Andrew Fishergate* (ed. G. Stroud and R. L. Kemp). York Archaeological Trust.

25. Rogers, J. The human skeletons. In *St Oswalds Priory* (ed. Caroline Heighway). CBA research report (forthcoming). Council for British Archaeology.

26. Waldron, T. (1991). Prevalence and distribution of OA in a population from Georgian and early Victorian London. *Annals of the Rheumatic Diseases*, 50, 301–7.

27. Rogers, J. The palaeopathology. (1993). In *Excavations in Trowbridge, Wiltshire 1977 and 1986–1988* (ed. A.H. Graham and S.M. Davies). Wessex Archaeology Report No. 2.

28. Jurmain, R.D. and Kilgore, L. (1995) Skeletal evidence of osteoarthritis, a palaeopathological perspective. *Annals of the Rheumatic Diseases*, 54, 443–50.

29. Rogers, J. and Dieppe, P. (1994). Is tibio-femoral osteoarthritis in the knee joint a new disease? *Annals of the Rheumatic Diseases*, 53, 612–13.

30. Merbs, C.F. (1983). *Patterns of activity-induced pathology in a Canadian Innit population*, p. 92. National Museums of Canada, Ottawa.

31. Molleson, T. (1993). The human remains. In *Poundbury, vol. 2*, (monograph series, no. 11) Dorset Natural History and Archaeological Society.

32. Jurmain, R.D. (1991). Degenerative changes in peripheral joints as indicators of mechanical stress: opportunities and limitations. *International Journal of Osteoarchaeology*, Nos 3 and 4, 247–52.

33. Waldron, H.A. and Cox, M. (1989). Occupational arthropathy evidence from the past. *British Journal of Industrial Medicine*, 46, 420–2.

34. Lim, K., Rogers, J., Shepstone, L., and Dieppe, P. (1995). The evolutionary origins of OA: a comparative skeletal study of hand disease in two primates. *Journal of Rheumatology*, 22:11, 2132–4.

35. Rogers, J., Lim, K., Shepstone, L., and Turnquist, J. (1996). Distribution of knee OA in human and macaque skeletons. *American Journal of Physical Anthropology*, supplement 22, 202.

36. Dieppe, P.A. and Rogers, J. (1985). Two dimensional epidemiology. *British Journal of Rheumatology*, 24, 310–12.

37. Boyleston, A., Wiggins, R., and Roberts, C. *The human skeletons in the Anglo–Saxon cemetery at Castledyke South, Barton on Humber* (ed. G. Drinkall and M. Foreman) (forthcoming).

38. Rogers, J., Watt, I., and Dieppe, P. (1995). The relationship between osteophytosis and OA in joints of the hand. *British Journal of Rheumatology*, 34, supplement, 132.

7 | *Pathogenesis of osteoarthritis*

7.1 Introduction: the concept of osteoarthritis as failure of the diarthrodial joint

Kenneth Brandt, L. Stefan Lohmander, and Michael Doherty

Our view of osteoarthritis (OA) and its pathogenesis continues to change. OA was previously considered a 'degenerative' disease, the inevitable accompaniment of ageing, with 'wear and tear' the principle pathogenetic mechanism. Now, OA is increasingly viewed as a metabolically active, dynamic process including both destruction and repair, that may be triggered by a variety of biochemical as well as mechanical insults. Any view of OA needs to take into account the following general observations:

1. *The phylogenetic and evolutionary preservation of OA*. Study of ancient skeletal remains suggests that OA has been present throughout the evolution of mankind[1-4]. The equivalent process of OA is found also in other animals with diarthrodial joints in which the epiphyses fuse in the adult[5-7]. Archaeological evidence supports the evolutionary antiquity of the condition in many species[3,4], including dinosaurs[8].

2. *The dynamic nature of the OA process.* Pathologically, OA is characterised by often exuberant new bone (osteophyte) formation, synovial hyperplasia, and capsular thickening. Although focal loss of hyaline cartilage is a cardinal feature, the chondrocytes, at least initially, multiply their numbers and increase their activity[9]; formation of new cartilage is evident at the joint margins (where it undergoes enchondral ossification to form osteophyte) and in synovium (as growing osteochondral bodies). The biochemical changes in OA cartilage differ from those of aging alone and include an increased turnover of many matrix components[10], and expression of chondroitin epitopes that are normally evident in young (growth) cartilage[11]. These features alone negate use of the term 'degenerative joint disease', suggesting more a generalized attempt by all joint components to produce new tissue in response to insults.

3. *The discordance between structural change, symptoms, and disability*. It is striking that clinical and radiographic evidence of OA may often be present without symptoms or compromised function[12-14]. This is particularly frequent at certain sites, such as finger joints, but is not uncommon even in large weight-bearing joints.

4. *The good outcome for many cases of symptomatic OA*. Although the effects of OA on an individual may be dramatic[15], OA is not inevitably progressive. Many OA patients have phases or 'flares' of symptoms, and eventual slow resolution of pain and stiffness. This is particularly likely for finger joints affected by nodal OA[16], but may also occur at hips and knees[17,18]. Although symptoms may resolve, the structural changes of OA persist and stabilize. Replacement of lost hyaline cartilage does not occur, but in rare cases radiographs may show 'improvement', with remodeling of bony contours and limited fibrocartilage replacement, which may manifest as an increase in interbone distance (Fig. 7.1)[19].

Such observations are all readily accommodated by the perspective of OA as a potential repair process in response to joint insult and cartilage destruction (Fig. 7.2)[9,20]. A variety of insults could trigger the need to repair. Once initiated, all the tissues in the joint are involved in what may be considered an adaptive response[9,20,21]. Increased metabolic activity by cartilage,

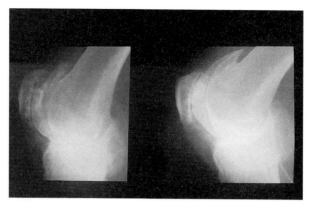

Fig. 7.1 Knee radiographs of a 68-year-old patient, taken 3 years apart, showing remodeling. During this time her symptoms had improved.

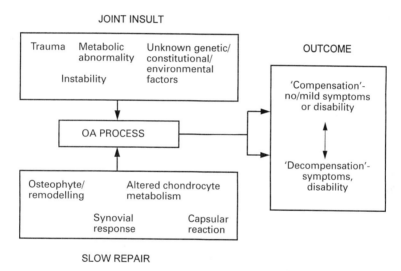

Fig. 7.2 Schematic representation of OA as a repair process triggered by a variety of insults and showing variable outcome.

new bone formation, and remodeling of the joint might help keep pace with tissue loss and better redistribute mechanical forces across the compromised joint; capsular thickening would tend to sustain joint stability. The outcome would depend on the balance between the severity and chronicity of the insult, and the effectiveness of the repair response. In many instances the repair might rectify the adverse effects of the insult ('compensated OA'), but in some cases overwhelming insult or poor tissue response would lead to 'decompensated' OA, with symptoms, disability, and progression of structural damage. Such a scenario would explain the *marked heterogeneity* of OA with different sites of involvement, different numbers of joints affected, and marked variability of outcome. If OA

were, in general, a slow but successful repair process, this would also explain its frequent presence in the absence of symptoms or impaired function, its generally benign natural history, and its widespread presence in man and other animals. If such a perspective is correct, the idea of OA as a single 'disease' is replaced by OA as a *'process'*, with diverse triggers and outcomes. A number of consequences require emphasis:

1. Although these triggers share a common phenotypic expression as 'OA', the way in which they insult the joint may vary greatly and may involve hereditary, constitutional, metabolic, endocrine, environmental, or biomechanical mechanisms. (Fig. 7.3).

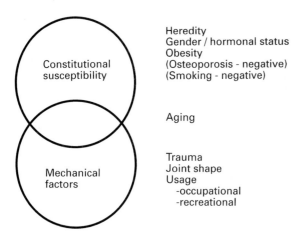

Heredity
Gender / hormonal status
Obesity
(Osteoporosis - negative)
(Smoking - negative)

Aging

Trauma
Joint shape
Usage
   -occupational
   -recreational

Fig. 7.3 Possible risk factors for development of OA.

2. The site of primary insult may be any tissue in the joint (bone, cartilage, synovium, capsule, ligament, muscle), since all are essential to its health and integrity.

3. Risk factors and mechanisms involved in development of OA need not be the same as those that determine progression or non-progression.

4. Caution must be exercised in extrapolating knowledge of the pathogenesis of OA from one joint site to another, or from one clinical form or model of OA, to OA in general.

The rationale for dividing the heterogeneous group of OA into more homogeneous subsets is to better identify these individual triggers and mechanisms. Although subsets may be defined in various ways, for example, by radiographic appearance (*atrophic* versus *hypertrophic*[22]) and by the presence of florid clinical inflammation[23] and calcium crystals (pyrophosphate arthropathy[24], apatite-associated arthropathy[25,26]), separation at least according to the *site* and *number* of joints affected appears important[27]. Caveats to defining such subsets, however, include: the occurrence of different subsets at different sites within the same individual; evolution from one subset to another; and interaction between primary (hereditary, constitutional) and secondary (mechanical) forms of OA[28].

An intriguing aspect of OA that remains unexplained is its *site specificity*. Only certain synovial joints show a high prevalence of OA (Fig. 7.4), with others being relatively spared. One hypothesis to explain this distribution relates to man's evolution[29]. Joints that have

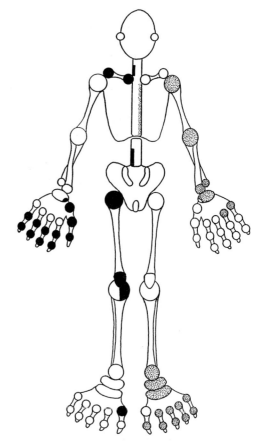

Fig. 7.4 The distribution of OA in man. Common target sites for OA are shown on the left (black). Relatively spared sites of involvement are shown on the right (stippled).

undergone major change in orientation and function, to permit our bipedal gait and associated liberation of the upper limb, may not yet have adapted to their new functional requirements: they may be underdesigned (that is, have poor functional reserve), and thus more frequently require a reparative response in the face of insult. The distribution of OA in man and other animals is consistent with this theory, though further testing of the hypothesis is clearly problematic. Within individual joints, there is additional specificity with respect to sites of maximal cartilage loss. For large joints, this most commonly occurs at sites of maximum load bearing, supporting the importance of physical factors. Although this biomechanical explanation fits the majority of cases of large joint OA, topographical variation certainly occurs and has been used as a basis for subset classification. For example, at the hip, superior (lateral, intermediate, medial), axial, and medial patterns of femoral head migration are recognized and have been attributed different associations[30].

The strong association between *aging* and OA prevalence, for all sites of involvement, also remains unexplained. Certain aspects of OA are virtually confined to the elderly, for example, marked calcium crystal deposition (calcium pyrophosphate, carbonate substituted apatite), involvement of atypical sites (glenohumeral joint, radiocarpal joint), and rapidly destructive OA of large joints (hip, knee, glenohumeral joint). The mechanism underlying these striking age associations might relate to the age-related decline in muscle function, impairment of joint proprioception, reduction of vascular supply, and nutrition of joint tissues, or reduced regenerative potential of connective tissue. All of these might lower resilience to insult, tip a compensated OA joint toward decompensation, and favor more rapid progression and poor outcome. There is certainly a dramatic decline with aging in the biomechanical properties of cartilage matrix[31], probably caused by subtle but cumulative changes in the structure of collagens, proteoglycans, and matrix proteins. The effect of aging on both normal and OA tissues certainly deserves further study.

A variety of biochemical and biomechanical triggers and mechanisms have been studied in OA, particularly with respect to the cartilage. It is often difficult, however, to disentangle deleterious initiating factors from events linked to tissue response, especially when studying established, particularly end-stage, disease. Physical and biomechanical factors, though usefully separated in test systems, are likely to be inexorably linked and interdependent *in vivo*. Sharp polarization between them is likely to be artificial. Furthermore, we should not assume an 'all-or-none', or linear response, for initiating or perpetuating triggers. For example, we know that a certain amount of regular loading is required for the health of both cartilage and bone, and that too little or too much loading may both result in cartilage fibrillation and thinning[32]. Such U-shaped response curves may cause problems for the unwary.

In this section, the individual component tissues of the joint are considered. The ways in which they are affected by, or contribute to, the OA process are detailed. Historically, the principal research focus has been on hyaline articular cartilage, with bone the second competing tissue of interest. However, as will be seen, all intracapsular and periarticular tissues are now coming under scrutiny, as the interdependence of joint tissues is realised. Although dedicated to individual tissues, behind every chapter are the perspectives of the integrated joint and the diversity of mechanisms that may result in OA joint failure.

References

1. Ruffer, M.A. and Rietti, A. (1911). On osseous lesions in ancient Egyptians. *Journal of Pathology and Bacteriology*, **16**, 439–65.
2. Rogers, J., Watt, I., and Dieppe, P. (1981). Arthritis in Saxon and medieval skeletons. *British Medical Journal*, **283**, 1668–70.
3. Jurmain, R.D. and Kilgore, L. (1995). Skeletal evidence of osteoarthritis: a palaeopathological perspective. *Annals of the Rheumatic Diseases*, **54**, 443–50.
4. Hutton, C. (1987). Generalised osteoarthritis: an evolutionary problem. *The Lancet* **1**, 1463–5.
5. Fox, H. (1939). Chronic arthritis in wild mammals. *Tr Am Phil Soc* **31**, 71–148.
6. Bennett, G.A. and Bauer, W. (1931). A systematic study of the degeneration of articular cartilage in bovine joints. *American Journal of Pathology*, **7**, 399–414.
7. Sokoloff, L. (1956). Natural history of degenerative joint disease in small laboratory animals. *Archives of Pathology*, **62**, 118–28.
8. Rothschild, B. (1990). Radiological assessment of osteoarthritis in dinosaurs. *Annals of Carnegie Museum*, **59**, 295–301.
9. Bland, J.H. and Cooper, S.M. (1984). Osteoarthritis: a review of the cell biology involved and evidence for reversibility. Management rationally related to known genesis and pathophysiology. *Seminars in Arthritis and Rheumatism*, **14**, 106–33.
10. Hammerman, D. (1989). The biology of osteoarthritis. *New England Journal of Medicine*, **320**, 1322–30.
11. Caterson, B., Mahmoodian, F., Sorrell, J.M., Hardingham, T.E., Bayliss, M.T., Carney, S.L., *et al.* (1990). Modulation of native chondroitin sulphate structure in tissue development and in disease. *Journal of Cell Science*, **97**, 411–17.
12. Lawrence, J.S., Bremner, J.M., and Bier, F. (1966). Osteoarthrosis: prevalence in the population and relationship between symptoms and X-ray changes. *Annals of the Rheumatic Diseases*, **25**, 1–23.
13. Davis, M.A., Ettinger, W.H., Neuhaus, J.M., Barclay, J.D., and Segal, M.R. (1992). Correlates of knee pain among US adults with and without radiographic knee osteoarthritis. *Journal of Rheumatology*, **19**, 1943–9.
14. Hadler, N.M. (1992). Knee pain is the malady – not osteoarthritis. *Annals of Internal Medicine*, **116**, 598–9.
15. Atkinson, J.P. (1996). A remembrance of Fred, the lowland gorilla. *Arthritis and Rheumatism*, **39**, 891–3.
16. Patrick, M., Aldridge, S., Hamilton, E., Manhire, A., and Doherty, M. (1989). A controlled study of hand function in nodal and erosive osteoarthritis. *Annals of the Rheumatic Diseases*, **48**, 978–82.
17. Danielsson, L.G. (1964). Incidence and prognosis of coxarthrosis. *Acta Orthopedica Scandinavica*, **supplement 64**, 1–114.

18. Hernborg, J.S. and Nilsson, B.E. (1977). The natural course of untreated osteoarthritis of the knee. *Clinical Orthopoedics and Related Research*, **123**, 130–7.

19. Perry, Gh., Smith, M.J.G., and Whiteside, C.G. (1972). Spontaneous recovery of the joint space in degenerative hip disease. *Annals of the Rheumatic Diseases*, **31**, 440–8.

20. Radin, E.L. and Burr, D.B. (1984). Hypothesis: joints can heal. *Seminars in Arthritis and Rheumatism*, **13**, 293–302.

21. Mankin, H.J. (1974). The reaction of cartilage to injury and osteoarthritis. *New England Journal of Medicine*, **291**, 1285–92.

22. Solomon, L. (1983). Osteoarthritis, local and generalised: a uniform disease? *Journal of Rheumatology*, **10** (**supplement 9**), 13–15.

23. Ehrlich, G. (1972). Inflammatory osteoarthritis: I. The clinical syndrome. *Journal of Chronic Diseases*, **25**, 317–28.

24. Doherty, M. and Dieppe, P.A. (1988). Clinical aspects of calcium pyrophosphate dihydrate crystal deposition. *Rheum Dis Clin N Am* **14**, 395–414.

25. Dieppe, P.A., Doherty, M., MacFarlane, D.G., Hutton, C.W., Bradfield, J.W., and Watt, I. (1984). *British Journal of Rheumatology*, **23**, 84–91.

26. Halverson, P.B., McCarty, D.J., Cheung, H., and Ryan, L.M. (1984). Milwaukee shoulder syndrome: eleven additional cases with involvement of the knee in seven (basic calcium phosphate deposition disease). *Seminars in Arthritis and Rheumatism*, **14**, 36–44.

27. Kellgren, J.H. and Moore, R. (1952) Generalised osteoarthritis and Heberden's nodes. *British Medical Journal*, **1**, 181–7.

28. Doherty, M., Watt, I., and Dieppe, P.A. (1983). Influence of primary generalised osteoarthritis on development of secondary osteoarthritis. *The Lancet*, **2**, 8–11.

29. Hutton, C. (1987). Generalised osteoarthritis: an evolutionary problem. *The Lancet* **2**, 1463–5.

30. Ledingham, J., Dawson, S., Preston, B., Milligan, G., and Doherty, M. (1992). Radiographic patterns and associations of osteoarthritis of the hip. *Annals of the Rheumatic Diseases*, **51**, 1111–16.

31. Kempson, G.E. (1991). Age-related changes in the tensile properties of human articular cartilage: a comparative study between the femoral head of the hip joint and the talus of the ankle joint. *Biochimica et Biophysica Acta*, **1075**, 223–30.

32. Buckwalter, J.A. (1995). Osteoarthritis and articular cartilage use, disuse and abuse: experimental studies. *Journal of Rheumatology*, **22**, 13–15.

7.2   Articular cartilage

7.2.1   Biochemistry and metabolism of normal and osteoarthritic cartilage

Dick Heinegård, Michael Bayliss, and Pilar Lorenzo

The clinical diagnosis of osteoarthritis (OA), as is described elsewhere in this book, depends on symptoms like pain, radiographic detection of joint space narrowing as a result of articular cartilage loss, and in many cases the presence of osteophytes. These alterations summarize some of the characteristic features of degenerative joint disease, for example, progressive destruction of the cartilage paralleled by attempted repair responses such as osteophyte formation. Although these diagnostic features appear late in the disease, it is apparent that molecular events occur long before alterations can be observed macroscopically, or even at the microscopical level. This lack of means for the early detection of conditions leading to joint destruction in OA has hampered development of effective therapy.

In the development of joint destruction it is clear that degradation of matrix constituents and their removal from the cartilage has to occur. It is also likely that any such process will elicit a response in the chondrocytes attempting to repair the matrix defect that develops. Therefore, the early alterations in cartilage which might be expected as the OA process develops should include an increased synthesis of some matrix components, to compensate for the increased degradation. It is, however, unlikely that these molecular events will occur in all tissue compartments simultaneously. Since the composition of the tissue compartments — pericellular (closest to the cells), territorial, interterritorial (furthest away from the cells) — and of different zones of cartilage — surface, middle, deep — show distinct differences at the molecular level, it is plausible that processes may start in one compartment and only later involve other compartments. Furthermore, it is possible that the cells have better means of sensing and compensating for matrix changes in their immediate environment and, therefore, are better fit to adequately deal with destructive events in the pericellular and territorial matrix.

This chapter deals with alterations in matrix composition with aging of normal cartilage, and the distinctly different alterations observed during the development of OA. The characterization of such changes will not only help us to identify targets for future therapeutic intervention, but will also provide the diagnostic tools that are required for identifying and monitoring those patients that will be subject to therapy.

An understanding of such alterations depends on the knowledge of the components that form the tissue and their individual functional roles. There are several groups of such macromolecular constituents, which are described below.

Collagen

The major structural element of the articular cartilage is the collagen network. This is formed from the major component in cartilage, that is, a large number of collagen II molecules assembled to form collagen fibers. This very tightly regulated assembly process occurs outside the cells and requires a modification of the proform of collagen secreted by the chondrocyte. Thus, specific proteolytic enzymes remove N- as well as C-terminal extensions. After removal of the extensions, the collagen molecules can associate to form fibers in a very specific manner[1]. The processed collagen molecule consists of three protein chains, forming a classical triple helical structure. This is a very compact, tightly held together functional molecule which is some 3000 Å long and only 15 Å thick. The peptide backbone is resistant to proteolysis, since it is protected by the side chain constituents of its amino acid residues. Each end of this processed molecule, however, retains a few amino acids, forming a telopeptide structure different from the rest (Fig. 7.5). Lysine residues in this telopeptide participate in cross-link formation between neighboring collagen molecules, which further stabi-

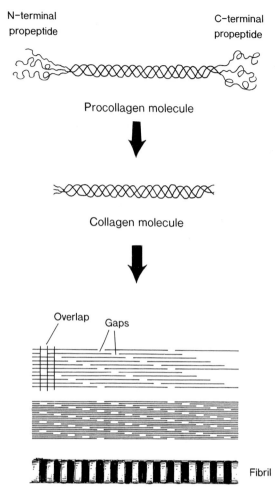

Fig. 7.5 Extracellular processing of collagen. Collagen is secreted in a proform that is cleaved by specific proteinases to a collagen molecule largely consisting of very compact and stable triple helical regions, with non-triple helical short telopeptides in both N- and C-terminal ends. These collagen molecules are then, in a highly organized way, assembled in several steps to form the collagen molecule. Covalent cross-links are formed over a period of years, involving lysine residues in the telopeptides. (From Mikael Wendel's PhD thesis on 'Skeletal Tissue Proteins', Lund, 1994.)

lizes the fibers. They constitute new stable derivatives called pyridinolines and are uniquely found in such cross-linked collagen. Another feature, which is unique to collagens, are the hydroxyproline residues constituting some 10 per cent of the total. They are essential for the stability of the collagen molecule, as are the hydroxylysine residues.

The collagen II that makes up the bulk of these fibers (Fig. 7.6) is specific for cartilage, but the fibers are

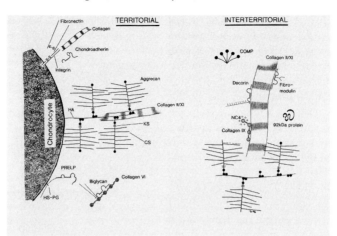

Fig. 7.6 Schematic illustration of the constituents of cartilage matrix. The spatial relationships of the various constituents to the chondrocyte, that is, their presence in the territorial (close to the cell) or inter-territorial matrix (furthest away from the cell) is shown and the macromolecular organization of matrix molecules is indicated.

more complex than they appear, in that they contain an additional collagen — collagen XI — also unique for cartilage. Current knowledge indicates that the collagen XI, which represents a few per cent of the total collagen, may have a role in determining the thickness of the collagen II fibers[1,2]. It is quite apparent that the growth of these fibers is very tightly regulated and differs between compartments. Thus, the thinnest fibers of the tissues occur in the territorial matrix close to the cells in the superficial parts of the articular cartilage. There is a gradual increase in fiber thickness distant from the cells, towards the interterritorial matrix. In general, fiber thickness also increases in all compartments, going from the superficial zones of the articular cartilage to the deep zones (Fig. 7.7). For example, the thickness of the fibers actually increases by a factor of about four from the thinnest fibers found in the superficial territorial compartment, to those thickest in the deep interterritorial compartment (see Fig. 7.7). The fibers run in preferred different directions in different parts of the articular cartilage. Thus, those in the most superficial parts run parallel to the surface, while those in the deep parts run perpendicular. In an intermediate part of the cartilage, fibers run in different directions (Fig. 7.7).

It is not known today what are the exact factors governing the assembly of the collagen molecules into fibers, resulting in these specific dimensions. It may involve a series of other constituents of the collagen fibrillar network, for example, the collagen IX, (Fig. 7.6). The collagen IX molecule contains the classical triple helical structure organized in three different collagenous domains, interrupted by non-triple helical

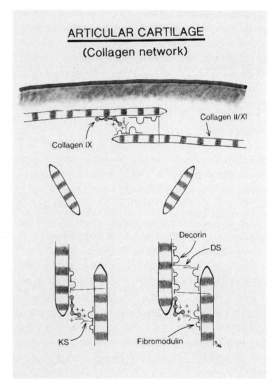

Fig. 7.7 Schematic illustration of the organization of the collagen network in cartilage. The superficial region of the cartilage contains collagen fibers arranged parallel to the surface, while the deepest, major part of the tissue contains fibers arranged perpendicular to the surface. In the intermediate zone, the fibers run in different directions. A number of other matrix macromolecules are bound at the surface of the collagen fiber. These appear to have important roles in 'knitting' together the collagen fibers to form a network, essential for counterbalancing the swelling pressure of the proteoglycans.

domains, that is, the NC-1,2,3, and 4 being the N-terminal, as is illustrated in Fig. 7.6. It has been shown that the collagen IX molecule is bound to the collagen II fiber surface in the tissue. This binding is stabilized by covalent cross-links[3], thus creating a fiber where no more collagen II molecules can be added to increase the fiber thickness and, thereby, the strength of the collagen II fiber itself — unless the collagen IX is removed by proteolysis.

It is of interest to note that its NC-4 domain is rather cationic, thereby providing areas along the collagen fiber of high positive-charge density (Figs 7.6 and 7.7).

Proteoglycans

The major non-collagenous component in articular cartilage is aggrecan. This very large molecule (Fig. 7.8) consists of a central protein core of some 2000 amino acids with several distinct domains and different functions. Those which are functionally most important are the chondroitin sulfate domains, CS1 and CS2 (Fig. 7.8) carrying a very large number of negatively charged glycosaminoglycan chains of chondroitin sulfate[4]. These chains occur as clusters in the CS2 domain, but are more randomly distributed in the CS1 domain, which has its own characteristic structure. There are some 100 such chains, each consisting of an average 40–50 disaccharide units with two negatively-charged groups in the form of sulfate on the N–acetyl galactosamine and carboxyl of the glucuronic acid. Thus, these two domains (CS1 and CS2) contribute some 8000–10 000 negatively-charged groups to the molecules, all fixed to the protein core via one end of the chondroitin sulfate chains. An extended protein domain next to the chondroitin sulfate (CS1) region, (Fig. 7.8), has a rather specific repeat structure[5] and carries a number of unique keratan sulfate chains. This domain is likely to confer special properties to the molecule, since the very closely spaced keratan sulfate chains provide a rather special structure. Another domain with important functional properties is the N-terminal hyaluronan binding domain, G1[4]. This confers on the aggrecan molecule the ability to specifically interact with hyaluronan. This mechanism is used to link a large number of such aggrecan molecules to one molecule of hyaluronan, forming a very high molecular weight complex, as illustrated in Fig. 7.9. Although the binding of aggrecan to hyaluronan is tight — almost as strong as that between antigen and antibody — an additional protein stabilizes the complex by binding both to the hyaluronan and to the G1 domain of the aggrecan[4]. This link-protein has many structural features similar to the G1 domain of aggrecan. Other globular domains have less well-

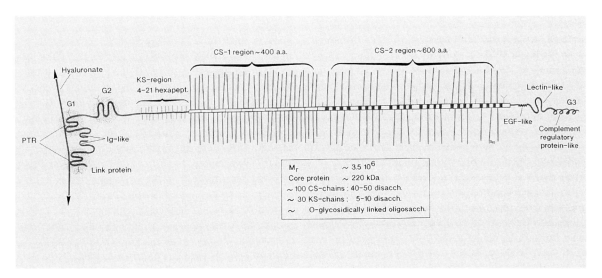

Fig. 7.8 Schematic illustration of the aggrecan molecule. A central core protein is substituted with some 100 glycosaminoglycans chains of chondroitin sulfate (CS) and keratan sulfate (KS). These chains consist of characteristic repeat disaccharides with negatively-charged sulfate and uronic acid carboxyl groups. The average chondroitin sulfate (CS) chain contains some 80–100 charged groups. Specific domains of the aggrecan include an N-terminal hyaluronate binding domain (G1), a homologous G2 domain, a keratan sulfate-rich region, two distinct regions of polypeptide repeats carrying the chondroitin sulfate chains and C-terminal EGF-like domain, a lectin homology domain, and a complement regulatory protein-like domain. Some molecules lack the C-terminal domain as a result of proteolytic cleavage.

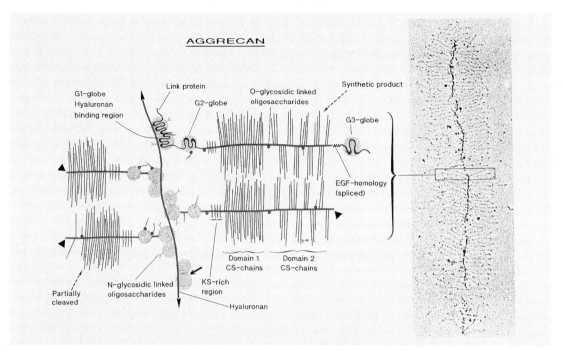

Fig. 7.9 Illustration of the proteoglycan aggregate. Several aggrecan molecules are bound, via their N-terminal end which contains a specific hyaluronate-binding domain, to an extremely long hyaluronate molecule. This results in a very large complex, with several hundred thousand fixed-charge groups, that creates osmotic gradient and swelling pressure. The appearance of the molecule upon electron microscopy, after rotatory shadowing, is shown on the right. The central filament represents hyaluronate decorated with globular link protein and hyaluronate-binding domains of the aggrecan molecules, seen as side chain filaments. The structure of the aggrecan molecule changes with age, such that most molecules have been cleaved in their C-terminal domain and are, therefore, shorter, as indicated by arrowheads in the figure. The ultimate retained cleavage product is the HABr (arrow) bound to HA, together with link protein. (Matthias Mörgelin kindly provided the E-M picture.)

defined properties. For example, the G2 domain is homologous with the major part of the G1 domain, yet its function is unknown. Similarly, the C-terminal, G3-domain, contains sequences homologous to epidermal growth factor (EGF), complement regulatory component, and a lectin[4], but their functions are not clear.

The basic structural features of aggrecan described above have been determined largely from studies of molecules purified from young animal cartilage. It is clear that a structure of this kind has the potential to generate aggregates of widely varying composition and molecular weight, to suit the mechanical and physicochemical properties of cartilage from different sources. These molecular changes are a consequence of biosynthetic and catabolic events, regulated by many cellular and extracellular processes. The extent to which these occur within articular cartilage, however, is not uniform and factors such as species, site (which joint), zone (through the cartilage depth), tissue compartment (pericellular, territorial, and interterritorial), and region of the joint (topographical distribution), all dictate

specific qualitative and quantitative changes in e.g. aggrecan structure[6]. However, it is the age of the individual that appears to have the most profound effect on the composition, stoichiometry, and stability of aggregates. Nowhere is this more evident than in normal human articular cartilage, and the schematic shown in Fig. 7.9 illustrates the main structural changes that occur during maturation and aging of the tissue. These mainly consist of an increased polydispersity and heterogeneity in the molecular size of individual aggrecan molecules, brought about by extracellular proteolytic cleavage of their core proteins. This may be confined to regions within the CS domain, but, with advancing age, an increased concentration of the G1 domain is observed, confirming that proteolytic modification of aggrecan can also be extensive (Fig. 7.9)[7,8]. The average size of the hyaluronan polymer also decreases with age. Thus, structural changes in both major components of the aggregate decrease its size in adult cartilage. Furthermore, studies have indicated that there is an age-related decrease in the concentration of link protein relative to aggrecan, suggesting that aggregation may be less effective in adult cartilage[9]. Although these structural changes may give the impression of a molecular system that is degenerating during aging, it is important to appreciate that this is not the case and that they provide normal, mature cartilage with the properties that enable it to survive the changing biochemical and biophysical environment to which it is exposed. It should also be noted that the biosynthesis, the composition, and the structure of aggrecan in human osteoarthritic cartilage is very different to that of adult normal cartilage: that is, OA is not an obligatory consequence of cartilage aging.

The aggregates represent an important structural unit, a key function of which is to provide a stable environment of high fixed-charge density, essential for imbibing and retaining water in the tissue by the high osmotic swelling pressure created. As is discussed in Chapter 7.2.2, there are sites in the aggrecan molecules that are very sensitive to cleavage by proteinases. Consequently, during normal and pathological turnover of cartilage matrix, proteoglycan fragments are released into the synovial space[10,11]. One such cleavage point is between G1 and G2 domains[12]. Upon this cleavage, the fragment generated, although large, is not held as tightly in the tissue and can diffuse out of the matrix. During normal turnover this process is controlled and tissue homeostasis is maintained, but in OA it leads to the disruption of the aggregate organization, loss of the fixed-charge groups from the tissue, and, thereby, reduction of its water-imbibing properties.

Matrix proteins

A set of molecules that are much less abundant in the cartilage are the non-collagenous matrix proteins. These include some proteins that are also proteoglycans by virtue of containing one, or a small number, of glycosaminoglycan side chains of keratan sulfate or chondroitin sulfate/dermatan sulfate (discussed below). In some instances, our understanding of the functions of these proteins is still emerging, while in other cases the proteins have only just been identified. However, from their specific distribution in the cartilage, it appears that they do have different functions and could serve as indicators for different metabolic processes in the tissue.

A major family of such proteins are the leucine-rich repeat proteins (LRR-proteins). These are made up from a central domain of characteristic repeats of some

25 amino acids[13,14]. Thus, ten to eleven repeats are surrounded by sets of disulfide loops, and in most cases there is an N-terminal as well as a C-terminal extension. The central leucine-rich repeat domain exposes a surface of so-called 'β-sheet' structures, that are classically known to participate in protein-protein interactions. Indeed, most of the members of this family of proteins bind specifically to other constituents in the matrix and contribute to the structural network, (Fig. 7.6). Thus, the central domain represents at least one structural feature for which, in several cases, functions can be assigned. In addition, the N-terminal extension peptide in some cases has glycosaminoglycan chains attached to it and, in other cases, it contains repeated tyrosine sulfate residues[15], (Fig. 7.6). Other structures of the N-terminal part range from a basic repeat sequence, adapted for interactions with, for example, heparin (PRELP)[14], to a molecule lacking this terminal extension altogether[16]. Decorin was the first in this series of molecules to be structurally defined[17]. It contains one side chain, slightly different from the traditional chondroitin sulfate chains found in aggrecan, such that the glucuronic acid residue is often exchanged for iduronate within the chain sequence. This side chain can adopt more complex secondary structures and it appears quite likely that it can form specific interactions with other molecules in the tissue, including dermatan sulfate chains (as indicated in Figs 7.6 and 7.7).

Thus, four members of this family — decorin, fibromodulin, lumican, and biglycan — have been shown to be able to interact with collagens. In most cases, these interactions include many different types of collagens, where the triple helical domain always appears involved. In the case of biglycan, interaction appears to be restricted to collagen VI (Hedbom, Timpl, Heinegård, unpublished observation), but its role in the collagen VI fibrillar network is not known. Decorin, fibromodulin, and lumican can also form specific protein-protein interactions, via the leucine-rich repeat region to various collagens, including collagen II found in cartilage. From electron microscopy data, as well as from studies *in vitro*, it appears that at least fibromodulin[18] and decorin[19,20,21] bind to distinct sites on the collagen and are found in the tissue localized along the collagen fibers, as is indicated schematically in Figs 7.6 and 7.7. Thus, one of the functional domains, that is, the LRR, forms one interacting site with the collagen, while another may be represented by the negatively-charged glycosaminoglycan chains that appear to be capable of either directly interacting with different collagen fibers and/or interacting with other components along the collagen. An example of such a component is the basic NC-4 domain extending from the collagen fibers, which may participate in ionic interactions with the acidic glycosaminoglycan chains of decorin, indicated in Figs 7.6 and 7.7.

Molecules, like chondroadherin may provide feedback information to the cells by interacting with a receptor, the integrin $\alpha 2 \beta 1$, on the chondrocyte surface (Camper, Lundgren-Åkerlund, Heinegård, unpublished observation). In this way, chondroadherin may have a role in maintaining normal tissue homeostasis. There are also a number of other integrins on the chondrocyte, such as those specific for collagens (primarily $\alpha 1 \beta 1$, but also $\alpha 2 \beta 1$) and those recognizing fibronectin ($\alpha 5 \beta 1$). At this stage, the exact role of these interactions is not known, although some preliminary evidence[22] indicates that chondroadherin may be involved in the regulation of cell proliferation. Chondroadherin shows high expression in the lower region of the growth plate between the zone of proliferating chondrocytes and the hypertrophic zone. It is also expressed in articular cartilage, where it is found primarily in the deeper one-third of the tissue (Shen, Heinegård, Sommarin, unpublished observation).

Another molecule which has the potential to interact at the cell surface is PRELP; it contains a domain specifically designed for binding to heparin / heparan sulfate[14]. This could influence reactions and interactions at the cell surface of the chondrocyte where heparan sulfate appears to be exclusively found in cartilage[23]. A possible role could be to modulate effects of fibroblast growth factor (FGF), which has potent effects on chondrocyte metabolism and which depends on heparin / heparan sulfate chains for its activity.

There are a number of other cartilage matrix proteins. Among those that are synthesized by chondrocytes, but little found in normal cartilage, is fibronectin. There is, however, a specific splice variant found in cartilage[24,25], and it has been shown that chondrocytes produce an increased amount of fibronectin in, for example, OA[26].

Another abundant cartilage macromolecule which has unique structural features is COMP[27], (Fig. 7.6). The protein is made up of five identical subunits, linked together close to their N-terminus, via a so-called heptad repeat which is stabilized by disulfide bonds. Each chain is terminated at the C-terminal end with a globular structure, giving the molecule an appearance like a bouquet of tulips, (Fig. 7.6). Interestingly,

COMP shows a pronounced homology to the thrombospondin family, one of which (the trimeric Thrombospondin-1) has been demonstrated as a protein in cartilage also[28]. Although very little is known about the function of COMP or thrombospondin in cartilage, it is likely that they can interact specifically with other matrix molecules, particularly in view of the five and three subunits respectively, which provide the potential for multimeric interactions. To date, no interacting partner has been identified, although it is clear that COMP retention in the tissue depends on divalent ions, since the molecule can be efficiently extracted with EDTA[29,30].

Some information on putative roles for COMP can be obtained from its localization. It is particularly enriched in growth cartilage, where it is synthesized and deposited by proliferating chondrocytes in the cell territorial matrix. COMP expression is very low in immature cartilage[31], but it increases as the articular cartilage develops and, in mature articular cartilage, it is primarily deposited in the inter-territorial compartment in the superficial zone of the tissue[31].

Further evidence indicating that COMP has important biological properties is obtained from mutations identified in the calcium-binding domain of the molecule, which results in severe growth disturbances, that is, pseudo-achondroplasia or severe epiphyseal dysplasias[32]. Thus, it may be that COMP is required for appropriate control of cell growth and proliferation.

The 92 kDa protein is a novel protein with little homology to previously described molecules. It consists of a single polypeptide chain, but the primary sequence of the molecule does not provide any indication of its function. It is interesting, however, that the protein is primarily localized in the mid-zones of the mature cartilage, in the interterritorial matrix furthest from the chondrocyte (Lorenzo and Heinegård, unpublished observation).

An interesting protein that appears unique for cartilage, albeit not present in normal articular cartilage, is CMP. This protein contains three identical subunits, each of about 50 kDa[33]. Its role in the tissue is not defined, but it contains von Willebrand factor (vWF) motifs typical for proteins with collagen-binding properties[34].

There are also a number of other proteins in cartilage whose functions have not been clearly defined. One of these is the matrix-Gla protein which was originally isolated from bone[35]. Hypertrophic chondrocytes express collagen X that appears to form a network around the cells[36]. Also, the hypertrophic chondrocytes express one of the more prominent bone proteins, for example, BSP[31]. This is of relevance in joint disease, where it appears that some of the chondrocytes develop to become hypertrophic in later stages of the OA disease.

Altered expression and abundance of the matrix proteins in disease

OA is largely a clinical diagnosis by patient history, X-ray, often joint instability, and pain. Since these features are only present late in the process and only then lead to patient awareness, very little is known about the early events in OA. Therefore, many studies of articular cartilage in OA have been focused on samples obtained at joint replacement surgery. Unfortunately, a misconception has made several investigators draw erroneous conclusions from studies of cartilage with a fairly normal appearance, which is retained in severely affected joints. It is now becoming increasingly clear that there is no normal cartilage in a diseased joint. Thus, an understanding of the early events in human OA, which may be amenable to therapeutic intervention, will only emerge from studies of other sources of diseased cartilage, that is, from non-symptomatic joints with very minor, early focal lesions.

We have recently been able to obtain such samples from knee joints of patients undergoing amputation due to tumor in the extremities. Some of these samples from non-symptomatic patients have shown very early fibrillation and, in some cases, slight surface erosion. We could use these cartilage samples to quantitate changes in matrix constituents and also to identify altered metabolic events. It turns out that the tissue with slight surface fibrillation shows metabolic alterations similar to those in normal-looking cartilage from a severely affected joint, indicating that the biochemical abnormality affects all areas of the joint cartilage, and that these samples represent different stages of the same degenerative process (Lorenzo, Bayliss, Heinegård, unpublished observation).

Collagen

One of the early events in osteoarthritic disease appears to be an increasing volume of the tissue: that is, it swells. This can only be accomplished if the tensile properties of the collagen network become impaired, thereby preventing this structural element from resisting the swelling pressure generated by the osmotic properties of the aggrecan molecules. Thus, one of the early events in OA has to involve processes affecting the collagen network, although not necessarily the structure of the collagen fibers themselves. As is discussed below, this may emanate from processes affecting the molecules associated with the collagen fibril surface which are important for maintaining the network properties outlined in Figs 7.7 and 7.10.

Some of the initial alterations in OA, however, are found with regard to aggrecan molecules.

Aggrecan

Early in development of osteoarthritic joint disease, the level of aggrecan in the tissue appears to change. These data are mostly inferred from histochemical studies, by staining with metachromatic and/or cationic dyes, that is, Toluidine blue, Safranin-O, or Ruthenium red. In our hands, however, although we see a pronounced reduction and altered distribution of such staining, the total amount of aggrecan in the tissue does not decrease (Lorenzo, Bayliss, Heinegård, unpublished observation). At the same time, in other studies, we have shown a substantial release of proteoglycan fragments into synovial fluid in early OA[37]. Thus, it seems likely that early in OA the proteoglycans which are lost from the tissue are replaced by the chondrocytes, to give an unchanged overall tissue content. The altered histological staining pattern possibly indicates a redistribution of aggrecan in the various compartments, as a consequence of different rates of synthesis and degradation in each region of the tissue. It is of particular interest to note that similar alterations in staining can be obtained by simply immobilizing a joint[38].

Another factor to take into account is that an early event in OA is tissue swelling, that is, increased tissue volume. It may be that the increased aggrecan synthesis reported does not result in higher concentrations of proteoglycans; the total amount is higher, but present in a larger volume of tissue.

As is discussed in Chapter 7.2.2, there is accumulating information on the character of the cleavage of aggrecan occurring in joint disease and, therefore, also the character of fragments of molecules released to the surrounding synovial fluid.

Matrix non-collagenous proteins

We have identified alterations in the metabolism of various matrix proteins occurring early in joint disease. A consistent finding is increased synthesis of COMP, the 92 kDa protein, an uncharacterized 39 kDa protein, and also, but to a lower extent, of fibronectin (Lorenzo, Bayliss, and Heinegård, unpublished observations). Similar observations, albeit of more pronounced alterations, were made in late disease, indicating that early changes are indeed part of the OA process. From studies of the distribution of the proteins in the cartilage, it appears that COMP is expressed by a novel population of cells in the deeper layers of the cartilage, and that these cells also express a high level of the 92 kDa protein (Lorenzo, Bayliss, and Heinegård, unpublished observations). These findings may, therefore, be an indication that some of the earliest responses in the OA process are initiated in the deeper layers of the cartilage rather than in the superficial zones.

It should be stressed, however, that at this stage of the disease we also find some surface fibrillation. This may result from degradation of the molecules linking the collagen fibrils, which interferes with their stability. This would result in a mechanically impaired collagen network, which in turn may yield surface fibrillations when the tissue is mechanically loaded (Fig. 7.10).

At the same time, we find alterations in the level of several matrix constituents. Thus, particularly the level of PRELP appears to decrease, whereas that of fibromodulin and decorin increases (Lorenzo, Bayliss, and Heinegård, unpublished observation). These increases would be consistent with an altered surface of the collagen fibrils and, therefore, altered tensile properties. It may be that their distribution in the tissue is altered, failing in providing the adequate properties in the various compartments.

It is apparent that studies of such early events in the cartilage will provide very important information on the nature of the initial process. It is possible that any attempt at therapeutically providing an overall stimulation of metabolism may not alter the progression of the OA process. It may prove optimal to combine an approach to prevent degradation with therapeutically induced stimulation of synthesis of a particular set of macromolecules by, for example, growth factors, to optimize the attempted repair.

One factor that should be considered in terms of modulating the progression of joint disease, is the situ-

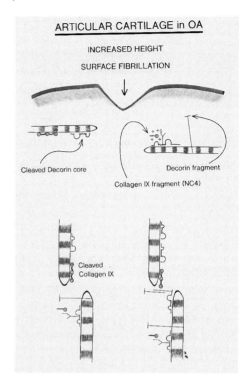

Fig. 7.10 Putative mechanisms for cartilage swelling in joint disease. The molecules putatively linking neighboring collagen fibrils may be cleaved in early stages of joint disease, allowing these fibrils to slip and displace in relation to one another. Such a process would explain early swelling, due to loss of the collagen counterbalance to the swelling pressure of the fixed-charge groups on aggrecan, and early fibrillation of the articular surface.

ation with regard to the load of the joint. It is quite possible that the load produced by normal activity of the individual may be harmful to the chondrocyte, when the tissue properties have been modified by early events in the disease. It is apparent from published data from *in vitro* studies that the chondrocyte metabolism in the tissue can be extensively modulated by mechanical load[39,40]. Therefore, future directions should include studies of effects of mechanical load on the damaged cartilage.

References

1.   van der Rest, M. and Garrone, R. (1991). Collagen family of proteins. *FASEB Journal*, 5, 2814–23.
2.   Mendler, M., Eich-Bender, S.G., Vaughan, L., Winterhalter, K.H., and Bruckner, P. (1989). Cartilage

contains mixed fibrils of collagen types II, IX and XI. *Journal of Cell Biology*, **108**, 191–7.

3. Eyre, D.R., Apon, S., Wu, J-J., Ericsson, L.H., and Walsh, K.A. (1987). Collagen type IX: evidence for covalent linkages to type II collagen in cartilage. *FEBS Letter*, **220 (2)**, 337–41.

4. Heinegård, D. and Oldberg, Å. (1989). Structure and biology of cartilage and bone matrix non-collagenous macromolecules. *FASEB Journal*, **3**, 2042–51.

5. Antonsson, P., Oldberg, Å., and Heinegård, D. (1989). The keratan sulfate enriched region of bovine cartilage proteoglycan consists of a consecutively repeated hexapeptide motif. *Journal of Biological Chemistry*, **264**, 16170–3.

6. Bayliss, M.T., Venn, G., Maroudas, A., and Ali, S.Y. (1983). Composition and structure of proteoglycans in different layers of human articular cartilage. *Biochemical Journal*, **209**, 387–400.

7. Roughley, P.J., Whilte, R.J., and Poole, A.R. (1985). Identification of a hyaluronic acid-binding protein that interferes with the preparation of high-buoyant-density proteoglycan aggregates from human articular cartilage. *Biochemical Journal*, **231**, 683–98.

8. Bayliss, M.T. (1990). Proteoglycan structure and metabolism during maturation and ageing of human articular cartilage. *Biochemical Society Transactions*, **18**, 799–802.

9. Hardingham, T.E. and Bayliss, M.T. (1990). Proteoglycans of articular cartilage: changes in ageing and in joint disease. *Seminars in Arthritis and Rheumatism*, **20 (No. 3, supplement 1)**, 12–33.

10. Inerot, S., Heinegård, D., Audell, L., and Olsson, S.-E. (1978). Articular cartilage proteoglycans in aging and osteoarthrosis. *Biochemical Journal*, **169**, 143–56.

11. Heinegård, D. and Saxne, T. (1991). Molecular markers of processes in cartilage in joint disease. *British Journal of Rheumatology*, **30**, 21–4.

12. Sandy, J.D., Plaas, A.H.K., and Koob, T.J. (1995). Pathways of aggrecan processing in joint tissues. Implications for disease mechanism and monitoring. *Acta Orthopaedica Scandinavica*, **66 (supplement 266)**, 26–32.

13. Kobe, B. and Deisenhofer, J. (1994). The leucine-rich repeat: a versatile binding motif. *Trends in Biochemical Science*, **19 (10)**, 415–21.

14. Bengtsson, E., Neame, P.J., Heinegård, D., and Sommarin, Y. (1995). The primary structure of a basic leucine-rich repeat protein, PRELP, found in connective tissues. *Journal of Biological Chemistry*, **270**, 25639–44.

15. Antonsson, P., Heinegård, D., and Oldberg, Å. (1991). Post-translational modifications of fibromodulin. *Journal of Biological Chemistry*, **266**, 16859–61.

16. Neame, P., Sommarin, Y., Boynton, R., and Heinegård, D. (1994). The structure of a 38 kDa leucine-rich protein (chondroadherin) isolated from bovine cartilage. *Journal of Biological Chemistry*, **269**, 21547–54.

17. Krusius, T. and Ruoslahti, E. (1986). Primary structure of an extracellular matrix proteoglycan core protein deduced from cloned cDNA. *Proceedings of the National Academy of Sciences, USA*, **83**, 7683–7.

18. Hedlund, H., Mengarelli-Widholm, S., Heinegård, D., Reinholt, F., and Svensson, O. (1994). Fibromodulin – distribution and association with collagen. *Matrix Biology*, **14**, 227–32.

19. Pringle, G. and Dodd, C. (1990). Immunoelectron microscopic localization of the core protein of decorin near the d and e bands of tendon collagen fibrils by use of monoclonal antibodies. *Journal of Histochemistry and Cytochemistry*, **38**, 1405–11.

20. Fleischmajer, R., Fisher, L., MacDonald, D., Jacobs Jr, L., Perlish, J., and Termine, J. (1991). Decorin interacts with fibrillar collagen of embryonic and adult human skin. *Journal of Structural Biology*, **106**, 82–90.

21. Hedbom, E. and Heinegård, D. (1993). Binding of fibromodulin and decorin to separate sites on fibrillar collagens. *Journal of Biological Chemistry*, **268**, 27307–12.

22. Sommarin, Y., Larsson, T., and Heinegård, D. (1989). Chondrocyte-matrix interactions. Attachment to proteins isolated from cartilage. *Experimental Cell Research*, **184**, 181–92.

23. Sommarin, Y. and Heinegård, D. (1986). Four classes of cell associated proteoglycans in suspension cultures of articular cartilage chondrocytes. *Biochemical Journal*, **233**, 809–18.

24. Wurster, N.B. and Lust, G. (1989). Molecular and immunologic differences in canine fibronectins from articular cartilage and plasma. *Archives of Biochemistry and Biophysics*, **269**, 32–45.

25. Bennett, V.D., Pallante, K.M., and Adams, S.L. (1991). The splicing pattern of fibronectin mRNA changes during chondrogenesis resulting in an unusual form of the mRNA in cartilage. *Journal of Biological Chemistry*, **266**, 5918–24.

26. Wurster, N.B. and Lust, G. (1982). Fibronectin in osteoarthritic canine articular cartilage. *Biochemical and Biophysical Research Communications*, **109**, 1094–101.

27. Oldberg, Å., Antonsson, P., Lindblom, K., and Heinegård, D. (1992). COMP (Cartilage Oligomeric Matrix Protein) is structurally related to the Thrombospondins. *Journal of Biological Chemistry*. **267**, 22346–22350.

28. Miller, R.R. and McDevitt, C.A. (1988) Thrombospondin is present in articular cartilage and is synthesized by articular chondrocytes. *Biochemical and Biophysical Research Communications*, **153**, 708–14.

29. Hedbom, E., Antonsson, P., Hjerpe, A., Aeschlimann, D., Paulsson, M., Rosa-Pimentel, E., *et al.* (1992). Cartilage matrix proteins: an acidic oligomeric protein (COMP) detected only in cartilage. *Journal of Biological Chemistry*, **267**, 6132–6.

30. DiCesare, P.E., Mörgelin, M., Carson, C.S., Pasumarti, S., and Paulsson, M. (1995). Cartilage oligomeric matrix protein: Isolation and characterization from human articular cartilage. *Journal of Orthopaedic Research*, **13**, 422–8.

31. Shen, Z., Heinegård, D., and Sommarin, Y. (1994). Distribution and expression of cartilage oligomeric matrix protein and bone sialoprotein show marked changes during rat femoral head development. *Matrix Biology*, **14**, 773–81.

32. Briggs, M.D., Hoffman, S.M. G., King, L.M., Olsen, A.S., Mohrenweiser, H., Leroy, J.G., *et al.* (1995). Pseudoachondroplasia and multiple epiphyseal dysplasia due to mutations in the cartilage oligomeric matrix protein gene. *Nature Genetics*, **10**, 330–6.

33. Paulsson, M. and Heinegård, D. (1981). Purification and structural characterization of a cartilage matrix protein. *Biochemical Journal*, **197**, 367–75.

34. Kiss, I., Deak, F., Holloway Jr., R.G., Delius, H., Mebust, K.A., Frimberger, E., *et al.* (1989). Structure of the gene for Cartilage Matrix Protein, a modular protein of the extracellular matrix. *Journal of Biological Chemistry*, **264**, 8126–34.

35. Hale, J., Fraser, J., and Price, P. (1988). The identification of Matrix Gla Protein in cartilage. *Journal of Biological Chemistry*, **263**, 5820–4.

36. LuValle, P., Daniels, K., Hay, E.D., and Olsen. B.R. (1992). Type X collagen is transcriptionally activated and specifically localized during sternal cartilage maturation. *Matrix*, **12**, 404–13.

37. Dahlberg, L., Ryd, L., Heinegård, D., and Lohmander, S. (1992). Proteoglycan fragments in joint fluid. Influence of arthrosis and inflammation. *Acta Orthopedica Scandinavica*, **63**, 417–23.

38. Palmoski, M., Perricone, E., and Brandt, K.D. (1979). Development and reversal of a proteoglycan aggregation defect in normal canine knee cartilage after immobilization. *Arthritis and Rheumatism*, **22**, 508–17.

39. Sah, R., Grodzinsky, A., Plaas, A., and Sandy, J. (1992). Effects of static and dynamic compression on matrix metabolism in cartilage explants. In *Articular cartilage and osteoarthritis* (ed. K. Kuettner, *et. al.*), pp. 373–92. Raven Press, New York.

40. Larsson, T., Aspden, R., and Heinegård, D. (1991). Effects of mechanical load on cartilage matrix biosynthesis *in vitro*. *Matrix*, **11**, 388–94.

7.2.2 Proteolytic degradation of normal and osteoarthritic cartilage matrix

John D. Sandy and Michael W. Lark

Introduction

The unique macromolecular matrix organization of articular cartilage, confers on the tissue the capacity to effectively transmit compressive and shear forces across the joint space. Compressive resistance is conferred largely by the high concentration of aggrecan in the tissue, whereas resistance to shear and tensile force is a function of the type II collagen network[1]. In the healthy mature joint, articular cartilage function is maintained by the homeostatic activities of the resident chondrocytes, which both synthesize and degrade this complex mixture of matrix proteins, glycoproteins, and proteoglycans. Once the adult cartilage matrix is established, some components, such as intercellular type II collagen, are relatively stable and probably undergo only limited remodeling during adult life[2]. On the other hand, other components, such as aggrecan located in the pericellular space, appear to undergo very active turnover[3,4]. The biomechanical and cell biological processes which orchestrate these turnover events are, therefore, central to the maintenance of tissue function. For each molecular species, the rate of synthesis, secretion, and matrix deposition must be appropriately balanced with the rate of degradation and removal. In addition, many matrix macromolecules (such as the heterotypic assemblies of type II and type IX collagen) are composite structures, so that the turnover of individual components must also be coordinated by the chondrocytes.

Proteinases which degrade the range of cartilage matrix proteins are obviously central players in these turnover events. Under normal homeostatic conditions, matrix macromolecules will be subject to attack by one or more proteinases which may possess a high degree of specificity for sites within that molecule. The end result of the proteolytic cascade will be the removal or modification of the protein in such a way that effective replacement with newly synthesised molecules can occur.

In osteoarthritis (OA), it appears that this proteolytic turnover of matrix gradually overwhelms the normal control mechanisms, so that cellular attempts to maintain matrix composition finally fail. The loss of control over this process can apparently be initiated by one or more of the predisposing conditions for OA – aging, genetic abnormality, altered biomechanics, or joint trauma. Just how these factors initiate the degenerative process at the cellular level, and which matrix components and proteinases are critically involved in the destruction of the cartilage, remains to be elucidated. In this chapter we will summarize current knowledge in this area, with particular emphasis on recent interesting developments in the control and molecular details of the proteolysis of aggrecan in cartilage.

Proteinases in cartilage or other joint tissues: the problem of clearly establishing a role for any proteinase in cartilage degradation

There is substantial evidence[5] from both animal and human tissue studies for the presence of a wide spectrum of proteinases in articular cartilage, chondrocytes, and other synovial joint tissues and cell types. It is not surprising that serine proteinases such as plasmin, cysteine proteinases such as cathepsin B and calpain, the aspartic proteinase cathepsin D, and matrix metalloproteinases such as MMP1 and MMP3, have all been identified as components of these joint tissues.

However, the complex nature of the cell biological processes involved in the control of the gene expression, synthesis, activation, and inhibition of proteinases, has made it very difficult to draw firm conclusions about the role of any individual enzyme in specific catabolic events in cartilage. The demonstration of the presence of an mRNA for a proteinase, or even the presence of the secreted enzyme in the cartilage matrix, cannot alone be taken as evidence for activity *in situ*. MMPs, for example, are generally secreted in inactive zymogen forms which require activation, and the activated enzymes may be rapidly inhibited by interaction with naturally occurring tissue inhibitors (TIMPs). In this regard, it has been shown that the treatment of human articular cartilage with recombinant human IL-1 results in cartilage resorption and, at the same time, the over-expression of plasminogen activators[6] and also pro-MMP3[7]. Whilst such correlative studies set an important framework for examining the precise role of such proteinases in matrix catabolism, they clearly stop short of directly demonstrating such a role for any particular proteinase. In the same way, immunohistochemical localization of MMP3 protein in normal and human OA cartilage[8] has revealed a strong correlation between the tissue content and precise localization of MMP3, and

the extent of tissue destruction; likewise, it has been shown that there are elevations of both MMP1 and MMP3 in joint fluids of patients with both inflammatory and non-inflammatory joint disease[51,52]. However, the majority of this enzyme protein is secreted into the joint space in an inactive form. Together, these studies indicate that there are elevations in MMPs in joints of patients with joint disease; however, they do not demonstrate that these enzymes are responsible for the tissue destruction.

Interestingly, studies employing both *in situ* hybridization[7] and immunolocalization[8] of MMP3 in normal human cartilage have indicated that this proteinase, when expressed, is enriched in the superficial zones of the tissue. This pattern of distribution may indicate that MMP3 has an important role in the turnover of matrix components, such as small proteoglycans, which may be concentrated in the superficial layer of the tissue and specifically involved in organizing the tangential collagenous weave of this region of the tissue. In the same way, detailed cytochemical and histochemical analysis for cathepsin B, of human OA femoral head cartilage[9] has suggested a role for this enzyme in sustaining the chronicity of the disease, since particularly high levels of protein were observed at sites within regenerating cartilage. Again, however, in the absence of evidence that products of cathepsin B activity are present in these sites, the extent of cathepsin B involvement in matrix degradation remains unknown.

Synthetic inhibitors and their effects on cartilage catabolism

In the absence of methods which can directly demonstrate the products of individual proteinases in cartilage matrix *in situ*, the role of a particular enzyme can be examined by evaluating the effect of well characterized proteinase inhibitors on specific catabolic processes. The extent to which these data can be reliably interpreted depends critically on the careful experimental demonstration that the inhibitors are exerting effects solely through inhibition of proteinase action, and not through general cytotoxicity.

A number of well-controlled studies have been done recently in this area. Interleukin-1-stimulated degradation of aggrecan in bovine nasal septum cartilage cultures was found to be sensitive to inhibition by a lipophilic peptidyl diazomethane inactivator of cysteine endopeptidases   (benzyloxycarbonyl-Tyr-Ala-CHN2) and a lipophilic epoxidyl peptide proinhibitor (trans-epoxysuccinyl-leucylamido-(3-methyl)butane ethyl ester) of cysteine proteinases[10]. The levels of these inhibitors, which were effective in blocking aggrecan release (1–10 μM), had no measurable effect on general metabolic parameters, such as protein synthesis, nor on the activity of the IL-1 signal transduction pathway in fibroblasts. It was concluded that one or more of the lysosomal cysteine proteinases (cathepsins B, L, and S) mediate the IL-1 effect on aggrecan degradation. In a subsequent study[11], the same system was assessed for its sensitivity to a cathepsin B-specific inhibitor (N-(L-3-trans-propylcarbamoyloxirane-2-carbonyl)-L-isoleucyl-L-proline) and its methyl ester, and both compounds were shown to be inhibitory. In addition, a metalloproteinase inhibitor (peptide hydroxamate, BB94) was found to inhibit this process. A detailed analysis of the effects of these compounds on general metabolic activity and on IL-1 transduction pathways led to the conclusion that the inhibitory effects could not be explained by cytotoxicity, and that a proteolytic cascade involving cysteine proteinases (probably cathepsin B) and MMPs is involved in aggrecan catabolism, under these conditions.

In a similar study, but with human articular cartilage explants[12], it was shown that IL-1 treatment promoted type II collagen degradation (determined immunohistochemically) and aggrecan degradation. Addition of a peptidylhydroxamate MMP inhibitor (R,S-N-(2-(hydroxyamino)2-oxyethyl)-4-methyl-1-oxypentyl-L-leucyl-L-phenylalaninamide) effectively reduced the degradation of both matrix components and with no detectable cytotoxic effects. Since the IL-1 addition was accompanied by the increased release of proMMPs, and this process was not affected by the MMP inhibitor, it was concluded that MMPs (such as MMP1 and MMP3) must account for aggrecan release and collagen degradation, under these conditions.

This series of inhibitor studies[10-12] clearly indicates that the degradation of aggrecan and collagen, induced by IL-1 treatment of cartilage explants, involves the action of matrix metalloproteinases. However, detailed structural analysis of the catabolic products is required to determine which MMPs specifically are involved, and to what extent these MMPs function to activate other proteinases or act directly on matrix components. In this regard, it is very significant that the products of aggrecan catabolism isolated from IL-1-treated cartilage explants do not appear to be generated by any of the MMPs which are known to be induced by IL-1

treatment[13]. This unexpected finding is discussed in detail below.

Detection of proteolytic degradation products in situ: the search for direct evidence of the activity of a specific proteinase in cartilage matrix

In order to obtain information on the nature of the proteinases which are directly involved in the degradation of specific matrix components, a number of laboratories have recently begun to carry out structural studies on catabolic products present in articular cartilage, meniscal cartilage, intraarticular ligaments, and synovial fluids. This precise structural characterization has become possible because of the recent availability of the amino acid sequences of many cartilage matrix proteins, acquired through cDNA techniques. Sequence information has, in turn, allowed for direct structural identification of products by N-terminal and C-terminal analysis, and also the generation of immunoreagents (monoclonal and polyclonal) which can identify products based on internal sequences and the 'new' N-terminal or C-terminal sequences (neoepitopes) generated following proteolytic cleavage. Many of the advances in this area relate to aggrecan degradation and Fig. 7.11 provides a summary of the recently described immunoreagents which are being applied to studies in this area.

Link protein degradation

Direct evidence for involvement of an MMP in the degradation of human cartilage link protein *in vivo* was obtained when the smallest link protein species present in the tissue was isolated and N-terminally sequenced[14]. The sequence predicted a cleavage *in situ* at the histidine 16-isoleucine 17 bond — a bond which was also found to be cleaved by a purified cartilage MMP, and later shown to be cleaved by recombinant MMP3[15]. It was concluded that an MMP with this cleavage specificity must have been active in the tissue *in vivo*, in order for this product to be present in extracts. Generation and application[15] of a monoclonal

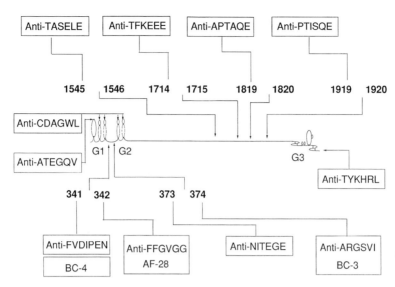

Fig. 7.11 Antibodies to aggrecan epitopes. The terminology in use for immunoreagents currently applied to structural analysis of aggrecan and its degradation products. The preparation and use of antisera to internal sequences (anti-CDAGWL, anti-ATEGQV, and anti-TYKHRL) is described in [32] and [35]. Antisera to C-terminal sequences within the CS-domain (anti-TASELE, anti-TFKEEE, anti-APTAQE, anti-PTISQE) are described in [32] and [40]. Antisera to C-terminal sequences within the interglobular domain (anti-FVDIPEN and anti-NITEGE) are described in [30] and [35]. The monoclonal antibody BC-3, which recognizes the N-terminal of ARGSVI, and the antibody BC-4, which recognizes the C-terminal of FVDIPEN, are described in [48]. The monoclonal antibody AF-28, which recognizes the N-terminal of FFGVGG, is described in [55]. The figure also depicts the human aggrecan residue numbers for the amino acids on each side of the cleavage sites recognized by the respective antibodies.

antibody, CH-3, which detects the new N-terminus of the MMP3-degraded form of link protein, showed that this form is most abundant in immature cartilages, consistent with a role for MMP3 or closely related MMPs in cartilage remodeling during growth. Interestingly, the small degraded link protein which accumulates with age in human articular cartilage was not detected by antibody CH-3, suggesting that proteinases in addition to MMPs are responsible for link protein proteolysis in mature cartilages. The identity of the other proteinases which generate degraded forms of link protein in cartilage remains unknown.

Collagen degradation

The major collagen fibrillar network of articular cartilage is composed of a heterotypic assembly of collagen types II, IX, and XI. The proteinases responsible for the normal turnover and remodeling of these composite structures, or their degradation in OA, are not yet clearly identified[16]. Whilst interstitial collagenase (MMP1) is almost certainly involved in the turnover of

actively remodeling collagenous matrices, such as that in the hypertrophic zone of the growth plate[17], the extent to which MMP1 acts in the slow remodeling of mature articular cartilage collagens is unclear. However, there is now some direct evidence[18] for remodeling *in vivo*, since a population of partially degraded type II collagen has been identified as a normal component of mature human cartilage with a monoclonal antibody (COL2-3/4m). This immunoreagent was prepared by immunization of mice with an ovalbumin-coupled 21 amino acid peptide (Gly-Lys-Val-Gly-Pro-Ser-Gly-Ala-Hyp-Gly-Glu-Asp-Gly-Arg-Hyp-Gly-Pro-Hyp-Gly-Pro-Gln) from the glycine-rich repeat region of the triple helical domain of human type II collagen. The epitope recognized by this antibody is exposed to some extent in normal tissue, but becomes more accessible following proteolysis and 'unwinding' of the triple helix. The proteinase responsible for this has not been conclusively identified, but given the resistance of the collagen helix to general proteolytic attack, and the apparently unique capacity of MMP1 to degrade the triple helix and generate this epitope *in vitro*, it appears that MMP1 may be involved.

This conclusion is also supported by the finding[19] that activation of endogenous tissue MMPs with aminophenyl mercuric acetate, increases the reactivity of the tissue to the antibody COL2-3/4m. Further, exposure of human cartilage to IL-1 increased the level of this epitope in the pericellular regions of the tissue, and this increase could be prevented by treatment with a specific MMP inhibitor[12]. This epitope can be detected in normal aged cartilage. However, its content is increased several-fold in OA samples[18]. It seems likely, therefore, that the proteinase responsible is active to a limited extent in normal cartilage, but that this activity is upregulated in OA cartilage.

A possible role for MMP3 in cartilage collagen degradation has been suggested by recent studies with recombinant enzyme[20]. In solution incubations, MMP3 cleaves the telopeptide region of type II collagen and the triple helical region of type IX collagen. Similar results were obtained on incubation of cartilage explants with this enzyme[21]. These results predict that MMP3, which appears to degrade a proportion of the aggrecan in cartilage matrix *in vivo*[22], also has the capacity to at least partially depolymerize the type II/type IX collagen network. In this regard it is very significant that the swelling of cartilage, which is an established hallmark of early OA change[23], can be reproduced by MMP3 treatment of cartilage explants[21]. On the other hand, the MMP3 knockout mouse[25] appears to develop normally, suggesting that MMP3 is not essential in mouse development. There may, therefore, exist a redundancy in the MMP family of proteinases, such that the functions of MMP1 and MMP3

can be readily achieved by other MMPs, as necessary. In this regard, MMP2 has now been shown[26] to be as effective as MMP1 in cleaving at the MMP1 site within the triple helical domain of type I collagen fibrils.

Aggrecan degradation by MMPs

In an approach similar to that used for link protein described above[14], direct evidence has also now been obtained for the involvement of MMPs in the degradation of aggrecan in human articular cartilage[22]. Aggrecan preparations from both macroscopically normal and OA human cartilages were analyzed for the presence of degraded forms of the G1 domain of aggrecan, which are retained in the tissue in association with hyaluronan. Isolation and sequencing of the C-terminal peptides of these G1 species showed a proportion, maybe 10 per cent of the total, to terminate at asparagine 342. This finding directly predicts that there is a cleavage of aggrecan *in vivo* at the asparagine 341 – phenylalanine 342 bond (see Fig. 7.12 for location). Evidence that this cleavage results from MMP activity was obtained by incubation of purified human aggrecan with recombinant human MMP3. This showed that the asparagine 341—phenylalanine 342 bond was cleaved by MMP3, although subsequent studies[27-29] have shown that a wide spectrum of metalloproteinases (MMPs-1,2,3,7,8,9,13) also display high activity towards this site in the aggrecan core protein. Furthermore, it has been shown that even with complete elimination of MMP3 in the knockout mouse,

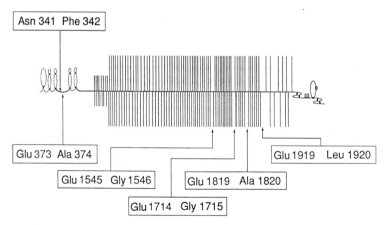

Fig. 7.12 Aggrecan cleavage sites for metalloproteinases and aggrecanase. The diagram of aggrecan shows the location of the major metalloproteinase cleavage site (asn 341- phe 342) above and the five different aggrecanase cleavage sites below. The long vertical lines on the aggrecan diagram denote the position of serine residues which are likely substituted with CS, and show how the aggrecanase cleavage sites in the CS domain are apparently located in 'gap' regions between clusters of CS chains.

there is still cleavage of aggrecan at this site in both collagen-induced and proteoglycan-induced arthritis[25], consistent with multiple members of the MMP family having the capacity to generate this cleavage *in vivo*.

It can, therefore, be concluded that a proportion of the aggrecan in both normal and OA human cartilage has been degraded *in vivo*, by one or more of the MMPs listed above. This observation has now also been confirmed by the generation and characterization[30] of an antiserum (anti-FVDIPEN), which can detect the G1 domain with a C-terminal of asparagine 341 (see Fig. 7.11 for epitope location). This species has now been detected by immunohistochemistry of human OA and RA cartilages[31], and on Western blots of human OA cartilages and synovial fluids[32]. In addition, Western analysis of human synovial fluids with antibody AF-28 (see Fig. 7.11 for epitope location) has also identified fragments which bear an N-terminus of phenylalanine 342[55], consistent with the predicted *in vivo* cleavage of the asparagine 341—phenylalanine 342 bond[22].

Aggrecan degradation by aggrecanase within the interglobular domain

MMP-dependent cleavage of the asparagine 342—phenylalanine 343 bond does not, however, fully explain the pathways of aggrecan degradation which occur in cartilage *in vivo*. A substantial proportion of the metabolic pool of aggrecan which is degraded and released into the synovial fluid, under normal conditions and in both early and late stage OA (and in inflammatory joint diseases), is degraded by a proteinase which cleaves instead the glutamate 373—alanine 374 bond of the interglobular domain[33,34]. The proteinase responsible for this has not yet been identified, but it is now widely referred to as aggrecanase. The locations of the MMP-sensitive and aggrecanase-sensitive sites in human aggrecan are shown in detail in Fig. 7.12.

If cleavage of the aggrecan molecule by MMPs at the asparagine 341-phenylalanine 342 bond was the major site of aggrecan cleavage *in vivo*, then the diffusible chondroitin sulfate-rich products released into the synovial fluid should carry an N-terminus of phenylalanine 342. Such products do not, however, appear to achieve high concentrations in synovial fluids. Instead, N-terminal analysis of fluid products has consistently

shown the major chondroitin sulfate-rich products to bear an N-terminus of alanine 374. This finding predicts cleavage at the glutamate 373—alanine 374 bond of aggrecan *in vivo*, at a site which is 32 amino acid residues on the C-terminal side of the MMP cleavage site. Cleavage at this site within the interglobular domain of aggrecan, without concomitant cleavage at the asparagine 341—phenylalanine 342 bond, would be expected to generate aggrecan G1 domain with a C-terminus of glutamate 373 (see Fig. 7.12). This species has indeed been identified, with antiserum anti-NITEGE (Fig. 7.11), in human OA articular cartilage extracts and synovial fluids[32], and by immunohistochemistry of normal, OA, and RA human cartilage samples[31]. This result directly demonstrates that a proportion of aggrecan is cleaved *in vivo* at the aggrecanase site, without cleavage at the MMP site.

Taken together, the analysis of cartilage and synovial fluid samples suggests that while aggrecanase is centrally involved in aggrecan degradation by normal and OA chondrocytes *in vivo*, MMP-dependent cleavage of a proportion of molecules also occurs. The relative importance of these two proteinase activities in the steady-state turnover of aggrecan, or in the accelerated catabolism of aggrecan seen in OA, remains to be determined. In this regard, a central role for aggrecanase is supported by a group of studies from different laboratories[35–38] which have shown that the initial, and quantitatively major, products of catabolism in IL-1 or RA-induced cartilage explants and chondrocyte culture systems result from aggrecanase activity alone. These explant studies have also shown that aggrecanase has the capacity to cleave aggrecan at four sites within the CS-bearing region of aggrecan, in addition to the glutamate 373—alanine 374 site (see Fig. 7.12). Inspection of the sequences around these sites shows that a common feature of aggrecanase-sensitive bonds is the presence of a glutamate residue in the P1 position, on the N-terminal side of the scissile bond.

Aggrecan degradation by aggrecanase within the CS attachment regions

Characterization of aggrecan in extracts of normal human articular cartilage from young and old individuals[39,53], and from OA and RA patients[40], has revealed the presence of up to 12 different core species bearing the G1 domain. These species range in size, from

380kDa, down to 35kDa, and appear to represent a spectrum of proteolytic products with different C-terminals, which range from full-length aggrecan, down to fragments generated by cleavage within the G1 domain. Whilst Western analysis[32] suggests that species of 62kDa and 52kDa in these samples terminate at glutamate 373 (aggrecanase product) and asparagine 341 (MMP product) respectively, the C-terminii for all of the other species remain unknown. Identification of these C-terminal sequences should provide a basis on which to identify all, or most, of the proteinases involved in aggrecan degradation *in vivo*. The recent production of antisera (anti-TASELE, anti-TFKEEE, anti-APTAQE, anti-PTISQE) designed to identify aggrecanase-generated products with C-terminals of glutamate 1545, glutamate 1714, glutamate 1819, and glutamate 1919, respectively (see Fig. 7.11), has now made an approach to this question possible[32].

What is aggrecanase?

The activity termed 'aggrecanase' has not yet been identified. The finding[41] that native and recombinant MMP8 can cleave the glutamate 373-alanine 374 bond in solution incubations with aggrecan core, suggests that aggrecanase may be an MMP, and this is supported by the findings that aggrecan catabolism in explant cultures can also be completely inhibited by non-cytotoxic MMP-specific inhibitors[11,19]. On the other hand, all of the MMPs which have been tested thus far, including MMP8, show a distinct preference for the asparagine 341—phenylalanine 342 bond, instead of the glutamate 373—alanine 374 bond. Moreover, the aggrecanase cleavage takes place in induced arthritis in the MMP3 knockout mouse, supporting the *in vitro* data that MMP3 is not responsible for the aggrecanase cleavage[25]. Further, in cell culture systems where aggrecanase degrades aggrecan following induction with IL-1 or RA, the active proteinase exclusively degrades the glutamate 373—alanine 374 bond, and there is no evidence for concomitant cleavage of the asparagine 341—phenylalanine 342 bond[35]. Aggrecanase in cell cultures would, therefore, appear to be incapable of cleaving the asparagine 341—phenylalanine 342 bond, a cleavage site which is highly sensitive to cleavage by the known MMPs.

In order to further investigate the nature of aggrecanase in cartilage, tissue has been treated with aminophenylmercuric acetate to activate endogenous MMPs. Under these conditions, the aggrecan matrix was extensively degraded, but analysis of the CS-rich products by N-terminal analysis[22], and of the G1 domain by Western analysis[19], showed that the only proteinases which were activated were MMPs which, as expected, cleaved the asparagine 341—phenylalanine 342 bond. There was, however, no evidence for aggrecanase products in these experiments, suggesting that, if aggrecanase is an MMP, it is not readily activated by APMA. The result also shows that the expected specificity of the MMPs for the asparagine 341—phenylalanine 342 bond is retained when the enzymes degrade aggrecan in the tissue microenvironment, suggesting that the cleavage specificity of MMPs is unlikely to be altered by the conditions of substrate presentation, pH, or other physicochemical parameters which may only operate in intact cartilage tissue.

On the other hand, the possibility that aggrecanase is a membrane-associated proteinase, which is normally activated at or near the cell surface, is supported by the finding that in IL-1 stimulated systems, only membrane-permeable cysteine proteinase inhibitors are effective[10,11], and also that the aggrecanase-dependent process can be readily prevented by bafilomycin A1[42]. Bafilomycin A1 is a selective inhibitor of lysosomal acidification, and the inhibitory effect of this compound suggests that maintenance of acidity, perhaps to allow intracellular cysteine proteinase-dependent activation of aggrecanase, is a critical step in aggrecanase function. In this regard, it may be relevant that a new group of membrane-type MMPs, which appear to be activated intracellular and which probably function primarily at cell surfaces, has now been described[43,44].

Whilst aggrecanase appears to be responsible for the accelerated release of aggrecan fragments from cartilage seen in human OA and inflammatory joint diseases[33,34], it is clearly not an activity which is exclusively associated with joint degeneration. An analysis of a range of bovine joint tissues, including cartilage, meniscus, ligaments, and tendons, taken during fetal development[32,45], has shown that fibrous and fibro-cartilagenous matrices accumulate the aggrecanase-generated G1 domain which terminates at glutamate 373. Aggrecanase, therefore, appears to be highly expressed *in vivo* by cells of a more fibroblastic phenotype which are present in collagen-rich matrices during development, and in tissues which do not accumulate high concentrations of aggrecan. Indeed, primary cultures of tendon fibroblasts have been shown to degrade aggrecan at the glutamate 373—alanine 374 bond, when cultured in alginate beads with exogenously supplied aggrecan[46]. Also significant in this regard is the finding that an analysis of *in vivo* degradation products, isolated from bovine brain, suggest that an aggrecanase-like activity is responsible for brevican turnover in brain development[47]. Brevican is an aggregating proteoglycan of brain which exhibits a general structural homology to aggrecan, but which is very sparsely substituted with chondroitin sulfate. These observations, therefore, suggest that 'aggrecanases' may be responsible for the controlled degradation of different aggregating proteoglycans in a range of tissues and situations.

Summary and conclusions

Our understanding of the precise pathways involved in the proteolytic degradation of cartilage matrix components is very limited. The available data suggests that proteinases from all groups (aspartic, cysteine, metallo, and serine) will play some role in the process. Some proteinases, such as cathepsin B and plasmin, may contribute by activating the proforms of other enzymes. Cathepsin D may be active in low pH microenvironments which may exist near the chondrocyte surface, or in regions of very high aggrecan concentration. The MMPs would appear to be most suited to proteolysis of matrix in the intercellular space between chondrocytes. Whilst it has been widely stated[5,7,8,12,18,21,49,50] that collagenase (MMP1), gelatinases (MMP2 and 9), and stromelysin (MMP3), probably play central roles in cartilage degradation, the evidence for this remains indirect. The possibility that new members of the MMP family, such as the membrane-type MMPs[43] or others, yet to be described, will be responsible for these processes cannot be excluded at present. The group of membrane-type MMPs appear particularly interesting in relation to aggrecanase activity in the pericellular space, since these proteinases are activated by intracellular processing at a furin site[44], and this process may be sensitive to the membrane-permeable inhibitors which interfere with the aggrecanase cascade[10,11,24]. Identification of aggrecanase should open new avenues for research in this area.

Finally, in relation to OA, it is important to note that excessive degradation of the major matrix components, aggrecan, and type II collagen, may represent a relatively late stage in the development of the OA lesion. The initial events, which result in tissue swelling and chondrocyte cloning, may involve excessive degradation of minor matrix components, such as the minor

collagens and small proteoglycans which are required for matrix stabilization and integrity. The proteinases responsible for these proteolytic events may represent the best targets for therapeutic intervention in this crippling disease.

Acknowledgments

This work was supported by grants (to John Sandy) from the Shriners of North America and Merck and Co.

References

1. Buckwalter, J., Hunziker, E., Rosenberg, L., Coutts, R., Adams, M., and Eyre, D. (1988). Articular cartilage: injury and repair. In *Injury and repair of the musculoskeletal soft tissues* (ed. S.Y. Woo and J. Buckwalter), pp. 405–25. American Academy of Orthopedic Surgeons.

2. Eyre, D.R. (1995). Collagen structure and function in articular cartilage. Metabolic changes in the development of osteoarthritis. In *Osteoarthritic disorders* (ed. K. Kuettner and V. Goldberg) pp. 281–90. American Academy of Orthopedic Surgeons. Park Ridge, Illinois.

3. Sandy, J.D. (1992). Extracellular metabolism of aggrecan. In *Articular cartilage and osteoarthritis* (ed. K. Kuettner, *et al.*), pp. 21–33. Raven Press, Ltd., New York.

4. Mok, S.S., Masuda, K., Hauselmann, H.J., Aydelotte, M.B., and Thonar, E.J-M.A. (1994). Aggrecan synthesised by mature bovine chondrocytes suspended in alginate. Identification of two distinct metabolic matrix pools. *Journal of Biological Chemistry*, **52**, 33021–7.

5. Woessner, J.F. (1995). Imbalance of proteinases and their inhibitors in osteoarthritis. In *Osteoarthritic disorders* (ed. K. Kuettner and V. Goldberg), pp. 281–90. American Academy of Orthopedic Surgeons.

6. Campbell, I.K., Piccoli, D.S., Butler, D.M., Singleton, D.K., and Hamilton, J.A. (1988). Recombinant human interleukin-1 stimulates human articular cartilage to undergo resorption and human chondrocytes to produce both tissue- and urokinase-type plasminogen activator. *Biochimica et Biophysica Acta*, **967**, 183–94.

7. Nguyen, Q., Mort, J.S., and Roughley, P.J. (1992). Preferential mRNA expression of prostromelysin relative to procollagenase and *in situ* localization in human articular cartilage. *Journal of Clinical Investigation*, **89**, 1189–97.

8. Okada, Y., Shinmei, M., Tanaka, O., Naka, K., Kimura, A., Nakanishi, I., *et al.* (1992). Localization of MMP3 (stromelysin) in osteoarthritic cartilage and synovium. *Laboratory Investigation*, **66**, 680–90.

9. Baici, A., Horler, D., Lang, A., Merlin, C., and Kissling, R. (1995). Cathepsin B in osteoarthritis: zonal variation

of enzyme activity in human femoral head cartilage. *Annals of the Rheumatic Diseases*, **54**, 281–8.

10. Buttle, D.J. and Saklatvala, J. (1992). Lysosomal cysteine endopeptidases mediate IL-1-stimulated cartilage proteoglycan degradation. *Biochemical Journal*, **287**, 657–61.

11. Buttle, D.J., Handley, C.J., Ilic, M.Z., Saklatvala, J., Mrata, M., and Barrett, A.J. (1993). Inhibition of cartilage proteoglycan release by a specific inactivator of cathepsin B and an inhibitor of MMPs. Evidence for two converging pathways of chondrocyte-mediated proteoglycan degradation. *Arthritis and Rheumatism*, **36**, 1709–17.

12. Mort, J.S., Dodge, G.R., Roughley, P.J., Liu, J., Finch, S.J., Dipasquale, G., *et al.* (1993). Direct evidence for active MMPs mediating matrix degradation in IL-1 stimulated human articular cartilage. *Matrix*, **13**, 95–102.

13. Sandy, J.D., Neame, P.J., Boynton, R.E., and Flannery, C.R. (1991). Catabolism of aggrecan in cartilage explants- identification of a major cleavage site within the interglobular domain. *Journal of Biological Chemistry*, **266**, 8683–5.

14. Nguyen, Q., Murphy, G., Roughley, P.J., and Mort, J.S. (1989). Degradation of proteoglycan aggregate by a cartilage metalloproteinase. Evidence for the involvement of stromelysin in the generation of link protein heterogeneity *in situ*. *Biochemical Journal*, **259**, 61–7.

15. Hughes, C.E., Caterson, B., White, R.J., Roughley, P.J., and Mort, J.S. (1992). Monoclonal antibodies recognizing protease-generated neoepitopes from cartilage proteoglycan degradation. Application to studies on human link protein cleavage by stromelysin. *Journal of Biological Chemistry*, **267**, 16011–14.

16. Hembry, R.M., Bagga, M.R., Dingle, J.T., Page, Thomas P., and Reynolds, J.J. (1994). Metalloproteinase production by rabbit articular cartilage; comparison of the effects of IL-1a *in vitro* and *in vivo*. *Virchow's Archiv.* **425**, 413–24.

17. Gack, S., Vallon, R., Schmidt, J., Grigoriadis, A., Tuckerman, J., Schekel, J., *et al.* (1995). Expression of interstitial collagenase during skeletal development of the mouse is restricted to osteoblast cells and hypertrophic chondrocytes. *Cell Growth and Differentiation*, **6**, 759–67.

18. Hollander, A.P., Heathfield, T.F., Webber, C., Iwata, Y., Bourne, R., Rorabeck, C., *et al.* (1994). Increased damage to Type II collagen in osteoarthritic articular cartilage detected by a new immunoassay. *Journal of Clinical Investigation*, **93**, 1722–32.

19. Bonassar, L.J., Stinn, J.L., Paguio, C.G., Frank, E.H., Moore, V.L., Lark, M.W., *et al.* (1996) Activation and inhibition of endogenous matrix metalloproteinases in articular cartilage: effects on composition and biophysical properties. *Arthritis and Rheumatism*, **333**, 359–67.

20. Wu, J.J., Lark, M.W., Chun, L.E., and Eyre, D.R. (1991). Sites of stromelysin cleavage in collagen types II, IX, X and XI of cartilage. *Journal of Biological Chemistry*, **266**, 5625–8.

21. Bonassar, L.J., Frank, E.H., Murray, J.C., Paguio, C.G., Moore, V.L., Lark, M.W., *et al.* (1995). Changes in cartilage composition and physical properties due to

stromelysin degradation. *Arthritis and Rheumatism*, **38**, 173–83.

22. Flannery, C.R., Lark, M.W., and Sandy, J.D. (1992). Identification of a stromelysin cleavage site within the interglobular domain of human aggrecan. Evidence for proteolysis at this site *in vivo* in human articular cartilage. *Journal of Biological Chemistry*, **267**, 1008–14.

23. Maroudas, A. (1976). Balance between swelling pressure and collagen tension in normal and degenerate cartilage. *Nature*, **260**, 808–9.

24. Buttle, D.J., Bramwell, H., and Hollander, A.P. (1995). Proteolytic mechanisms of cartilage breakdown: a target for arthritis therapy? *Journal of Clinical Pathology: Molecular Pathology*, **48**, M167–77.

25. Mudgett, J.S., Chartrain, N.A., Christen, A., McDonnell, J., Shen, C.F., Kawka, D.W., *et al.* (1995). Collagen-induced arthritis in the stromelysin-1 (MMP3) knock-out mouse. *Transactions of the Orthopedic Research Society*, **20**, 148.

26. Aimes, R.T. and Quigley, J.P. (1995). Matrix metalloproteinase-2 is an interstitial collagenase. *Journal of Biological Chemistry*, **270**, 5872–6.

27. Flannery, C.R. and Sandy, J.D. (1993). Aggrecan catabolism in cartilage: studies on the nature of a novel proteinase (aggrecanase) which cleaves the Glu373-Ala374 bond of the interglobular domain. *Orthopedic Transactions*, **17**, 677.

28. Fosang, A.J., Last, K., Knauper, V., Neame, P.J., Murphy, G., Hardingham, T.E., *et al.* (1993). Fibroblast and neutrophil collagenases cleave at two sites in the aggrecan interglobular domain. *Biochemical Journal*, **295**, 273–6.

29. Flannery, C.R. and Sandy, J.D. (1995). Identification of MMP-13 as the major matrix metalloproteinase expressed by chondrocytes during retinoic acid-induced matrix catabolism. *Transactions of the Orthopedic Research Society*, **20**, 102.

30. Lark, M.W., Williams, H., Hoernner, L.A., Weidner, J., Ayala, J.M., Harper, C.F., *et al.* (1995). Quantification of a matrix metalloproteinase generated aggrecan G1 fragment using monospecific anti-peptide serum. *Biochemical Journal*, **307**, 245–52.

31. Bayne, E.K., Donatelli, S.A., Sargeant, J., Singer, I.I., Lark, M.W., Hoernner, L.A., *et al.* (1995). *Transactions of the Orthopedic Research Society*, **20**, 328.

32. Sandy, J.D., Plaas, A.H.K., and Koob, T.J. (1995). Pathways of aggrecan processing in joint tissues-implications for disease mechanism and monitoring *Acta Orthopedica Scandinavica*, **supplement 266**, **66**, 22–5.

33. Sandy, J.D., Flannery, C.R., Neame, P.J., and Lohmander, S.F. (1992). The structure of aggrecan fragments in human osteoarthritic synovial fluid. Evidence for the involvement in osteoarthritis of a novel proteinase which cleaves the glu 373- ala 374 bond of the interglobular domain. *Journal of Clinical Investigation*, **89**, 1512–16.

34. Lohmander, S.L., Neame, P.J., and Sandy, J.D. (1993). The structure of aggrecan fragments in human synovial fluid. Evidence that aggrecanase mediates cartilage degradation in inflammatory joint disease, joint injury and osteoarthritis. *Arthritis and Rheumatism*, **36**, 1214–22.

35. Lark, M.W., Gordy, J.T., Weidner, J.R., Ayala, J., Kimura, J.H., Williams, H.R., *et al.* (1995). Cell-mediated catabolism of aggrecan : Evidence that cleavage at the 'aggrecanase' site (glu³⁷³—ala³⁷⁴) is a primary event in proteolysis of the interglobular domain. *Journal of Biological Chemistry*, **270**, 2550–6.

36. Ilic, M.Z., Handley, C.J., Robinson, H.C., and Mok, M.T. (1992). Mechanism of catabolism of aggrecan. *Archives of Biochemistry and Biophysics*, **294**, 115–22.

37. Plaas, A.H.K., Sandy, J.D. (1993). A cartilage explant system for studies on aggrecan structure, biosynthesis and catabolism in discrete zones of the mammalian growth plate. *Matrix*, **13**, 135–47.

38. Loulakis, P., Shrikhande, A., Davis, G., and Maniglia, C.A. (1992). N-terminal sequences of proteoglycan fragments isolated from medium of IL-1 treated articular cartilage cultures. Putative sites of enzymic cleavage. *Biochemical Journal*, **284**, 589–93.

39. Vilim, V. and Fosang, A.J. (1994). Proteoglycans isolated from dissociative extracts of differently aged human articular cartilage: characterization of naturally occurring hyaluronan-binding fragments. *Biochemical Journal*, **304**, 887–94.

40. Cs-Szabo, G., Roughley, P.J., Plaas, A.H.K., and Glant, T.T. (1995). Large and small proteoglycans of osteoarthritic and rheumatoid articular cartilage. *Arthritis and Rheumatism*, **38**, 660–8.

41. Fosang, A.J., Last, K., Neame, P.J., Murphy, G., Knauper, V., Tschesche, H., *et al.* (1994). Neutrophil collagenase (MMP-8) cleaves at the aggrecanase site E373-A374 in the interglobular domain of cartilage aggrecan. *Biochemical Journal*, **304**, 347–51.

42. Yocum, S.A., Lopresti-Morrow, L.L., Gabel, C.A., Milici, A.J., and Mitchell, P.G. (1995). Bafilomycin A1 inhibits IL-1 stimulated proteoglycan degradation by chondrocytes without affecting stromelysin synthesis. *Archives of Biochemistry and Biophysics*, **316**, 827–35.

43. Takino, T., Sato, H., Yamamoto, E., and Seiki, M. (1995). Cloning of a human gene potentially encoding a novel matrix metalloproteinase having a C-terminal transmembrane domain. *Gene*, **155**, 293–8.

44. Pei, D. and Weiss, S.J. (1995). Furin dependent intracellular activation of the human stromelysin-3 zymogen. *Nature*, **3375**, 244–7.

45. Koob, T.J., Hernandez, D.J., Gordy, J.T., and Sandy, J.D. (1995). Aggrecan metabolism in bovine meniscus: role of aggrecanase in normal development. *Transactions of the Orthopedic Research Society*, **20**, 3.

46. Sandy, J.D., Garcia, K., Gordy, J., and Plaas, A. (1995). Aggrecanase-mediated cleavage of aggrecan by cultured fibroblasts. *Transactions of the Orthopedic Research Society*, **20**, 331.

47. Yamada, H., Watanabe, K., Shimonaka, M., and Yamaguchi, Y. (1994). Molecular cloning of brevican, a novel brain proteoglycan of the aggrecan/versican family. *Journal of Biological Chemistry*, **269**, 10119–26.

48. Hughes, C.E., Caterson, B., Fosang, A.J., Roughley, P.J., and Mort, J.S. (1995). Monoclonal antibodies that specifically recognize neoepitope sequences generated by 'aggrecanase' and matrix metalloproteinase cleavage of aggrecan: application to catabolism *in situ* and *in vitro*. *Biochemical Journal*, **305**, 799–804.

49. Fosang, A.J., Last, K., Brown, L., Jackson, D.C., and Gardiner, P. (1995). Identification of metalloproteinase-derived aggrecan fragments with FFGVG N-terminal sequence in human synovial fluids. *Transactions of the Orthopedic Research Society*, **20**, 4.

50. Vincenti, M.P., Clark, I.M., and Brinckerhoff, C.E. (1994). Using inhibitors of metalloproteinases to treat arthritis. Easier said than done? *Arthritis and Rheumatism*, **37**, 1115–26.

51. Poole, A.R. (1995). In *Osteoarthritic disorders* (ed. K. Kuettner and V. Goldberg), pp. 247–60. American Academy of Orthopedic Surgeons.

52. Walakowits, L.A., Moore, V.L., Bhardwaj, N., Gallick, G.S., and Lark, M.W. (1991). Detection of high levels of stromelysin and collagenase in synovial fluids from patients with rheumatoid arthritis and post-traumatic knee injury. *Arthritis and Rheumatism*, **35**, 35–42.

53. Lohmander, L.S., Hoernner, L.A., and Lark, M.W. (1993). Metalloproteinases, tissue inhibitor and proteoglycan fragments in knee synovial fluid in human OA. *Arthritis and Rheumatism*, **36**, 181–9.

54. Ilic, M.Z., Mok, M.T., Williamson, O.D., Campbell, M.A., Hughes, C.E., and Handley, C.J. (1995). Catabolism of aggrecan by explant cultures of human articular cartilage in the presence of retinoic acid. *Archives of Biochemistry and Biophysics*, **322**, 22–30.

55. Fosang, A.J., Last, K., Gardiner, P., Jackson, D.C., and Brown, L. (1995). Development of cleavage-site specific monoclonal antibody for detecting metalloproteinase-derived aggrecan fragments: detection of fragments in synovial fluids. *Biochemical Journal*, **310**, 337–43.

7.2.3   Articular cartilage regeneration
Jenny A. Tyler and Ernst B. Hunziker

Introduction

The function of articular cartilage is to provide a smooth, frictionless articulating surface which can undergo rapid, reversible compression; evenly distribute an applied load; and minimize contact stress on the underlying bone. The ability of cartilage to behave as a viscoelastic tissue, in terms of deformation and hydraulic permeability, relies on the interaction between the aggregating proteoglycans and the composite collagen fibril network in the mid and deeper zones[1]. One essential feature is the fixed negative charge of the glycosaminoglycans which become hydrated, creating a considerable swelling pressure. The tensile strength of the cross-linked collagen restrains and limits expansion of the tissue. Mature cartilage is avascular and aneural. The highly specialized matrix, therefore, also acts as a selective permeability barrier, particularly in the superficial zone, and determines which molecules enter the tissue to reach the cells. The anisotropic appearance, biochemistry, and function of the distinct zones, characteristic of mature cartilage, are rigorously maintained throughout life by the resident chondrocytes and are essential for efficient functioning of the joint[2]. The success or failure of cartilage repair depends to a large extent on the ability of the repair cells to reestablish a hyaline cartilage with physiological mechanical properties.

There are two main types of injury to articular cartilage. The first is acute and transient, involving loss of proteoglycan and other non-collagenous material from the tissue. Many environmental influences induce this type of matrix depletion including abnormal mechanical loading, local infection, anti-inflammatory drugs, and synovial membrane disruption[3–5]. The outcome is usually complete recovery and restoration of a functional matrix, provided that the stimulus inducing increased degradation and decreased synthesis of proteoglycan is not prolonged, and the collagen network is not disrupted. These reversible processes can, therefore, be thought of as a continuous active remodeling, controlled by the chondrocyte, to restore the balance of matrix equilibrium. The second type of injury involves

mechanical severing of the collagen fibers accompanied by a significant loss of cells and occurs due to fracture, frictional abrasion, and penetrating lesions. The outcome is extremely variable depending on the volume/surface area of the defect and whether the subchondral bone or other peri-articular tissues are involved, but in general such cartilage lesions are usually irreversible and do not heal successfully[2,6].

Osteoarthritis (OA) results from a failure of chondrocytes within the joint to maintain the balance between synthesis and degradation of the extracellular matrix. The condition is heterogeneous with ill-defined pathogenesis although genetic, environmental, and mechanical influences have been implicated as initiating factors. Extensive studies on the regulation of chondrocyte metabolism by growth factors and cytokines supports the idea that the relative concentration of such mediators, or an altered response of the cells during degeneration, may determine the rate of progress and final outcome of this syndrome[4]. In OA, for reasons that are not understood, the initial transient loss of proteoglycan persists, despite increased synthesis, and progresses to the irreversible loss of collagen and cells within focal regions of the cartilage and later, to more extensive lesions involving the subchondral bone. The only predictably effective treatment for the resulting pain and disability in an osteoarthritic hip or knee is removal of both damaged and healthy cartilage from the surface of the affected joint, and replacement with a prosthesis. The procedure restores a fairly normal range of pain-free motion and is considered to be very successful for elderly patients[7]. However, total joint arthroplasties have a limited lifespan and will not support the unlimited heavy loading or vigorous use required to provide a quality of life demanded by younger patients[8]. Alternative treatments are, therefore, eagerly sought. As an interim measure, a variety of surgical techniques (described in Chapter 8) have been examined including grafting fresh or cryopreserved perichondrial or periosteal tissues; osteotomy to correct angular deformity; interposing flaps of soft tissue over the damaged area; and introducing a variety of materials such as carbon fiber, Dacron, and Teflon micromesh to strengthen the fibrocartilage formed following perforation of subchondral bone.

This chapter seeks to outline the way in which specific growth factors and matrices have been used to encourage cartilage repair by the chondrocyte. It is not intended to be a comprehensive review of the literature on this topic but serves to provide representative examples of novel, practical approaches that are being explored to optimize, in the first instance, a durable recovering of damaged cartilage and, eventually, true regeneration of this specialized tissue.

Factors contributing to the restoration of durable cartilage

It is well known that lesions which penetrate through cartilage into the subchondral bone induce a healing response that follows a typical pattern. Experimentally, the response has been documented by many researchers[9–11] and is described in detail by Shapiro *et al.* for full-thickness defects in the distal femur of the rabbit[12]. Inflammatory and premesenchymal cells are readily recruited from the marrow space, a fibrin clot forms, and locally released growth factors induce migration, replication, and matrix formation that leads to a rapid and complete resurfacing of the defect with scar tissue (Fig. 7.13(a)). This material is remodeled in one to two weeks to form a covering which resembles cartilage, based on the presence of chondrocytes and a proteoglycan-rich matrix which stains heavily with Safranin O. By eight weeks, the upper portion of the defect contains good-looking cartilage with subchondral bone below the level of the tidemark (Fig. 7.13(b)), and this appearance can persist for up to six months (Fig. 7.13(c)).

The clinical equivalent of these experiments, namely arthroscopic debridement[13] and the introduction of Pridie drill holes into subchondral bone[14,15], is frequently performed as a palliative surgical treatment for knee OA. The risk / benefit ratio is very favorable as the procedure has been said to provide considerable symptomatic relief of pain, albeit for short periods of time. However, no data from controlled prospective trials is available to substantiate those claims. Unfortunately, the repair tissue created by these spontaneous events is mechanically inferior. Within six months to one year, (Fig. 7.13(d)), surface fibrillation, loss of proteoglycan and, eventually, deep fissures lead to overt disintegration of the repair tissue[16,17].

There are a number of reasons for this mechanical failure. Residual chondrocytes surrounding the defect do not participate in the repair process, so there are no collagen fibers which span across the interface between new and old cartilage. Integration is further impaired because neither fibrin nor incoming cells can stick well to the cartilage edges due to the antiadhesive nature of some of the matrix proteins, particularly decorin and biglycan[18,19]. Treatment of the defect surface with enzymes such as chondroitinase or trypsin to deplete, transiently, the cartilage of the small proteoglycans has been shown to improve adhesion of both cells[19] and implanted collagen gels[20]. However, the main obstacle with repair induced in this manner is the inability of the new cells to remodel the scar tissue and develop hyaline cartilage with the typical specialized zonal arrangement of matrix. Unfortunately, we do not have a clear understanding of how these discrete zones are formed during normal development, although graded exposure to solutes from the synovial fluid, differential mechanical loading, and oxygen tension have all been implicated in creating the correct localized environment. Recent experience also suggests that the origin of the cells recruited to induce repair is of critical importance in determining the final ratio of fibrocartilage to hyaline cartilage in the restored tissue. The extreme variability in the success of spontaneous healing induced by debridement procedures from a few months to many years, therefore, probably depends to a large extent on the chance proportion of appropriate stem cells introduced into the defect in different patients. To address these deficiencies, much research is presently focused on the design of novel matrices and the use of biological glues, specific growth factors, and methods of optimizing recruitment of the correct type of cell.

Design of matrices

The introduction of materials such as carbon fiber, Dacron, and Teflon into joints to strengthen repair tissue has been practised for many years[21,22]. Recent advances in biomaterial science mean that specific matrices can now be designed to modify and guide the repair process[23,24]. Matrix scaffolds can be made from a variety of polymers or copolymers including glycolates, lactates, alginates, collagens, and acrylates. They can be used to restore the contour of a damaged joint, to provide resilience to compression and tensile strength, to deliver cells and growth factors to a defect site, enhance cell migration, and create a template for matrix deposition. The pore size and rate of degradation can be controlled by varying the degree of

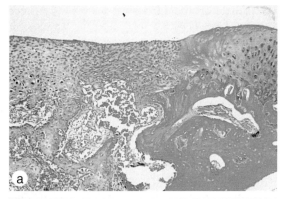

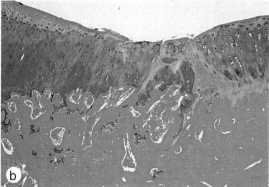

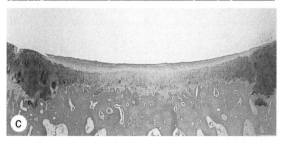

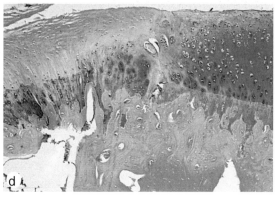

crosslinking and final form of the product[25-27]. Biocompatibility, with regard to cell attachment and growth, can be improved by making the surface of the structure slightly hydrophilic[28], and mechanical properties, comparable in terms of initial modulus to those of natural cartilage, can be incorporated into the hydrogel composites[29]. The matrix design will, therefore, vary for different applications.

Synthetic polymers

One recent report documented the use of a mixture of poly(ethyl) methacrylate polymer and tetrahydrofurfuryl monomer to form a xerogel that continued to imbibe fluid from the surrounding tissues, over a period of several months, following implantation into osteochondral (3 mm diameter) defects in the femoral condyle of mature rabbits. The heterocyclic methacrylate polymer set *in situ* and swelled slightly, ensuring a continuous interface and tight fit with the surrounding bone. Fluid uptake encouraged adsorption of matrix proteins, growth factors, and cells from the bone. An important point to note from this report[30] is that optimal cartilage formation which endured to the end of the eight-month study was obtained by placing the polymer slightly below the surface of the subchondral bone. If the polymer was set lower, it became surrounded by bone and no cartilage grew over the surface; if the polymer was set higher, the cartilage covering was incomplete. One interpretation of this data is that the presence of such a hydrophilic polymer (containing up to 34 per cent water at equilibrium) may have provided a firm but resilient base that protects the growing cartilage from repeated compression. The

Fig. 7.13 Spontaneous repair induced by bleeding. Photomicrographs illustrating spontaneous repair of full-thickness defects in the femur of mature rabbits (18 months, 5 kg) drilled through to the subchondral bone and left without treatment: (a) 10 days; (b) 8 weeks; (c) 24 weeks; (d) 48 weeks after creation. The resin embedded sections have been processed with Safranin O dye which stains proteoglycans red. (a) At 10 days, repair tissue still consists largely of undifferentiated mesenchymal cells, but there is already evidence of cartilage formation (red-stained tissue) just below the surface at the far left. (b) At 8 weeks, hyaline cartilage has formed within the defect (red-stained tissue). (c) At 24 weeks, integrity of the repair tissue is still maintained. (d) At 48 weeks, repair tissue shows signs of degeneration, and its affinity for Safranin O is markedly reduced. From Shapiro *et al.*[12], with permission from the authors and the publisher.

surface properties of the polymer may also have encouraged adhesion and growth of mesenchymal cells from the synovial tissue and fluid, giving rise to an increased population of cells capable of differentiating into hyaline cartilage while suppressing an influx of cells from the bone, some of which favour the formation of fibrocartilage.

Polylactate and polyglycolate have also been extensively used, singly and as co-polymers, to provide a scaffold for seeded cells. The resulting structures are fairly hydrophobic and require a surface hydrophilic coating to establish sufficient cells to lay down a cartilagenous matrix. The original studies by Langer, Vacanti, *et al.* proved that bovine or human chondrocytes seeded onto polyglycolic acid (PGA) mesh could form cartilage in tissue culture that was maintained when implanted subcutaneously into athymic mice[31–33]. The matrix determined the final shape of the cartilage which could be grown on a large scale in bioreactors[34,35]. Metabolites of these products sometimes create a very acidic environment *in vivo* that may cause adverse tissue reactions. However, the procedure is very useful for creating cartilage plugs *in vitro* that can be used for *in vivo* grafting.

Manufacture of cartilage plugs for in vivo *grafting*

Chondrogenic autografts and osteochondral allografts have the advantage that the replacement is confined only to the damaged site on the joint surface, leaving the less affected surrounding cartilage intact. Clinical[36–39] and experimental[40–43] studies using perichondrial and periosteal grafts have shown that these tissues have considerable potential to repair large cartilage defects. However, shortage of suitable tissue and lack of efficient means to coordinate fresh donors and recipients has prevented the procedure becoming more widely available. A search for alternative supplies of suitable tissue has encouraged the development of techniques to manufacture cartilage for grafting.

One recently described system[44] involved seeding rabbit chondrocytes on to PGA scaffolds which were allowed to attach for 48 hours, then placed in a closed bioreactor and kept for several weeks under conditions of continuous pressurized fluid flow to maintain diffusion throughout the growing cartilage plug. Such systems offer a considerable advantage to overcome the mass transfer limitations of conventional static tissue

culture facilities, allowing the formation of cartilage (1 cm diameter) up to 4 mm thick. The ability to apply controlled shear stresses on the developing tissue should also encourage optimal chondrocyte differentiation *in vitro*. In the near future, specifically designed functional cartilage implants could be made to order within a few weeks, from suitable allogenic donor cells. Such materials are, of course, subject to the same problems connected with transport and storage as freshly isolated natural cartilage and osteochondral grafts[45–47]. Storage in culture media at 4 °C helps maintain viability of the chondrocytes for up to 28 days[48], but indefinite storage at subzero temperatures is not possible, at present, as the cells do not survive a freeze / thawing process. Finding a means to achieve restoration of cell function following freezing 3–5 mm thick cartilage plugs is the focus of much active research.

Collagenous polymers

Type I collagen-based matrices are the most versatile of polymers. They are biodegradable, with little foreign body reaction, and can be spun into fibers and woven into fabrics, braids, and meshes, or presented as a powder sponge or gel[49–51]. Experiments to repair defects using collagen preparations alone have proved very disappointing and, in general, are less successful than simple fibrin induced by bleeding. However, major advances are being made using collagen as a scaffold for seeding transplanted cells and as a carrier for growth factors.

Identification of cells with optimal chondrogenic potential

One approach to increasing the number of cells with chondrogenic potential, at the site of repair, has been to isolate suitable cells, replicate them in culture, and implant them at high density into the cartilage defect *in vivo*[52]. Many experimental, and a few clinical, studies have been reported using either committed fully differentiated chondrocytes or mesenchymal prechondrogenic cells derived from periosteum or bone marrow. Clear differences have been noted in the behavior of these different cell types during the repair process.

Chondrocytes as donor cells

Articular cartilage, characteristically, has a very low ratio of cells to matrix. Differentiated mature chondrocytes, when isolated by enzyme dispersal from the tissue, therefore, have to be taken through several cycles of replication to provide sufficient cells for transplantation[53-55]. Traditionally, the most rapid cell growth is achieved by growing chondrocytes as adherent monolayers in the presence of serum. However, during this process they become flattened and modulate into a non-specific fibroblastic-like cell capable of producing very little cartilage-specific matrix[56]. Such cells, transplanted alone, therefore, do not produce durable hyaline cartilage tissue. Modulated chondrocytes, when replanted in suspension as non-adherent rounded cells, or seeded within a gel matrix, slowly regain the ability to express and lay down Type II collagen and aggrecan[57], although the efficiency of this reversibility decreases with the number of subcultures. Mixing cells with a gel matrix prior to transplantation is, therefore, likely to be more successful. Mature chondrocytes modulated to a fibroblastic form in culture are very different from the fibroblastic mesenchymal cells derived from the bone marrow, synovium, or periosteum. They are not multipotential and have a very limited capacity to remodel mesenchymal scar tissue, or to form into calcified cartilage or bone *in vitro* and *in vivo*. Experimental studies placing articular chondrocytes, resuspended in a Type I collagen gel, into cartilage-bone defects, clearly showed a rapid formation of cartilage matrix from the surface to the base of the hole, well below the level of the subchondral bone. However, even after six months, there was no remodeling of the lower part of the cavity to form bone in either the patellar groove or medial femoral condyle[58] of the rabbit knee. The repair tissue, therefore, disintegrated and failed, partly because the mechanical loading on the new cartilage plug was different to the surrounding cartilage on a bony base, but also because there was no evidence of integration around the edges of the defect. Other reports[59], describing the use of chondrocytes to fill large osteochondral cavities in the knee of horses, involved also a considerable influx of cells from the subchondral bone which did give rise to a bony layer within the defect. However, only two-thirds of the newly restored matrix remained at the end of the one-year study, with a high proportion of fibrocartilage present.

A similar, but more complex, procedure was used to fill defects in the knee of experimental rabbits[60,61] and as a clinical treatment in patients[62]. The patients (mean age 27; range 14 to 48 years) had discrete focal cartilage defects down to, but not through, the subchondral bone with disabling symptoms including locking, localised pain, swelling, and retropatellar crepitus. Thirteen of the defects on the femoral condyle were due to trauma, and three due to osteochondritis dissecans; one of the defects on the patellar facet was due to trauma, and seven to chondromalacia patellae (grade IV). Cartilage slices (300–500 mg) were obtained, through an arthroscope, from a minor load-bearing area on the upper medial femoral condyle of the damaged knees, and the chondrocytes, released by collagenase digestion, were cultured as adherent monolayers in the presence of serum to increase cell numbers. The cartilage lesions (mean area 3.1 cm^2; range 1.6–6.5 cm^2) were excised to remove any abnormal looking tissue, but were not drilled through to the bone. A periosteal flap, taken from the proximal medial tibia, was placed with the cambial layer, towards the cavity, and sutured to the surrounding normal cartilage. The modulated chondrocytes were resuspended at high density and injected under the flap into the defect space. A reassuring point to note from this study was that many of the patients gained symptomatic relief from the treatment for up to 16 months. Biopsy samples demonstrated the presence of cartilage-like material in the center of the repair tissue, from histological analysis of stained sections and immunoreactivity to Type II collagen. These were judged to be fair to moderate in treatment of femoral lesions, and poor for defects in the patella. Unfortunately, it is not possible to conclude from these experiments whether the chondrocytes, or the periosteal cells, made the major contribution to produce the new cartilage matrix. It is also not clear whether it is an advantage to encourage cells from the bone in cases where committed chondrocytes are used as the main source of cells. Penetration into the bone serves to introduce matrix and growth factors into the defect as well as precursor cells. The use, in future experiments, of an implanted matrix to ensure complete filling of the cavity, as well as added growth factors to stabilize and promote redifferentiation of the chondrocytes, may help to clarify these points and enhance the success of this type of repair. It may be that transplanted chondrocytes will be most useful for the repair of lesions confined to the cartilage, which do not have access to the bone cavity. However, the problems with poor integration remain.

Osteochondral progenitor cells as donors

Osteochondral progenitor cells, which form hyaline cartilage when transplanted into full-thickness defects, can be isolated from both bone marrow and periosteum[40–43,63–65]. Cells which readily attached were isolated by Wakitani *et al.*[65], either from total nucleated cells present in samples extracted from the marrow, or from collagenase digests of periosteum and selected, by growing them to confluence as adherent monolayers for two weeks. Prior to use, the mesenchymal cells were resuspended within a type I collagen gel, then transplanted into large defects 3 mm deep, with a surface area of 3×6 mm, in the weight-bearing region of the medial femoral condyle of the same rabbit from which the cells were obtained. Within two weeks these progenitor cells had differentiated into chondrocytes. The upper half of the defect contained a matrix that showed intense metachromatic staining with toluidine blue. After four weeks, the thickness of this upper layer of cartilage had decreased, although still thicker than the preexisting cartilage, and was hyaline-like in appearance. At 12 weeks, the repair cartilage was now thinner than the original tissue and, in some areas, the metachromatic staining of the matrix was faint or absent. At the end of the study, 24 weeks after transplantation, the repaired surface remained smooth but was very thin, with some loss of matrix staining. Tissue derived from enriched periosteal cells was less successful overall, with an irregular surface. When tested with an indentor, both this covering and the repair cartilage derived from enriched bone marrow cells was less compliant (more stiff) than the fibrous repair cartilage formed with collagen alone, but was still more compliant than the original normal cartilage.

In all the groups, the subchondral bone was efficiently and completely replaced up to the level of the overlaying cartilage. The osteochondral progenitor cells, therefore, not only differentiated into chondrocytes but, in the deeper half of the defect, the cartilage was then vascularized and replaced by bone in a process comparable with endochondral ossification[66]. Caplan *et al.*, therefore, refer to these pluripotential progenitor cells as 'mesenchymal stem cells', as they can become chondrogenic or osteogenic according to the local environment *in vitro* and *in vivo*, and can be distinguished from hemopoietic cells by adherence in tissue culture. Identification of the specific growth factors which promote lineage progression, differentiation, and maturation of these connective tissue cells to form bone, cartilage, muscle, tendons, ligaments, or meniscus is the focus of research in many laboratories.

One long-term goal of matrix design is to utilize such knowledge to manipulate directly the recruitment of predetermined cell types from a non-specific source. RGD or other peptide sequences specifying particular cell attachments could be attached to the matrix[67–69] or, alternatively, antagonists could be introduced to prevent the attachment of inappropriate cells. An improved understanding of the ligands that promote specific cell migration and attachment of precursor cells in different lineages will, undoubtedly, allow this to be realized in the future. Collagen and other matrix products avidly bind growth factors and have already proved invaluable as carriers of bone inductive materials for the treatment of very large bone defects and difficult fractures, the repair of spinal fusions, and for guided tissue regeneration in peridontal surgery[70–74]. It should be possible, therefore, to utilize our present knowledge of the way mesenchymal cells and chondrocytes respond to growth factors, to induce the regeneration of cartilage in a similar manner.

Transforming growth factors

Mature chondrocytes and their precursors produce and respond to a wide range of growth factors which are classified into groups and subgroups based on amino acid sequence homology; isoforms are sometimes also classified according to the specificity of their biological activity and affinity for different cell surface receptors. Extensive studies on the response of chondrocytes to these factors have been described in detail elsewhere[75–79]. In general terms, basic fibroblast growth factors (bFGF-1–9), epidermal growth factors (EGF-1–6), platelet-derived growth factors (PDGF-1 and 2), insulin-like growth factors (IGF-1 and 2), transforming growth factors (TGF-β 1–5), and bone morphogenic proteins (BMP-1–8) have all been shown to regulate different aspects of cell migration and replication in tissue culture, or during development, at all stages of differentiation. They also regulate and modify the action of each other in the induction of chondrogenic differentiation and maintenance of the differentiated phenotype. IGFs, BMPs, and TGFs can also promote the synthesis and decrease the degradation of cartilage matrix in mature articular chondrocytes and maintain the differentiated phenotype[78,80–83]. However, only TGFs and BMPs are chondrogenic in the sense that they can induce the transformation of mesenchymal precursor cells into chondrocytes, which will either then form articular cartilage or progress through the stages of endochondral ossification to hypertrophy, calcify, and form bone[84–87].

The members of this TGF-β supergene family which also includes cartilage-derived morphogenic proteins (CDMP-1 and -2), activins, inhibins, and the Mullerian inhibiting substances (MIS) share significant but varying degrees of sequence homology with the prototype TGF-β1. Growth factors from this family that have been identified in cartilage and bone are listed in Table 7.1; alternative names commonly used for identical proteins are shown in parenthesis. The most related isoforms, which have more than 75 per cent homology, are written in the same box; while the subgroups share between 35 and 60 per cent homology, as shown[88,89].

One major difference between the BMP and TGF isoforms is that BMPs (and CDMPs) can directly induce bone at non-skeletal sites, *in vivo*, the dimensions of the new tissue being defined by the volume of matrix implanted. The rat ectopic assay system was used initially by Urist[84] and later by Wang[90], Reddi[87], Sampath[91] *et al.* to identify, isolate, and purify the different types of BMP. TGF-βs, when implanted subcutaneously, do not induce bone but form a fibrous,

sclerotic callous[92]. Topical application of BMPs and TGF-βs *in vivo* to skeletal sites such as calvariae[93] or full-thickness cartilage lesions[94] leads to rapid induction of bone formation. This suggests that BMPs can induce chondrogenic and osteogenic differentiation in stem cells very early in the lineage pathway, whereas TGF-βs probably can only act on cells at a later stage of differentiation. BMPs are pleitropic morphogens and exactly the same preparation of, for example, OP-1 (BMP-7) soaked in a type I collagen sponge that induces bone when placed in a fractured femur, will form dentine or ligamentous tissue when implanted at those specific sites *in vivo*. It would seem, therefore, that once differentiation has been initiated in a primary (probably common) stem cell, the local environmental conditions of oxygen tension, mechanical loading, vascular supply (or lack of) dictate the final pathway and tissue form that arises at that site.

Growth factors in the transforming growth factor family can be mitogenic, antiproliferative, chemotactic, or inductive. The biological effects vary dramatically with dose, duration of exposure, and state of differentiation of the target cell[95]. Apart from variations in relative potency, there are no qualitative differences in the range of biological effects on skeletal tissues among isoforms of TGF-β 1–5. However, the temporal and regional expression varies considerably. Mesenchymal cell cultures stimulated with retinoic acid induce production of β1 immediately, β2 after two to three days, and β3 at about six days[96]. Raloxifene (an antiestrogen) increases expression of β3 relative to β1 and β2, which decreases recruitment and resorption by osteoclasts[97]. β3 is found preferentially in perichondrium

Table 7.1   TGFβ superfamily

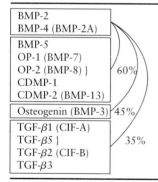

Growth factors from the TGF-β superfamily which have been identified in mammalian cartilage and bone. Isoforms shown within a box share more than 75% amino acid sequence homology and subgroups between 35%–60%, as shown. Alternative names for the same growth factor are given in parenthesis.

Abbreviations: BMP, bone morphogenic protein; OP, osteogenic protein; CDMP, cartilage-derived morphogenic protein; TGF, transforming growth factor; CIF, cartilage inducing factor.

and undifferentiated mesenchyme adjacent to sites of membraneous ossification; $\beta2$ is more evident in perichondrium, precartilaginous regions, transitional chondrocytes, and growth zones of long bones; whereas $\beta1$ is highly expressed by differentiated chondrocytes and osteoblasts, and is readily detected in mature cartilage and bone[98,99]. The exact physiological significance of these complex, multiple layers of regulation is not yet fully understood but clearly they provide a wonderful array of choices with which to fine tune chondrogenic differentiation. It could also be predicted that members of the TGF-β family should be the growth factor of choice to induce, surgically, biological regeneration of articular cartilage defects.

Induction of cartilage regeneration in superficial defects

The failure of articular cartilage to initiate healing, repair, and regeneration is not due to the lack of a source of suitable stem cells. Mesenchymal cells from the margin of synovial joints can differentiate to form hyaline cartilage and bone, and will always do so reproducibly and efficiently given appropriate stimulation. Almost all osteoarthritic knees show evidence of regenerated healthy cartilage covering osteophytes which have originated from such cells. The reason why a similar response does not occur within central cartilage defects on the medial tibial plateau is twofold. The cartilage matrix surrounding the defect is antiadhesive, so any floating or migrating stem cells cannot stick and there is no chemotactic signal from the site of injury because the chondrocytes are too sparse to release enough growth factor. Cartilage also has no access from the vascalature for macrophages, which usually enter a wound and mount a cascade of cytokine production to induce chemotaxis and attract repair cells. Hunziker and Rosenberg understood these basic limitations and circumvented them to provide the first evidence that the natural capacity of the joint to regenerate cartilage can be harnessed successfully[19,100]. Their experimental model used a staged delivery of growth factors within a biodegradable gel to attract stem cells from the synovial membrane at the margin of the joint. No transplantation of cells or tissue was involved. Five traumatic defects were created in the intercondylar groove and medial femoral condyle of mature Yucatan mini-pigs (mean age three years; weight 65 kg) and New Zealand white rabbits (mean

age 18 months; weight 5 kg) (Fig. 7.14(a)). Cell adhesion to the cartilage was improved by painting the surface with an enzyme solution that was washed away after four minutes. This caused a transient loss of proteoglycan to a depth of about 20 μm (Figs 7.14(b) and (c)).

The space to be repaired had to be defined by filling the defect with a biodegradable matrix; fibrin, collagen, and gelatin were all found to be suitable for this purpose *in vivo*. A low concentration (0.2–10 ng/ml) of a chemotactic/mitogenic growth factor, and a high concentration (200–1000 ng/ml) of a transforming growth factor encapsulated within multilamellar liposomes, were evenly dispersed throughout the gel. In many experiments, over a number of years, it was found that bFGF, PDGF, growth hormone (GH), epidermal growth factor (EGF), IGF-1, TGF-$\beta1$, $\beta2$, and $\beta3$ were all able to attract cells into the defect by about one week, and support replication to a high cell density to form a non-specific mesenchymal type tissue mass in two to three weeks (Fig. 7.14(e)). As those cells remodeled the gel, they also broke up the liposomes and became exposed to the high dose of transforming growth factor which switched them into a chondrogenic mode at three to four weeks Figure 7.14(f) shows partially switched cells in the lower half of the defect. By six weeks, a cartilage matrix of hyaline appearance — grossly and histologically — was formed within the defect Fig. 7.15. This matrix stained strongly with toluidene blue and was shown by immunohistochemistry to contain type II collagen. Animals examined 12 months after surgery showed no evidence of degeneration in defects that contained repaired cartilage, and good integration was observed with the surrounding cartilage; distinct zones, typical of mature tissue (Fig. 7.16), were maintained. However, all animals were given complete freedom of movement postoperatively and, sometimes, the gel fell out of the prepared lesions within the first week. This complication would obviously be easier to manage in patients who could be told to use the affected joint carefully for the first two weeks, after which time the migrating cells anchor the remodeled tissue in place. The use of biological adhesives (described below) may be beneficial in such circumstances.

In control experiments, no healing at all was observed in these mature animals, in defects that were left empty, although spontaneous cartilage repair is often seen in younger, immature animals. Topical application of growth factors with no gel encouraged multilayers of cells which filled about 10 per cent of the space (Fig. 7.14(d)). Defects filled with matrix alone contained fibroblast-like cells, but only at very low density, even one year after surgery. Increased cellularity, but still only fibroblast-like cells, were evident as a mesenchymal scar tissue if any of the growth factors were included just in the free, low dose form. Transformation into chondrocytes was seen only if liposomes were present that contained a growth factor from the TGF-β family (TGF-β1, β2, β3, BMP$_2$). If high doses (200–1000 ng ml) of IGF-1 were substituted, a much higher density of close packed cells was observed which remodeled the gel, but remained fibroblastic within a primitive scar tissue and did not form cartilage (Fig. 7.14(e)).

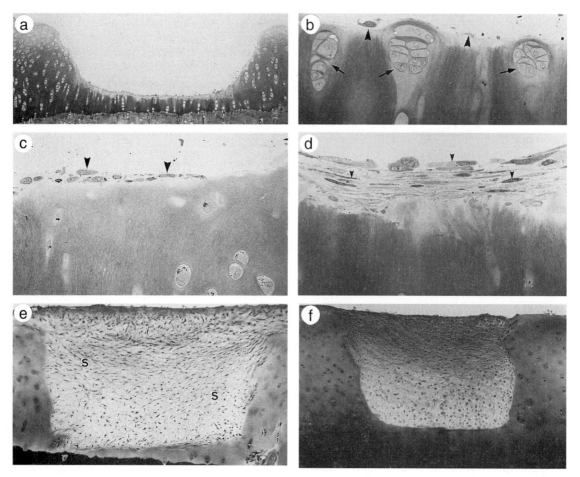

Fig. 7.14 The use of growth factors to induce chondrogenesis *in vivo*. Photomicrographs illustrating the appearance, at 4 weeks, of superficial articular cartilage defects that do not penetrate into the subchondral bone in the knee of: (a)-(d); mature rabbits (18 months; 5 kg); (e) and (f); adult mini-pigs (3 yr, 65 kg). (a) When left untreated, such defects did not heal as long as one year for after surgery. (b) Proliferating chondrocyte clusters were often seen at the edge of the defect but did not migrate into the space. (c) Adhesion of cells from the synovial fluid occurred following controlled removal of surface proteoglycans with chondroitinase AC. (d) Multilayers of such cells formed following the topical application of a mitogenic growth factor (IGF-1, TGF-β; 20 ng/ml), filling about 10% of the space. (e) Complete infilling with mesenchymal cells was achieved only if the defect was filled with a biodegradable matrix (fibrin, collagen, gelatin) containing the mitogenic growth factor. Those cells did not transform into chondrocytes. (f) A chondrogenic switch occurred 3–4 weeks after surgery if a growth factor from the TGF-β superfamily (200–1000 ng/ml), but not IGF-1, was placed in liposomes and included within the gel in addition to the free chemotactic mitogenic growth factor. The illustration shows the beginning of this switch in the lower half of the defect. (a)–(d): semi-thin resin embedded sections stained with toluidine blue; (e) and (f): thick, surface-polished saw cuts stained with basic fuchsin and McNeil's Tetrachrome.)

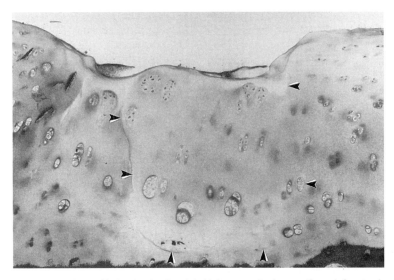

Fig. 7.15 Regeneration *in vivo* using a fibrin matrix. Partial thickness articular cartilage defect in the femur of a mini-pig (3 yr, 65 kg) after 6 weeks of treatment with a fibrin gel containing free TGF-β2 (5 ng ml) and liposome-encapsulated TGF-β2 (400 ng ml). Arrowheads denote the original edges of the defect. Fairly good integration has been achieved, but fibrin retracts on setting and is unsuitable for long-term repair. (The resin-embedded section is a thick, surface-polished saw cut, surface-stained with basic fuchsin and toluidene blue.)

Biological adhesives

Fibrin-based glues have been used extensively in experimental orthopedics to improve the adhesiveness of transplanted cells. In general, they have proved unsatisfactory and, in some cases, difficult to attach to the defect site[101,102] (Fig. 7.15). Recent experiments[103] demonstrated that transglutaminase had an improved adhesive strength, compared to fibrin, when tested on cartilage – cartilage bonding. Tissue transglutaminase is present naturally in cartilage where it plays a role in cross-linking matrices during maturation[104]. Increased amounts have also been detected whenever matrix is fixed within a lesion at sites of repair[105]. Cross-link formation is calcium-dependent and requires a peptide-bound glutamine residue as a substrate to accept an amino group from an adjacent lysine-containing peptide or from a synthetic polymer with a substituted amino group[106]. Type II collagen and fibronectin can both act as a glutaminyl substrate for the enzyme and also form stable cross-links with any lysine containing protein. Preliminary results demonstrated that coating superficial cartilage defects with transglutaminase, or incorporating it within the gel, improved the bonding between the implanted collagen/TGF-β matrix and the defect edges, and did not interfere with any stage of the regeneration process. This type of adhesive may, therefore, prove extremely useful to enhance the retention of matrices within defect sites that are shallow but with a large surface area.

Induction of cartilage regeneration in full-thickness defects

Great care needs to be exercised when introducing growth factors from the TGF-β superfamily into a joint to induce cartilage repair. High doses of free TGF-β, when delivered by intra-articular injection, have been shown to promote inflammation, synovial hyperplasia, and osteophyte formation[107–109]; BMPs, by definition, will induce bone formation at an ectopic site. Fortunately, all these growth factors can be made to bind so tightly to the implanted matrices that minimal leakage into the synovial cavity occurs. It is also important that bone formation, in response to these mediators, is not stimulated to the extent that it becomes stiffer than normal or extends up into the layers of cartilage. In patients where lesions penetrate the bone or where it is deemed appropriate to drill into the bone to ensure a firm anchorage, it may be desirable to use a lower concentration of TGF-β/BMP in the matrix below the level of the subchondral bone than that

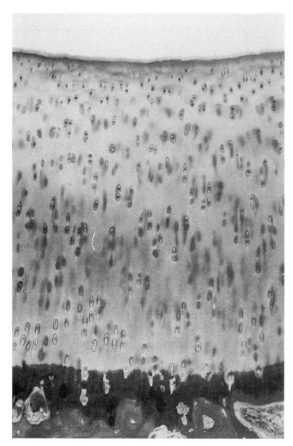

Fig. 7.16 Mature articular cartilage. Articular cartilage from the femur of a mature rabbit (18 m, 5 kg), showing typical zonal arrangement of the chondrocytes. (The resin-embedded section is a thick, surface-polished saw cut, surface-stained with basic fuchsin and toluidene blue.)

required for induction of cartilage formation. Alternatively, for the treatment of very large cavities where rapid bone formation is necessary, the use of a cell-excluding membrane such as a hyaluronic acid film or Teflon have proved successful experimentally in separating completely the two compartments[110]. This would enable optimal formation of cartilage and bone to be defined by the surgeon, and not left to chance.

Conclusion

Our present understanding of the basic principles involved in the successful induction of cartilage regeneration is such that this can now be achieved consistently in experimental model systems, and will now be

adapted for clinical use. The procedure is more demanding than those shortly to be introduced for the repair of bone and will, therefore, take longer to optimize. Ideally, the materials introduced will be delivered by arthroscopy, as a one-step intervention; will be natural products that degrade within a few weeks to be replaced by durable hyaline cartilage; and will be applicable to focal lesions characteristic of early OA as well as traumatic injuries. There is no question that, before long, such methods will enable us for the first time to intervene directly in the disease process, and to begin to slow down the progressive destruction of joint tissues in OA.

References

1. Mow, V.C., Setton, L.A., Guilak, F., and Ratcliffe, A. (1994) Mechanical factors in articular cartilage and their role in osteoarthritis. In *Osteoarthritic disorders* (ed. K.E.K Kuettner and V.M. Golderg), pp. 147–71. American Academy of Orthopedic Surgeons.
2. Hunziker, E.B. (1992). Articular cartilage structure in humans and experimental animals. In *Articular cartilage and osteoarthritis* (ed. K.E. Kuettner, R. Schleyerbach, J.G. Peyron, *et al.*), pp. 183–9. Raven Press, New York.
3. Helminen, H.J., Purvelin, J., Kiviranta, K., *et al.* (1987) Joint loading effects on articular cartilage. In *Joint loading, biology and health of articular structures* (ed. H.J. Helminen), pp. 1046–63. John Wright and Sons, Bristol.
4. Tyler, J.A. (1991). Cartilage degradation. In *Cartilage: molecular aspects* (ed. B. Hall and S. Newman), pp. 213–56. CRC Press, Boca Raton, FL.
5. Hess, E.V. and Herman, J.H. (1986). Cartilage metabolism and anti-inflammatory drugs in osteoarthritis. *American Journal Medicine*, **15**, 1–32.
6. Ghadially, F.N., Thomas I., Oryschak A.F., *et al.* (1977). Long-term results of superficial defects in articular cartilage: a scanning electron microscope study. *Journal of Pathology*, **121**, 213–17.
7. Charnley, J. and Cupic, Z. (1973). The nine- and ten-year results of low friction arthroplasty of the hip. *Clinical Orthopaedics*, **95**, 9–13.
8. Chandler, H.P., Resiuck, F.T., and Wilson, R.L. (1981). Total hip replacement in patients who are under the age of 30 at the time of arthroplasty. A five-year follow-up study. *Journal of Bone and Joint Surgery*, **63A**, 9–12.
9. Convery, F.R., Akeson, W.H., and Woo, S.LY. (1972). The repair of large osteochondral defects. An experimental study in horses. *Clinical Orthopaedics*, **82**, 253–62.
10. De Palma, A.F., McKeever, C.D., and Subin, D.K. (1966). Process of repair of articular cartilage demonstrated by histology and autoradiograph with tritiated thymidine. *Clinical Orthopaedics*, **48**, 229–42.
11. Mitchel, N. and Shepard, N. (1976). The resurfacing of adult rabbit articular cartilage by multiple perforations

through the subchondral bone. *Journal of Bone and Joint Surgery*, **58B**, 230–3.

12. Shapiro, F., Koide, S., and Glimcher, M.J. (1993). Cell origin and differentiation in the repair of full-thickness defects in articular cartilage. An experimental investigation in the rabbit. *Journal of Bone and Joint Surgery*, **75A** (4), 532–53.

13. Johnson, L.L. (1990). The sclerotic lesion: pathology and the clinical response to arthroscopic abrasion arthroplasty. In *Articular cartilage and knee joint function, basic science and arthroscopy* (ed. J.W. Ewing), pp. 319–33. Raven Press, New York.

14. Childers, E.C.J. and Ellwood, S.C. (1979). Partial chondrectomy and subchondral bone drilling for chondromalacia. *Clinical Orthopaedics*, **144**, 114–20.

15. Insall, J. (1974). The Pridie debridement operation for osteoarthritis of the knee. *Clinical Orthopaedics*, **32–B(3)**, 302–6.

16. Coletti, J.M. Jr, Akeson, W.H., and Woo, S.L-Y (1972). A comparison of the physical behaviour of normal articular cartilage and the arthroplasty surface. *Journal of Bone and Joint Surgery*, **54A**, 147–60.

17. Furukawa, T., Eyre, D.R., Koide, S., and Glimcher, M.J. (1980). Biochemical studies on repair cartilage resurfacing experimental defects in the rabbit knee. *Journal of Bone and Joint Surgery* **62A**, 79–89.

18. Lewandowska, K., Choi, H.U., Rosenberg, L.C., Zardi, L., and Culp, L.A. (1987). Fibronectin mediated adhesion of fibroblasts: inhibition by dermatan sulphate proteoglycan and evidence for a cryptic glycosaminoglycan-binding domain. *Journal of Cell Biology*, **105(3)**, 1443–54.

19. Rosenberg, L. and Hunziker, E.B. (1995). Cartilage repair in osteoarthritis: the role of dermatan sulphate proteoglycans. In *Osteoarthritic disorders* (ed. K.E. Kuettner and V.M. Goldberg), pp. 341–56. American Academy of Orthopedic Surgeons.

20. Mochizuki, Y., Goldberg, V.M., and Caplan, A.I. (1993). Enzymatical digestion for the repair of superficial articular cartilage lesions. In *Transactions of the 39th Annual Meeting, Orthopedic Research Society*, p. 728. San Francisco.

21. Brittberg, M., Faxen, E., and Peterson, L. (1994). Carbon fibre scaffolds in the treatment of early knee osteoarthritis. A propective 4-year follow-up of 37 patients. *Clinical Orthopaedics*, **307**, 155–64.

22. Messner, K. (1994). Durability of artificial implants for repair of osteochondral defects of the medial femoral condyle in rabbits. *Biomaterials*, **15(9)**, 657–64.

23. Thomson, R.C., Wake, M.C., Yaszemski, M.J., and Mikos, A.G. (1995). Biodegradable polymer scaffolds to regenerate organs. *Advances in Polymer Science*, **122**, 245–74.

24. Kohn, J. (1990). Current trends in the development of synthetic materials for medical applications. *Medical Developments Technology*, **1**, 34–8.

25. Thomson, R.C., Yaszemski, M.J., Powers, J.M., and Mikos, A.G. (1995). Fabrication of biodegradable polymer scaffolds to engineer trabecular bone. *Journal of Biomaterial Science. Polymer Edition*, **7(1)**, 23–38.

26. Yaszemski, M.J., Payne, R.G., Hayes, W.C., Langer, R.S., Aufdemorte, T.B., and Mikos, A.G. (1995). The ingrowth of new bone tissue and initial mechanical properties of a degrading polymeric composite scaffold. *Tissue Engineering*, **I(1)**, 41–52.

27. Kemp, P.D., Cavallaro, J.F., and Hastings, D.N. (1995). Effects of carboiimide crosslinking and bad environment on the remodelling of collagen scaffolds. *Tissue Engineering*, **1(1)**, 71–9.

28. Downes, S., Braden, M., Archer, R.S., Patel, M., Davy, K.W., and Swai, H. (1994). Modification of polymers for controlled hydrophilicity: the effect on surface properties. In *Surface properties of biomaterials* (ed. R. West and G. Batts), pp. 11–23. Butterworth-Heinemann Ltd., Oxford.

29. Corkhill, P.H., Fitton, J.H., and Tighe, B.J. (1993). Towards a synthetic articular cartilage. *Journal of Biomaterial Science, Polymer Edition*. **4(6)**, 615–30.

30. Downes, S., Archer, R.S., Kayser, M.V., Patel, M.P., and Braden, M. (1994). The regeneration of articular cartilage using a new polymer system. *Journal of Materials Science: Materials in Medicine*, **5**, 88–95.

31. Freed, L.E., Marquis, J.C., Vunjak-Novakovic, G., Emmanuel, J., and Langer, P. (1993). Composition of cell-polymer cartilage implants. *Biotechnology and Bioengineering*, **43**, 505–614.

32. Freed, L.E., Marquis, J.C., Nohria, A., Emmanuel, J., Mikos, A.G., and Langer, R. (1993). Neocartilage formation *in vitro* and *in vivo* using cells cultured on synthetic biodegradable polymers. *Journal of Biomedical Materials Research*, **27**, 11–23.

33. Vacanti, C.A., Kim, W., Schloo, B., Upton, J., and Vacanti, J.P. (1994). Joint resurfacing with cartilage grown from cell-polymer structures. *American Journal of Sports Medicine*, **22(4)**, 485–8.

34. Vacanti, C.A., Paige, K.T., Kim, W.S., Sakata, J., Upton, J., and Vacanti, J.P. (1994). Experimental tracheal replacement using tissue-engineered cartilage. *Journal of Paediatric Surgery*, **29(2)**, 201–4.

35. Freed, L.E., Vunjak-Novakovic, G., and Langer, R. (1993). Cultivation of cell-polymer cartilage implants in bioreactors. *Journal of Cellular Biochemistry*, **90(3)**, 355–74.

36. Brent, B. (1992). Auricular repair with autogenous rib cartilage grafts — two decades of experience with 600 cases. *Plastic Reconstructive Surgery*, **90(3)**, 355–74.

37. Czitrom, A.A., Langer, F., McKnee, N., and Gross, A.E. (1986). Bone and cartilage allotransplantation. A review of 14 years of research and clinical studies. *Clinical Orthopaedics*, **208**, 141–5.

38. Meyers, M.H., Akeson, W., and Convery, F.R. (1989). Resurfacing of the knee with fresh osteochondral allograft. *Journal of Bone and Joint Surgery*, **71(5)**, 704–13.

39. Girdler, N.M. (1993). Repair of articular defects with autologous mandibular condylar cartilage. *Journal of Bone and Joint Surgery (Br)*, **75** (5), 710–14.

40. Woo, S.L., Kwan, M.K., Lee, T.Q., Field, F.P., Kleiner, J.B., and Coutts, R.D. (1987). Perichondral autograft for articular cartilage. Shear modulus of neocartilage studied in rabbits. *Acta Orthopaedica Scandinavica*, **58(5)**, 510–15.

41. Homminga, G.A., Bulstra, S.K., Bounmeester, P.S., and van der Linden, A.J. (1990). Perichondral grafting for

cartilage lesions of the knee. *Journal of Bone and Joint Surgery (Br)*, **72** (6), 1003–7.

42. Coutts, R.D., Woo, S.L.-Y., Amiel, D., Von Schroeder, H.P., and Kwan, M.K. (1992). Rib perichondrial autografts in full-thickness articular cartilage defects in rabbits. *Clinical Orthopaedics*, **275**, 263–73.

43. Moran, M.E., Kim, H.K.W., and Slater, B.B. (1992). Biological resurfacing of full-thickness defects in patellar articular cartilage of the rabbit — Investigation of autogenous periosteal grafts subjected to continuous passive motion. *Journal of Bone and Joint Surgery*, **74**(5), 659–67.

44. Dunkelman, N.S., Zimber, M.P., LeBaron, R.G., Pavelec, R., Kwan, M., and Purchio, A.F. (1995). Cartilage production by rabbit articular chondrocytes on a polyglycolic acid scaffolds in a closed bioreactor system. *Biotechnology and Bioengineering*, **46**, 299–305.

45. Malinin, T.I., Wagner, J.L., Pita, J.C., and Lott, K. (1985). Hypothermic storage and cryopreservtion of cartilage. An experimental study. *Clinical Orthopaedics*, **197**, 15–26.

46. Muldrew, K., Hurtig, M., Novak, K., Schachar, N., and McGann, L.E. (1994). Localization of freezing injury in articular cartilage. *Cryobiology*, **31**(1), 31–8.

47. Malinen, T.I., Mnaymneh, W., Lott, K., and Hinkle, D.K. (1994). Cryopreservation of articular cartilage — ultrastructural observations and long-term results of experimental distal femoral transplantation. *Clinical Orthopedic Related Research*, **303**, 18–32.

48. Scharchar, N.S. and McGann, L.E. (1986). Investigations of low temperature storage of articular cartilage for transplantation. *Clinical Orthopaedics*, **208**, 146–50.

49. Cavallaro, J.F., Kemp, P.D., and Kraus, K.H. (1994). Collagen fabrics as biomaterials. *Biotechnology and Bioengineering*, **49**, 781–91.

50. Kato, Y.P. and Silver, F.H. (1990). Continuous collagen fibres: evaluation of biocompatibility and mechanical properties *Biomaterials*, **11**, 169–75.

51. Macready, N. and O'Reilly, S. (1995). Collagen as a biomaterial. *Inside Surgery*, **11**(2), 89–97.

52. Nevo, Z., Robinson, D., and Halperin, N (1992). The use of grafts composed of cultured cells for repair and regeneration of cartilage and bone. In *Bone: fracture, repair and regeneration* (ed. B.K. Hall), pp. 123–52. CRC Press, Boca Raton, FL.

53. Bentley, G. and Greer H. (1971). Homotransplantation of isolated epiphyseal and articular cartilage chondrocytes into joint surfaces of rabbits. *Nature*, **230**, 385–8.

54. Itay, S., Abramovici, A., and Nevo, Z. (1987). Use of cultured embryonal chick epiphyseal chondrocytes as grafts for defects in chick articular cartilage. *Clinical Orthopaedics*, **220**, 284–303.

55. Grande, D.A., Pitman, M.I., Peterson, L., Menche, D., and Klein, M. (1989). The repair of experimentally produced defects in rabbit articular cartilage by autologous chondrocyte transplantation. *Journal of Orthopaedic Research*, **7**, 208–18.

56. Benya, P.D., Padilla, S., and Nimni, M.E. (1978). Independent regulation of collagen types of chondrocytes during the loss of differentiated function in culture. *Cell*, **15**, 1313–21.

57. Benya, P.D. and Shaffer, J.D. (1982). Dedifferentiated chondrocytes re-express the differentiated collagen phenotype when cultured in agarose gels. *Cell*, **30** (1), 215–24.

58. Wakitani, S., Kimura, T., Hirocka, A., Ochi, T., Yoneda, M., Yasui, N., *et al.* (1989). Repair of rabbit articular surfaces with allograft chondrocytes embedded in collagen gel. *Journal of Bone and Joint Surgery (Br)*, **71**(1), 74–80.

59. Sams, A.E. and Nixon, A.J. (1995). Chondrocyte laden collagen scaffolds for resurfacing extensive articular cartilage defects. *Osteoarthritis and Cartilage*, **3**, 47–59.

60. Grande, D.A., Pitman, M.I., Peterson, L., Menche, D., and Klein, M. (1987). The repair of experimentally produced defects in rabbit articular cartilage by autologus chondrocyte transplantation. *Journal of Orthopaedic Research*, **7**, 208–18.

61. Brittberg, M., Nilson, A., Peterson, L., Lindahl, A., and Isaksson, O. (1989). Healing of injured rabbit articular cartilage after transplantation with autologously isolated and cultured chondrocytes. In *Bat Sheva Seminars on methods used in research on cartilagenous tissues*, Abstracts, Vol. 1, pp. 28–9. Israel, Tel Aviv.

62. Brittberg, M., Lindahl, A., Nilsson, A., Ohlsson, C., Isaksson, O., and Peterson, L (1994). Treatment of deep cartilage defects in the knee with autologous chondrocyte transplantation. *New England Journal of Medicine*, **331**(14), 879–95.

63. Benayahu, D., Kletter, Y., Zipori, D., and Wientroub, S. (1989). Bone marrow derived stromal cell line expresses osteoblastic phenotype *in vitro* and osteogenic capacity *in vivo*. *Journal of Cellular Physiology*, **140**, 1–7.

64. Haynesworth, S.E., Goshima, J., Goldberg, V.M., and Caplan, A.I. (1992). Characterisation of cells with osteogenic potential from human marrow. *Bone*, **13**, 81–8.

65. Wakitani, S., Goto, T., Pineda, S.J., Randel, G., Young, D.V.M., Mansour, J.M., *et al.* (1994). Mesenchymal cell-based repair of large full-thickness defects of articular cartilage. *Journal of Bone and Joint Surgery*, **76A**, 579–92.

66. Caplan, A.I. and Boyan, B.D. (1994). Endochondral bone formation: the lineage cascade. In *Bone* (ed. B. Hall), pp. 1–46. CRC Press, Boca Raton, FL.

67. Hubbell, J.A., Massia, S.P., and Drumheller, P.P. (1992). Surface-grafted cell-binding peptides in tissue engineering of the vascular graft. *Annals of the New York Academy of Science*, **665**, 253–8.

68. Lin, H.B., Garcia-Echeverria, C., Asakura, S., Sun, W., Mosher, D.F., and Cooper, S.L. (1992). Endothelial cell adhesion on polyurethanes containing covalently attached RGD peptides. *Biomaterials*, **13**, 905–14.

69. Loeser, R.F. (1994). Modulation of integrin-mediated attachment of chondrocytes to extracellular matrix proteins by cations, retinoic acid, and transforming growth factor β. *Experimental Cell Research*, **211**, 17–23.

70. Rutherford, R.B., Sampath, T.K., Renger, D.C., and Taylor, T.D. (1992). Use of bovine osteogenic protein to promote rapid osteointegration of endosseus dental implants. *International Journal of Oral Maxilofacial Implants*, **7**, 297–301.

71. Cook, S.D., Wolfe, M.W., Salkeld, S.L., and Renger, D.C. (1995). The effect of recombinant human osteogenic protein 1 on healing of large segmental bone defects in non-human primates. *Journal of Bone and Joint Surgery*, **77A**, 734–50.

72. Cook, S.D., Baffes, G.C., Wolfe, M.W., Sampath, T.K., and Renger, D.C. (1994). *In vivo* evaluation of recombinant osteogenic protein (rh OP-1) implants as a bone graft substitute for spinal fusions. *Spine*, **19**, 1655–63.

73. Muschler, G.F., Hyodo, A., Manning, T., Kambic, H., and Easley, K. (1994). Evaluation of human BMP-2 in a canine spiral fusion model. *Clinical Orthopaedics*, **308**, 229–40.

74. Ripamonti, U., Ma, S.S., van den Heever, B., and Reddi, A.H. (1992). Osteogenin, a bone morphogenic protein absorbed on porous hydroxyapetite substrate induces rapid bone differentiation in calvarial defects of adult primates. *Plastic Reconstructive Surgery*, **90**, 382–93.

75. Adolphe, M. and Benya, P. (1992). Different types of cultured chondrocytes: the *in vitro* approach to the study of biological regulation. In *Biological regulation of the chondrocytes* (ed. M. Adolphe), pp. 105–39. CRC Press.

76. Gospodarowicz, D., Ferrara, N., Schweigerer, L., and Neufeld, G. (1987). Structural characterisation and biological functions of fibroblast growth factor. *Endocrine Review*, **8**, 95–114.

77. Kato, Y. (1992). Roles of fibroblast growth factor and transforming growth factor β families in cartilage formation. In *Biological regulation of the chondrocyte* (ed. M. Adolphe), pp. 141–80. CRC Press, Boca Raton, FL.

78. Trippel, S.B. (1992). Role of insulin-like growth factors in the regulation of chondrocytes. In *Biological regulation of the chondrocyte* (ed. M. Adolphe), pp. 161–90. CRC Press, Boca Raton, FL.

79. Sporn, M.B., Roberts, A.B., Wakefield, L.M., and Assoian, R.K. (1986). Transforming growth factor β: biological function and chemical structure. *Science*, **233**, 532–4.

80. Morales, T.I. and Hascall, V.C. (1989). Factors involved in the regulation of proteoglycan metabolism in articular cartilage. *Arthritis and Rheumatism*, **32**, 1197–201.

81. Tyler, J.A. (1989). Insulin-like growth factor 1 can decrease degradation and promote synthesis of proteoglycan in cartilage exposed to cytokines. *Biochemical Journal*, **260**, 543–8.

82. Luyten, F.P., Yu Ym, Yanagishita, M., Vukicevic, S., Hammons, R.G., and Reddi, A.H. (1992). Natural bovine osteogenin and recombinant human bovine morphogenic protein 2B are equipotent in the maintenance of proteoglycan in bovine articular explant cultures. *Journal of Biological Chemistry*, **267**, 3691–5.

83. Luten, F.P., Chen, P., Paralkar, V., and Reddi, A.H. (1994). Recombinant bone morphogenic protein 4, transforming growth factor β and activin A enhance the cartilage phenotype of articular chondrocytes *in vitro*. *Experimental Cell Research*, **210**, 224–9.

84. Urist, M.R. (1983). Bone: formation by autoinduction. *Science*, **150**, 893.

85. Seyedin, S.M., Thompson, A.Y., and Bentz, H. Cartilage inducing factor A. (1986) Apparent identity to transforming growth factor β. *Journal of Biological Chemistry*, **261**, 5693–5.

86. Seyedin, S.M., Segarini, Pr., and Rosen, D.M. (1987). Cartilage inducing factor B is a unique protein structurally and functionally related to transforming growth factor β. *Journal of Biological Chemistry*, **262**, 1946–9.

87. Reddi, A.H. (1992). Regulation of cartilage and bone differentiation by bone morphogenetic proteins. *Current Opinion in Cell Biology*, **4**, 850–5.

88. Centrella, M., Horowitz, M.C., Wozney, J.M., and McCarthy, T.L. (1994). Transforming growth factor β gene family members and bone. *Endocrine Reviews*, **15**, 27–39.

89. Massagué, J., Attisano, L., and Wrana, J.L. (1994). The TGF β family and its composite receptors. *Trends in Cell Biology*, **4**, 172–8.

90. Wozney, J.M., Rosen, V., Celeste, A.J., Mitstock, L.M., Whitters, M.J., Kriz, R.W., *et al.* (1988). Novel regulators of bone formation: molecular clones and activities. *Science*, **242**, 1528–34.

91. Sampath, T.K., Maliakal, J.C., Hauschka, P.V., Jones, W.K., Sasak, H., Tucker, R.F., *et al.* (1992). Recombinant human osteogenic protein 1 (hOP-1) induces new bone formation *in vivo* with a specific activity comparable with natural bovine osteogenic protein and stimulates osteoblast proliferation and differentiation *in vitro*. *Journal of Biological Chemistry*, **267**, 20352–62.

92. Roberts, A.B., Sporn, M.B., Assoian, R.K., Smith, J.M., Roche, N.S., Wakefield, L.M., *et al.* (1986). TGFβ: rapid induction of fibrosis and angiogenesis *in vivo* and stimulation of collagen formation *in vitro*. *Proceedings of the National Academy of Sciences*, **83**, 4167–71.

93. Noda, M. and Camilliere, J.J. (1989). *In vivo* stimulation of bone formation by TGFβ. *Endocrinology*, **124**, 2291–4.

94. Beck, L.S., Amman, A.J., Aufdemorte, T.B., Deguzman, L., Xu, Y., Lee, W.P., *et al.* (1991). *In vivo* induction of bone by recombinant TGFβ 1. *Journal of Bone and Mineral Research*, **6**, 961–8.

95. Centrella, M., McCarthy, T.L., and Canalis, E. (1987). TGFβ is a bifunctional regulator of replication and collagen synthesis in osteoblast-enriched cell cultures from fetal rat bone. *Journal of Biological Chemistry*, **262**, 2869–74.

96. Gazit, D., Ebner, R., Kahn, A.J., and Derynck, R. (1993). Modulation of expression of cell surface binding of members of the TGF β superfamily during retinoic acid – induced osteoblastic differentiation of multipotential mesenchymal cells. *Molecular Endocrinology*, **7**, 189–98.

97. Yang, N.N., Hardikar, S., Kim, J., and Sato, M. (1993). Raloxifene and 'anti-estrogen' stimulates the effects of estrogen on inhibiting bone resorption through regulating TGFβ 3 expression on bone. *Journal of Bone and Mineral Research*, **8**, 118.

98. Schmid, P., Cox, D., Bilbe, G., Maier, R., and McMaster, G.K. (1991). Differential expression of TGFβ1, β2 and β3 genes during mouse embryogenesis. *Development*, **111**, 117–30.

99. Millan, F.A., Denhez, F., Kondaiah, P., and Akhurst, R.J. (1991). Embryonic gene expression of TFGβ1, β2

and β3 suggest different development functions *in vivo*. *Development*, **111**, 131–44.

100. Hunziker, E.B. and Rosenberg, L.C. (1995). Repair of partial thickness articular cartilage defects. (Cell recruitment from the synovium.) *Journal of Bone and Joint Surgery (Am.)*, **78A**, 721–33.

101. Hendrickson, D.H., Nixon, A.J., and Grande, D.A. (1994). Chondrocyte-fibrin matrix transplants for resurfacing extensive articular cartilage defects. *Journal of Orthopaedic Research*, **12**, 485–97.

102. Kaplonyi, G., Zimmerman, I., Frenyo, A.D., Farkas, T., and Nemes, G. (1988). The use of fibrin adhesive in the repair of chondral and osteochondral injuries. *Injury*, **19**, 267–72.

103. Jürgensen, K., Aeschlimann, D., Cavin, V., Genge, M., and Hunziker, E.B. (1995). A new biological glue for cartilage–cartilage interfaces: tissue transglutaminase. *Journal of Bone and Joint Surgery (Am)*, **79A**, 185–94.

104. Aeschliman, D., Wetterwald, A., Fleisch, H., and Paulsson, M. (1993). Expression of tissue transglutaminase in skeletal tissues correlates with events of terminal differentiation of chondrocytes. *Journal of Cell Biology*, **120**, 1461–70.

105. Upchurch, H.F., Conway, E., Patterson, M.K. Jr, and Maxwell, M.D. (1991). Localization of cellular transglutaminase on the extracellular matrix after wounding: characteristics of the matrix bound enzyme. *Journal of Cellular Physiology*, **149**, 375–82.

106. Folk, J.E. and Finlayson, J.S. (1977). The ε-(γ-glutamyl) lysine cross-link and the catalytic role of transglutaminase. *Advances in Protein Chemistry*, **31**, 1–133.

107. Allen, J.B., Manthey, C.L., and Hand, A.R. (1990). Rapid onset of synovial inflammation and hyperplasia induced by transforming growth factor β. *Journal of Experimental Medicine*, **171**, 231–47.

108. Elford, P.R., Graeber, M., and Ohtsu, A. (1992). Induction of swelling, synovial hyperplasia and cartilage proteoglycan loss upon intra-articular injection of TGFβ2 in the rabbit. *Cytokine*, **4**, 232–8.

109. Wahl, S.M. (1992). Transforming growth factor β in inflammation. A cause and a cure. *Journal of Clinical Immunology*, **12**, 61–74.

110. Hunziker, E.B. and Shenk, R.K. (1995). A differential treatment protocol for inducing cartilage and bone repair in full-thickness articular cartilage defects. *Transactions of the 41st Annual meeting of the Orthopaedic Research Society*, **20**, 170. Orlando, Florida.

7.2.4   Mechanical properties of normal and osteoarthritic articular cartilage
Van C. Mow and Lori A. Setton

Introduction

Articular cartilage forms a thin layer lining the articulating ends of all diarthrodial joints. The primary functions of this layer are to minimize contact stresses generated during joint loading, and to contribute to lubrication mechanisms in the joint[1-3]. When an external load is applied to the joint, the cartilage will deform to increase contact areas and local joint congruence. As a result, tensile, shear, and compressive stresses are generated in the cartilage layer in a spatially-varying distribution across the joint and through the cartilage thickness. The response of cartilage to these stresses can vary markedly, as a result of the specialized composition and structural organization of the tissue. Furthermore, the response of the tissue to an applied load will vary with time, giving rise to well-described viscoelastic behaviors, such as creep, stress relaxation, and energy dissipation (that is, hysteresis) (Fig. 7.17). These viscoelastic behaviors arise from

interstitial fluid flow through the porous matrix and from time-dependent deformation of the solid macromolecules in response to loading. Exudation and imbibition of the interstitial fluid play important roles in articular cartilage, not only by providing a mechanism for transport of nutrients[4], but also by providing the tissue with a mechanism which permits it to recover its initial dimensions after removal of a load, thereby resisting permanent deformation with joint loading[5]. This ability of cartilage to imbibe fluid, or swell, is important also for maintaining non-zero stresses in the material, when unloaded, giving rise to a 'pre-stress' which may be important in load-bearing[6-9].

Normal articular cartilage is able to withstand the large forces associated with weight bearing and joint motion over a lifetime. In osteoarthritis (OA), however, cartilage degeneration results in gross fibrillation of the articular surface, that is, the presence of cracks or fissures, with partial or complete loss of the tissue[10-12]. Additional signs of OA include an increase in cartilage

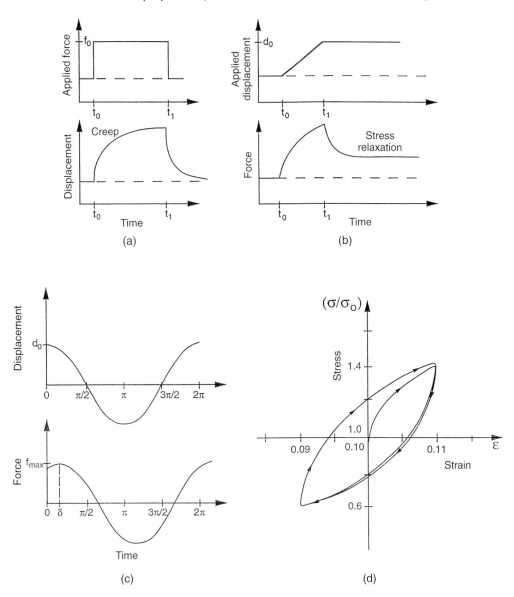

Fig. 7.17 Schematics of load-deformation behaviors of viscoelastic materials. (a) In a creep test, a step load (f_0) applied to a viscoelastic solid at t_0 results in a transient increase of deformation, or creep. In articular cartilage, this transient behavior is governed by the frictional forces generated as the interstitial fluid flows through the porous-permeable solid matrix, and by the frictional interactions between matrix macromolecules, such as proteoglycan and collagen. Removal of f_0 at t_1 results in recovery as shown. In articular cartilage, recovery occurs as a result of the elasticity of the solid matrix and fluid imbibition. (b) In a stress-relaxation test, a displacement is applied at a steady rate, or ramped from t_0 to t_1, until a desired level of compression is reached. This displacement results in a stress rise followed by a period of stress relaxation for $t > t_1$, until an equilibrium stress value is reached. In articular cartilage, the stress rise is due to the frictional forces of fluid flow and intermolecular interactions, and stress relaxation is due to fluid redistribution within the tissue, and to internal rearrangement of the molecular organization. (c) In dynamic testing, a steady oscillatory displacement, or force, may be applied to a linear viscoelastic material, which results in an oscillatory response which lags the input by a loss angle, δ. (d) In cyclic deformation, a hysteresis loop is always generated for dissipative materials. The area enclosed within the hysteresis loop is the energy dissipated (per unit volume of material) required to execute one cycle of deformation. For articular cartilage, the energy dissipated is largely due to the friction of fluid flow through the porous-permeable solid matrix. In shear, the energy dissipated is due to intermolecular friction among the main structural macromolecules (collagen and proteoglycans).

hydration, subchondral bone changes, osteophytosis, altered chondrocyte activity, and changes in the structure and composition of the proteoglycans (PG), collagen, and other macromolecules in the cartilage[10,13-23].

It is known that cartilage tends to 'soften' during degeneration and in OA. The goals of many studies of cartilage mechanics have been to determine the relationships between composition, structure, and material properties of normal articular cartilage, and to determine the changes in the material properties of cartilage associated with degeneration[24-31]. In this chapter, we provide an historical review of the study of structure-function relationships in normal articular cartilage and a contemporary understanding of how the mechanical function of the tissue may change in OA.

Composition and structure of articular cartilage

Articular cartilage may be considered to be a composite solid matrix which is saturated with water (Fig. 7.18). A detailed description of the composition and structure of articular cartilage is provided in Chapter 7.2.1. The water phase constitutes 65–85 per cent of the total tissue weight and is important in controlling many of the physical properties of the tissue[7,18,27,32,33]. The dominant structural components of the solid matrix, by composition, are the collagen molecules (about 75 per cent of dry tissue weight) and the negatively-charged proteoglycans (PGs) (about 20–30 per cent of dry

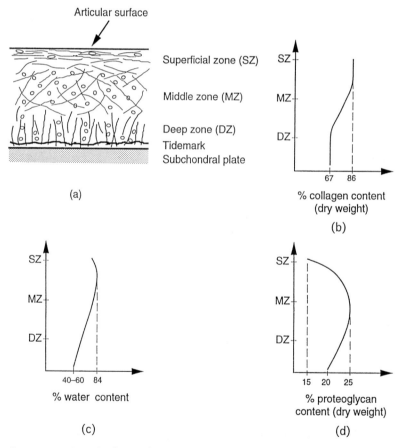

Fig. 7.18 (a) Schematic representation of collagen ultrastructure within a sagittal plane of articular cartilage. The superficial tangential zone (SZ) is a region of densely-packed collagen fibers. In the middle zone (MZ), the collagen fibers are more loosely packed and are randomly orientated in the sagittal plane. In the deep zone (DZ), the collagen fibers assemble in larger bundles prior to insertion into the calcified zone across the tidemark. (b) The distribution of collagen per unit dry weight of cartilage, as a function of depth from the articular surface. Note the concentration of collagen throughout the depth reflects the collagen ultrastructural organization. (c) The distribution of water content (total weight minus dry weight/total weight) as a function of depth from the articular surface. (d) The distribution of proteoglycan content per unit dry weight of cartilage as a function of depth from the articular surface.

tissue weight). Collagen molecules assemble to form small fibrils and larger fibers, with an orientation and dimension that varies through the depth of the cartilage[34]. The PGs of articular cartilage consist of large numbers of aggregating macromolecules, known as 'aggrecan'. A single aggrecan molecule consists of a protein core to which numerous glycosaminoglycans (GAG) are attached. The GAGs in cartilage consist of repeating disaccharide units, each of which contains at least one negatively-charged ionic group (for example, COO or SO_3^-). These charged groups confer a net negative charge for the aggrecan in solution and in the tissue, which has been quantified as a 'fixed charge density'[35]. Most aggrecan molecules are bound to a long chain of hyaluronan to form the large PG aggregates of $50–100 \times 10^6$ daltons. The large size and complex structure of the aggregates serve to immobilize and restrain the PGs within the interfibrillar space, forming the 'solid matrix' of articular cartilage[36,37]. There are numerous additional molecular species (for example, types XI and IX collagen, biglycan, decorin) which contribute to the organization and function of the cartilage. A more complete description of these species and their function is given in other chapters of this book.

The solid matrix of articular cartilage has a highly specific ultrastructure, consisting of successive 'zones', from the surface to the subchondral bone interface (see Fig. 7.18)[23,34,38,39]. Collagen fibers, in the most superficial zone, are densely packed and oriented parallel to the surface. The surface zone is characterized also by a relatively low PG content and a lower permeability to fluid flow[18,39,40]. In the middle, or transitional zone, the collagen fibers are distributed randomly[41,42] or are radially oriented[34,43], and the PG content varies from 10–25 per cent of the dry weight. In this region, there exists a relatively high swelling pressure and high water content[18,23,33]. In the deep zone, adjacent to the subchondral bone, the PG content is again lower, and the collagen fibers are larger and exist in 'bundles' which are oriented perpendicular to the bony interface[34,42].

The mechanical behavior of articular cartilage is governed by a complex set of interactions between the constituents of the tissue, which occur at every scale, from the submicroscopic to the macroscopic. The physical response of cartilage to applied forces or deformation involves physical and chemical interactions between collagen, PGs, non-collagenous proteins, dissolved ions, and interstitial water. The chondrocytes must ultimately maintain the composition and structure of the extracellular matrix[4], and provide for the biomechan-

ical function of the cartilage layer over the lifetime of the joint. In OA, however, the chondrocytes are no longer able to maintain homeostasis. Numerous changes occur in the composition and structure of the matrix molecules, and in intermolecular interactions, which give rise to changes in the mechanical properties of the cartilage. In the following sections, we will review the mechanical behaviors of normal articular cartilage in tension, shear, compression, and swelling; and describe the changes associated with aging, degeneration, and OA.

Mechanics of articular cartilage

Tension

When cartilage is loaded or stretched in tension, the collagen fibrils and entangled PG molecules align and stretch along the axis of loading (Fig. 7.19). For small deformations, when the tensile stress in the specimen is relatively small, a 'toe-region' is seen in the stress-strain curve, due primarily to realignment of the collagen network, rather than to stretching of the collagen fibers. With larger deformation, the collagen fibers are stretched, and generate a larger tensile stress, due to the stiffness of the fibrils themselves[44–46]. The proportional-

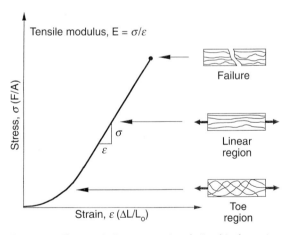

Fig. 7.19 Characteristic stress-strain relationship for articular cartilage in a steady strain-rate tensile experiment. As cartilage is pulled in tension, the stress increases non-linearly in the toe region as randomly-oriented collagen fibers align with the direction of loading. In the linear region, the tensile stress increases linearly as the collagen fibers are stretched, until failure occurs. Note: A and L_0 are the initial cross-sectional area and length of the specimen, respectively. F and ΔL are the tensile force and change in length, respectively, and ε and σ are the tensile strain and stress, respectively.

ity constant in the 'linear' region of the tensile stress-strain curve is known as the 'Young's modulus'. This modulus is a measure of the flow-independent, or intrinsic stiffness of the collagen-PG solid matrix, and depends on the density of collagen fibers, fiber diameter, the type or amount of collagen cross-linking, and the strength of ionic bonds and frictional interactions between the collagen network and the more labile PG network[24,29,47,48].

The tensile modulus of cartilage may be determined from the stress-strain relationship at equilibrium, or using constant strain-rate data from quasi-static tests conducted at very low strain-rates. In general, the tensile modulus of normal cartilage varies from 5 MPa to 25 MPa, depending on the location on the joint surface (for example, high versus low weight-bearing regions), and the depth and orientation of the test specimen, relative to the surface. For skeletally mature tissue, the surface zone of articular cartilage is much stiffer than middle and deep zone cartilage, and the tensile stiffness is greater in samples oriented parallel to the local 'split-line' direction at the surface[24,29,44–46].

In human cartilage, the tensile modulus, stiffness, and failure stress, correlate with the collagen content, and the ratio of collagen to PG[24,44]. After treatment with elastase, to disrupt collagen cross-linking, a reduction was observed in the tensile stiffness and failure stress of up to 99 per cent, demonstrating that collagen cross-linking and fibrillar organization are significant determinants of the tensile properties of cartilage[44,47,49]. In contrast, no significant correlations have been observed between the failure or intrinsic tensile properties and the PG content of the cartilage[24,43,44,48,49]. Significant changes in viscoelastic behavior, however, have been observed after enzymatic extraction of GAGs, including a significant increase in the rate of collagen alignment and, therefore, the rate of deformation, or creep, of cartilage samples in tension[48]. Apparently, mechanical friction between the PG and collagen fibers retards the rate of deformation of cartilage in tension, and so contributes to the transient, rather than intrinsic, properties of the solid matrix. In summary, these studies point to a more significant role for collagen than for PG in governing the intrinsic tensile stress-strain behavior and failure behavior of articular cartilage.

Tensile properties have been obtained for human cartilage with evidence of fibrillation, and for OA cartilage obtained from joint arthroplasty. Table 7.2 presents a summary of data from one such study of the tensile properties of normal, fibrillated, and OA human articular cartilage[24]. Decreases in the tensile modulus of femoral groove cartilage were observed, both in samples from patients with OA, and samples with only mild fibrillation obtained from non-arthritic subjects. Importantly, grossly normal cartilage adjacent to degenerated areas exhibited decreased tensile stiffness and failure stress, similar in magnitude to those of the OA tissue[44]. Apparently, the disorganization, or 'loosening', of the fibrillar network, which occurs with degeneration, is manifest as a significant decrease in both the tensile stiffness and tensile strength of cartilage. Age-related changes have also been reported, including a decrease in tensile stiffness and fracture stress of cartilage from surface and deep zones[29,45]. In general, these age-related and other non-progressive degenerative changes are less severe than OA changes. Aging changes have been attributed to alterations in collagen density or structure, which may be distinct from the 'unwinding', fibrillation, or loss of collagen cross-linking associated with OA[11]. This is consistent with recent studies which demonstrate that collagen fibers in normal cartilage from aged individuals do not significantly increase in diameter and, therefore, maintain a constant molecular density with aging[50].

In conclusion, the changes in cartilage mechanics, with OA, appear to be secondary to structural changes in the collagen network. Many questions remain unanswered, however, about the mechanisms for these differences in tensile properties of normal aging, non-progressive cartilage degeneration, and OA.

Shear

Articular cartilage responds to shearing forces by both stretching and deformation of the collagen fibers in the

Table 7.2 Equilibrium tensile modulus (mean ± SD) of normal, fibrillated, and osteoarthritic human articular cartilage[24]

Site sampled	Normal	Fibrillated	Osteoarthritic
Surface	7.79 (1.73)	7.15 (1.89)	1.36 (0.09)
Subsurface	4.85 (1.37)	7.47 (0.65)	0.85 (0.81)
Middle	4.00 (1.05)	4.90 (1.03)	2.11 (0.30)

All samples were harvested from the femoral condyle in an orientation parallel to the local split-line direction.

Unloaded

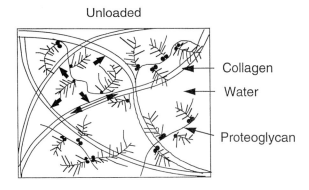

Collagen

Water

Proteoglycan

Pure shear

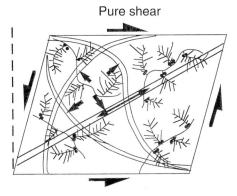

Fig. 7.20 When a block of material is sheared, stretching can occur throughout the material. Maximum stretch will occur in the 45° direction, i.e. the principal direction. This maximum tensile strain is equal in magnitude to the imposed shear strain. Therefore, when a block of articular cartilage is sheared, collagen fibers can be stretched by a significant amount. By comparing the magnitude of the tensile modulus and the shear modulus, the number of collagen fibers recruited to be stretched in this manner may be calculated to be only 5% to 10% of the fibers available within the tissue.

solid matrix (Fig. 7.20). Under conditions of pure shear, the tissue deforms with no change in volume and, therefore, with no significant interstitial pressure gradient or fluid flow through the matrix[51-54]. Viscoelastic effects, such as creep, stress-relaxation, and hysteresis, arise in shearing as a result of the frictional interactions between the collagen and PGs in the matrix. Shear studies of articular cartilage have been performed under equilibrium, transient, or dynamic conditions to characterize the intrinsic, or flow-dependent, shear behaviours of the material[51-56]. The equilibrium shear modulus for normal human, bovine, and canine articular cartilage has been found to vary from 0.05 to 0.25 MPa.

Dynamic shear experiments are used to quantify the dissipation resulting from frictional interactions between macromolecules in the matrix. Values for the dynamic shear modulus of healthy cartilage are in the range of 0.2 to 2.0 MPa, and will vary with both frequency and magnitude. The loss angle for cartilage in shear is a measure of the matrix dissipation, with loss angles of 0° corresponding to a perfectly elastic material, and 90° to a perfectly dissipative material. The values for the loss angle of healthy articular cartilage similarly depend on frequency and magnitude, but generally are in the range of 9°–15°. Several studies have reported decreases in the dynamic shear modulus of bovine cartilage of as much as 50 per cent, after experimental depletion of the PG content[51,54]. In contrast, increases in the dynamic shear modulus have been observed in cartilage, after incubation with formaldehyde, which promotes cross-linking of the collagen network[51]. While the shear behavior of cartilage clearly depends on both collagen and PG molecular species, the relatively small loss angle and large shear modulus suggest that the collagen fibers may be the dominant determinant of the behavior of articular cartilage in shear. PGs may contribute significantly to the shear stiffness of cartilage, however, by generating a large swelling pressure which 'inflates' the collagen network, and thus provides for a tensile pre-stress in the network[54]. This pre-stress may be important in permitting the collagen network to function to resist shear.

Few shear studies have been reported for fibrillated or OA cartilage from humans. Hayes and Mockros[55] observed that degenerated cartilage was significantly more compliant in shear than normal cartilage, and attributed this to loss of the articular surface and of 'ground substance' (that is, decreased PG content). The observed changes are consistent with trends demonstrated for the shear behavior of bovine cartilage, after depletion of PG or collagen[51,54]. Direct evidence of a role for either collagen or PG in these degeneration-induced changes has yet to be confirmed by studies of human cartilage with OA in the shear configuration.

Compression

When cartilage is loaded in compression, volumetric changes can occur due to exudation and / or redistribution of fluid within the tissue. These effects give rise to significant time-dependent viscoelastic behaviors, such as creep and stress relaxation[37,57]. Furthermore, movement of the interstitial fluid is accompanied by very high drag forces between the fluid and the solid matrix, and very high interstitial fluid pressures[7,37]. Therefore, articular cartilage will creep in response to a *constant* compressive load, that is, its compressive deformation will increase with time until an equilibrium value is reached (Fig. 7.17(a)). Similarly, if a *constant* displacement is imposed on the cartilage sample, a transient decrease in compressive stress will occur to a constant value at equilibrium (Fig. 7.17(b))[7,37]. At equilibrium, no fluid flow or pressure gradients exist, and the entire load is borne by the solid matrix. The compressive modulus of cartilage may be obtained from the relationship between compressive stress and strain at equilibrium (for example, H_A or E), which has been shown to be linear under conditions of small strain[7,37]. Upon removal of the compressive load, articular cartilage will 'recover' its initial dimensions, largely through the elasticity of the solid matrix, and imbibition and redistribution of fluid within the interstitium[5,37,57,58]. While the dominant, dissipative mechanism for the compressive viscoelastic effects in cartilage is the drag associated with interstitial fluid flow through the permeable solid matrix, flow-independent interactions between macromolecules of the solid matrix may also contribute[40,51-54].

Fluid movements are governed by the hydraulic permeability of the solid matrix (k), which is related to the apparent size and connectivity of its pore structure[7,18,35,37,39,57,59]. The PG concentration affects tissue permeability, because negative charges will impede hydraulic fluid flow[18,60]. In addition, the hydraulic permeability is related to the volumetric deformation of the tissue during compression, because of the changes in fixed charge density and apparent pore size associated with tissue compaction[59,61]. As a result, both the transient and equilibrium compressive behaviors of cartilage exhibit a dependence on PG content, as demonstrated experimentally with *in situ* indentation and uniaxial, confined compression testing (Fig. 7.21)[28,29,49,62-64].

The compressive creep behavior of cartilage has been analyzed with a constitutive model incorporating both a fluid and a solid phase to describe the flow-dependent viscoelasticity[37]. This biphasic model has served as an important tool for determining the material properties of articular cartilage from compression tests[27,65-67]. In addition, the biphasic theory provides a framework for interpreting and predicting the effects of flow-dependent phenomena in cartilage, under more complex loading and geometric configurations[1]. The theoretical predictions of the compressive creep and stress-relaxation experiments have been obtained, and mater-

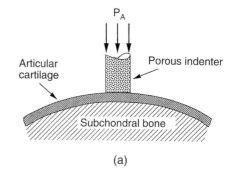

(a)

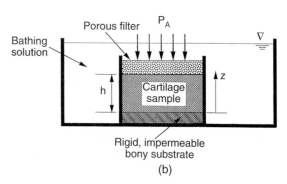

(b)

Fig. 7.21 Schema of two configurations frequently used to study the compressive behavior of articular cartilage. (a) In the biphasic indentation configuration, a compressive load (P_A) is applied to the cartilage surface through a rigid porous-permeable and flat-ended circular indenter, as shown. The porous-permeable indenter allows fluid exudation to occur freely into the indenter tip and, therefore, creep of the cartilage layer. The kinetics of creep are rate-limited by interstitial fluid flow and exudation and, therefore, tissue permeability. This test, along with the biphasic indentation theory, permits the determination of the aggregate modulus H_A, Poisson's ratio, ν_s, and hydraulic permeability, k. (b) In the confined compression configuration, a load (P_A) is applied onto the cartilage sample via a rigid porous-permeable loading platen. The side walls are assumed to be smooth, impermeable, and rigid, thereby preventing lateral expansion and fluid flow. This yields a uniaxial or one-dimensional test. This test, along with the biphasic confined compression creep theory, permits the determination of the aggregate modulus H_A, and hydraulic permeability, k.

ial properties have been determined from the experimental data[27,65-67]. Values for the equilibrium compressive modulus ($H_A = 0.4$–1.0 MPa) for normal cartilage vary with the location on the joint surface, and between species. The hydraulic permeability in articular cartilage ($k = 0.5$–5.0×10^{-15} m⁴/N-sec) is extremely small, indicating that very large interstitial fluid pressures and drag-induced dissipations occur in normal articular cartilage, during compressive loading. These mechanisms for fluid pressurization and flow-dependent energy dissipation provide an efficient method to shield the solid matrix of cartilage from the high stresses and strains associated with joint loading, as the pressurized fluid component provides for the majority of load-bearing in the cartilage layer [1,3].

Values for the compressive modulus, determined using the biphasic theoretical analyses, correlate with both the hydration and GAG content of articular cartilage[3,27], pointing to the importance of the physicochemical properties of the negatively charged PGs in influencing the compressive behaviors of cartilage. During compression, the fixed-charge density will increase, resulting in an increased swelling pressure and propensity of the cartilage to imbibe fluid. This elevated swelling pressure is associated with an apparent stiffening of the cartilage matrix in compression. Therefore, biological factors which contribute to a lower fixed-charge density, such as a higher water or lower GAG content, will give rise to a tissue which is more compliant in compression.

Little is known of the compressive behavior of human articular cartilage with degeneration or OA. Articular cartilage with surface fibrillation, pitting, or fraying is more compliant in *in situ* indentation and confined compression tests[5,30,55]. The compressive modulus of human patellar cartilage has also been found to decrease with increasing severity of degeneration, as defined by both the histochemical and morphological grading schemes[27]. In the same study, the compressive modulus of this cartilage was also found to decrease with advancing age, a factor which was difficult to isolate from severity of degeneration. Hydraulic permeability, in contrast, had not been found to vary with either age or degeneration. The compressive modulus and hydraulic permeability are known to depend strongly on the hydration of the tissue, which may not vary significantly with age. In summary, it is the changes associated with OA, such as fibrillation, increased hydration, and decreased PG content, which serve to compromise the compressive properties of articular cartilage.

Recently, a constitutive model for articular cartilage was developed to incorporate the effects of PG-associated negative charge groups. This model, the triphasic theory[68], provides for explicit mathematical relationships between the material coefficients of cartilage and the fundamental physicochemical parameters, such as hydration (as measured by porosity), reference fixed charge density, and the drag coefficients between water and solid or between ions and water[60]. This theory has been used to quantify experimental observations of a direct relationship between the hydraulic permeability and water content of articular cartilage[18,27,69]. According to triphasic theory predictions, the hydraulic permeability of articular cartilage will vary with the square of the porosity, pointing to the importance of hydration in governing fluid flow, ion transport, and all other transient deformational phenomena related to hydraulic permeability. The high level of agreement between the experimental data and predictions based on the triphasic theory offers promise that the fundamental mechanisms underlying the physical behaviors of normal, degenerated, and OA cartilage can be elucidated with use of this material model.

Swelling

Changes in the hydration of articular cartilage, or 'edema', are among the first effects to be detected in cartilage degeneration and in OA[18,23,28,32]. With aging, a slight decrease in hydration occurs, so that swelling may be one of the few characteristics that distinguish age-related degeneration from OA[58,70]. For this reason, an understanding of the mechanisms which underlie cartilage swelling are of great interest.

Swelling in cartilage arises from the presence of a high density of negatively charged PG molecules. Each PG-associated negative charge requires a 'mobile' counter-ion (for example, Na^+) to maintain electroneutrality within the interstitium, giving rise to an imbalance of mobile ions between interstitium and the external solution. This excess of mobile ions generates an osmotic pressure[6,35,71] which contributes to the swelling pressure in the tissue. Because the PG molecules in cartilage are constrained to occupy a small volume[36], the fixed charges on the PGs will interact and give rise to an inter-charge repulsive force which contributes to the swelling pressure[3,68]. These ionic interactions are modulated by the counter-ion concentration in the interstitial fluid (and, therefore, by the ion concentration in the external solution). With an increasing concentration of interstitial ions, the osmotic pressure and charge-to-charge interactions will decrease, resulting in an overall decrease in swelling pressure of the cartilage.

At equilibrium, the swelling pressure in articular cartilage will be balanced by tensile forces generated in the collagen network[6] and by the stresses developed in the solid matrix[68]. Therefore, the solid matrix is in a state of pre-stress, even when unloaded[8,68]. This balance between swelling pressure and matrix stress determines the dimensions and hydration of the cartilage in the unloaded state. Thus, changes in the internal swelling pressure arising from altered GAG or counter-ion concentrations result in changes in the dimensions of the tissue and in its hydration. In addition, variations in GAG concentration and matrix stiffness throughout the cartilage (see 'Composition and structure of articular cartilage', p. 110) will cause non-uniform swelling throughout the tissue, and will give rise to a 'warping' or 'curling' effect *ex situ*[72,73].

Cartilage imbibes water in hypotonic salt solution, and loses water in hypertonic salt solutions[6,57,74]. The amount of fluid imbibition has been shown to increase in human cartilage after treatment with collagenase to digest the collagen network[48,74]. Furthermore, human cartilage with signs of fibrillation has been found to imbibe more fluid than grossly normal tissues from human ostearthritic joints[70,75]. Thus, integrity of the collagen network is important for resisting the swelling pressures in articular cartilage, with the result that a damaged collagen network is associated with increased hydration.

Quantification of water imbibition after equilibration in a bath, as described above, has been used extensively to study changes in cartilage swelling with aging and with OA[18,27,70,74,75]. Additional studies have focused on measurements of *in situ* water content of normal, aging, and OA cartilage, rather than water weight gain after excision and equilibration. With a method to measure cartilage weight immediately after excision from the bone, cartilage from grossly normal femoral heads was found to have a lower water content than cartilage from femoral heads with OA[70,75]. An important finding was that grossly normal cartilage from sites adjacent to those with 'coarse' fibrillation had a hydration similar to that of cartilage with 'fine' fibrillation. These results suggest that the elevated water content of OA cartilage is very sensitive to collagen network damage, corroborating earlier findings of increased hydration in cartilage after digestion with collagenase[74].

The swelling behaviors of articular cartilage also vary with orientation of the tissue, due to anisotropy of the matrix. With a method to measure dimensional swelling changes in cartilage, strips of bovine cartilage were found to swell to a greater extent in the thickness dimension, than in length or width, when bathed in solutions of varying ion concentrations[72]. More recently, our own studies of dimensional swelling effects have demonstrated that the greatest magnitude of swelling strain occurs in the deepest zone of cartilage

in the length dimension, with virtually no swelling strains at the surface[73]. The differences in swelling strain between surface and deep zones are consistent with differences in tissue organization and composition (Fig. 7.18).

Swelling behaviors of cartilage have also been studied using the isometric tension, or compression, experiment[25,72,76–78]. In these tests, samples of cartilage are held at a fixed length with a tensile or compressive strain offset, and are subjected to a change in the ionic environment of the bathing solution. The transient force response will increase with a change from physiological saline (0.15M NaCl) to a hypotonic solution, indicating an increase in interstitial swelling pressure. The ratio of equilibrium stresses in varying osmotic environments, and the time constant of stress decay, have been quantified for cartilage in tension and in compression. Importantly, these studies have demonstrated that the transient swelling behaviors are highly dependent on the ratio of collagen to PG, and on PG concentration alone, a dependence which reflects the fundamental mechanism for swelling in articular cartilage[25].

Important changes have been reported in the isometric swelling behavior of normal, fibrillated, and OA human knee articular cartilage[25,78], including a decrease in the isometric stress in physiological saline relative to that in hypotonic saline, indicating that the tissue is less able to resist a large, interstitial swelling pressure. In addition, the transient swelling behavior of the fibrillated and OA cartilage changed, as evidenced by a more rapid stress response to a change in the ionic conditions. The changes were significantly greater in OA cartilage. These results support the prevailing hypothesis that the integrity of the collagen and PG networks is essential for maintaining both the equilibrium and transient swelling behaviors of the cartilage. Few additional studies have been performed on human OA cartilage to confirm whether disruption of the collagen-PG network is responsible for the swelling change.

An experimental canine model of cartilage degeneration: transection of the anterior cruciate ligament

While studies of human OA have advanced our understanding of the altered mechanics of cartilage in the OA joint, they provide little information on the temporal progression of degeneration, particularly in the earliest stages of the disease. Studies of experimentally induced cartilage degeneration in animal models, however, provide a means of tracking the time sequence of these early events[79–81]. In addition, they permit isolation of the aging factor from the degenerative process of OA, which has proved to be a major problem in studies of human OA. Many experimental models of cartilage degeneration have been based on altered joint mechanics, including single or repetitive impact loading[21,82–84], and damage to ligaments or menisci[78,81,85,86]. In models which involve damage to ligaments or menisci, inhibition of these force-attenuating mechanisms will alter both the magnitude and distribution of forces applied to the cartilage surface *in vivo*. The canine anterior cruciate ligament (ACL) transection model of joint instability and OA has been the model most widely used in studies of degenerative changes in articular cartilage[13,16,17,19,22,26,56,69,79,87–90].

After ACL transection, morphological changes in the articular cartilage include fibrillation of the articular surface, early loss of PG and collagen fibril organization, increased cellularity, degeneration of the meniscus, thickening of the joint capsule, and osteophytosis[87,89–91]. Biochemical and metabolic changes in the articular cartilage include increases in hydration, and in PG and collagen synthesis and breakdown[13,92,93], and alterations in the molecular structure of the PGs[13,16,17,19,87,91]. Many of these changes occur within the first few weeks after the surgical injury and may be accelerated by interruption of sensory input from the joint[94]. Finally, there is evidence that the changes in the canine knee after ACL transection are progressive, and eventually mimic those observed in end-stage human OA[79]. In this section, we review the ACL transection model of OA, and focus on the associated changes in cartilage biomechanics in the tensile, compressive, shear, and swelling configurations.

Tension

In an early study of ACL transection in the canine knee, decreases in the equilibrium tensile modulus of the articular cartilage were observed as early as two weeks after surgery[31]. More recently, studies of the tensile behavior of articular cartilage from beagle and greyhound knees — performed 6, 12, and 16 weeks after transection of the ACL[69,88] (Table 7.3) – showed a significant decrease in the tensile modulus of the surface zone (average about 64 per cent of control values), independent of site on the joint surface. In addition, site-matched cartilage hydration was greater, and the collagen content lower, in cartilage from cruciate-deficient dogs, than from controls[19,69,88]. Also, there was evidence of an 11 per cent decrease in the collagen cross-link density, suggesting an accelerated turnover of the collagen network at the articular surface[88].

Shear

The mechanical behaviors of articular cartilage, after ACL transection, were also studied in shear in the greyhound knee[56]. A large decrease in the dynamic shear modulus was seen six weeks after surgery (average about 56 per cent of control values), with little evidence of change from 6–12 weeks. Evidence of an increase in the loss angle (a measure of viscous dissipation), suggests that increased inter-molecular frictional dissipation may exist in the experimental cartilage (that is, loosening of the collagen-PG solid matrix). Hydration also increased after surgery (Fig. 7.22), a finding which was correlated with the decrease in dynamic shear modulus. Consistent with the results of the tensile study of cartilage in this model (see above), the changes in shear behavior support the concept of a disruption in the collagen-PG matrix that is not unlike that observed in human OA cartilage (see 'Mechanics of articular cartilage: shear', p. 112).

Table 7.3 Equilibrium tensile modulus (mean ± SD) of cartilage from dogs subjected to anterior cruciate ligament transection (ACLT)

	Greyhound[71]		Beagle[86]
Interval after ACLT	Femoral groove	Femoral condyle	Femoral condyle
Control	27.4 (8.4)	23.3 (8.5)	15.5 (4.5)
6 weeks	23.3 (8.7)	13.2 (4.4)	–
12 weeks	12.5 (2.9)	6.7 (2.5)	–
16 weeks	–	–	8.6 (5.0)

All cartilage was harvested from the surface and subsurface zones parallel to the split-line direction.

Table 7.4 Compressive properties (mean ± SD) of greyhound knee articular cartilage, 6 weeks and 12 weeks after transection of the anterior cruciate ligament (ACLT)[71]

	Control	6 weeks after ACLT	12 weeks after ACLT
k ($\times 10^{-15}$m^4/Ns)			
Covered	2.4 (1.3)	2.6 (0.4)	4.1 (1.0)[*]
Uncovered[†]	5.0 (1.7)	5.8 (0.4)	6.3 (1.0)[*]
H_A (MPa)			
Covered	0.56 (0.19)	0.31 (0.10)[*]	0.42 (0.10)[*]
Uncovered	0.49 (0.19)	0.34 (0.09)[*]	0.36 (0.07)[*]
μ_S (MPa)			
Covered	0.25 (0.08)	0.14 (0.03)[*]	0.19 (0.05)[*]
Uncovered	0.23 (0.07)	0.17 (0.04)[*]	0.18 (0.04)[*]
ν_s			
Covered	0.07 (0.10)	0.08 (0.07)	0.09 (0.06)
Uncovered	0.05 (0.08)	0.00 (0.00)	0.04 (0.04)
Thickness (mm)			
Covered	0.85 (0.17)	0.85 (0.11)	0.94 (0.24)
Uncovered[†]	1.7 (0.4)	1.5 (0.2)	1.4 (0.3)

Results of biphasic indentation testing of cartilage sites on the tibial plateau, covered or uncovered by the meniscus.
[*] significantly different from control, $p < 0.05$
[†] significantly different from covered sites, $p < 0.05$

Compression

In studies of the ACL transection model, decreases in the compressive modulus of canine cartilage were observed at some sites on the tibial plateau, at all time points, beginning with two weeks after surgery[26,31]. More recently, we have analyzed the compressive behavior of cartilage in the canine ACL transection model, using an indentation test and the biphasic theory[69]. Table 7.4 presents the compressive properties of greyhound knee cartilage from the tibial plateau, after ACL transection. Decreases in the compressive modulus were observed in cartilage from sites which are both covered and uncovered by the meniscus *in vivo* (average about 24 per cent of control values). These changes suggest a matrix which is more compliant and deformable in compression, consistent with the changes in human OA cartilage (see 'Mechanics of articular cartilage: compression', p. 113). Twelve weeks after surgery, a significant increase in hydraulic permeability was evident, which was correlated with an increase in hydration of the cartilage (Fig. 7.22). This increase in permeability is believed to be one of the most injurious changes in the mechanics of articular cartilage, after transection of the ACL, in that it results in increased matrix deformations and decreased hydrostatic pressures under physiological loading[1,7,40]. These changes will be associated with elevated magnitudes of fluid flow and exudation, as well as reductions in fluid

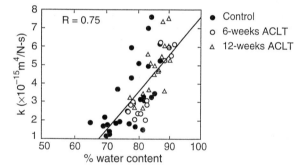

Fig. 7.22 Hydraulic permeability (k) of greyhound articular cartilage from the covered and uncovered regions of the tibial plateau, plotted against water content. Tissues samples were obtained from normal knee joints, and from the OA knees of dogs 6 weeks and 12 weeks after anterior cruciate ligament transection[69]. The line shown is a linear regression line at $R = 0.75$. However, the theoretically predicted quadratic function between permeability and tissue hydration works equally well in describing this set of experimental data (i.e. $k \sim \phi^2$)[60].

pressurization, as a mechanism for load support in the degenerating cartilage[1,3].

Swelling

Swelling studies of articular cartilage, after ACL transection, have uniformly reported an increase in hydration in comparison with controls[13,19,26,56,69,79,89–91]. After equilibration in physiological saline for 30, 60, or

90 minutes[26], hydration increased to a significant extent in all samples of OA cartilage from femoral and tibial sites. Differences in swelling between control and experimental cartilage were as great as 100 per cent. These findings are consistent with the concept that disruption of the solid network impairs the ability of the tissue to resist swelling, as observed in human OA cartilage (see 'Mechanics of articular cartilage: swelling', p. 115). The balance between swelling pressure and collagen network stress seems to be the determining factor for tissue hydration and swelling[6].

Summary

Precise quantitation of cartilage degeneration, and the exact relationship to the mechanical behaviour and function of diarthrodial joints, remains an elusive topic of study. Experimental models of joint instability have successfully recreated many of the changes in cartilage associated with OA, and so provide a basis for studying the sequence of events during progression of early articular cartilage degeneration. In both human joint degeneration and experimental models of joint instability, the earliest pathological changes in cartilage are the deterioration of the collagen network and increase in water content. These events appear to be focused at the articular surface. Further, the morphologic and compositional changes are associated with dramatic alterations in cartilage mechanics, including significant loss of the tensile, compressive and shear stiffnesses, and energy-storage capacity of the matrix; and an increase in the hydraulic permeability of the cartilage. While many studies point to disruption of the collagen-PG matrix as the initiating factor in progressive degeneration, it remains to be determined if this initial disruption is a direct result of mechanical forces or a product of altered chondrocyte activity, such as an increase in enzymatically-mediated matrix catabolism. With a better understanding of the time course of events in OA, more successful approaches to the prevention or treatment of cartilage degeneration and of OA may be developed.

Acknowledgments

This work was sponsored in part by grants from the National Institutes of Health (AR38733), the Veteran's Administration Medical Center, and the Whitaker Foundation (LAS).

References

1. Ateshian, G.A., Lai, W.M., Zhu, W.B., and Mow, V.C. (1994). An asymptotic solution for two contacting biphasic cartilage layers. *Journal of Biomechanics*, **127**, 1347–60.

2. Dowson, D. (1990). Bio-tribology of natural and replacement synovial joint. In *Biomechanics of diarthrodial joints* (ed. V.C. Mow *et al.*), pp. 305–45. Springer-Verlag, New York.

3. Mow, V.C., Ateshian, G.A., and Ratcliffe, A. (1992a). Anatomic form and biomechanical properties of articular cartilage of the knee joint. In *Biology and biomechanics of the traumatized synovial joint: the knee as a model* (ed. G.A.M. Finerman and F.R. Noyes), pp. 55–81. American Academy of Orthopedic Surgeons, Rosemont, Illinois.

4. Stockwell, R.A. (1979). *Biology of cartilage cells*. Cambridge University Press, Cambridge.

5. Sokoloff, L. (1966). Elasticity of aging cartilage. *Proceedings of the Federation of American Societies for Experimental Biology*, **25**, 1089–95.

6. Maroudas, A. (1976). Balance between swelling pressure and collagen tension in normal and degenerate cartilage. *Nature*, **260**, 1089–95.

7. Mow, V.C., Ratcliffe, A., and Poole, A.R. (1992b). Cartilage and diarthrodial joints as paradigms for hierarchical materials and structures. *Biomaterials*, **13**, 67–97.

8. Setton, L.A., Gu, W.Y., Lai, W.M., and Mow, V.C. (1992). Pre-stress in articular cartilage due to internal swelling pressure. *ASME Advances in Bioengineering*, **BED-22**, 485–8.

9. Setton, L.A., Gu, W.Y., Mow, V.C., and Lai, W.M. (1995b). Predictions of the swelling-induced pre-stress in articular cartilage. In *Mechanics of poroelastic media* (ed. A.P.S. Selvadurai), pp. 299–322. Kluwer Academic Publishers.

10. Mankin, H.J., and Brandt, K.D. (1992). Biochemistry and metabolism of cartilage in osteoarthritis. In *Osteoarthritis: diagnosis and medical/surgical management II* (ed. R.W. Moskowitz *et al.*), pp. 109–54. W.B. Saunders and Co, Philadelphia.

11. Meachim, G. and Emery, I.H. (1974). Quantitative aspects of patellofemoral cartilage fibrillation in Liverpool necropsies. *Annals of the Rheumatic Diseases*, **33**, 39–47.

12. Sokoloff, L. (1969). *Biology of degenerative joint disease*. University of Chicago Press, Chicago.

13. Carney, S.L., Billingham, M.E.J., Muir, H., and Sandy, J.D. (1984). Demonstration of increased proteoglycan turnover in cartilage explants from dogs with experimental arthritis. *Journal of Orthopaedic Research*, **2**, 201–6.

14. Eyre, D.R. (1995). Collagen structure and function in articular cartilage: metabolic changes in the develop-

ment of osteoarthritis. In *Osteoarthritic disorders* (ed. K.E. Kuettner and V.M. Goldberg), pp. 219–27. American Academy of Orthopedic Surgeons, Rosemont, Ilinois.

15. Hardingham, T.E. and Fosang, A. (1992). Proteoglycans: many forms and many functions. *FASEB Journal*, **6**, 861–70.

16. Manicourt, D.H. and Pita, J.C. (1988). Progressive depletion of hyaluronic acid in early experimental osteoarthritis. *Arthritis and Rheumatism*, **31**, 538–44.

17. Manicourt, D.H., Thonar, E.J., Pita, J.C., and Howell, D.S. (1989). Changes in the sedimentation profile of proteoglycan aggregates in early experimental canine osteoarthritis. *Connective Tissue Research*, **23**, 33–50.

18. Maroudas, A. (1979). Physicochemical properties of articular cartilage. In *Adult articular cartilage* (ed. M.A.R. Freeman), pp. 215–90. Pitman Medical, Kent, UK.

19. Muller, F.J., Setton, L.A., Howell, D.S., Mow, V.C., and Pita, J.C. (1994). Centrifugal and biochemical comparison of proteoglycan aggregates from articular cartilage in experimental models of joint disuse and joint instability. *Journal of Orthopaedic Research*, **43**, 146–8.

20. Poole, A.R. (1986). Proteoglycans in health and disease: structure and functions. *Biochemical Journal*, **236**, 1–14.

21. Radin, E.L., Ehrlich, M.G., Chernack, R., Abernethy, P., Paul, I.L., and Rose, R.M. (1978). Effect of repetitive impulsive loading on the knee joints of rabbits. *Clinical Orthopaedics*, **131**, 288–93.

22. Ratcliffe, A., Shurety, W., and Caterson, B. (1993). The quantitation of a native chondroitin sulfate epitope in synovial fluid and articular cartilage from canine experimental osteoarthritis and disuse atrophy. *Arthritis and Rheumatism*, **36**, 543–51.

23. Venn, M.F. and Maroudas, A. (1977). Chemical composition and swelling of normal and osteoarthritic femoral head cartilage. I. Chemical composition. *Annals of the Rheumatic Diseases*, **36**, 121–9.

24. Akizuki, S., Mow, V.C., Muller, F., Pita, J.C., Howell, D.S., and Manicourt, D.H. (1986). Tensile properties of knee joint cartilage. I. influence of ionic conditions, weight bearing, and fibrillation on the tensile modulus. *Journal of Orthopaedic Research*, **4**, 379–92.

25. Akizuki, S., Mow, V.C., Muller, F., Pita, J.C., and Howell, D.S. (1987). Tensile properties of human knee joint cartilage. II: influence of weight bearing, and tissue pathology on the kinetics of swelling. *Journal of Orthopaedic Research*, **5**, 173–86.

26. Altman, R.D., Tenenbaum, J., Latta, L., Riskin, W., Blanco, L.N., and Howell, D.S. (1984). Biomechanical and biochemical properties of dog cartilage in experimentally induced osteoarthritis. *Annals of the Rheumatic Diseases*, **43**, 83–90.

27. Armstrong, C.G. and Mow, V.C. (1982). Variations in the intrinsic mechanical properties of human articular cartilage with age, degeneration, and water content. *Journal of Bone and Joint Surgery*, **64A**, 88–94.

28. Hirsch, C. (1944). A contribution to the pathogenesis of chondromalacia of the patella. *Acta Chiriurgica Scandinavica – Supplementum*, **83**, 1–106.

29. Kempson, G.E. (1975). Mechanical properties of articular cartilage and their relationship to matrix degradation and age. *Annals of the Rheumatic Diseases*, **34(Suppl 2)**, 111–13.

30. Kempson, G.E., Freeman, M.A.R., and Swanson, S.A.V. (1971). The determination of a creep modulus for articular cartilage from indentation tests on the human femoral head. *Journal of Biomechanics*, **4**, 239–50.

31. Myers, E.R., Hardingham, T.E., Billingham, M.E.J., and Muir, H. (1986). Changes in the tensile and compressive properties of articular cartilage in a canine model of osteoarthritis. *Transactions of the Orthopaedic Research Society*, **11**, 231.

32. Mankin, H.J. and Thrasher, A.Z. (1975). Water content and binding in normal and osteoarthritic human cartilage. *Journal of Bone and Joint Surgery*, **57A**, 76–80.

33. Torzilli, P.A., Rose, D.E., and Dethmers, D.A. (1982). Equilibrium water partition in articular cartilage, *Biorheology*, **19**, 519–26.

34. Clark, J.M. (1991). Variation of collagen fiber alignment in a joint surface: a scanning electron microscope study of the tibial plateau in dog, rabbit, and man. *Journal of Orthopaedic Research*, **9**, 246–57.

35. Maroudas, A. (1968). Physiochemical properties of cartilage in the light of ion-exchange theory. *Biophysical Journal*, **8**, 575–95.

36. Hascall, V.C. and Hascall, G.K. (1983). Proteoglycans. In *Cell biology of extracellular matrix*, (2nd edn) (ed. Elizabeth D. Hay), Chap. 2 Plenum Press, New York.

37. Mow, V.C., Kuei, S.C., Lai, W.M., and Armstrong, C.G. (1980). Biphasic creep and stress relaxation of articular cartilage in compression: theory and experiments. *Journal of Biomechanical Engineering*, **102**, 73–84.

38. Mow, V.C., Lai, W.M., and Redler, I. (1974). Some surface characteristics of articular cartilage, part I: a scanning electron microscopy study and a theoretical model for the dynamic interaction of synovial fluid and articular cartilage. *Journal of Biomechanics*, **7**, 449–56.

39. Muir, H., Bullough, P., and Maroudas, A. (1970). The distribution of collagen in human articular cartilage with some of its physiological implication. *Journal of Bone and Joint Surgery*, **52B**, 554–63.

40. Setton, L.A., Zhu, W.B., and Mow, V.C. (1993b). The biphasic poroviscoelastic behavior of articular cartilage: role of the surface zone in governing the compressive behavior. *Journal of Biomechanics*, **26**, 581–92.

41. Aspden, R.M. and Hukins, D.W.L. (1981). Collagen organization in articular cartilage determined by X-ray diffraction, and its relationship to tissue function, *Proceedings of Royal Society of London*, **212B**, 299–307.

42. Redler, I., Zimny, M.L., Mansell, J., and Mow, V.C. (1975). The ultrastructural and biomechanical significance of the tidemark of articular cartilage. *Clinical Orthopaedics and Related Research*, **112**, 357–62.

43. Broom, N.D. and Silyn-Roberts, H. (1990). Collagen-collagen versus collagen-proteoglycan interactions in the determination of cartilage strength. *Arthritis and Rheumatism*, **33**, 1512–17.

44. Kempson, G.E., Muir, H., Pollard, C., and Tuke, M. (1973). The tensile properties of the cartilage of human

femoral condyles related to the content of collagen and glycosaminoglycans. *Biochimica Biophysica Acta*, **297**, 456–72.

45. Roth, V. and Mow, V.C. (1980). The intrinsic tensile behavior of the matrix of bovine articular cartilage and its variation with age. *Journal of Bone and Joint Surgery*, **62A**, 1102–17.

46. Woo, S.L.-Y., Akeson, W.H., and Jemmott, G.F. (1976). Measurements of non-homogeneous directional mechanical properties of articular cartilage in tension. *Journal of Biomechanics*, **9**, 785–91.

47. Schmidt, M.B., Schoonbeck, J.M., Mow, V.C., Eyre, D.R., and Chun, L.E. (1987). The relationship between collagen crosslinking and the tensile properties of articular cartilage. *Transactions of the Orthopaedic Research Society*, **12**, 134.

48. Schmidt, M.B., Mow, V.C., Chun, L.E., and Eyre, D.R. (1990). Effects of proteoglycan extraction on the tensile behavior of articular cartilage. *Journal of Orthopaedic Research*, **8**, 353–63.

49. Kempson, G.E., Tuke, M.A., Dingle, J.T., Barrett, A.J., and Horsfield, P.H. (1976). The effects of proteolytic enzymes on the mechanical properties of adult human cartilage. *Biochimica et Biophysica Acta*, **428**, 741–60.

50. Wachtel, E., Maroudas, A., and Schneiderman, R. (1995). Age-related changes in collagen packing of human articular cartilage. *Biochemica et Biophysica Acta*, **1243**, 239–43.

51. Hayes, W. and Bodine, A. (1978). Flow-independent viscoelastic properties of articular cartilage matrix. *Journal of Biomechanics*, **11**, 407–19.

52. Simon, W.H., Mak, A.F., and Spirt A. (1990). The effect of shear fatigue on bovine articular cartilage. *Journal of Orthopaedic Research*, **8**, 86–93.

53. Spirt, A.A., Mak, A.F., and Wassell, R.P. (1989). Nonlinear viscoelastic properties of articular cartilage in shear. *Journal of Orthopaedic Research*, **7**, 43–9.

54. Zhu, W.B., Mow, V.C., Koob, T.J., and Eyre, D.R. (1993). Viscoelastic shear properties of articular cartilage and the effects of glycosidase treatment. *Journal of Orthopaedic Research*, **11**, 771–81.

55. Hayes, W.C. and Mockros, L.F. (1971). Viscoelastic properties of human articular cartilage. *Journal of Applied Physiology*, **31**, 562–8.

56. McCutchen, C.W. (1962). The frictional properties of animal joints. *Wear*, **5**, 1–17.

57. Setton, L.A., Mow, V.C., and Howell, D.S. (1995a). Changes in the shear properties of canine knee cartilage resulting from anterior cruciate transection. *Journal of Orthopaedic Research*, **13**, 473–82.

58. Linn, F.C. and Sokoloff, L. (1965). Movement and composition of interstitial fluid of cartilage. *Arthritis and Rheumatism*, **8**, 481–94.

59. Lai, W.M. and Mow, V.C. (1980). Drag-induced compression of articular cartilage during a permeation experiment. *Biorheology*, **17**, 111–23.

60. Gu, W.Y., Lai, W.M., and Mow, V.C. (1993). Transport of fluid and ions through a porous-permeable charged-hydrated tissue, and streaming potential data on normal bovine articular cartilage. *Journal of Biomechanics*, **26**, 709–23.

61. Mansour, J.M. and Mow, V.C. (1976). The permeability of articular cartilage under compressive strain and at high pressures. *Journal of Bone and Joint Surgery*, **58A**, 509–16.

62. Bader, D.L., Kempson, K.E., Egan, J., Gilbey, W., and Barrett, A.J. (1992). The effects of selective matrix degradation on the short-term compressive properties of adult human articular cartilage. *Biochimica et Biophysica Acta*, **1116**, 147–54.

63. Kempson, G.E., Muir, H., Swanson, S.A.V., and Freeman, M.A.R. (1970). Correlations between stiffness and the chemical constituents of cartilage on the human femoral head. *Biochimica et Biophysica Acta*, **215**, 70–7.

64. Stahurski, T.M., Armstrong, C.G., and Mow, V.C. (1981). Variation of the intrinsic aggregate modulus and permeability of articular cartilage with trypsin digestion. *ASME Biomechanics Symposium*, **AMD-43**, 137–40.

65. Athanasiou, K.A., Rosenwasser, M.P., Buckwalter, J.A., Malinin, T.I., and Mow, V.C. (1991). Interspecies comparisons of *in situ* intrinsic mechanical properties of distal femoral cartilage. *Journal of Orthopaedic Research*, **9**, 330–40.

66. Athanasiou, K.A., Agarwal, A., Muffoletto, A., Dzida, F.J., Constantinides, G., and Clem, M. (1995). Biomechanical properties of hip cartilage in experimental animal models. *Clinical Orthopaedics and Related Research*, **316**, 254–66.

67. Mow, V.C., Gibbs, M.C., Lai, W.M., Zhu, W., and Athanasiou, K.A. (1989a). Biphasic indentation of articular cartilage — part II. A numerical algorithm and an experimental study. *Journal of Biomechanics*, **22**, 853–61.

68. Lai, W.M., Hou, J.S., and Mow, V.C. (1991). A triphasic theory for the swelling and deformation behaviors of articular cartilage. *Journal of Biomechanical Engineering*, **113**, 245–58.

69. Setton, L.A., Mow, V.C., Muller, F.J., Pita, J.C., and Howell, D.S. (1994a). Mechanical properties of canine articular cartilage are significantly altered following transection of the anterior cruciate ligament. *Journal of Orthopaedic Research*, **12**, 451–63.

70. Grushko, G., Schneiderman, R., and Maroudas, A. (1989). Some biochemical and biophysical parameters for the study of the pathogenesis of osteoarthritis. A comparison between the process of aging and degeneration in human hip cartilage. *Connective Tissue Research*, **19**, 149–76.

71. Donnan, F.G. (1924). The theory of membrane equilibria. *Chemical Reviews*, **1**, 73–90.

72. Myers, E.R., Lai, W.M., and Mow, V.C. (1984). A continuum theory and an experiment for the ion-induced swelling behavior of articular cartilage. *Journal of Biomechanical Engineering*, **106**, 151–8.

73. Setton, L.A., Tohyama, H., Lai, W.M., Guilak, F., and Mow, V.C. (1994b). Experimental measurement of the *in vitro* curling behavior of articular cartilage. *ASME Advances in Bioengineering*, **BED-28**, 135–6.

74. Maroudas, A. and Venn, M. (1977). Chemical composition and swelling of normal and osteoarthritic femoral head cartilage. II. Swelling. *Annals of the Rheumatic Diseases*, **36**, 399–406.

75. Brocklehurst, R., Bayliss, M.T., Maroudas, A., Coysh, H.L., Freeman, M.A.R., Revell, P.A., and Ali, S.Y. (1984). The composition of normal and osteoarthritic articular cartilage from human knee joints. *Journal of Bone and Joint Surgery*, **66A**, 95–106.

76. Eisenberg, S.R. and Grodzinsky, A.J. (1987). The kinetics of chemically induced non-equilibrium swelling of articular cartilage and corneal stroma. *Journal of Biomechanical Engineering*, **109**, 79–89.

77. Grodzinsky, A.J., Roth, V., Myers, E.R., Grossman, W.D., and Mow, V.C. (1981). The significance of electromechanical and osmotic forces in the non-equilibrium swelling behavior of articular cartilage in tension. *Journal of Biomechanical Engineering*, **103**, 221–31.

78. Takei, T., Myers, E.R., and Mow, V.C. (1984). Quantitation of tensile and swelling behavior of mildly fibrillated human articular cartilage. *Transactions of the Orthopaedic Research Society*, **9**, 365.

79. Brandt, K.D., Braunstein, E.M., Visco, D.M., O'Conner, B., Heck, D., and Albrecht, M. (1991). Anterior (cranial) cruciate ligament transection in the dog: a bona fide model of osteoarthritis, not merely of cartilage injury and repair. *Journal of Rheumatology*, **18**, 436–46.

80. Moskowitz, R.W. (1992). Experimental models of osteoarthritis. In *Osteoarthritis: diagnosis and medical-/surgical management II* (ed. R.W. Moskowitz *et al.*), pp. 213–32. W.B. Saunders and Co, Philadelphia.

81. Pritzker, K.P.H. (1994). Animal models of osteoarthritis: processes, problems and prospects. *Annals of the Rheumatic Diseases*, **53**, 406–20.

82. Armstrong, C.G., Mow, V.C., and Wirth, C.R. (1985). Biomechanics of impact-induced microdamage to articular cartilage: a possible genesis for chondromalacia patella. In *The knee*, Symposium on Sports Medicine (ed. G.A.M. Finerman), pp. 70–84. C.V. Mosby, St Louis, Missouri.

83. Radin, E.L. and Paul, I.L. (1971). Response of joints to impact loading. I: *in vitro* wear. *Arthritis and Rheumatism*, **14**, 356–62.

84. Thompson, R.C., Oegema, T.R., Lewis, J.L., and Wallace, L. (1991). Osteoarthrotic changes after acute transarticular load, an animal model. *Journal of Bone and Joint Surgery*, **73A**, 990–1001.

85. Moskowitz, R.W., Davis, W., and Sammarco, J. (1973). Experimentally induced degenerative joint lesions following partial meniscectomy in the rabbit. *Arthritis and Rheumatism*, **16**, 397–405.

86. Pond, M.J. and Nuki, G. (1973). Experimentally induced osteoarthritis in the dog. *Annals of the Rheumatic Diseases*, **32**, 387–8.

87. Dunham, J., Shackleton, D.R., Nahir, A.M., Billingham, M.E.J., Bitensky, L., Chayen, J., *et al.* (1985). Altered orientation of GAGs and cellular changes in the tibial cartilage in the first two weeks of experimental OA. *Journal of Orthopaedic Research*, **3**, 258–68.

88. Guilak, F., Ratcliffe, A., Lane, N., Rosenwasser, M.P., and Mow, V.C. (1994). Mechanical and biochemical changes in the superficial zone of articular cartilage in a canine model of osteoarthritis. *Journal of Orthopaedic Research*, **12**, 474–84.

89. McDevitt, C. and Muir, H. (1976). Biochemical changes in the cartilage of the knee in experimental and natural osteoarthritis in the dog. *Journal of Bone and Joint Surgery*, **58B**, 94–101.

90. McDevitt, C., Gilbertson, E., and Muir, H. (1977). An experimental model of osteoarthritis: early morphological and biochemical changes. *Journal of Bone and Joint Surgery*, **59B**, 24–35.

91. Sandy, J.D., Adams, M.E., Billingham, M.E.J., Plaas, A., and Muir, H. (1984). *In vivo* and *in vitro* stimulation of chondrocyte biosynthetic activity in early experimental osteoarthritis. *Arthritis and Rheumatism*, **27**, 388–97.

92. Ratcliffe, A., Beauvais, P.J., and Saed-Nejad, F. (1994). Differential levels of aggrecan aggregate components in synovial fluids from canine knee joints with experimental osteoarthritis and disuse. *Journal of Orthopaedic Research*, **12**, 464–73.

93. Eyre, D.R., McDevitt, C.A., Billingham, M.E.J., and Muir, H. (1980). Biosynthesis of collagen and other matrix components by articular cartilage in experimental osteoarthritis. *Biochemical Journal*, **188**, 823–37.

94. O'Connor, B.L., Visco, D.M., Brandt, K.D., Myers, S.L., and Kalasinski, L.A. (1992). Neurogenic acceleration of osteoarthrosis. *Journal of Bone and Joint Surgery*, **74A**, 367–76.

7.2.5   Response of the chondrocyte to mechanical stimuli

Alan J. Grodzinsky, Young-Jo Kim, Michael D. Buschmann, A. Minerva Garcia, Thomas M. Quinn, and Ernst B. Hunziker

Introduction

Articular cartilage functions as a weight-bearing, wear-resistant material in synovial joints. Cartilage is subjected to a wide range of static and dynamic loading conditions, with peak stress amplitudes reaching 10–20 MPa (100–200 atmospheres) during activities such as stair climbing[1]. The ability of cartilage to withstand compressive, tensile, and shear forces depends critically on the composition and structural integrity of its extracellular matrix (ECM). The maintenance of a functionally intact ECM requires the chondrocyte-mediated synthesis, assembly, and degradation of proteoglycans, collagens, non-collagenous proteins and glycoproteins, and other matrix molecules[2]. The regulation of these metabolic processes *in vivo* appears to involve a combination of cell biological and physical mechanisms.

Clinical observations and animal studies *in vivo* suggest that joint loading and motion can induce a wide range of metabolic responses in cartilage[3]. *Immobilization* or reduced loading can cause profound decreases in aggrecan synthesis and content[4-7] and a resultant softening of the tissue[8]. In contrast, aggrecan concentration is often higher in areas of habitually loaded cartilage[9], and can be further increased by *dynamic* loading or remobilization of a joint[4,10,11], with concomitant restoration of biomechanical properties[8]. More severe *static*[12], *impact*[13], or strenuous exercise loading[14]. can cause cartilage degradation with osteoarthritic changes[14,15]. Thus, while some degree of normal joint loading appears to promote structural adaptation, abnormal mechanical forces predispose cartilage to degeneration[16].

The cell biological and biophysical transduction mechanisms by which chondrocytes respond to mechanical stimuli are not fully understood and are difficult to identify *in vivo*. Complexities include quantifying the biomechanics of loading, and distinguishing between direct effects of loading on cartilage metabolism and indirect (for example, loading-induced systemic) effects. An understanding of the cellular transduction mechanisms is further complicated by the important and complex role of the ECM and chondrocyte-ECM interactions[17]. Thus, the use of isolated chondrocytes devoid of matrix may not be appropriate for testing hypotheses on mechanisms[17]; conclusions would have to be interpreted with caution. As a result, cartilage explant systems and chondrocyte / gel-substrate culture systems have become increasingly important in the study of chondrocyte response to loading, since chondrocyte phenotypic expression and cell-matrix structure is preserved in these model systems.

Many physical phenomena which occur in cartilage during loading *in vivo* have been identified and quantified *in vitro*: compression of cartilage results in deformation of cells and extracellular matrix[18-21], hydrostatic pressure gradients, fluid flow, streaming potentials and currents[22-24]; and physiochemical changes including altered matrix water content, fixed charge density, mobile ion concentrations, and osmotic pressure[25-29]. Any of these mechanical, chemical, or electrical phenomena may modulate matrix metabolism (Fig. 7.23). An understanding of the spatial distribution of these forces and flows within cartilage, during compression, has been aided by the development of theoretical models for the mechanical[30,31], physicochemical[32,33], and electromechanical[34] behavior of cartilage. Such models can provide a useful framework for correlating the spatial distributions of biosynthesis and physical stimuli that occur within cartilage explants during compression[24,35]. Below, we review the results of studies designed to quantify the nature and kinetics of chondrocyte metabolic response to known mechanical stimuli, and then highlight recent *in vitro* studies designed to explore mechanotransduction mechanisms.

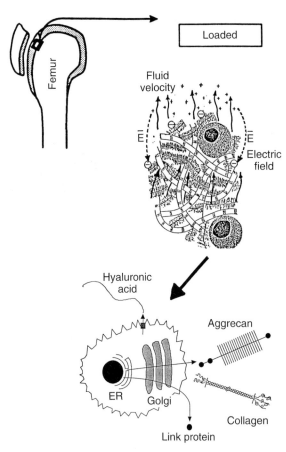

Fig. 7.23 Schematic of fluid flows and electric fields caused by dynamic compression of cartilage, which can modulate cell synthesis of matrix macromolecules including aggrecan, link protein, hyaluronan, and collagen (data from[42]).

Effects of static / dynamic compression on matrix synthesis

Geometrically defined cartilage explants can be maintained *in vitro* in a stable and controlled biochemical and physical environment, suitable for testing the effects of mechanical stimuli on biosynthesis[36]. Calf and adult bovine cartilage explants have been most commonly used; they can attain steady-state levels of aggrecan synthesis[37], loss, and aggregation with hyaluronan and link protein[38], suitable for studying perturbations caused by applied mechanical stimuli. Investigators have also used human[39], canine[40], and other tissue sources.

The application of mechanical compression directly to cartilage explants, using a range of amplitudes and

frequencies, has been motivated by the physiologically relevant loading parameters used in animal studies. The qualitative trends seen in these animal studies have been substantiated and amplified using explant models: (1) static compression has been shown to significantly inhibit biosynthesis of proteoglycans and proteins[27,39–43], while (2) dynamic compression can markedly stimulate matrix production[42,44–49]. The response to dynamic compression, however, depends on compression frequency. For example, biosynthesis in 3 mm diameter explants was not affected by low strain amplitude (1–4 per cent) unconfined compression at low frequency (<0.001 Hz), while aggrecan and protein synthesis in these same explants were stimulated by compression at higher frequencies (0.01–1 Hz)[42] (Fig. 7.24(a)). Chondrocytes cultured in agarose also exhibited inhibition of synthesis in response to static compression and stimulation of synthesis under 0.01–1 Hz dynamic compression[50], but only after the cells had synthesized and deposited *de novo* a dense extracellular matrix.

Several physical mechanisms (that is, the physical and chemical signals) may regulate the chondrocyte metabolic response to these static and dynamic compression regimes. Static compression has been shown to reduce the rate of transport of macromolecules, due to reduced average ECM pore size[41]; change local ion concentrations, including pH, in the pericellular matrix, via the Donnan effect[27–29]; and alter cell and nucleus structure[20,21,51]. Dynamic compression can additionally superimpose fluid flows, pressure gradients, and streaming currents or potentials[22–24]. *In vitro* explant systems have the potential to be quantitative and specific in relating mechanical and biological parameters; selected examples are described in more detail below.

Kinetics of proteoglycan and protein biosynthetic response to compression

Measurements of the rate at which chondrocytes can sense and respond to mechanical stimuli can give insight regarding intracellular biosynthetic pathways and extracellular processing times. Previous studies have revealed that the inhibition of biosynthesis during static compression can occur as rapidly as one hour after application of compression[42,52]. Recovery of biosynthesis after release of static compression can be

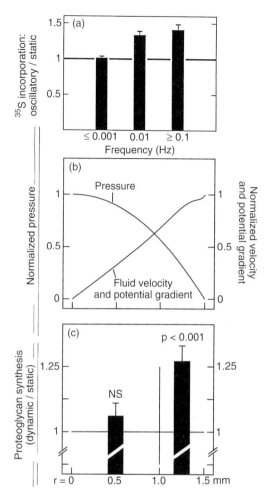

Fig. 7.24 (a) Effect of compression frequency on proteoglycan synthesis in cartilage explants; (b) normalized profiles of intratissue fluid velocity, streaming potential field, and hydrostatic pressure as a function of radial position within 3 mm diameter cartilage disks subjected to dynamic compression at 0.1 Hz (from [24]); (c) measured proteoglycan synthesis (^{35}S-sulfate incorporation) in the 2 mm diameter core and the outer ring of 3 mm diameter disks compressed at 0.1 Hz, relative to statically held controls (data from [24,49]).

onment with increasing durations of static compression; protein synthesis may be initially blocked. Over time, the concentration of enzymes necessary for glycosylation may decrease, and hence, the longer the time necessary for recovery of aggrecan synthesis with increased duration of compression. Compression-induced changes in cell and matrix morphology may also become less reversible with increased duration of compression.

Regarding intracellular processing, the intracellular aggrecan core protein *pool size* was observed to decrease by 50 per cent in response to a 25 per cent static compression, whereas the *intracellular rate of processing* of core protein into proteoglycan was unaffected by compression[53]. In contrast, four hours after release of a 50 per cent static compression, core protein pool size remained significantly decreased, and the rate of intracellular processing into proteoglycan was two-fold slower[53]. Extracellular processing of newly-synthesized aggrecan into proteoglycan aggregates has also been found to be sensitive to compression: the extracellular conversion of aggrecan to a form capable of binding with hyaluronan was delayed by static compression, in a dose-dependent manner that appeared related to the change in intratissue pH induced by compression[54]. Regarding dynamic compression, after cessation of a one-day dynamic compression (5 per cent sinusoidal strain amplitude at 0.1 Hz), proteoglycan synthesis returned to control levels after about 24 hours, while protein synthesis returned within a few hours (Kim Y.-J., unpublished results).

Forces and flows during dynamic compression: role of specific mechanical stimuli

To explore the effect of the dynamic component of compression on biosynthesis, Sah *et al.*[42] and Kim *et al.*[49] applied small amplitude, cyclic, unconfined compressions to cartilage disks, superimposed on a static offset compression. Experimental and control explants were subjected to the same level of static offset compression. Since low amplitude dynamic compression did not significantly alter the average water content or fixed charge density of the cartilage disks, there were negligible changes in the physiochemical status of the tissue[55]. In this manner, the effects of oscillatory deformation of cells and matrix, fluid flow, streaming potentials, and hydrostatic pressure could be explored

much slower, and depends on the duration and amplitude of the static compression prior to release[40,42,43,52]. After a two-hour static compression followed by release, aggrecan synthesis recovered fully in another two hours[42,52]. In contrast, after release of a 12-hour, 50 per cent static compression, 60 hours were necessary for biosynthesis to return to free-swelling levels[53]. The recovery of synthesis of link protein[53], fibronectin[40], and total protein synthesis[42] occurred more rapidly (also see below). These data suggest that cellular processes may be adapting to their new envir-

separately from physiochemical stimuli. The profiles of fluid velocity, streaming potential, and hydrostatic pressure, induced within cartilage by dynamic compression, will depend on the frequency of loading, specimen geometry, and the experimental loading configuration. At higher frequencies (for example, 1 Hz), there may be very little fluid exudation imbibition during each loading cycle, with elastic-like matrix deformation[56]. In contrast, at lower frequencies, fluid flow within the tissue may be much more significant during each cycle.

In these experiments[42,49], plane parallel, cylindrical disk specimens were compressed between fluid-impermeable platens used to simplify the loading configuration. However, even for this simple geometry, the spatial profiles of fluid velocity, and so on, are highly *non-uniform* within each disk. Theoretical analyses[24,30] show that at higher-loading frequencies, the hydrostatic pressure within the ECM is highest in the central region of the cartilage disk (Fig. 7.24(b)); however, the fluid velocity and streaming potential fields are highest near the radial periphery of the disk. Kim *et al.*[24] took advantage of these non-uniform profiles and hypothesized that spatially non-uniform mechanical stimuli would produce a corresponding spatially non-uniform biosynthetic response. This would enable a direct experimental test of the relative importance of oscillatory fluid flow, hydrostatic pressure, streaming potential, and cell deformation in modulating chondrocyte metabolism during dynamic compression, via measurement of the *frequency dependence* and the *spatial (radial) distribution* of newly-synthesized matrix macromolecules within the cartilage explant disks[24,49].

After dynamic compression of the 3 mm disks, the center 2-mm core of each disk was removed and the core and outer ring were analyzed separately for radio-label incorporation. While compression at frequencies between 0.002 and 0.01 Hz caused a stimulation of biosynthesis that was distributed throughout the core and outer ring of the disk, compression at 0.1 Hz caused a stimulation that was confined mainly to the outer ring (Fig. 7.24(c))[49]. (These radially dependent biosynthetic profiles were further confirmed by quantitative autoradiography[35].) These distributions in incorporation were then compared to theoretical estimates of the radial distribution of forces and flows within the matrix[24,49] (Fig. 7.24(b)). The observed biosynthetic patterns (Fig. 7.24(c)) most closely matched the radial dependence of fluid flow and its associated streaming potential, and cell deformation[24]. Thus, the stimulation of chondrocyte biosynthesis by *dynamic* mechanical

compression appeared associated mainly with changes in fluid flow, flow-induced streaming potentials, and/or cell shape, which were greatest near the disk periphery at higher frequencies (Fig. 7.24(b)), while hydrostatic pressure was probably less important.

Nevertheless, the slight biosynthetic stimulation in the central region, together with measured peak dynamic loads of about 0.5–1 MPa at the higher frequencies would be consistent with the possibility that hydrostatic pressure can stimulate biosynthesis[58]. With increasing frequency (strain rates), dynamic compression of cartilage would induce increasing levels of hydrostatic pressure within the tissue[30]. The effect of hydrostatic pressure on cartilage metabolism could be studied via mechanical compression of cartilage (as above), or more directly by pressurizing the fluid in a vessel containing chondrocytes or cartilage explants. The effects of hydrostatic pressure on chondrocyte activity in embryonic chicken, fetal mouse, bovine and human cartilage, and in rat chondrosarcoma cells have been reported[58–63]. In general, static or low frequency hydrostatic pressure caused a decrease in GAG synthesis, while higher frequency hydrostatic loading caused an increase in GAG synthesis. However, the effective threshold pressure for increased synthesis varied widely. In chick embryonic chondrocytes and fetal mouse cartilaginous long bone rudiments, cyclic pressures as low as 13 kPa[61,62,64] elicited a stimulatory response, while pressures on the order of 5 MPa[58–60] were needed to induce similar increases in matrix synthesis in bovine and human articular cartilage.

Compression-induced fluid flow and solute transport

Although fluid flow within the ECM may stimulate biosynthesis via several mechanisms, one possible mechanism may be related to increased convective transport of nutrients and growth factors[65]. Bernich *et al.*[66] observed that pressure-induced fluid flow through cartilage disks *in vitro* could greatly enhance the transport of glucose and other small nutrients through the tissue. Maroudas and coworkers measured the effects of static[67] and dynamic[65] compression on the partitioning and absorption of large and small molecules into cartilage, including radio-labeled BSA, IGF-I, urea, and sodium. They concluded that static compression affected the transport of large solutes more than that of small solutes, and that dynamic compression enhanced the desorption of large solutes much more than small solutes. If convective transport is an operative metabolic stimulant during dynamic compression of cartilage, it might act by (1) directly stimulating chondrocytes (for example, fluid shear at the cell surface[68]), or (2) altering the pericellular concentrations of macromolecular cytokines, growth factors, degradative enzymes, endogenous enzyme inhibitors, newly synthesized matrix macromolecules, or other nutrients[35].

Recently, Garcia *et al.* developed an approach to quantify the individual contributions of diffusion, convection, and electrical migration to the transport within cartilage of neutral and charged proteins, and lower MW solutes[69]. This approach allows direct measurement within each experiment of solute diffusion, convection (by application of an electric current to induce electro-osmotic fluid flow within the tissue (Fig. 7.25(a))), and electrical migration of charged solutes (which would occur in the presence of streaming potentials). Their results showed that convective enhancement of transport was particularly important for larger solutes. However, the effects of fluid convection became significant for solutes as small as 300–600 Da[69]. They further observed[70] that protein flux within cartilage could be greatly enhanced by fluid velocities relevant to physiologic mechanical loading. For example, transport of ^{125}I-IGF-1 and ^{125}I-rhTIMP-1 were enhanced by approximately 20- and 60-fold, respectively, above diffusion alone, by fluid velocities of about 1–2 μm per second. Fig. 7.25(b) shows the initial diffusive flux of IGF-1 across cartilage disks mounted in a transport chamber (from t = 590 to t = 745 minutes), followed by a 20-fold increase in flux at t = 745 minutes produced by application of electro-osmotic fluid flow within and across the cartilage disks[70].

Intracellular pathways: differential effects of compression on specific ECM macromolecules

The ability of the matrix to adapt to biomechanical demands is likely related to observations that the resident chondrocytes are capable of responding to specific physical stimuli within the tissue. Most studies of the effects of compression on cartilage biosynthesis *in vitro* have focused on total PG and protein synthesis using radiolabel precursors. However, some recent studies have begun to address the differential effects of compression on synthesis of specific matrix molecules, including biglycan and decorin[71,72], fibromodulin[71],

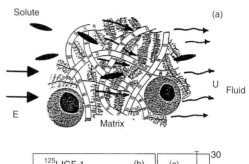

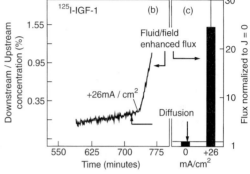

Fig. 7.25 (a) Macromolecular transport within cartilage ECM may be significantly affected by intratissue fluid flows (U) and compression-induced streaming potential fields (E); (b) diffusive transport of radiolabeled IGF-1 across disks of adult bovine cartilage (t=600–750 minutes); (c) electro-osmotically induced fluid velocities of ~1 μm/sec [within the physiologic range during dynamic compression, applied at t = 750 minutes in (b)], can augment diffusive transport by ~25-fold (data from [69] and [70]).

fibronectin[40], hyaluronan and link protein[53], and of ^{35}S-aggrecan and ^{3}H-collagen metabolism.

The three molecular components of the proteoglycan aggregate, for example, involve very different intracellular biosynthetic pathways. Link protein, a typical glycoprotein, undergoes a set of well-defined post-translational steps of N-linked oligosaccharide addition and trimming prior to its secretion from the cell. On the other hand, the post-translational processing of aggrecan core protein is spatially and temporally much more elaborate, requiring sequential addition of N-linked oligosaccharides, chondroitin sulfate (CS), O-linked oligosaccharides, and keratan sulfate (KS)[73]. (Synthesis of CS is initiated in the late endoplasmic reticulum and continued in the proximal regions of the Golgi complex[73], and KS is added to preformed O-linked oligosaccharides in the trans-Golgi in close spatial and temporal association[74,75].) In marked contrast to both aggrecan and link protein, hyaluronan does not involve a protein precursor. Rather, hyaluronan is synthesized at the plasma membrane by hyaluronate synthase and secreted directly into the extracellular matrix[76].

If mechanical stimuli were to elicit *differential* effects on the biosynthetic pathways of these molecules, significant insights could be gained concerning the intracellular mechanisms and extracellular processing that underlies chondrocyte response to compression. With this motivation, Kim *et al.*[53,71] studied the effects of static compression and release of compression on synthesis of aggrecan, link protein, and hyaluronan (HA). The major findings were: (1) aggrecan and link protein synthesis were inhibited by static compression, but HA synthesis was unaffected (Fig. 7.26); (2) both aggrecan and total protein synthesis recovered to free-swelling levels by about three days after release of a 12-hour, 50 per cent static compression; however, link protein synthesis recovered fully eight hours after release of compression, aggrecan synthesis was still inhibited eight hours after release, and HA synthesis was unaffected by release of compression (see Fig. 7.26). The gradual but complete recovery of total protein and aggrecan synthesis after release of static compression, and the much more rapid recovery of link protein synthesis, suggested that the inhibitory effect of static compression was not due to cellular damage.

Furthermore, these data showed that static compression and release have differential effects on various cellular products.

The inability of static compression or compression/release to alter HA synthesis has important implications regarding hypotheses linking biosynthetic pathways to the effects of mechanically-generated cell and cell membrane deformation, and to connection between ECM and cytoskeletal structures. Unlike aggrecan and link protein synthesis, which require extensive intracellular processing, HA synthesis involves only the HA-synthase complex at the plasma membrane. There have been several studies with chondrocytes showing instances in which HA synthesis can continue, while CS synthesis is inhibited, such as that during treatment with IL-1[77] or Brefeldin[78,79]. These results suggest that the response of cartilage to compression/release is not a general inhibition or recovery of cellular activity, but appears to be part of a transduction mechanism which results in spatial and/or temporal alterations of specific pathways. Therefore, physiologic loading and unloading regimes over the long term might induce such differential effects on synthesis and accumulation of these matrix molecules *in vivo*, thereby resulting in significant alterations in matrix composition and functional properties.

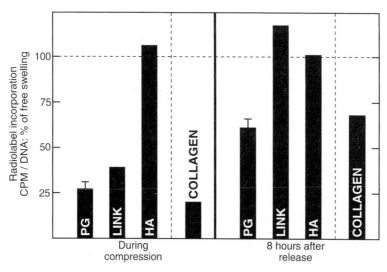

Fig. 7.26 (a) Biosynthetic rates of aggrecan, link protein, hyaluronan, and collagen during 12-hour static compression of calf cartilage explants to 50% of cut thickness, and (b) 8 hours after release of compression, normalized to that of free-swelling control disks (data from[53]).

Cellular mechanisms: biophysical, morphological, and biosynthetic correlates

Cell and nucleus deformation at equilibrium follows imposed tissue deformation

The effects of tissue compression on the deformation of the matrix, chondrocyte, and intracellular components have been studied to better understand the possible role of cell shape/deformation on chondrocyte signal transduction. Using Nomarski imaging[18,19], confocal microscopy[20], and stereology of explant specimens fixed after static and dynamic compression[21,35], investigators have found that compression applied to the surfaces of cartilage specimens causes a corresponding compression of the pericellular[19], as well as territorial and interterritorial[18,20,21,35], matrix, near and around the cells. In adult cartilage, columns of chondrocyte-containing chondrons appear compacted at all depths[18,19] with accompanying loss of pericellular matrix volume and water content. Recent studies[20,21,80] have shown that distinct changes in cell and nucleus shape are produced by compression imposed at tissue surfaces. In general, compression caused flattening of the cells in the direction of loading and a decrease in cell volume[20,21,51], and could also cause changes in cell surface area[21], nucleus volume and height[21,80], and nucleus surface area[21]. These changes vary with depth, the degree of anisotropy of the collagen network, and the age of the tissue.

Buschmann *et al.*[21] have directly examined whether such changes in cell and nucleus morphology are related to the changes in aggrecan biosynthesis caused by static compression. Cartilage explant disks were radiolabeled during compression, fixed in the compressed state (Fig. 7.27), and subsequently processed for quantitative autoradiography[81] and light microscopy-based stereological estimations[21]. Analysis of light microscope images was used to measure ^{35}S-sulfate autoradiography grain density (associated with incorporation of newly synthesized proteoglycans into the matrix). They found a general inhibition of total aggrecan synthesis with increasing static compression levels, and a compression-induced spatial gradient in aggrecan synthesis which was not present in free-swelling disks. This spatial inhomogeneity appeared to be directly related to mechanical boundary conditions

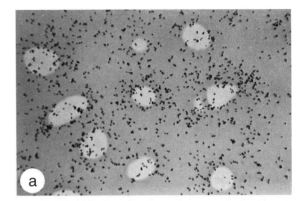
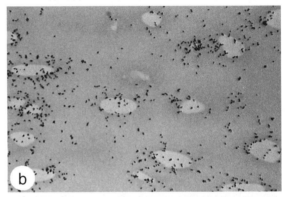
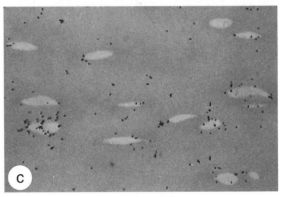

Fig. 7.27 Light micrographs of autoradiography sections. Cartilage disks were labeled during 12-hour compression and fixed in the compressed state: (a) free swelling at 1.5 mm thick; compressed to (b) 1.0 mm and (c) 0.75 mm. ^{35}S-sulfate incorporation into aggrecan results in silver grains; digitized images were used to quantitate aggrecan synthesis. Micrographs taken from similar regions were used for stereological evaluation (from[21]).

and the manner in which the load was applied and, therefore, may represent a spatially specific functional adaptation to mechanical loading. Stereological measurements at the center of disks showed a reduction in cell and nucleus volume, surface area, and radii in the vertical direction of compression. Horizontal radii were unchanged, however, consistent with the observation of minimal radial expansion of the explant disks in (unconfined) compression[21]. Thus, vertical and horizontal cell dimensions in compressed tissue followed deformations imposed at the tissue surfaces. These correlated changes in biosynthesis and stereological parameters[21] suggest that alterations in cell and nuclear structure may be an important mode by which chondrocytes can detect and respond to changes in the mechanical environment.

As described above, proteoglycan synthesis is generally decreased by static compression, while dynamic compression can stimulate synthesis. Quantitative autoradiography has enabled investigators to characterize the spatial profiles of aggrecan biosynthesis within the tissue, caused by dynamic[35,57], as well as static[21] compression. Quinn[35,82] recently extended these methods to quantify the spatial distributions of incorporated radiolabel around individual cells, within 3 mm diameter by 1 mm thick explant disks, that had been subjected to static or dynamic compression (Fig. 7.28). ^{35}S-sulfate autoradiography grain density was measured (with about 1 μm resolution) in the cell-associated and further removed matrix, as a function of distance from the cell membrane and angular orientation around centrally sectioned cells. Systematic random sampling[83] over the entire cross-section of explant disks allowed for the identification of trends associated with cell populations from particular explant locations.

Analysis of compressed cartilage disks revealed that the spatial distribution of newly synthesized proteoglycans incorporated around individual chondrocytes, was strongly influenced by the orientation of mechanical compression which was applied to the whole disk in the thickness direction. Static compression decreased the content of newly synthesized proteoglycans found in both the cell-associated and further removed matrices of cells in the central region of explant disks (Fig. 7.28(a)(iii)), compared to that in free-swelling controls (FSW) (Fig. 7.28(a)(i)). However, cells near the radial edge (outer 25 per cent of the 3 mm diameter cross-section) of statically compressed explants (Fig. 7.28(a)(iv)), where anisotropic matrix deformations would be maximum, exhibited a pronounced directional character with respect to inhibition of cell-associated proteoglycan incorporation, which was not

evident near the center of compressed explants (Fig. 7.28(a)(iii)), nor in free-swelling samples (Fig. 7.28(a)(ii)). At the radial edge, the deposition of newly synthesized proteoglycans was inhibited significantly at the 'north' and 'south' poles of the cells (that is, in the axial direction of compression) (Fig. 7.28(a)(iv)) compared to free-swelling controls (Fig. 7.28(a)(ii)), but not significantly altered around the 'equators' of the flattened cells (Fig. 7.28(a)(iv)). Figure 7.28 (b) shows the effect of dynamic compression at 0.1 Hz on the distribution of newly synthesized proteoglycans around cells. Previous studies at the tissue level (Fig. 7.24(c)) had shown that proteoglycan synthesis was stimulated at this frequency predominantly in the outer radial ring of 3 mm diameter explants. At the cell level, Quinn found that this stimulation of proteoglycan synthesis was manifested by a marked increase in the content of newly synthesized proteoglycans in the cell-associated matrix of these cells (Fig. 7.28(b)(iv)). The increased content at the 'equators' was not that different from the 'poles'. In contrast, cells in the central region of dynamically compressed disks (Fig. 7.28(b)(iii)) showed little change in content of newly synthesized proteoglycans, consistent with the lack of stimulation in the central region at the tissue level (Fig. 7.24(c)). These microscale data highlight the complexity of the chondrocyte's micromechanical and biochemical environment, and suggest the importance of fluid flows in the pericellular matrix during dynamic compression (Fig. 7.25), as well as mechanical deformations, as potential mediators of metabolic activity.

Comparison of changes in aggrecan synthesis at the center of cartilage disks, to changes in cell and nucleus structure at the same location, showed that aggrecan synthesis was reduced simultaneously with reductions in cell and nucleus volumes, surface areas, and vertical radii[21]. Based on these data alone, however, it is difficult to establish a direct cause and effect relationship between biosynthesis and any one structural parameter. Nevertheless, the distinct correlation between changes in aggrecan synthesis, and general cell and nucleus structure, serves to highlight a number of potentially important control points and molecular mechanisms which may link synthesis to structure of the cell or nucleus[21]. The chondrocyte / extracellular-matrix interface bears integrin[84,85] and hyaluronan receptors[86]. The cytoplasmic domain of integrin receptors is linked directly to the cell cytoskeleton and possesses a tyrosine kinase activity[87]. Mechanical perturbations at the cell membrane may, therefore, be

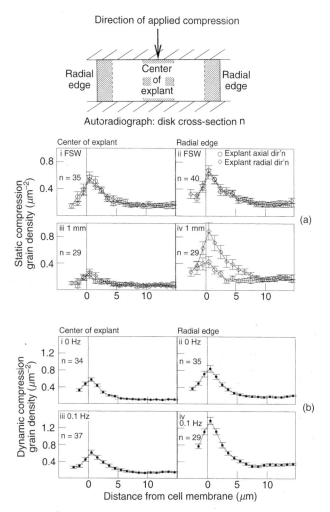

Fig. 7.28 Autoradiography grain density in histological sections taken from calf articular cartilage explants subjected to (a) static and (b) dynamic mechanical loads. For the ^{35}S-sulfate radiolabel used, autoradiography grain density was directly proportional to the volume density of PGs which were synthesized during compression and appeared at the indicated distances from the the cell membrane (positive distances represent extracellular points). (a) Radiolabel was introduced during static compression to 1 mm ((a) (iii), (iv)) and compared to free-swelling (FSW) controls (a) (i), (ii). Data for cell populations located near the explant center (inner 25% of the 1.5 mm disk radius; (a) (i), (iii) are plotted alongside data for cells located at the disk radial edge (outer 25% of disk radius; (a) (ii), (iv) (b) Radiolabel was introduced during dynamic compression at 0.1 Hz (b) (iii), (iv) and compared to 0 Hz controls held within the same device. Data for cell populations located near the explant center (inner 25% of the 1.5 mm disk radius; (b) (i), (iii) are plotted alongside data for cells located at the disk radial edge (outer 25% of disk radius; (b) (ii), (iv) (data from[82]).

transduced mechanically or chemically to alter biosynthesis at various levels. Cell deformation can be directly translated to nuclear deformation[21,80]. Although it is not known whether this nuclear deformation involves biochemical mediation by the cell, it is possible that it is primarily controlled by the mechanics of the cytoskeleton[88] and nucleoskeleton[89]. Nuclear size has also been shown to increase in response to growth factor stimulation[90], and one potential regulatory point

may be nucleocytoplasmic transport regulated by nuclear pore complexes[91]. Potential mechanical regulation of biosynthesis at the transcriptional level, through deformation of chromatin structure, may be related to the finding of reduced nucleus volume under compression. In the case of static compression, net volume reduction of the nucleus may lead to a more condensed chromatin state and inhibition of biosynthesis, while dynamic oscillatory compression which can stimulate biosynthesis may induce local cell and nucleus expansion[57].

Response of isolated chondrocytes to mechanical stimuli

There is increasing interest in the transplantation of chondrocytes and chondrocyte-seeded matrices for regeneration of cartilage in OA, and the repair of cartilage defects caused by acute injury. An understanding of the chondrocyte response to physiologic loading will be the key to the ultimate long term success of such approaches. The use of isolated chondrocytes in the study of metabolic response to load must be approached with caution, however, because of the important role of the natural ECM[17] in signal transduction and in transmitting the external load to the cell and intracellular components. Thus, agarose and alginate gel culture has been used by investigators, as model systems complementary to the intact explant, for exploring the physical mechanisms that may regulate cartilage cell behavior[50,51,92]. Agarose[93–95] and alginate[96,97] culture has been used to study chondrocyte phenotypic expression, proliferation, and ability to accumulate a PG-rich extracellular matrix during long-term culture. Chondrocytes in long-term agarose culture can synthesize and assemble a mechanically functional matrix[98]. After several weeks in culture, by which time a dense ECM had been deposited within the agarose, the chondrocytes responded to regimes of static and dynamic compression[50] in a manner similar to that in cartilage explants[42]. However, matrix deposition in this case had occurred under free-swelling conditions. The possibility that the composition and quality of the newly developed matrix could be significantly altered by continuous compression during *long-term* culture remains, and would provide a useful system to study chondrocyte biosynthetic and catabolic responses to compression.

Mechanical loading and cartilage degradation

In OA, cartilage matrix composition is altered substantially, considerably weakening the tissue to the extent that mechanical wear from joint motion can result in erosion of cartilage down to the bone surface[99].

Cartilage matrix molecules are susceptible to degradation by several classes of proteinases[100]. The role of enzymatic degradation in OA is under intense investigation, but is not completely understood. It has been suggested[101] that families of enzymes, including metalloproteinases[102], serine proteinases[103], and a novel 'aggrecanase'[104] contribute to cartilage degradation in OA. It is known[105] that a portion of the aggrecan G1 domain of aggrecan that accumulates in human cartilage is associated with matrix metalloproteinase activity. However, the aggrecan fragments that are present in the synovial fluid of early and late post-traumatic arthritis[104] and inflammatory arthritis[106] contain the cleavage site consistent with 'aggrecanase' activity.

The role of mechanical agents in the degradation of cartilage *in vivo* has recently been reviewed[107]. It is clear that acute mechanical overload can cause severe cartilage damage[13,15]. Recent studies *in vitro* have simulated the effects of controlled impact loads on cartilage explants to assess matrix fissuring, chondrocyte viability, and damage to the collagen network[108,109]. Other than such acute destruction, the mechanisms by which mechanical forces in the joint may contribute to specific catabolic pathways for matrix degradation remain to be elucidated. It is possible that mechanical compression could alter enzymatic pathways and, thereby, the forms of the catabolic fragments of aggrecan, link protein, hyaluronan, and collagen. In this regard, it is important to distinguish between the direct effects of mechanical load in disrupting cartilage matrix and mechanical stimulation of cell-mediated catabolic pathways. For example, high amplitude cyclic compression of cartilage explants has been found to produce a dose-dependent sustained release of aggrecan and collagen fragments, resulting in tissue swelling[110], as well as increased release of aggrecan G1 domain fragments[82]. Analysis of the specific cleavage sites associated with such released macromolecular fragments[111] can give insight as to whether compression has induced 'mechanically novel' catabolic fragments, or has simply accelerated the loss of fragments found during normal turnover of matrix. Further research in these areas will be essential for a more complete understanding of the chondrocyte response to mechanical loads.

Acknowledgments

Supported in part by NIH Grant AR33236. The authors thank Drs. Eliot Frank, John Sandy, and Anna Plaas for critical contributions to this work.

References

1. Hodge, W.A., Fijan, R.S., Carlson, K.L., Burgess, R.G., Harris, W.H., and Mann, R.W. (1986). Contact pressures in the human hip joint measured *in vivo*. *Proceedings of the National Academy of Science*, **83**, 2879–83.
2. Heinegard, D. and Oldberg, A. (1989). Structure and biology of cartilage and bone matrix non-collagenous macromolecules. *FASEB*, **3**, 2042–51.
3. Helminen, H.J., Kiviranta, I., Tammi, M., Saamanen, A.M., Paukkonen, K., and Jurvelin, J. (ed.) (1987). *Joint loading*. Wright, Bristol.
4. Caterson, B. and Lowther, D.A. (1978). Changes in the metabolism of the proteoglycans from sheep articular cartilage in response to mechanical stress. *Biochimica et Biophysica Acta*, **540**, 412–22.
5. Palmoski, M.J., Perricone, E., and Brandt, K.D. (1979). Development and reversal of a proteoglycan aggregation defect in normal canine knee cartilage after immobilization. *Arthritis and Rheumatism*, **22**, 508–17.
6. Kiviranta, I., Jurvelin, J., Tammi, M., Saamanen, A-M., and Helminen, H.J. (1987). Weight bearing controls glycosaminoglycan concentration and articular cartilage thickness in the knee joints of young beagle dogs. *Arthritis and Rheumatism*, **30**, 801–9.
7. Behrens, F., Kraft, E.L., and Oegema, T.R. (1989). Biochemical changes in articular cartilage after joint immobilization by casting or external fixation. *Journal of Orthopaedic Research*, **7**, 335–43.
8. Jurvelin, J., Kiviranta, I., Saamanen, A-M., Tammi, M., and Helminen, H.J. (1989). Partial restoration of immobilization-induced softening of canine articular cartilage after remobilization of the knee (stifle) joint. *Journal of Orthopaedic Research*, **7**, 352–8.
9. Slowman, S.D. and Brandt, K.D. (1986). Composition and glycosaminoglycan metabolism of articular cartilage from habitually loaded and habitually unloaded sites. *Arthritis and Rheumatism*, **29**, 88–94.
10. Salter, R.B. (1993). *Continuous passive motion*. Williams and Wilkins, Baltimore, MD.
11. Kiviranta, I., Tammi, M., Jurvelin, J., Saamanen, A.M., and Helminen, H.J. (1988). Moderate running exercise augments glycosaminoglycans and thickness of articular cartilage in the knee joint of young beagle dogs. *Journal of Orthopaedic Research*, **6**, 188–95.
12. Gritzka, T.L., Fry, L.R., Cheesman, R.L., and Lavigne, A. (1973). Deterioration of articular cartilage caused by continuous compression in a moving rabbit joint. *Journal of Bone and Joint Surgery*, **55A**, 1698–1720.
13. Radin, E.L., Martin, R.B., Burr, D.B., Caterson, B., Boyd, R.D., and Goodwin, C. (1984). Effects of mechanical loading on the tissues of the rabbit knee. *Journal of Orthopaedic Research*, **2**, 221–34.
14. Säämämen, A-M., Kiviranta, I., Jurvelin, J., Helminen, H.J., and Tammi, M. (1994). Proteoglycan and collagen alterations in canine knee articular cartilage following 20 km daily running exercise for 15 weeks. *Connective Tissue Research*, **30**, 191–201.
15. Thompson, R.C., Oegema, T.R., Lewis, J.L., and Wallace, L. (1991). Osteoarthrotic changes after acute transarticular load: an animal model. *Journal of Bone and Joint Surgery*, **73A**, 990–1001.
16. Arokoski, J., Kiviranta, I., Jurvelin, J., Tammi, M., and Helminen, H.J. (1993). Long-distance running causes site-dependent decrease of cartilage glycosaminoglycan content in the knee joints of beagle dogs. *Arthritis and Rheumatism*, **36**, 1451–9.
17. Muir, H. (1995). The chondrocyte, architect of cartilage. *BioEssays*, **17(12)**, 1039–48.
18. Broom, N.D. and Myers, D.B. (1980). A study of the structural response of wet hyaline cartilage to various loading situations. *Connective Tissue Research*, **7**, 227–37.
19. Poole, C.A. (1993). The structure and function of articular cartilage matrices. In *Joint Cartilage degradation* (ed. J.F. Woessner, Jr and D.S. Howell), pp. 1–35. Dekker, New York.
20. Guilak, F., Ratcliffe, A., and Mow V.C. (1995). Chondrocyte deformation and local tissue strain in articular cartilage: a confocal microscopy study. *Journal of Orthopaedic Research*, **13**, 410–21.
21. Buschmann, M.D., Hunziker, E.B., Kim, Y-J., and Grodzinsky, A.J. (1996). Altered aggrecan synthesis correlates with cell and nucleus structure in statically compressed cartilage. *Journal of Cell Science*, **109**, 499–508.
22. Mow, V.C., Kuei, S.C., Lai, W.M., and Armstrong, C.G. (1980). Biphasic creep and stress relaxation of articular cartilage in compression: theory and experiments. *Journal of Biomechanical Engineering*, **102**, 73–84.
23. Frank, E.H. and Grodzinsky, A.J. (1987). Cartilage electromechanics — I. electrokinetic transduction and the effects of electrolyte pH and ionic strength. *Journal of Biomechanics*, **20**, 615–27.
24. Kim, Y-J., Bonassar, L.J., and Grodzinsky, A.J. (1995). The role of cartilage streaming potential, fluid flow and pressure in the stimulation of chondrocyte biosynthesis during dynamic compression. *Journal of Biomechanics*, **28**, 1055–66.
25. Maroudas, A. (1979). Physicochemical properties of articular cartilage. In *Adult articular cartilage*, (2nd edn) (ed. M.A.R. Freeman), pp. 215–90. Pitman, Tunbridge Wells, England.
26. Grodzinsky, A.J. (1983). Electromechanical and physicochemical properties of connective tissue. *CRC Critical Reviews in Bioengineering*, **9**, 133–99.
27. Gray, M.L., Pizzanelli, A.M., Grodzinsky, A.J., and Lee, R.C. (1988). Mechanical and physicochemical determinants of the chondrocyte biosynthetic response. *Journal of Orthopaedic Research*, **6**, 777–92.
28. Urban, J.P.G., Hall, A.C., and Gehl, K.A. (1993). Regulation of matrix synthesis rates by the ionic and osmotic environment of articular chondrocytes. *Journal of Cellular Physiology*, **154**, 262–70.
29. Boustany, N.N., Gray, M.L., Black, A.C., and Hunziker, E.B. (1995). Correlation between the synthetic activity and glycosaminoglycan concentration in epiphesial cartilage raises questions about the regulatory role of interstitial pH. *Journal of Orthopaedic Research*, **13**, 733–9.
30. Armstrong, C.G., Lai, W.M., and Mow, V.C. (1984). An analysis of the unconfined compression of articular

cartilage. *Journal of Biomechanical Engineering*, **106**, 165–73.

31. Mak, A.F. (1986). Unconfined compression of hydrated viscoelastic tissues: a biphasic poroviscoelastic analysis. *Biorheology*, **23**, 371–83.

32. Eisenberg, S.R. and Grodzinsky, A.J. (1987). The kinetics of chemically induced non-equilibrium swelling of articular cartilage and corneal stroma. *Journal of Biomechanical Engineering*, **109**, 79–89.

33. Lai, W.M., Hou, J.S., and Mow, V.C. (1991). A triphasic theory for the swelling and deformation behaviors of articular cartilage. *Journal of Biomechanical Engineering*, **113**, 245–58.

34. Frank, E.H. and Grodzinsky, A.J. (1987). Cartilage electromechanics – II. a continuum model of cartilage electrokinetics and correlation with experiments. *Journal of Biomechanics*, **20**, 629–39.

35. Quinn, T.M., Grodzinsky, A.J., Buschmann, M.D., Kim, Y.-J., and Hunziker, E.B. (1997). Mechanical compression alters proteoglycan synthesis and matrix deformation around individual cells in cartilage explants. *Journal of Cell Science*, (submitted).

36. Sah, R.L.Y., Grodzinsky, A.J., Plaas, A.H.K., and Sandy, J.D. (1992). Effects of static and dynamic compression on matrix metabolism in cartilage explants. In *Articular cartilage and osteoarthritis* (ed. K.E. Kuettner, R. Schleyerbach, J.G. Peyron, and V.C. Hascall), pp. 373–92. Raven Press, New York.

37. Hascall, V.C., Morales, T.I., Hascall, G.K., Handley, C.J., and McQuillan, D.J. (1983). Biosynthesis and turnover of proteoglycans in organ culture of bovine articular cartilage. *Journal of Rheumatology*, **10S**, 45–52.

38. Hardingham, T. and Bayliss, M. (1990). Proteoglycans of articular cartilage: changes in aging and in joint disease. *Seminars in Arthritis and Rheumatology*, **20,S**, 12–33.

39. Schneiderman, R., Kevet, D., and Maroudas, A. (1986). Effects of mechanical and osmotic pressure on the rate of glycosaminoglycan synthesis in the human adult femoral head cartilage: an *in vitro* study. *Journal of Orthopaedic Research*, **4**, 393–408.

40. Burton-Wurster, N., Vernier-Singer, M., Farquhar, T., and Lust, G. (1993). Effect of compressive loading and unloading on synthesis of total protein, proteoglycan, and fibronectin by canine cartilage explants. *Journal of Orthopaedic Research*, **11**, 717–29.

41. Jones, I.L., Klamfeldt, D.D.S., and Sandstrom, T. (1982). The effect of continuous mechanical pressure upon the turnover of articular cartilage proteoglycans *in vitro*. *Clinical Orthopaedics*, **165**, 283–9.

42. Sah, R.L., Kim, Y.-J., Doong, J.H., Grodzinsky, A.J., Plaas, A.H.K., and Sandy, J.D. (1989). Biosynthetic response of cartilage explants to dynamic compression. *Journal of Orthopaedic Research*, **7**, 619–36.

43. Guilak, F., Meyer, B.C., Ratcliffe, A., and Mow, V.C. (1994). The effects of matrix compression on proteoglycan metabolism in articular cartilage explants. *Osteoarthritis and Cartilage*, **2**, 91–101.

44. Palmoski, M.J. and Brandt, K.D. (1984). Effects of static and cyclic compressive loading on articular carti-

lage plugs *in vitro*. *Arthritis and Rheumatism*, **27**, 675–81.

45. Copray, J.C.V.M., Jansen, H.W.B., and Duterloo, H.S. (1985). Effects of compressive forces on proliferation and matrix synthesis in mandibular condylar cartilage of the rat *in vitro*. *Archives of Oral Biology*, **30**, 299–304.

46. Larsson, T., Aspden, R.M., and Heinegard, D. (1991). Effects of mechanical load on cartilage matrix biosynthesis *in vitro*. *Matrix*, **11**, 388–94.

47. Korver, T.H., van de Stadt, R.J., and Kiljan, E. (1992). Effects of loading on the synthesis of proteoglycans in different layers of anatomically intact articular cartilage *in vitro*. *Journal of Rheumatology*, **19**, 905–12.

48. Parkkinen, J.J., Lammi, M.J., Helminen, H.J., and Tammi, M. (1992). Local stimulation of proteoglycan synthesis in articular cartilage explants by dynamic compression *in vitro*. *Journal of Orthopaedic Research*, **10**, 610–20.

49. Kim, Y-J., Sah, R.L-Y., Grodzinsky, A.J., Plaas, A.H.K., and Sandy, J.D. (1994). Mechanical regulation of cartilage biosynthetic behavior: Physical stimuli. *Archives of Biochemistry and Biophysics*, **311**, 1–12.

50. Buschmann, M.D., Gluzband, Y.A., Grodzinksy, A.J., and Hunziker, E.B. (1995). Mechanical compression modulates matrix biosynthesis in chondrocyte/agarose culture. *Journal of Cell Science*, **108**, 1497–1508.

51. Freeman, P.M., Natarajan, R.N., Kimura, J.H., and Andriacchi, T.P. (1994). Chondrocyte cells respond mechanically to compressive loads. *Journal of Orthopaedic Research*, **12**, 311–20.

52. Gray, M.L., Pizzanelli, A.M., Lee, R.C., Grodzinsky, A.J., and Swann, D.A. (1989). Kinetics of the chondrocyte biosynthetic response to compressive load and release. *Biochimica et Biophysica Acta*, **991**, 415–25.

53. Kim, Y-J., Grodzinsky, A.J., and Plaas, A.H.K. (1996). Compression of cartilage results in differential effects on biosynthetic pathways for aggrecan, link protein, and hyaluronan. *Archives of Biochemistry and Biophysics*, **328**, 331–40.

54. Sah, R.L., Grodzinsky, A.J., Plaas, A.H.K., and Sandy, J.D. (1990). Effects of tissue compression on the hyaluronate binding properties of newly synthesized proteoglycans in cartilage explants. *Biochemical Journal*, **267**, 803–8.

55. Sah, R.L., Kim, Y-J., and Grodzinsky, A.J. (1990). The effect of mechanical compression on cartilage metabolism. In *Methods for cartilage Research* (ed. A. Maroudas and K.E. Kuettner), pp. 116–19. Academic Press, New York.

56. Eberhardt, A.W., Keer, L.M., Lewis, J.L., and Vithoontien, V. (1990). An analytical model of joint contact. *Journal of Biomechanical Engineering*, **112**, 407–13.

57. Buschmann, M.D., Kim, Y-J., Hunziker, E.B., and Grodzinksy, A.J. (1995). Stimulated aggrecan synthesis correlates with expansive solid matrix strain and increased fluid flow in dynamically compressed cartilage. *Transactions of the Combined Orthopaedic Research Societies of the USA, Japan, and Canada*, **2**, 117.

58. Hall, A.C., Urban, J.P.G., and Gehl, K.A. (1991). The effects of hydrostatic pressure on matrix synthesis in articular cartilage. *Journal of Orthopaedic Research*, 9, 1–10.

59. Kimura, J.H., Schipplein, O.D., Kuettner, K.E., and Andriacchi, T.P. (1985). Effects of hydrostatic loading on extracellular matrix formation. *Transactions of the Orthopaedic Research Society*, 10, 365.

60. Lippiello, L., Kaye, C., Neumata, T., and Mankin, H.J. (1985). *In vitro* metabolic response of articular cartilage segments to low levels of hydrostatic pressure. *Connective Tissue Research*, 13, 99–107.

61. van Kampen, G.P.J., Veldhuijzen, R., Kuijer, R., van de Stadt, R.J., and Schipper, C.A. (1985). Cartilage response to mechancial force in high-density chondrocyte cultures. *Arthritis and Rheumatism*, 28, 419–24.

62. Veldhuijzen, J.P., Huisman, A.H., Vermeiden, J.P.W., and Prahl-Andersen, B. (1987). The growth of cartilage cells *in vitro* and the effect of intermittent compressive force. a histological evaluation. *Connective Tissue Research*, 16, 187–96.

63. Parkkinen, J.J., Ikonen, J., Lammi, M.J., Laakkonen, J., and Tammi, M. (1993). Effects of cycle hydrostatic pressure on proteoglycan synthesis in cultured articular chondrocytes and cartilage explants. *Archives of Biochemistry and Biophysics*, 300, 458–65.

64. Klein-Nulend, J., Veldhuijzen, J.P., and Burger, E.H. (1986). Increased calcification of growth plate cartilage as a result of compressive force *in vitro*. *Arthritis and Rheumatism*, 29, 1002–9.

65. O'Hara, B.P., Urban, J.P.G., and Maroudas, A. (1990). Influence of cyclic loading on the nutrition of articular cartilage. *Annals of the Rheumatic Diseases*, 49, 536–9.

66. Bernich, E., Rubenstein, R., and Bellin, J.S. (1976). Membrane transport properties of bovine articular cartilage. *Biochimica et Biophysica Acta*, 448, 551–61.

67. Cohen, S., Snir, E., Schneiderman, R., and Maroudas, A. (1993). Solute transport in cartilage: Effect of static compression. *Transactions of the Orthopaedic Research Society*, 18, 622.

68. Smith, R.L., Donion, B.S., Gupta, M.K., Mohtai, M., Das, P., Carter, D.R., *et al.* (1995). Effects of fluid-induced shear on articular chondrocytes morphology and metabolism *in vitro*. *Journal of Orthopaedic Research*, 13, 824–31.

69. Garcia, A.M., Frank, E.H., Grimshaw, P.E., and Grodzinsky, A.J. (1996). Contributions of fluid convection and electrical migration to transport in cartilage: relevance to loading. *Archives of Biochemistry and Biophysics*, 333, 317–25.

70. Garcia, A.M., Lark, M.W., Trippel, S.B., and Grodzinsky, A.J. (1996). Transport of TIMP and IGF-1 in cartilage: Contributions of fluid flow and electrical migration. *Transactions of the Orthopaedic Research Society*, 21, 12.

71. Kim, Y-J., Grodzinsky, A.J., Plaas, A.H.K., and Sandy, J.D. (1992). The differential effects of static compression on the synthesis of specific cartilage matrix components. *Transactions of the Orthopaedic Research Society*, 17, 108.

72. Visser, N.A., van Kampen, G.P.J., de Koning, M.H.M.T., and van der Korst, J.K. (1994). The effects of loading on the synthesis of biglycan and decorin in intact mature articular cartilage *in vitro*. *Connective Tissue Research*, 30, 241–50.

73. Hascall, V.C., Heinegard, D.K., and Wight, T.N. (1991). Proteoglycans: metabolism and pathology. In *Cell Biology of Extracellular matrix*, (2nd edn) (ed. E.D. Hay), pp. 149–75. Plenum Press, New York.

74. Lohmander, L.S., Hascall, V.C., Yanagishita, M., Kuettner, K.E., and Kimura, J.H. (1986). Post-translational events in proteoglycan synthesis: kinetics of synthesis of chondroitin sulfate and oligosaccharides on the core protein. *Archives of Biochemistry and Biophysics*, 250, 211–27.

75. Thonar, E. J-M., Lohmander, L.S., Kimura, J.H., Fellini, S.A., Yanagishita, M., Hascall, V.C., *et al.* (1983). Biosynthesis of O-linked oligosaccharides on proteoglycans by chondrocytes from the swarm rat chondrosarcoma. *Journal of Biological Chemistry*, 258, 11564–70.

76. Prehm, P. (1984). Hyaluronate is synthesized at plasma membranes. *Biochemical Journal*, 220, 597–600.

77. Morales, T.I. and Hascall, V.C. (1989). Effects of interleukin-1 and lipopolysac-charides on protein and carbohydrate metabolism in bovine articular cartilage organ cultures. *Connective Tissue Research*, 10, 255–75.

78. Wong-Palms, S. and Plaas, A.H.K. (1995). Glycosaminoglycan addition to proteoglycans by articular chondrocytes — evidence for core protein-specific pathways. *Archives of Biochemistry and Biophysics*, 319, 383–92.

79. Calabro, A. and Hascall, V.C. (1994). Differential effects of Brefeldin on chondroitin sulfate and hyaluronan synthesis in rat chondrosarcoma cells. *Journal of Biological Chemistry*, 269, 22764–70.

80. Guilak, F. (1995). Compression-induced changes in the shape and volume of the chondrocyte nucleus. *Journal of Biomechanics*, 28(12), 1529–41.

81. Buschmann, M.D., Maurer, A.M., Berger, E., and Hunziker, E.B. (1996). A method of quantitative autoradiography for the spatial localization of proteoglycan synthesis rates in cartilage. *Journal of Histochemistry and Cytochemistry*, 44, 423–31.

82. Quinn, T.M. (1996). *Articular cartilage: matrix assembly, mediation of chondrocyte metabolism, and response to compression*. PhD Thesis, MIT, Cambridge, M assachusetts.

83. Gundersen, H.J. (1988). The nucleator. *Journal of Microscopy*, 151, 3–21.

84. Durr, J., Goodman, S., Potocnik, A., and von der Mark, K. (1993). Localization of β-1-integrins in human cartilage and their role in chondrocyte adhesion to collagen and fibronectin. *Experimental Cell Research*, 207, 235–44.

85. Enomoto, M., Leboy, P.S., Menko, A.S., and Boettiger, D. (1993). β-1 Integrins mediate chondrocyte interaction with type-I collagen, type-II collagen, and fibronectin. *Experimental Cell Research*, 205, 276–85.

86. Knudson, C.B. and Knudson, W. (1993). Hyaluronan-binding proteins in development, tissue homeostasis and disease. *FASEB Journal*, 7, 1233–41.

87. Burridge, K., Turner, C.E., and Romer, L.H. (1992). Tyrosine phosphoylation of paxillin and pp125[FAK] accompanies cell adhesion to extracellular matrix: a role in cytoskeletal assembly. *Journal of Cell Biology*, **119**, 893–903.

88. Sims, J.R., Karp, S., and Ingber, D.E. (1992). Altering the cellular mechanical force balance results in integrated changes in cell, cytoskeletal and nuclear shape. *Journal of Cell Science*, **103**, 1215–22.

89. Spector, D.L. (1993). Macromolecular domains within the cell nucleus. *Reviews in Cell Biology*, **9**, 265–315.

90. Ingber, D.E., Madri, J.A., and Folkman, J. (1987). Endothelial growth factors and extracellular matrix regulate DNA synthesis through modulation. *In Vitro Cellular and Developmental Biology*, **23**, 387–94.

91. Pante, N. and Aebi, U. (1993). The nuclear pore complex. *Journal of Cell Biology*, **122**, 977–84.

92. Lee, D.A. and Bader, D.L. (1995). The development and characterization of an *in vitro* system to study strain-induced cell deformation in isolated chondrocytes. *In Vitro Cellular and Developmental Biology*, **31**, 828–35.

93. Benya, P.D. and Shaffer, J.D. (1982). Dedifferentiated chondrocytes re-express the differentiated collagen phenotype when cultured in agarose gels. *Cell*, **30**, 215–24.

94. Sun, D., Aydelotte, M.B., Maldonado, B., Kuettner, K.E., and Kimura, J.H. (1986). Clonal analysis of the population of chondrocytes from the swarm rat chondrosarcoma in agarose culture. *Journal of Orthopaedic Research*, **4**, 427–36.

95. Aydelotte, M.B. and Kuettner, K.E. (1993). Heterogeneity of articular chondrocytes and cartilage matrix. In *Joint cartilage degradation* (ed. J.F. Woessner, Jr and D.S. Howell), pp. 37–66. Dekker, New York.

96. Häuselmann, H.J., Aydelotte, M.B., Schlumacher, B.L., Kuettner, K.E., Gitelis, S.H., and Thonar, E. J-M. A. (1992). Synthesis and turnover of proteoglycans by human and bovine adult articular chondrocytes cultured in alginate beads. *Matrix*, **12**, 116–29.

97. Mok, S.S., Masuda, K., Häuselmann, H.J., Aydelotte, M.B., and Thonar, E.J-M.A. (1994). Aggrecan synthesized by mature bovine chondrocytes suspended in alginate. *Journal of Biological Chemistry*, **269**(52), 33021–7.

98. Buschmann, M.D., Gluzband, Y.A., Grodzinsky, A.J., Kimura, J.H., and Hunziker, E.B. (1992). Chondrocytes in agarose culture synthesize a mechanically functional extracellular matrix. *Journal of Orthopaedic Research*, **10**, 745–58.

99. Bullough, P.G. (1992). The pathology of osteoarthritis. In *Osteoarthritis* (ed. R.W. Moskowitz, D.S. Howell, V.M. Goldberg, and H.J. Mankin), pp. 39–70. W.B. Saunders, Philadelphia.

100. Nagase, H. and Woessner, Jr, J.F. (1993). Role of endogenous proteinases in the degradation of cartilage matrix. In *Joint cartilage degradation* (ed. J.F. Woessner, Jr and D.S. Howell), pp. 159–86. Dekker, New York.

101. Ehrlich, M.G., Mankin, H.J., and Treadwell, B.V. (1973). Acid hydrolase activity in osteoarthritic and normal human cartilage. *Journal of Bone and Joint Surgery*, **55A**, 1068–76.

102. Nguyen, Q., Murphy, G., Roughly, P.J., and Mort, J.S. (1989). Degradation of proteoglycan aggregate by a cartilage metalloprotease. *Biochemical Journal*, **259**, 61–7.

103. Kempson, G.E., Tuke, M.A., Dingle, J.T., Barrett, A.J., and Horsfield, P.H. (1976). The effects of proteolytic enzymes on the mechanical properties of adult human articular cartilage. *Biochimica et Biophysica Acta*, **428**, 741–60.

104. Sandy, J.D., Flannery, C.R., Neame, P.J., and Lohmander, L.S. (1992). The structure of aggrecan fragments in human synovial fluid. *Journal of Clinical Investigation*, **89**, 1512–16.

105. Flannery, C.R., Lark, M.W., and Sandy, J.D. (1991). Identification of a stromelysin cleavage site within the interglobular domain of human aggrecan. *Journal of Biological Chemistry*, **267**, 1008–14.

106. Lohmander, L.S., Neame, P.J., and Sandy, J.D. (1993). The structure of aggrecan fragments in human synovial fluid. *Arthritis and Rheumatism*, **36**, 181–9.

107. Evans, C.H. and Brown, T.D. (1993). Role of physical and mechanical agents in degrading the matrix. In *Joint cartilage degradation* (ed. J.F. Woessner, Jr and D.S. Howell), pp. 187–208. Dekker, New York.

108. Jeffrey, J.E., Gregory, D.W., and Aspden, R.M. (1995). Matrix damage and chondrocyte viability following a single impact load on articular cartilage. *Archives of Biochemistry and Biophysics*, **322**(1), 87–96.

109. Farquhar, T., Xia, Y., Burton-Wurster, N., Jelinski, L., and Lust, G. (1995). Latent weakening of articular cartilage after impact loading, revealed by ionic stress and by MR imaging. *Transactions of the Orthopaedic Research Society*, **20**, 195.

110. Sah, R.L., Doong, J.Y.H., Grodzinsky, A.J., Plaas, A.H.K., and Sandy, J.D. (1991). Effects of compression on the loss of newly synthesized proteoglycans and proteins from cartilage explants. *Archives of Biochemistry and Biophysics*, **286**, 20–9.

111. Bonassar, L.J., Sandy, J.D., Lark, M.W., Plaas, A.H.K., Frank, E.H., and Grodzinsky, A.J. (1997). Inhibition of cartilage degradation and changes in physical properties induced by IL-1β and Retinoic Acid using matrix metalloproteinase inhibitors. *Archives of Biochemistry and Biophysics*, **344**, 404–12.

7.2.6   Crystals and osteoarthritis
H. Ralph Schumacher Jr

A potentially important, but still inadequately investigated, aspect of articular cartilage and other articular tissues is their tendency to form calcium-containing crystals. These crystals precipitate in the extracellular matrix of the cartilage and can be released into the joint space. Calcium deposition in cartilage as a feature of osteoarthritis (OA) was noted in autopsy specimens by Bennet *et al.* as early as 1942[1]. These deposits, which were hematoxyphilic on routine staining of histologic sections with hematoxylin/eosin, were located in the menisci and were probably apatite. Radiographic evidence of cartilage calcification (chondrocalcinosis) was described by Zitnan and Sitaj in their extensive studies in Czechoslovakia[2] (Fig. 7.29). Subsequently, McCarty and coworkers[3] ascertained that the calcium deposits were crystals of calcium pyrophosphate dihydrate (CPPD). Deposition of CPPD crystals occurs in some families[4] and in some diseases associated with OA, but was soon recognized to occur commonly also with age[5]. The increased prevalence of CPPD deposition with age makes it likely that the CPPD crystal will have some impact on OA. This chapter addresses several aspects of calcium crystal deposition in relation to OA.

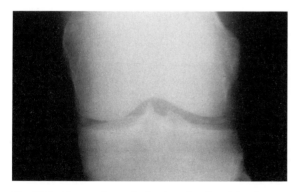

Fig. 7.29   Knee radiograph showing chondrocalcinosis, manifested by calcification in medial and lateral menisci. This radiograph shows no evidence of osteoarthritis.

Types of crystals seen in OA and their prevalence, as determined by various techniques

Several reports have described CPPD and apatite crystals, together or separately, in synovial fluid from patients with knee OA[6–8]. We found at least one of these types of crystals in samples of synovial fluid from 60 per cent of 100 consecutive patients with OA who had knee effusions[6]. Eighteen per cent of the specimens contained apatite alone (defined by the presence of 2+ alizarin red positive chunks and confirmed by electronmicroscopy), 13 per cent contained CPPD, and 29 per cent of the samples had both types of calcium crystals. The proportion of OA subjects whose synovial fluid contained crystals rose with increasing radiographic severity of OA, so that synovial fluid from all nine patients with grade 4 OA contained crystals. Crystals were more common in patients who had previously received an intra-articular steroid injection than in those who had not; however, those patients also had more severe OA. Other investigators have found CPPD and/or apatite in as many as 71 per cent of synovial effusions from patients with OA[7].

The technique for identification of CPPD crystals in synovial fluid is fairly standardized, with examination of drops of the fluid by compensated polarized light microscopy (Fig. 7.30). Tiny crystals can easily be missed by this method, but their detection can be facilitated by electron microscopy[9], centrifugation of the synovial fluid, with examination of the pellet, or special extraction techniques[10,11]. A recent extraction study by Swan *et al.*[10] has suggested that the proportion of OA fluids that contain crystals may be much higher than generally recognized[10]. Whether the presence of a large crystal load has a measurable effect on the manifestations of OA or the rate of progression of the disease has not been studied, but seems possible.

Identification of apatites is more difficult than identification of CPPD. We employ the alizarin red S

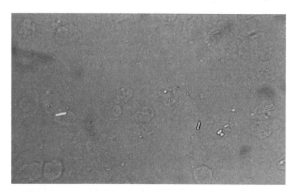

Fig. 7.30 Rod-shaped, square, or rhomboid-shaped birefringent CPPD crystals in synovial fluid cells. (400× polarized light.)

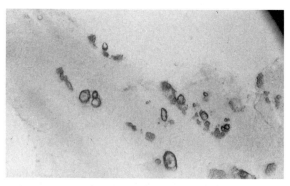

Fig. 7.31(a) Fragment of tissue obtained by centrifugation of synovial fluid, showing shiny but non-birefringent clumps of apatite crystals. (400× light microscopy.)

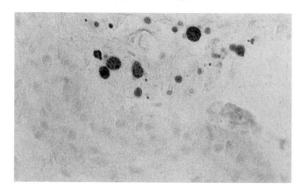

Fig. 7.31(b) Alizarin red S darkly staining similar apatite clumps in a fragment of synovial tissue. (400× light microscopy.)

stain as a clinical screening technique[12], but require transmission electron microscopy with elemental analysis and/or X-ray or electron diffraction, to confirm the presence of apatite. Fourier transform infrared analysis may also be used for this purpose. Centrifugation of the synovial fluid sample to concentrate the crystalline material increases the yield when the volume of the effusion is large (Fig. 7.31). Halverson successfully uses a ^{14}C disodium etidronate binding assay[13] to quantitate apatite in synovial fluid.

Of necessity, studies of synovial fluid crystals examine only the subset of patients with OA who have a joint effusion, and only those joints, such as the knee, from which synovial fluid can readily be extracted. In a study in which biopsies of articular cartilage were obtained from metacarpophalangeal (MCP) joints of patients without joint effusions, who had a distinctive form of OA secondary to hemochromatosis, crystals of apatite and/or CPPD were detected by electron-microscopy in all specimens examined. This was true even in three cases in which no evidence of calcification was present radiographically or on examination of the cartilage by light microscopy[14].

Ali has described the presence of a potentially important crystal, suspected to be Whitlockite (see p. 139), in OA cartilage[15,16]. To date, other crystals, such as oxalate and calcium carbonate, have not been detected in OA joints. It has been suggested that in gouty subjects who have Heberden's nodes, monosodium urate crystals are seen more frequently in the nodes than would be expected by chance[17]. There is no evidence, however, that this represents anything more than preferential deposition of the monosodium urate crystal in an altered matrix, that is, urate crystal deposition is not considered to be a primary factor in OA.

However, gout should be kept in mind as a complication of OA and is a cause of secondary OA.

Cholesterol crystals have been detected in some chronic OA joint effusions and appear to result from the release of lipids from cell membranes. They have not been identified as a significant factor in the course of the disease. Various lipids are present in cartilage matrix and cells, however, and may deserve further study.

Are crystals only a late result of OA or can they be an early finding?

Most studies of crystals in OA joints are, as might be expected, performed on samples from patients who are already symptomatic or have advanced disease when the sample of synovial fluid is obtained. In virtually all such reports, the proportion of OA patients in whom apatite crystals are detected increases with the severity of OA[6,7]. The pathogenesis of OA in these cases, that is, whether the presence of the crystal is a result of more severe disease or contributes to it, is unknown.

There is some suggestion that crystals may be present very early in the course of OA — before the disease is clinically detectable. Ali, who has performed extensive studies on apatite and other crystals in articular cartilage, has reported the presence of a calcium phosphate crystal with distinctive square morphology, consistent with Whitlockite, and has noted these crystals even in normal cartilage from relatively young persons[15,16]. Others have not followed up on these observations.

In our studies of articular cartilage obtained at autopsy[18], in which radiographs of the cartilage were obtained *ex vivo*, calcification was more common when anatomic evidence of OA was present, but cartilage from 7.8 per cent of subjects with minimal or no pathologic changes of OA also exhibited calcification. Ninety-three per cent of cartilage samples classified as showing definite OA stained positively for calcium with alizarin S and Von Kossa stains, while 24 per cent of those with minimal or no OA also showed such staining.

We recently examined samples of articular cartilage from cruciate-deficient dogs at an early stage of OA[19]. Although we saw no evidence of CPPD crystals, alizarin red-positive material was present in the synovial fluid only six weeks after cruciate ligament section — long before any overt morphologic evidence of OA had developed. Electron microscopic studies of pellets, obtained after centrifugation of the synovial fluid, showed apatite-like crystals in membranous arrays, suggesting that cell membranes were the initial site of deposition. The origin of these arrays is now under investigation. The above findings suggest that apatite and other calcium phosphates may be present at a much earlier stage in OA than is generally recognized.

Morphologic studies of familial chondrocalcinosis have shown clearly that deposition of CPPD crystals in the midzone of the articular cartilage and in the meniscus may antedate any clinical evidence of OA[4]. Metabolic changes in chondrocytes and matrix occur in association with this crystal deposition process[20-22]. The concentration of inorganic pyrophosphate is increased in synovial fluid from patients with OA (as it is in samples from subjects with CPPD disease)[23].

Levels tend to correlate with the severity of radiographic joint degeneration. How these changes relate to the early metabolic changes in OA cartilage requires further study.

Because CPPD crystal deposition is very common in patients with advanced OA, further study is needed to determine whether the mechanism of crystal formation in OA is the same as that in idiopathic CPPD deposition disease. Interestingly, the distribution of joint involvement in primary CPPD deposition disease is somewhat different from that in primary OA. For example, wrist and metacarpophalangeal joint involvement are more common in CPPD disease than in OA[24].

Deposition of apatite crystals in the midzone and deeper zone of articular cartilage has been produced in rabbits by chronic oral administration of dihydrotachysterol[25]. Although degenerative changes were noted in the chondrocytes, morphologic changes of OA were not seen over a 90-day period of observation[25]. It would be informative to follow such animals for a longer period. In short-term studies in the same rabbit model, intra-articular injection of ferrous chloride after dihydrotachysterol administration resulted in synovial deposition of apatite, but no overt evidence of OA.

The pathogenesis of crystal deposition in cartilage is still under study. Additional investigations of the earliest phases of crystal deposition are needed. As noted below, morphologic and biochemical changes occur in the articular cartilage matrix with crystal deposition. Some studies have shown nucleation of CPPD or apatites on matrix vesicle-like structures and collagen fibers within the cartilage[9,25,26]. Clearly, both structures may calcify, but the primary sites of calcification *in vivo* and the sequence of crystal deposition are unclear.

How might crystals affect the course of OA?

An interesting speculation, supported by studies of Hayes *et al.*[27], is that crystals, by virtue of their hardness, have a deleterious mechanical effect on articular cartilage. The wear of plugs of normal equine cartilage was tested in the presence or absence of monoclinic 1×5 μm CPPD crystals, large hydroxyapatite clumps, or 50–100 μm orthorhombic calcium pyrophosphate tetrahydrate. Each of these crystals resulted in an increase in the release of sulfate from the cartilage into the lubricant solution, reflecting loss of integrity of the extracellular matrix of the tissue. It would be of interest to similarly test cartilage which contained crystals within its matrix, and other particulate material, such as cartilage wear fragments.

In a longitudinal radiographic study of patients with chondrocalcinosis and OA, although the intensity of calcium deposition increased with time, this did not seem to predict progression of changes of OA[28]. Over a mean duration of observation of 4.6 years, only 27 per cent exhibited progression of joint symptoms and 16 per cent had more advanced radiographic changes of OA. The most common sign of radiographic progression was an increase in osteophytosis. No correlation was observed between the extent of calcification and progression of arthropathy.

It is now generally accepted that inflammation is a component of OA[29,30], although details concerning the cells and cell products involved, the temporal relationship of inflammation to the changes in cartilage and subchondral bone, and the relation of joint inflammation to crystals all require further study. Synovial fluid from patients with OA tends to contain a slightly higher cell count than normal synovial fluid, even though the total white cell count is less than $2000/mm^3$ and is often considered 'non-inflammatory'. Evidence of synovial membrane inflammation is common in OA, at least at the time the patient presents with symptoms[29,30]. Whether this inflammation is due, in part, to the presence of crystals is unknown.

Efforts to show that the presence of apatite crystals increases the intensity of joint inflammation as reflected by the synovial fluid analysis, have not shown a positive correlation in OA. In fact, we noted a tendency for the synovial fluid leukocyte count to be lower in samples of synovial fluid from OA patients in which apatite crystals were detected, than in samples which did not contain crystals[6,31] (Table 7.5). In contrast to apatite, CPPD crystals seem to be associated with an increase in the synovial fluid leukocyte count in patients with OA[32].

We have also tested the acute phlogistic response to CPPD, apatite, and a mixture of these two crystals in the rat subcutaneous air pouch model[32]. On a weight basis, the synthetic apatites caused much less inflammation, as measured by the leukocyte count and levels of protease, prostaglandin E_2, and tumor necrosis factor-α (TNF-α), than CPPD or the mixture (Fig. 7.32). Recently, Fam et al. injected CPPD crystals into rabbits in which OA had been induced by partial lateral meniscectomy and section of the fibular collateral and sesamoid ligaments[33]. While the CPPD concentrations used were considerably higher than those usually present in human OA, the severity of inflammation and of pathologic changes in the cartilage were both more severe in CPPD-injected knees, than in the OA knees which were not injected with a crystal load. The findings tend to support a role for the crystals in the pathogenesis of the more severe OA associated with the presence of the crystals[34].

Even in the absence of overt inflammation, as detected by synovial fluid analysis, CPPD or apatite crystals may have a chronic effect in the joint after they have been phagocytized by synovial cells. Cheung has shown that synovial cells cultured in vitro with apatite or CPPD, release collagenase, neutral protease, and prostaglandins[35]. The low grade, largely mononuclear

Table 7.5 Mean and standard deviations of the leukocyte counts, differential leukocyte percentages, and absolute leukocyte counts among the non-inflammatory synovial fluid (SF), divided by nature of crystalline materials contained[32]

Group and No. of specimens	SF cells					
	WBC / mm³	PMN	L	Mo	Macro	SLC
1 MSU (15)		25 ± 23%	14 ± 6%	43 ± 13%	7 ± 5%	14 ± 10%
	677 ± 693	(278 ± 428*)	(71 ± 80)	(268 ± 317)	(38 ± 43)	(74 ± 96)
2 CPPD alone		12 ± 16	18 ± 10	52 ± 17	6 ± 4	12 ± 10
or ± AP-like (14)	300 ± 127	(48 ± 74)	(55 ± 69)	(146 ± 69)	(16 ± 13)	(34 ± 34)
3 AP-like (8)		12 ± 15	15 ± 9	51 ± 8	7 ± 5	16 ± 12
	13 ± 96	(10 ± 14)	(20 ± 26)	(66 ± 47)	(12 ± 13)	(24 ± 35)
4 No crystals		11 ± 13	22 ± 12	50 ± 12	6 ± 5	12 ± 8
(62)	319 ± 308	(38 ± 84)	(81 ± 134)	(153 ± 146)	(19 ± 27)	(29 ± 27)
5 Whole group		13 ± 16	20 ± 11	49 ± 13	6 ± 5	12 ± 9
(100)	365 ± 398	(78 ± 201)	(74 ± 115)	(164 ± 177)	(21 ± 28)	(36 ± 47)

WBC = leukocyte counts / mm³; ± = differential leukocyte percentages; * = absolute leukocyte counts / mm³; MSU = monosodium urate; CPPD = calcium pyrophosphate dihydrate; AP = apatite-like clumps; PMN = polymorphonuclear leukocyte; L = lymphocyte; Mo = monocyte; Macro = macrophage or large phagocytic mononuclear cell; SLC = type B synovial lining cell; No = number in group.

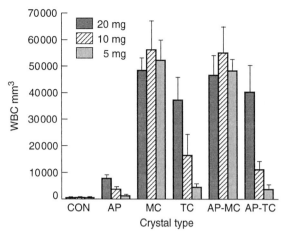

Fig. 7.32 Leukocyte counts induced by injections of single types and mixed calcium containing crystals. CON = control, AP = apatite, MC = monoclinic CPPD, TC = triclinic CPPD, AP-MC = mixture of apatite and monoclinic CPPD, AP-TC = mixture of apatite and triclinic CPPD. CPPD crystals (especially monoclinic CPPD) produced higher leukocyte counts than apatite crystals (p < 0.01). Leukocyte counts of mixed crystals were predominantly determined by CPPD crystals. (Reprinted, with permission, from reference 32.)

cell inflammation seen in OA certainly could be driven, in part, by crystals. Even in the absence of symptoms or signs of acute inflammation, phagocytized crystals of CPPD (Fig. 7.33) and apatite (Fig. 7.34) can be found in mononuclear cells in synovial fluid from patients with OA. This is analogous to the phagocytosis of monosodium urate (MSU) crystals by mononuclear cells in interim gout, in which the phenomenon may contribute to bone lysis (tophi)[36]. Notably, we found that patients in whom both apatite and CPPD were

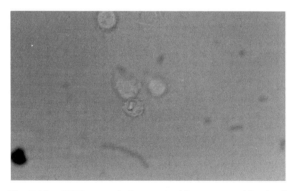

Fig. 7.33 CPPD crystal phagocytized by a synovial fluid cell in a non-inflammatory fluid from a patient with osteoarthritis. Routine light microscopy of wet preparation. (Magnification ×400)

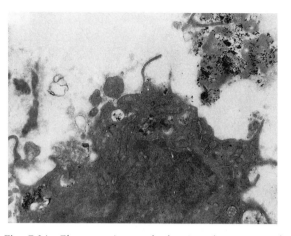

Fig. 7.34 Electron micrograph showing phagocytosis of clumps of apatite crystals by a mononuclear cell. Extracellular apatite is coated by protein-like material. N = nucleus of synovial fluid cell. (Magnification ×10, 000)

present within synovial fluid leukocytes tended to have more severe radiographic evidence of OA[18] than patients whose joint fluid did not show evidence of intracellular crystals. In the most destructive forms of OA, such as the Milwaukee shoulder syndrome and similar rapidly destructive arthritis of the hip or knee[37,38], virtually all samples of joint fluid which have been examined here contained apatites and/or CPPD.

What are the implications for clinicians and researchers of crystal deposition in OA?

Would removal of crystals make a difference in the progression of OA or in the associated symptoms? In the distinctive, destructive OA of the Milwaukee shoulder syndrome, tidal irrigation of the joints of two patients resulted in symptomatic improvement which was sustained for approximately 10 months[39]. Tidal irrigation has also been used in patients with knee OA with some evidence of temporary benefit[40,41], although the beneficial effect could be due not only to removal of crystals but of other debris, enzymes, cytokines, and other mediators of inflammation. Until methods are developed to dissolve crystals or prevent their formation, it may be difficult to define their role in OA. If subsets of patients with OA in whom crystals are present could be identified, clinical comparisons could be made.

Tetracyclines, which have been proposed as disease-modifying agents in both OA and rheumatoid arthritis[42,43], bind avidly to apatites. Could this binding serve to retain the drug in phagocytic vacuoles after ingestion of apatites, resulting in a more prolonged effect of the drug on cartilage metalloprotease levels? Hydroxychloroquine has also been considered in treatment of OA. In an experimental model, we have shown that this antimalarial decreases protease levels and may inhibit CPPD crystal-induced inflammation[44]. In clinical trials of disease-modifying drugs for OA, the presence of crystals and of low-grade synovial inflammation are variables that will require consideration.

Intra-articular injection of depot corticosteriod preparations is widely used for symptomatic treatment of OA, although the effectiveness of this treatment is controversial. Two studies suggest that injection of depot corticosteroids can cause periarticular calcification[45,46], although neither study focused on OA. These findings raise the possibility that synovial fluid crystal deposition may be increased by steroid injection. If so, this might be a relative contraindication to this form of treatment. On the other hand, our own limited experience suggests that OA patients whose synovial fluid contains alizarin-positive material, may respond better to an intra-articular steroid injection than OA patients whose synovial fluid does not contain such material[47]. Among OA patients treated with ibuprofen and an intra-articular injection of triamcinolone hexacetonide, those whose synovial fluid contained alizarin red positive material had significantly better improvement in stiffness and tended to have less pain, than those whose synovial fluid did not contain alizarin-positive deposits.

Whether the presence of crystals delineates a subset of OA patients who would respond better to an NSAID than to acetaminophen is unknown. Although acetaminophen is often effective in the symptomatic treatment of OA[48,49], it is clear that some patients obtain better pain relief with an NSAID than with acetaminophen[50]. Because NSAIDs carry considerably more risk than acetaminophen in patients with OA, it is important to determine if, and/or when, the anti-inflammatory effects of those agents are useful in OA.

References

1. Bennet, G.A., Waine, H., and Bauer, W. (1942). Changes in the knee joint at various ages with particular reference to the nature and development of degenerative joint disease. Commonwealth Fund, New York.

2. Zitnan, D. and Sitaj S. (1976). Natural course of articular chondrocalcinosis. *Arthritis and Rheumatism*, **19**, 363–90.

3. McCarty, D.J. (1977). Calcium pyrophosphate dihydrate crystals deposition disease (pseudogout syndrome) — clinical aspects. *Clinics in the Rheumatic Diseases*, **3**, 61–89.

4. Reginato, A.J., Schumacher, H.R., and Martinez, V.A. (1974). The articular cartilage in familial chondrocalcinosis: light and electron microscopic study. *Arthritis and Rheumatism*, **17**, 977–92.

5. Ellman, M.H. and Levin, B. (1975). Chondrocalcinosis in elderly persons. *Arthritis and Rheumatism*, **18**, 43–7.

6. Gibilisco, P.A., Schumacher, H.R., Hollander, J., and Soper, K.A. (1985). Synovial fluid crystals in osteoarthritis. *Arthritis and Rheumatism*, **28**, 511–15.

7. Halverson, P. and McCarty, D.J. (1986). Patterns of radiographic abnormalities associated with basic calcium phosphate and CPPD crystal deposition in the knee. *Annals of the Rheumatic Diseases*, **45**, 603–5.

8. Dieppe, P.A., Doyle, D.V., Huskisson, E.C., Willoughby, D.A., and Crocker, P.R. (1978). Mixed crystal deposition and osteoarthritis. *British Medical Journal*, **21**, 150.

9. Beutler, A., Rothfuss, S., Clayburne, G., Sieck, M., and Schumacher, H.R. (1993). Calcium pyrophosphate dihydrate crystal deposition in synovium. Relationship to collagen fibers and chondrometaplasia. *Arthritis and Rheumatism*, **369**, 704–15.

10. Swan, A., Chapman, B., Heap, P., *et al.* (1994). Submicroscopic crystals in osteoarthritis synovial fluids. *Annals of the Rheumatic Diseases*, **53**, 467–70.

11. Swan, A.J., Heywood, B.R., and Dieppe, P.A. (1992). Extraction of calcium containing crystals from synovial fluids and articular cartilage. *Journal of Rheumatology*, **19**, 1763–73.

12. Paul, H., Reginato, A.J., Schumacher, H.R. (1983). Alizarin red S staining as a screening test to detect calcium compounds in synovial fluid. *Arthritis and Rheumatism*, **26**, 191–200.

13. Halverson, P.B. and McCarty, D.J. (1979). Identification of hydroxyapatite crystals in synovial fluid. *Arthritis and Rheumatism*, **22**, 389–95.

14. Schumacher, H.R. (1982). Articular cartilage in the degenerative arthropathy of hemochromatosis. *Arthritis and Rheumatism*, **25**, 1460–8.

15. Ali, S.Y., Rees, J.A., and Scotchford, C.A. (1992). Microcrystal deposition in cartilage and in osteoarthritis. *Bone and Mineral*, **17**, 115–18.

16. Scotchford, C.A. and Ali, S.Y. (1995). Magnesium whitlockite deposition in articular cartilage: a study of 80 specimens from 70 patients. *Annals of the Rheumatic Diseases*, **54**, 339–44.

17. Lally, E.V., Zimmerman, B., Ho, G., and Kaplan, S.R. (1989). Urate-mediated inflammation in nodal osteoarthritis: clinical and roentgenographic correlations. *Arthritis and Rheumatism*, **32**, 86–90.

18. Gordon, G.V., Villanueva, T., Schumacher, H.R., and Gohel, V. (1984). Autopsy study correlating degree of osteoarthritis, synovitis and evidence of articular calcification. *Journal of Rheumatology*, **11**, 681–6.

19. Schumacher, H.R., Rubinow, A., Rothfuss, S., Weiser, P., and Brandt, K. (1994). Apatite crystal clumps in synovial fluid are an early finding in canine osteoarthritis. *Arthritis and Rheumatism*, 37 (**supplement**), S346 (abstract).

20. Rachow, J.W. and Ryan, L.M. (1988). Adenosine triphosphate pyrophosphohydrolase and neutral inorganic pyrophosphatase in pathologic joint fluids. *Arthritis and Rheumatism*, 28, 1283–8.

21. Pattrick, M., Hamilton, E., Hornby, J., and Doherty, M. (1991). Synovial fluid pyrophosphate and nucleoside triphosphate pyrophosphatase: comparison between normal and diseased and between inflamed and non-inflamed joints. *Annals of the Rheumatic Diseases*, 50, 214–18.

22. Krankendonk, S., Ryan, L., Buday, M., Llynch, K., and Derfus, B. (1994). Human osteoarthritic vesicles generate both monoclinic calcium pyrophosphate dihydrate and apatite crystals *in vitro*. *Journal of Bone and Joint Surgery*, 18, 502–3.

23. Silcox, D.C. and McCarty, D.J. (1974). Elevated inorganic pyrophosphate concentrations in synovial fluids in osteoarthritis and pseudogout. *Journal of Laboratory and Clinical Medicine*, 83, 518–31.

24. McCarty, D.J. (1993). Calcium pyrophosphate dihydrate crystal deposition disease. In *Primer on the rheumatic diseases* (10th edn). (ed. H.R. Schumacher), pp. 219–22. Arthritis Foundation, Atlanta

25. Reginato, A.J., Schumacher, H.R., and Brighton, C.T. (1982). Experimental hydroxyapatite synovial and articular cartilage calcification. Light and electron microscopic studies. *Arthritis and Rheumatism*, 25, 1239–49.

26. Derfus, B., Steinberg, M., Mandel, N., et al. (1995). Characterization of an additional articular cartilage vesicle fraction that generates calcium pyrophosphate dihydrate crystals *in vitro*. *Journal of Rheumatology*, 22, 1514–19.

27. Hayes, A., Harris, B., Dieppe, P.A., and Clift, S.E. (1993). Wear of articular cartilage: the effect of crystals. *Proceedings of the Institute of Mechanical Engineering*, 207, 41–58.

28. Doherty, M., Dieppe, P., and Watt, I. (1993). Pyrophosphate arthropathy: a prospective study. *British Journal of Rheumatology*, 32, 189–96.

29. Lindblad, S. and Hedors, E. (1987). Arthroscopic and immunohistological characterization of knee joint synovitis in osteoarthritis. *Arthritis and Rheumatism*, 30, 1081–8.

30. Schumacher, H.R. (1995). Synovial inflammation, crystals and osteoarthritis. *Journal of Rheumatology*, 22, 101–3.

31. Louthrenoo, W., Sieck, M., Clayburne, G., Rothfuss, S., and Schumacher, H.R. (1991). Supravital staining of cells in non-inflammatory synovial fluids: analysis of the effects of crystals on cell populations. *Journal of Rheumatology*, 18, 409–13.

32. Watanabe, W., Baker, D.G., and Schumacher, H.R. (1992). Comparison of the acute inflammation induced by calcium pyrophosphate dihydrate, apatite and mixed crystals in the rat air pouch model of a synovial space. *Journal of Rheumatology*, 19, 1453–7.

33. Fam, A.G., Morava-Protzner, I., Purcell, C., Young, B.D., Bunting, P.S. and Lewis, A.J. (1995). Acceleration of experimental lapine osteoarthritis by calcium pyrophosphate microcrystalline synovitis. *Arthritis and Rheumatism*, 38, 201–10.

34. Ledingham, J., Regan, M., Jones, A., and Doherty, M. (1995). Factors affecting radiographic progression of knee osteoarthritis. *Annals of the Rheumatic Diseases*, 54, 53–8.

35. Cheung, H.S., Halverson, P.B., and McCarty, D.J. (1981). Release of collagenase, neutral protease and prostaglandins from cultured mammalian synovial cells by hydroxyapatite and calcium pyrophosphate dihydrate crystals. *Arthritis and Rheumatism*, 24, 1338–44.

36. Agudelo, C. and Schumacher, H.R. (1973). The synovitis of acute gouty arthritis: a light and electron microscopic study. *Human Pathology*, 4, 265–79.

37. McCarty, D.J., Halverson, P.B., Carrera, G.J., Brewer, B.J., and Kozin, F. (1981). 'Milwaukee shoulder' — association of microspheroids containing hydroxyapatite crystals, active collagenase and neutral protease with rotator cuff defects. I: clinical aspects. *Arthritis and Rheumatism*, 24, 464–73.

38. Zakraoui, L., Schumacher, H.R., Rothfuss, S., Sieck, M., and Clayburne, G. (1996). Idiopathic destructive arthropathies: clinically light, and election microscopic studies. *Journal of Clinical Rheumatology*, 2, 9–17.

39. Caporal, R., Rossi, S., and Montecucco, C. (1994). Tidal irrigation in Milwaukee shoulder syndrome (letter). *Journal of Rheumatology*, 21, 1781–2.

40. Chang, R.W., Falconer, J., Stulberg, D., et al. (1993). A randomized controlled trial of arthroscopic surgery versus closed needle joint lavage for patients with osteoarthritis of the knee. *Arthritis and Rheumatism*, 36, 289–96.

41. Ike, R.W., Arnold, W.J., Rothschild, E.W., and Sha, L. (1992). Tidal irrigation cooperating group: tidal irrigation versus conservative medical management in patients with osteoarthritis of the knee: a prospective randomized trial. *Journal of Rheumatology*, 19, 772–9.

42. Brandt, K.D. (1995). Toward pharmacologic modification of joint damage in osteoarthritis. *Annals of Internal Medicine*, 122, 874–5.

43. Greenwald, R. (1995). Tetracyclines may be therapeutically beneficial in rheumatoid arthritis, but not for the reasons you might think. *Journal of Clinical Rheumatology*, 1, 185–9.

44. Meng, Z.H., Branigan, P., Park, J., Rao, J., Baker, D.G., and Schumacher, H.R. (1995). Hydroxychloroquine inhibits matrix metalloprotease production in experimental calcium pyrophosphate dihydrate crystal induced inflammation in the rat subcutaneous air pouch. *Arthritis and Rheumatism*, (**Suppl. 9**), S244 (abstract).

45. McCarty, D.J. (1972). Treatment of rheumatoid joint inflammation with triamcinolone hexacetonide. *Arthritis and Rheumatism*, 15, 157–73.

46. Hardin, J.G. Jr, Greilier, J.M., and Andriopouls, N. (1976). Controlled study of long-term effects of 'total hand' injection: a preliminary report (abstract). *Arthritis and Rheumatism*, 19, 800–1.

47. Schumacher, H.R., Stineman, M.G., Magge, S., Huppert, A., Rahman, M. (1996). The association between synovial fluid and treatment response in osteoarthritis. *Internal Medicine*, **4**, 25–34.

48. Bradley, J.D., Brandt, K.D., Katz, B.P., Kolasinski, L.A., and Ryan, S.I. (1992). Treatment of knee osteoarthritis: relationship of clinical features of joint inflammation to the response to a non-steroidal anti-inflammatory drug or pure analgesic. *Journal of Rheumatology*, **19**, 1950–4.

49. Bradley, J.D., Brandt, K.D., Katz, B.P., Kalasinski, L.A., and Ryan, S.I. (1991). Comparison of an anti-inflammatory dose of ibuprofen and analgesic dose of ibuprofen, and acetaminophen in the treatment of patients with osteoarthritis of the knee. *New England Journal of Medicine*, **325**, 87–91.

50. Williams, H.J., Ward, J.R., Egger, M.J., *et al.* (1993). Comparison of naproxen and acetaminophen in a two-year study of treatment of osteoarthritis of the knee. *Arthritis and Rheumatism*, **36**, 1196–1206.

7.3   Subchondral bone

David B. Burr

Osteoarthritis (OA) is not only a disease of cartilage, but affects all tissues of the joint. As the name suggests, the bone below the articular cartilage is an integral part of the disease process. As such, it is worthwhile to review its physical properties and involvement in the disease process as a basis to evaluate treatments for OA that are directed at the bony changes, as well as at the destruction of the articular cartilage.

The subchondral plate

Morphology

The subchondral plate is comprised of the subarticular mineralized tissues. It extends from the tidemark (junction of the calcified and uncalcified cartilage) to the beginning of the marrow space (Fig. 7.35). It includes

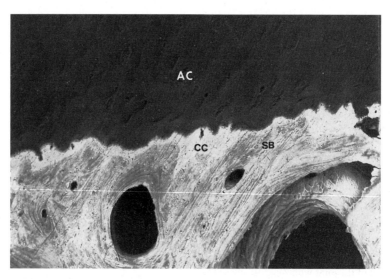

Fig. 7.35   Backscattered electron microscopic image from the infero-medial portion of the human femoral head. The calcified cartilage (CC) is clearly demarcated from the articular cartilage (AC) and the adjacent subchondral bone (SB). (Original magnification 100×)

both calcified cartilage and the lamellar subchondral cortical bone that underlie and support the articular cartilage (Fig. 7.35). Although collagen fibers are continuous between the layers of articular hyaline cartilage and calcified cartilage, continuity has not been demonstrated at the osteochondral junction[1,2]. Therefore, the osteochondral junction may represent a region of weakness, particularly to shear stresses. The subchondral plate supports the articular cartilage, directs loads to the diaphyseal cortex[3], and may be a source of nutrients to the deeper layers of the hyaline cartilage, especially during growth[4].

The thickness of the subchondral bone varies normally by species[5], age[6], body weight, location[2] and function, and changes in joint disease. The thickness of subchondral bone on the convex side of a joint is generally fairly constant, but on the concave side is much greater in the central weight-bearing area than toward the margins (Fig. 7.36)[2,6], suggesting that plate thickness is determined by weightbearing. This possibility is supported by the positive association between the thicknesses of subchondral bone, trabecular bone, and articular cartilage[7]. Most estimates of the thickness of subchondral bone of the tibial plateau are between 0.1–2.0 mm,[6] although thicknesses up to 3.0 mm have been reported in the weightbearing region of the tibial plateau in older individuals[2].

Subchondral bone is highly vascular (Fig. 7.37), although many of the vessels do not reach the calcified cartilage and, except in disease, none penetrates to the articular cartilage[2,4]. The vascular pores average about

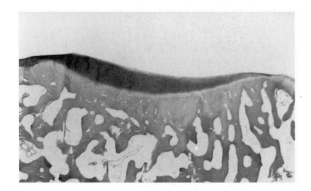

Fig. 7.36 Proximal tibial condyle of a New Zealand white rabbit, showing thicker subchondral bone below the central weight-bearing portion of the joint with thinning toward the joint periphery, where the overlying articular cartilage is also thinner. (Stained with Safranin O. Original magnification. 2.5×)

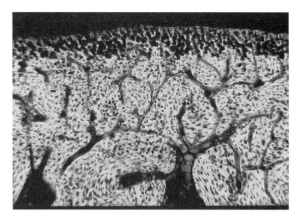

Fig. 7.37 Vascular tree in subchondral bone of the proximal tibia of a normal rabbit. Note the extensive anastomoses among the vessels. (Stained with Villanueva's tetrachrome. Original magnification 125×)

89 μm in diameter, ranging from more than 100 μm where extensions of the marrow cavity with lining cells penetrate, to 10–30μm vascular (Haversian) canals surrounded by concentric lamellae. The distribution and numbers of these spaces may vary across the joint. Although the vascularity of the subchondral plate generally increases in OA, it does not change with age alone[2,8]. Vascular perfusion of the plate may, in fact, decline until about the age of 70[9], when increases associated with normal degenerative changes occur.

Whether these vascular spaces provide a nutritional pathway for the cartilage is unclear[10], but the absence of vascular loops and failure to observe vessels penetrating the tidemark suggest that they do not function in a nutritional capacity. They may be more important to nutrition in younger individuals, in whom diffusion of hydrogen ions into articular cartilage from subchondral bone can be detected, than in adults, in whom no diffusion is evident[4]. If hydrogen does not diffuse, it is unlikely that larger molecules, for example, O_2, amino acids, and glucose, would do so. The observation that subchondral avascular necrosis is associated with articular cartilage deterioration in youth but not in adults[11,12] supports the idea. More likely, the vessels supply the bone, providing a means for repairing and replacing the cortical bone and calcified cartilage of the subchondral plate through normal remodeling processes. This is important in the rapid densification of subchondral bone after joint overload[13] and the bony sclerosis in joints affected by OA.

Unmyelinated nerve fibers are present in subchondral bone[14], but nerves have not been identified in the calcified cartilage. Subchondral cysts in equine femoral heads and fetlocks fail to elicit much of a pain response, suggesting that most of the nerves in subchondral bone may be vasomotor rather than nociceptive[15]. Recently, nerve fibers which were shown immunohistochemically to contain substance P (a neuropeptide that acts as both a vasodilator and a neurotransmitter in sensory nerves) and free nerve endings, were identified in Haversian canals of the normal subchondral plate[16], although SP-reactive fibers were not detected in either hyaline articular cartilage or calcified cartilage. Another neurotransmitter and vasodilator, calcitonin gene-related peptide (CGRP), is also frequently associated with blood vessels in bone near the epiphysis[17]. 5-Hydroxytryptamine, a neurotransmitter that acts as a vasoconstrictor, has also been identified in subchondral bone[18].

Remodeling

Remodeling of the subchondral region during development results in calcification of the zone of hypertrophic cartilage in the growth plate, providing a transition between cartilage and the primary spongiosa. After maturity, remodeling of the plate probably functions to maintain joint congruity and reduce joint stresses in overloaded regions. Remodeling in the calcified bed is one of the earliest biological reactions to repetitive impulsive loading and to single impact injury of the canine knee[19].

Measurements of normal remodeling in the human subchondral plate are rare, because of the difficulty of sampling non-diseased bone. Little is known, therefore, about normal turnover rates, except what can be inferred by extension from animal studies or from bone scintigraphy. In animals, bone turnover in the subchondral plate is very rapid prior to closure of the growth plate, and slows significantly with age[20]; it is likely that bone remodeling in the human subchondral plate follows a similar pattern. Also, because bone responds to strain and high levels of strain tend to depress the activation of new sites of bone turnover, it is likely that the rate of remodeling is less in weight-bearing regions of a joint than in less loaded areas, although differences have not been detected in various regions of tibial subchondral bone in animal studies[5]. However, a lower remodeling rate would increase the mean tissue age in the weight-bearing areas and would be reflected in a greater amount of mineralized bone underlying the weight-bearing areas, as found in the normal human elbow[21]. The situation may be reversed in end-stage OA, in which remodeling appears to be more active in weight-bearing areas of the femoral head[22].

Rates of mineral apposition in the human femoral head range from 0.81–3.66 μm per day[23]. The lower value is comparable to the normal rate in cortical bone, but the upper is 2–3 times greater. Higher rates occur on eburnated surfaces of OA femoral heads than in the subchondral bone underlying intact cartilage, and rates in osteopenic regions are slightly lower than those in sclerotic regions[23]. Consistent with this, fewer osteoclasts are present in osteopenic regions than in sclerotic regions of bone.

In a murine model of spontaneous OA, bone formation rates were as high as 3.57 μm per day in the early stages, and fell to 1.42–2.14 μm per day when the disease was advanced, compared to a rate of 0.71 μm per day in normal controls[24]. The normal appositional rate in mice is similar to that in human iliac crest, and can probably be taken as a reasonable estimate of normal bone remodeling in humans. Interestingly, the increase in bone formation rate was seen only in regions underlying cartilage degeneration; appositional rates in regions of bone underlying normal cartilage adjacent to focal OA cartilage lesions were normal[24]. Significant variations in remodeling parameters have been noted between medial and lateral tibial condyles, across each condyle, and at various distances from the joint surface[25].

High rates of bone turnover may reduce the stiffness of subchondral bone even though the bone itself increases in thickness[26]. Grynpas *et al.*[22] reported both a thicker subchondral plate (compared to young and old normals) and abnormally low mineralization of subchondral bone in femoral heads from patients with OA. Hypomineralization can be explained by an increased rate of turnover, in which osteoid volume and thickness and the rate of bone resorption are increased, but porosity is not. This can occur in the absence of an imbalance between formation and resorption.

In contrast, others[27,28] have reported low bone formation and resorption activity in human knee OA, or have been unable to detect increased alkaline phosphatase activity[29]. These differences probably reflect the stage of the disease, with rapid formative processes early in the disease, reflected by the presence of woven bone[28], and substantial slowing of bone turnover in late-stage disease, when sclerosis is apparent. This is consistent with the increased uptake of radioactive tracers early in the disease process[47] and the finding that uptake is greater when OA develops rapidly than when it develops more slowly[30]. However, OA is a focal process, and the bone below degenerating cartilage may exhibit a combination of regions of high bone turnover (both formation and resorption), cystic degeneration, and osteophytosis[31].

Most studies of bone turnover in the human subchondral plate have been performed in samples obtained at surgery from patients with end-stage OA. This is a poor source of material for study of the pathophysiology of joint breakdown. Changes detected in the subchondral bone may be secondary to the cartilage deterioration or to a reduction in weightbearing. However, normal human tissue from younger individuals who have not developed full-thickness cartilage loss is difficult to obtain.

Mechanical properties

Subchondral bone is viscoelastic, that is, it deforms less, or becomes stiffer, when loading is rapid than when loading is more gradual. Deformation of the bone increases the contact area under load and minimizes stresses within the cartilage. When cartilage deformation under an impact load is limited, the contact area is minimized and high stresses can be generated in the cartilage matrix. This is one reason that impact loading is detrimental to cartilage integrity.

Bone is a better shock absorber than articular cartilage, which is too thin to be effective in this capacity[3,32,33]. By attenuating force through joints, the bone underlying the articular surface can protect the cartilage from damage caused by excessive loads. Nonetheless, load transfer from the articular surface to the diaphyseal cortex creates large shear stresses in the subchondral bone[3], particularly under the edges of the contact region. However, because of the undulations at the tidemark and osteochondral junction (Fig. 7.38), the calcified cartilage bed transforms these shear stresses into compressive and tensile stresses[34], which cartilage is better able to withstand. The calcified cartilage also helps minimize shear stresses by providing an intermediate layer less stiff than the subchondral bone[35].

The presence of the subchondral bone also raises the injury threshold for articular cartilage by constraining radial deformation of the cartilage under load[34,36]; if the cartilage is unconstrained a 50 per cent increase in cartilage deformation will cause vertical fissures[36]. In the presence of attached subchondral bone, fissures are less likely to develop. Cartilage can withstand about 2.5–5 times the peak deformation caused by the load generated by walking, suggesting that the subchondral bone provides a large safety factor and has great capac-

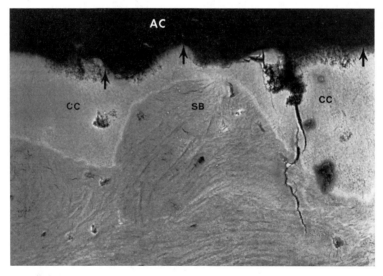

Fig. 7.38 Backscattered electron microscopic image from the infero-medial portion of a human femoral head, showing sharp undulations at the osteochondral junction and gentler undulations at the tidemark (arrows). Areas near the tidemark appear to be undergoing calcification. AC = articular cartilage; CC = calcified cartilage; SB = subchondral bone. (Original magnification 400×)

Table 7.6 Force attenuation in joints[1]

Tissue	Attenuation (%)
Subchondral bone	30
Cortical bone	30–35
Cartilage	1–3
Joint capsule / synovium	35
Synovial fluid	0

[1]Reference 33

ity to protect cartilage from all but the most severe impact injuries.

Normal subchondral bone attenuates loads through the joint to a greater degree than either articular cartilage or periarticular soft tissues[33,37]. In normal joints, subchondral bone absorbs 30–50 per cent of the load through the joint, while cartilage attenuates only 1–3 per cent (Table 7.6)[33,38]. When subchondral bone becomes sclerotic, however, it is less able to absorb and dissipate the energy of impact, increasing the force transmitted through the joint. Because of this, OA knees absorb only about 50 per cent of the load absorbed by normal knees[38].

The mechanical properties of the subchondral bone depend largely on its thickness and vary, therefore, from location to location. Although subchondral bone is morphologically similar to lamellar bone of the cortex, it is not as stiff as diaphyseal cortical bone[39]. Both strength and stiffness increase exponentially with apparent density and mineral content, so that a small increase in apparent density signifies a much larger increase in stiffness. However, because the rapid turnover of bone in early OA increases the amount of osteoid present in the subchondral bone[22,27] and reduces overall mineralization[31], subchondral bone in OA may actually be osteopenic. The younger mean tissue age[22], and the observation that much of this new bone is woven[28], may account for some observations of decreased hardness, elastic modulus, and strength of subchondral bone in OA[26,29,40,41].

Subchondral bone in osteoarthritis

The relationship of bone density to OA

Although there are reports to the contrary[42], many clinical observations suggest that osteopenic women do not develop severe OA[43]. OA and osteoporosis tend to be mutually exclusive[44,45]. Fewer than 1 per cent of the population have coexisting OA and osteoporosis[44].

Severe OA is not usually seen on femoral heads removed after femoral neck fracture, and bone density in subjects with OA of the hip is greater than normal for their age group[46]. In subjects with joint pain of OA, the risk of hip fracture is only one-third as great as in those without pain[47], while the incidence of hip fracture in mothers of children with OA is only half as great as that in the general population of comparable age and gender[48]. In the Framingham Study[49], mean bone density of the proximal femur was 5–9 per cent higher in women with grade 1–2 OA than in those without OA; men showed similar, but statistically insignificant, patterns.

It should be noted that the above studies included only subjects with established OA. Whether increased bone density antedated, or was secondary to, joint deterioration cannot be answered by clinical studies. Although few studies have examined whether bone density is causally related to OA in a site-specific fashion, Milgram and Jasty[50] approached this question in an analysis of 21 patients with osteopetrosis. Although only three of their subjects were over 40 years old, all had OA of the hip and knee. Casden *et al.* also noted a high prevalence of hip OA in osteopetrotic adults[51]. These studies do not establish that the increase of density of the osteopetrotic bone caused the regeneration of the overlying cartilage, because the bony deformation which occurs in osteopetrosis[52] may alter loading conditions and directly cause cartilage degeneration.

The inverse relationship between osteoporosis and OA may reflect a generalized qualitative difference in bone in the two conditions. Growth hormone levels are elevated in patients with OA compared to those with osteoporosis[53]. Growth hormone stimulates the synthesis of insulin-like growth factor-I (IGF-I) and may be responsible for the higher IGF levels found in iliac crest bone of subjects with OA of hand joints[54]. IGF stimulates bone formation by enhancing bone cell growth and differentiation. The presence of increased levels of growth factors in bone at a distance from the site of joint deterioration suggests that persons who will develop OA may be predisposed to develop bone that is more dense and stiffer than normal as a result of a remodeling imbalance that favors bone formation.

Many of the clinical studies which have concluded that an inverse relationship exists between OA and osteoporosis have failed to account for possible confounding factors, such as physical activity, obesity and race. For example, obesity, a well-known risk factor for knee OA (see Chapter 2), is itself associated with an increase in bone density. Furthermore, the samples used in clinical studies that have demonstrated an inverse relationship between osteoporosis and OA were not random, but were subject to selection bias because only those with clinical manifestations of OA were identified as subjects[46,55,56]. In some cases, appropriate controls for age and sex were omitted[46,57], the sample sizes were extremely small[57,58], or the diagnosis of OA was based on self-report of joint pain without radiographic conformation[59,60].

Bone density in relation to common risk factors for OA

The fact that occupational or sports-related overuse of a joint, and obesity, both predispose to OA (see Chapter 2), suggests that physical joint loads contribute to OA. Bone is more responsive to mechanical load than cartilage, and is known to become more dense under increased loads. However, most studies have not measured bone density in joints, either site-specifically or longitudinally, prior to the development of clinically apparent OA.

It is possible that metabolic pathways exist which predispose to joint deterioration. Controlling for serum cholesterol and uric acid concentrations, diabetes, body fat distribution, and blood pressure does not reduce the relationship between obesity and OA. On this basis, Davis *et al.*[61] suggested that obesity exerts a mechanical, rather than a metabolic effect by causing joint overload. However, these investigators did not measure serum estradiol levels, even though obese women have higher levels of endogenous estrogen. After menopause, adipose tissue is the main source of estrone, via conversion from androstenedione. Estrogens are known to maintain bone mass and to have an effect on cartilage through nuclear receptors[62], but whether they exert a protective[63] or detrimental effect on the development of OA[64] is unknown. Because estrogen stimulates release of transforming growth factor-β (TGF-β)[65] and IGF[66] from human bone cells, increased bone formation

stimulated by TGF-β and IGF could provide a causal link between obesity, increased density of subchondral bone, and OA. A metabolic predisposition to OA would help explain the higher incidence of OA in women than in men, even when obesity and physical activity have been controlled[67].

OA is more prevalent in blacks than in whites, particularly among women[67]. The basis for this racial difference is not clear, but blacks have a higher bone mass and slower bone turnover than whites[68], resulting in a higher mean skeletal tissue age. This provides another possible explanation for the association between OA and an increase in the density of subchondral bone.

Thus, all three risk factors for OA discussed above, that is, physical activity, obesity, and race, either cause or are coincidentally associated with high bone density, implying a causal link between bone density and OA. However, studies showing temporal topographic relations between subchondral bone changes and the development of OA are needed to prove cause and effect.

The importance of subchondral bone in the pathogenesis of OA: initiation versus progression

Radin *et al.*[69] proposed that subchondral bone changes initiate progressive joint degeneration. They suggested that impulsive loading of joints increases the density and stiffness of subchondral bone, which is then less able to attenuate and distribute forces through the joint[70]. This increases the stresses in the articular cartilage, promoting degeneration.

However, cartilage damage does not always lead to full-thickness cartilage loss[71]. The initiation of cartilage damage, and its progression to full thickness loss (that is, OA), may involve distinct pathophysiologic mechanisms. Radin and Rose[70] proposed that *initiation* of cartilage fibrillation is caused by steep stiffness gradients in the underlying subchondral bone. When inhomogeneity in density, or stiffness of the subchondral bone, is present, cartilage overlying the less dense bone will deform more than that over the bone of greater density. This differential deformation 'stretches' the cartilage at the edge of the joint contact area, generating stresses that can tear the cartilage and initiate joint deterioration. *Progression* to full-thickness loss, they contended[70], occurs only in the presence of continued impulsive loading over an already stiffened subchondral plate.

The hypothesis that stiffened subchondral bone alone drives the destruction of the overlying articular cartilage has not been supported by finite element models. Mathematical modeling studies[32] show that even substantial increases in subchondral bone density will cause only modest increases in mechanical stress in the overlying cartilage. The amount of stiffening of subchondral bone required to significantly increase cartilage stresses was well beyond normal expectations. This suggests that, although stiffened subchondral bone might play an important part in the OA process, it is insufficient to account for articular cartilage destruction.

Nevertheless, there is consensus that end-stage OA is characterized by remodeling of the calcified tissues of the joint and subchondral sclerosis. Disagreements arise about whether these changes are primary, occur simultaneously with, or are secondary to, deterioration of the cartilage.

In several animal models of OA an increase in density of subchondral bone occurs early in the process that eventually leads to full-thickness cartilage loss[13]. For example, after a nine-week period of impulsive loading in rabbits, which resulted in a 15 per cent increase in bone volume, progressive changes in articular cartilage, leading to complete disorganization of the articular surface, followed within six months[13].

Such studies do not establish a cause-and-effect relationship between subchondral bone changes and cartilage deterioration. However, subchondral bone of the medial tibial plateau thickens well before development of cartilage fibrillation in cynomolgus monkeys who develop OA spontaneously[72], in which fibrillation is mainly limited to areas of cartilage overlying thickened subchondral bone. Similarly, when the tibia is angulated by 30°, cartilage deterioration in rabbits[73] corresponds both spatially and temporally to the increase in density of the subchondral bone; in regions in which the subchondral plate is not thickened, the cartilage remains normal. In mice with advanced OA, cartilage overlying sclerotic bone breaks down, while cartilage over adjacent areas of normal bone density remains intact[24]. These studies suggest that subchondral sclerosis may be a necessary precondition for progression to full-thickness cartilage loss.

The contention that an increase in density of subchondral bone may be necessary for progression of OA is supported also by changes that occur in canine knee joints after transection of the anterior cruciate ligament. In this model, bone volume in the subchondral plate is increased within 18 months, but full-thickness loss of cartilage does not develop for more than four years. However, mild histologic changes of OA are evident in the cartilage months before significant subchondral thickening is apparent. Therefore, subchondral plate changes must not be required *for initiation* of OA in this model, although stiffening of subchondral bone may be necessary for *progression* to full-thickness loss of cartilage[74].

The role of the calcified cartilage and advancement of the tidemark in OA

Calcified cartilage provides a layer of intermediate stiffness between the articular cartilage and subchondral bone[1,34]; its elastic modulus is more than 10 times lower than that of subchondral bone[35]. The normal undulating structure of the interfaces between the calcified and non-calcified cartilage (the tidemark), and between the calcified cartilage and underlying subchondral bone (osteochondral junction) (Fig. 7.38), transforms shear stresses into tensile and compressive stresses which are less destructive to cartilage[34].

Focal advance of the tidemark leads to thinning of the overlying hyaline articular cartilage (Fig. 7.39)[75], while concurrent advancement and thickening of the subchondral bone can maintain[76], or thicken[77,78], the zone of calcified cartilage, compromising the normal proportionality between the articular and calcified cartilage. Green *et al.*[76] found mild fibrillation of cartilage associated with as many as eight reduplications of the tidemark, although reduplication also occurs in non-fibrillated and non-weight-bearing areas[79]. A small degree of tidemark advancement can profoundly increase mechanical stress focally in the overlying articular cartilage, and could contribute to cartilage loss in OA. However, although most data shows an association between tidemark advancement and cartilage fibrillation[80], both changes could represent independent effects of aging, rather than a cause-and-effect mechanism for progression of OA[76].

The advantage afforded by maintenance of the relative thickness of the layers of calcified cartilage and hyaline cartilage with respect to the integrity of the articular surface remains unknown. However, the ratio of thickness of articular to calcified cartilage in normal joints (approximately 10:1) is usually very highly maintained[78].

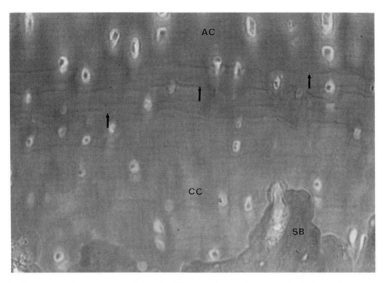

Fig. 7.39 Tidemark duplication in the proximal tibia of a New Zealand white rabbit. At least six tidemarks are clearly visible. AC = articular cartilage; CC = calcified cartilage; SB = subchondral bone. (Stained with Safranin O. Original magnification 98×)

Repair of damage to subchondral bone

Patients in whom subchondral damage can be visualized by magnetic resonance imaging immediately after a high-impact knee injury, often develop overt cartilage loss within six months, even if the cartilage is arthroscopically normal immediately after the injury[81]. This supports the concept that damage to the subchondral tissues without overt damage to articular cartilage may lead to OA.

Microfractures in the subchondral bone may stimulate remodeling, accounting for increased vascularity and the presence of granulation tissue in degenerating joints[82]. Microcracks, averaging 56 μm in length, occur routinely in calcified cartilage from non-diseased femoral heads of middle-aged humans[83,84], and are associated with foci of vascular remodeling in OA cartilage (Fig. 7.40). Single or repetitive high-impact loads cause microcracks in calcified cartilage[19,85], which are followed by focal remodeling of the subchondral bone and deterioration of the overlying articular cartilage. This provides evidence that microdamage in calcified cartilage can play a role in the pathogenesis of OA, secondary to joint trauma. It is not known whether similar processes are implicated in the development of OA in the absence of overt joint trauma, nor has it been demonstrated satisfactorily that articular cartilage

itself is not damaged during the acute loading episode. It cannot be stated with certainty, therefore, that damage to calcified cartilage or subchondral bone *causes* deterioration of the overlying cartilage. Repair of microcracks requires vascular invasion from the subchondral bone, so it is probably necessary for the crack to penetrate to the osteochondral junction for repair to occur, unless some unknown form of cellular signaling exists.

Vascular changes in subchondral bone in OA

In both clinical and experimental studies[1,9,86], OA is associated with increased vascularity of the subchondral plate and calcified cartilage. Chondromalacia patellae is associated with a 10 per cent increase in the number of arterial capillaries[18]. This increased vascularity suggests that the subchondral plate is attempting to adapt or maintain joint geometry through normal remodeling as the OA joint becomes less congruent[9]. Foci of vascular invasion in calcified cartilage are osteon-like remodeling units, led by a tunneling resorption front of multinucleated chondroclast/osteoclastic cells (Fig. 7.41). Recent electron microscopic studies of vascular canals[1] confirm the cutting cone-like structure of these vascular invasion foci.

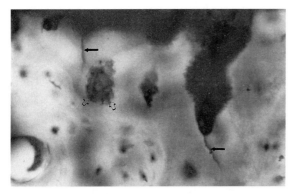

(a)

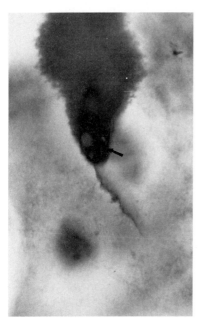

(b)

Fig. 7.40 Microcracks (closed arrows) present *in vivo* in the calcified cartilage of the human femoral head. Both sections were stained *en bloc* with basic fuchsin. (a) The crack on the right is associated with a resorption front, while the one on the left is associated with a vascular bud containing chondroclasts (open arrows). (Original magnification 156×) (Used with permission from reference 84. Copyright 1993, American Medical Association) (b) Higher magnification view showing chondroclasts leading the resorption front that is repairing a microcrack. (Original magnification 312×) (Used with permission from Burr, D.B. and Schaffler, M.B. (1995). The involvement of subchondral mineralized tissues in osteoarthrosis: quantitative microscopic evidence. (*Microscopy Research and Technique*, © 1997 John Wiley & Sons, Inc)

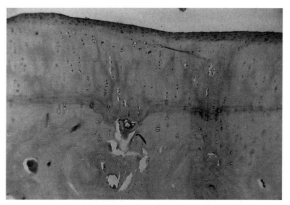

Fig. 7.41 Vascular invasion (arrows) of the calcified and articular cartilage in the proximal tibia of a sheep. Note that tidemark duplication is present. (Stained with Safranin O. Original magnification 98×) (Used with permission from Burr, D.B. and Schaffler, M.B. (1995) The involvement of subchondral mineralized tissues in osteoarthrosis: quantitative microscopic evidence. (*Microscopy Research and Technique*, © 1997 John Wiley & Sons, Inc)

melysin[87], and to dissociate these proenzymes from complexes with metalloproteinase inhibitors[88]. Production of angiogenesis factors by chondrocytes is associated with cartilage resorption and calcification in the growth plate[89], leading to speculation that a similar relationship may occur in OA. Levels of angiogenesis factors in the synovial fluid[90] are increased in about two thirds of all patients with OA. Failure of the chondrocytes to produce a sufficient concentration of protease inhibitors, which will also prevent vascular ingrowth, has been proposed as a pathogenetic factor in OA[91], but cause and effect have not yet been established[89]. The presence of high levels of angiogenesis factors in the hypertrophic zone of the growth plate has led to speculation that vascular ingrowth in OA may be a process of renewed endochondral ossification[89], but the processes are quite different morphologically, in that chondrocytes do not appear to become hypertrophic or apoptotic in OA.

Although remodeling may be beneficial in OA by increasing the joint contact area and thereby reducing stress on the cartilage, it is commonly held that vascular invasion of calcified cartilage is a critical component in the progression of OA[1,9,77]. Deep fibrillation and fissuring of the cartilage matrix occur focally, with increased vascular invasion of the calcified bed[79]. In the calcified cartilage, vascular invasion of the calcified region, renewed mineralization around the regions of new vascular ingrowth, thickening of the calcified carti-

Vascular ingrowth in OA may be associated with angiogenesis factors, which are known to activate matrix-neutral metalloproteinases, such as prostro-

lage, and focal reduplication of the tidemark are hallmarks of the OA process[9,18,20,76,77]. The increased remodeling probably accounts for some observations of hypomineralization of the subchondral tissues in OA[22] because it reduces the mean tissue age. These findings give rise to the hypothesis that the fate of articular cartilage is not determined solely by stiffening of subchondral bone but, rather, by remodeling processes in both subchondral bone and calcified cartilage that cause alterations of the cartilage biologically and mechanically.

Vascular invasion of the subchondral plate may also be a cause of joint pain in OA, by creating intraosseous hypertension, either as a result of arterial hyperplasia[92] or reduced venous return[93]. Vessels within the bone may become engorged, particularly during rest, and cause aching of the joint. The association between increased intra-articular pressure and increased osseous pressure[94] provides a mechanism for this pathway.

Effects of pharmacologic agents on subchondral bone in OA

Agents that reduce bone turnover could theoretically inhibit development of progressive OA by preserving joint architecture[95]. Bisphosphonates[95-97], which inhibit the activation of new remodeling sites in bone, result secondarily in an increase in density of the subchondral plate. If, as suggested above, dense subchondral bone is responsible for progressive OA, agents that reduce bone turnover should not prove very effective in this disease. However, intra-articular injection of etidronate (ethane diphosphonate, Didronel®) was found to reduce the severity of joint pathology in the canine cruciate-deficiency model of OA (Altman, R., unpublished observation). Whether bisphosphonates are effective in reducing sclerosis of bone or destruction of the overlying cartilage in humans with OA has not yet been studied.

Pharmacologic agents for OA which are designed to act on bone, ideally should increase turnover without causing a large loss of bone through an imbalance between resorption and formation. Agents that prevent thickening of subchondral bone may be more beneficial than those that tend to preserve joint architecture. Finally, it should be kept in mind that the changes in joint architecture that occur in OA are not primary, but secondary, and represent an attempt by the joint to adapt to changing loads. To prevent this attempt at adaptation is more likely to intensify the pathologic changes of OA than to alleviate them.

References

1. Bullough, P.G. (1981). The geometry of diarthrodial joints, its physiologic maintenance, and the possible significance of age-related changes in geometry-to-load distribution and the development of osteoarthritis. *Clinical Orthopaedics and Related Research*, **156**, 61–6.
2. Clark, J.M. and Huber, J.D. (1990). The structure of the human subchondral plate. *Journal of Bone and Joint Surgery*, **72B**, 866–73.
3. Hayes, W.C., Swenson L.W. Jr, and Schurman, D.J. (1978). Axisymmetric finite element analysis of the lateral tibial plateau. *Journal of Biomechanics*, **11**, 21–33.
4. Ogata, K., Whiteside, L.A., and Lesker P.A. (1978). Subchondral route for nutrition to articular cartilage in the rabbit. *Journal of Bone and Joint Surgery*, **60A**, 905–10.
5. Armstrong, S.J., Read, R.A., and Price, R. (1995). Topographical variation within the articular cartilage and subchondral bone of the normal ovine knee joint: a histological approach. *Osteoarthritis and Cartilage*, **5**, 25–33.
6. Milz, S. and Putz, R. (1994). Quantitative morphology of the subchondral plate of the tibial plateau. *Journal of Anatomy*, **185**, 103–10.
7. Noble, J. and Alexander K. (1985). Studies of tibial subchondral bone density and its significance. *Journal of Bone and Joint Surgery*, **67a**, 295–302.
8. Woods, C.G., Greenwald, A.S., and Haynes, D.W. (1970). Subchondral vascularity in the human femoral head. *Annals of the Rheumatic Diseases*, **29**, 138–42.
9. Lane, L.B., Villacin, A., and Bullough, P.G. (1977). The vascularity and remodelling of subchondral bone and calcified cartilage in adult human femoral and humeral heads. *Journal of Bone and Joint Surgery*, **59B**, 272–8.
10. Greenwald, A.S. and Haynes, D.W. (1969). A pathway for nutrients from the medullary cavity to the articular cartilage of the human femoral head. *Journal of Bone and Joint Surgery*, **51B**, 747–53.
11. McKibbin, B. and Holdsworth, F.W. (1966). The nutrition of immature joint cartilage in the lamb. *Journal of Bone and Joint Surgery*, **48B**, 793–803.
12. Zahir, A. and Freeman, M.A.R. (1972). Cartilage changes following a single episode of infarction of the capital femoral epiphysis in the dog. *Journal of Bone and Joint Surgery*, **54A**, 125–36.
13. Radin, E.L., Martin, R.B., Burr, D.B., Caterson, B., Boyd, R.D., and Goodwin, C. (1984). Effects of mechanical loading on the tissues of the rabbit knee. *Journal of Orthopaedic Research*, **2**, 221–34.
14. Milgram, J.W. and Robinson, R.A. (1965). An electron microscopic demonstration of unmyelinated nerves in the Haversian canals of the adult dog. *Bulletin of the Johns Hopkins Hosp.*, **117**, 163–73.

15. Nixon, A.J., Adams, R.M., and Teigland, M.B. (1988). Subchondral cystic lesions (osteochondrosis) of the femoral heads in a horse. *Journal of the American Veterinary Medical Association*, **192**, 360–2.

16. Nixon A.J. and Cummings, J.F. (1994). Substance P immunohistochemical study of the sensory innervation of normal subchondral bone in the equine metacarpophalangeal joint. *American Journal of Veterinary Research*, **55**, 28–33.

17. Bjurholm, A., Kreicbergs, A. Brodin, E., and Schultzberg, M. (1988). Substance P- and CGRP-immunoreactive nerves in bone. *Peptides*, **9**, 165–71.

18. Badalamente, M.A. and Cherney S.B. (1989). Periosteal and vascular innervation of the human patella in degenerative joint disease. *Seminars in Arthritis and Rheumatism*, **18**, 61–6.

19. Thompson, R.C., Oegema, T.R., Lewis, J.L., and Wallace L. (1991). Osteoarthrotic changes after acute transarticular load. *Journal of Bone and Joint Surgery*, **73A**, 990–1001.

20. Lemperg, R. (1971). The subchondral bone plate of the femoral head in adult rabbits. I. Spontaneous remodeling studied by microradiography and tetracycline labeling. *Virchows Archives*, **352**, 1–13.

21. Eckstein F., Muller-Gerbl, M., Steinlechner, M., Kierse R., and Putz, R. (1995). Subchondral bone density in the human elbow assessed by computed tomography osteoabsorptiometry: a relation of the loading history of the joint surfaces. *Journal of Orthopaedic Research*, **13**, 268–78.

22. Grynpas, M.D., Alpert, B., Katz, I., Lieberman, I., and Pritzker, K.P.H. (1991). Subchondral bone in osteoarthritis. *Calcified Tissue International*, **49**, 20–6.

23. Amir, G., Pirie, C.J., Rashad, S., and Revell, P.A. (1992). Remodelling of subchondral bone in osteoarthritis: a histomorphometric study. *Journal of Clinical Pathology*, **45**, 990–2.

24. Benske, J., Schunke, M., and Tillmann, B. (1988). Subchondral bone formation in arthrosis. Polychrome labeling studies in mice. *Acta Orthopaedica Scandinavica*, **59**, 536–41.

25. Shimuzu, M., Tsuji, H., Matsui H., Katoh, Y., and Sano A. (1993). Morphometric analysis of subchondral bone of the tibial condyle in osteoarthrosis. *Clinical Orthopaedics and Related Research*, **293**, 229–39.

26. Miyanaga, Y. (1979). Mechanical behavior of the subchondral bone in experimentally induced osteoarthritis. *Journal of the Japanese Orthopaedic Association*, **53**, 681–95.

27. Havdrup, T., Hulth, A., and Telhag, H. (1976). The subchondral bone in osteoarthritis and rheumatoid arthritis of the knee. *Acta Orthopaedica Scandinavica*, **47**, 345–50.

28. Christensen, P., Kjaer, J., Melsen, F., Nielsen H.E., Sneppen, O., and Vang, P-S. (1982). The subchondral bone of the proximal tibial epiphysis in osteoarthritis of the knee. *Acta Orthopaedica Scandinavica*, **53**, 889–95.

29. Lereim, P., Linde, A., and Goldie, J.F. (1975). The presence of alkaline phosphatase in the subchondral bone of the medial tibial condyle in the normal state and in osteoarthritis and rheumatoid arthritis. *Archiv für Orthopädische und Unfall-chirurgie*, **83**, 181–5.

30. Danielsson, L.G., Dymling, J-F., and Heripret, G. (1963). Coxarthrosis in man studied with external counting of [85]Sr and [47]Ca. *Clinical Orthopaedics and Related Research*, **31**, 184–99.

31. Jeffery, A.K. Osteogenesis in the osteoarthritic femoral head: a study using radioactive ^{32}P and tetracycline bone markers. *Journal of Bone and Joint Surgery*, **55B**, 262–72.

32. Brown, T.D., Radin, E.L., Martin, R.B., and Burr, D.B. (1984). Finite element studies of some juxtarticular stress changes due to localized subchondral stiffening. *Journal of Biomechanics*, **17**, 11–24.

33. Radin, E.L., Paul, I.L., and Lowy, M. (1970). A comparison of the dynamic force transmitting properties of subchondral bone and articular cartilage. *Journal of Bone and Joint Surgery*, **52A**, 444–56.

34. Redler, I., Mow, V.C., Zimny, M.L., and Mansell, J. (1975). The ultrastructure and biomechanical significance of the tidemark of articular cartilage. *Clinical Orthopaedics and Related Research*, **112**, 357–62.

35. Mente, P. and Lewis, J. (1992). Elastic modulus of calcified cartilage. *Transactions of the Orthopaedic Research Society*, **17**, 212.

36. Finlay, J.B. and Repo, R.U. (1978). Cartilage impact *in vitro*: effect of bone and cement. *Journal of Biomechanics*, **11**, 379–88.

37. Jacob, H.A.C., Huggler, A.H., Dietschi, C., and Schreiber, A. (1976). Mechanical function of subchondral bone as experimentally determined on the acetabulum of the human pelvis. *Journal of Biomechanics*, **9**, 625–7.

38. Hoshino, A. and Wallace, W.A. (1987). Impact-absorbing properties of the human knee. *Journal of Bone and Joint Surgery*, **69B**, 807–11.

39. Brown T.D. and Vrahas, M.S. (1984). The apparent elastic modulus of the juxtarticular subchondral bone of the femoral head. *Journal of Orthopaedic Research*, **2**, 32–8.

40. Lereim, P., Goldie, I., and Dahlberg, E. (1974). Hardness of the subchondral bone of the tibial condyles in the normal state and in osteoarthritis and rheumatoid arthritis. *Acta Orthopaedica Scandinavica*, **45**, 614–27.

41. Zysset, P.K., Sonny, M., and Hayes, W.C. (1994). Morphology-mechanical property relations in trabecular bone of the osteoarthritic proximal tibia. *Journal of Arthroplasty*, **9**, 203–16.

42. Healey, J.H., Vigorita, V.J., and Lane, J.M. (1985). The coexistence and characteristics of osteoarthritis and osteoporosis. *Journal of Bone and Joint Surgery*, **67A**, 586–92.

43. Dequeker, J. (1985). The relationship between osteoporosis and osteoarthritis. *Clinics in the Rheumatic Diseases*, **11**, 271–96.

44. Pogrund, H., Rutenberg, M., Makin, M., Robin, G., Menczel, J., and Steinberg, R. (1982). Osteoarthritis of the hip joint and osteoporosis: a radiological study in a random population sample in Jerusalem. *Clinical Orthopaedics and Related Research*, **164**, 130–5.

45. Verstraeten, A., van Ermen, H., Haghebaert, G., Nijs, J., Geusens, P., and Dequeker, J. (1991). Osteoarthrosis

retards the development of osteoporosis. *Clinical Orthopaedics and Related Research*, **264**, 169–77.

46. Foss, M.V.L. and Byers, P.D. (1972). Bone density, osteoarthrosis of the hip, and fracture of the upper end of the femur. *Annals of the Rheumatic Diseases*, **31**, 259–64.

47. Cumming, R.G. and Klineberg, R.J. (1993). Epidemiological study of the relation between arthritis of the hip and hip fractures. *Annals of the Rheumatic Diseases*, **52**, 707–10.

48. Astrom, J. and Beertema, J. (1992). Reduced risk of hip fracture in the mothers of patients with osteoarthritis of the hip. *Journal of Bone and Joint Surgery*, **74B**, 270–1.

49. Hannan, M.T., Anderson, J.J., Zhang, Y., Levy, D., and Felson, D.T. (1993). Bone mineral density and knee osteoarthritis in elderly men and women. The Framingham Study. *Arthritis and Rheumatism*, **36**, 1671–80.

50. Milgram, J.W. and Jasty, M. (1982). Osteopetrosis. A morphological study of twenty-one cases. *Journal of Bone and Joint Surgery*, **64A**, 912–29.

51. Casden, A.M., Jaffe, F.F., Kastenbaum, D.M., and Bonar S.F. (1989). Osteoarthritis associated with osteopetrosis treated by total knee arthroplasty. *Clinical Orthopaedics and Related Research*, **247**, 202–7.

52. Sokoloff, L. (1990). Relationship of bone and cartilage in osteoarthritis. In: *Bone morphometry* (ed. H.E. Takahashi), pp. 274–7. Nishimura Co. Ltd, Niigata.

53. Dequeker, J., Burssens, A., and Bouillon R. (1982). Dynamics of growth hormone secretion in patients with osteoporosis and in patients with osteoarthritis. *Hormone Research*, **16**, 353–6.

54. Dequeker, J., Mohan, S., Finkelman, R.D., Aerssens, J., and Baylink, D.J. (1993). Generalized osteoarthritis associated with increased insulin-like growth factor types I and II and transforming growth factor B in cortical bone from the iliac crest. *Arthritis and Rheumatism*, **36**, 1702–8.

55. Byers, P.D., Contemponi, C.A., and Farkas, T.A. (1970). A postmortem study of the hip joint including the prevalence of the fractures of the right side. *Annals of the Rheumatic Diseases*, **29**, 15–31.

56. Dequeker, J., Goris, P., and Uytterhoeven, R. (1983). Osteoporosis and osteoarthritis (osteoarthrosis). Anthropometric distinctions. *Journal of the American Medical Association*, **249**, 1448–51.

57. Schnitzler, C.M. (1979). Bone formation, bone resorption and bone mineralisation in osteoarthritis and osteoporosis. *Journal of Bone and Joint Surgery*, **61B**, 257.

58. Roh, Y.S., Dequeker, J., and Mulier, J.C. (1974). Bone mass in osteoarthrosis measured *in vivo* by photon absorption. *Journal of Bone and Joint Surgery*, **56A**, 587–91.

59. Jones, G., Nguyen, T., Sambrook, P.N., Lord, S.R., Kelly, P.J., and Eisman, J.A. (1995). Osteoarthritis, bone density, postural stability, and osteoporotic fractures: a population based study. *Journal of Rheumatology*, **22**, 921–5.

60. Cumming, R.G. and Klineberg, R.J. (1993). Epidemiological study of the relation between arthritis of the hip and hip fractures. *Annals of the Rheumatic Diseases*, **52**, 707–10.

61. Davis, M.A., Ettinger, W.H., and Neuhaus, J.M. (1988). The role of metabolic factors and blood pressure in the association of obesity with osteoarthritis of the knee. *Journal of Rheumatology*, **15**, 1827–32.

62. Tsai, C-L. and Liu T-K. (1992). Up-regulation of estrogen receptors in rabbit osteoarthritic cartilage. *Life Sciences*, **50**, 1727–35.

63. Hannan, M.T., Felson, D.T., Anderson, J.J., Naimark, A., and Kannel, W.B. (1990). Estrogen use and radiographic osteoarthritis of the knee in women. *Arthritis and Rheumatism*, **33**, 525–32.

64. Rosner, I.A., Goldberg, V.M., and Moskowitz, R.W. (1986). Estrogens and osteoarthritis. *Clinical Orthopaedics and Related Research*, **213**, 77–83.

65. Oursler, M.J., Cortese, C., Keeting, P., Anderson, M.A. Bonde, S.K., and Riggs, B.L. (1991). Modulation of transforming growth factor-β production in normal human osteoblast-like cells by 17-β estradiol and parathyroid hormone. *Endocrinology*, **129**, 3313–20.

66. Ernst, M. and Rodan, G.A. (1991). Estradiol regulation of insulin-like growth factor-I expression in osteoblastic cells: evidence for transriptional control. *Molecular Endocrinology*, **5**, 1081–9.

67. Anderson, J.J. and Felson, D.T. (1988). Factors associated with osteoarthritis of the knee in the First National Health and Nutrition Examination Survey (HANES I). *American Journal of Epidemiology*, **128**, 179–89.

68. Kleerekoper, M., Nelson, D.A., Peterson, E.L., Flynn, M.J., Pawluszka, A.S., Jacobsen, G. *et al.* (1994). Reference data for bone mass, calciotropic hormones, and biochemical markers of bone remodeling in older (55–75) postmenopausal white and black women. *Journal of Bone and Mineral Research*, **9**, 1267–76.

69. Radin, E.L., Paul, I.L., and Rose, R.M. (1972). Mechanical factors in osteoarthritis. *Lancet*, **1**, 519–22.

70. Radin, E.L. and Rose, R.M. (1986). Role of subchondral bone in the initiation and progression of cartilage damage. *Clinical Orthopaedics and Related Research*, **213**, 34–40.

71. Meachim, G. (1963). The effect of scarification on articular cartilage in the rabbit. *Journal of Bone and Joint Surgery*, **45B**, 150–61.

72. Carlson, C.S., Loeser, R.F., Jayo, M.J., Weaver, D.S., Adams, M.R., and Jerome, C.P. (1994). Osteoarthritis in cynomolgus macaques: a primate model of naturally occurring disease. *Journal of Orthopaedic Research*, **12**, 331–9.

73. Wu, D.D., Burr, D.B., Boyd, R.D., and Radin, E.L. (1990). Bone and cartilage changes following experimental varus or valgus tibial angulation. *Journal of Orthopaedic Research*, **8**, 572–85.

74. Dedrick, D.K., Goldstein, S.A., Brandt, K.D., O'Connor, B.L., Goulet, R.W., and Albrecht, M. (1993). A longitudinal study of subchondral plate and trabecular bone in cruciate-deficient dogs with osteoarthritis followed up for 54 months. *Arthritis and Rheumatism*, **36**, 1460–7.

75. Karvonen, R.L., Negendank, W.G., Teitge, R.A., Reed, A.H., Miller, P.R. and Fernandez-Madrid, F. (1994). Factors affecting articular cartilage thickness in osteoarthritis and aging. *Journal of Rheumatology*, **21**, 1310–18.

76. Green, W.T., Martin, G.N., Eanes, E.D., and Sokoloff, L. (1970). Microradiographic study of the calcified layer of articular cartilage. *Archives of Pathology*, **90**, 151–8.

77. Lane, L.B. and Bullough, P.G. (1980). Age-related changes in the thickness of the calcified cartilage zone and the number of tidemarks in adult human articular cartilage. *Journal of Bone and Joint Surgery*, **62B**, 372–5.

78. Muller-Gerbl, M., Schulte, E., and Putz, R. (1987). The thickness of the calcified layer in different joints of a single individual. *Acta Morphologica Neerlando–Scandinavica*, **25**, 41–9.

79. Meachim, G. and Allibone, R. (1984). Topographical variation in the calcified zone of the upper femoral articular cartilage. *Journal of Anatomy*, **139**, 341–52.

80. Hulth, A. (1993). Does osteoarthrosis depend on growth of the mineralized layer of cartilage? *Clinical Orthopaedics and Related Research*, **287**, 19–24.

81. Vellet, A.D., Marks, P.H., Fowler, P.J., and Munro, T.G. (1991). Occult post-traumatic osteochondral lesions of the knee: prevalence, classification, and short-term sequelae evaluated with MR imaging. *Radiology*, **178**, 271–6.

82. Trueta, J. (1963). Studies on the etiopathology of osteoarthritis of the hip. *Clinical Orthopaedics and Related Research*, **31**, 7–19.

83. Sokoloff, L. (1993). Microcracks in the calcified layer of articular cartilage. *Archives of Pathology and Laboratory Medicine*, **117**, 191–5.

84. Mori, S., Harruff, R., and Burr, D.B. (1993). Microcracks in articular calcified cartilage of human femoral heads. *Archives of Pathology and Laboratory Medicine*, **117**, 196–8.

85. Vener, M.J., Thompson, R.C., Lewis, J.L., and Oegema, T.R. (1992). Subchondral damage after acute transarticular loading: An *in vitro* model of joint injury. *Journal of Orthopaedic Research*, **10**, 759–65.

86. Farkas, T., Boyd, R.D., Schaffler, M.B., Radin, E.L., and Burr, D.B. (1987). Early vascular changes in rabbit subchondral bone after repetitive impulsive loading. *Clinical Orthopaedics and Related Research*, **219**, 259–67.

87. Weiss, J.B., Hill, C.R., Davis, R.J., McLaughlin, B., Sedowofia, K.A., and Brown R.A. (1983). Activation of procollagenase by low molecular weight angiogenesis factor. *Bioscience Report*, **3**, 171–7.

88. Weiss, J.B., Odedra, R., and McLaughlin, B. (1987). Low molecular mass angiogenic factors. In *Micro-circulation: an update*, vol. 2 (ed. M. Tsuchiya), pp. 777–80. Elsevier, Amsterdam.

89. Brown, R.A. and Weiss, J.B. (1988). Neovascularisation and its role in the osteoarthritic process. *Annals of the Rheumatic Diseases*, **47**, 881–5.

90. Brown, R.A., Tomlinson, I.W., Hill, C.R., Weiss, J.B., Phillips, P., and Kumar, S. (1983). Relationship of angiogenesis factor in synovial fluid to various joint diseases. *Annals of the Rheumatic Diseases*, **42**, 301–7.

91. Stephens, R., Ghosh, P., and Taylor, T. (1979). The pathogenesis of osteoarthritis. *Medical Hypotheses*, **5**, 809–16.

92. Harrison, M.H.M., Schajowicz, F., and Trueta, J. (1953). Osteoarthritis of the hip: A study of the nature and evolution of the disease. *Journal of Bone and Joint Surgery*, **35B**, 598–626.

93. Arnoldi, C.C., Linderholm, H., and Muussbichler, H. (1972). Venous engorgement and intraosseus hypertension in osteoarthritis of the hip. *Journal of Bone and Joint Surgery*, **54B**, 409–21.

94. Bunger, C., Djurhuus, J.C., Sorensen, S.S., and Lucht, U. (1981). Intraosseus pressure in the knee in relation to stimulated joint effusion, joint position and venous obstruction. *Scandinavian Journal of Rheumatology*, **10**, 283–8.

95. Francis, M.D., Hovancik, K., and Boyce, R.W. (1989). NE-58095: a diphosphonate which prevents bone erosion and preserves joint architecture in experimental arthritis. *International Journal of Tissue Reactions*, **11**, 239–52.

96. Osterman, T., Kippo, K., Lauren, L., Hannuniemi, R., and Sellman, R. (1995). Effect of clodronate on established collagen-induced arthritis in rats. *Inflammation Research*, **44**, 258–63.

97. Markusse, H.M., Lafeber, G.J.M., and Breedveld, F.C. (1990). Bisphosphonates in collagen arthritis. *Rheumatology International*, **9**, 281–3.

7.4   Synovium

7.4.1   Synovial mediators of cartilage damage and repair in OA

Wim B. van den Berg, Peter M. van der Kraan, and Henk M. van Beuningen

Introduction

Although, by definition, osteoarthritis (OA) is not a prominent inflammatory condition, some degree of synovial hypertrophy and fibrosis is seen in the majority of symptomatic cases, whereas a moderate, but focal chronic synovitis has been noted in about 20 per cent of surgically resected specimens. Previously considered as a boring, 'degenerative' disease, a consequence of trauma or aging, OA is now increasingly viewed as a deranged reparative process, with potential for intervention when key events or mediators can be properly defined. The present chapter will summarize the current status of mediators and processes described in the synovial tissue of osteoarthritic conditions, with a focus on cytokines, enzymes, and growth factors. To put the relevance of the synovial reaction in perspective, the next paragraph will first briefly deal with OA characteristics and potential pathogenic pathways.

Role of synovial reaction in OA pathogenesis

OA is defined as a focal lesion of the articular cartilage, combined with a hypertrophic reaction (sclerosis) in the subchondral bone and new bone formation (osteophytes) at the joint margins. The overall picture resembles a failure in attempt at repair. It is a longstanding debate whether the initiating process originates in the bone or in the cartilage. This discussion is further complicated by the heterogeneous character of the ill-defined condition of OA. It is generally accepted that OA may occur as a consequence of multiple causes, ranging from blunt joint trauma, biomechanical overloading, inborn or acquired joint incongruency and genetic defects in matrix components or assembly, to

an imbalance of synovial homeostasis. Probably, the joint has only a limited capacity to react to various insults and, in fact, the osteoarthritic lesion may reflect a common endpoint. On the other hand, it seems likely that the synovial reaction and mediators involved may be different in the initial stages of the various forms. As an illustration of complexity, meniscal damage or ligament rupture causes an abrupt shift in biomechanical loading of cartilage and bone, but it also generates an attempted repair reaction in the damaged tissue, be it ligamentous or cartilaginous in nature. It is now recognized, from studies in the anterior cruciate ligament transection model in dogs, that the first changes in the articular cartilage reflect a hypertrophic reaction, with enhanced synthesis of matrix and increase in content[1]. This is followed by a stage of increased matrix turnover, with net depletion of matrix components, and, finally, damage and loss of the collagen network. The hypertrophic stage clearly precedes the occurrence of the lesional stage, with its characteristic focal loss of cartilage.

There is no doubt that in late stages of OA the synovial reaction is sustained at least, in part, by wear particles and crystals released from the damaged cartilage. These triggers will stimulate synovial macrophages and fibroblasts, resulting in generation of a broad range of inflammatory mediators, resembling those found in inflammatory joint disease such as rheumatoid arthritis (RA). This may even include an immune reaction, under conditions where the individual loses its tolerance against autoantigens from the cartilage (Fig. 7.42). The general concept in OA puts major emphasis on direct activation of cartilage and bone, with minor involvement of the synovium. This may include a reaction of the chondrocyte to altered matrix stresses, for instance, due to shifts in loading or local trauma, resulting in the generation of chondrocyte mediators, which then act in the cartilage in an autocrine or paracrine fashion. In addition, diffusion to

Processes in the OA joint

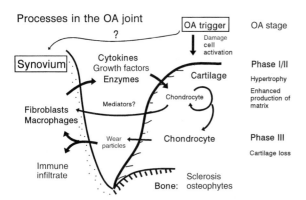

Fig. 7.42   Processes in osteoarthritic cartilage and synovial tissue.

the synovium may occur, triggering synovial fibroblasts and macrophages, and contributing to perpetuation of the process. As an alternative hypothesis, direct activation and mediator generation may occur in the synovium as a consequence of disturbed homeostasis, for instance, following unsuccessful and, therefore, continued attempt at repair of ruptured ligaments, with sustained generation of growth factors. Although direct proof for the latter pathway in OA is lacking at the moment, it is now generally accepted that excessive growth factor generation is the underlying cause of tissue fibrosis in some kidney and liver diseases, and scar formation in skin[2]. This principle is called the 'dark side of tissue repair' and may apply to OA as well.

Cytokines in OA / RA synovium

It is generally accepted that both TNFα and IL-1 are dominant cytokines in the synovial tissue of patients with RA. Evidence is accumulating that IL-1 is by far a more destructive mediator for the articular cartilage than TNFα[3,4], but TNFα is considered as an important driving force of IL-1 production[5]. IL-1 is also produced in considerable quantities in OA synovial tissues and this may be a major source, apart from IL-1 originating from the articular cartilage, of the increased IL-1 levels in OA synovial fluid[6,7]. Of importance, IL-1 appears to be the driving force for the production of destructive enzymes (collagenase, stromelysin), and IL-6 in OA synovial tissue[8]. This is suggested by the marked inhibition of enzyme and IL-6 levels upon culture of OA synovium in the presence of IL-1 receptor antagonist (IL-1ra). The exact role of IL-6 has yet to be defined. It is considered as an upregulator of the expression of tissue inhibitor of metalloproteinase (TIMP) in synovial cells, and a pivotal stimulus of acute phase protein production by the liver. This includes several enzyme inhibitors, suggesting an important role in negative feedback control. On the other hand, IL-6 is considered a major factor in bone destruction. Its role as a potent stimulator of B cell growth seems of minor importance in OA.

Recent studies tried to identify the cellular source of the cytokines in both OA and RA, using immunohistochemistry on tissue specimens. In fact, most investigations were focused on RA synovial tissue, and OA synovial tissue was generally included as a control, in an attempt to identify disease-specific factors. Bearing in mind that the bulk of the studies refer to tissue obtained at late stages of the disease, at the time of surgery, it is demonstrated that most cytokines can be found in both OA and RA synovium. Differences, if present, are mainly quantitative and not qualitative in nature. A selection of destructive cytokines and regulators is summarized in Table 7.7, reflecting the general

Table 7.7   Synovial cytokines in OA and RA; relative abundance and major function

	OA	RA	References	Major functions
IL-1	++	+++	6,7,10	Potent inducer of extracellular matrix destruction and matrix synthesis inhibition.
IL-1RA	+++	++	6,16,17	Inhibitor of IL-1 actions.
TNFα	+	+++	7,9,10	Induces matrix destruction and inhibits matrix synthesis. Less potent than IL-1. Induces IL-1 production.
sTNF-R	++	++	20,21	Inhibits TNFα.
LIF	++	+++	11	Involved in synthesis inhibition of extracellular matrix components.
IL-6	++	+++	7,22,23	Upregulates TIMP and IL-RA.
IL-4	–	+	15	Inhibits production of TNFα and Il-1. Upregulates IL-1RA.
IL-10	+	++	13,14	Inhibits TNFα production.
IL-8	++	++	24,25	Attracts inflammatory cells to the joint.
MCP-1	++	++	24	Attracts inflammatory cells to the joint.

– to +++ refers to relative abundance in OA and RA.

feeling of relative abundance in RA synovium. There is a tendency that TNFα is less abundant in OA synovium, whereas both IL-1α and IL-1β can be found in considerable quantities. This seems in accordance with significant levels of TNFα in synovial fluid samples of most RA patients, whereas TNFα was found only in a few OA samples[7,9,10].

Leukemia inhibitory factor (LIF) is a relatively new cytokine, showing cartilage-destroying activity. It has been claimed that this is a separate action, not mediated through generation of IL-1 and/or TNFα[11,12]. LIF can be induced by numerous cytokines and its relative role in OA remains to be identified.

In terms of localization of cytokines, expression seems more abundant in the lining layer in RA as compared with OA, but this must be viewed in relation to the more pronounced hypertrophy of the lining in RA. A final conclusion on differences in localization is furthermore hampered by the large variation in patterns found in different biopsies from the same patient.

Apart from absolute levels of destructive mediators, it is of crucial importance to obtain information on the balance with natural inhibitors or regulators. TNFα and IL-1 production is under the control of cytokines like IL-4, IL-10 and IL-13. First studies in RA synovium reveal the apparent absence of IL-4, whereas IL-10 is present in variable amounts[13–15]. Information on these molecules in OA synovium is virtually lacking.

The action of the cytokines TNFα and IL-1 is under the control of cytokine-specific soluble receptors, which can be shedded from connective tissue and leucocytes. In addition, Il-1 is balanced by the presence of IL-1 receptor antagonist (IL-1ra). Clear evidence is presented that IL-1ra gene expression and protein is abundant in OA synovia[16,17]. This antagonist is mainly found in the lining cells, and less so in the sublining. The inhibitor seems also more abundant in OA, as compared with RA synovium. However, it must be borne in mind that a 1000-fold excess of antagonist over IL-1 is needed to fully block the IL-1 activity[18,19], making it doubtful whether the observed levels of IL-1ra are sufficient to really contribute to control. On the other hand, it cannot be excluded that levels in close vicinity of cells can be extremely high.

Enzymes/inhibitors in OA synovium

As stated on p. 00, IL-1 and TNFα can increase the production of proteases in synovial tissue and may be responsible for the enhanced levels of collagenase, stromelysin, and plasminogen activators found in human OA synovium. In experimental canine OA, a coordinate synthesis was noted of IL-1 and stromelysin[26]. Moreover, in human OA synovium a correlation was demonstrated between the amount of inflammatory cells and neutral protease levels[27]. In line with this, expression of stromelysin and collagenase was less prominent in OA synovium, as compared with RA synovium[28,29]. Tissue inhibitor of metalloproteinase (TIMP) was easily detectable in both synovia, and levels were clearly enhanced above normal. Although the ratio protease/inhibitor was higher in RA, an unfavourable imbalance was also found in OA, suggestive for a role of these enzymes in tissue destruction.

Despite the clear presence, there is still doubt about the dominant involvement of stromelysin in cartilage destruction. This is mainly due to the abundant appearance of proteoglycan breakdown epitopes in OA cartilage and synovial fluid, not fitting with preferential cleavage sites of this enzyme[30]. In reference to the detected aggrecan epitopes, the putative enzyme involved in the destruction is now called aggrecanase, although an enzyme displaying this particular cleavage could not be identified in either arthritic cartilage or synovium. It remains to be seen whether we really deal with a new enzyme, or an activity displayed by a peculiar combination of known enzymes.

Anyway, most of the stromelysin generated by IL-1 will be in the inactive form, needing additional proteolytic activation. A potential role in activation has been attributed to the plasminogen-plasmin activator system[31,32]. Plasminogen activator inhibitors 1 and 2 (PAIs) are found in increased quantities in RA synovium, but not in OA synovium.

Recently, increasing attention has been given to other classes of enzymes. Cathepsins were found in elevated quantities in OA synovium, including the subtypes B, L, and D. The level of their specific natural inhibitors was not different in OA and normal synovium[33,34]. Moreover, cathepsins seem important in activation of latent proteases[35]. A selection of enzymes detected in OA is summarized in Table 7.8. Further details on the role of the various enzyme systems will be addressed in other chapters of this book.

Growth factors in OA synovium

In a broad sense, cytokines are defined as peptide regulatory factors that are produced by cells and act on cells, often in close vicinity. In that respect, the

Table 7.8 Dominant synovial tissue proteinases and inhibitors in OA

Protease	References	Characteristics
Collagenase (MMP-1)	28,29,36	Produced by macrophage and fibroblast-like synoviocytes[30]. Amount correlates with inflammation[23]. Synthesized as an inactive pro-enzyme.
Stromelysin (MMP-3)	27,36,37	Produced by macrophage and fibroblast-like synoviocytes[30]. Amount appears to be correlated with inflammatory cell infiltration. Synthesized in an inactive proform. Preferential cleavage site VDIPEN.
Tissue inhibitor of metalloproteinases (TIMP)	28,29,36	Produced by macrophage and fibroblast-like synoviocytes[30]. Inhibits metalloproteinases.
Aggrecanase	30	Enzyme not identified. Preferential cleavage site NITEGE.
Plasminogen activator (PA)	31,32	Activates plasminogen.
Plasminogen activator inhibitor (PAI)	31,32	Inhibits plasminogen activator.
Cathepsins	33,34	Normally lysozomal enzymes.
Calpain	38	Normally an intracellular enzyme but found in synovial fluid in OA.
Calpastatin	38	Inhibits calpains, detected in synovial fluid.

definition includes the various growth regulating mediators. However, for the moment, most authors will categorize part of the classical lymphokines and monokines under the heading 'cytokines', including a group of interleukins with clear growth-promoting activity on leucocytes, omitting yet another category of 'real' growth factors. On historical grounds, these growth factors are named after their dominant or initial mode of action, target tissue, or cellular origin. Many of these so-called growth factors can also be produced by the synovial tissue and often have a characteristic impact on synovial cells, as well as on cartilage and bone. Table 7.9 comprises a selection of growth factors, found in increased quantities in OA synovium and implicated directly or indirectly in cartilage damage and/or repair.

The colony-stimulating factors (CSFs) have their main action on bone marrow cells, stimulating hematopoietic differentiation, but are also implicated in bone resorption, through stimulation of osteoclast generation. In synovial tissue, their main action is probably the activation of granulocyte and/or macrophage function, whereas recent data also demonstrate activation of chondrocytes (including enhanced production of IL-8). GM-CSF is a major factor in inflamed synovium of RA patients, although increased levels are also found in most OA synovial samples. Of interest, expression of both M-CSF and G-MCSF can be markedly enhanced in cultures of synovial fibroblasts upon exposure to IL-1, but only M-CSF seems constitutively expressed[39], implicating GM-CSF in acute

Table 7.9 Synovial tissue growth factors in OA; detection of protein and / of message

Growth factor	References	Characteristics
Macrophage-colony stimulating factor (M-CSF)	39	Constitutively expressed by OA fibroblasts. Augments functional activities of monocytes and macrophages.
Granulocyte-macrophage colony stimulating factor (GM-CSF)	39	Activates granulocytes and macrophages.
Transforming growth factor β (TGFβ)	43,50	Chemotactic for fibroblasts and inflammatory cells. Induces fibrosis. Modulates proteoglycan and collagen synthesis in synovium and cartilage.
Insulin-like growth factor I and II (IGF)	47	Increases chondrocyte anabolism. Mitogenic for fibroblasts.
Fibroblast growth factor (FGF)	40,41	Mitogenic for fibroblasts. Modulates proteoglycan metabolism in cartilage.
Epidermal growth factor (EGF)	51	Mitogenic for fibroblasts. Modulates proteoglycan metabolism in cartilage.
Platelet-derived growth factor (PDGF)	41	Mitogenic for fibroblasts. Modulates proteoglycan metabolism in cartilage.

inflammatory episodes, and M-CSF to be more important in sustained activation.

A second category of growth factors comprises PDGF, FGF, EGF, and TGFβ; all having potent mitogenic activity for synovial fibroblasts and inducing activation of cell function. The latter may include enhanced production of destructive enzymes and generation of cytokines such as IL-1 and LIF. These factors probably contribute to the fibrotic reaction seen in OA synovial tissue. In contrast, the same set of growth factors may be involved in cartilage repair, through stimulation of chondrocyte proliferation and cartilage matrix synthesis. The relative importance of the latter action must of course be viewed in terms of local production of similar factors by the chondrocyte itself. Both basic FGF (bFGF) as well as acidic FGF (Heparin binding GF) are found in synovial lining and sublining cells, and expression is higher in RA, as compared to OA synovium[40]. The same holds for expression of PDGF[41].

A factor of particular interest, but of highly pleiotropic nature, is TGFβ. It is a potent chemotactic factor, attracting inflammatory phagocytes to the synovial tissue. In addition, it is a strong stimulus for fibroblast proliferation. However, it is rather unique amongst the growth factors in that it inhibits enzyme release and stimulates the production of enzyme inhibitors such as TIMP[42]. This effect is found with synovial cells as well as chondrocytes. In that respect, TGFβ may be viewed as an important feedback regulator of local tissue damage, following inflammatory episodes in the synovium. Finally, it stimulates matrix production by activated chondrocytes. Of importance, TGFβ is produced in a latent form, linked to latency-associated peptide (LAP). Activation, with uncoupling from LAP, may occur under acidic conditions or by proteases. It is commonly accepted that most tissues, including synovium and cartilage, contain large amounts of latent TGFβ, which may become activated upon insults. Apart from TGFβ production by activated cells, these stores of latent TGFβ probably have a major impact on the response of a particular tissue. Significant levels of (active) TGFβ are found in synovial fluid samples of both RA and OA patients, and enhanced production of TGFβ is demonstrated in synovial tissue of such patients[43]. Major cell sources include macrophages and fibroblasts, and strong TGFβ immunostaining is noted in pannus tissue, at close vicinity to the articular cartilage. Of importance, in fibrotic areas exclusive expression of TGFβ is noted, in contrast to the dominant coexpression with cytokines such as IL-1 and TNFα at sites containing inflammatory infiltrates[44]. Unfortunately, such immunolocalization studies do not discriminate between latent and active TGFβ and the impact in the process of RA and OA remains largely to be identified.

A last category of important growth factors is that of the IGFs. Insulin-like growth factors, as the name implies, are growth factors which are abundant in serum and share some properties with insulin. IGF-II is an abundant factor in the embryonic stage, whereas IGF-I is the dominant factor in adult life. However, it cannot be excluded that IGF-II becomes of relevance under pathological conditions or at repair sites often showing embryonic elements. IGF-I is a potent stimulator of chondrocyte proteoglycan synthesis and inhibits proteoglycan breakdown[45]. In that sense, it is an important homeostatic factor for cartilage and it was found that IGF-I is the main anabolic stimulus for chondrocyte proteoglycan present in serum and synovial fluid[46]. Since serum contains high levels of IGF-I, originating from the liver, it is commonly thought that the bulk of the IGF in synovial fluid is coming from the circulation. However, normal chondrocytes do make IGFs and recently, expression of both IGF-I and IGF-II message was demonstrated in synovium and subsynovium of OA patients[47]. The action of IGFs is under the control of IGF-binding proteins, which can also be produced by chondrocytes. Cells isolated from OA cartilage make enhanced levels of IGF-bps[48], but information on *in situ* production by OA synovial tissue is lacking.

Effects of synovial mediators on cartilage

As mentioned above, various cytokines, enzymes, and growth factors are found in increased quantities in OA synovium and can have a direct impact on cartilage and chondrocyte function. Although absolute levels of particular mediators may be indicative of their role, the net effect is mainly determined by the balance of synergizing, counteracting, and regulating mediators. The pattern of cartilage destruction is quite different in OA, as compared to RA, yet enhanced production of numerous mediators can be found in both synovial tissues and differences, if present, seem mainly quantitative and not qualitative. This suggests that other, yet unidentified, factors are of pivotal importance, or that other aspects determine the particular cartilage

Table 7.10 Cytokines in cartilage metabolism

Category	Mediator
Destructive cytokines	IL-1α, IL-1β, TNFα, TNFβ, LIF, (TGFβ)
Modulatory cytokines	IL-4, IL-6, IL-10, IL-13, TGFβ
Growth factors, chondrogenic factors...	IGF-1, PDGF, FGF, TGFβ1,2,3, BMPs...,

response, such as local inhibitors or typical receptor expression patterns on chondrocytes in RA or OA cartilage.

In terms of their most characteristic effect on chondrocytes, cytokines can be broadly categorized in three classes: destructive cytokines, regulatory cytokines, and anabolic factors (Table 7.10). As a prime example of a destructive cytokine, IL-1 induces enhanced protease release, and inhibits chondrocyte proteoglycan and collagen synthesis. Regulatory factors like IL-4 and IL-10 inhibit IL-1 production and enhance production of IL-ra, providing a 'double hit' to control the destructive action of IL-1. Finally, factors from the anabolic category, such as IGF-1 and TGFβ, do not really interfere with IL-1 production or action, but in fact display opposing activity—stimulation of proteoglycan and collagen synthesis, and suppression of protease action, the latter by inhibition of release and / or upregulation of inhibitors. This plain counteraction further underlines the importance of balances of the various factors.

Other members of the anabolic group worth mentioning are FGF and PDGF, which show stimulation of proteoglycan synthesis on top of the IGF-I effect[52], and may contribute to cartilage repair by stimulation of chondrocyte proliferation. However, a critical understanding of their role is complicated by a seemingly complex interaction with IL-1. It was demonstrated that previous exposure of chondrocytes to FGF enhances the subsequent protease release after IL-1[53]. PDGF also seems to stimulate IL-1 dependent protease release, but reduces IL-1 mediated inhibition of proteoglycan synthesis[54]. These observations are conceivable with the notion that some growth factors can both potentiate repair, as well as enhance breakdown. More recently, a series of bone morphogenic proteins (BMPs) and specific chondrogenic factors were cloned. We are now confronted with a rapidly growing list of members showing more or less selective anabolic effects on chondrocytes. It is yet unclear how these latter factors balance IL-1 effects, and whether production of such factors by the synovial tissue makes a significant contribution to cartilage homeostasis and repair.

Involvement of mediators in OA cartilage pathology

To obtain insight in key factors in OA cartilage pathology, it is imperative to identify the critical changes in the articular cartilage, and to try to fit these patterns with actions of particular mediators or combinations of mediators. Under normal condition, cartilage maintains its homeostasis by a regulated balance of synthesis and degradative events. In theory, cartilage pathology may arise from local overproduction of destructive mediators or a shortage of controlling mediators, including inhibitors and anabolic growth factors. Moreover, a shift in responsiveness of the chondrocyte to these mediators may contribute to loss of homeostasis. There is no doubt that the OA chondrocyte displays an altered phenotype, which remains present after at least a number of cell passages in culture. It is yet unclear whether this state reflects cause or outcome of the OA process (Fig. 7.43).

An intriguing observation in human OA cartilage is the enhanced sensitivity of the chondrocytes to undergo stimulation of proteoglycan synthesis by TGFβ. Normal cartilage does not show enhanced proteoglycan synthesis upon first exposure to TGFβ. Only after a number of days in culture, in particular in the presence of TGFβ, the chondrocytes start to show this profile, probably under a TGFβ-induced shift in phenotype[55,56]. The fact that OA chondrocytes already show

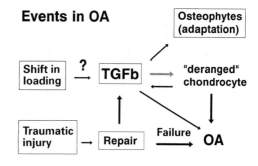

Fig. 7.43 Potential pathogenic mechanisms in osteoarthritis.

this pattern suggests previous exposure to TGFβ and critical involvement of this factor in the disease process. Further indication of a role of TGFβ in OA is provided by the marked upregulation of chondrocyte proteoglycan synthesis and induction of osteophytes in murine knee joints, upon repeated local injection of TGFβ[57]. Osteophytes are characteristic features in OA and it was observed that repeated local injection with another growth factor, IGF-I, does not induce these hallmarks. Finally, upon prolonged exposure to TGFβ, the femoral cartilage of the murine knee joint shows typical loss of proteoglycans close to the tidemark, and disorganization of chondrocyte spacing (Fig. 7.44). Enhanced TGFβ generation may result from continued biomechanical overload of chondrocytes or unsuccessful and, therefore, continued repair processes in either cartilage or ligamentous tissue. The outcome of continued TGFβ exposure is a shift in the subtypes of proteo-

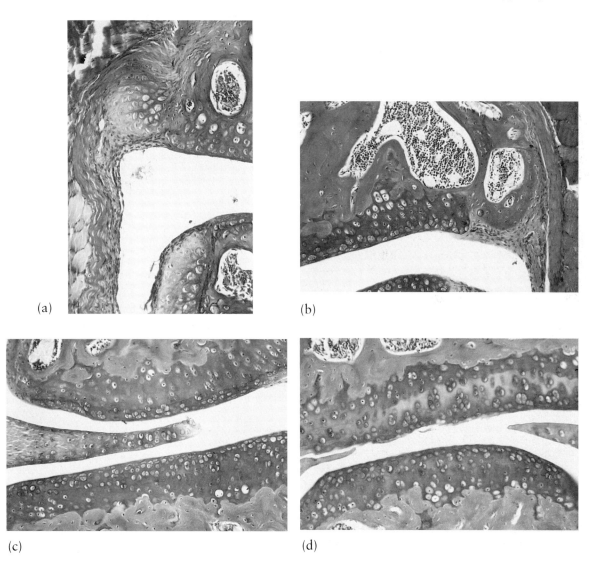

(a)

(b)

(c)

(d)

Fig. 7.44 Safranin O stained of sections of the murine knee joint after local TGFβ injection: (a) outgrowth of chondroid tissue at the joint margin at day three after the last of triple TGFβ injections, given on alternate days; (b) similar treatment, but four weeks later — note the maturation into a mature osteophyte, containing bone marrow; (c) control section of tibial plateau; (d) similar region one month after six TGFβ injections, given on alternate days — note the loss of proteoglycan staining and the irregular surface and spacing of chondrocytes.

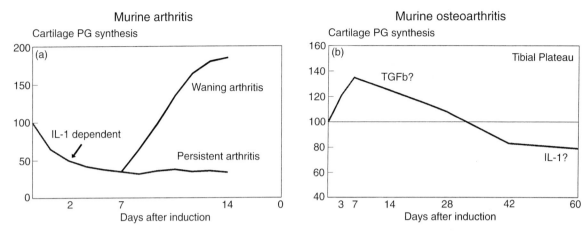

Fig. 7.45   Profile of chondrocyte proteoglycan synthesis in articular cartilage after induction of (a) joint inflammation or (b) osteoarthritis.

glycans made by the cartilage cells, probably resulting in impaired matrix assembly.

Although often suggested, a critical role of IL-1 in early stages of OA seems unlikely. Observation from inflammatory models show that chondrocyte proteoglycan synthesis is markedly inhibited shortly after induction of joint inflammation and remains suppressed in the presence of ongoing inflammation. Studies with neutralising antibodies and IL-1ra provided convincing evidence that IL-1 is the pivotal mediator of this suppression[3,58]. In marked contrast, chondrocyte proteoglycan synthesis is enhanced in early stages of experimental OA (Fig. 7.45). This is hardly compatible with a dominant role of IL-1, and at least suggests overkill by generation and / or activation of anabolic factors. An OA phenomenon which may be attributable to IL-1 is the shift in phenotype of the chondrocyte. After prolonged exposure to IL-1, the production of cartilage specific collagen types such as type II and type IX is reduced, whereas an increase in types I and III collagen is noted[59]. This shift may contribute to inadequate matrix repair.

Apart from overproduction of mediators, pathology may be linked to lack of action of anabolic growth factors. There is no evidence that IGF levels are limiting in synovial fluid of either OA or RA patients. However, in experimental joint inflammation IGF nonresponsiveness is noted in chondrocytes, compatible with the low level of proteoglycan synthesis in the arthritic chondrocytes. Moreover, production of aberrant, small proteoglycans has been demonstrated in arthritic cartilage and this could be mimicked in normal cartilage, in the absence of IGF[60]. Another

variant of improper IGF signalling seems to be present in OA cartilage. The chondrocytes make enhanced levels of IGF binding proteins, potentially limiting the homeostatic action of IGF. If this is the only disturbance in the IGF pathway, the lack of response may be overcome with high levels of IGF. This warrants therapeutic approaches with high doses of IGF-I. Of interest, steroids display actions similar to IGF[60] and low doses may be applied instead of IGF, to bypass problems related to disturbed IGF receptor signalling or inhibitory binding proteins.

Final remarks

Many of the effects described in the previous sections can be ascribed to factors coming from the synovial tissue, the articular cartilage, or from both sources. To further identify key factors and the relative importance of the synovial reaction, studies are needed in various stages of proper experimental OA models, using inhibitors selectively targeting synovial tissue or cartilage. As an example, treatment with neutralizing antibodies to cytokines or growth factors will selectively touch the synovial process, since antibody penetration of cartilage will be scant. By contrast, a smaller inhibitor such as IL-1ra will probably have sufficient access to both tissue compartments. In the near future, gene targeting, in combination with selective adhesion molecules, may provide a more elegant approach, offering interesting mechanistical tools and, hopefully, also therapeutic promises. Given the concept of failure in attempt at repair in OA, it is tempting to supply anabolic factors. However, too much growth factor may be pathologic, as suggested for TGFβ, whereas shifts in receptor expression on OA chondrocytes may skew growth factor responses. It is anticipated that characterization of new members of the BMPs and chondrogenic factors, in particular, may provide better tools for proper repair in due time.

References

1. Adams, M.E. and Brandt, K.D. (1991). Hypertrophic repair of canine articular cartilage in osteoarthritis after anterior cruciate ligament transection. *Journal of Rheumatology*, 18, 428–35.
2. Border, W.A. and Ruoslahti, E. (1992). Transforming growth factor-β in disease. The dark side of tissue repair. *Journal of Clinical Investigation*, 90, 1–7.
3. Van de Loo, A.A.J., Joosten, L.A.B., van Lent, P.L.E.M., Arntz, O.J., and van den Berg, W.B. (1995). Role of interleukin-1, tumor necrosis factor α, and interleukin-6 in cartilage proteoglycan metabolism and destruction. Effect of *in situ* blocking in murine antigen- and zymozan- induced arthritis. *Arthritis and Rheumatism*, 38, 164–72.
4. Probert, L., Plows, D., Kontogeorgos, G., and Kollias, G. (1995). The type I IL-1 receptor acts in series with TNF to induce arthritis in TNF-transgenic mice. *European Journal of Immunology*, 25, 1794–7.
5. Brennan, F.M., Chantry, D., Jackson, A., Maini, R., and Feldmann, M. (1989). Inhibitory effect of TNFα antibodies on synovial cell interleukin-1 production in rheumatoid arthritis. *Lancet*, i, 244–7.
6. Deleuran, B.W., Chu, C.Q., Field, M., Brennan, F.M., Katsikis, P., Feldmann, M., *et al.* (1992). Localization of interleukin-1α, type-1 interleukin-1 receptor and interleukin-1 receptor antagonist in the synovial membrane and cartilage / pannus junction in rheumatoid arthritis. *British Journal of Rheumatology*, 31, 801–9.
7. Farahat, M.N., Yanni, G., Poston, R., and Panayi, G.S. (1993). Cytokine expression in synovial membranes of patients with rheumatoid arthritis and osteoarthritis. *Annals of the Rheumatic Diseases*, 52, 870–5.
8. Pelletier, J.P., McCollum, R., Cloutier, J.M., and Martel-Pelletier, J. (1995). Synthesis of metalloproteinases and interleukin-6 (Il-6) in human osteoarthritic synovial membrane is an Il-1 mediated process. *Journal of Rheumatology*, Suppl 43, 109–14.
9. Chu, C.Q., Field, M., Feldmann, M., and Maini, R.N. (1991). Localization of tumor necrosis factor alpha in synovial tissue and at the cartilage pannus junction in patients with rheumatoid arthritis. *Arthritis and Rheumatism*, 34, 1125–32.
10. Miller, V.E., Rogers, K., and Muirden, K.D. (1993). Detection of tumour necrosis factor α and interleukin-1 β in the rheumatoid and osteoarthritic cartilage / pannus junction by immunohistochemical methods. *Rheumatology International*, 13, 77–82.
11. Lotz, M., Moats, T., and Villiger, P.M. (1992). Leukemia inhibitory factor is expressed in cartilage and synovium and can contribute to the pathogenesis of arthritis. *Journal of Clinical Investigation*, 90, 888–96.
12. Bell, M.C. and Carroll, G.J. (1995). Leukemia inhibitory factor (LIF) suppresses proteoglycan synthesis in porcine and caprine cartilage explants. *Cytokine*, 7, 137–41.
13. Katsikis, P.D., Chu, C.Q., Brennan, F.M., Maini, R.N., and Feldmann, M. (1994). Immunoregulatory role of IL-10. *Journal of Experimental Medicine*, 179, 15–17.
14. Cush, J.J., Splawski, J.B., Thomas, R., McFarlin, J.E., Schulze-Koops, H., Davis, L.S. *et al.* (1995). Elevated interleukin-10 levels in patients with rheumatoid arthritis. *Arthritis and Rheumatism*, 338, 96–104.
15. Miossec, P., Naviliat, M., Dupuy D'Angeac, A., Sany, J., and Banchereau, J. (1990). Low levels of interleukin-4 and high levels of transforming growth factor β in rheumatoid synovitis. *Arthritis and Rheumatism*, 33, 1180–7.
16. Firestein, G.S., Berger, A.E., Tracey, D.E., Chosay, J.G., Chapman, D.L., Paine, M.M., *et al.* (1992). Il-1 receptor antagonist protein production and gene expression in rheumatoid and osteoarthritis synovium. *Journal of Immunology*, 149, 1054–62.
17. Fujikawa, Y., Shingu, M., Torisu, T., and Masumi, S. (1995). Interleukin-1 receptor antagonist production in cultured synovial cells from patients with rheumatoid arthritis and osteoarthritis. *Annals of the Rheumatic Diseases* 54, 318–20.
18. Arend, W.P. (1991). Interleukin 1 receptor antagonist. A new member of the interleukin 1 family. *Journal of Clinical Investigation*, 88, 1445–51.
19. Smith, R.J., Chin, J.E., Sam, L.M., and Justen, J.M. (1991). Biologic effects of an interleukin-1 receptor antagonist protein on interleukin-1-stimulated cartilage erosion and chondrocyte responsiveness. *Arthritis and Rheumatism*, 34, 78–83.
20. Roux-Lombard, P., Punzi, L., Hasler, F., Bas, S., Todesco, S., and Gallati, H., *et al.* (1993). Soluble tumor necrosis factor receptors in human inflammatory synovial fluids. *Arthritis and Rheumatism*, 36, 485–9.
21. Steiner, G., Studnicka-Benke, A., Witzmann, G., Höfler, E., and Smolen, J. (1995). Soluble receptors for tumor necrosis factor and interleukin-2 in serum and synovial fluid of patients with rheumatoid arthritis, reactive arthritis and osteoarthritis. *Journal of Rheumatology*, 22, 406–12.
22. Guerne, P.A., Zuraw, B.L., Vaughan, J.H., Carson, D.A., and Lotz, M. (1989). Synovium as a source for interleukin-6 *in vitro*. Contribution to local systemic manifestations of arthritis. *Journal of Clinical Investigation*, 83, 585–92.
23. Field, M., Chu, C., Feldmann, M., and Maini, R.N. (1991). Interleukin-6 localisation in the synovial membrane in rheumatoid arthritis. *Rheumatology International*, 11, 45–50.
24. Seitz, M., Loetscher, P., Dewald, B., Towbin, H., Ceska, M., and Baggiolini, M. (1994). Production of interleukin-1 receptor antagonist, inflammatory chemotactic proteins, and prostaglandin E by rheumatoid and

osteoarthritic synovium. Regulation by IFN-gamma and Il-4. *Journal of Immunology*, **15**, 2060–5.

25. Verburgh, C.A., Hart, M.H.L., Aarden, L.A., and Swaak, A.J.G. (1993). Interleukin-8 (Il-8) in synovial fluid of rheumatoid and non-rheumatoid joint effusions. *Clinical Rheumatology*, **12**, 494–9.

26. Pelletier, J.P., Faure, M.P., DiBattista, J.A., Wilhelm, S., Visco, D., and Martel-Pelletier, J. (1993). Coordinate expression of stromelysin, interleukin-1, and oncogene proteins in experimental osteoarthritis. *American Journal of Pathology*, **142**, 95–105.

27. Okada, Y., Shinmei, M., Tanaka, O., Naka, K., Kimura, A., Nakanishi, I., *et al.* (1992). Localization of matrix metalloprotease 3 (stromelysin) in osteoarthritic cartilage and synovium. *Laboratory Investigation*, **66**, 680–90.

28. Firestein, G.S., Paine, M.M., Littman, B.H. (1991). Gene expression (collagenase, tissue inhibitor of metalloproteinases, complement, and HLA-DR) in rheumatoid arthritis and osteoarthritis synovium. *Arthritis and Rheumatism*, **34**, 1094–1105.

29. Clark, I.M., Powell, L.K., Ramsey, S., Hazleman, B.L., and Cawston, T.E. (1993). The measurement of collagenase, tissue inhibitor of metalloproteinase (TIMP), and collagenase-TIMP complex in synovial fluids from patients with osteoarthritis and rheumatoid arthritis. *Arthritis and Rheumatism*, **36**, 372–9.

30. Lohmander, L.S., Neame, P.J., and Sandy, J.D. (1993). The structure of aggrecan fragments in human synovial fluid. *Arthritis and Rheumatism*, **36**, 1214–1222.

31. Saxne, T., Lecander, I., and Geborek, P. (1993). Plasminogen activators and plasminogen activator inhibitors in synovial fluid. Difference between inflammatory joint disorders and osteoarthritis. *Journal of Rheumatology*, **20**, 91–6.

32. Pelletier, J.P., Mineau, F., Faure, M.P., and Martel-Pelletier, J. (1990). Imbalance between the mechanisms of activation and inhibition of metalloproteinases in the early lesions of experimental osteoarthritis. *Arthritis and Rheumatism*, **33**, 1466–76.

33. Martel-Pelletier, J., Cloutier, J.M., and Pelletier, J.P. (1990). Cathepsin B and cysteine protease inhibitors in human osteoarthritis. *Journal of Orthopaedic Research*, **8**, 336–44.

34. Keyszer, G.M., Heer, A.H., Kriegsmann, J., Geiler, T., Trabandt, A., Keysser, M., *et al.* (1995). Comparative analysis of cathepsin L, cathepsin D, and collagenase messenger RNA expression in synovial tissues of patients with rheumatoid arthritis and osteoarthritis, by *in situ* hybridisation. *Arthritis and Rheumatism*, **38**, 976–84.

35. Buttle, D.J., Handley, C.J., Ilic, M.Z., Saklatvala, J., Murata, M., and Barrett, A.J. (1993). Inhibition of cartilage proteoglycan release by a specific inactivator of cathepsin B and an inhibitor of matrix metalloproteinases. *Arthritis and Rheumatism*, **36**, 1709–17.

36. McCachren, S.S. (1993). Expression of metalloproteinases and metalloproteinase inhibitor in human arthritic synovium. *Arthritis and Rheumatism*, **36**, 1085–93.

37. Zafarullah, M., Pelletier, J.P., Cloutier, J.M., and Martel-Pelletier, J. (1993). Elevated metalloproteinase and tissue inhibitor of metalloproteinase mRNA in human osteoarthritic synovia. *Journal of Rheumatology*, **20**, 693–7.

38. Suzuki, K., Shimizu, K., Hamamoto, T., Nakagawa, Y., Hamakubo, T., and Yamamuro, T. (1990). Biochemical demonstration of calpains and calpastatin in osteoarthritic synovial fluid. *Arthritis and Rheumatism*, **33**, 728–32.

39. Seitz, M., Loetscher, P., Fey, M.F., and Tobler, A. (1994). Constitutive mRNA and protein production of macrophage colony-stimulating factor but not of other cytokines by synovial fibroblasts from rheumatoid arthritis and osteoarthritis patients. *British Journal of Rheumatology*, **33**, 613–19.

40. Nakashima, M., Eguchi, K., Aoyagi, T., Yamashita, I., Ida, H., Sakai, M., *et al.* (1994). Expression of basic fibroblast growth factor in synovial tissues from patients with rheumatoid arthritis. Detection by immunohistochemical staining and *in situ* hybridisation. *Annals of the Rheumatic Diseases*, **53**, 45–50.

41. Remmers, E.F., Sano, H., Lafyatis, R., Case, J.P., Kumkumian, G.K., Hla, T., *et al.* (1991). Production of platelet derived growth factor B chain (PDGF-B/c-sis) mRNA and immunoreactive PDGF B-like polypeptide by rheumatoid synovium: coexpression with heparin binding acidic fibroblast growth factor. *Journal of Rheumatology* **18**, 7–13.

42. Wright, J.K., Cawston, T.E., and Hazleman, B.L. (1991). Transforming growth factor beta stimulates the production of the tissue inhibitor of metalloproteinases (TIMP) by human synovial and skin fibroblasts. *Biochimica et Biophysica Acta*, **1094**, 207–10.

43. Chu, C.Q., Field, M., Abney, E., Zheng, R.Q.H., Allard, S., Feldmann, M., *et al.* (1991). Transforming growth factor-β1 in rheumatoid synovial membrane and cartilage/pannus junction. *Clinical and Experimental Immunology*, **86**, 380–6.

44. Chu, C.Q., Field, M., Allard, S., Abney, E., Feldmann, M., and Maini, R.N. (1992). Detection of cytokines at the cartilage / pannus junction in patients with rheumatoid arthritis: implications for the role of cytokines in cartilage destruction and repair. *British Journal of Rheumatology*, **31**, 653–61.

45. Tyler, J.A. (1991). Insulin-like growth factor can decrease degradation and promote synthesis of proteoglycan in cartilage exposed to cytokines. *Biochemical Journal*, **260**, 543–8.

46. Schalkwijk, J., Joosten, L.A.B., van den Berg, W.B., van Wijk, J.J., van de Putte, L.B.A. (1989). Insulin-like growth factor stimulation of chondrocyte proteoglycan synthesis by human synovial fluid. *Arthritis and Rheumatism*, **32**, 66–71.

47. Keyszer, G.M., Heer, A.H., Kriegsmann, J., Geiler, T., Keysser, C., Gay, R.E., *et al.* (1995). Detection of insulin-like growth factor I and II in synovial tissue specimens of patients with rheumatoid arthritis and osteoarthritis. *Journal of Rheumatology*, **22**, 275–81.

48. Doré, S., Pelletier, J.P., DiBattista, J.A., Tardif, G., Brazeau, P., Martel-Pelletier, J.M. (1994) Human osteoarthritic chondrocytes possess an increased number of insulin-like growth factor I binding sites but are unresponsive to its stimulation. *Arthritis and Rheumatism*, **37**, 253–63.

49. Falus, A., Lakatos, T., and Smolen, J. (1992). Dissimilar biosynthesis of interleukin-6 by different areas of synovial membrane of patients with rheumatoid arthri-

tis and osteoarthritis. *Scandinavian Journal of Rheumatology*, 21, 116–19.

50. Fava, R., Olsen, N., Keski-Oja, J., Moses, H., and Pincus, T. (1989). Active and latent forms of transforming growth factor β in synovial effusions. *Journal of Experimental Medicine*, 169, 291–6.

51. Farahat, M.N., Yanni, G., Poston, R., and Panayi, G.S. (1993). Cytokine expression in synovial membranes of patients with rheumatoid arthritis and osteoarthritis. *Annals of the Rheumatic Diseases*, 52, 52, 870–5.

52. Verschure, P.J., Joosten, L.A.B., van der Kraan, P.M., and van den Berg, W.B. (1994). Responsiveness of articular cartilage from normal and inflamed mouse knee joints to various growth factors. *Annals of the Rheumatic Diseases*, 53, 455–60.

53. Chandrasekhar, S. and Harvey, A.K. (1989). Induction of interleukin-1 receptors on chondrocytes by fibroblast growth factor: A possible mechanism for modulation of interleukin-1 activity. *Journal of Cell Physiology*, 138, 236–46.

54. Smith, R.J., Justen, J.M., Sam, L.M., Rohloff, N.A., Ruppel, P.L., Brunden, M.N., *et al.* (1991). Platelet-derived growth factor potentiates cellular responses of articular chondrocytes to interleukin-1. *Arthritis and Rheumatism*, 34, 697–706.

55. Lafeber, F.P.J.G., van der Kraan, P.M., Huber-Bruning, O., van der Berg, W.B., and Bijlsma, J.W.J. (1993). Osteoarthritic human cartilage is more sensitive to

transforming growth factor β than is normal cartilage. *British Journal of Rheumatology*, 32, 281–6.

56. Inoue, H., Kato, Y., Iwamoto, M., Hiraki, Y., Sakuda, M., and Suzuki, F. (1989). Stimulation of proteoglycan synthesis by morphological transformed chondrocytes grown in the presence of fibroblast growth factor and transforming growth factor-beta. *Journal of Cell Physiology*, 138, 329–37.

57. Van Beuningen, H.M., van der Kraan, P.M., Arntz, O.J., and van den Berg, W.B. (1994). Transforming growth factor-β1 stimulates articular cartilage chondrocyte proteoglycan synthesis and induces osteophyte formation in the murine knee joint. *Laboratory Investigation*, 71, 279–90.

58. Van de Loo, A.A.J., Arntz, O.J., Otterness, I.G., and van den Berg, W.B. (1992). Protection against cartilage proteoglycan synthesis inhibition by anti-interleukin-1 antibodies in experimental arthritis. *Journal of Rheumatology*, 19, 348–56.

59. Goldring, M.B., Birkhead, J., Sandell, I.J., Kimura, T., and Krane, S.M. (1988). Interleukin-1 suppresses expression of cartilage-specific types II and IX collagen and increases type I and II collagens in human chondrocytes. *Journal of Clinical Investigation*, 82, 2026–37.

60. Verschure, P.J., van der Kraan, P.M., Vitters, E.L., and van den Berg, W.B. (1994). Stimulation of proteoglycan synthesis by triamcinolone acetonide and insulin-like growth factor-1 in normal and arthritic murine articular cartilage. *Journal of Rheumatology*, 21, 920–6.

7.4.2 Synovial physiology in the context of osteoarthritis
Jo C.W. Edwards

Physiology, as a branch of physical science, must deal with processes definable in dimensions of mass, length, and time. Unfortunately, osteoarthritis (OA) belongs to a disease nomenclature yet to be assimilated into this framework. A number of only partly interdependent processes are amalgamated into the single concept of a disease, although we are spared the ultimate pseudo-concept of 'disease activity'. Perhaps not surprisingly, arguments about the pathophysiology of OA often go round in circles. Nevertheless, OA can reasonably be broken down into a few central, physical concepts, including the loss of articular hyaline cartilage under the influence of load, formation of new cartilage and bone at the perimeter of an articular surface, and the accumulation of excess hyaluronan-rich synovial fluid. Pain is also important, since patients described as having OA frequently differ from others in their age

group only in that they complain of pain. Pain may not be measurable in an objective sense, but its electrical and biochemical correlates are.

A number of questions can be asked about the role of synovial physiology in these processes, but perhaps the following are of specific interest:

1. Does failure of the provision of nutrition to chondrocytes by synovium contribute to cartilage loss?

2. Does failure of efficient lubrication of articular surface by synovial fluid contribute to cartilage loss?

3. What factors determine changes in the volume and composition of synovial fluid?

4. What is the involvement of catabolic or anabolic factors from synovium in the development of cartilage loss and osteophytosis?

5. Does failure of the non-adhesive nature of synovial surface play a role?

6. What role does the neurophysiology of synovium play?

These questions are not easy to answer, largely because little is known of changes in synovial function in disease. Even where changes are known, their contribution to the pathogenesis of OA remains speculative. Thus, the following discussion must concentrate on current views of normal synovial function, with only cautious comment on the role of abnormal function in disease.

Structural elements in synovium

The detailed structure of synovium is reviewed elsewhere[1-3]. The essential elements of the tissue are a surface layer of cells (or intima), a superficial microvascular net, and a connective tissue substratum (or subintima) (Fig. 7.46). These elements are variable, and at any one point one or more may be absent. Thus, intimal cells may rest directly on adjacent muscle, fibrous synovium may lack an intimal layer, and some areas of the tissue, including smaller villi, are avascular.

The intimal cells and matrix

The intimal cell layer comprises both macrophages and synovial intimal fibroblasts (SIF) (Fig. 7.47). The macrophages behave much as macrophages do else-

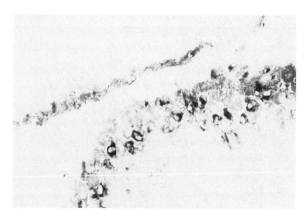

Fig. 7.47 Normal human synovial intima stained for macrophage non-specific esterase (black) and with DAF, which marks the SIF (red).

where, although in inflamed tissue they tend to express immunoglobulin receptor FcγRIII, which is specifically implicated in the binding of immune complexes, rather than FcγRI[4,5]. SIF are highly specialized[6], as detailed in Table 7.11. This list is not exhaustive and is likely to expand over the next few years. Many of the activities of these cells relate to control of tissue cohesion, and the regulation of synovial fluid volume and composition, as discussed in more detail below.

The intimal extracellular matrix is amorphous or finely fibrillar. It contains elements found in basement membrane, including laminin and collagen type IV[3], but, probably because of the absence of entactin, which links other basement membrane components together (Zvaifler, verbal communication), no true basement membrane is present. This is of key importance to the filtering properties of the intima[7].

The vascular net

Immediately beneath the intimal cells lies a rich net of capillaries[8-10]. These capillaries have fenestrations which tend to face the synovial cavity lumen. About 100–200 microns further into the tissue is a net of venules, arterioles, and lymphatics. This vascular net occurs in the synovium of both joints and tendon sheaths[11].

The subintima

Synovial subintima may appear unspecialized, being either fatty, areolar, or fibrous[1]. However, its bland appearance may hide specialized properties of two types. Synovium has to move and deform constantly[12,13]. A thin collagenous layer is often present

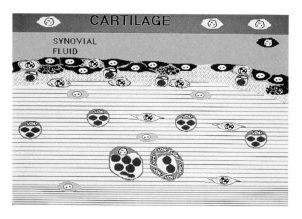

Fig. 7.46 Diagrammatic representation of the structural elements of synovium. Synovial intimal fibroblasts (SIF) are shown as dark blue, stromal fibroblasts as pale blue, and macrophages are outlined in red. Capillaries and mast cells (purple granules) are present just beneath the intima, with larger vessels deeper in the subintima.

Table 7.11   Specialized properties of Synovial Intimal Fibrosis

High levels of enzyme activity or content
    Uridine diphosphoglucose dehydrogenase (UDPGD)
    Hyaluronan synthase

Prominent cell surface molecule expression
    Vascular cell adhesion molecule-1 (VCAM-1)
    Complement decay-accelerating factor (DAF)
    CD44 (hyaluronan receptor)
    $\beta 1$ integrins ($\alpha 3,5,6$)

Synthesis of pericellular matrix molecules
    Hyaluronan
    Collagen types IV and VI
    Laminin
    Chondroitin-6-sulphate rich proteoglycan (C-6-S)
    Fibronectin
    Fibrillin

immediately beneath the intima, which may play an important role in the integrity of the tissue surface. Looser layers and fatty islands may be important in allowing deformation in specific planes.

The subintima may also provide a reservoir of fibroblasts which can be recruited to replace damaged SIF. The histogenetic relationship between subintimal fibroblast and SIF remains uncertain, but a number of strands of evidence suggest that subintimal cells will take on the specialized features of SIF when at a tissue surface[3,6,14]. Fibroblasts present in other types of loose connective tissue will not do this. This inherent specialization of synovial fibroblasts may relate to their derivation from interzone tissue, which, in the early embryo, is continuous with perichondrium. Perichondrium gives rise to stromal cells which populate bone marrow, some of which share features with SIF, including expression of the adhesion molecule VCAM-1 and high activity of the enzyme uridine diphosphoglucose dehydrogenase (UDPGD).

Functional correlates

The functions of synovium are often misunderstood, perhaps because of inappropriate analogies between biological and manmade joints, and between synovial tissue and other mesenchymal tissues or epithelia. Biological joints do not interlock, relying entirely on tensile forces in ligaments and tendons for stability[12]. There are a number of reasons why it may be disadvantageous to pack biological joints with large volumes of fluid, and as a result, joints are packed with a viscoplastic solid (synovium) enveloped by structures under tension. It is unlikely that any manmade material would withstand this environment. Perhaps because there has been no need to find out what would be needed to design such a material, the properties of synovium as a deformable packing remain unrecorded.

The intimal layer appears to represent a hybrid between mesenchyme and epithelium. Havers[15] suggested that synovium acted as an exocrine gland but failed to address the fact that synovial cavities have no exit. The exchange of water and solutes across the synovial surface is quite unlike the secretory activity of a gland, and is probably closer to the situation in the vitreous rather than the aqueous humor of the eye.

With these caveats in mind, it may be useful to focus on certain specific functions of relevance to the processes encompassed by OA.

Chondrocyte nutrition

Mature articular hyaline cartilage is avascular. Nutrition must occur by diffusion either across the articular surface or from subchondral bone. There has been considerable discussion about the contribution of these two routes[16,17]. The consensus is that solutes chiefly, if not exclusively, arrive via the articular surface. This is consistent with the fact that large areas of articular cartilage surface are closely apposed to synovial tissue carrying a dense superfical capillary net; relatively small areas being apposed to another cartilage surface in most joints (Figs 7.48 and 7.49). The distance between articular cartilage surface and synovium is generally 40–100 microns (Mead, unpublished), which is a trivial diffusion gap in contrast to the thickness of the cartilage itself. Thus, large areas of articular cartilage have a readily available source of nutrition.

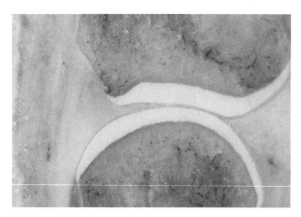

Fig. 7.48 Human interphalangeal joint sectioned at –70° C to show apposition of synovium to much of the articular cartilage surface, separated by a thin film of synovial fluid.

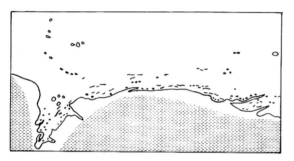

Fig. 7.49 Diagrammatic montage from micrographs of whole joint section showing distribution of small vessels in the synovium of a normal human interphalangeal joint. Vessels shown as black dots. Cartilage shown as hatched area.

Other areas of the articular surface have less good access to solutes derived from synovium. These include areas in apposition to another articular surface, and areas in apposition to fibrous structures such as menisci or similar avascular discs, as found in the distal interphalangeal joints. Some of these articular surface areas will only be distant from synovium in some positions of the joint, coming into close apposition with synovium in other positions[12]. The areas with most limited direct access to synovium are probably the central parts of relatively immobile joints, as in the tarsus, and contact areas on convex articular surfaces. The latter often remain in close apposition to another articular surface throughout the range of motion of the joint.

These 'at risk' areas may gain nutrition via two routes. Synovial fluid may be a major route, but it is essential to note that it is possible to describe a pathway for cartilage nutrition which does not require the presence of fluid. Diffusion through cartilage itself, from the perimeter of the joint, is likely to be inefficient, since many mil-

limetres may need to be traversed by nutrients. However, if the joint is moved, even the areas of articular surface which never come into apposition with synovium will come into apposition with cartilage which has more direct access to nutrition, and exchange of nutrients across the articular surfaces may occur[12].

The alternative route through synovial fluid is often assumed, but has both advantages and disadvantages. In a static joint, diffusion through the fluid has no advantage over diffusion through solid tissue. Indeed, the fluid acts as a diffusion gap. However, if the joint is moved, fluid which has been replenished with nutrients by contact with synovium will be drawn across the articular surfaces. Isometric muscle contraction may also contribute to synovial fluid movement by squeezing the fluid film out from between central articular contact points, with subsequent recoil.

A further possibility is raised by a fascinating analysis of synovial fluid dynamics made by Levick[7], which suggests that convection currents are created in synovial fluid, even at rest, by simultaneous bidirectional flow across the synovial surface. At points close to capillaries, efflux into the joint space may occur, while influx into the synovium is occurring at sites distant (in terms of tens of microns) from capillaries. This may be facilitated by the siting of capillary fenestrations on the aspect closest to the tissue surface. It is likely that directional flow in and out of the joint space also occurs cyclically during activity (Fig. 7.50). The suggestion that fluid flux in and out of cartilage during load-bearing contributes to solute flux has not been supported by experiment[18].

The problem with the synovial fluid route is the very small volume involved. A film of fluid 40 microns thick will provide a limited source of solutes for a 2 mm

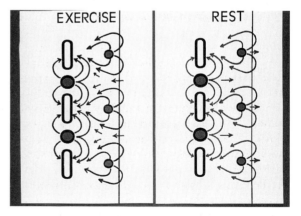

Fig. 7.50 Predicted bidirectional flow across the synovial surface. Vertical line = tissue surface, solid circles = blood vessels, open ellipses = lymphatics, arrows = flow.

thick layer of cartilage on either side (dilution factor ×
100). The more a joint is moved, the less important this
volume effect becomes. However, chondrocyte nutrition is likely to be most limited during periods of
immobility, and fluid-based transport may be of little
value in this context.

The critical question relating to chondrocyte nutrition is the level of nutrient availability required to
allow chondrocytes to survive and maintain their
matrix. Viable chondrocytes can be retrieved from
cadavers several days after death, suggesting that they
are resistant to low levels of nutrition. However, the
level of nutrition required for long-term viability at
body temperature has yet to be established.

The above notwithstanding, it may useful to consider
conditions which might lead to reduced chondrocyte
nutrition, because this could play a role in unexplained
cartilage loss in some joints. The subchondral plate may
be more permeable to solutes in youth, than in maturity[16], and subchondral plate closure could contribute to
chondrocyte undernutrition in joints with relatively
limited synovial accessibility for central cartilage areas,
such as the hip. There may also be a reduction in synovial vascularity with age. No formal analysis has been
reported. However, our own experience of normal synovial tissue has been that the rich capillary net seen in
children is much less consistent in patients over 50 years.

Excess synovial fluid volume, for any reason, will
increase the diffusion gap between synovium and cartilage, in static joints. However, this may be offset by the
presence of a larger reservoir of solutes within the fluid
compartment.

Perhaps the factor most likely to reduce chondrocyte
nutrition is immobility. Studies of immobilised joints in
animals have shown changes in chondrocyte metabolism and, in at least one system, structural cartilage
damage[19]. However, it is not clear that these observations can be extrapolated to man. In the clinical
context, long-term immobility does not appear to be
associated with cartilage loss on a regular basis.

Synovectomy might be expected to lead to undernutrition of chondrocytes, particularly in the short term,
with the development of a diffusion barrier due to
fibrin clot on the exposed tissue surface. Again, experience suggests that although cartilage damage in
inflammatory arthritis may progress after synovectomy,
early ischemic damage does not occur[20].

Perhaps the lesson from current information is that
chondrocytes will survive most changes in synovial
physiology, including the acid test of synovial removal.
It may be that the subintimal vascular net is required
more for synovial intimal cell than chondrocyte viabil-

ity. It is of note that tenosynovium carries a superficial
capillary net of comparable density and fenestration to
that seen in joints, despite the absence of cartilage
requiring nourishment[11]. However, there remains the
possibility that low levels of nutrition contribute to cartilage failure in some cases.

Lubrication

A full analysis of the mechanisms of joint lubrication is
not possible here. The reader is directed to a review by
Unsworth[21] which addresses the complexities of the
issue with both skill and sympathy for the lay, but
patient, reader. In very simple terms, synovial intimal
cells add to interstitial fluid a range of solutes with
complementary roles in lubrication. A glycoprotein,
known as lubricin, has been described, which produces
a concentration-dependent reduction in the coefficient
of friction between cartilage surfaces[22]. Synovial fluid
phospholipids may also contribute to lubrication, but
this remains contentious[23]. Hyaluronan probably contributes by conferring non-Newtonian properties to
synovial fluid, which ensure the maintenance of a fluid
film during high-load, low-speed motion[21].

The critical question is whether a failure of the lubricating mechanism between articular surfaces encourages irreversible structural damage to cartilage. The
relationship between lubrication and wear is complex.
Long-distance runners do not have major problems
with joint wear, suggesting that under normal circumstances, shear forces at articular surfaces are low
enough to avoid any significant damage to cartilage
collagen. However, following intra-articular fracture,
even when well reduced, cartilage wear nearly always
supervenes, suggesting that if the cartilage surface
structure is abnormal, normal lubricating mechanisms
are inadequate to prevent wear. The critical factor may
be the maintenance of fluid film, or hydrodynamic,
lubrication. As long as a fluid film is present, and any
surface irregularities do not make contact, wear is
likely to be minimal[21]. If contact occurs, wear may
occur and, once established, may generate increased
irregularity and consequent acceleration of damage.

In terms of a primary role for disordered lubrication
in cartilage loss, all that can be said is that in patients
with established cartilage loss the synovial fluid
hyaluronan content is normal, if not increased (see
below on fluid volume control). Changes in glycoprotein lubricants, such as lubricin, do not appear to
have been described. In inflammatory joint disease,
synovial fluid hyaluronan levels are lower. This could
contribute to cartilage damage, but would be difficult

to disentangle from other mechanisms. Moreover, in seronegative spondarthropathies, inflammatory fluid of low hyaluronan content may be present in a joint for many weeks without any subsequent evidence of articular cartilage damage.

Control of synovial fluid volume

The maintenance of a low, but measurable, volume of synovial fluid is probably of importance to chondrocyte nutrition, cartilage lubrication, and cushioning of synovial tissue from deforming forces during movement. It is more useful to think of synovial fluid as a liquid extracellular matrix than as a secretion. Water and electrolytes pass through the synovial space from capillary to lymphatic, just as in solid connective tissue (Fig. 7.50). The locally synthesized component which, for synovial fluid, chiefly means hyaluronan, turns over much more slowly, with a half-life of about 20 hours[24]. There is no active transport and, although there may be bidirectional flow across the synovial surface, the net flux over a long period is always zero.

Connective tissue water content is determined by a balance between forces controlling water influx and efflux. Hydrostatic pressure in capillaries and venules encourages influx. Efflux, via the lymphatics, is encouraged by intermittent compression of the tissue from the actions of muscles, and possibly arteriolar pulsation, but is discouraged by the tendency of extracellular matrix to retain a certain amount of water. In the absence of inflammation, the volume tends to remain constant with major changes in perfusion, suggesting that equilibrium is dependent on the hydrophilic properties of the tissue matching the forces tending to expel fluid into lymphatics. This equilibrium is probably narrowly defined, since matrix components such as hyaluronan show exponentially increasing osmotic pressure with increasing concentration[24].

Synovial fluid volume control can be seen in broadly similar terms. The volume is that which is retained by the hydrophilic action of hyaluronan. However, synovial fluid differs from other connective tissue fluid in that it is free flowing, and could potentially be expelled *en masse* into the lymphatics. There appears to be a simple but subtle mechanism for preventing this, proposed several years ago, but recently confirmed experimentally by Levick[7]. The synovial intimal matrix has a porosity which allows solutes as large as proteins to pass without significant hindrance. However, hyaluronan is so large that its diffusion will be significantly impeded by the intimal matrix. More importantly, if muscle contraction acts to squeeze synovial fluid out of

the joint cavity, hyaluronan molecules will impact in the intimal matrix and impede the passage not only of themselves, but also of water (Fig. 7.51). This is because the impacted hyaluronan reduces the effective porosity of the matrix to the size of the interstices of the hyaluronan molecule. The same thing happens if you try to force synovial fluid through a millipore filter — an unrewarding activity! In a sense, synovial fluid exploits the properties of both a fluid and a gel.

If synovial fluid volume is dependent on the amount of hyaluronan present in the cavity, long-term control of volume must depend on the rates of hyaluronan synthesis and clearance. It has been assumed for a long time that SIF are the chief source of synovial fluid hyaluronan, and this is supported by the cytochemical demonstration of their high UDPGD activity[25]. UDPGD activity is necessary for the provision of UDP-glucuronate for the formation of the repeating glucuronate/n-acetylglucosamine disaccharides of hyaluronan, and may be rate limiting, at least under some conditions[26].

The factors regulating the rate of hyaluronan synthesis by SIF *in vivo* are not known. It seems likely that stresses at the synovial surface might stimulate synthesis. Increased hyaluronan production would be likely to increase the cushioning effect of synovial fluid on synovium, thus reducing such stresses and providing a homeostatic feedback system. However, it is of interest that in knee joints of sheep, immobilized for five months by external fixation, UDPGD activity in SIF was not significantly reduced (Pitsillides and Skerry, unpublished observations).

The issue is of some clinical interest, because most patients with cartilage loss, and many with evidence of osteophytosis alone, have an increased synovial fluid volume with a normal or high hyaluronan concentra-

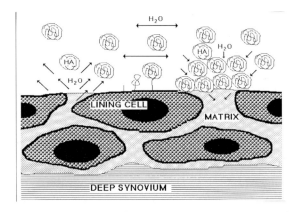

Fig. 7.51 Diagrammatic representation of the pathways of fluid flux from blood vessels (red lumen) to lymphatics (white lumen) during exercise and rest.

tion. This suggests that abnormal mechanical forces do encourage excess hyaluronan production through whatever means. However, increased amounts of hyaluronan in such joints could also be due to reduced rates of clearance. This might occur if the density of the synovial intimal matrix filter was increased as a result of fibrosis. Studies of OA and rheumatoid arthritic joints indicate that hyaluronan clearance is lower in the former[27], but the relationship to normality is uncertain. Clearance in rheumatoid joints may be increased owing to breakdown of tissue surface integrity under the influence of matrix proteases.

An interesting phenomenon relates to the very high concentrations of hyaluronan found in the fluid within ganglia (20 mg/ml; Pitsillides, unpublished) and, presumably, in cystic herniations seen with Heberden's nodes containing semisolid jelly-like material. It may be that in such cases hyaluronan is forced into a blind space from a communicating joint or tendon sheath, and that under these conditions normal homeostasis fails.

A state of inadequate synovial fluid volume has not been described but would be an obvious risk factor for failure of hydrodynamic lubrication and cartilage wear. It is doubtful whether current techniques would be capable of identifying such a state, but subtraction techniques on sequential MR imaging, after gadolinium injection, may be capable of resolving even small volumes of synovial fluid.

Synovial non-adherence

Perhaps the most fundamental of all synovial functions is to maintain, in the face of inflammatory or mechanical injury, a plane of discontinuity within connective tissue which allows movement to occur between, rather than within, tissue elements. The alternative scenario is that of the fibrous joint, such as the intervertebral disc, in which movement occurs by viscoplastic deformation of soft tissue. In man, fibrous joints are largely restricted to sites of relatively infrequent or limited movement, although the frog knee is a fibrous or fibrovesicular joint!

The maintenance of a plane of discontinuity, or synovial space, appears to relate to special properties of synovial fibroblasts. From a very early stage in embryonic development, the tissue interposed between skeletal cartilage elements, and destined to become synovium, is distinguished by prominent expression of the hyaluronan receptor, CD44[28]. At a stage just before the synovial cavity forms, a line of cells at the site of imminent separation shows high activity of UDPGD. It has been proposed that joint cavity formation is facili-

tated by an interaction between local excess hyaluronan and cell bound CD44. *In vitro*, the presence of low levels of hyaluronan CD44 promotes cell-cell adhesion, but at high levels of hyaluronan, adhesion is inhibited[29]. This is explained on the basis of CD44 molecules on separate cells, binding to the same hyaluronan molecules at low hyaluronan levels, but the formation of discrete hyaluronan 'halos' around each cell in the presence of hyaluronan excess. This antiadhesive effect of high concentrations of hyaluronan probably continues to operate in the mature synovial joint.

At a stage when the embryonic joint has yet to form a cavity, the cells destined to become intimal fibroblasts (SIF) are identifiable by their expression of complement decay-accelerating factor (DAF), which is the molecule recognized by the monoclonal antibody mab67[30-32] (Fig. 7.47). DAF is expressed at low levels on blood cells and endothelium. It is expressed at much higher levels on the cells lining internal body surfaces such as synovial intima, Bowman's capsule, and amniotic epithelium. It is also present on the outermost layer of fetal, but not adult, epidermis. All of these structures require to be non-adherent. It seems likely that DAF prevents adhesion by inhibiting complement-mediated damage to a specialized surface layer of cells during the inflammatory response to injury.

The other molecule associated with adhesion, seen at exceptionally high levels on SIF, is vascular cell adhesion molecule-1 (VCAM-1)[33-34]. This molecule binds to the $\alpha4\beta1$ integrin on mononuclear leucocytes. Two possible roles for VCAM-1 on SIF can be identified. Firstly, it may provide a mechanism for allowing $\alpha4\beta1$ integrin negative polymorphonuclear leucocytes to enter the synovial fluid during inflammation, while retaining monocytes and lymphocytes within the tissue. This may allow killing of pathogens, followed by clearance of debris by macrophages retained at the intimal surface. A second, more subtle possibility, is that by enmeshing synovial intimal macrophages with their VCAM-1 bearing dendrites, SIF regulate the interaction of $\alpha4\beta1$ integrin on the macrophages with another ligand in the matrix, namely fibronectin. Binding of cells to fibronectin may be an early stage in the formation of inflammatory adhesions.

Failure of the antiadhesive properties of SIF is likely to be of relevance to cartilage damage only when this occurs secondarily to pannus formation in inflammatory joint disease. It may also be relevant to adhesive capsulitis of the shoulder. However, the molecules involved in non-adhesion may play a role in synovial inflammation, whether primary or secondary.

Synovitis and soluble mediators

OA gets its name from the formation of new bone associated with load bearing cartilage loss. It had been known as hypertrophic arthritis, to distinguish it from inflammatory or atrophic arthritis in which osteopenia predominates. The changes in bone density seen in these types of arthritis may well relate to cytokines and growth factors secreted by resident or immigrant synovial cells. This subject is considered in detail in the preceding chapter, and will not be enlarged upon here. However, it may be worth noting the possible implication of some of the factors discussed, in terms of non-adhesion in the genesis of synovitis.

Apparently fortuitously, SIF resemble the follicular dendritic cells of germinal centres, not only in being fibroblast-like cells with branching dendrites, but in their prominent coexpression of VCAM-1 and DAF[35]. Both molecules are likely to favour local survival of lymphocytes. The ways in which synovial fibroblasts interact with lymphocytes remain to be elucidated, but the presence of these molecules in synovium may go some way to explain the tendency for lymphocytes to accumulate in synovium, not only in rheumatoid disease but also, to a lesser degree, in the synovium of patients with primary cartilage or bone abnormalities.

Synovial innervation

Synovium is well supplied with thinly myelinated and unmyelinated nerve fibers[36]. These nerves appear to be involved chiefly in vasomotor regulation and pain sensation. Vasomotor control is achieved by post-ganglionic adrenergic neurons. Pain is mediated through unmyelinated C fibers.

Normal perception of joint movement is attributed to sensory nerves beyond the synovium, in the capsule and musculotendinous units. However, when synovium is inflamed, sensitization of pain fibers by prostanoids and other inflammatory mediators leads to a sensation of pain on movement.

Abnormalities of synovial innervation could contribute to the damage to cartilage and bone seen in neuropathic joints. However, exposure to excessive trauma may relate more to absence of pain sensation in supportive ligaments. In rheumatoid arthritis, the superficial synovium is deficient in pain fibers[37], but joint movement is associated with pain, and there seems to be no clear indication that synovial denervation contributes to secondary cartilage damage.

Although unmyelinated C fibers have an afferent function in terms of pain sensation, they can also have an efferent function. They contain neuropeptides, such as substance P, which is synthesized in the cell body in the dorsal root ganglion. Discharge of substance P from peripheral fibers may modulate the sensation of pain and contribute to the control of inflammation, including the regulation of vascular tone. A single nerve fiber can, therefore, modulate its own stimulation by what is known as the axon reflex. Both substance P and calcitonin gene-related peptide are known to be involved in this process. It has been suggested that neurophsyiological mechanisms may play a considerable role in inflammatory joint disease[36], although their role in cartilage loss or local hyperostosis, as in Heberden's nodes, has not been explored to the same extent.

Summary

Although synovial function is essential to that of articular cartilage, there is relatively little evidence to suggest that abnormalities of synovium have a role in load bearing cartilage loss or osteophytosis, except when they occur secondary to primary inflammatory disease. It is tempting to speculate that synovial fibrosis might lead to undernutrition of chondrocytes in the hip with advancing age, or that inadequate synovial fluid volume might contribute to chondromalacia patellae. However, the secondary role of synovium in joint effusions and pain is more clearly established, and it is here that therapeutic avenues are likely to be open.

As with changes in cartilage, the study of processes within synovium and synovial fluid is still hampered by the low resolution of non-invasive imaging techniques. However, with the current rate of advance of modalities such as MRI, perhaps we can look forward to an era in which analysis of synovial pathophysiology becomes of direct clinical relevance.

References

1. Key, J.A. (1932). The synovial membrane of joints and bursae. *Special cytology*, vol. 2, pp. 1055–76. P.B. Hoeber Inc., New York.

2. Edwards, J.C.W. (1987). Structure of synovial lining. In *The synovial lining in health and disease*, (pp. 31–40) Chapman and Hall, London.

3. Revell, P.A., Al-Saffar, N., Fish, S., and Osei, D. (1995). Extracellular matrix of the synovial intimal cell layer. *Annals of the Rheumatic Diseases*, 54, 404–7.

4. Bröker, B., Edwards, J.C.W., Fanger, M., and Lydyard, P. (1990). The prevalence and distribution of macrophages

bearing FcRI, FcRII and FcRIII in synovium. *Scandinavian Journal of Rheumatology*, **19**, 123–35.

5. Athanasou, N. (1995). Synovial macrophages. *Annals of the Rheumatic Diseases*, **54**, 392–4.

6. Edwards, J.C.W. (1995). Synovial intimal fibroblasts. *Annals of the Rheumatic Diseases*, **54**, 395–7.

7. Levick, J.R. (1995). Fluid movement across synovium in healthy joints: role of synovial fluid macromolecules. *Annals of the Rheumatic Diseases*, **54**, 417–23.

8. Davies, D.V. and Edwards, D.A.W. (1948). The blood supply of the synovial membrane and intra-articular structures. *Annals of the Royal College of Surgeons*, **2**, 142–56.

9. Stevens, C.R., Blake, D.R., Merry, P., Revell, P.A., and Levick, I.R. (1991). A comparative study by morphometry of the microvasculature in normal and rheumatoid synovium. *Arthritis and Rheumatism*, **34**, 1508–13.

10. Wilkinson, L.S. and Edwards, J.C.W. (1989). Microvascular distribution in normal human synovium. *Journal of Anatomy*, **167**, 129–36.

11. Neal, C., Read, N., Goodwyn, D., and Edwards, J.C.W. (1989). Fenestration of tenosynovial capillaries. *British Journal of Rheumatology*, **28**, 31–3.

12. Edwards, J.C.W. (1987). Functions of synovial lining. In *The synovial lining in health and disease*, pp. 41–74. Chapman and Hall, London.

13. Simkin, P. (1993). Biology of the joints. In *Mechanics of human joints*. (V. Wright and E.L. Radin), pp. 3–26. Marcel Dekker, New York.

14. Edwards, J.C.W. (1994). The nature and origins of synovium. *Journal of Anatomy*, **184**, 493–501.

15. Havers, C. (1691). *Osteologia nova*. Samuel Smith, London.

16. Ogata, K., Whiteside, L.A., and Lesker, P.A. (1978). Subchondral route for nutrition to articular cartilage in the rabbit. Measurement of diffusion with hydrogen gas *in vivo*. *Journal of Bone and Joint Surgery (Am)*, **60A**, 905–10.

17. Berry, J.L., Thaeler-Oberdoerster, D.A., and Greenwald, A.S. (1986). Subchondral pathways to the superior surface of the human talus. *Foot-Ankle*, **7**, 2–9.

18. O'Hara, B.P., Urban, J.P., and Maroudas, A. (1990). Influence of cyclic loading on the nutrition of articular cartilage. *Annals of the Rheumatic Diseases*, **49**, 536–9.

19. Meyer-Carrive, I. and Ghosh, P. (1992). Effects of tiaprofenic acid on cartilage proteoglycans in the rabbit joint immobilisation model. *Annals of the Rheumatic Diseases*, **51**, 448–55.

20. Paus, A.C. and Pahle, J.A. (1991). Evaluation of knee joint cartilages and menisci in patients with chronic inflammatory joint diseases. A prospective arthroscopic study before, six and twelve months after open synovectomy. *Scandinavian Journal of Rheumatology*, **20**, 252–61.

21. Unsworth, A. (1993). *Lubrication of human joints*. *Mechanics of human joints*. (V. Wright and E.L. Radin), pp. 137–62. Marcel Dekker, New York.

22. Swann, D.A., Silver, F.H., Slayter, H.S., Stafford, W., and Shore, E. (1985). The molecular structure and lubricating activity of lubricin isolated from bovine and human synovial fluids. *Biochemical Journal*, **225**, 195–201.

23. Williams, P.F., Powell, G.L., and LaBerge, M. (1993). Sliding friction analysis of phosphatidylcholine as a boundary lubricant for articular cartilage. *Proceedings of the Institute of Mechanical Engineers H.*, **207**, 59–66.

24. Laurent, T.C., Laurent, U.B.G., and Fraser, J.R.E. (1995). Functions of hyaluronan. *Annals of the Rheumatic Diseases*, **54**, 429–32.

25. Wilkinson, L.S., Pitsillides, A.A., Worrall, J.G., and Edwards, J.C.W. (1992). Light microscopic characterisation of the fibroblastic synovial lining cell (synoviocyte). *Arthritis and Rheumatism*, **35**, 1179–84.

26. McGarry, A. and Gahan, P.B. (1985). A quantitative cytochemical study of UDPDglucose: NAD oxidoreductase activity during stelar differentiation in Pisum sativum L.C. Meteor. *Histochemistry*, **83**, 551–4.

27. Pitsillides, A.A., Will, R., Bayliss, M.T., and Edwards, J.C.W. (1994). Changes in synovial fluid hyaluronan associated with intra-articular corticosteroid injection. *Arthritis and Rheumatism*, **37**, 1030–8.

28. Edwards, J.C.W., Wilkinson, L.S., Jones, H.M., Soothill, P., Henderson, K.J., Worrall, J.G., et al. (1994). The formation of human synovial joint cavities: a possible role for hyaluronan and CD44 in altered interzone cohesion. *Journal of Anatomy*, **185**, 355–67.

29. Underhill, C.B. and Dorfman, A. (1978). The role of hyaluronic acid in intercellular adhesion in cultured mouse cells. *Experimental Cell Research*, **117**, 155–64.

30. Medof, M.E., Walter, E.I., Rutgers, J.L., Knowles, D.M., and Nussenzweig, V. (1987). Identification of the complement decay accelerating factor on epithelium and glandular cells and in body fluids. *Journal of Experimental Medicine*, **165**, 848–64.

31. Stevens, C.R., Mapp, P.I., and Revell, P.A. (1990). A monoclonal antibody (Mab 67) marks type B synoviocytes. *Rheumatology International*, **10**, 103–6.

32. Edwards, J.C.W. and Wilkinson, L.S. (1996). Distribution in human tissues of the synovial lining associated epitope recognised by monoclonal antibody 67. *Journal of Anatomy*, **188**, 119–27.

33. Morales, Ducret, J., Wayner, E., Elices, M.J. et al. (1992). a4/b1 integrin (VLA-4) ligands in arthritis: Vascular cell adhesion molecule expression in synovium and on fibroblast-like synoviocytes. *Arthritis and Rheumatism*, **149**, 1424–31.

34. Wilkinson, L.S., Edwards, J.C.W., Poston, R., and Haskard, D.O. (1993). Cell populations expressing VCAM-1 in normal and diseased synovium. *Laboratory Investigation*, **68**, 82–8.

35. Edwards, J.C.W. and Cambridge, G. (1995). Is rheumatoid arthritis a failure of B cell death in synovium? *Annals of the Rheumatic Diseases*, **54**, 696–700.

36. Mapp, P.I. (1995). Innervation of synovium. *Annals of the Rheumatic Diseases*, **54**, 398–403.

37. Gronblad, M., Kontinnen, Y.T., Korkala, O., Liesi, P., Hukkanen, M., and Polak, J. (1988). Neuropeptides in the synovium of patients with rheumatoid arthritis and osteoarthritis. *Journal of Rheumatology*, **15**, 1807–10.

7.5   Innervation of the joint and its role in osteoarthritis

Joel A. Vilensky

Joint innervation and its role in joint disease

The classical view pertaining to the relationship between the nervous system and joints is that neural elements simply transmit sensation, both noxious and proprioceptive, to the central nervous system (CNS). However, recent data suggest that some of the pain associated with osteoarthritis (OA) may *originate* in the CNS, rather than in the joint or periarticular tissues, and that the CNS may participate in the pathogenesis of the disease.

Joint receptors and nerves

Articular nerves consist of myelinated and unmyelinated sensory afferent axons, and sympathetic efferent axons. The myelinated axons convey sensations from mechanoreceptors (afferent neurons that transmit impulses in response to mechanical deformation), and range in diameter from 2–17 μm[1,2,3]. Their conduction velocity varies directly with size[4]. The unmyelinated fibers consist of very small (less than 2 μm) sensory fibers from widely distributed free nerve endings, which transmit sensations of pain[5], and sympathetic efferent fibers, which regulate blood flow (Table 7.12)[3]. Most of the free receptors are inactive during normal circumstances; they do not respond to movement, but show activity upon abnormal deformation or exposure to chemical agents, for example, inflammatory mediators[2]. Stimulation of free nerve endings is associated with the conscious perception of pain[5].

Although the morphologic and physiologic response characteristics of joint mechanoreceptors (Fig. 7.52; Table 7.12) have been well established, the function of these receptors is controversial. For example, Schaible and Grubb[6] recently questioned whether there is any conscious perception of information other than pain from joints, whereas other studies imply that information from joints is important for movement and position sense[2,7]. Nevertheless, it is well accepted that

mechanoreceptors contribute to the generation of postural and protective muscular reflexes. For example, upon excessive ligament stretch, Golgi tendon organ-like endings (Table 7.12) are thought to stimulate antagonistic muscles, that is, those with actions that would reduce the stretch, thereby protecting the joint. Other mechanoreceptors contribute to postural and protective reflexes less directly, via the muscle spindle system[2], which functions to maintain muscle tone with changes in muscle length, and to provide the CNS with proprioceptive information.

The majority of studies of knee joint afferents have found them to be active only near the extremes of the normal range of motion, suggesting that they act primarily to protect the joint from hyperflexion, hyperextension, over-rotation, and so on. However, Johansson *et al.*[2] concluded that the amount of time needed for impulses from these afferents to activate muscular contractions that could provide such protection is too long to prevent the potentially damaging movement. They suggested, alternatively, that mechanoreceptors assure joint stability by acting continuously to regulate muscle tension around joints. Johansson *et al.*[2] noted that this hypothesis, which emphasizes the sensory role of knee joint ligaments, explains why surgical treatment of anterior cruciate ligament (ACL) deficiency is often disappointing, that is, sensory feedback from the joint is modified by the injury, or the ligament repair or reconstruction (see p. 184).

Joint pain

Intrinsic mechanisms

In the presence of joint inflammation, afferent fibers exhibit increased sensitivity. Under these conditions normally innocuous movements generate increased neural activity, which is presumably perceived as pain. The increase in neural impulses is generated by greater reactivity in the receptors that normally respond to the

Table 7.12 Characteristics of articular receptors[1,2,3]

Type	Morphology	Parent nerve fiber	Location	Characteristics	Function
Ruffini endings	Thinly encapsulated, globular structures	Small myelinated (6–9 μm)	Joint capsule, medial meniscus, cruciate ligaments	Low threshold, slowly adapting	Static and dynamic mechanoreceptors, transmit information on joint position, intra-articular pressure, amplitude and velocity of movement
Pacinian corpuscles	Thickly encapsulated corpuscles	Medium myelinated (9–12 μm)	Joint capsule, medial meniscus, cruciate ligaments	Low threshold, rapidly adapting (inactive in immobile joint and when joint is moving at constant speed)	Dynamic mechanoreceptors, signal acceleration or deceleration
Golgi tendon organ-like endings (similar to structure in muscle tendons)	Thinly encapsulated fusiform corpuscles	Large myelinated (13–17 μm)	Ligaments, medial meniscus	High threshold, slowly adapting (inactive in immobile joints)	Dynamic mechanoreceptors, signal tension in ligaments, especially at extreme range of movement
Free nerve endings	Network of fine nerve fibers	Myelinated (2.5 μm) and unmyelinated (< 2 μm)	Throughout most articular tissues (but not articular cartilage and synovial membrane)	Very high threshold, non-adapting	Nociceptors, mechanoreceptors and chemoreceptors (respond to mechanical deformation and chemical agents, e.g., inflammatory mediators)

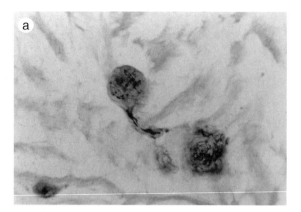

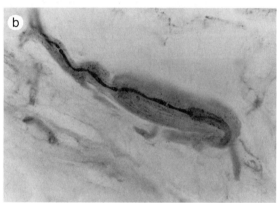

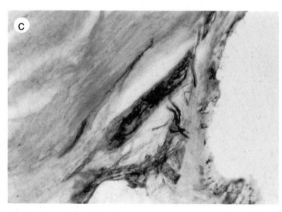

Fig. 7.52 Photomicrographs of mechanoreceptors. (a) Two Ruffini endings splitting from a single axon. Note dense neuronal arborization within the thin, spheroidal capsules. (b) Pacinian corpuscle. Note the dense capsule of circumferential lamellae surrounding a single nerve fiber. (c) Golgi tendon organ-like ending. Note the thin, elongated capsule enclosing neuronal arborization. The differing morphology reflects differing functional characteristics (see Table 7.12)[5]. (Magnification: ×147.)

innocuous movements, and by activation of nociceptors, which normally do not respond to these movements (hyperalgesia)[6,8]. Additionally, joints appear to contain 'silent nociceptors,' which become mechanosensitive only after the development of local inflammation[6]. Pain from diseased joints is often induced or increased when the joint is 'loaded' (weight bearing) and moving, although joint pain may occur in the immobile or unloaded joint ('rest pain')[6]. Presumably, rest pain results from the response of joint nociceptors to increased pressure or inflammatory mediators, or from an increase in the sensitivity of spinal or supraspinal neurons (see p. 179). Because abolition or inhibition of the sensitizing process within the joint may provide a means to reduce pain, some of the possible causes of this increased sensitivity are discussed below.

Intraarticular pressure

Normally, only a small quantity of synovial fluid can be aspirated from the human knee joint[9], whereas large quantities can be aspirated from diseased joints. This increase in volume is associated with an increase in pressure (as much as 36 mm Hg, compared to 0 mm Hg in the normal joint at rest)[9], which may enhance the sensitivity of joint afferents. However, experimentally induced joint distention initially produced mainly feelings of 'tightness' in normal and arthritic knees. Additional distention resulted in sensations of pain, but such sensations rapidly diminished after a few seconds. Twenty-four hours later many of the patients indicated that their knees felt 'much better' than before the experimentally induced distention[9]. Thus, reduction of pressure alone does not appear to explain why aspiration of synovial fluid from inflamed joints may result in a reduction in pain.

Inflammatory mediators

A variety of inflammatory mediators (prostaglandins, thromboxanes, leukotrienes, kinins, and others) are found in synovial fluid from diseased joints. When these mediators are injected locally into joints, joint afferents show an enhanced response to pressure or chemical stimuli[6]. Furthermore, afferents in inflamed joints react more strongly to injection of prostaglandin than those in normal joints; thus, some substance

Plates

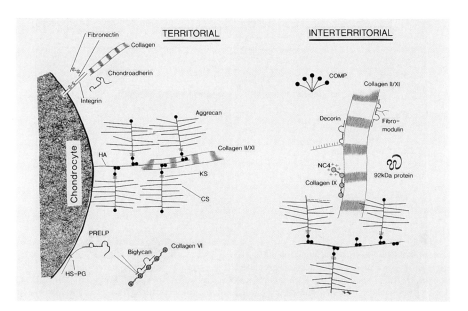

Fig. 7.6 Schematic illustration of the constituents of cartilage matrix. The spatial relationships of the various constituents to the chondrocyte, that is, their presence in the territorial (close to the cell) or inter-territorial matrix (furthest away from the cell) is shown and the macromolecular organization of matrix molecules is indicated.

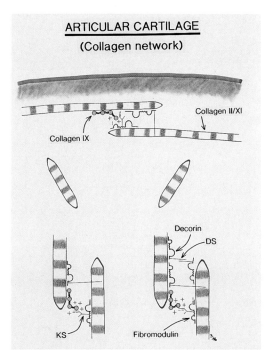

Fig. 7.7 Schematic illustration of the organization of the collagen network in cartilage. The superficial region of the cartilage contains collagen fibers arranged parallel to the surface, while the deepest, major part of the tissue contains fibers arranged perpendicular to the surface. In the intermediate zone, the fibers run in different directions. A number of other matrix macromolecules are bound at the surface of the collagen fiber. These appear to have important roles in 'knitting' together the collagen fibers to form a network, essential for counterbalancing the swelling pressure of the proteoglycans.

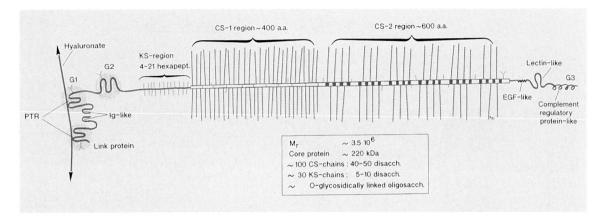

Fig. 7.8 Schematic illustration of the aggrecan molecule. A central core protein is substituted with some 100 glycosaminogly-cans chains of chondroitin sulfate (CS) and keratan sulfate (KS). These chains consist of characteristic repeat disaccharides with negatively-charged sulfate and uronic acid carboxyl groups. The average chondroitin sulfate (CS) chain contains some 80–100 charged groups. Specific domains of the aggrecan include an N-terminal hyaluronate binding domain (G1), a homologous G2 domain, a keratan sulfate-rich region, two distinct regions of polypeptide repeats carrying the chondroitin sulfate chains and C-terminal EGF-like domain, a lectin homology domain, and a complement regulatory protein-like domain. Some molecules lack the C-terminal domain as a result of proteolytic cleavage.

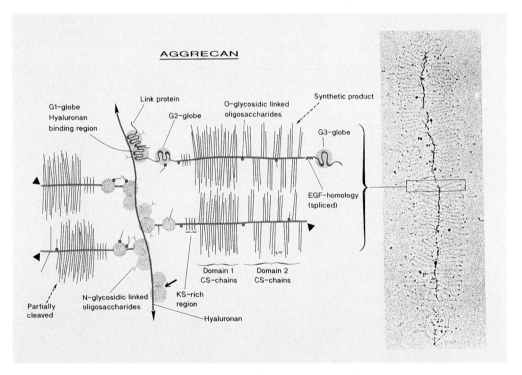

Fig. 7.9 Illustration of the proteoglycan aggregate. Several aggrecan molecules are bound, via their N-terminal end which contains a specific hyaluronate-binding domain, to an extremely long hyaluronate molecule. This results in a very large complex, with several hundred thousand fixed-charge groups, that creates osmotic gradient and swelling pressure. The appearance of the molecule upon electron microscopy, after rotatory shadowing, is shown on the right. The central filament represents hyaluronate decorated with globular link protein and hyaluronate-binding domains of the aggrecan molecules, seen as side chain filaments. The structure of the aggrecan molecule changes with age, such that most molecules have been cleaved in their C-terminal domain and are, therefore, shorter, as indicated by arrowheads in the figure. The ultimate retained cleavage product is the HABr (arrow) bound to HA, together with link protein. (Matthias Mörgelin kindly provided the E-M picture.)

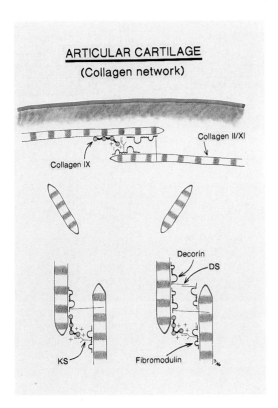

ARTICULAR CARTILAGE
(Collagen network)

Collagen IX

Collagen II/XI

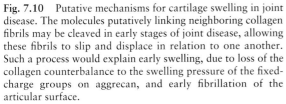

Decorin

DS

KS

Fibromodulin

Fig. 7.10 Putative mechanisms for cartilage swelling in joint disease. The molecules putatively linking neighboring collagen fibrils may be cleaved in early stages of joint disease, allowing these fibrils to slip and displace in relation to one another. Such a process would explain early swelling, due to loss of the collagen counterbalance to the swelling pressure of the fixed-charge groups on aggrecan, and early fibrillation of the articular surface.

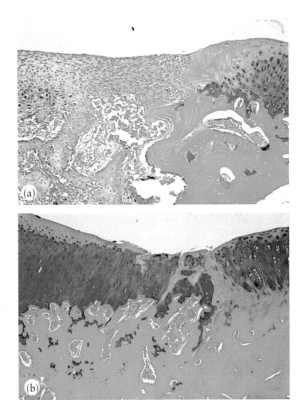

(a)

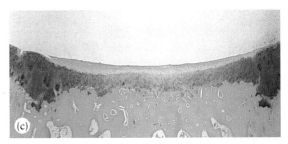

(b)

(c)

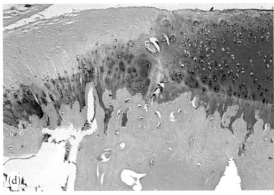

(d)

Fig. 7.13 Spontaneous repair induced by bleeding. Photomicrographs illustrating spontaneous repair of full-thickness defects in the femur of mature rabbits (18 months, 5 kg) drilled through to the subchondral bone and left without treatment: (a) 10 days; (b) 8 weeks; (c) 24 weeks; (d) 48 weeks after creation. The resin embedded sections have been processed with Safranin O dye which stains proteoglycans red. (a) At 10 days, repair tissue still consists largely of undifferentiated mesenchymal cells, but there is already evidence of cartilage formation (red-stained tissue) just below the surface at the far left. (b) At 8 weeks, hyaline cartilage has formed within the defect (red-stained tissue). (c) At 24 weeks, integrity of the repair tissue is still maintained. (d) At 48 weeks, repair tissue shows signs of degeneration, and its affinity for Safranin O is markedly reduced. From Shapiro et al.[12], with permission from the authors and the publisher.

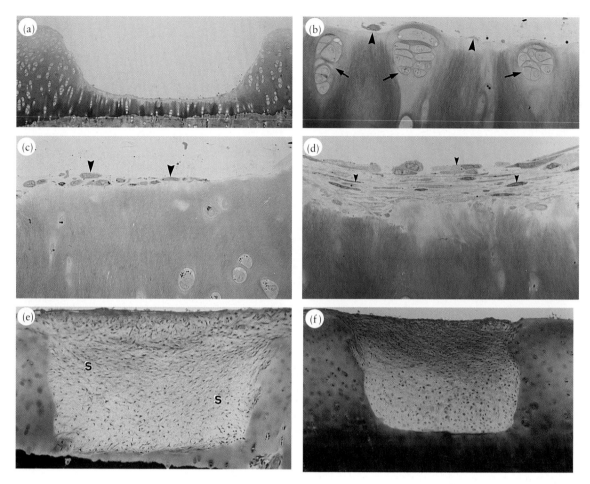

Fig. 7.14 The use of growth factors to induce chondrogenesis *in vivo*. Photomicrographs illustrating the appearance, at 4 weeks, of superficial articular cartilage defects that do not penetrate into the subchondral bone in the knee of: (a)-(d); mature rabbits (18 months; 5 kg); (e) and (f); adult mini-pigs (3 yr, 65 kg). (a) When left untreated, such defects did not heal for as long as one year after surgery. (b) Proliferating chondrocyte clusters were often seen at the edge of the defect but did not migrate into the space. (c) Adhesion of cells from the synovial fluid occurred following controlled removal of surface proteoglycans with chondroitinase AC. (d) Multilayers of such cells formed following the topical application of a mitogenic growth factor (IGF1, TGFβ; 20 ng/ml), filling about 10% of the space. (e) Complete infilling with mesenchymal cells was achieved only if the defect was filled with a biodegradable matrix (fibrin, collagen, gelatin) containing the mitogenic growth factor. Those cells did not transform into chondrocytes. (f) A chondrogenic switch occurred 3–4 weeks after surgery if a growth factor from the TGF β superfamily (200–1000 ng/ml), but not IGF1, was placed in liposomes and included within the gel in addition to the free chemotactic mitogenic growth factor. The illustration shows the beginning of this switch in the lower half of the defect. (a)–(d): semi-thin resin embedded sections stained with toluidine blue; (e) and (f): thick, surface-polished saw cuts stained with basic fuchsin and McNeil's Tetrachrome.)

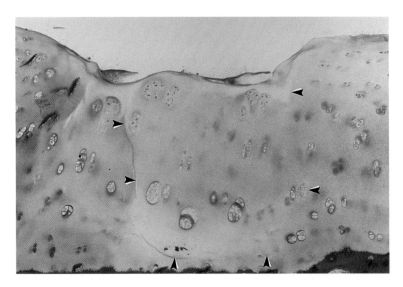

Fig. 7.15 Regeneration *in vivo* using a fibrin matrix. Partial thickness articular cartilage defect in the femur of a mini-pig (3 yr, 65 kg) after 6 weeks of treatment with a fibrin gel containing free TGFβ2 (5 ng ml) and liposome-encapsulated TGFβ2 (400 ng ml). Arrowheads denote the original edges of the defect. Fairly good integration has been achieved, but fibrin retracts on setting and is unsuitable for long-term repair. (The resin-embedded section is a thick, surface-polished saw cut, surface-stained with basic fuchsin and toluidene blue.)

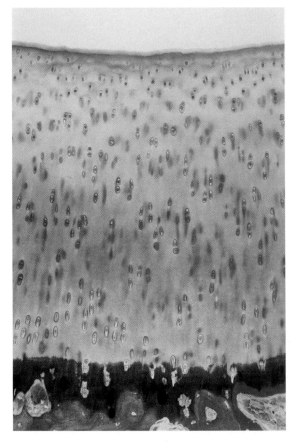

Fig. 7.16 Mature articular cartilage. Articular cartilage from the femur of a mature rabbit (18 m, 5 kg), showing typical zonal arrangement of the chondrocytes. (The resin-embedded section is a thick, surface-polished saw cut, surface-stained with basic fuchsin and toluidene blue.)

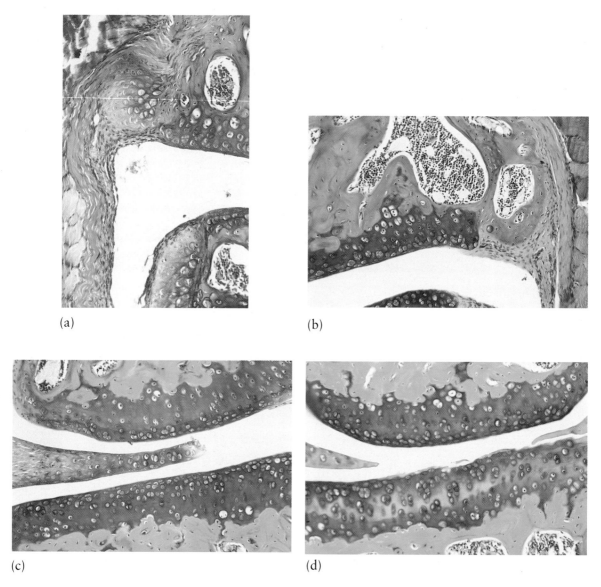

Fig. 7.44 Safranin O stained of sections of the murine knee joint after local TGFβ injection: (a) outgrowth of chondroid tissue at the joint margin at day three after the last of triple TGFβ injections, given on alternate days; (b) similar treatment, but four weeks later — note the maturation into a mature osteophyte, containing bone marrow; (c) control section of tibial plateau; (d) similar region one month after six TGFβ injections, given on alternate days — note the loss of proteoglycan staining and the irregular surface and spacing of chondrocytes.

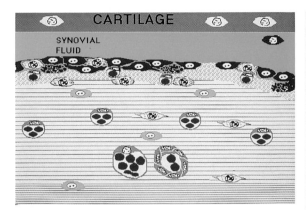

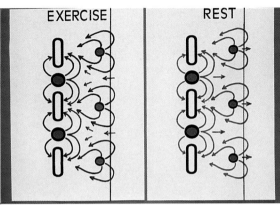

Fig. 7.46 Diagrammatic representation of the structural elements of synovium. Synovial intimal fibroblasts (SIF) are shown as dark blue, stromal fibroblasts as pale blue, and macrophages are outlined in red. Capillaries and mast cells (purple granules) are present just beneath the intima, with larger vessels deeper in the subintima.

Fig. 7.51 Diagrammatic representation of the pathways of fluid flux from blood vessels (red lumen) to lymphatics (white lumen) during exercise and rest.

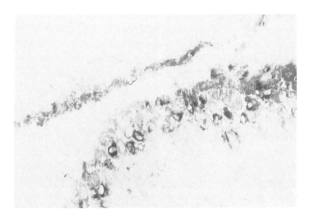

Fig. 7.47 Normal human synovial intima stained for macrophage non-specific esterase (black) and with DAF, which marks the SIF (red).

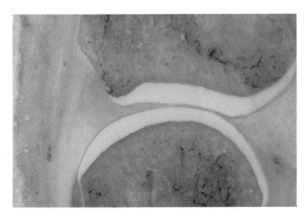

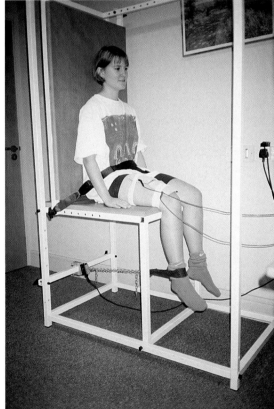

Fig. 7.48 Human interphalangeal joint sectioned at −70° C to show apposition of synovium to much of the articular cartilage surface, separated by only a very thin film of synovial fluid.

Fig. 7.58 Equipment used for measuring isometric quadriceps strength and twitch superimposition.

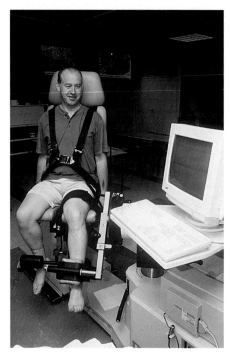

Fig. 7.59 Equipment used for measuring isokinetic quadriceps strength.

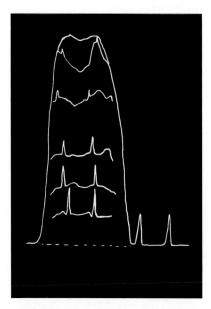

Fig. 7.60 Typical trace from a subject performing variable strength muscle contractions whilst receiving constant superimposed percutaneous twitches.

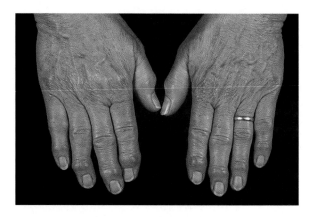

Fig. 8.4 Hand involvement in generalized nodal OA, with typical Heberden's and Bouchard's nodes.

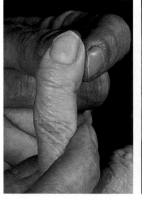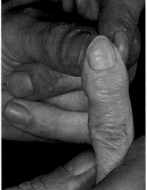

Fig. 8.5 Instability of the DIPJ in erosive OA.

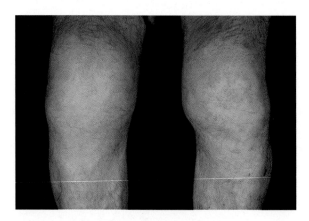

Fig. 8.7 Pyrophosphate arthropathy presenting as acute synovitis of the knee.

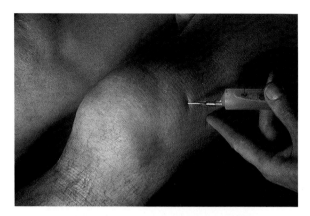

Fig. 8.8 Turbid synovial fluid obtained during an acute attack of acute pyrophosphate arthropathy.

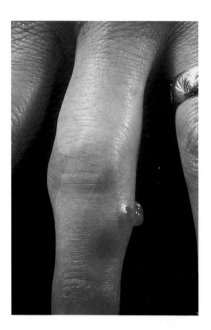

Fig. 8.14 Mucous cyst exuding hyaluronan-rich jelly extending distally.

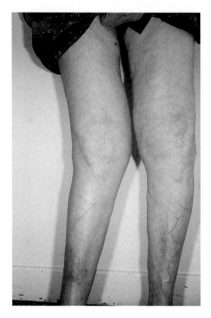

Fig. 8.9 Chronic pyrophosphate arthropathy in the knee of an elderly lady, with marked valgus deformity of the right knee.

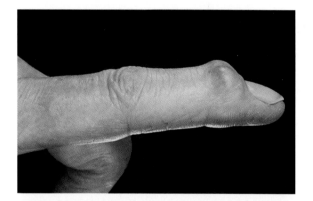

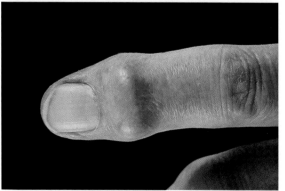

Fig. 8.15 Typical posterolateral swelling of the DIPJ.

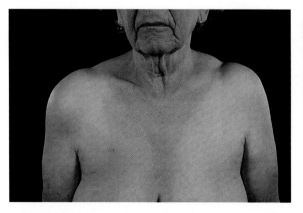

Fig. 8.12 Large, cool effusion in a 'Milwaukee shoulder' (apatite-associated arthropathy).

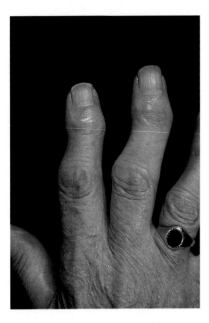

Fig. 8.16   Ulnar deviation at the DIPJs; radial deviation at the DIPJs.

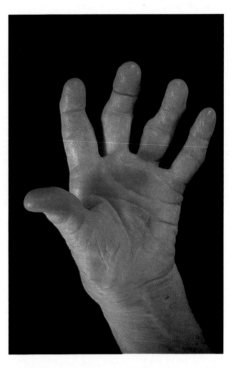

Fig. 8.18   Squaring of the 1st CMCJ due to osteophyte, remodeling and subluxation, with consequent wasting of the thenar muscles.

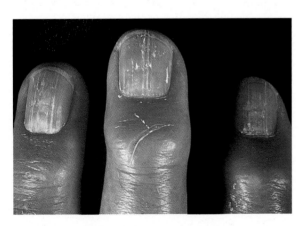

Fig. 8.17   'Heberden's nodes nails' with longitudinal and transverse nail ridging.

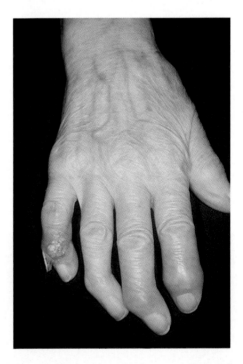

Fig. 8.19   A discharging gouty tophus in an elderly lady with pre-existing nodal OA.

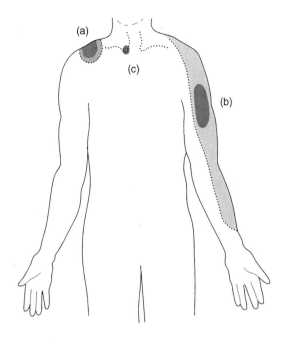

Fig. 8.20 Pattern of pain around the shoulder from OA of: (a) acromioclavicular joint; (b) glenohumeral joint; (c) sterno-clavicular joint.

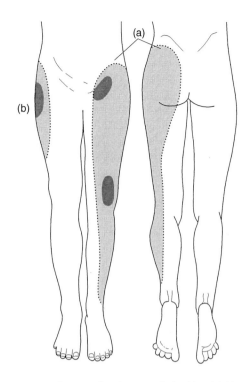

Fig. 8.23 Radiation of pain around the hip: (a) hip OA; (b) trochanteric bursitis.

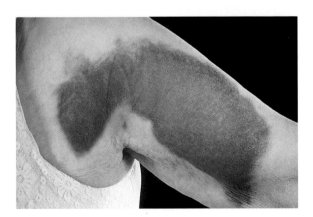

Fig. 8.21 Extensive bruising of the upper arm due to rupture of the shoulder joint — 'epaule senile haemorrhagique'.

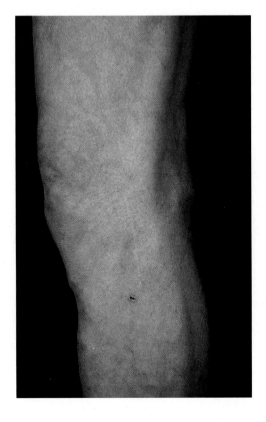

Fig. 8.26 Swelling due to a popliteal cyst complicating knee OA.

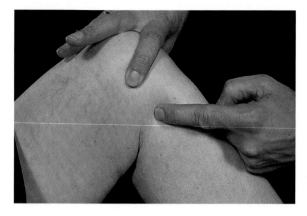

Fig. 8.27 A common periarticular tender site at the knee; the left index finger is placed over the medial joint line and the right index finger over the inferior insertion of the medial collateral ligament.

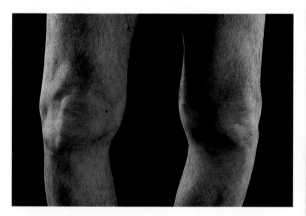

Fig. 8.28 Typical varus deformity with knee OA.

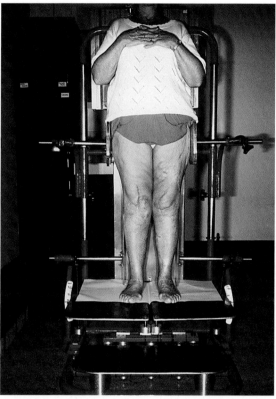

Fig. 8.31 Positioning device for ensuring reproducibility of radiographic positioning for knee radiography.

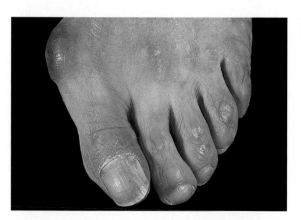

Fig. 8.29 Hallux valgus due to OA of the 1st MTPJ.

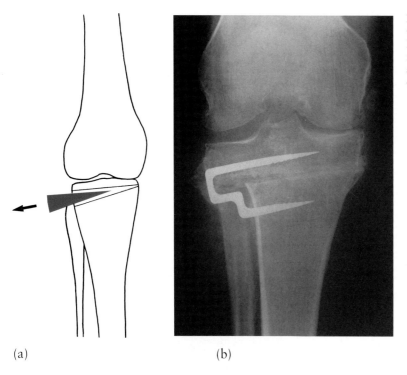

Fig. 9.17 Tibial valgus osteotomy for OA of the medial compartment of the knee: (a) schematic drawing, showing resection of bone wedge; (b) postoperative radiograph showing closed osteotomy.

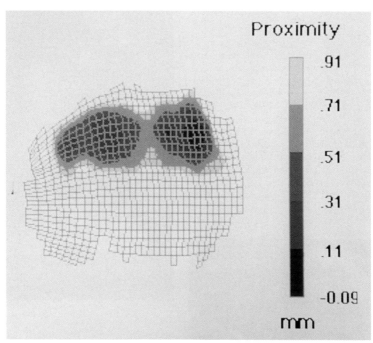

Fig. 11.43 Surface-contact mapping with MRI. Map of *in situ* contact areas for the patellar cartilage of the amputated knee shown in Fig. 11.38. MR images were segmented manually, and geometric models of the articular surfaces of the patellofemoral joint were generated from the contour curves, using parametric bicubic B-spline representations. Contact areas between the B-spline geometric models were determined by the proximity method[46] and depicted in intervals of 0.2 mm. In this example, the contact areas of the patellar cartilage on the femoral cartilage are shown in shades of orange.

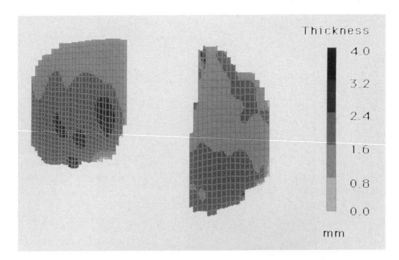

Fig. 11.45 Mapping cartilage thickness with MRI. B-spline geometric model of the tibial cartilage of the knee shown in Fig. 11.38 was generated using the same method as for *in situ* contact area mapping (Fig. 11.43). Regional cartilage thicknesses (perpendicular to the cartilage-bone interface) are depicted at intervals of 0.8 mm and shown in shades of orange.

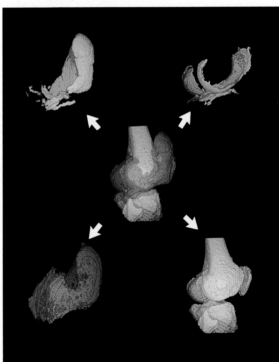

Fig. 11.46 3D analysis of different articular structures in the knee. 3D surface renderings (posterolateral view) of cartilage (yellow), thickened synovium (transparent red), effusion (blue), and bones (white) of an OA knee. The individual articular components are shown surrounding a central composite image. The 3D images were reconstructed using the magnetization-transfer subtraction image data for the knee shown in Fig. 11.39. The volume of each articular component can be determined by summing the voxels within its 3D reconstructed image. (Reproduced from *Osteoarthritic disorders* (ed. K.E. Kuethner and V.M. Goldberg) (1995). American Academy of Orthopaedic Surgeons, Rosemont, IL; with permission.)

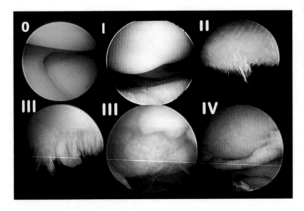

Fig. 11.55 Depth of articular cartilage lesions according to the classification proposed by Beguin and Locker[15]. (b) Examples: chondroscopy; 2.7 mm arthroscope; local anesthesia. Reading from left to right: grade 0 = normal medial femorotibial compartment; grade I = swelling of the lateral femoral condyle; grade II = 'velvet-like' aspect of the patella; grade III = 'crab-meat-like' aspect of the patella; grade III = deep ulceration of the medial femoral condyle; grade IV = exposure of subchondral bone of the medial femoral condyle.

present in inflamed tissue increases the susceptibility of nociceptors to the effects of prostaglandins[10].

Non-steroidal anti-inflammatory drugs (NSAIDs) have been shown to decrease afferent activity in acute and chronic models of joint disease[6]. The ability of NSAIDs to reduce inflammation is associated with inhibition of prostaglandin synthesis[11]. Analgesic effects are often attributed to a local reduction of hyperalgesia, resulting from the decrease in prostaglandin synthesis in the periphery and in the spinal cord[11,12]. The lack of efficacy of NSAIDs in some patients with arthritis may relate, in part, to the fact that only a proportion of joint afferents are sensitive to increased prostaglandin levels. For example, when prostaglandin E_2 was injected into the cat knee via the saphenous artery, only about 60 per cent of the tested fibers from free nerve endings showed direct excitation and/or sensitization to movement and/or chemical stimulation with bradykinin[8].

Autonomic (sympathetic) nervous system

Joints receive sympathetic innervation, which regulates blood flow in articular arteries. Blood flow increases after elimination of sympathetic innervation and decreases when articular nerves are electrically stimulated[6]. However, chronically inflamed rat knees do not show vasoconstriction upon saphenous nerve stimulation, suggesting that the inflammatory process reduces the effectiveness of sympathetic transmission, either by changes in postsynaptic receptor sites, depletion of neurotransmitters, or degeneration of postsynaptic fibers[13].

Chemical sympathectomy (by injection of guanethidine, which destroys postganglionic sympathetic neurons) has been shown to reduce the severity of adjuvant-induced arthritis in rats. This procedure reduces sympathetic activity which, in an innervated joint, may exacerbate arthritis by facilitating access to the joint cavity of cells and mediators, or impeding clearance of inflammatory mediators[14]. In patients with rheumatoid arthritis (RA) or OA, lumbar sympathectomy effectively reduced intractable knee and hip pain. The improvement was attributed to denervation of afferents that travel in the lumbar sympathetic trunks[15].

Activation of the sympathetic system by noise or emotional stimuli exacerbates pain in arthritis patients. Thus, it is possible that persistent sympathetic stimulation is a component of pain in some arthritis cases, providing another possible explanation of why NSAIDs do not provide satisfactory analgesia in all patients[16].

Spinal mechanisms

Hyperexcitability

The spinal cord is not a passive element in arthritis. Neugebauer and Schaible[17], in studies on cats, recorded from neurons in the spinal cord below the level of a complete transection before and after development of experimentally induced acute inflammation of the knee. Inflammation enhanced the responses of neurons to innocuous movements, and activity of neurons that previously had not been activated by these movements could now be demonstrated. The area of skin over which some neurons responded also increased. These reactions demonstrate neuronal hyperexcitability, which presumably contributes to sensations of pain. At the cellular level, neuronal hyperexcitability is associated with increased spontaneous activity, reduced threshold for activation, augmented responses to repetitive stimulation, and expansion of dorsal root neuron receptive fields[18,19]. Neuronal hyperexcitability associated with inflammation may be related initially to the release in the spinal cord of high concentrations of the excitatory amino acids aspartate and glutamate, and the neuropeptide, substance P, by dorsal horn neurons. These effects have been shown to trigger a cascade of cellular changes, for example, increased expression of the proto-oncogenes, *c-fos* and *c-jun*, that alter the response of the neuron to external stimuli[18].

Descending and segmental inhibition

Serotoninergic descending systems in the spinal cord modulate pain[20]. Concentrations of tryptophan, serotonin, and 5-hydroxyindoleacetic acid (an intermediate in the synthesis of serotonin from tryptophan) have been shown to be elevated in the spinal cord of rats with experimentally induced polyarthritis[6]. Descending noradrenergic inhibitory systems also appear to be activated in polyarthritic rats[21]. The persistence of joint pain in patients with arthritis suggests that these inhibitory systems are insufficient to nullify the continuous afferent barrage that presumably occurs.

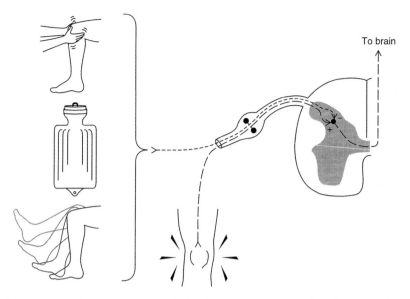

Fig. 7.53 Schematic illustration of how cutaneous stimulation (massage, heat, range of motion exercise) can inhibit transmission of nociceptive impulses from a diseased knee. The cutaneous afferent neuron makes an inhibitory synapse on the spinal neuron receiving excitatory (nociceptive) impulses from the joint, blocking transmission of the nociceptive (pain) sensation.

Physical stimuli such as superficial or deep heat, massage, and range-of-motion exercise reduce pain because cutaneous afferent impulses inhibit transmission of articular nociceptive impulses in the spinal cord (Fig. 7.53)[22]. It may be possible to pharmacologically activate similar spinal interneuronal mechanisms of pain inhibition. Spinal cord levels of gamma-aminobutyric acid (GABA), an interneuronal inhibitory neurotransmitter, have been shown to increase after induction of arthritis in rats. Activation of this system in the presence of inflammation, presumably to counteract pain, may explain why the GABA agonist, baclofen, has not been effective as a therapeutic analgesic in chronic pain. Nevertheless, additional information on this system may provide a basis for a novel approach to relieving arthritis pain[23].

Neuropeptides and neurogenic inflammation

Increased release of neuropeptides from afferent fibers in joints occurs in arthritis, and may contribute to the development of joint disease by producing vasodilatation, resulting in increased blood flow to the joint and plasma extravasation in the innervated tissue[24,6]. Afferent fibers containing substance P and calcitonin gene-related peptide (CGRP) are commonly found in articular tissues, particularly in association with vascular structures. However, the presence of such fibers not associated with blood vessels suggests that release of these neuropeptides is also directly involved in inflammatory processes, that is, 'neurogenic inflammation'[7]. Lam and Ferrell[25] found that experimentally induced acute joint inflammation was reduced by 44 per cent in animals pretreated with capsaicin, which depletes substance P from nerve endings, and by 93 per cent when pretreated with the substance P antagonist, d-Pro[4],d-Trp[7 9 10]-SP(4–11). Neurogenic inflammation occurs partly as a result of the promotion by neuropeptides, including substance P, of inflammatory cell chemotaxis, neutrophil activation, mast cell degranulation, and fibroblast proliferation — all of which are components of the inflammatory process in joints[25].

McDougall *et al.*[26] recently reported that chronically inflamed rat knees, one and three weeks after intraarticular injection of Freund's complete adjuvant, failed to show a dose-dependent vasodilatation in response to topical substance P application. Apparently, substance P receptors are either grossly modified or inactivated by the inflammatory process. Loss of this neurovascular control mechanism may contribute to the degenerative changes that accompany inflammatory joint disease.

Substance P levels have been shown to be higher in synovial fluid of patients with OA, RA, Reiter's syndrome and post-traumatic arthritis than in the plasma of normal subjects. Substance P levels were also significantly higher in synovial fluid than in the plasma of the respective patient groups, except for the group with Reiter's syndrome[27]. However, Kidd *et al.*[28]. questioned the bioactivity of substance P in synovial fluid; thus, higher levels may not be directly related to joint pain.

Arthritis can also result in an increase in the substance P content of the spinal cord. Oku *et al.*[29] found that in polyarthritic rats, innocuous movement of the inflamed ankle joint produced a significant increase in the spinal release of substance P. Recently, Neugebauer *et al.*[30] reported that intraspinal release of substance P occurred when noxious pressure, but not light pressure, was applied to the knee of normal rats, and suggested that substance P may be contained only in high-threshold mechanoreceptors or 'silent nociceptors' (initially mechano-insensitive receptors). In cats with experimentally induced arthritis, substance P was released in the spinal cord after application of innocuous light pressure to the inflamed knee, but not when the same stimulus was applied to a normal joint[31].

Calcitonin gene-related peptide (CGRP), another neuropeptide released from afferent nerves, also may contribute to the development and/or severity of some types of arthritis[32]. In the spinal cord, release of CGRP in the spinal cords of rats and cats was increased within the first few hours after induction of knee joint inflammation, presumably contributing to the generation of inflammation-evoked changes of sensitivity of spinal cord neurons and, therefore, to perception of joint pain[32].

Inhibition of the local effects of neuropeptides may be of therapeutic value. Topical application of capsaicin (which depletes substance P from nerve endings; see p. 180) in patients with knee OA may reduce joint pain[33] (see Chapter 9.7). However, Matucci-Cerinic *et al.*[33] noted that chronic administration of capsaicin may enhance chemotaxis, and increase collagenase production and synoviocyte proliferation.

Release of substance P from knee afferents can be inhibited by opioid receptor agonists[34]. Accordingly, low doses of intraarticular morphine produced greater pain relief after knee arthroscopy than the same dose given intravenously. None of the patients who received intraarticular morphine experienced any of the side effects associated with systemic administration[35]. Some neuropeptides (for example, somatostatin) inhibit the action of substance P in joints and in the spinal cord. Somatostatin has been shown to be an effective analgesic in cancer[36,37], cluster headaches[38], RA[39], and psoriatic arthritis[40]. With respect to therapeutic reduction in levels of substance P in the joint or spinal cord, it should be noted that substance P levels in cerebrospinal fluid of patients with chronic pain are low, rather than high[41], suggesting that there is not a direct relationship between substance P levels and chronic pain.

Supraspinal mechanisms and perception of pain

Afferents from joints enter the spinal cord via dorsal roots and have extensive projections within the cord. Information from joint afferents is conveyed to the brain via the dorsal column, spinothalamic, spinoreticular, and spinocerebellar pathways. This information reaches the cerebellum, reticular formation, and thalamus[1].

Electrophysiological studies of the thalamus (ventrobasal and intralaminar regions) and somatosensory cortex in rats with adjuvant-induced arthritis have shown that, compared to normal rats, few cells respond to intense joint stimulation, whereas many respond to innocuous stimuli[42,43,44]. Gautron and Guilbaud[42] suggested that this abnormal response could result from failure of some central inhibitory process, or from neuronal hyperexcitability associated with the development of peripheral inflammation (see p. 176).

The finding that development of arthritis results in marked changes in the way the CNS responds to joint stimulation (that is, modification in the response of neurons) indicates that the perception of arthritis pain is a dynamic process that is influenced by past experience, rather than simply an instantaneous response to afferent noxious input[18]. Clearly, greater understanding of this process is essential for optimal treatment of chronic arthritis pain.

Neuromuscular mechanisms

Neuropathic joints

Ligaments alone cannot prevent joint dislocation during strenuous activity, when forces can exceed the mechanical strength of the ligament[2]. Thus, coordinated muscular activity has an important role in protecting joints. Two important questions pertain to this joint protection mechanism: are joint afferents an integral part of the protective mechanisms? And, if so, how is the information transmitted by joint afferents used to protect joints?

Table 7.13 Diseases and conditions associated with neuropathic arthropathy (Charcot joints)[46]

Alcoholic peripheral neuropathy
Amyloidosis
Arachnoiditis
Arachnoidosis
Congenitial insensitivity to pain
Diabetic peripheral neuropathy
Familial dysautonomia (Riley–Day syndrome)
Familial interstitial hypertrophic polyneuropathy (Dejerine–Sottas disease)
Hereditary sensory radicular neuropathy
Injury to spinal cord or peripheral nerves
Leprosy
Multiple sclerosis
Myelomeningocele
Pernicious anemia (subacute, with spinal cord degeneration)
Peroneal muscle atrophy (Charcot–Marie–Tooth disease)
Spina bifida with meningomyelocele
Steroid injections (systemic and intraarticular)
Syringomyelia
Tabes dorsalis
Tuberculosis
Tumors (spinal cord or peripheral nerve)
Uremia

The presence of neuropathic (Charcot) joints suggests that the answer to the first question is affirmative. Neuropathic joint disease is a destructive arthropathy usually associated with disorders affecting peripheral nerves (Table 7.13; Fig. 7.54)[45]. Presumably, in the conditions listed in Table 7.13, as a result of a loss of

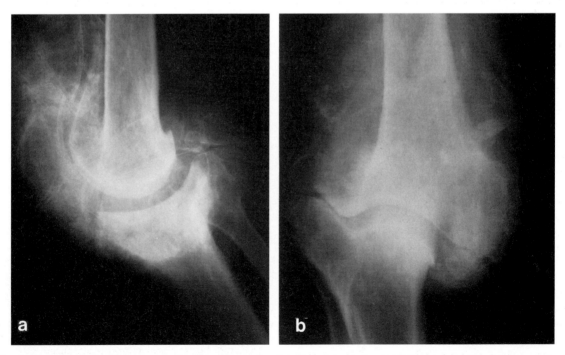

Fig. 7.54 Lateral (a) and anteroposterior (b) radiographs of the knee of a patient with Charcot arthropathy as a result of syphilis. Note gross deformity, dislocation, extensive osteophyte formation, marked bony remodeling, and synovial osteochondromatosis.

sensation, the joint is subjected to mechanical trauma, which initiates a cycle ultimately leading to joint destruction[46]. However, an alternative hypothesis[47] for the etiology of Charcot joints suggests that joint degeneration occurs because circulatory changes (hyperemia) lead to rapid bone resorption by osteoclasts. These circulatory changes are initiated by a neural 'reflex' usually associated with dorsal root disease (for example, syphilis), spinal cord disease (for example, syringomyelia), or nerve-trunk disease (for example, diabetes). The circulatory effects may account for the observation that a normal joint may completely break down within six weeks in a bedridden person, having been subjected to no activity and, therefore, no trauma[47]. Neuropathic joints are most commonly seen today in the mid- and forefoot of patients with diabetes mellitus[48].

Patients with neuropathic joint disease may present with a single, painless, swollen, deformed joint with no history of injury. Less often, they have polyarticular disease, resulting from insensitivity in more than one joint, as can occur in tabes dorsalis[49]. Although most patients with a neuropathic joint show a reduced response to deep pain and proprioception, as many as one-third have pain in the involved joint at the time of presentation[45]. Accordingly, it has been suggested that loss of proprioception, rather than loss of nociception is the critical element leading to the development of a Charcot joint[50].

Joint protection

Despite the intuitive logic, upon close examination, a definitive relationship between peripheral sensory neuropathy and joint disease is not evident. Many patients with peripheral sensory disorders do not develop joint problems. For example, only 0.1 per cent of diabetics (5 per cent of those with clinically identifiable peripheral sensory neuropathy), 5 per cent of tabetics, and 25 per cent of those with syringomyelia develop neuropathic joint disease[46,51]. Often, it is not until the occurrence of a significant episode of joint trauma that the patient with a peripheral sensory disorder develops a Charcot joint[52]. Further, Charcot joints are more common in patients who are physically active and are usually not found in spastic patients, presumably because spasticity 'splints' the limb, thereby protecting it from excessive joint displacement[53].

Also suggesting that impaired sensation, by itself, does not result in joint degeneration are experiments in which dogs undergo extensive unilateral hindlimb deafferentation resulting from L4–S1 dorsal root ganglionectomy. These dogs showed no evidence of knee OA for as long as 16 months after surgery, despite the fact that the deafferented knee was grossly hyperextended at paw contact (Fig. 7.55)[54,55]. However, if the ACL is transected two weeks after the dog has been subjected to knee deafferentation, knee joint degeneration proceeds very rapidly and may be evident upon gross examination as soon as three weeks after ACL transection (Fig. 7.56)[56]. These data strongly emphasize the important role of peripheral sensory nerves in protecting injured or unstable joints, but not normal joints. It would appear that one of the factors accounting for the fact that *all* individuals with peripheral sensory neuropathy do not develop neuropathic arthropathy is the absence of joint injury. Notably, Slowman-Kovacs *et al.*[57] described three patients with diabetic neuropathy in whom minor trauma to the foot or ankle resulted in neuropathic arthropathy within three to six weeks. They suggested that these patients represent a human counterpart to the canine studies, with the diabetic neuropathy serving as the functional equivalent of deafferentation and the injury as the equivalent of transection of the ACL.

Despite the fact that joints, if used in a relatively normal manner, can maintain their integrity in the

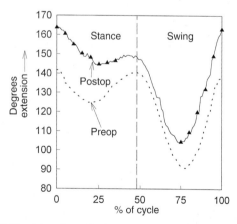

Fig. 7.55 Mean knee displacement patterns for one stride of six dogs preoperatively (preop) and six months after the dorsal roots of spinal segments L4–S1, inclusive, had been severed (postop) to deafferent the ipsilateral hindlimb. The curves begin at touchdown of the paw (0% of the gait cycle), and the cycle is divided into two major components (stance and swing phases). Postoperatively, the knee is significantly more extended than normal at many points during the cycle ($p < 0.05$; denoted by triangles). Despite this increase in extension, which is approximately 20° at touchdown, these dogs do not develop OA.[55,56]

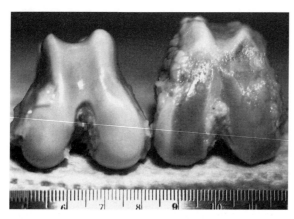

Fig. 7.56 Left and right distal femora of a dog in which the left dorsal roots of spinal segments L4–S1, inclusive, had been severed to deafferent the ipsilateral hindlimb, and in which the ipsilateral ACL had been transected two weeks later. The medial and lateral condyles of the femur of the unstable knee show extensive full-thickness loss of articular cartilage, with exposure of the subchondral bone, and extensive osteophytosis. The right femur is normal. In this model of OA gross pathological changes may be evident as early as three weeks after ACL transection.[56]

absence of sensory innervation, afferent nerves clearly influence muscle activity around joints. This is intuitively apparent in Hilton's law[58], which states that nerves that supply joints also supply innervation to the muscles crossing that joint and the skin overlying the insertion of those muscles. Externally applied pressure to the knee and ankle joint in animals, as well as passive joint movement, can induce reflex contraction in muscles that cross these joints[2]. However, studies on the effects of joint movement are contradictory; some indicating that moving a joint into extension facilitates flexor muscles, and moving it into flexion facilitates extensors, whereas other studies suggest that extension stimulates extensors and flexion facilitates flexors[46].

Proprioceptive ability is reduced in patients with ACL deficiency[59] or with knee OA[50], suggesting that lack of, or abnormal, proprioceptive feedback might permit excessive or inappropriate loading of the joint. Thus, decreased proprioception in OA or ACL-deficient patients, and in elderly non-arthritic individuals who also show impairment of joint position sense[50], may initiate or accelerate joint degeneration. Similarly, a reduction in quadriceps muscle strength occurs after an ACL tear (even after correction is made for the decrease in muscle cross-sectional area)[60], or after the development of knee OA[61], implying that changes occurred in afferent input, leading to deficits in motor unit activation[60,61]. In contrast, Co et al.[62] found no

discernible proprioceptive differences between the affected and normal limb in humans who had undergone autologous ACL reconstruction, suggesting that mechanoreceptors in the intact ACL are not essential for knee proprioception.

Several studies have shown changes in the activity patterns of muscles around the ACL-deficient knee during gait (for example, earlier onset of contraction of lateral hamstrings and medial gastrocnemius), compared to controls[63,64]. However, Peat et al.[65] reported that the electromyographic patterns of lower limb muscles of patients who underwent unilateral total knee replacement were similar to those of controls, suggesting that knee mechanoreceptors do not play a critical role in muscle coordination during gait, and are, therefore, not essential to joint protection during gait. Figure 7.57 summarizes some aspects of the relationship between the nervous system and joints, including protection of the joint by muscle activity.

CNS programming

O'Connor and Brandt[46] presented an alternative to the prevailing idea that joint protection is dependent on muscular reflexes triggered by joint receptors. They suggested that joint protection mechanisms are incorporated within the movement coordinating programs that are embedded in spinal cord circuitry and, therefore, are not dependent on continuous ipsilateral sensation. Such a programmed system of movement control has been well demonstrated for locomotor behavior in mammals, in which the spinal cord can generate stepping patterns in the absence of all movement-related afferent feedback[66]. O'Connor and Brandt[46] speculated that with normal joint movements, the programmed patterns confine joint excursion and load within a safe range, preventing joint damage.

Although the hypothesis of O'Connor and Brandt[46] suggests that sensory input is not essential for joint protection in an intact joint under normal conditions, sensation would become very important in an injured joint where the programmed movement patterns might no longer be appropriate and result in joint damage. O'Connor and Brandt[46] also suggested that it is possible for the nervous system to learn new patterns to protect an unstable joint, and that development of these patterns depends temporarily on sensory input from the affected joint. As discussed above, canine knee joints subjected to ACL transection soon after ipsilateral deafferentation show signs of damage as early as three weeks after ACL transection[56]. However,

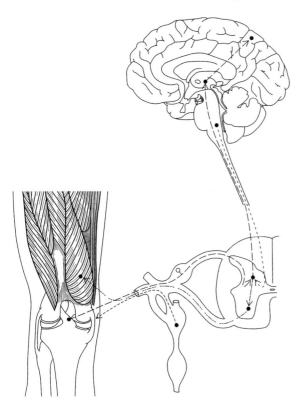

Fig. 7.57 Schematic drawing of some aspects of joint neurology. An afferent fiber from the anterior cruciate ligament synapses in the dorsal horn of the spinal cord, with impulses from the fiber subsequently being transmitted, via a reflex arc, to a motoneuron, which innervates the vastus medialis, potentially 'protecting' the joint, and to the cortex via the thalamus. Impinging on the dorsal horn synapse is a descending fiber from the brainstem, which modulates (inhibits pain transmission to the cortex). A sympathetic fiber, to control blood flow, travels from a sympathetic ganglion to the knee joint capsule. An important component, not shown, is the release of neuropeptides (e.g., substance P) by the afferent fiber, both in the joint and spinal cord.

dogs subjected to ACL transection in which ipsilateral deafferentation was delayed for 52 weeks developed only mild OA, which was no more severe than in neurologically intact dogs that had undergone ACL transection at the same time[54]. O'Connor et al.[54] concluded that in the dogs in which deafferentation had been delayed, the CNS initially used ipsilateral sensation to acquire the ability to protect the unstable joint from breakdown, and that these new protective kinematic patterns eventually became programmed into the CNS, which then no longer depended upon sensation to protect the joint. Thus, the unstable joint of these dogs

was still protected by the neuromuscular system, despite the absence of ipsilateral sensation.

O'Connor et al.[54] also raised the issue of whether OA might develop in persons who have normal peripheral sensation but whose movement programs are inappropriate, perhaps as a result of a CNS lesion, and suggested that it might be possible to reprogram the CNS to protect unstable joints. Interestingly, CNS reprogramming is thought to occur in humans with ACL deficiency[67]. During gait, these individuals tend to avoid quadriceps contraction when the knee is nearly fully extended, preventing an abnormally large anterior displacement of the tibia on the femur. Andriacchi[67] suggested that the rhythmic nature of this adaptation and its transfer to the contralateral limb indicate that it is not a response to afferent input made during each step, but one which is incorporated into the CNS program for walking.

Microklutziness

In an intriguing study, Radin et al.[68] attempted to demonstrate how minor neuromuscular incoordination might be a causative factor in the development of knee OA in humans. They compared the gait of humans who had intermittent activity-related knee pain and were, therefore, considered to be 'preosteoarthrotic', to that of age-related controls. Kinematic and kinetic analyses showed that the involved limb of the knee pain group contacted the ground faster and harder, and showed a more rapid rise in the ground reaction force immediately after heel-strike, than that of the controls. The authors considered this sequence of events to represent repetitive impulsive loading of the knee joint, which has been shown to result in the development of OA in animal studies. The authors referred to this pattern of incoordination as 'microklutziness', and considered it to represent minor incoordination within the neuromuscular system. It should be emphasized that no evidence was provided that the experimental group had, or subsequently developed, OA. Nevertheless, the presence of 'microklutziness' might explain why Charcot arthropathy develops in some patients with sensory neuropathy, but not in others.

Conclusion

Joint afferents may contribute to the development of arthritis through excessive release in joint tissues of neuropeptides and other inflammatory mediators. This process, increased intraarticular pressure, and changes in articular blood flow presumably modify joint neurophysiology, resulting in hyperexcitability in these afferents and joint pain.

Hyperexcitability of joint afferents apparently triggers hyperexcitability in spinal and supraspinal neurons, establishing a mechanism whereby joint pain may no longer be directly dependent on the presence of the originating stimulus, but rather becomes a response based on past experience and, therefore, not susceptible to a peripherally acting analgesic — that is, pain becomes the disease.

Joint afferents also transmit information to the CNS that may be used to coordinate muscle activity that protects joints from potentially damaging movements. This is clearly the case for injured joints, but protective mechanisms for normal joints may be an integral part of the programmed movement patterns embedded in the neuronal circuitry within the CNS. Nevertheless, reduced or abnormal joint proprioception, due to joint injury or OA, may initiate or accelerate joint degeneration. Similarly, CNS or peripheral nervous system lesions that affect muscle coordination have the potential to initiate or exacerbate joint injury. Successful treatment of arthritis and arthritis pain may need to address the contributions of the nervous system to the development of joint disease.

Acknowledgments

Dr Brian O'Connor provided the photographs of the joint receptors and canine knee joints, Dr Ethan Braunstein provided the radiographs of the patient with Charcot arthropathy, and Ms Roberta Shadle drew the illustrations.

References

1. Johansson, H. and Sjölander, P. (1993). The neurophysiology of joints. In *Mechanics of human joints: physiology, pathophysiology, and treatment* (ed. V. Wright and E.L. Radin), pp. 243–90. Marcel Dekker, New York.
2. Johansson, H., Sjölander, P., and Sojka, P. (1991). Receptors in the knee joint ligaments and their role in the biomechanics of the joint. *Biomedical Engineering*, 18, 341–68.
3. Wyke, B. (1981). The neurology of joints: a review of general principles. *Clinics in Rheumatic Diseases*, 7, 223–39.
4. Freeman, M.A.R. and Wyke, B. (1967). The innervation of the knee joint. An anatomical and histological study in the cat. *Journal of Anatomy*, 101, 505–32.
5. Zimny, M.L. and Wink, C.S. (1991). Neuroreceptors in the tissues of the knee joint. *Journal of Electromyography and Kinesiology*, 1, 148–57.
6. Schaible, H-G. and Grubb, B.D. (1993). Afferent and spinal mechanisms of joint pain. *Pain*, 55, 5–54.
7. Marshall, K.W. and Chan, A.D.M. (1993). Neurogenic contributions to degenerative and inflammatory arthroses. *Current Opinion in Orthopedics*, 4, 48–55.
8. Schaible, H-G. and Schmidt, R.F. (1988). Excitation and sensitization of fine articular afferents from cat's knee joint by prostaglandin E$_2$. *Journal of Physiology*, 403, 91–104.
9. Jayson, M.I.V. and Dixon, A.S.J. (1970). Intra-articular pressure in rheumatoid arthritis of the knee. I. Pressure changes during passive joint distension. *Annals of the Rheumatic Diseases*, 29, 261–5.
10. Heppelmann, B., Schaible, H-G., and Schmidt, R.F. (1985). Effects of prostaglandins E1 and E2 on the mechanosensitivity of group III afferents from normal and inflamed cat knee joints. *Advances in Pain Research and Therapy*, 9, 91–101.
11. Abramson, S.B. (1992). Treatment of gout and crystal arthropathies and uses and mechanisms of action of non-steroidal anti-inflammatory drugs. *Current Opinion in Rheumatology*, 4, 295–300.
12. Malmberg, A.B. and Yaksh, T.L. (1992). Hyperalgesia mediated by spinal glutamate or substance P receptor blocked by spinal cyclooxygenase inhibition. *Science*, 257, 1276–9.
13. McDougall, J.J., Karimian, S.M., and Ferrell, W.R. (1994). Alteration of substance P-mediated vasodilation and sympathetic vasoconstriction in the rat knee joint by adjuvant-induced inflammation. *Neuroscience Letters*, 174, 127–9.
14. Levine, J.D., Dardick, S.J., Roizen, M.F., Helms, C., and Basbaum, A.I. (1986). Contribution of sensory afferents and sympathetic efferents to joint injury in experimental arthritis. *The Journal of Neuroscience*, 6, 3423–9.
15. Herfort, R.A. (1957). Extended sympathectomy in the treatment of chronic arthritis. *The Journal of the American Geriatric Society*, 6, 904–15.
16. Wong, H.Y. (1993). Neural mechanisms of joint pain. *Annals of Academy of Medicine (Singapore)*, 4, 646–50.
17. Neugebauer, V. and Schaible, H-G. (1990). Evidence for a central component in the sensitization of spinal neurons with joint input during development of acute arthritis in cat's knee. *Journal of Neurophysiology*, 64, 299–311.
18. Coderre, T.J., Katz, J., Vaccarino, A.L., and Melzack, M. (1993). Contribution of central neuroplasticity to pathological pain: review of clinical and experimental evidence. *Pain*, 52, 259–85.
19. Konttinen, Y.T., Kemppinen, P., Segerberg, M., Hukkanen, M., Rees, R., Santavirta, S., *et al.* (1994). Peripheral and spinal neural mechanisms in arthritis, with particular reference to treatment of inflammation and pain. *Arthritis and Rheumatism*, 37, 965–82.
20. Burt, A.M. (1993). *Textbook of neuroanatomy.* W.B. Saunders, Philadelphia.

21. Weil-Fugazza, J., Godefroy, F., Manceau, V., and Besson, J.M. (1986). Increased norepinephrine and uric acid levels in the spinal cord of arthritic rats. *Brain Research*, **374**, 190–4.

22. Melzack, R. and Wall, P.D. (1965). Pain mechanisms: a new theory. *Science*, **150**, 971–9.

23. Malcangio, M. and Bowery, N.G. (1994). Spinal cord SP release and hyperalgesia in monoarthritic rats: involvement of the GABAb receptor system. *British Journal of Pharmacology*, **113**, 1561–6.

24. Khoshbaten, A. and Ferrel, W.R. (1990). Responses of blood vessels in the rabbit knee to acute joint inflammation. *Annals of the Rheumatic Diseases*, **49**, 540–4.

25. Lam, F.Y. and Ferrell, W.R. (1989). Inhibition of carrageenan induced inflammation in the rat knee joint by substance P antagonist. *Annals of the Rheumatic Diseases*, **48**, 928–32.

26. McDougall, J.J., Karimian, S.M., and Ferrell, W.R. (1995). Prolonged alteration of vasoconstrictor and vasodilator responses in rat knee joints by adjuvant monoarthritis. *Experimental Physiology*, **80**, 349–57.

27. Marshall, K.W., Chiu, B., and Inman, R.D. (1990). Substance P and arthritis: analysis of plasma and synovial fluid levels. *Arthritis and Rheumatism*, **33**, 87–90.

28. Kidd, B.L., Cruwys, S., Mapp, P.I., and Blake, D.R. (1993). Sympathetic nervous system in chronic joint pain. *Annals of the Rheumatic Diseases*, **52**, 552.

29. Oku, R., Satoh, M., and Takagi, H. (1987). Release of substance P from the spinal dorsal horn is enhanced in polyarthritic rats. *Neuroscience Letters*, **74**, 315–19.

30. Neugebauer, V., Schaible, H-G., Weiretter, F., and Freudenberger, U. (1994). The involvement of substance P and neurokinin-1 receptors in the responses of rat dorsal horn neurons to noxious but not to innocuous mechanical stimuli applied to the knee joint. *Brain Research*, **666**, 207–15.

31. Schaible, H-G., Jarrott, B., Hope, P.J., and Duggan, A.W. (1990). Release of immunoreactive substance P in the cat spinal cord during development of acute arthritis in the cat's knee: a study with antibody bearing microprobes. *Brain Research*, **529**, 214–23.

32. Schaible, H-G., Freudenberger, U., Neugebauer, V., and Stiller, R.U. (1994). Intraspinal release of immunoreactive calcitonin gene-related peptide during development of inflammation in the joint *in vivo* — a study with antibody microprobes in cat and rat. *Neuroscience*, **62**, 1293–1305.

33. Matucci-Cerinic, M., McCarthy, G., Lombardi, A., Pignone, A., and Partsch, G. (1995). Neurogenic influences in arthritis: potential modification by capsaicin. *Journal of Rheumatology*, **22**, 1447–1449.

34. Yaksh, T.L. (1988). Substance P release from knee joint afferent terminals: modulation by opioids. *Brain Research*, **458**, 319–24.

35. Stein, C., Comisel, K., Haimerl, E., Yassouridis, A., Lehrberger, K., Herz, A., *et al.* (1991). Analgesic effect of intraarticular morphine after arthroscopic knee surgery. *New England Journal of Medicine*, **325**, 1123–6.

36. Chrubasik, J., Meynadier, J., Blond, S., Scherpereel, P., Ackerman, E., Weinstock, M., *et al.* (1984). Somatostatin: a potent analgesic. *Lancet*, **11**, 1208–9.

37. Smith, S., Lowell, A., Roberts, J., Oates, J.A., and Pincus, T. (1990). Resolution of musculoskeletal symptoms in carcinoid syndrome after treatment with the somatostatin analog octreotide. *Annals of Internal Medicine*, **112**, 66–8.

38. Sicuten, F., Geppetti, P., Marabini, S., and Lembeck, F. (1984). Pain relief by somatostatin in attacks of cluster headaches. *Pain*, **18**, 359–65.

39. Matucci-Cerinic, M. and Marabini, S. (1988). Somatostatin treatment for pain in rheumatoid arthritis: a double blind versus placebo study in knee involvement. *Medical Science Research*, **16**, 233–4.

40. Matucci-Cerinic, M., Pignone, A., Lotti, T., Partsch, G., Livi, R., and Cognoni, M. (1992). Gold salts and somatostatin: a new clinical combined analgesic treatment for psoriatic arthritis. *Drugs under Experimental and Clinical Research*, **18**, 53–61.

41. Almay, B.G.L., Johansson, F., Von Knorring, L., Le Greves, P., and Terenius, L. (1988). Substance P in CSF of patients with chronic pain syndromes. *Pain*, **33**, 3–9.

42. Gautron, M. and Guilbaud, G. (1982). Somatic responses of ventrobasal thalamic neurones in polyarthritic rats. *Brain Research*, **237**, 459–71.

43. Kayser, V. and Guilbaud, G. (1984). Further evidence for changes in the responsiveness of somatosensory neurons in arthritic rats: a study of the posterior intralaminar region of the thalamus. *Brain Research*, **323**, 144–7.

44. Lamour, Y., Guilbaud, G., and Willer, J.C. (1983). Altered properties and laminar distribution of neuronal responses to peripheral stimulation in the Sml cortex of the arthritic rat. *Brain Research*, **273**, 183–7.

45. Sequeira, W. (1994). The neuropathic joint. *Clinical and Experimental Rheumatology*, **12**, 325–37.

46. O'Connor, B.L. and Brandt, K.D. (1993). Neurogenic factors in the etiopathogenesis of osteoarthritis. *Rheumatic Disease Clinics of North America*, **19**, 581–605.

47. Johnson, L.C. (1964). Morphologic analysis in pathology: the kinetics of disease and general biology of bone. In *Bone biodynamics* (ed. H.M. Frost), pp. 543–654. Little Brown and Company, Boston.

48. Ellman, M.A. (1993). Neuropathic joint disease (Charcot joints). In *Arthritis and allied conditions* (ed. D.J. McCarthy and W.J. Kropman), pp. 1407–25. Lea and Febiger, Philadelphia.

49. Beetham, W.P., Kaye, R.L., and Polley, H.F. (1963). Charcot's joints: a case of extensive polyarticular involvement and discussion of certain clinical and pathologic features. *Annals of Internal Medicine*, **58**, 1002–12.

50. Barrett, D.S., Cobb, A.G., and Bentley, G. (1991). Joint proprioception in normal, osteoarthritic and replaced knees. *Journal of Bone and Joint Surgery*, **73B**, 53–6.

51. Steindler, A. (1931). The tabetic arthropathies. *Journal of the American Medical Association*, **96**, 250–6.

52. Johnson, J.T.H. (1967). Neuropathic fractures and joint injuries. *The Journal of Bone and Joint Surgery*, **49-A**, 1–30.

53. Bruckner, F.E. and Howell, A. (1972). Neuropathic joints. *Seminars in Arthritis and Rheumatism*, **2**, 47–69.

54. O'Connor, B.L., Visco, D.M., Brandt, K.D., Albrecht, M., and O'Connor, A.B. (1993). Sensory nerves only temporarily protect the unstable canine knee joint from osteoarthritis. *Arthritis and Rheumatism*, **36**, 1154–63.

55. Vilensky, J.A., O'Connor, B.L., Brandt, K.D., Dunn, E.A., and Rogers, P.I. (1994). Serial kinematic analysis of the canine knee after L4–S1 dorsal root ganglionectomy: implications for the cruciate deficiency model of osteoarthritis. *The Journal of Rheumatology*, **21**, 2113–17.

56. O'Connor, B.L., Palmoski, M.J., and Brandt, K.D. (1985). Neurogenic acceleration of degenerative joint lesions. *Journal of Bone and Joint Surgery*, **67-A**, 562–71.

57. Slowman-Kovacs, S., Braunstein, E.M., and Brandt, K.D. (1990). Rapidly progressive Charcot arthropathy following minor joint trauma in patients with diabetic neuropathy. *Arthritis and Rheumatism*, **33**, 412–17.

58. Hilton, J. (1863). *Lectures on rest and pain*. Bell, London.

59. Barrack, R.L., Skinner, H.B., and Buckley, S.L. (1989). Proprioception in the anterior cruciate deficient knee. *American Journal of Sports Medicine*, **17**, 1–6.

60. Elmqvist, L-G., Lorentzon, R., Johansson, C., and Fugl-Meyer, A.R. (1988). Does a torn anterior cruciate ligament lead to change in the central nervous drive of the knee extensors? *European Journal of Applied Physiology*, **58**, 203–7.

61. Hurley, M.V. and Newman, D.J. (1993). The influence of arthogenous muscle inhibition on quadriceps

62. Co, F.H., Skinner, H.B., and Cannon, W.D. (1993). Effect of reconstruction of the anterior cruciate ligament on proprioception of the knee and the heel strike transient. *Journal of Orthopaedic Research*, **11**, 696–704.

63. Lass, P., Kaalund, S., leFever, S., Arendt-Nielsen, L., Sinkjær, T., and Simonsen, O. (1991). Muscle coordination following rupture of the anterior cruciate ligament. *Acta Orthopaedica Scandinavica*, **62**, 9–14.

64. Sinkjær, T. and Arendt-Nielsen, L. (1991). Knee stability and muscle coordination in patients with anterior cruciate ligament injuries: an electromyographic approach. *Journal of Electromyography and Kinesiology*, **1**, 209–17.

65. Peat, M., Woodbury, M.G., and Ferkul, D. (1984). Electromyographic analysis of gait following total knee arthroplasty. *Physiotherapy Canada*, **36**, 68–72.

66. Grillner, S. (1985). Neurobiological bases of rhythmic motor acts in vertebrates. *Science*, **228**, 143–9.

67. Andriacchi, T.P. (1990). Dynamics of pathological motion: applied to the anterior cruciate deficient knee. *Journal of Biomechanics*, **23**(Supplement 1), 99–105.

68. Radin, E.L., Yang, K.H., Riegger, C., Kish, V.L., and O'Connor, J.J. (1991). Relationship between lower limb dynamics and knee joint pain. *Journal of Orthopaedic Research*, **9**, 398–405.

7.6   Muscle in osteoarthritis
Sheila O'Reilly and Adrian Jones

Introduction

The role of muscle in osteoarthritis (OA) remains unclear despite some recent important advances. Muscles provide the power required to move synovial joints. In addition, they act as stabilizers in conjunction with other intra-articular and periarticular structures. At some joints, such as the shoulder, they are the key stabilizer. Clearly, any changes to muscle strength or integrity may influence joint function and may have an important bearing on the osteoarthritic joint.

Assessing the role of muscle is constrained by the ability to measure it. The first part of this chapter, therefore, focuses on the various methods of assessing muscle, and their relative merits and pitfalls. It is important to remember that OA is primarily a problem of the elderly. Changes in muscle due to aging must, therefore, be understood, and these are briefly discussed. Finally, the current knowledge on muscle in OA is reviewed with reference to the pathophysiological changes, and their relevance to pain and disability. The role of exercise in OA is covered elsewhere, but therapeutic intervention is intimately linked to future research in muscle and is, therefore, considered at the end of the chapter. Much of the research both in normal subjects and patients with OA has focused on the quadriceps mechanism and the knee, although limited findings with regard to other muscle groups will be discussed.

Assessment of muscle

Muscle function

Dynamic versus static measurements

Muscle is capable of producing both force and movement (change of length). Static measurements are of force produced at a constant muscle length, that is, there is no movement of the limb (lever arm). Dynamic measures allow the muscle to change length and guage force generated and/or velocity of contraction. Muscle can alter its length by shortening (concentric contraction) or by lengthening (eccentric contraction). All measurements, whether static or dynamic, have disadvantages and there is no consensus as to which is preferable.

Isometric strength

This is the only possible measure of static strength, that is, iso = constant, metric = movement. It can be measured subjectively using a simple grading method such as the MRC scale (Table 7.14). This may be adequate in a clinical setting, but insensitive as a research method. Use of a simple strain gauge held by the examiner is more precise and still inexpensive. When measuring large muscles, such as the quadriceps, it is important to ensure constant positioning of the limbs and immobilization of other muscle groups. For the quadriceps, researchers have designed specialized chairs, an example of which is shown (Fig. 7.58)[1]. Isometric equipment is, nevertheless, inexpensive in comparison with dynamic apparatus. The technique is also easy to perform both for the examiner and subject, and since confined to one muscle or muscle group is relatively simple to interpret.

The main disadvantage is that as a non-dynamic measure it may equate poorly with normal muscle function and structure. Whilst there is some evidence for correlation between isometric strength and muscle

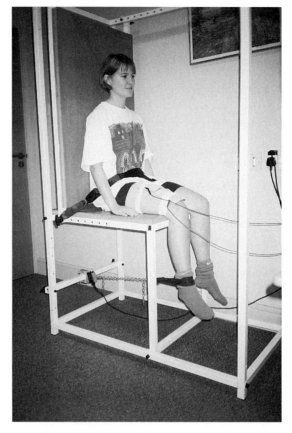

Fig. 7.58 Equipment used for measuring isometric quadriceps strength and twitch superimposition.

fiber composition[2], the relationship is greater for dynamic measures[3]. In addition, although there is agreement between isometric and isokinetic strength (dynamic) at low velocity, the relationship is less good at higher velocities[4].

Isotonic strength

This is a dynamic assessment involving constant resistance (tonic = weight) and measurement of angular

Table 7.14 Medical Research Council grading scale[*] for muscle strength using manual resistance

Grade	Description
5	Normal power against resistance
4	Reduced power against resistance
3	Power sufficient for motion against gravity but not additional resistance
2	Power sufficient to move limb only with gravity abolished
1	Flicker of contraction but no motion
0	No visible contraction

[*]Grades are commonly qualified in clinical practice using +/– signs

velocity. As such it is a measure of 'speed' rather than 'strength' and correlates poorly with isometric strength. It is less reliable than other dynamic measures and is not widely used, other than in sports training.

Isokinetic strength

Isokinetic devices measure torque (angular force) developed at a constant velocity. In practice, a variety of velocities are used, but most commonly 30 °/sec, 60 °/sec, 90 °/sec, and 120 °/sec. If the velocity is maintained at 0 °/sec the result should be identical to isometric torque. Such devices or dynamometers are reliable, and are becoming increasingly used for research purposes (Fig. 7.59). Unlike isometric devices, however, they are expensive and not widely available in a clinical setting. Maintaining constant velocity is not a 'functional' movement and, as such, may be less pleasant to perform. Another potential disadvantage is the large volume of data obtained for different angular velocities. There is no consensus as to which velocity is most appropriate and interpretation between and even within studies can be difficult.

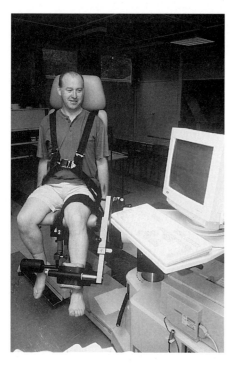

Fig. 7.59 Equipment used for measuring isokinetic quadriceps strength.

Explosive power

This is the ability of muscle to perform work over short periods of time (one second or less). It measures changes in both force and speed of shortening, and is measured in Watts (force × velocity). Since less restraints are made, it may be more functional; measurement of two-legged jumping power on a force plate has been the traditional method. Clearly, this may be difficult and potentially unsafe for elderly people, particularly with OA or other joint disorders. More recently, a technique for measuring power utilization in a single-leg extension has been developed[5]. This correlates well with functional activities such as stair climbing. Since it involves more than one muscle group (hip and knee extensors), results may be more difficult to interpret than non-dynamic measures, particularly in terms of response to interventions. Technique is important for this method and, hence, there may be a learning effect which may again pose a problem for intervention studies.

Single versus composite measures

For some areas of the musculoskeletal system it may be difficult to isolate individual muscles and more appropriate to use a composite action. In the hand, for example, whilst strength of adductor pollicis can be measured[1], it is more typical to measure grip strength[6]; a movement involving finger and thumb flexion, thumb opposition, and wrist extension and pronation. For other areas, such as proximal limbs, it may be more appropriate, particularly in a research setting, to isolate muscle groups such as the quadriceps or biceps. The choice of measurement clearly depends on the feasibility and ease of technique, in addition to the purpose of measurement — clinical or research. In certain situations it may also be relevant to compare strength of opposing muscle groups (agonist/antagonist ratio), particularly in a rehabilitation setting where outcome may depend on improving strength in both groups[7].

Voluntary versus involuntary measures

All measures of muscle strength, whether static or dynamic, require voluntary effort on the part of the subject. As such, they will be influenced greatly by lack of compliance or effort. This can be overcome to some extent by verbal encouragement[8], but even with this it can never be assumed that maximal effort is achieved.

For the last thirty years researchers have attempted to overcome this problem, although there are still few techniques available and these are not often utilized.

The first technique developed induces muscle tetany by direct electrical stimulation of a nerve, with measurement of subsequent maximal contraction. For large muscles, such as the quadriceps, however, this degree of contraction is painful and potentially harmful. This technique has had very limited use in OA sufferers. Normal subjects are generally reported to fully activate their muscles[1]. Not surprisingly, very limited data is available on OA patients.

The second option uses the technique of twitch superimposition[9]. Percutaneous stimulation is applied in order to cause a small proportion of muscle to contract (Fig. 7.58). The same degree of stimulation is then applied to the muscle when the subject is 'maximally' contracting. The magnitude of the twitch is inversely proportional to the amount of muscle not already contracting. The predicted strength (MVCp) can then be calculated from the formula of Bigland–Ritchie[10].

Formula for calculating maximal predicted muscle strength (MVC_p) from measured muscle strength (MVC_m), twitch height at rest (t_0) and twitch height during measured muscle contraction (t_m):

$$MVC_p = \frac{MVC_m \times t_0}{\left(t_0 - t_m\right)}$$

Figure 7.60 shows a typical trace obtained from the quadriceps muscle with variations in effort. Maximal voluntary strength is expressed as a percentage of predicted strength to give a measure of activation or inhibition of the muscle. If this technique is to be applied to the OA population, it is vital to know the degree of activation in normal subjects and the reproducibility in both normal subjects and patients with OA. Early work suggested 100 per cent activation occurred in normal volunteers. In fact, 'normal' subjects were excluded from analysis if not fully activating; subsequent attribution was to undiagnosed knee pathology[9]. More recent studies concerning fibromyalgia have demonstrated lack of activation of up to 15 percent in normal subjects[11]. Further work is, therefore, needed to determine the 'normal range' for muscle inhibition. Data concerning reproducibility of this technique is sparse. The technique is not confined to the quadriceps, with results published for the biceps, adductor pollicis, and even the erector spinal muscles of the back. This

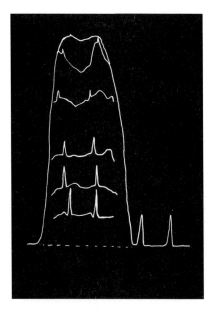

Fig. 7.60 Typical trace from a subject performing variable strength muscle contractions whilst receiving constant superimposed percutaneous twitches.

technique cannot, however, decipher the cause for any incomplete activation. It may be due to lack of effort, possibly mediated by pain or other factors; or it may be due to true inhibition of the quadriceps, a phenomenon known as 'arthrogenous inhibition' and possibly neuronally mediated[12]. This will be explained more fully in later sections.

The third method of measuring activation of the quadriceps involves the H-reflex. This is a monosynaptic reflex and is analogous to a tendon jerk. It produces a small muscle contraction in response to low intensity stimulation of a mixed nerve. This muscular response can be measured by surface electromyography[13]. A measured decline in the H-reflex amplitude can be used to measure activation. This has the advantage that activation is measured directly, rather than as a function of voluntary effort and is, therefore, more likely to represent 'true' arthrogenous inhibition. The technique, however, is complicated and its use is, therefore, limited.

Electromyography

Electromyography (EMG) can be used to study gross differences in activity, particularly between muscles. It may be of value in studying a limb in functional activities such as rising from a chair, or in examining the contribution of muscles in a muscle group such as the quadriceps. It cannot, however, accurately quantitate forces generated. Recordings can be made using either surface or needle electrodes. Surface electrodes have the advantage that they are better tolerated and easier to apply, but readings are clearly influenced by position and subject movement. EMG is also of value in detecting spontaneous muscle activity and changes associated with myopathy or neuropthy.

Imaging

Several imaging techniques are available including ultrasound scanning, computerised tomography (CT), and dual-energy X-ray absorptiometry (DEXA). Magnetic resonance imaging (MRI) can provide detailed anatomy of muscles, and newer associated techniques can examine biological processes in muscle.

Cross-sectional imaging

Ultrasound scanning[14], CT[15], and MRI[16] can all be used to determine cross-sectional area of muscle. Of these, MRI is most precise, since it is better able to differentiate muscle from soft tissues; both CT and MRI have good reproducibility[16,17]. In single time point studies, cross-sectional area correlates well with strength. This relationship, however, varies greatly within individuals, thereby limiting its use as a predictor of strength[18]. Results from intervention studies to improve strength confirm the limits of the relationship. Increases in strength are comparably greater, and more rapidly achieved, than increases in muscle area[16]. Suggested factors to account for this include learning effects, change in neural drive[19], and changes in fiber type or structure[20].

Dual-energy X-ray absorptiometry

Although primarily used for measuring bone mineral density, DEXA can also measure tissue composition and, hence, arrive at estimates of lean muscle mass, fat, and bone[21]. Its role in muscle measurements in OA patients is unknown.

Magnetic resonance spectroscopy (MRS) and other in vivo biochemical techniques

MRI, by providing information on spatial positioning of electrons, can provide excellent anatomical informa-tion. MRS spectroscopy is an extension of this which utilizes other atoms, such as phosphorus[22]; this enables study of the biochemical activity of muscle, such as high energy phosphate metabolism. Other, as yet research techniques, involve *in vivo* spatial monitoring of radiotracer activity, such as positron emission tomographic (PET) and single positron emission computerised tomographic scanning.

Histochemical studies

Although the techniques described above may provide information on the biochemistry and physiology of muscle, muscle biopsy, with histochemical staining, remains an important investigation. Muscle tissue is easily achieved by means of closed percutaneous needle biopsy or by open biopsy. As a diagnostic tool, it is well established. In a research setting, it is possible to measure fiber composition and size, particularly in relation to physical performance. Fibers have been classified as fast twitch (type II), which can be subdivided into types a, b, and c; or slow twitch (type I)[23]. In normal individuals, high proportions of fast twitch fibers are associated with better dynamic performance[3]. Serial biopsies may be used to monitor fiber response to training, although caution is required in interpretation, due to variation in fiber size within an individual.

Changes in muscle with aging

Prevalence of OA, both in terms of symptoms and structural change, is known to increase with aging, making it essentially a disease of the elderly population. It is, therefore, important to consider the changes in muscle, both structural and functional, that occur with aging to decide if these may be implicated in the aetiopathogenesis of OA.

Cross-sectional studies have shown reduction in muscle strength with age in both men and women[24,25]. This reduction occurs in isokinetic as well as isometric strength[26], a finding which is not confined to the quadriceps[27]. Longitudinal studies are less conclusive, with some demonstrating progressive decline after the age of 70[28] and others suggesting preservation of strength[29]. This discrepancy may relate to differences in activity between study populations and it is likely that a decline in strength continues into 'old' old age. Muscle weakness correlates with impaired function[30] and walking velocity[31]. Presence of quadriceps weakness can predict those most likely to fall[32] — a finding suggesting weakness as a cause of functional problems, rather than an effect.

Muscle wasting may, in part, explain decline in strength[33]. Muscle biopsy specimens from elderly populations demonstrate decreases in the percentage of type II fibers (that is, relatively less fast twitch fibers as well as a preferential reduction in their size[34]). The former may predominate[35], which would to some extent explain the discrepancy in muscle mass and strength found in the elderly.

Changes in muscle in OA

Evidence for weakness in OA

The importance of maintaining strength in addition to joint mobility in OA has long been stressed. It is surprising, therefore, that the evidence for muscle weakness in OA is only now emerging and remains somewhat unclear. Muscle wasting in OA was first reported in the nineteenth century[36]. Muscle strength was not assessed until much more recently. Again, this work has focused on the knee, with several studies demonstrating quadriceps weakness in OA patients, as compared to age- and sex-matched controls[37,38]. The findings are similar for isometric and isokinetic measurements, and also for endurance or fatiguability. The importance of this weakness and its relationship to symptoms has subsequently been examined in a community setting[39]. Poor quadriceps strength in this population was a more relevant factor for disability than radiological severity of OA. This led to the hypothesis of weakness contributing to joint dysfunction, and hence provoking symptoms. Earlier work, however, had suggested that muscle strength could only partially explain disability[40]. It is important to remember that psychological factors influence pain and disability in OA[41]. Such factors are likely to impair voluntary effort during strength testing[8], thus confounding the association. This has been supported in two recent hospital-based studies[42,43]; the latter confirming the association of poor muscle activation with tendency to anxiety and depression. This relationship is currently being examined in a community setting, results suggesting that even adjusting for poor activation and psychological variables, quadriceps weakness remains associated with pain and disability[44].

Whilst attention has tended to focus on the quadriceps (Q) mechanism, some researchers have examined hamstring (H) strength to derive the Q/H ratio. This ratio is preserved in OA patients, as compared with age-matched controls, suggesting that the hamstring mechanism may be important[45,46]. Research in terms of other joints or muscle groups is sparse, although there is some evidence for muscle fatiguability in cervical spine OA[47].

The underlying cause for this predisposition to weakness with OA is not fully understood; several mechanisms are likely to play a role. Two of these, altered muscle structure and arthrogenic inhibition, are considered in more detail below. It should be stressed, however, that these will interrelate and are unlikely to occur in isolation.

Weakness and alterations in muscle structure/size

Early studies of histology in joint disorders suggested alterations in fiber size and proportion of fiber type[48], which was partly determined by age and degree of mobility. With hip OA, the changes of selective atrophy of type II fibers has been demonstrated, which is independent of age and may be related to disuse[49]. The relative increase in type I fibers, since they are less responsive to stimulation, may serve to increase the stiffness of the muscle. This has led to the hypothesis that this change may be an adaptive mechanism for an osteoarthritic joint with altered biomechanics[50]. Alternatively, it may be that a higher than normal percentage of type I fibers may render the joint more susceptible to developing OA, possibly by altering its shock-absorbing potential and dynamic function. Some evidence for this comes from the work of Radin *et al.*, who detected minor gait abnormalities in 'pre-osteoarthrotic' subjects[51]. This 'microklutziness' causes repetitive impulse loading, which in animal models is known to provoke OA change. These 'preosteo-arthrotic' subjects had knee pain but no radiological features of OA and it is, therefore, only speculative that they would develop definite OA. Many of the assumptions relating to human OA remain speculative.

The cause for loss of muscle fibers, assuming it is not simply a response to disuse, is unknown. In animals, there is some evidence for mediation by loss of neurotrophic factors[52]. Support for this in humans comes from a study demonstrating increased muscle protein degradation in patients with OA, which can be reduced by percutaneous stimulation[53]. Prior to stimulation, the rates of synthesis and degradation were increased, with a net imbalance in favor of degradation leading to atrophy. Following stimulation, the degradative pathway was ablated.

Weakness and arthrogenic inhibition

The concept of reflex inhibition has long been recognized[52] and is inhibition of the muscle, probably neuronally mediated, in response to some change within the joint or surrounding structures. Patients undergoing meniscectomy have provided a useful model for study, with reduced activation (up to 70 per cent) of the quadriceps demonstrated postoperatively using EMG[12]. Such findings have been confirmed with more sophisticated techniques, such as twitch superimposition. Pain may not be an important mediator in this inhibition[54], suggesting it is not simply due to lack of effort. Inhibition is greater if an effusion is present; it can also be provoked in a normal subject by infusing fluid into the knee to create an effusion[13], an effect which is lessened by prior injection of intra-articular anesthetic[55]. The early findings of Harding, that dorsal root section prevents muscle atrophy, (as demonstrated by experimental inflammation in animal models), adds further support for this being neurally mediated[56]. Possible mechanisms have been comprehensively reviewed[57], but remain largely theoretical, and the role of pain (possibly unperceived) has not been discounted. It is likely that whatever its underlying mechanism, it is intimately linked to muscle wasting and weakness.

The existence of arthrogenic inhibition in established OA is less clear. Varying degrees of inhibition have been demonstrated with chronic knee effusions[58], but this inhibition is not altered by joint aspiration[59]. Some workers have demonstrated inhibition in all patients with early OA[60]; its presence partially diminished by rehabilitation. Other work, on hospital-referred subjects, suggests inhibition to be more variable, with 36 per cent of knee OA subjects demonstrating more than 20 percent inhibition[43]. To some extent, this may depend on whether the OA is related to previous trauma. From ongoing work in the community, inhibition is more apparent in subjects with knee pain, compared to those pain free, irrespective of the presence of structural change[61]. Whilst arthrogenous inhibition may occur in OA, the contribution of pain and/or psychological factors on voluntary effort cannot be overlooked. As yet, there is no practical way to assess the importance of each.

Future directions and implications for therapy

The role of muscle in OA is clearly an important one. Much of the work on muscle function and dysfunction remains at a preliminary stage, although many groups are now exploring this area. A key question is whether muscle dysfunction may worsen, or even precipitate, structural change. Likewise, more information in terms of effects on pain and disability is required.

Muscle would seem to be an obvious therapeutic target in OA. Certainly, strategies to improve strength are in worldwide use, despite being of unproven efficacy. Large intervention trials are now under way at several centers and will potentially elucidate further the place of muscle in OA.

Further work on 'inhibition' in OA is clearly needed and, in particular, the degree to which this may be influenced by structural, physiological, and psychological factors. This would be relevant both in the interpretation of previous studies and in the development of new therapeutic strategies.

References

1. Edwards, R.H.T., Young, A., Hosking, G.P., and Jones, D.A. (1977). Human skeletal muscle function: description of tests and normal values. *Clinical Science*, **52**, 283–90.
2. Tesch, P. and Karlsson, J. (1978). Isometric strength performance and muscle fibre distribution in man. *Acta Physiologica Scandinavica*, **103**, 47–51.
3. Thorstenssen, A., Grimsby, G., and Karlsson, J. (1976). Force velocity relations and fiber composition in human knee extensor muscles. *Journal of Applied Physiology* **40**, 12–16.
4. Knapik, J.J. and Ramos, M.U. (1980). Isokinetic and isometric torque relationships in the human body. *Archives of Physiological and Medical Rehabilitation* **61**, 64–7.
5. Bassey, J. and Short, A. (1990). A new method for measuring power output in a single leg extension: feasibility, reliability and validity. *European Journal of Applied Physiology* **60**, 385–90.
6. Spiegel, J.S., Paulus, H.E., Ward, N.B., Spiegel, T.M., Leake, B., and Kane, R.L. (1987). What are we measuring? An examination of walk time and grip strength. *Journal of Rheumatology*, **14**, 80–6.
7. Calmels, P. and Minaire, P. (1995). A review of the agonist / antagonist muscle pairs ratio in rehabilitation. *Disability and Rehabilitation*, **17**, 265–76.
8. Ikai, M. and Steinhaus, A.H. (1961). Some factors modifying the expression of human strength. *Journal of Applied Physiology*, **16**, 157–63.
9. Rutherford, O.M., Jones, D.A., and Newham, D.J. (1986). Clinical and experimental application of the percutaneous twitch superimposition technique for the study of human muscle activation. *Journal of Neurology, Neurosurgery and Psychiatry*, **49**, 1288–91.
10. Bigland-Ritchie, B., Furbish, F., and Woods, J.J. (1986). Neuromuscular transmission and muscle activation in

human post-fatigue ischaemia. *Journal of Physiology*, 377, 76–P.

11. Nørregaard, J., Bülow, P.M., Vestergaard-Poulsen, P., Thomsen, C., and Danneskiold-Sansøe, B. (1995). Muscle strength, voluntary activation and cross-sectional area in patients with fibromyalgia. *British Journal of Rheumatology* 34, 925–31.

12. Stokes, M. and Young, A. (1984). The contribution of reflex inhibition to arthrogenous muscle weakness. *Clinical Science* 67, 7–14.

13. Spencer, J.D., Hayes, K.C., and Alexander, I.J. (1984). Knee joint effusion and quadriceps reflex inhibition in man. *Archives of Physiological and Medical Rehabilitation*, 65, 171–7.

14. Ikai, M. and Fukunaga, T. (1968). Calculation of muscle strength per unit cross-sectional area by means of ultrasonic measurement. *Internationale Zeitschrift for Angewande Physiologie Einschliesslich Arbeitphysiologie*, 26, 26–32.

15. Haggmark, T., Jansson, E., and Svane, B. (1978). Cross-sectional area of the thigh muscle in man measured by computed tomography. *Scandinavian Journal of Clinical Laboratory Investigation*, 38, 355–60.

16. Narici, M.V., Roi, G.S., Landoni, L., Minetti, A.E., and Cerretelli, P. (1989). Changes in force, cross sectional area and neural activation during strength training and detraining of the human quadriceps. *European Journal of Applied Physiology*, 59, 310–19.

17. Jones, D.A. and Rutherford, O.M. (1987). Human strength training: the effects of three different regimes and the nature of the resultant changes. *Journal of Physiology* 391, 1–11.

18. Maughan, R.J., Watson, J.S., and Weir, J. (1983). Strength and cross-sectional area of human skeletal muscle. *Journal of Physiology*, 338, 37–49.

19. Moritani, T. and deVries, H.A. (1979). Neural factors versus hypertrophy in the time course of muscle strength gain. *American Journal of Physiology and Medicine*, 58, 115–30.

20. Hakkinen, K., Komi, P.V., and Tesch, P. (1985). Changes in isometric force and relaxation time, electromyographic and muscle fibre characteristics of human skeletal muscle during strength training and detraining. *Acta Physiologica Scandinavica*, 125, 573–85.

21. Fuller, N.J., Laskey, M.A., and Elia, M. (1992). Assessment of the composition of major body regions by dual-energy X-ray absorptiometry (DEXA), with special reference to limb muscle mass. *Clinical Physiology* 12, 253–66.

22. Edwards, R.H., Gibson, H., Roberts, N., Clague, J.E., and Martin, P.A. (1992). Magnetic resonance spectroscopy and imaging of muscle: a physiological approach. *International Journal of Sports Medicine* 13 (supplement 1), 143–6.

23. Gollnick, P.D., Armstrong, R.B., Saubert, C.W., Piehl, K., Saltin, B. (1972). Enzyme activity and fiber composition in skeletal muscle of untrained and trained men. *Journal of Applied Physiology* 33, 312–19.

24. Young, A., Stokes, M., and Crowe, M. (1984). Size and strength of the quadriceps muscles of old and young women. *European Journal of Clinical Investigation*, 14, 282–7.

25. Young, A., Stokes, M., and Crowe, M. (1985). The size and strength of the quadriceps muscles of old and young men. *Clinical Physiology*, 5, 145–54.

26. Murray, M.P., Gardner, G.M., Mollinger, L.A., and Sepic, S.B. (1980). Strength of isometric and isokinetic contractions: knee muscles of men aged 20 to 86. *Physical Therapy*, 60, 412–19.

27. Pearson, M.B. and Bassey, E.J. (1985). Muscle strength and anthopometric indices in elderly men and women. *Age and Ageing*, 14, 49–54.

28. Aniansson, A., Sperling, L., Rundgren, A., and Lehnberg, E. (1983). Muscle function in 75-year-old men and women: a longitudinal study. *Scandinavian Journal of Rehabilitation Medicine*, (supplement 9), 92–102.

29. Grieg, C.A., Botella, J., and Young, A. (1993). The quadriceps strength of healthy elderly people re-measured after eight years. *Muscle Nerve*, 16, 6–10.

30. Ensrud, K.E., Nevitt, M.C., Yunis, C., Cauley, J.A., Seeley, D.G., Fox, K.M., et al. (1994). Correlates of impaired function in older women. *Journal of the American Geriatric Society*, 42, 481–9.

31. Chang, R.W., Dunlop, D., Gibbs, J., and Hughes, S. (1995). The determinants of walking velocity in the elderly. *Arthritis and Rheumatism*, 38, 343–50.

32. Lipsitz, L.A., Nakajima, I., Gagnon, M., Hirayama, T., Connelly, C.M., Izumo, H., et al. Muscle strength and fall rates among residents of Japanese and American nursing homes: an international cross-cultural study. *Journal of the American Geriatric Society*, 42, 953–9.

33. Frontera, W.R., Hughes, V.A., Lutz, K.J., and Evans, W.J. (1991). A cross-sectional study of muscle strength and mass in 45- to 75-year-old men and women. *Journal of Applied Physiology*, 71, 644–50.

34. Larsson, L., Grimby, G., and Karlsson, J. (1979). Muscle strength and speed of movement in relation to age and muscle morphology. *Journal of Applied Physiology*, 46, 451–6.

35. Lexell, J., Henriksson-Larsén, K., Winblad, B., and Sjöström, M. (1983). Distribution of different fibre types in human skeletal muscles, effect of aging studied in whole muscle cross-sections. *Muscle Nerve*, 6, 588–95.

36. Adams, R. (1857). *A treatise on rheumatic gout or chronic rheumatic arthritis of all joints*, Churchill, London.

37. Nodesjö, L.O., Nordgren, B., Wigren, A., and Kolstad, K. (1983). Isometric strength and endurance in patients with severe rheumatoid arthritis or osteoarthritis in the knee joints. *Scandinavian Journal of Rheumatology*, 12, 152–6.

38. Ekdahl, C., Andersson, S.V., and Svensson, B. (1989). Muscle function of the lower extremities in rheumatoid arthritis and osteoarthrosis. *Journal of Clinical Epidemiology*, 42, 947–54.

39. McAlindon, T.E., Cooper, C., Kirwan, J.R., and Dieppe, P.A. (1993). Determinants of disability in knee osteoarthritis. *Annals of the Rheumatic Diseases*, 52, 258–62.

40. Lankhorst, G.J., Van de Stadt, R.J., and Van der Korst, J.K. (1985). The relationships of functional capacity, pain, and isometric and isokinetic torque in

osteoarthrosis of the knee. *Scandinavian Journal of Rehabilitation Medicine*, **17**, 167–72.

41. Summers, M.N., Haley, W.E., Reveille, J.D., and Alarcón, G.S. (1988). Radiographic assessment and psychological variables as predictors of pain and functional impairment in osteoarthritis of the knee or hip. *Arthritis and Rheumatism*, **31**, 204–9.

42. Dekker, J., Tola, P., Aufdemkampe, G., and Winkers, M. (1993). Negative affect, pain and disability in osteoarthritis patients: the mediating role of muscle weakness. *Behavioral Research and Therapy* **31**, 203–6.

43. Jones, A.C., Regan, M., and Doherty, M. (1995). Determinants of arthrogenic inhibition in knee osteoathritis. *British Journal of Rheumatology*, **34** (**supplement 1**), 134.

44. O'Reilly, S.C., Jones, A.C., Muir, K.M., and Doherty, M. (1996). Quadriceps strength and depression are important factors in knee pain and associated disability. *British Journal of Rheumatology*, **35** (**supplement 1**), 135.

45. Hall, K.D., Hayes, K.W., and Falconer, J. (1993). Differential strength decline in patients with osteoarthritis of the knee: revision of a hypothesis. *Arthritis Care Research*, **6**, 89–96.

46. Tan, J., Balci, N., Sepici, V., and Gener, F.A. (1995). Isokinetic and isometric strength in osteoarthrosis of the knee. *American Journal of Medical Rehabilitation*, **74**, 364–9.

47. Gogia, P.P. and Sabbahi, M.A. (1994). Electromyographic analysis of neck muscle fatigue in patients with osteoarthritis of the cervical spine. *Spine*, **19**, 502–6.

48. Staudte, H.W. and Brussatis, F. (1977). Selective changes in size and distribution of fibre types in vastus muscle from cases of different knee joint affections. *Zeitschrift Fur Rheumatologie*, **36**, 143–60.

49. Širca, A. and Sušec-Micieli, M. (1980). Selective type II fibre muscular atrophy in patients with osteoarthritis of the hip. *Journal of Neurological Science*, **44**, 149–59.

50. Martin, T.P., Lori, A.G., Hoeppner, P., Blevins, F.T., and Coutts, R.D. (1990). Properties of muscle fibres from the vastus lateralis or gluteus medius associated with an osteoarthritic joint. *Canadian Journal of Rehabilitation*, **4**, 151–7.

51. Radin, E.L., Yang, K.H., Riegger, C., Kish, V.L., and O'Connor, J.J. (1991). Relationship between lower limb dynamics and knee joint pain. *Journal of Orthopaedic Research*, **9**, 298–405.

52. Harding, A.E.B. (1929). An investigation into the cause of arthritic muscle atrophy. *Lancet* **1**, 433–4.

53. Gibson, J.N.A., Morrison, W.L., Scrimgeour, C.M., Smith, K., Stoward, P.J., and Rennie, M.J. (1989). Effects of therapeutic percutaneous electrical stimulation of atrophic human quadriceps on muscle composition, protein synthesis and contractile properties. *European Journal of Clinical Investigation*, **19**, 206–12.

54. Shakespeare, D.T., Stokes, M., Sherman, K.P., and Young, A. (1985). Reflex inhibition of the quadriceps after meniscectomy: lack of association with pain. *Clinical Physiology*, **5**, 137–44.

55. de Andrade, J.R., Grant, C., and Dixon, A. (1965). Joint distension and reflex muscle inhibition in the knee. *Journal of Bone and Joint Surgery (AM)*, **47**, 313–22.

56. Harding, A.E.B. (1929). An investigation into the cause of arthritic muscle atrophy. *Lancet*, **1**, 433–4.

57. Young, A. (1993). Current issues in arthrogenous inhibition. *Annals of the Rheumatic Diseases*, **52**, 829–34.

58. Fahrer, H., Rentsch, H.U., Gerber, N.J., Beyer, Ch., Hess, Ch., and Grünig, B. (1988). Knee effusion and reflex inhibition of the quadriceps: a bar to effective training. *Journal of Bone and Joint Surgery (Br)*, **70-B**, 635–8.

59. Jones, D.W., Jones, D.A., and Newham, D.J. (1987). Chronic knee effusion and aspiration: the effect on quadriceps inhibition. *British Journal of Rheumatology*, **26**, 370–4.

60. Hurley, M.V. and Newham, D.J. (1993). The influence of arthrogenous muscle inhibition on quadriceps rehabilitation of patients with early, unilateral osteoarthritic knees. *British Journal of Rheumatology*, **32**, 127–31.

61. O'Reilly, S.C., Jones, A.C., Muir, K.M., and Doherty, M. (1995). Knee pain quadriceps weakness and muscle activation in the community. *British Journal of Rheumatology*, **34** (**supplement 2**), 45.

8 | Clinical features of osteoarthritis and standard approaches to the diagnosis

8.1 Signs, symptoms, and laboratory tests

Sheila O'Reilly and Michael Doherty

This chapter focuses on the common clinical presentations of osteoarthritis (OA). General aspects of the symptoms and signs of OA, and the varying patterns and associations are discussed; the features of OA at individual joint sites are then detailed. Atypical features and presentations, particularly relating to serious complications, are briefly highlighted. Finally, the merits and pitfalls of routine investigations are addressed.

General clinical features

OA is a complex, heterogeneous process that may be triggered by diverse constitutional and environmental factors. It is, therefore, not surprising that the clinical presentation of OA is extremely variable in terms of timing of onset, pattern of involvement, and severity. Equally variable are the prognosis and outcome in different patients, and at different joint sites. Despite this heterogeneity, a number of generalizations about OA can be made:

- no primary extra-locomotor manifestations
- usually only one or a few joints are problematic
- slow evolution of symptoms and structural change
- strong age association — uncommon before middle age

- often poor correlation between symptoms, disability, and degree of structural change
- symptoms and signs predominantly relate to joint damage rather than inflammation.

For example, although rare conditions that predispose to OA may have non-locomotor manifestations, the changes of OA are confined to one system. Symptoms and signs of OA are usually slow to evolve, mainly relate to joint damage, and uncommonly present before middle age. Although polyarticular involvement is common, usually only one or a few joints present clinical problems at any one time.

The main clinical features of OA are *symptoms* (predominantly pain and stiffness), *functional impairment*, and *signs*. It has long been noted that there is often marked discordance between these three, especially for smaller joints affected by OA[1]. In a clinical setting, therefore, only a good clinical history and examination, and consideration of the patient as a whole, will permit determination of the specific factors relating to pain and disability in that individual.

Symptoms of OA

Common symptoms of OA are listed in Table 8.1

Table 8.1 Common symptoms and signs of OA

Symptoms	Signs	
Pain	Crepitus	
Stiffness	Restricted movement	
Alteration in shape	Tenderness	– joint line
Functional impairment		– periarticular
± anxiety, depression	Bony swelling	
	Deformity	
	Muscle wasting / weakness	
	± effusions, increased warmth	
	± instability	

Pain

This is the dominant symptom in OA and the usual reason for seeking medical opinion. Initially, it is typically aching in nature, related to joint use, and relieved by rest. Such 'mechanical' pain is reputed to differentiate OA from inflammatory arthropathies, though formal studies only confirm the diversity of pain descriptors within each disease and the overlap between them[2]. As OA progresses, pain may become more persistent and occur also at rest and at night. Interference with restorative sleep may further compound pain severity through associated fatigue and lack of well-being.

The correlation between pain and degree of structural OA change is closest at the hip, then the knee, and is worst for hand and spinal apophyseal joints. At any site, however, joints with severe radiographic change are more likely to be painful than those with mild or no change (Fig. 8.1). A circadian pattern is

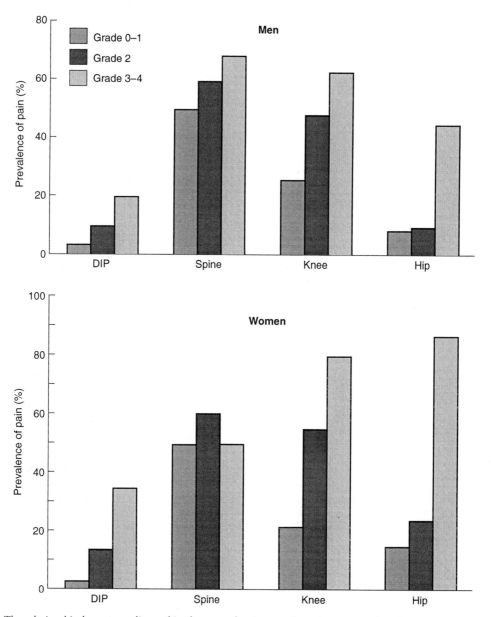

Fig. 8.1 The relationship between radiographic change and pain at various sites. Data taken from a population survey in Northern England[57].

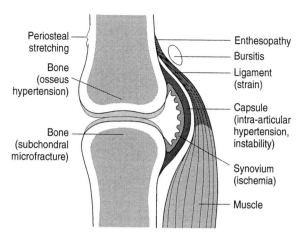

Fig. 8.2   Potential sites and mechanisms of local pain generation in OA.

demonstrable in many sufferers[3]. Women may be more likely to report pain, though the strength of this relationship varies between studies and between joints[4,5]. Pain reporting correlates strongly with psychological variables such as anxiety and depression[6,7].

The mechanisms of pain production in OA remain unclear. The OA process may affect all intracapsular and periarticular tissues of the synovial joint, resulting in many possible causes of pain (Fig. 8.2). Cartilage itself is aneural, but there is rich sensory innervation in other joint tissues. Raised intraosseous pressure, presumably secondary to venous obstruction, is well-documented in large joint OA[8] and is a suggested major cause of nocturnal pain. This 'bony' pain is often associated with severe structural change and poor prognosis. Periosteal stretching by bone proliferation, and subchondral microfractures may also contribute to pain. Intra-articular hypertension caused by synovial hypertrophy, excess fluid, or mechanical derangement may stimulate capsular mechanoreceptors, and ischemia from mild synovitis may excite synovial nociceptors. Periarticular involvement is common around OA joints but is often overlooked as a cause of pain[9]. Bursitis, enthesopathy, tendinitis, and ligamentous strain probably result from altered mechanical loading across the joint due to remodeling, inflammation, and pain. Myalgia and cramps may accompany OA, and muscle weakness itself may indirectly contribute to pain (suggested by the demonstrable reduction in pain following training[10]).

Stiffness

For patients, 'stiffness' may vary in meaning from slowness of joint movement, to pain on initial move-

ment such as getting up from a chair. Early morning stiffness, often interpreted as a measure of inflammation, is occasionally severe, but most patients complain more of inactivity stiffness or 'gelling' later in the day. Stiffness is generally short lived, compared to the more prolonged, often generalized stiffness of inflammatory arthropathy; a duration of less than 30 minutes forms part of the American College of Rheumatology (ACR) diagnostic criteria for OA[11].

Anxiety and depression

Anxiety and depression are common in patients with OA; they are important in their own right, in addition to the amplifying effects on pain perception and level of disability[6]. Closely allied to anxiety and depression is fibromyalgia, which, like OA, predominates in women and shows increasing prevalence with age[12,13]. Fibromyalgia may amplify the symptoms and disability of OA or be the principal cause of pain. It is important to recognize, since it is typically unresponsive to analgesics and requires a different treatment approach.

Altered joint shape, deformity

Obvious bony swelling and deformity may be a source of distress for some patients. This is particularly common with Heberden's nodes and hand OA, which may be thought unsightly.

Functional impairment

OA contributes greatly to overall disability in the community[14], with knee OA the greatest contributor. Disability may include poor mobility, difficulty with activities of daily living, social isolation, and loss of work opportunities with consequent financial concerns. Subsequent handicap is determined by the circumstances and aspirations of the individual. Like pain, it is a common reason for seeking medical advice. A number of validated instruments are available to assess self-reported disability and dimensions relating to general health status and quality of life. The explanation for disability and functional loss is not always clear. Pain is an important contributor and muscle weakness appears to correlate well with disability at the knee[15]. Reduced range of joint movement may be a principal feature or a contributor to overall disability. As with pain, the extent of disability is influenced by accompanying psychological factors, although it may be impossible to differentiate causation and consequence.

Signs of OA

Common examination findings in OA are listed in Table 8.1. Many of these signs, particularly those of joint damage and remodeling, are incorporated into classification or diagnostic criteria for individual joints. Their usefulness is influenced by agreement of their presence. Several studies confirm only moderate agreement between assessors for most of these signs, crepitus appearing the least reproducible[16,17]. Despite this caveat, certain signs are helpful in clinical assessment.

Crepitus

Coarse crepitus, accompanying an irregular joint surface, conducts well through bone and air. It is typically palpable over a wide area of the joint, and felt throughout the range of movement; in gross cases it may be clearly audible. Although a key feature in criteria, course crepitus is a non-specific sign of joint damage.

Tenderness

Tenderness to palpation along the joint-line ('capsular/joint-line tenderness') suggests a capsular/intracapsular origin of pain. Point tenderness away from the joint-line suggests a periarticular lesion; pain on resisted active movements and/or stress tests may further localize the involved structure. Periarticular lesions (bursitis, enthesopathy) commonly accompany large joint (knee, hip) OA. They may be the principal cause of pain and are often readily amenable to local treatment.

Reduced range of movement

This is extremely common in OA joints. More important than the precise reduction in movement, however, is the accompanying loss of function. This requires separate assessment of screening movements for activities of daily living to compliment self-reported disability. Reduced movement mainly results from osteophyte encroachment, remodeling, and capsular thickening, but may be accentuated by effusion and soft tissue swelling.

Deformity and instability

Deformity is a sign of advanced OA, with severe cartilage loss, osteophyte, remodeling, and bone attrition.

Although deformities at individual sites may be highly characteristic of OA, none are specific. Instability is an uncommon late sign that may accompany severe deforming OA at certain sites (for example, the knee). Most commonly, however, capsular thickening maintains stability as OA slowly progresses. Local traumatic instability (for example, cruciate rupture) may, of course, be a predisposing factor and predate signs of OA.

Muscle wasting and weakness

Wasting is often a difficult sign, particularly in the elderly or obese patient. When present, it is global, affecting all muscles that act over the affected joint. Assessment of muscle weakness around a painful joint is problematic (see Chapter 7.6).

Increased warmth and effusions

Varying degrees of synovitis, evidenced by warmth, synovial thickening, effusion, and stress pain, may accompany or predate signs of joint damage. Such inflammatory signs are most evident at the knee and during the early development stage of nodal finger interphalangeal OA. Effusions at the knee have been suggested as a risk factor for progression[18]. Large, warm effusions are uncommon, and the possibility of alternative pathology or associated calcium crystal deposition should be considered.

Clinical patterns ('subsets') of OA

Several attempts have been made to subdivide the broad spectrum of OA, in order to better define causative factors, and to determine natural history and prognosis. The earliest classification, by recognized etiology, into *primary* or *secondary* OA, largely proved unhelpful because: (1) it still left a large primary group in whom the predisposing factors were unclear; and (2) there is frequent overlap between the two, as shown, for example, by a higher prevalence of post-meniscectomy 'secondary' OA in subjects with predisposition to 'primary' nodal OA[19].

Division according to known predisposing factors (for example, dysplasia, collagenosis, Perthe's) has been retained but principally relates to atypical and early-onset OA (see later). Further division of the larger 'primary' OA group is often according to:

- the joint site involved
- the number of joints involved (one, few, many)
- associated intra-articular calcium crystal deposition
- presence of marked clinical inflammation
- the radiographic bone response (atrophic, hypertrophic).

Although 'subsets' differing in several such features have emerged, it is important to note there are no sharp distinctions. The above features change with time, so that one subset may evolve into another, and different subsets may exist at different sites within an individual. Most useful, perhaps, is simple division by site and number of involved joints. Risk factors for development and progression are increasingly attributed to specific sites or to polyarticular involvement. The common patterns (Fig. 8.3) will be described, since their recognition has some relevance for patient education and prognosis.

Nodal generalized OA

This pattern, recognized since the nineteenth century, has been well characterized[20]. It is probably the most common, easily recognized, and best accepted subset. Its characteristics are as follows:

- marked familial predisposition
- female preponderance
- typical onset in middle age with hand symptoms and signs
- multiple Heberden's, with or without Bouchard's, nodes
- polyarticular finger interphalangeal OA
- good functional outcome for hand OA
- later predisposition to OA of the knee (less frequently hip and other joints).

Presentation is usually in middle age (forties, fifties) with symptoms of pain, stiffness, and swelling in one or a few finger interphalangeal joints (IPJs). Gradually, more joints are recruited, resulting in a stuttering onset of hand IPJ polyarthritis ('monoarthritis multiplex'). Hand symptoms can persist for several years, but usually settle to leave the firm posterolateral swellings of Heberden's (distal IPJ) and Bouchard's (proximal IPJ) nodes, and typical radial or ulnar deviations (Fig. 8.4). Mild knee symptoms may accompany this slow evolution of hand OA, but it is usually in later life (sixties, seventies) that other joints become problematic. The knee is, by far, the commonest large joint involved, typically with medial and patellofemoral compartment OA. The hip and other joints (gleno-

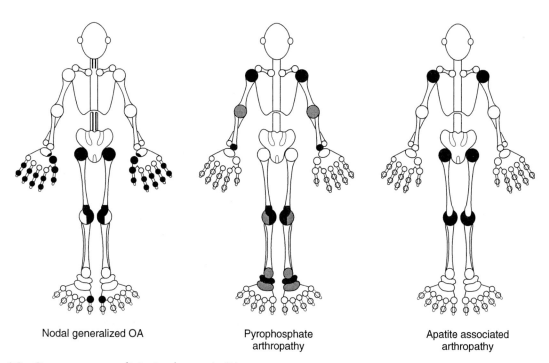

Nodal generalized OA   Pyrophosphate arthropathy   Apatite associated arthropathy

Fig. 8.3   Common patterns of joint involvement in OA.

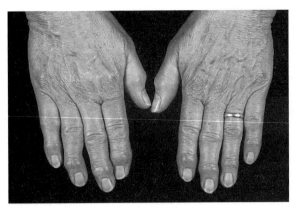
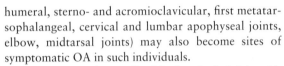

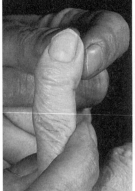
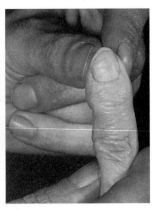

Fig. 8.4   Hand involvement in generalized nodal OA, with typical Heberden's and Bouchard's nodes.

Fig. 8.5   Instability of the DIPJ in erosive OA.

humeral, sterno- and acromioclavicular, first metatarsophalangeal, cervical and lumbar apophyseal joints, elbow, midtarsal joints) may also become sites of symptomatic OA in such individuals.

The existence of generalized (polyarticular) OA, with nodal change the marker of the subset, is supported by several studies[20,21]. Additional support for nodal generalized OA as a subset with strong constitutional, possibly autoimmune[22], predisposition comes from the following observations:

- symmetry of hand involvement[23].
- strong genetic predisposition[24].
- high prevalence of IgG rheumatoid factor positivity[25]
- biochemical differences in chondroitin sulphation from non-nodal large joint OA[26].

The problem arises, however, of when to apply the label 'nodal OA'. There are no agreed diagnostic criteria and the occurrence of just one, or a few Heberden's nodes with limited interphalangeal OA is a common, often asymptomatic finding in the elderly. One study[27] suggested a further division of 'non-nodal generalized OA', with involvement of more proximal than distal interphalangeal joint involvement, and a more equal sex distribution, than nodal OA. Clearly, distinction between nodal and non-nodal polyarticular OA is often blurred.

Erosive ('inflammatory') OA

The presence of radiographic erosions in addition to more typical 'degenerative' changes in hands prompted differentiation of this subset from nodal OA[28,29].

Affected IPJs may become unstable (Fig. 8.5) and, occasionally, even ankylosed (Fig. 8.6) — both of which are further distinguishing features from the more common nodal OA. Its inflammatory nature and equal involvement of proximal and distal IPJs may suggest rheumatoid arthritis. Radiographic erosions, however, are subchondral not marginal, and classically evolve to a 'gulls wing' appearance combining subchondral erosion with proliferative bone remodeling (Fig. 8.6). Unlike nodal OA, it does not predispose to generalized OA, but is less favourable with regard to hand function[30].

Existence of this subset, however, is disputed; some authors view it merely as severe involvement within the spectrum of nodal OA[31]. Progression to seropositive rheumatoid arthritis in some patients[32], further undermines its credibility as a discrete subset of OA.

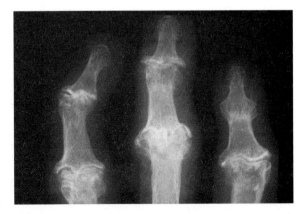

Fig. 8.6   Typical radiographic features in erosive OA with 'gull's wing' deformities and ankylosis of one DIPJ.

Crystal associations

Deposition of calcium crystals [calcium pyrophosphate dihydrate (CPPD) and basic calcium phosphates — mainly carbonate substituted hydroxyapatite] is a common accompaniment to the OA process, and shows a strong association with age. Crystal identification is mainly via examination of synovial fluid, though gross deposits may show on radiographs as chondrocalcinosis (usually, but not inevitably CPPD) and, less commonly, as calcification in synovium, capsule, or periarticular structures (tendon, bursae). Whether they have a pathological role in OA remains uncertain[33]. Their presence, however, has been used as a means of defining certain clinical presentations and subsets of OA.

Pyrophosphate arthropathy

Acute pyrophosphate arthropathy ('pseudogout') typically presents as acute monoarthritis in an elderly patient. The knee is the usual target site (Fig. 8.7), but almost any joint may be involved. Most episodes are spontaneous, though direct trauma or stress response to intercurrent illness may be triggering factors. Pain is severe, and there may be an accompanying systemic response with pyrexia and mild confusion. Examination reveals florid synovitis with marked tenderness, warmth, effusion, and restricted movement with stress pain. Overlying erythema is common and the principal differential diagnosis is sepsis. Aspirated synovial fluid is inflammatory (turbid, low viscosity, high cell count — that is, more than 90 per cent polymorphs) (Fig. 8.8) and often blood-stained. Diagnosis is confirmed by identification of CPPD crystals in syn-

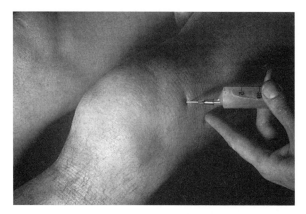

Fig. 8.8 Turbid synovial fluid obtained during an acute attack of acute pyrophosphate arthropathy.

ovial fluid, and exclusion of sepsis by Gram stain and culture. Attacks are self-limiting and usually resolve within one to two weeks. The mechanism of the attack is thought to be 'shedding' of preformed CPPD crystals from their origin in fibro- and hyaline cartilage. This is the one clear instance where CPPD crystals cause inflammation and arthropathy.

Acute attacks may occur alone, but often superimpose on chronic symptomatic arthropathy. *Chronic pyrophosphate arthropathy* (CPPD deposition and structural joint change) also mainly targets knees, especially of elderly women (Fig. 8.9). Other common sites

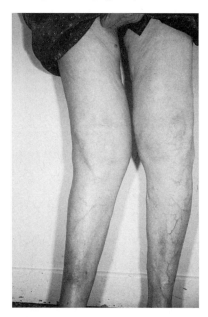

Fig. 8.9 Chronic pyrophosphate arthropathy in the knee of an elderly lady, with marked valgus deformity of the right knee.

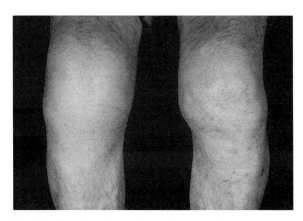

Fig. 8.7 Pyrophosphate arthropathy presenting as acute synovitis of the knee.

are shoulders, wrists, elbows, and metacarpophalangeal joints. Clinical and radiographic features are essentially those of OA, but possible distinctions that have been emphasized include:

- marked predominance in elderly women
- atypical distribution (glenohumeral, elbow, radiocarpal, and metacarpophalangeal joints are not common target sites for OA)
- frequent marked inflammatory component (especially at knees, glenohumeral, and radiocarpal joints)
- frequent 'hypertrophic' radiographic appearance with prominent osteophyte, cysts, and osteochondral bodies (Fig. 8.10)
- CPPD crystals in synovial fluid, with or without chondrocalcinosis and calcification of articular structures on radiographs
- association with rapidly progressive hip OA[34], and tendency to radiographic progression at the knee[35].

Many elderly OA patients with CPPD, however, have coexisting nodal OA and no clinical or radiographic features to set them apart from non-crystal associated OA. Joint damage (for example, meniscectomy) is known to predispose both to localized OA and to localized CPPD deposition[36]. Furthermore, at the knee, synovial fluid positivity for CPPD increases with the severity and compartmental extent of radiographic OA[37]. It therefore seems likely that CPPD, in the context of OA, is more commonly a marker of the extent of the OA process (that is, joint tissue response to insult) than for a subset of OA with a specific pathogenesis.

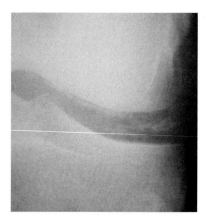

Fig. 8.11 Isolated chondrocalcinosis at the knee, with involvement of hyaline cartilage and fibrocartilage (Reproduced with the kind permission of Mosby-Year Book Inc).

Isolated chondrocalcinosis due to CPPD deposition may occur without the structural changes of OA, as a common age-related phenomenon, particularly at the knee (Fig. 8.11). It may be asymptomatic, or result in acute pseudogout. Chondrocalcinosis *per se* is rare below age 55 and, particularly if florid and polyarticular, should lead to consideration of either familial CPPD deposition, which is uncommon but described in most countries[38], or predisposing metabolic disease[39] (Table 8.2). Pseudogout, arthralgia, or incidental radiographic chondrocalcinosis may be the initial presentation of metabolic disease. Although rare, recognition is important since it may have therapeutic implications and, in the case of hemochromatosis, require screening of asymptomatic relatives.

Less common syndromes that may arise in the context of widespread chronic pyrophosphate arthropathy include: acute tendinitis (Achilles, triceps, flexor digitorum), rarely with tendon rupture; tenosynovitis (hand flexors, extensors); and bursitis (olecranon, infrapatellar, retrocalcaneal).

Apatite-associated arthropathy ('Milwaukee shoulder syndrome')

Like CPPD, 'apatite' (carbonate substituted hydroxyapatite, tricalcium phosphate, octacalcium phosphate) crystals can often be identified in OA fluids and joint tissues. The origin of the apatite remains unclear, though most evidence suggests it predominantly forms within cartilage, rather than being shed from subchondral bone[40]. Again, the chance of finding basic calcium crystals in knee OA fluids increases with age, and with extent and severity of OA change[37]. However, the

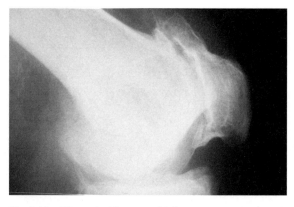

Fig. 8.10 The typical hypertrophic bone response in chronic pyrophosphate arthropathy.

Table 8.2 Metabolic diseases associated with CPPD deposition

	Chondrocalcinosis	Pseudogout	Chronic arthropathy
Hyperparathyroidism	Yes	Yes	No
Hemochromatosis	Yes	Yes	Yes
Hypophosphatasia	Yes	Yes	Yes
Hypomagnesemia	Yes	Yes	No
Hypothyroidism	Probably	No	No
Gout	Possibly	Possibly	No
Wilson's disease	Possibly	No	No
Acromegaly	Possibly	No	No

finding of plentiful apatite aggregates in synovial fluid and tissue has been linked to arthropathy, showing the following features:

- confinement to elderly subjects, predominantly women over 75
- localization to one or a few large joints (shoulder, hip, knee)
- subacute onset; rapid, painful progression; poor outcome
- large cool effusions (Fig. 8.12); marked instability
- 'atrophic' radiographic appearance with marked attrition of cartilage and bone (Fig. 8.13).

As with chronic pyrophosphate arthropathy, there is considerable overlap with less extreme forms of progressive OA. Furthermore, concurrence of CPPD and apatites is common ('mixed crystal deposition'), and association with progressive, destructive knee OA is suggested[41]. However, the poor specificity of calcium crystals for distinctive arthropathy (other than pseudogout) questions their use as a marker for joint *disease*.

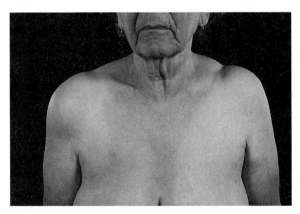

Fig. 8.12   Large, cool effusion in a 'Milwaukee shoulder' (apatite-associated arthropathy).

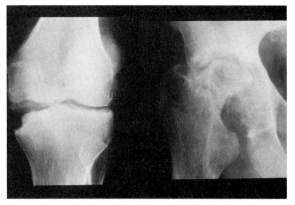

Fig. 8.13   Marked bone atrophy at the hip and knee in a patient with apatite-associated arthropathy.

Further work is required to establish their usefulness as markers of varying aspects of the OA *process*.

OA secondary to other disease

A history of severe trauma or intra-articular mechanical derangement is, by far, the most common attributable cause of localized 'secondary' OA. Generalized hypermobility is common and may be found on examination of even an elderly patient with OA, though its putative association with generalized OA[42] remains unconfirmed. There is recent evidence to suggest an association between hypermobility in the hand and localized OA[43]. A number of defined diseases may insult synovial joints and lead to non-inflammatory arthropathy with radiographic features predominantly of OA. Despite some overlap, for clinical purposes they are best grouped according to presentation (Table 8.3). Many are rare, and present additional clinical or radiographic features that suggest the diagnosis. Endemic and inherited conditions generally cause young-onset, polyarticular OA that is clearly unusual. Conditions that present later in life with pauciarticular OA,

Table 8.3   Principal diseases predisposing to OA

Generalized, mainly polyarticular OA
(Spondylo-) epiphyseal dysplasias
Collagenoses (e.g. Stickler syndrome – progressive hereditary arthro-opthalmopathy)
Ochronosis
Hemochromatosis
Wilson's disease
Endemic OA (e.g. Kashin–Beck disease, Malmad disease)

Pauciarticular, large-joint OA
1 Knee
Epiphyseal dysplasia
Osteonecrosis (mainly medial femoral condyle)
Acromegaly
Neuropathic (Charcot) joint (classically syphilis)
2 Hip
Acetabular dysplasia
Perthes disease
Slipped femoral epiphysis
Osteonecrosis
3 Shoulder
Neuropathic (Charcot) joint (mainly syringomyelia)
Osteonecrosis (proximal humerus)
4 Elbow
Neuropathic (Charcot) joint (mainly syringomyelia)
Osteonecrosis (distal humerus)
5 Wrist
Neuropathic (Charcot) joint (mainly syringomyelia)
6 Finger interphalangeal joints
Thiemann's disease
7 Hindfoot / midfoot
Neuropathic (Charcot) joint (mainly diabetes)

---

however, may more easily be missed. In general, features that should lead to consideration of a predisposing disease include:

- premature-onset OA (under 45 years)
- atypical distribution (for example, prominent metacarpophalangeal and radiocarpal OA in hemochromatosis)
- short stature, abnormal body habitus, short digits
- premature-onset chondrocalcinosis (under 55 years)
- florid polyarticular chondrocalcinosis (any age).

As has already been emphasized for pain causation, only a broad-based consideration of the whole patient will permit delineation of potential predisposing disease.

Clinical features of OA at specific sites

Predilection for OA to target certain joints is striking. This limited distribution remains unexplained, though one hypothesis suggests that joints which have changed function in recent evolutionary history are still 'under-designed', with little mechanical reserve, for their new functions and, therefore, more commonly 'fail' in the face of joint insult[44]. Nevertheless, because of the high prevalence of OA, even involvement of more 'protected' joint sites by OA is not uncommon. Trauma, in particular, may result in OA at almost any site.

Hand and wrist

The hand and wrist comprise many small joints acting together as a functional unit. OA selectively targets only certain of these joints, the pattern differing according to gender[45], with women showing more common, more widespread, and more severe involvement. Although theories abound, the reasons for this remain unclear.

Proximal and distal IPJ involvement predominates in women and typically starts around middle age with symptoms of pain, stiffness, and swelling, slowly affecting one IPJ after another. Initially, there may be features of articular and periarticular inflammation, with

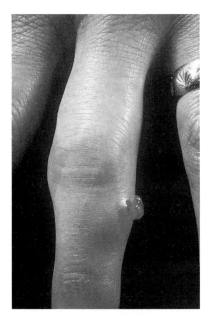

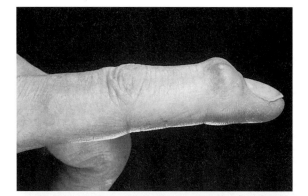

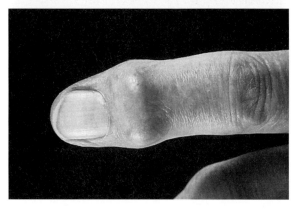

Fig. 8.14 Mucous cyst exuding hyaluronan-rich jelly extending distally.

Fig. 8.15 Typical posterolateral swelling of the DIPJ.

redness and warmth. Mucous cysts, containing hyaluronan-rich jelly, form on the superolateral aspect of the IPJs and may spread quite a distance proximally or, less commonly, distally from the joint (Fig. 8.14). These herald the characteristic firm Heberden's (distal IPJ) and Bouchard's (proximal IPJ) nodes (Fig. 8.15). Fully established nodes may remain as discrete posterolateral swellings, or merge to form a posterior bar. Once fully developed, pain and stiffness usually subside and outcome, with respect to hand function, is usually excellent[30]. Concomitant to node formation is gradual evolution of focal OA in the underlying IPJs. This may result in fixed flexion and highly characteristic fixed lateral (ulnar or radial) deviation, especially of distal IPJs — the ends of the fingers usually pointing towards the longitudinal axis of the hand (Fig. 8.16). Florid distal IPJ involvement may result in longitudinal nail ridging ('Heberden's nodes nails'; Fig. 8.17). Despite sometimes gross deviation, IPJ instability is not a feature; if present, 'erosive' OA changes are likely to be seen on the radiograph. Similarly, ankylosis, usually limited to just one or two IPJs, is a rare late consequence of erosive OA. Compared to nodal OA, symptoms of erosive OA are often more chronic, and late functional outcome less good.

First carpometacarpal joint (1st CMCJ) or thumbbase disease may occur alone or in the context of nodal generalized OA. It is generally more problematic than IPJ OA, causing pain on usage — maximal over the

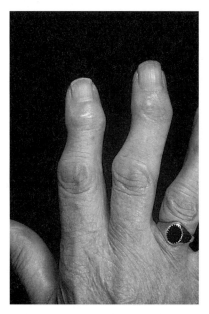

Fig. 8.16 Ulnar deviation at the DIPJs; radial deviation at the DIPJs.

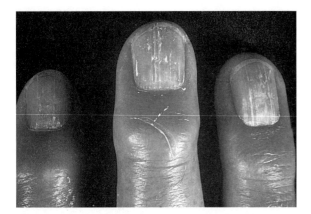

Fig. 8.17 'Heberden's nodes nails' with longitudinal and transverse nail ridging.

joint itself, but often radiating distally towards the thumb and proximally to the wrist and distal forearm (sometimes causing confusion with carpal tunnel syndrome). Common problems with daily activities include doing up buttons, lifting saucepans, opening jars, and writing. Examination may reveal localized tenderness; restricted, painful, weak thumb movements (with or without crepitus); and difficulty with fine precision pinch. Any muscle wasting globally affects thenar muscles, unlike the selective involvement of opponens, abductor pollicis, and flexor pollicis with median nerve entrapment. In advanced OA, characteristic 'squaring' occurs due to osteophyte, remodeling, and subluxation (Fig. 8.18). The scaphotrapezoid joint is an integral part of the thumb-base unit and is also commonly affected by OA, either alone or together with the 1st CMCJ. Pain is discrete, with little or no radiation; and tenderness, the principal examination finding, is well localized. Palpable osteophyte and subluxation are rare.

The radiocarpal joint may develop 'secondary' OA following wrist trauma/fracture, but it is also a common site for chronic pyrophosphate arthropathy, particularly in the elderly. Pain and tenderness are well localized to the joint-line, and signs of synovitis may be marked. Isolated median, or combined median and ulnar nerve entrapment may complicate pyrophosphate arthropathy at this site, relating more to soft tissue inflammation than articular derangement[46]. Involvement of the midcarpal articulation is a less common finding, again usually in association with CPPD deposition in elderly subjects.

A clinical problem that may arise in hands of elderly patients with longstanding nodal OA is superimposed

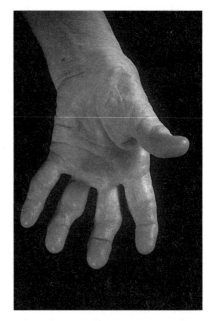

Fig. 8.18 Squaring of the 1st CMCJ due to osteophyte, remodeling and subluxation, with consequent wasting of the thenar muscles.

tophaceous gout, secondary to chronic diuretic therapy. This presents with chronic or subacute pain and swelling of finger joints, and may be mistaken for exacerbation or 'reactivation' of nodal OA. Typical acute attacks with lower limb predominance may be absent, and the diagnosis may be missed until the 'infected nodes' discharge pus and white material (Fig. 8.19).

Elbow

Elbow OA is uncommon in the absence of predisposing trauma or disease, but may occur as a site of CPPD deposition and in the context of nodal OA. Isolated 'primary' OA of the elbow is described in men in association with metacarpophalangeal OA[47]. Pain is predominant at the elbow but may radiate distally into the forearm. Any, or all, of the three articulations may be involved. Reduced flexion and extension, often with fixed flexion, is usual with humeroulnar involvement, and pronation/supination may be restricted with proximal radio-ulnar OA. Crepitus and synovitis are occasionally marked. The outcome of elbow OA is usually good; function is generally retained and symptoms are often limited to a few years.

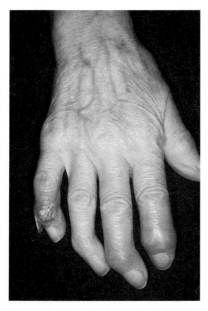

Fig. 8.19 A discharging gouty tophus in an elderly lady with pre-existing nodal OA.

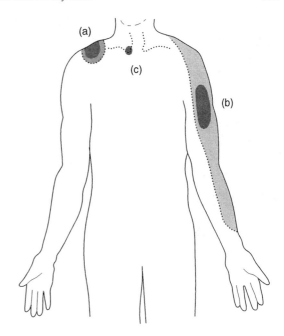

Fig. 8.20 Pattern of pain around the shoulder from OA of: (a) acromioclavicular joint; (b) glenohumeral joint; (c) sternoclavicular joint.

Shoulder

The acromioclavicular joint (ACJ) is commonly affected by OA. Pain is well localized (Fig. 8.20) and experienced mainly on abduction and elevation of the arm. Examination reveals localized tenderness, often with bony swelling, and crepitus on shrugging the shoulder; typically, there is a painful superior arc and pain on reaching for the opposite shoulder (or on forced passive abduction). Associated rotator cuff pathology and/or subacromial bursitis, however, commonly coexist to present a more complex collection of regional symptoms and signs.

The glenohumeral joint (GHJ) is rarely affected by OA, except in elderly women, in whom it is a common cause of shoulder pain and disability[48]. Examination reveals anterior joint-line tenderness and equally restricted active and passive movement; external rotation and abduction are the earliest and most severely affected movements. Global wasting of deltoid and rotator cuff muscles may give a bony prominence to the shoulder ('squaring') and scapula. Crepitus may be palpable anteriorly, or around the acromion, if there is superior humeral migration and subacromial impingement. Again, coexisting rotator cuff disease and subacromial bursitis may amplify the disability and complicate the clinical picture.

More severe, rapidly progressive OA of the GHJ may associate with plentiful synovial fluid apatite ('Milwaukee shoulder') and/or CPPD crystals (see p. 00). Clinically, large effusions may be present either anteriorly (filling in the normal depression below the clavicle and lateral to deltoid) or, more commonly, anterolaterally (due to cuff rupture and free communication between the GHJ cavity, subacromial and subdeltoid bursae). Joint rupture may result in acute exacerbation of symptoms, followed by wide bruising around the upper arm — 'epaule senile haemorrhagique'[49] (Fig. 8.21). Marked instability, and occasional secondary subluxation or even dislocation may result. The outcome of such painful, debilitating arthritis is poor.

The sternoclavicular joint is a common site for signs of OA (bony swelling, crepitus) in older subjects but rarely gives rise to symptoms. If present, pain is well localized to the joint. Pain, particularly if progressive and associated with warmth, soft tissue swelling, or erythema should lead to aspiration and consideration of sepsis and crystals (CPPD).

Hip

Attempts have been made to classify hip OA in various ways, according to recognized preceding disease

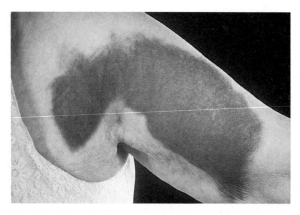

Fig. 8.21 Extensive bruising of the upper arm due to rupture of the shoulder joint — 'epaule senile haemorrhagique'.

(primary/secondary), bilaterality/unilaterality, presence of generalized OA, distribution of OA within the joint, or radiographic appearance. No classification has been entirely successful and there may be considerable overlap between patterns. The most widely used system is radiographic division by anatomic site (Fig. 8.22)[50]. *Superior pole OA* is the commonest form and includes all types of OA secondary to structural abnormality. This is the characteristic pattern in men and is often unilateral at presentation. It may result in superolateral or superomedial femoral head migration. *Medial pole OA* is far less common and predominates in women; it

is more likely to be bilateral at presentation and less likely to progress with (axial) femoral migration. A *concentric* pattern, associated with generalized OA, is also described[51], though nodal OA probably more strongly associates with medial pole OA. However characterized, there is usually striking symmetry of radiographic features in patients with bilateral hip OA. In up to 30 per cent of patients, categorization according to anatomic site proves impossible ('indeterminate' pattern;[18,52]).

The hip shows the best correlation between symptoms and radiographic change. Pain from the hip is typically felt maximally deep in the anterior groin (femoral nerve), but may be referred over a wide area including the lateral thigh and buttock (sciatic nerve), anterior thigh and knee (obturator nerve), and as far down the leg as the ankle (Fig. 8.23). Occasionally, pain is maximally felt at the knee, with little proximal discomfort; unlike pain arising from the knee, this referred pain is poorly localized over a wide area, involves the distal thigh, and may be partially relieved by rubbing. Pain is initially felt on walking, but later occurs at rest and subsequently at night. Stiffness is common, and patients may have particular difficulty

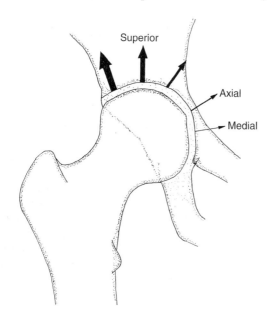

Fig. 8.22 Patterns of femoral migration around the OA hip; the arrows indicate relative frequency of each pattern.

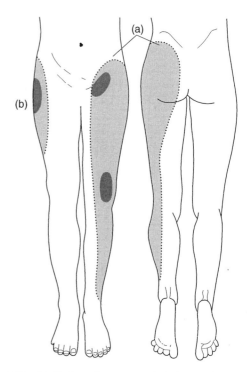

Fig. 8.23 Radiation of pain around the hip: (a) hip OA; (b) trochanteric bursitis.

with bending to put on socks, tights, and shoes; walking, manoeuvring stairs, and getting in and out of cars becomes increasingly difficult. In women, painful hip abduction during intercourse may be an added problem.

The principal examination finding is painful restriction of hip movement (both active and passive), with internal rotation in flexion, the first and most severely affected. Hip, but not knee movement, will reproduce referred pain. Anterior groin tenderness, lateral to the femoral pulsation, is common; pain and tenderness over the greater trochanter, worse when lying on that side, implies secondary trochanteric bursitis; an antalgic gait is usual. In advanced cases, wasting of gluteal and anterior thigh muscles may be apparent, with a Trendelenburg gait due to abductor weakness. A fixed flexion, external rotation deformity is the most usual end-stage result, with compensatory exaggerated lumbar lordosis and pelvic tilt. Ipsilateral leg shortening follows severe joint attrition and superior femoral migration.

Knee

The medial tibiofemoral (MTF), lateral tibiofemoral (LTF) and patellofemoral (PF) compartments share the same capsule, making the knee the largest synovial joint. This is a major target site for OA, showing associations with age, female gender, obesity, nodal OA, and CPPD deposition. As with the hip, categorization can be made by compartmental involvement. The MTF compartment is most commonly affected in terms of radiographic change (Fig. 8.24)[53], though with increasing imaging of the PF joint (Fig. 8.25) it is apparent that this is another common site, and one that may correlate more closely with symptoms[54]. Mono-

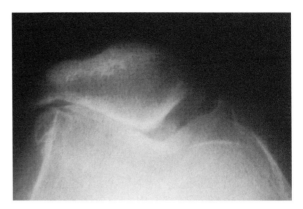

Fig. 8.25 Skyline radiograph of the knee showing severe patellofemoral OA with osteophyte and joint space narrowing.

compartmental (MTF or PF) and bicompartmental (MTF and PF) involvement is most common. Isolated 'primary' LTF OA is rare, but the LTF compartment becomes increasingly involved as OA progresses (associating with synovial fluid CPPD and apatite[37]). Knee involvement is usually bilateral and symmetrical, particularly in women. If strictly unilateral (mainly younger men), it is usually 'secondary' to mechanical insult / trauma such as meniscectomy.

Pain is well localized to the originating compartment. MTF OA gives anteromedial pain, mainly on walking. PF OA causes anterior knee pain, worse on negotiating stairs/inclines, and progressive aching on prolonged sitting that is relieved by standing and 'stretching' the legs. Well-circumscribed pain, felt away from the joint line, suggests a periarticular lesion; posterior pain usually indicates a complicating popliteal cyst (Fig. 8.26). Stiffness and 'gelling' are common at this site, particularly after sitting. Loss of function, especially for walking and bending, may result in major disability. Common complaints of 'giving way' mainly relate to altered patella tracking from quadriceps weakness, severe PF OA, or altered load bearing.

Examination commonly reveals coarse crepitus with joint-line tenderness (MTF, LTF) and/or pain on PF stressing. Flexion and extension are usually restricted and painful, and weakness of the quadriceps may result in quadriceps 'lag' (that is, more passive than active extension against gravity). Periarticular tenderness is common, particularly on the medial tibia below the MTF line (Fig. 8.27). Point tenderness at this site, with reproduction of pain on valgus stressing, suggests enthesopathy of the inferior insertion of the medial collateral ligament. More widespread tenderness, with warmth and soft-tissue swelling, suggests anserine bur-

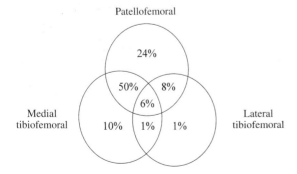

Fig. 8.24 Venn diagram showing patterns of compartmental disease in OA of the knee.

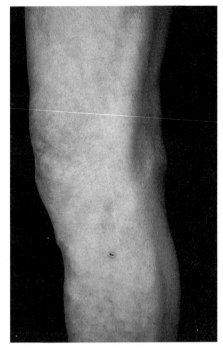

Fig. 8.26   Swelling due to a popliteal cyst complicating knee OA.

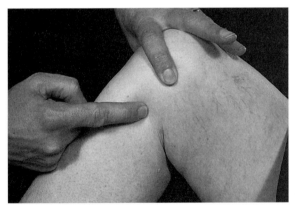

Fig. 8.27   A common periarticular tender site at the knee; the left index finger is placed over the medial joint line and the right index finger over the inferior insertion of the medial collateral ligament.

sitis (both lesions may coexist and distinction is often difficult). Tender medial fat pads are also common, especially in obese women. Signs of synovitis (warmth, effusions, synovial swelling, stress pain) are variable but modest effusions are not uncommon. Quadriceps muscle wasting is frequently present but often difficult to detect in the older patient. With time, bony swelling

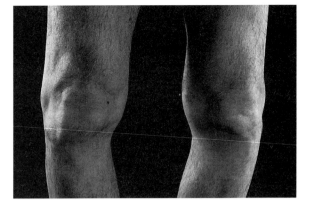

Fig. 8.28   Typical varus deformity with knee OA.

may be palpable and visible, especially along the anterior V-shaped contour of the bony ridges of the femoral condyles. Severe MTF OA may result in varus angulation as the typical deformity of OA (Fig. 8.28), often accompanied by some degree of fixed flexion. Valgus deformity, however, is not rare, particularly with extensive tricompartmental disease and associated calcium crystal deposition. Varus and valgus are best assessed standing; fixed flexion is best assessed lying on the couch. The gait is often antalgic; lateral 'thrust' during stance phase may occur with an unstable knee. Instability is not a usual consequence but may occur in advanced, destructive OA, or as a predisposing cause.

Foot and ankle

OA of the first metatarsophalangeal joint (MTPJ) is common but often asymptomatic. The usual deformity is hallux valgus, often with rotational deformity of the big toe (Fig. 8.29). Abnormal mechanical stress from

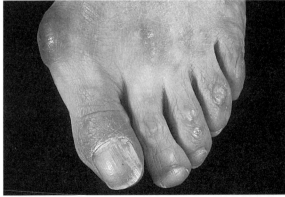

Fig. 8.29   Hallux valgus due to OA of the 1st MTPJ.

inappropriate footwear may encourage this deformity (it is rare in people who do not wear shoes) as may metatarsus primus varus. Secondary problems, which cause most symptoms, include medial fibrotic bursitis ('bunion') and cross-over toes. Hallux rigidus is less common and associates with large dorsal osteophytes which limit extension and thus interfere with the toe-off phase of walking.

OA changes, and nail dystrophy, similar to those in the hand, may affect the toe interphalangeal joints but are uncommon[55]. Osteophytes may develop in the talonavicular or calcanoecuboid joints, and, if large, may cause difficulties getting into shoes, and pain and stiffness when walking on uneven surfaces. Ankle and subtalar involvement is uncommon unless related to severe injury or preexisting structural abnormality; CPPD deposition may, however, occur at this site, especially in men.

Spine

'Degenerative' change in the spine is almost invariable and particularly targets the lower cervical and lower lumbar segments. By definition, OA is limited to the apophyseal (facet) synovial joints. However, apophyseal joint OA often, though not invariably, coexists with changes (for example, narrowing, osteophyte, disc protrusion) in nearby intervertebral joints, although the relationship between the two remains unclear. Such changes are often asymptomatic, though overall back pain is more common in those with radiographic 'degeneration'[56].

Lumbar spine OA may associate with chronic or intermittent 'mechanical' pain, usually aggravated by movement or standing. Although predominantly close to the spine, pain is often diffuse with radiation to the buttocks or leg. Cervical involvement similarly causes diffuse pain, maximal in the neck, but often radiating to the shoulder, the occiput, or down the arms. Pain is typically provoked by neck movements. The clinical picture is often complicated by pain and stiffness from coexisting ligamentous and muscular strains. Pain radiation down limbs from lower cervical or lower lumbar spine structures requires differentiation from pain due to root entrapment (Table 8.4).

Compared to peripheral joints, examination of the spine is generally unhelpful in differentiating periarticular from articular pain. Findings may include local segmental tenderness (centrally over interspinous ligaments, paracentrally over apophyseal joints), local muscle spasm, and painful reduced movement. Tenderness over the posterior ilio-lumbar ligament region, iliac crest, or occipital ridge are common, suggesting enthesopathy. A neurological examination and examination for hyperalgesic tender sites (with negative control sites) may be required in patients with an appropriate history suggesting root entrapment, spinal stenosis, or fibromyalgia.

Warning symptoms and signs

Acute or subacute synovitis

'Flares' of OA are common in terms of temporary exacerbation of pain and stiffness, and may be accompanied by signs of mild to modest synovitis. However, florid acute or subacute synovitis, especially if accompanied by marked erythema, should not be attributed to OA, and always requires urgent investigation for an alternative cause. A common superimposed acute problem is crystal synovitis (pseudogout; less commonly urate gout), which usually causes pain and signs that are at their worst within just 24–48 hours. Sepsis, however, should always be a concern (though rheumatoid arthritis and oral steroid therapy are stronger risk factors in adults than joint damage *per se*). Sepsis is

Table 8.4 Comparison between radiated axial pain and root entrapment

	Radiated	Root
Pain		
Maximal over or close to the spine	Yes	No
Clearly related to neck / back movement	Yes	No
Follows a dermatomal distribution	No	Yes
Eased by rubbing	Yes	No
Altered sensation		
Normal or hyperaesthetic	Yes	No
Reduced	No	±
Reduced power	No	±
Impaired reflexes	No	±

most commonly subacute in onset. Progressive pain and stiffness, additive joint involvement (for example, a flare in a 1st MTPJ, followed by flares in the ipsilateral ankle and then knee), and accompanying night sweats or malaise should always suggest sepsis, especially in a compromised OA patient (for example, with diabetes, renal impairment). In all such instances it is vital to aspirate the joint and examine fluid for sepsis (gram stain and culture) and crystals (compensated polarised microscopy). Sepsis and pseudogout may coexist and *both* investigations are mandatory.

Rapid progression

Rapidly worsening pain, or subacute onset of severe pain, is unusual in OA. Its occurrence should lead to consideration of osteonecrosis or fracture. Osteonecrosis most commonly occurs at the distal medial femoral condyle and femoral head, causing pain on weight bearing but also often marked ('bone') pain at night. Fracture pain is mainly noticed during weight bearing. Bone malignancy (mainly secondary deposits from lung, breast, prostate; or myeloma) adjacent to an OA joint may also cause progressive nocturnal and, eventually, persistent bone pain which is well localized and poorly correlates with joint movement. All three pathologies may be apparent on the plain radiograph; if not, however, a radionuclide scan is a useful and sensitive second investigation.

Locking

Sudden, painful, marked restriction on usage, usually lasting very briefly before spontaneously 'unlocking', strongly suggests an internal mechanical derangement. It is mainly limited to the knee and elbow. Osteochondral bodies, formed as part of the OA process, or a torn meniscus at the knee, are the usual causes. A history of recurrent, troublesome locking should lead to further investigation with a view to possible surgical intervention.

Usefulness and pitfalls of investigations

Radiology

The radiographic changes in OA are fully covered in Chapter 8.2. The main uses of plain radiographs in OA are:

- to support the clinical diagnosis of OA
- to further assess the degree of structural change and chondrocalcinosis
- to assess progression of structural change in large joints.

Although very helpful in these respects, the poor correlation between X-ray changes and symptoms has already been emphasized. Furthermore, radiographic OA is common in the older population and may be an incidental finding of little relevance to pain causation (for example, from a periarticular lesion or bone malignancy). Radiographs cannot, therefore, replace a sound history and clinical examination to answer the question 'why does this patient have pain at this site at this point in time?' Over-reliance on the radiograph for clinical decision-making should be avoided.

By comparison to radiographs, other imaging techniques are rarely required for clinical assessment of OA. MRI is particularly useful for soft tissue pathology, intracapsular derangement, and osteonecrosis; and bone scintigraphy for osteonecrosis, stress fracture, or suspected malignancy.

Laboratory tests

Blood and urine tests have no role in diagnosis of OA. Their main use is to confirm or exclude metabolic disease that predisposes to 'OA' or chondrocalcinosis (Table 8.5). Screening for disease is only justified in the situations of young-onset OA or chondrocalcinosis, florid polyarticular chondrocalcinosis, or presence of

Table 8.5 Initial biochemical investigations for metabolic disease predisposing to chondrocalcinosis or atypical, young-onset OA

Test	Disease
Serum ferritin, liver function	Hemochromatosis, Wilson's disease
Calcium, alkaline phosphatase	Hyperparathyroidism, hypophosphatasia
Serum magnesium	Hypomagnesemia
Thyroid function	Hypothyroidism
Urine homogentisic acid	Ochronosis

other suggestive clinical or radiographic features[39]. Routine screening in older subjects, other than for measurement of calcium level and thyroid function (done for other reasons in this age group) is unrewarding and not recommended. As yet, there are no biochemical 'markers' of OA for diagnosis or assessment of severity, progression, or prognosis (Chapter 8.3).

Although inflammatory markers and autoimmune profile are often undertaken to exclude inflammatory arthropathy these tests are imperfect in this respect. OA itself does not trigger a readily detected acute phase response. Elevations of erythrocyte sedimentation rate (ESR), C reactive protein, and plasma viscosity may, however, occur in a patient with OA from unrelated disease in other systems, or from the mild non-specific elevation (mainly ESR) that is common in the elderly. Such tests, therefore, do not exclude a clinical diagnosis of OA. Acute pseudogout may cause a marked acute phase response, sometimes equivalent to that of septic arthritis, and only synovial fluid analysis allows correct diagnosis. Rheumatoid factors (especially IgM, low titres) are non-specific and can occur in otherwise normal subjects; their presence, therefore, does not exclude OA as the clinical problem. Similarly, elevated serum uric acid associates with obesity, diuretic use, and renal impairment (common in many OA patients) and is of little diagnostic use; gout is only confirmed by finding urate crystals in synovial fluid or tophus aspirate.

Synovial fluid analysis

Synovial fluid in OA is generally 'non-inflammatory' with retained viscosity, low turbidity, and low cell count (mainly mononuclear). However, these features show wide variation and no diagnostic specificity. The main clinical value of synovial fluid analysis is:

(1) to confirm presence of CPPD crystals (to explain acute synovitis and chondrocalcinosis);

(2) to exclude sepsis in an acutely swollen OA joint, and;

(3) to confirm possible coexisting urate gout.

In conclusion, only a comprehensive history and examination of the patient, focusing on both the locomotor symptoms and the person will allow accurate diagnosis and assessment of OA. Investigations are helpful in only a few defined situations.

References

1. Cobb, S., Merchant, W.R., and Rubin, T. (1957). The relation of symptoms to osteoarthritis. *Journal of Chronic Disease*, 5, 197–204.
2. Helliwell, P.S. (1995). The semeiology of arthritis: discriminating between patients on the basis of their symptoms. *Annals of the Rheumatic Diseases*, 54, 924–6.
3. Bellamy, N., Sothern, R.B., and Campbell, J. (1990). Rhymic variation in pain perception in osteoarthritis of the knee. *Journal of Rheumatology*, 17, 364–72.
4. Lawrence, R.C., Everett, D., and Hochberg, M.C. (1990). Arthritis. In *Health status and well-being of the elderly: national health and nutrition examination — I:epidemiologic follow-up survey* (ed. R. Huntley and J. Cornoni-Huntley), pp. 136–51. Oxford University Press, New York.
5. Davis, M.A. (1981). Sex differences in reporting osteoarthritic symptoms: a sociomedical approach. *Journal of Health and Social Behaviour*, 23, 298–310.
6. Summers, M.N., Haley, W.E., Reveille, J.D., and Alarcon, G.S. (1988). Radiographic assessment and psychological variables as predictors of pain and functional impairment in osteoarthritis of the knee or hip. *Arthritis and Rheumatism*, 31, 204–9.
7. Davis, M.A., Ettinger, W.H., Neuhas, J.M., Barclay, J.D., and Segal, M.R. (1992). Correlates of knee pain among US adults with and without radiographic knee osteoarthritis. *Journal of Rheumatology*, 19, 1943–9.
8. Arnoldi, C.C., Lemperg, R.K., and Linderholm H. (1975). Intraosseous hypertension and pain in the knee. *Journal of Bone and Joint Surgery*, 57B, 360–3.
9. Merrit, J.L. Soft tissue mechanisms of pain in osteoarthritis. (1989). *Seminars in Arthritis and Rheumatism*, 18 (supplement 2), 51–6.
10. Fisher, N.M., Gresham, G., and Prendergast, D.R. (1993). Effects of a quantitative progressive rehabilitation program applied unilaterally to the osteoarthritic knee. *Archives of Physical Medicine and Rehabilitation*, 74, 1319–26.
11. Altman, R. (1991). Classification of disease:osteoarthritis. *Seminars in Arthritis and Rheumatism*, 20 (supplement 2), 40–7.
12. Croft, P., Rigby, A.S., Boswell, R., Schollum, J., and Silman, S. (1993). The prevalence of chronic widespread pain in the general population. *Journal of Rheumatology*, 20, 710–13.
13. Wolfe, F., Ross, K., Anderson, J., Russell, I.J., and Hebert, L. (1995). The prevalence and characteristics of fibromyalgia in the general population. *Arthritis and Rheumatism*, 38, 19–28.
14. Badley, E.M. (1995). The effect of osteoarthritis on disability on health care use in Canada. *Journal of Rheumatology*, 22 (supplement 43), 19–22.
15. McAlindon, T.E., Cooper, C., Kirwan, J.R., and Dieppe, P.A. (1993). Determinants of disability in osteoarthritis of the knee. *Annals of the Rheumatic Diseases*, 52, 258–62.
16. Cushnaghan, J., Cooper, C., Dieppe, P., Kirwan, J., and McAlindon, T. (1990). Clinical assessment of osteoarthritis of the knee. *Annals of the Rheumatic Diseases*, 49, 768–70.

17. Jones, A., Hopkinson, N., Pattrick, M., Berman, P., and Doherty, M. (1992). Evaluation of a method for clinically assessing osteoarthritis of the knee. *Annals of the Rheumatic Diseases*, **51**, 243–5.

18. Ledingham, J., Dawson, S., Preston, B., Milligan, G., and Doherty, M. (1992). Radiographic patterns and associations of osteoarthritis of the hip. *Annals of the Rheumatic Diseases*, **51**, 1111–16.

19. Doherty, M., Watt, I., and Dieppe, P. (1983). Influence of primary generalised osteoarthritis on development of secondary osteoarthritis. *Lancet*, **1**, 8–11.

20. Kellgren, J.H. and Moore, R. (1952). Generalised osteoarthritis and Heberden's Nodes. *British Medical Journal*, 181–7.

21. Hochberg, M.C., Lane, N.E., Pressman, A.R., Genant, H.K., Scott, J.C., and Nevitt, M.C. (1995). The association of radiographic changes of osteoarthritis of the hand and hip in elderly women. *Journal of Rheumabiogy*, **22**, 2291–4.

22. Doherty, M., Pattrick, M., and Powell, R. (1990). Nodal generalised osteoarthritis an autoimmune disease. *Annals of the Rheumatic Diseases*, **49**, 1017–20.

23. Egger, P., Cooper, C., Hart, D.J., Doyle, D.V., Coggon, D., and Spector, T.D. (1995). Patterns of joint involvement in osteoarthritis of the hand: the Chingford study. *Journal of Rheumatology*, **22**, 1509–13.

24. Stecher, R.M. (1995). Heberden's Nodes. A clinical description of osteoarthritis of the finger joints. *Annals of Rheumatic Diseases*, **14**, 1–10.

25. Hopkinson, N.D., Powell, R.J., and Doherty, M. (1992). Autoantibodies, immunoglobulins and Gm allotypes in nodal generalized osteoarthritis. *British Journal of Rheumatology*, **31**, 605–8.

26. Yaqub, R., Fawthrop, F., Bayliss, M., and Doherty, M. (1995). Levels of chondroitin sulphate (CS) and Keratan sulphate (KS) epitopes, glycosaminoglycans (GAGS) and hyaluronan in normal knee synovial fluid (SF). *British Journal of Rheumatology*, **34** (supplement 1), 103.

27. Acheson, R.M. and Collart, A.B. (1975). New Haven Survey of joint diseases. XVII. Relationships between some systemic characteristics and osteoarthrosis in a general population. *Annals of the Rheumatic Diseases*, **34**, 379–87.

28. Ehlich, G.E. (1972). Inflammatory osteoarthritis: I. The clinical syndrome. *Journal of Chronic Diseases*, **25**, 317–28.

29. Peter, J.B., Pearson, C.M., and Marmor, L. (1966). Erosive osteoarthritis of the hands. *Arthritis and Rheumatism*, **9**, 365–88.

30. Pattrick, M., Aldridge, S., Hamilton, E., Manhire, A., and Doherty, M. (1989). A controlled study of hand function in nodal and erosive osteoarthritis. *Annals of the Rheumatic Diseases*, **48**, 978–82.

31. Cobby, M., Cushnaghan, J., Creamer, P., and Watt, I. (1990). Erosive osteoarthritis: is it a separate disease entity? *Clinical Radiology*, **42**, 258–63.

32. Ehlich, G.E. (1975). Osteoarthritis beginning with inflammation: definitions and correlations. *Journal of the American Medical Association*, **232**, 157–9.

33. Doherty, M. and Dieppe, P. (1988). Clinical aspects of calcium pyrophosphate crystal deposition. *Rheumatic Disease Clinics of North America*, **14**, 395–414.

34. Menkes, C.J., Decraemere, W., Postel, M., and Forest, M. (1985). Chondrocalcinosis and rapid destruction of the hip. *Journal of Rheumatology*, **12**, 130–3.

35. Ledingham, J.M., Regan, M., Jones, A., and Doherty, M. (1995). Factors affecting radiographic progression of knee osteoarthritis. *Annals of the Rheumatic Diseases*, **54**, 53–8.

36. Doherty, M., Watt, I., and Dieppe, P.A. (1982). Localised chondrocalcinosis in post-meniscectomy knees. *Lancet*, **1**, 1207–10.

37. Pattrick, M., Hamilton, E., Wilson, R., Austin, S., and Doherty, M. (1993). Association of radiographic changes of osteoarthritis, symptoms, and synovial fluid particles in 300 knees. *Annals of the Rheumatic Diseases*, **52**, 97–103.

38. Doherty, M., Hamilton, E., Henderson, J., Misra, H., and Dixey, J. (1991). Familial chondrocalcinosis due to calcium pyrophosphate dihydrate crystal deposition in English families. *British Journal of Rheumatology*, **30**, 10–15.

39. Jones, A.C., Chuck, A.J., Arie, E.A., Green, D.J., and Doherty, M. (1992). Diseases associated with calcium pyrophosphate deposition disease. *Seminars in Arthritis and Rheumatism*, **22**, 188–202.

40. Dieppe, P.A., Doherty, M., MacFarlane, D.G., Hutton, C.W., Bradfield, J.W., and Watt, I. (1984). Apatite-associated destructive arthritis. *British Journal of Rheumatology*, **23**, 84–91.

41. Dieppe, P.A., Campion, G., and Doherty, M. (1988). Mixed crystal deposition. *Rheumatic Disease Clinics of North America*, **14**, 415–26.

42. Bird, H.A., Tribe, C.R., and Bacon, P.A. (1978). Joint hypermobility leading to osteoarthritis and chondrocalcinosis. *Annals of the Rheumatic Diseases*, **37**, 203–11.

43. Jónsson, H., Valtysdóttir, S.T., Kjartansson, O., and Brekkan, A. (1996). Hypermobility associated with osteoarthritis of the thumb base: a clinical and radiological subset of hand osteoarthritis. *Annals of the Rheumatic Diseases*, **55**, 540–3.

44. Hutton, C.W. (1987). Generalized osteoarthritis: an evolutionary problem? *Lancet*, **1**, 1463–5.

45. Acheson, R.M., Chan, Y., and Clemett, A.R. (1970). New Haven survey of joint diseases. XII: distribution and symptoms of osteoarthrosis in the hands with reference to handedness. *Annals of the Rheumatic Diseases*, **29**, 275–86.

46. Pattrick, M., Watt, I., Dieppe, P.A., and Doherty, M. (1988). Peripheral nerve entrapment at the wrist in pyrophosphate arthropathy. *Journal of Rheumatology*, **15**, 1254–7.

47. Doherty, M. and Preston, B. (1989). Primary osteoarthritis of the elbow. *Annals of the Rheumatic Diseases*, **48**, 743–7.

48. Chard, M. and Hazelman, B. (1987). Shoulder disorders in the elderly. *Annals of the Rheumatic Diseases*, **46**, 684–9.

49. de Seze, S., Babault, A., and Ramdon, S. (1968). L'epaule senile hemorrhagique. *L'Actualite Rhumatologique*, **1**, 107–15.

50. Pearson, J.R. and Riddell, D.M. (1962). Idiopathic osteoarthritis of the hip. *Annals of the Rheumatic diseases*, **21**, 31–7.

51. Solomon, L. (1976). Patterns of osteoarthritis of the hip. *Journal of Bone and Joint Surgery*, **41**, 118–25.

52. Croft, P., Cooper, C., Wickham, C., and Coggon, D. (1992). Is the hip involved in generalised osteoarthritis? *British Journal of Rheumatology*, **31**, 325–8.

53. Ledingham, J.M., Regan, M., Jones, A., and Doherty, M. (1993). Radiographic patterns and associations of osteoarthritis of the knee in patients referred to hospital. *Annals of the Rheumatic Diseases*, **52**, 520–6.

54. McAlindon, T.E., Snow, S., Cooper, C., and Dieppe, P.A. (1992). Radiograpic patterns of osteoarthritis of the knee joint in the community: the importance of the patellofemoral joint. *Annals of the Rheumatic Diseases*, **51**, 844–9.

55. McKendry, R.J. Nodal osteoarthritis of the toes. (1986). *Seminars in Arthritis and Rheumatism*, **16**, 126–34.

56. Symmons, D.P.M., van Hemert, A.M., Vandenbroucke, J.P., and Valkenburg, H.A. (1991). A longitudinal study of back pain and radiological changes in the lumbar spines of middle aged women. II. Radiological findings. *Annals of the Rheumatic Diseases*, **50**, 162–6.

57. Lawrence, J.S. (1977). Osteoarthrosis. In *Rheumatism in populations*, pp. 98–155. Heinemann, London.

8.2   Plain radiographic features of osteoarthritis

Frank M. Jewell, Iain Watt, and Michael Doherty

The plain radiograph remains a key investigation in the clinical management of osteoarthritis (OA). It is particularly helpful for:

(1) diagnosis — showing characteristic structural changes typical of OA and absence of features of alternative arthropathies (for example, inflammatory erosive disease);

(2) assessment of the severity of structural change;

(3) identification of associated chondrocalcinosis.

In interpreting the radiographs a number of important caveats need to be remembered, most importantly:

(1) the common discordance between symptoms, disability, and degree of structural OA change — for determination of symptom causation, the radiograph is no substitute for a thorough history and examination;

(2) requirement of optimal views and techniques — for example, in certain joints the assessment of joint space narrowing requires stressed (loaded) views;

(3) lack of specificity of individual radiographic features;

(4) difficulties with quantification of OA changes — the radiograph is relatively insensitive for detection of early OA and minor progression of cartilage and bone change (as may be required for intervention studies; see Chapter 11.5);

(5) a static, not dynamic, assessment — the radiograph provides an anatomical record of prior OA change; scintigraphy and magnetic resonance imaging (MRI) are more informative of current dynamic, physiological change.

The radiograph does, however, provide a readily available, safe, and cost-effective means of assessing gross OA change. For clinical decision-making purposes it is a sufficiently reliable, informative investigation of joint structure such that other imaging modalities are infrequently required.

In this chapter, the individual radiographic features of OA will be described and explained. The characteristic changes and important complications encountered at target sites will then be illustrated.

Radiographic features of OA

The radiological features of OA are most easily understood in terms of the underlying pathology[1]. The simplest concept involves initiation of OA within cartilage and bone at points of high stress. Focal cartilage degeneration ensues, with associated attrition of the underlying subchondral bone. Elsewhere in the joint, stress shielding occurs and a reparative process characterized by new bone formation ensues. The disease is thus characterized by simultaneous occurrence of destructive changes and attempts at repair.

The four main radiographic features of OA are joint space narrowing, subchondral sclerosis and subchon-

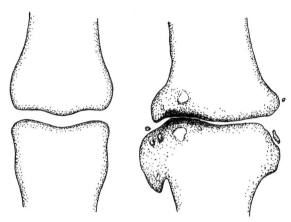

Fig. 8.30   Diagram of a normal (left) and OA (right) joint, showing focal joint space narrowing, adjacent subchondral sclerosis, marginal osteophyte, cysts, and osteochondral bodies typical of OA.

dral cyst formation which represent destruction, and osteophytosis which represents attempted repair (Fig. 8.30). In addition, other features such as osteochondral body formation, synovial abnormalities, and crystal deposition may be observed.

Joint space narrowing

Loss of cartilage is a cardinal feature of OA. It is usually focal and tends to predominate at sites of maximum load-bearing within individual joints. The focal thinning of cartilage is an important observation that allows differentiation of OA from other arthropathies, such as rheumatoid arthritis, which commonly cause generalized cartilage loss. There are exceptions to this, such as diffuse cartilage loss occurring in the small phalangeal joints of the hand and, occasionally, in the ankle joint.

Cartilage is not imaged directly on conventional radiographs, but hyaline cartilage thickness can be estimated from the width of the joint space. This assumes that opposing joint surfaces are in contact and may require weight bearing or stress views to ensure this is so. The inability to demonstrate the internal structure of hyaline cartilage means that advanced pathological changes such as focal ulceration can be present without any change in joint space width[2]. Such insensitivity is not a practical problem in diagnostic terms because other features of OA are usually present. However, there is a significant problem when joint space width is used as a marker of disease progression. In addition to the lack of sensitivity to focal pathologi-

cal change within the cartilage, there are technical problems related to precision and accuracy in the assessment of joint space width. Errors arise from technical aspects of image production and radiographic positioning of the patient. Image quality will determine the smallest change in joint space width that can be detected. This is compromised by geometric distortion arising from the X-ray source, variable spatial resolution of film/screen combinations, and reduced contrast from X-ray scatter within the patient. In practice, these can be minimized by using X-ray tubes with a small focal spot, use of non-screen film, and a Bucky grid to reduce scatter. However, there are compromises to be made and methods vary depending on the joint to be imaged. The variability in patient positioning is important as even small alterations may cause considerable error in joint space width measurement. Custom-built adjustable positioning apparatus can be used to standardize patient position for studies of disease progression (Fig. 8.31). The method can be further refined using computerized analysis of digital

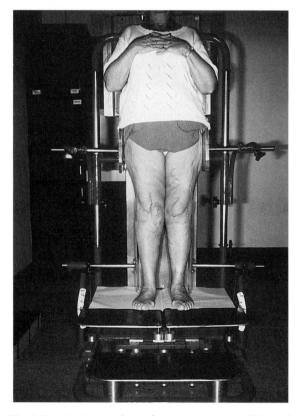

Fig. 8.31   Positioning device for ensuring reproducibility of radiographic positioning for knee radiography.

images. In dedicated hands, measurements with a precision of a few per cent can be obtained. However, the rate of progression of disease is so slow that detection of change in a short time scale of a few months is unrealistic using current methodology. Quantitative methods using macroradiography show more promise[3].

Subchondral sclerosis

Changes in the thickness and biomechanical properties of hyaline cartilage during the evolution of OA cause increased transmission of forces to the subchondral bone. Initially, the bone responds with increased local blood flow and deposition of new bone on existing trabeculae. Eventually, this physiological response is overwhelmed. Trabecular microfractures, and then macroscopic bony collapse, may ensue. This progression is identified on plain radiographs by development of subchondral sclerosis at the sites of maximal stress. In time, frank bony collapse can be visualized. In general, subchondral sclerosis does not develop until cartilage thinning is recognizable. Areas of a joint denuded of hyaline cartilage are usually associated with a striking degree of adjacent radiographic subchondral bony sclerosis. The surface of the denuded zone appears smooth and polished to the orthopedic surgeon or pathologist. This is referred to in pathological terms as eburnation. Remodeling of the subchondral bone can result in grooving of the articular surface.

Physiological trabecular condensation may occur at some sites and must not be confused with the pathological sclerosis of OA (Fig. 8.32); it may be seen in the lateral aspect of the acetabulum in the hip, and sometimes in the medial tibial plateau of the knee. Support for a physiological response may be gained from recognition of a normal joint space width, and clinical evidence of increased joint stress, such as an active lifestyle and increased body mass.

Subchondral cyst formation

Subchondral cysts are a typical feature of OA but they are also seen in other arthropathies. They are known by a multitude of other names including geodes, synovial cysts, and necrotic pseudocysts. The plethora of descriptions reflects the absence of a definitive account of their causation. The term 'cyst' is most commonly used but is strictly erroneous because these cavities are not lined by epithelium. They occur within areas of bony sclerosis at sites of increased pressure transmis-

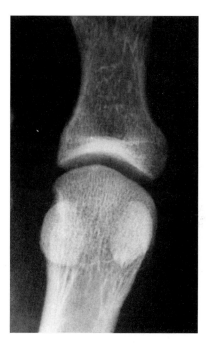

Fig. 8.32 Normal subchondral trabecular condensation at the base of the proximal phalanx in the first metatarsophangeal joint.

sion. Two mechanisms of formation are postulated and they are not necessarily mutually exclusive. The synovial fluid intrusion mechanism envisages the passage of synovial fluid from the joint cavity to the subchondral bone via fissured or ulcerated cartilage, with pressure necrosis of trabeculae allowing cavitation. The bony contusion theory postulates direct subchondral bony injury as a consequence of diminished hyaline cartilage, with cavities forming secondary to traumatic bony necrosis.

Radiographically, the cysts occur in areas of increased joint stress and are associated with bony sclerosis and joint space narrowing (Fig. 8.33). Communication with the articular surface can occasionally be demonstrated. They may be multiple, but are rarely more than 2 cm in diameter. Larger cysts raise the possibility of an accompanying disorder such as rheumatoid arthritis or a crystal arthropathy. If typical associated radiographic features are not present, then a wider differential diagnosis for subchondral cyst formation should be considered (Table 8.6).

Osteophyte formation

Osteophytes are the hallmark of OA. These bony outgrowths occur most commonly at the margins of

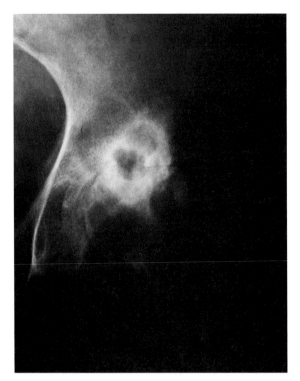

Fig. 8.33 Prominent subchondral cysts in the acetabular roof of an osteoarthritic hip.

osteoarthritic joints, by a process of enchondral ossification at the junction of hyaline cartilage and synovium / periosteum. The stimulus causing metaplasia of synovium into cartilage and subsequent osteophyte growth is unknown, but may be related to reduced stress transmission consequent on changes elsewhere in the joint[4]. Teleologically, osteophytes can be regarded as an attempt at repair and redistribution of abnormal joint loading. One way of achieving this is by tighten-

ing up of capsular laxity and minimizing the unloading of peripheral hyaline cartilage.

Osteophytes are most easily recognized radiographically as bony excrescences at joint margins tangential to the X-ray beam. It is easily forgotten that marginal osteophytes consist of continuous lips of new bone formation around the edges of a joint. Viewed *en face* they may be seen as bands of sclerosis or even mimicking cartilage calcification. Osteophytes may develop early in the evolution of OA and can be seen prior to reduction in joint space width. They can arise in unusual sites such as the intercondylar notch in the knee, where they are easily confused with loose bodies. These central osteophytes arise from enchondral ossification of residual islands of hyaline cartilage and are sometimes referred to as 'stud' or 'button' osteophytes. Certain joints demonstrate new bone formation from periosteum in contradistinction to enchondral ossification of peripheral and central osteophytes. Such periosteal osteophytes form along the femoral neck in OA of the hip. This phenomenon is known as 'buttressing' and is regarded as a response to altered mechanical stresses across the joint (see Fig. 8.30).

There is rarely any problem identifying osteophytes on conventional radiographs. Care must be taken not to confuse the normal age-related remodeling of joint anatomy, which results in squaring of usually rounded articular margins, with true osteophytes. Traction from joint capsules and ligamentous attachments may also result in bony spur formation, but these should not be confused with osteophyte.

Osteochondral bodies

Disintegration of the joint surface in OA results in chondral or osteochondral fragments breaking free into the joint space. These osteochondral bodies may be

Table 8.6   Causes of subchondral bone lucency

---

1 Arthropathies
　　Osteoarthritis
　　Rheumatoid arthritis
　　Metabolic disorders (Gout and hemochromatosis)
　　Hemophilia
2 Synovial proliferation
　　Pigmented villonodular synovitis
　　Amyloid
3 Miscellaneous (usually solitary)
　　Non-neoplastic cysts (post-traumatic cysts and intraosseous ganglion)
　　Benign bone tumors (chondroblastoma and giant cell tumor)
　　Malignant bone tumors (myeloma and metastases)
　　Tuberculosis

---

loose or may become incorporated into the synovium. They may alter in size and appearance by a process of resorption or accretion. Alternatively, chondroid metaplasia may occur *de novo* in the synovium with subsequent ossification. The composition of such bodies is also variable; many show features of partial enchondral ossification, others may be more irregular and consist of dense bone only.

Radiographically, osteochondral bodies occur in the presence of established features of OA (Fig. 8.34). They may vary in size and position, and can disappear completely. They often gravitate to characteristic sites within individual joints and may sometimes be difficult to visualize due to overlapping bony structures. They may even migrate into adjacent bursae such as a popliteal cyst.

Care must be taken not to confuse osteochondral bodies with normal anatomical structures such as the fabellum behind the knee, or anatomical variants such as unfused accessory ossification sites. Other pathological conditions may give rise to osteochondral bodies, including osteochondritis dissecans or synovial osteochondromatosis. The former occurs in young people without accompanying radiographic features of OA; the latter is a metaplastic condition of synovium. Enormous numbers of uniformly small cartilaginous bodies may be produced, in contrast to OA in which a small number of variably sized osseous bodies are usually seen.

Calcification

Calcification of fibrocartilage and hyaline cartilage is commonly associated with OA joints (Fig. 8.35). Such calcification can occur in isolation as an asymptomatic incidental finding and is increasingly common with old age. When it occurs with OA, the reparative response may be quite florid, and result in a rather hypertrophic form of OA known as pyrophosphate arthropathy. Such an association may indicate a poorer prognosis for the joint. This is particularly the case in the knee and hip where joint destruction may be rapid. The deposited calcium salt is usually calcium pyrophosphate, although crystals of hydroxyapatite may coexist. This subject is dealt with in more detail in Chapter 7.2.6. Chondrocalcinosis also occurs more frequently in certain metabolic conditions[5], and a summary of related conditions is shown in Table 8.7. Conventional

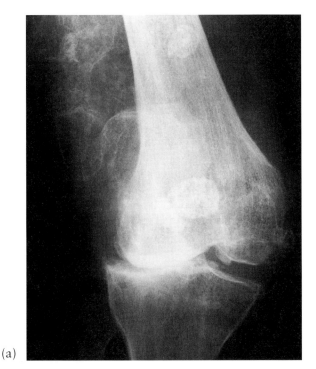
(a)

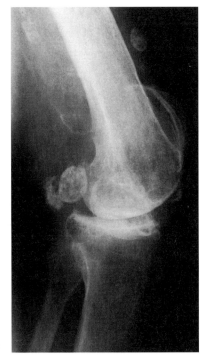
(b)

Fig. 8.34(a) and (b). Multiple large osteochondral bodies in a patient with severe OA of the medial compartment of the knee. There is associated varus deformity and subluxation of the patella.

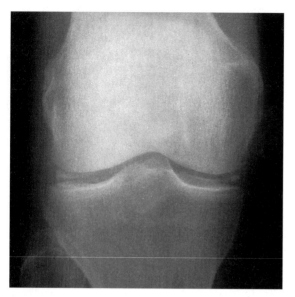

Fig. 8.35   Chondrocalcinosis is present in both menisci in the knee.

radiographs are insensitive at demonstrating chondrocalcinosis, although improved detection rates can be achieved with macroradiography. Crystal shedding and cartilage attrition may result in some variability in the degree of cartilage calcification present at any one time.

In addition to cartilage, other structures such as synovium, capsule, entheses and, occasionally, bursae may calcify.

Additional features of advanced OA

Pathological studies demonstrate synovial thickening with some features of chronic inflammation in OA. The consensus view is that these synovial abnormalities have no role in the pathogenesis of OA and simply

reflect a secondary response of the synovium to joint damage. This response varies in intensity and may lead to the formation of a joint effusion.

Asymmetrical loss of cartilage may result in altered joint mechanics and acceleration of joint damage. Deformity ensues, resulting in stretching of joint capsules and ligaments, as well as major functional impairment.

Extensive regional osteonecrosis of subchondral bone may occur rarely; the condition is not detected initially on plain radiographs. Subsequently, extensive subchondral bony collapse may be seen. Typical sites include the femoral head and the medial femoral condyle (Fig. 8.36). Idiopathic osteonecrosis in this setting is associated with OA but can also occur in its absence.

Characteristics of OA in individual joints

Interphalangeal joints

OA in the interphalangeal (IP) joints is usually symmetrical, involving multiple joints. The typical patient is a middle-aged female with predominantly distal interphalangeal (DIP) joint involvement. Proximal IP joints may be affected, but only rarely in isolation, and association with DIP OA is the rule (Fig. 8.37).

Typical radiographic features include joint space narrowing and marginal osteophytes. In comparison with inflammatory arthropathies, in which erosions occur at joint margins, OA involves the full width of the articular surface. Diffuse joint space narrowing occurs, with congruent undulating articular surfaces creating the 'seagull' sign. Marginal osteophytes are prominent and are easily detected clinically due to the paucity of over-

Table 8.7   Conditions associated with chondrocalcinosis

1 Familial predisposition (usually polyarticular with variable degrees of arthropathy)
2 Previous joint insult (mono- or pauci-articular chondrocalcinosis: following meniscectomy or surgery for osteochondritis dissecans etc.)
3 Osteoarthritis (calcium pyrophosphate dihydrate crystal deposition with or without radiographic chondrocalcinosis)
4 Metabolic disorders (polyarticular chondrocalcinosis)
   – hyperparathyroidism
   – hemochromatosis (arthropathy in addition to chondrocalcinosis)
   – hypophosphatasia
   – hypomagnesemia
   – hypothyroidism
   – gout, acromegaly, familial hypocalciuric hypercalcemia

Note: Florid polyarticular chondrocalcinosis or chondrocalcinosis occurring before age 60 should always lead to consideration of metabolic or familial predisposition.

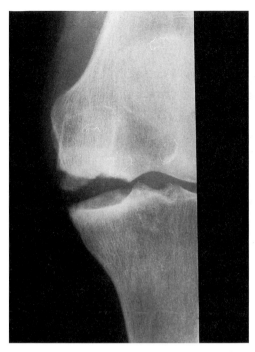

Fig. 8.36 Osteonecrosis of the medial femoral condyle is demonstrated and results in frank destruction and fragmentation of the subchondral bone and articular surface.

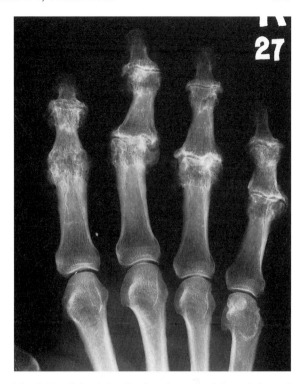

Fig. 8.37 OA of the distal and proximal interphalangeal joints. Note the characteristic grooving of the distal articular surface and horizontal subluxation. (c) A radiograph of DIP joints of a patient with psoriasis showing marginal erosions. (d) A radiograph of a patient with erosive OA demonstrating central destruction of hyaline cartilage.

lying soft tissue. They are associated with Heberden's nodes in the DIP joints and Bouchard's nodes in the PIP joints. When deformity occurs it is usually in the form of radial or ulnar deviation, compared to flexion extension deformities in rheumatoid arthritis.

Metacarpophalangeal joints

Involvement of the metacarpophalangeal (MCP) joints with OA is unusual in the absence of involvement of the DIP and PIP joints. The typical features of OA are present and the loss of joint space may be diffuse in a similar fashion to the IP joints. Osteophytes and subchondral cysts are usually more prominent on the radial aspect of the metacarpal head, though the reason for this is unclear. MCP joint OA of the thumb can occur without accompanying changes in the IP joints. Middle and index finger MCPJ OA may be seen as a result of a lifetime of sustained heavy labour (Fig. 8.38).

The differential diagnosis of MCP joint OA is usually straightforward when multiple joints in the hand are involved. When MCP joints are affected in relative isolation then other diagnoses should be con-

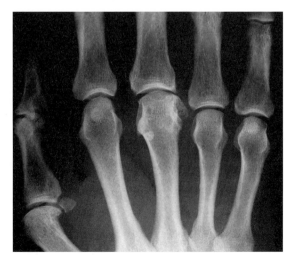

Fig. 8.38 OA of the third MCP joint. Note the extensive marginal osteophytes and asymmetric loss of joint space.

sidered. In particular, hemochromatosis has a predilection for MCP joint involvement. It may manifest hook-like osteophytes, identical to those seen in OA. However, hemochromatosis produces multiple small subchondral cysts in several MCP joints and may occur at a relatively young age (less than 55 years), whilst OA creates larger and fewer geodes. Corroborating evidence of a crystal arthropathy may be found elsewhere in the hand, for example, chondrocalcinosis of the triangular ligament with radiocarpal arthropathy. There may also be involvement of other joints less frequently affected by OA, such as the ankle.

Wrist and carpus

The most commonly affected joints in the carpus are the carpometacarpal (CMC) joint of the thumb and the scapho-trapezium (ST) articulation. The CMC joint demonstrates typical features of OA and is usually seen in association with multiple DIP joint involvement. Initially, the radiographic abnormalities are confined to the trapezium-metacarpal joint. Progression to include the remaining articulations of the trapezium may occur, especially involvement of the ST joint. Isolated OA of the ST joint is not uncommon. The main features are joint space narrowing and subchondral sclerosis (Fig. 8.39). Osteophytes are not often visualized on conventional radiographs; there are no atypical radiographic features of OA in these joints. Radial subluxation of the metacarpal may be a feature of CMC joint OA in the thumb.

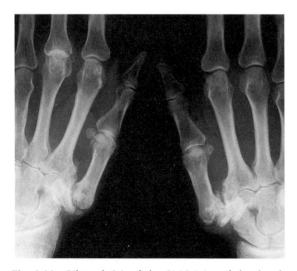

Fig. 8.39   Bilateral OA of the CMC joint of the thumb, demonstrating joint space loss with subchondral sclerosis.

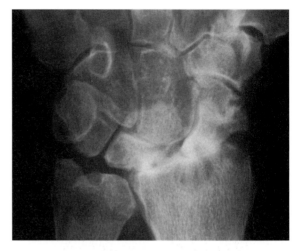

Fig. 8.40   Severe radiocarpal OA associated with non-union of a fracture of the waist of the scaphoid.

OA in the remainder of the carpus and the wrist joint is unusual in the absence of a history of trauma or avascular necrosis. Certain patterns of joint arthritis may be recognized from the radiographs. For example, instability associated with scaphoid fractures may result in radio-scaphoid arthritis (Fig. 8.40). This may progress to involve intercarpal joints and, ultimately, scapho-lunate advanced collapse (SLAC). Another example is the occurrence of radiocarpal and midcarpal joint OA in conjunction with chondrocalcinosis: these are the features of pyrophosphate arthropathy.

Elbow

OA of the elbow is relatively unusual in the absence of trauma or other internal mechanical derangement. Typical features of repair and destruction are noted as in other joints. All three compartments may be involved but there is usually more severe change in the humero-radial compartment. Elbow OA may occur in association with MCPJ OA, particularly in middle-aged men[6]. Patients with OA may complain of 'locking', caused by loose osteochondral bodies (Fig. 8.41). The reduced degree of freedom imposed by a hinge joint means that very small osteochondral fragments can cause severe functional problems. Such small loose bodies may be difficult to identify on routine radiographs. They are usually found in the olecranon recess of the joint cavity and may require further imaging such as air arthrography, CT, or MRI to confirm their presence.

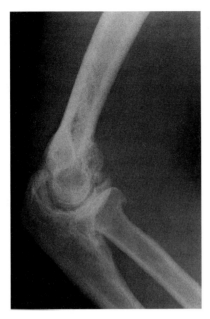

Fig. 8.41 Lateral radiograph demonstrating OA of the elbow. Features include marginal osteophytes, joint space narrowing, and a loose osteochondral body projected over the anterior aspect of the joint.

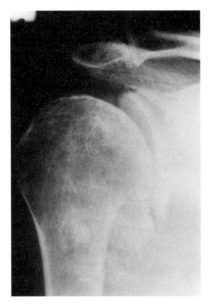

Fig. 8.42 A frontal view of the shoulder demonstrating OA of the glenohumeral joint. Note the prominent inferior humeral head osteophyte and asymmetrical joint space loss. There is also OA of the acromioclavicular joint is also present.

Shoulder

Several pathological processes may occur in the shoulder region. OA of the acromioclavicular (AC) joint is very common with increasing age. Conversely, primary OA of the glenohumeral joint is much less frequent. However, it is not uncommon for a pre-existing condition such as rotator cuff disease to be present, which predisposes to gleno-humeral joint OA. Radiographic features include localized thinning of articular cartilage, initially in the postero-superior portion of the glenoid and humeral head. This corresponds to the area of contact at the point of maximal joint loading in abduction. Subchondral sclerosis and cyst formation is seen. Osteophytes may be identified around the glenoid margin; humeral head osteophytes are typically seen inferomedially in the region of the anatomical neck (Fig. 8.42). They are demonstrated to best advantage if the arm is held in external rotation. Calcification of the hyaline cartilage of the humeral head and the fibrocartilage of the glenoid labrum may also be seen. In some cases, OA may progress as a more atrophic form, with destruction of the femoral head as the prominent feature and little accompanying regenerative bony change. These are the features of AADA (apatite

associated destructive arthropathy) or 'Milwaukee' shoulder.

Signs of previous trauma or associated rotator cuff disease may be detected (Fig. 8.43). Indirect evidence of rotator cuff disease includes the presence of possible sources of impingement (for example, the presence of ACJ OA with inferior acromial osteophytes), sclerosis, and cortical irregularity of the rotator cuff insertion on the greater tuberosity and superior migration of the humeral head. Caution is advised in the use of measurements of the width of the subacromial space in the assessment of rotator cuff disease. Estimates will vary depending on the angle of the X-ray beam. Ideally, the subacromial space is optimally visualized with approximately 15° of caudal angulation of the beam. In such cases, the normal subacromial space should measure at least 8 mm in width. Generalized thinning of articular cartilage, in the presence of eburnation and osteophytosis, should raise the possibility of secondary reparative OA, following a previous inflammatory arthropathy such as rheumatoid arthritis.

Hip

OA of the hip exhibits all the cardinal signs mentioned earlier in the chapter. The variation in the pattern of radiographic abnormalities suggests that patients with

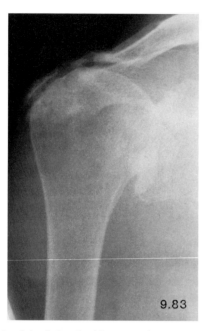

9.83

Fig. 8.43 OA of the shoulder, secondary to rotator cuff disease. Rupture of the cuff has allowed superior migration of the humeral head with subsequent pressure erosion of the acromion and lateral end of the clavicle.

OA of the hip form a heterogeneous group who may share different precipitating factors. These radiographic patterns will be described without discussion of etiology. Individual radiographic features of OA will then be considered, with a discussion of some important points in differential diagnosis.

The hemispherical head of the femur articulates with the cup-shaped acetabulum in a ball and socket configuration. However, the articular cartilage of the acetabulum is horseshoe-shaped, rather than hemispherical, because of the presence of the acetabular notch. This deficiency, and the presence of acetabular anteversion, means that hyaline cartilage is distributed predominantly superolaterally and posteromedially (alternatively referred to as inferomedially). The pattern of joint space narrowing in OA may, thus, vary depending on the precise location of focal hyaline cartilage loss. Such patterns are more easily appreciated early in the development of OA. Classification may be more difficult in established arthritis.

The most common site of joint space narrowing is in the superior weight-bearing portion of the joint. Superolateral migration is the most common pattern in both sexes and is usually unilateral[7]. It incorporates superior joint space narrowing and lateral migration of the femoral head, with accompanying widening of the posteromedial joint space. The associated features of OA such as cyst formation, osteophytosis, and sclerosis are predominantly superolateral. This pattern of migration is seen in dysplastic hips (Fig. 8.44(a)). Superomedial migration is more commonly seen in women and is often bilateral (Fig. 8.44(b)). Superior joint space narrowing occurs with resorption along the superolateral aspect of the femoral head, and osteophytosis along the femoral neck and medial/inferior aspect of the femoral head. This process results in apparent medial slipping of the femoral head.

Posteromedial migration (Fig. 8.44(c)) of the femoral head is usually bilateral and more common in women. It is difficult to explain selective joint space narrowing in a zone of low stress — variations in acetabular design, increased varus angulation of the femoral neck, and association with generalized OA have been considered, but no definite answer exists. The radiographic appearances include narrowing of the posteromedial joint space, with associated preservation or widening of the lateral joint space width. Lateral and medial osteophytosis may occur.

Axial migration includes features of the previously described patterns and results in concentric loss of hyaline cartilage (Fig. 8.44(d)). Associated features of OA are present and mild protrusio acetabuli may occur. It is less common than the other patterns of migration.

Florid osteophytosis is easily identified on routine images of the hip. However, even well-established osteophytosis can be missed if insufficient attention is paid to analyzing the radiograph. Concentric femoral head marginal osteophytes may be indicated by innocuous and easily overlooked zones of sclerosis. Acetabular osteophytes are seen along the posterior acetabular margin and can be made inconspicuous by the overlying femoral head. Central osteophytes are seen adjacent to the fovea on the femoral head and around the margin of the acetabular notch.

Subchondral cyst formation in OA of the hip may be a more prominent feature than in other joints. Cysts may occur on both sides of the joint and can occur early in the disease process. Such cysts may be very large and are sometimes the earliest feature in the acetabular roof.

Calcification may be seen in the acetabular labrum and is associated with calcification of the symphysis pubis.

OA of the hip is routinely assessed using frontal views only; weight-bearing radiographs are not com-

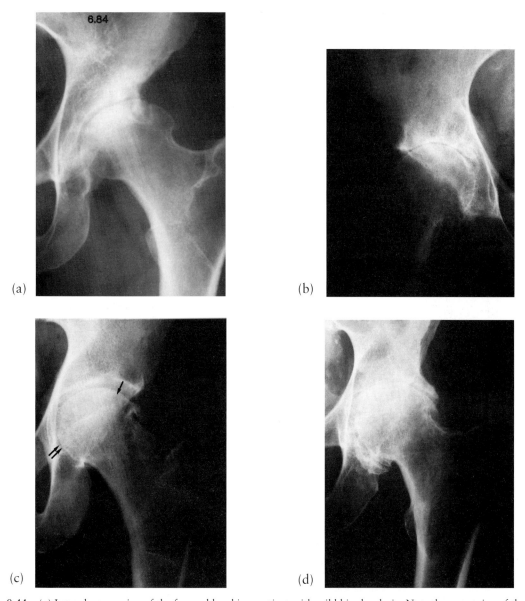

Fig. 8.44 (a) Lateral uncovering of the femoral head in a patient with mild hip dysplasia. Note the narrowing of the lateral joint space, subchondral cyst formation, and 'collar' osteophyte around the femoral head. (b) Typical changes of OA in the superior and medial aspects of the hip joint. There is almost complete loss of hyaline cartilage with prominent acetabular cysts. (c) Posteromedial OA of the hip. Note the relative widening of the superolateral joint space (arrow) caused by loss of postero-medial joint space width (double arrow). (d) Concentric joint space narrowing with florid reparative features of OA.

monly performed. Lateral views may assist in detecting postero-inferior OA. If required, further detail of the distribution of cartilage loss can be determined using CT.

The differential diagnosis of OA in the older age group is not usually a problem. More careful consideration is required in premature OA, rapidly progressive disease, and when OA is secondary to previous

inflammatory arthropathy or synovial disorder. These difficulties are considered in a later section (see p. 234).

Knee

The knee is the joint most commonly affected by OA. It is a complex joint which endures considerable mechanical stresses in the course of life. Many factors causing alteration in the mechanical forces acting through the knee can predispose to OA. The usual features of OA are demonstrated, but the distribution of change may vary and can provide clues to the underlying cause.

The **tibio-femoral compartments** consist of medial and lateral joint spaces. In OA it is the medial compartment which is usually worst affected, though both may be involved and, occasionally, medial and lateral compartments may be equally affected (Fig. 8.45). Osteophytosis is usually prominent and may be the earliest radiological sign of OA. Osteophytes are most easily identified at the articular margins of the tibia on the frontal view and along the margins of the femoral condyles on the lateral view. Central osteophytes arising from the mesial articular margins of the femoral condyles and the tibial spines are also seen. A prominent anterior intercondylar tibial bump may develop (Parson's third intercondylar spine; see Fig. 8.46)[8]. Joint space narrowing may be severe and can result in direct apposition of femoral and tibial bone surfaces. Subchondral sclerosis and loss of hyaline cartilage occur concomitantly, with sclerosis usually more pronounced on the tibial aspect of the joint. Subchondral cysts are less common than in the hip and usually occur in the tibia rather than the femur.

The **patellofemoral compartment** is affected as commonly, if not more so, than the medial tibio-femoral compartment[9]. The patella possesses two articular facets, medial and lateral. The lateral facet is broader and is much more commonly the site of OA. This is related to the higher transmitted forces arising from the valgus configuration of the normal knee. Joint space

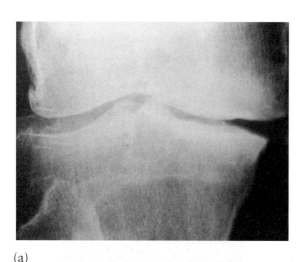

(a)

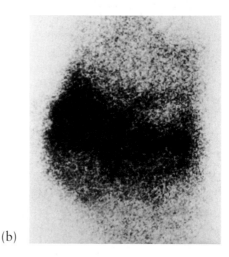

(b)

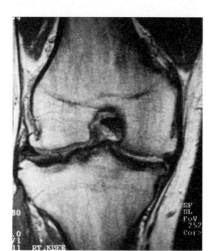

(c)

Fig. 8.45 OA of the knee is illustrated using different imaging modalities in order to demonstrate typical features and to highlight some of the shortcomings of plain radiographs. (a) Typical OA affecting both tibiofemoral compartments of the right knee. Marginal osteophytes are present in addition to subchondral sclerosis and joint space narrowing medially. (b) A late-phase bone scan of the same knee demonstrates markedly increased uptake of radionuclide in the subchondral bone of both compartments, especially on the lateral side. The discrepancy in the findings of the two studies illustrates the limitations of plain radiographs in deriving physiological information. (c) A coronal T1 weighted magnetic resonance image of the knee shows osteophyte, subchondral sclerosis, and joint space narrowing more clearly than the plain radiograph. In addition, the distribution of cartilage loss is evident in the medial joint compartment, the menisci can be assessed, and ligamentous integrity can be evaluated.

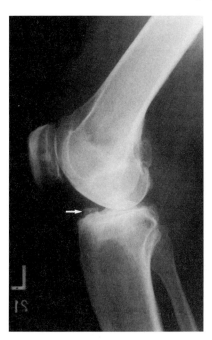

Fig. 8.46 Parson's bump is indicated on this lateral view of the knee (arrow).

narrowing, subchondral sclerosis, and osteophyte formation occur (Fig. 8.47). Lateral subluxation of the patella is a common feature. Joint space narrowing may be difficult to judge on a lateral view, particularly when a joint effusion is present. Eventually, bony apposition may occur between the patella and the anterior cortex of the lower femur. Anterior scalloping of the femur ensues as a result of pressure erosion (Fig. 8.48). Osteophytic lipping is readily identified at the upper and lower poles of the patella and is sometimes quite florid.

Additional features of OA such as joint deformity secondary to ligamentous laxity and osteochondral body formation are often seen in the knee. The fabellum possesses hyaline cartilage and articulates with the posterior surface of the lateral femoral condyle. It may develop features of OA such as sclerosis and osteophyte formation, and may enlarge as an early feature of OA.

Calcification is detected on knee radiographs with increasing frequency in older age groups. Approximately seven per cent of octogenerians will demonstrate articular calcification on knee X-rays. The most common site is in the menisci, where it may appear rather globular, followed by the hyaline cartilage, where it usually has a linear distribution. More rarely, calcification may also be noted in the synovium and ligamentous attachments.

The knee is anatomically and biomechanically complex. Consequently, the routine frontal and lateral

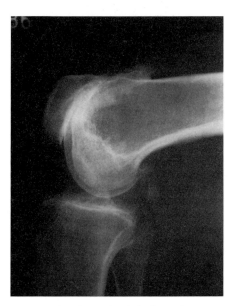

Fig. 8.47 Lateral radiograph of the knee showing marked loss of patellofemoral joint space width, subchondral sclerosis, and marginal osteophytes.

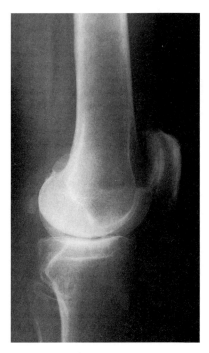

Fig. 8.48 Lateral radiograph of the knee demonstrating pressure erosion on the anterior surface of the lower femur in patellofemoral joint arthritis.

views do not provide all the information required by clinicians for assessing disease severity and planning treatment. Specific specialized radiographic views have been developed to derive additional information.

Weight-bearing views

Routine radiographs of the knee are obtained with the patient lying on an X-ray table. Such radiographs may understimate the extent of hyaline cartilage loss and the degree of angular deformity in the joint. Antero-posterior weight-bearing views allow simultaneous imaging of both knees, and more realistic assessment of lateral subluxation and varus/valgus deformity (Fig. 8.49). It has been estimated that weight-bearing views may result in an additional two to five milli-metres of joint space narrowing in affected tibiofemoral compartments[10]. Lateral weight-bearing views are not usually performed because they are technically more difficult and add no useful additional information.

'Skyline' views

The X-ray beam passes through the patellofemoral joint from below, with the knee held in thirty degrees of flexion (Merchant's view). This method affords excellent assessment of patellofemoral joint space separately for both medial and lateral facets. Focal loss of hyaline cartilage, horizontal displacement of the patella, subchondral cysts, and marginal osteophytes are easily assessed (Fig. 8.50).

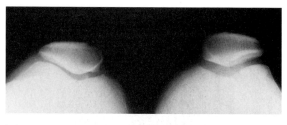

(a)

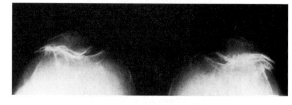

(b)

Fig. 8.50 Merchant's view of the patellofemoral joints. Early lateral facet OA is demonstrated in (a). Advanced OA with prominent grooving of the articular surfaces is shown in (b).

Tunnel views

Frontal radiographs acquired with the knee in flexion permit improved visualization of the intercondylar notch region. This may be advantageous in the evaluation of central osteophytes or in localizing possible loose osteochondral bodies.

Stress views

Joint laxity cannot be assessed on routine views. When the full extent of ligamentous laxity is required then manual stress applied during acquisition of the radiograph can provide an objective measure. In practice, these views are not often requested.

Load line views

The net vector of forces transmitted through the lower limb passes through the femoral head and the centre of the ankle mortise. The usual arrangement is for this line to intersect the knee in the intercondylar region. Abnormal skeletal design, in the form of developmental bone dysplasia or malunited fractures, may result in excess transmission of forces to one of the tibiofemoral condyles and predispose to OA. Long-leg films, which include both legs from hip to ankle, allow direct assessment of the load line (Fig. 8.51). This is particularly

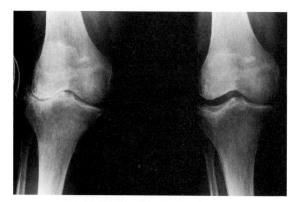

Fig. 8.49 Two views of the same knee with medial compartment OA in the standing (left) and supine (right) positions. These images convincingly demonstrate how non-weight-bearing views may underestimate loss of hyaline cartilage and deformity.

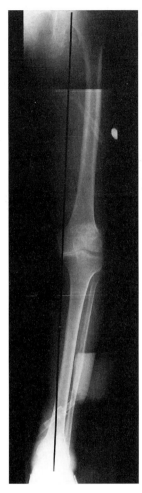

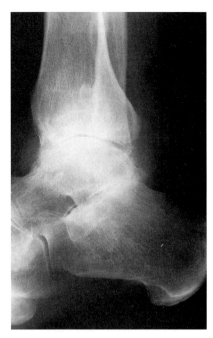

Fig. 8.52 Severe OA of the ankle is demonstrated on this lateral radiograph, with accompanying changes in the subtalar joint. The patient had suffered a previous ankle fracture.

Fig. 8.51 A long-leg frontal radiograph shows the load line passing medial to the intercondylar region because of the varus deformity caused by medial joint compartment OA.

useful in pre operative assessment of angular deformity, prior to osteotomy or joint replacement.

Ankle

OA of the ankle is unusual in the absence of predisposing factors. The most common reason is a previous fracture, particularly if the ankle mortise is involved. Abnormal biomechanics following subtalar fusion may also result in secondary OA.

The typical features of OA are seen on ankle radiographs. Reduction in joint space width may be diffuse rather than focal (Fig. 8.52); Joint space narrowing is more easily appreciated on weight-bearing views but these are not routinely performed. Marginal osteo-

phytes are readily recognized on frontal and lateral projections. Care must be taken not to mistake true osteophyte from capsular tug lesions and talar beaking seen in abnormal subtalar joint motion.

Great toe metatarsophalangeal joint

OA of the first metatarsophalangeal (1st MTP) joint is very common. This reflects the considerable mechanical forces transmitted through the joint during ambulation. OA at this site also occurs in young people in their second or third decade. The reason for this is not clear but may be caused by unrecognized chondral or osteochondral trauma. In older patients, hallux valgus deformity, associated with metatarsus primus varus, may result in OA.

Radiographic changes include joint space narrowing, sclerosis, marginal osteophytosis, and valgus deformity (Fig. 8.53). Osteophytes are most prominent over the dorsal surface of the metatarsal head and are best demonstrated on a lateral standing view of the foot. Osteophytes are also seen around the margins of the sesamoid bones. Medial and lateral sesamoids articulate with the planter surface of the first metatarsal head and are seen to good advantage on tangential views of the flexed forefoot.

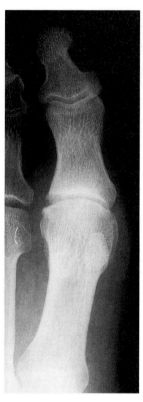

Fig. 8.53   OA of the great toe MTP joint. Features include asymmetric joint space narrowing with osteophytes, modest subchondral sclerosis, and small geodes.

Posterior facet joint OA in the spine

Posterior facet joint OA becomes more frequent with increasing age and is commonly associated with spondylotic change but not invariably. Facet joint OA is often seen at different levels from the associated degenerate disc disease. Other predisposing factors to facet joint OA include scoliosis and trauma. Facet joint configuration is variable between patients and at different levels in the spine. As a result, routine antero-posterior and lateral views visualize the joints with differing degrees of success, at different spinal levels. Facet joints are also curved in space so that the X-ray beam is tangential to only a small portion of the joint in any single projection. In spite of these caveats, OA of the facet joints can be identified. Joint space narrowing and osteophytosis may not always be detected, but the accompanying sclerosis usually is. This is most commonly seen in the lower lumbar spine at L5/S1 (Fig. 8.54(a)). Optimal assessment of the facet joints requires computed tomography (Fig. 8.54(b)).

Patterns of OA

OA is not a simple condition. Testimony to this statement are the variations in the pattern of multiple joint involvement, the variable natural history of OA progression, and differences in the response of individual joints. Each of these factors will be considered in turn.

Patterns of joint involvement

Kellgren and Moore[11] described a particular pattern of joint involvement in idiopathic (primary) OA. Typically, the other joints involved, in patients with Heberden's nodes, included the proximal interphalangeal joints of the hand, the thumb carpometacarpal joint, the great toe metatarsophalangeal joint, the spinal apophyseal joints, and the knees. This pattern was more common in middle-aged women. Subsequently, a non-nodal (that is, not associated with Heberden's nodes) type, favouring involvement of wrists and hips in men, was described[12]. It is generally accepted that subgroups of polyarticular forms of OA exist, although epidemiological studies do not all agree on the exact details of joint involvement and sex predilection[13].

Another described variant of polyarticular OA is inflammatory or erosive OA[14]. This condition afflicts middle-aged females. It is usually rapid in onset, with clinical features of an inflammatory arthropathy involving the distal interphalangeal joints of the hands symmetrically, and the CMC joint of the thumb and trapezio-scaphoid articulation on the radial aspect of the hand. The radiological features include joint space narrowing, sclerosis, and marginal osteophytes. In addition, erosive changes are seen which characteristically involve the central portion of the joint at sites of hyaline cartilage thinning (Fig. 8.55). Periosteal new bone formation may accompany erosive change and, eventually, bony ankylosis can occur. Following ankylosis, the proliferative bony response abates, and osteophytes and sclerosis may disappear. These radiographic changes are most commonly seen in the distal interphalangeal joints. Other sites such as the MTP and IP joints of the feet, knees, hips, and spinal apophyseal joints may be symptomatic, but radiographic erosions are unusual. The relationship of erosive OA to non-erosive OA is unclear. The remarkably similar pattern of joint involvement in the hand in both disorders, and variability in the degree of erosive change on radiographs, suggest that erosive

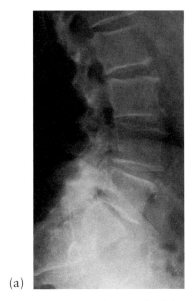
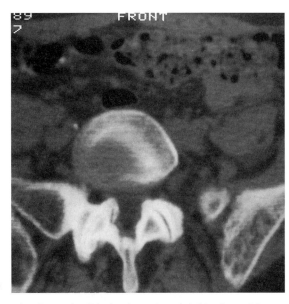

(a)   (b)

Fig. 8.54   Facet joint OA at the L5 S1 level shown (a) on a lateral radiograph of the lumbar spine, and (b) using axial computed tomography, which demonstrates joint space narrowing, sclerosis, and marginal osteophyte formation.

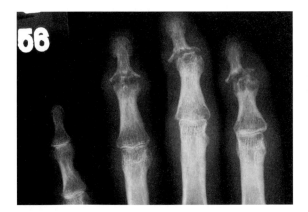

Fig. 8.55   Erosive OA in the DIP joints, showing prominent erosive changes in addition to the usual features of OA.

OA represents one extreme of a continuum of joint response[15].

A particular pattern of joint involvement is seen in pyrophosphate arthropathy in which features of OA are associated with chondrocalcinosis. In addition to OA of weight-bearing joints such as the knees and hips, OA is seen more frequently, and with greater severity than normal, in less commonly affected joints such as the radiocarpal, elbow, and glenohumeral articulations. Furthermore, the presence of chondrocalcinosis in the knee is associated with more severe OA of the patellofemoral joint.

Natural history of disease progression

The natural history of OA varies considerably between different joints and different people. As a generalization, most patients demonstrate slow radiographic progression, with little change over many years. Disease progression tends to occur more rapidly in smaller joints, with the slowest rate of change observed in the knee. Disease activity may also be episodic, with changes over several months followed by a long period of stabilization during which no discernible radiographic progression may occur.

These observations hinder the use of radiographs for quantitative assessment of disease activity. Kellgren and Lawrence[16] developed a grading system for OA which remains the standard reference for defining radiographic severity. Common to grading systems in other arthropathies, such as rheumatoid arthritis, these methods are insensitive to small changes in disease status. Furthermore, the divisions between disease stages are arbitrary. This is a particular problem in OA because disease progression may be very slow. Alternative methods of quantifying disease progression using reproducible radiographic techniques and sophisticated bone texture analysis are discussed elsewhere[17].

Variations in the response of individual joints

The degree of reparative response in OA joints varies between individuals; it may also vary within a particular individual at different times. This phenomenon has given rise to the concept of hypertrophic and atrophic forms of OA, though in practice considerable overlap occurs and a spectrum of activity can be demonstrated. Hypertrophs mount a vigorous reparative response and exhibit florid osteophytosis, with marked sclerosis and frequent osteochondral body formation. Atrophs have poorly developed osteophytes and sclerosis. They are associated with joint effusions containing the biochemical products of subchondral bone attrition. Such individuals are commonly elderly and female. This phenomenon reflects the variability in the response of joints to insult and contributes to the heterogeneity of the OA population. It also complicates radiographic assessment of disease activity.

Considerations in the differential diagnosis of OA

Recognition of the typical features of OA on a radiograph should not signify completion of the diagnostic process. In most cases, a diagnosis of primary OA will be correct. However, consideration should be given to the available clinical and radiographic clues, so that secondary OA and coexistent medical conditions are not overlooked. This approach will be illustrated in the following scenarios.

Premature OA

Premature OA may be defined (somewhat arbitrarily) as occurring before 55 years of age. It may occur without any discernible predisposing factors. Patients may give a family history of premature OA, perhaps reflecting abnormal matrix architecture. OA in a young adult patient involving a single joint should prompt a search for a predisposing factor. Evidence of previous fracture, surgery, or osteochondritis dissecans may be visible on the radiograph. Modeling deformities may

indicate previous insults such as slipped femoral capital epiphysis or Perthe's disease in the hip.

Early OA involving multiple joints may be caused by developmental disorders such as multiple epiphyseal dysplasia, or an endocrine disorder such as acromegaly. Mild dysplastic change is easily overlooked (see Fig. 8.44(a)). The presence of chondrocalcinosis in the setting of premature OA should suggest the possibility of hemochromatosis.

Secondary reparative OA

Osteopenia and diffuse loss of joint space width, in the presence of typical features of OA, should raise the possibility of secondary osteoarthritic change following a previous inflammatory arthropathy such as rheumatoid arthritis or septic arthritis (Fig. 8.56). The reparative features of OA may be so florid as to obscure evidence of a pre-existing articular disorder; this may occur in gouty arthritis and hemophilia. Both conditions produce geodes which may be confused with subarticular cysts associated with OA.

Rapidly progressive OA

Rapidly progressive OA of the hip can occur in elderly patients after a prolonged period of stabilization and without any obvious precipitating cause (Fig. 8.56). However, this event is infrequent and warrants serious consideration of other disorders. These include avascular necrosis of the femoral head, occult infection, neuroarthropathy, and previously unrecognized crystal

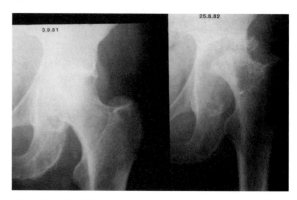

Fig. 8.56 Rapid destruction of the hip joint is demonstrated in this female patient over a twelve-month period. No precipitating cause was found.

arthropathy. Radiographic evidence of avascular necrosis may be present, such as flattening and ill definition of the cortex of the sclerosed femoral head. Chondrocalcinosis in the hip joint, or symphysis, may suggest crystal-associated arthropathy. Joint infection in the elderly may be indolent, and the usual features of an aggressive inflammatory disorder such as intense osteopenia and erosions may be absent.

Severe pain

Severe pain in a joint with radiographic features of OA should stimulate a search for complications or alternative diagnoses. A rare complication of knee OA is osteonecrosis of the medial femoral condyle. Initial radiographs may be normal or show subtle subchondral lucency with ill definition of the cortical margin. Substantial bony collapse may ensue. The presence of a joint effusion should raise the possibility of infection or acute crystal arthropathy such as pseudogout. Severe pain in the hands of elderly patients with nodal OA of the interphalangeal joints should raise the possibility of superimposed gout: this may be induced by diuretic therapy. Radiographic clues include the presence of soft tissue tophi, erosions, and florid osteophytosis in addition to the usual features of OA.

Erosive change

The presence of erosions alongside features of OA in the hands may cause confusion with other erosive arthropathies. In fact, the characteristic symmetrical DIP distribution, coupled with the presence of central rather than marginal erosive change, means that erosive OA is readily distinguished from other erosive arthropathies such as rheumatoid arthritis and psoriasis (Fig. 8.57)[18]. It should not be forgotten that radiological features of specific arthropathies may take time to develop. There may be clinical pointers to rheumatoid arthritis or gout in patients with OA, and such patients may present prior to the development of characteristic X-ray changes.

Summary

The plain radiograph remains the dominant imaging modality in the diagnosis and assessment of OA. The basic features of OA have been described, along with specific findings in individual joints. The radiographic features amount to a history of the response of the joint to previous insults. Different patterns of disease, involvement of different joint compartments, and variation in rate of disease progression testify to the heterogeneity of this fascinating disorder.

References

1. Resnick, D. (1995). *Diagnosis of bone and joint disorders* (3rd edn), 1263–371. W.B. Saunders, Philadelphia.
2. Buckland-Wright, J.C. (1994). Quantitative radiography of osteoarthritis. *Annals of the Rheumatic Diseases*, **53**, 268–75.
3. Buckland-Wright, J.C., Macfarlane, D.G., and Lynch, J. (1992). Relationship between joint space width and subchondral sclerosis in the osteoarthritic hand: a quantitative microfocal radiographic study. *Journal of Rheumatology*, **19**, 788–95.
4. Thompson, R.C. and Bassett, R.C. (1970). Histological observations on experimentally induced degeneration of articular cartilage. *Journal of Bone and Joint Surgery (Am)*, **52**, 435–43.
5. Jones, A.C., Chuck, A.J., Arie, E.A., Green, D.J., and Doherty, M. (1992). Diseases associated with calcium pyrophosphate deposition disease. *Seminars in Arthritis and Rheumatism*, **22**, 188–202.
6. Doherty, M. and Preston, B. (1989). Primary osteoarthritis of the elbow. *Annals of the Rheumatic Diseases*, **48**, 743–7.
7. Ledingham, J., Dawson, S., Milligan, G., and Doherty, M. (1992). Radiographic patterns and associations of osteoarthritis of the hip. *Annals of the Rheumatic Diseases*, **51**, 1111–16.
8. Brossman, J., White, L.M., Stabler, A., Preidler, K.W., Andresen, R., Haghighi, P. *et al.* (1996). Enlargement of the third intercondylar tubercle of Parsons as a sign of osteoarthritis of the knee — a paleopathologic and radiographic study. *Radiology*, **198**, 845–9.
9. Ledingham, J., Regan, M., Jones, A., and Doherty, M. (1993). Radiographic patterns and associations of osteoarthritis of the knee in patients referred to hospital. *Annals of the Rheumatic Diseases*, **52**, 520–6.
10. Leach, R.E., Gregg, T., and Siber, F.J. (1970). Weight bearing radiography in osteoarthritis of the knee. *Radiology*, **97**, 265–8.
11. Kellgren, J.H. and Moore, R. (1952). Generalised osteoarthritis and Heberden's nodes. *British Medical Journal*, **1**, 181–7.
12. Kellgren, J.H., Lawrence, J.S., and Bier, F. (1963). Genetic factors in generalised osteoarthritis. *Annals of the Rheumatic Diseases*, **22**, 237–54.
13. Buchanon, W.W. and Park, W.M. (1983). Primary generalised osteoarthritis: definition and uniformity. *Journal of Rheumatology*, **10**(supplement 9), 4.

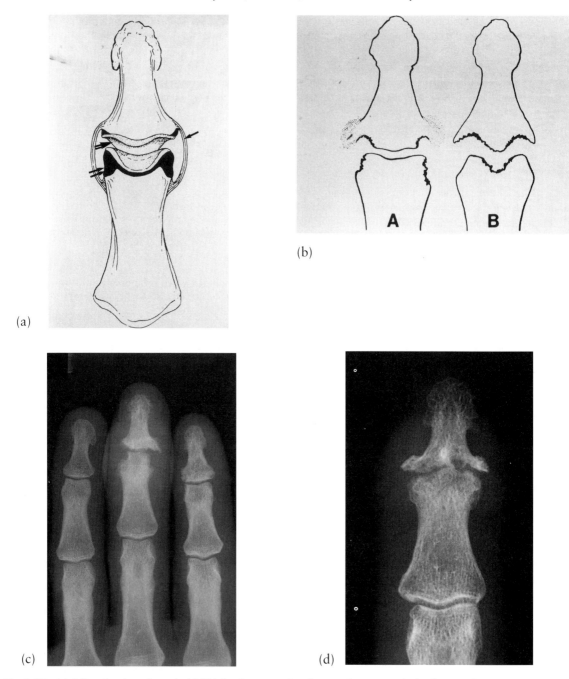

Fig. 8.57 (a) A line drawing of a typical DIP joint demonstrating the capsule (arrow), the hyaline cartilage (open arrow), and the bare area between the attachment of the synovium and the margin of the articular surface (double arrow). (b) Typical distribution of erosive change occurring within the bare area in inflammatory arthropathies, such as psoriasis, is shown on the left (A). The usual central pattern of joint destruction in OA, corresponding to hyaline cartilage, is shown on the right (B). (Figures 8.57 (a) and (b) are produced with permission from Martel[18]).

14. Crain, D.C. (1961). Interphalangeal osteoarthritis characterised by painful inflammatory episodes resulting in deformity of the proximal and distal articulations. *Journal of the American Medical Association*, **175**, 1049–53

15. Cobby, M., Cushnaghan, J., Creamer, P., Dieppe, P.A., and Watt, I. (1990). Erosive osteoarthritis: is it a separate disease entity? *Clinical Radiology*, **42**, 258–63.

16. Kellgren, J.H. and Lawrence, J.S. (1957). Radiological assessment of osteoarthritis. *Annals of the Rheumatic Diseases*, **16**, 494–501.

17. Lynch, J.A., Hawkes, D.J., and Buckland-Wright, J.C. (1991). Analysis of texture in macroradiographs of osteoarthritic knees using fractal signature. *Physics in Medicine and Biology*, **36**, 709–22.

18. Martel, W., Stuck, K.J., Dworin, A.M., and Hylland, R.G. (1980). Erosive osteoarthritis and psoriatic arthritis: a radiologic comparison in the hand, wrist and foot. *American Journal of Roentgenology*, **134**, 125–35.

8.3   The natural history and prognosis of osteoarthritis

Cyrus Cooper and Elaine Dennison

Introduction

Osteoarthritis (OA) is the most frequent joint disorder in the world today[1]. The term describes a complex disease process in which a combination of systemic and local mechanisms result in characteristic pathological and radiological changes. These abnormalities are often, but not always, associated with symptoms and disability. OA has been recognized in all human populations which have been examined to-date, and can be found in skeletal remains from periods in evolution as far back as Neolithic times[2]. It also occurs in several animal species, particularly the dog and horse. Despite this ubiquity, our understanding of the etiology, clinical features, and natural history of OA remains incomplete. This chapter reviews three aspects of the disorder: (1) approaches to definition; (2) measurement of OA and descriptive epidemiological characteristics of the disorder; and (3) the rate and determinants of progression.

Definition

The subdivision of arthritic conditions into discrete pathological entities is a relatively recent phenomenon in the history of medicine[3]. Earlier this century, pathologists differentiated between two broad groups of arthritis: atrophic and hypertrophic. Atrophic disorders were characterized by synovial inflammation with erosion of cartilage and bone, and came to include rheumatoid and septic arthritis. The hypertrophic group were never subdivided, however, and gradually became synonymous with what is now termed OA. The term thus encompasses a large and heterogeneous spectrum of idiopathic joint disorders.

Any working definition of OA entails consideration of pathologic, radiologic, and clinical components[4]. The key pathological feature is focal destruction of articular cartilage, which is followed by changes in subchondral bone. Cartilage denudation increases the stress borne by underlying bone, resulting in microfractures and cyst formation in areas of increased intra-articular pressure. Consequent reparative changes in bone include bony sclerosis and osteophyte formation. The precise relationship between these features of the disorder remain unclear. Osteophyte, for example, is often found in the lower limb joints of elderly people without evidence of cartilage loss or diffuse subchondral sclerosis. In practical terms, however, studies of the natural history of OA depend upon assessment of radiological and clinical indices which purport to represent these underlying pathological changes. In recent years, these have been supplemented by a number of other process markers of the disorder, for example, biochemical markers and novel imaging techniques. The strengths and weaknesses of these approaches will now be discussed.

Radiographic assessment of OA

The radiographic features currently used to assess OA were originally selected to measure various aspects of cartilage loss and subchondral bone reaction. Although several radiographic grading systems have been proposed over the last 15 years, most epidemiologic studies have utilised the Empire Rheumatism Council system, first described over three decades ago[5]. This system, developed by Kellgren and Lawrence, assigns one of five grades (0–4) to OA at various joint sites: knee, hip, hand, and spine. Grading is performed by comparing the index radiograph with reproductions in a radiographic atlas. The criteria for increasing severity of OA are shown in Table 8.8 and relate to the assumed sequential appearance of osteophytes, joint space loss, subchondral sclerosis, and cyst formation.

Epidemiological studies support the notion that any radiographic grading system for OA should be joint specific. The age- and sex-specific prevalence of OA, the individual risk factors for the disorder, and the relationship between radiographic change and symptoms are all known to differ according to joint site. There are, however, two important caveats to the use of this overall grading system. First, inconsistencies in the descriptions of radiographic features of OA by Kellgren and Lawrence themselves, have led to studies being performed using criteria which are discordant[6]. Second, the prominence awarded to the osteophyte at all joint sites remains controversial. To address these issues, recent studies have broken up this overall radiographic grading system into its component features, quantified each feature more precisely, and assessed the reproducibility and clinical correlates of each. These studies have been attempted for OA at the knee, hip, and hand.

For the knee, each of joint space narrowing, osteophyte, and the overall Kellgren and Lawrence grade showed good within-observer reproducibility, but the scoring of osteophyte was most closely associated with knee pain[7]. At the hip, comparison of joint space narrowing, osteophyte, sclerosis, and an overall grading system suggested that measurement of joint space was more reproducible than that of osteophyte, sclerosis, or the composite score, and was the most closely associated with reported hip pain[8]. Finally, in the hand, joint space narrowing, osteophyte, and overall Kellgren / Lawrence grade can all be assessed reproducibly, but osteophyte appears to be more closely associated with pain[9]. Although these findings require confirmation by future studies, it is clear that a need exists for a standardized approach to the categorization of individual radiographic features at these different joint sites. Recent atlases of standard radiographs have helped in ensuring a more consistent approach to the grading of individual features and permit greater extrapolation between the results of different studies.

Radiographic measures also remain a cornerstone in the assessment of the progression of OA. A consensus meeting of the American Academy of Orthopedic Surgeons, the National Institutes of Health, and the World Health Organisation has recently produced recommendations for the use of radiographic measures for this purpose[10]. Careful attention must be paid to patient positioning and to inclusion of views which permit assessment of different compartments of a joint. Thus, assessment of the knee requires a weight-bearing view in the anteroposterior projection, as well as views to include the patellofemoral compartment (either supine lateral or skyline). For the hip joint, progression should be recorded for joint space narrowing, both by millimetre measurements of the interbone distance and

Table 8.8   The Kellgren Lawrence grading system of OA

---

1 Radiologic features on which grades were based
   (a) Formation of osteophytes on the joint margins or, in the case of the knee joint, on the tibial spines
   (b) Periarticular ossicles; these are found chiefly in relation to the distal and proximal interphalangeal joints
   (c) Narrowing of joint cartilage associated with sclerosis of subchondral bone
   (d) Small pseudocystic areas with sclerotic walls, situated usually in the subchondral bone
   (e) Altered shape of the bone ends, particular in the head of the femur
2 Radiographic criteria for assessment of OA
   Grade 0   None   No features of OA
   Grade 1   Doubtful   Minute osteophyte, doubtful significance
   Grade 2   Minimal   Definite osteophyte, unimpaired joint space
   Grade 3   Moderate   Moderate diminution of joint space
   Grade 4   Severe   Joint space greatly impaired with sclerosis of subchondral bone

---

Reproduced from Spector *et al.*[6]

by visual grading (0–3 according to a standardized atlas). Femoral osteophytes are graded 0–3 and features such as subchondral bone cysts, sclerosis, attrition, and migration pattern can be recorded as present or absent. Radiographic features of knee disease should be recorded separately for the medial, lateral, and patellofemoral compartments. As with the hip, the narrowest point of the tibiofemoral joint space can be measured in millimetres, and both joint space narrowing and osteophyte can be graded 0–3 in all compartments. Although advanced techniques can be used to assist assessment of the radiographs, for example, digitization of the images with computerized methods for the assessment of interbone distance or osteophyte, these techniques remain research tools and have not yet superseded radiographic assessment by eye.

Clinical assessment

The major symptoms of OA in a joint are:

- use-related pain
- stiffness
- loss of movement.

Major signs are:

- bony swelling
- crepitus
- joint margin tenderness
- cool effusion
- decreased range of movement
- instability.

Pain is undoubtedly the most important symptom; it tends to be use-related and associated with stiffness after inactivity. There is a documented discrepancy between radiographic grade and reporting of pain (Fig. 8.58), and this relationship is influenced by gender and the joint site under consideration. In the earliest epidemiological studies, women were more likely to report pain than men, and the concordance between pain and radiographic damage was strongest for the hip and weakest for the hand. With more sophisticated methods of assessing OA, it became clear that there is a gradation between the severity of radiographic disease and the prevalence of symptoms in a given joint. This is illustrated in Table 8.9 which shows the progressively increasing prevalence of reported hip pain among men aged 60–75 years, according to the degree of joint space narrowing apparent on their

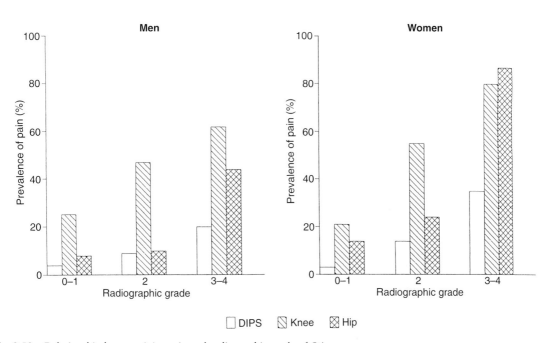

Fig. 8.58 Relationship between joint pain and radiographic grade of OA.

Table 8.9   Risk of reported hip pain according to degree of joint space narrowing among 60–75-year-old men

Minimum joint space (mm)	*OR for hip pain	95% CI
3.0+	1.0	–
2.0–2.4	1.6	1.1–2.3
1.5–1.9	2.2	1.4–3.6
1.0–1.4	5.1	2.3–11.4
< 1.0	12.2	3.3–45.7

*OR = odds ratio; CI = confidence interval
Data derived from Croft *et al.*[8]

pelvic radiographs. There are a number of potential mechanisms for pain in OA, including raised intraosseous pressure, inflammatory synovitis, periarticualr problems, periosteal elevation, muscle changes, and central neurogenic changes.

Among the clinical signs of OA, bony swelling of the affected joint and crepitus stand out as being highly repeatable[11] and discriminatory between OA and other joint disorders. The usefulness of other signs, for example, soft tissue swelling, instability, and joint margin tenderness in the diagnosis and monitoring of OA currently remains uncertain.

Assessment of clinical outcome in the disorder has been the subject of intensive research in the last decade. The properties of outcome measurement instruments in OA are important in determining the most appropriate methodology for studies; reliability, validity, and responsiveness to change are the three key criteria. The World Health Organisation currently recommend the use of either the Western Ontario and MacMaster Universities (WOMAC) OA index or the Lequesne algofunctional index for the monitoring of hip or knee OA[12,13]. These indices are statistically more efficient than a multiplicity of unidimensional measures, and appear to detect changes in pain and physical function with greater sensitivity than either the Stamford Health Assessment Questionnaire or Arthritis Impact Measurement Scales. The Lequesne index includes assessment of pain, stiffness, walking distance, and daily-living activities for the hip and knee. Both disease-specific instruments may be supplemented by generic health status measures, most widely used of which are the shortform 36 (SF-36), the Nottingham Health Profile, and Euroquol.

Other techniques for assessing natural history

There are other investigative modalities which may be of assistance in characterizing the natural history of OA. At the present time, these remain essentially research tools the use of which in routine clinical practice remains to be validated.

Radionuclide scintigraphy

Isotope scintigraphy using bone-seeking radionuclides such as 99m technetium labelled methylene or hydroxymethylene diphosphonate (HDP) is a sensitive means of assessing physiological change in bone and synovium. The main role of scintigraphy in OA is to distinguish the activity of different types of process in a joint[14]. Scintigraphy may also be a means of detecting change before it becomes apparent on plain radiography[15]. This predictive capacity has been demonstrated in studies of hand OA in which the bone scan may be active before radiographic change occurs and often reverts to normal at a time when well-marked osteophytes are present, implying an altered, inactive state of the joint[16]. Such studies have also shown that hand OA is a phasic phenomenon in which each joint follows its own course.

Scintigraphic studies of knee OA have pointed to the heterogeneity of this disorder[14]. In the tibiofemoral joint, different categories of abnormality have been detected (for example, a generalized pattern which correlates well with pain and function, and which can be suppressed by intra-articular corticosteroid injection).

Other patterns include tramline activity along the joint margin which is reported to correlate with subchondral bone sclerosis, and an extended pattern which appears to be a marker of severe disease.

Magnetic resonance imaging

Magnetic resonance imaging (MRI) provides high-contrast soft tissue images which can be produced in any spatial plane. Despite the advantages of high resolution and this ability to produce images in any desired plane, MRI is costly and relatively unavailable. Initial studies of MRI in OA have concentrated on the anatomic features of the disorder[17,18]. These studies have highlighted a number of occult pathologies in joints which were otherwise thought to have simple OA, for example, meniscal damage and local osteochondral defects in the knee. MRI has been correlated with scintigraphic findings in the knee, and has been used in animals to visualize acute changes in cartilage. In addition, it is the investigation of choice in evaluating osteonecrosis, bony infection, periarticular pathology (such as rotator cuff lesions), and some forms of algodystrophy.

Biochemical markers

There is continual turnover of the components of healthy cartilage, with increased synthesis and degradation occurring in disorders such as OA. Some of the products of this turnover can be detected in various body fluids[19,20]. Thus, proteoglycan molecules are cleaved by metalloproteinases synthesized by the chondrocyte. Fragments may then diffuse through the cartilage into the synovial fluid and the systemic circulation. Antibodies have been raised to various parts of the intact proteoglycan and collagen molecules, and to fragments produced during synthesis and degradation; these can be measured in OA. Components which can be reliably assayed include keratan sulphate, chondroitin sulphate, various collagen and procollagen fragments, and bone matrix proteins. There is increasing interest in the use of such biochemical marker assays to study the disease processes involved in OA. At present, however, none of the available markers can be specifically recommended as providing a measure of disease progression.

Epidemiology of OA

Prevalence

Most currently available information on the epidemiology of OA comes from population-based radiographic surveys. In earlier such studies, attention was focused on OA of the hand joints, or on generalized (polyarticular) OA. More recent studies from Europe and the United States classify rates for individual joints and permit comparison between them.

The prevalence of radiographic OA rises steeply with age at all joint sites. In a survey of 6585 inhabitants randomly selected from the population of a Dutch village[21], 75 per cent of women aged 65–70 years had OA of their DIP joints (Fig. 8.59). Despite the predilection for older age groups, it should be noted that even by 40 years of age 10–20 per cent of subjects had evidence of severe radiographic disease affecting their hands or feet. Knee disease appeared less frequent than hand and foot involvement. Population-based studies in the United States suggest comparable prevalence rates to those in Europe, rising from less than 1 per cent among people aged 25–34, to 30 per cent in those 75 years and above[22]. Both hand and knee disease appear to be more frequent in women than in men, although the female to male ratio varies among studies between 1.5 and over 4.0. Hip OA is less common than knee OA, and prevalence rates in men and women appear more similar. Some, but not all, studies have reported a male preponderance at this site[1].

Although OA is worldwide in its distribution, geographic differences in prevalence have been reported[23]. These are often difficult to interpret because of differences in sampling procedure and radiographic consistency. European and American data do not appear to differ markedly for hand and knee disease. However, hand involvement appears to be particularly frequent in Pima and Blackfoot Indian populations within the United States. Greater variation has been found in the distribution of hip OA, with low rates reported among African Negroes, Asian Indians, Hong Kong Chinese, and Japanese.

Incidence

The only available data on the incidence of OA have been collected in the United States. In a population-

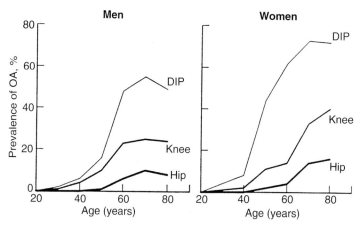

Fig. 8.59 Prevalence of radiographic OA in the hand, knee, and hip among Dutch men and women; data derived from Van Saase *et al.*[21].

based incidence study of hip and knee OA, using the medical record linkage system of the Mayo Clinic[24], age- and sex-adjusted rates for OA of the hip and knee were found to be 47.3 per 100 000 person-years (95 per cent confidence interval [CI] 27.8–66.8) and 163.8 per 100 000 person-years (95 per cent CI 127.1–200.6), respectively. Age-adjusted rates for OA of the hip and knee were similar for men and women. In men, the results showed a steadily increasing rate with age; in women, there was a plateau in incidence after the menopause.

Data from the Baltimore Longitudinal Study of Aging are available for the incidence of hand OA[25]. Among men aged 60 years and older, and incidence rate of 100 per 100 000 person-years was suggested. However, this analysis was restricted to a small group of male volunteers and was focused on radiographic hand disease, with no ascertainment of symptoms.

The most recent data to characterize the incidence of symptomatic hand, hip, and knee OA were obtained from the Fallon Community Health Plan, a health maintenance organization located in the north–east United States[26]. In this study, the age- and sex-standardized incidence rate of hand OA was 100 per 100 000 person-years (95 per cent CI 86–115), for hip OA, 88 per 100 000 person-years (95 per cent CI 75–101), and for knee OA, 240 per 100 000 person-years (95 per cent CI 218–262). The incidence of hand, hip, and knee disease increased with age, and women had higher rates than men, especially after the age of 50 years (Fig. 8.60); a levelling off occurred for both groups at all joint sites around the age of 80 years. By the age of 70–89 years, the incidence of symptomatic knee OA among women approached 1 per cent per year.

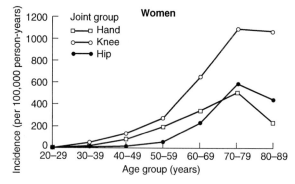

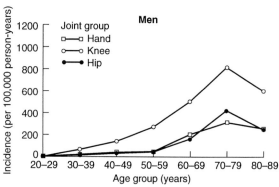

Fig. 8.60 Incidence of hand, hip, and knee OA with advancing age; data derived from Oliveria *et al.*[26]

The natural history of OA

Knee OA

The knee is a complex joint with three major compartments: the medial and lateral tibiofemoral joints, and the patellofemoral joint. Each of these areas can be affected by OA separately, or in any combination. Isolated medial compartment, or medial plus patellofemoral disease, are the commonest combinations[27] (Fig. 8.61).

Table 8.10 lists the studies which have examined the natural history of knee OA[28]. Disease evolution is slow, usually taking many years. However, there is evidence that once established, the condition can remain relatively stable, both clinically and radiologically, for a further period of several years. The correlation between the clinical outcome of knee OA and its radiographic course is not strong. In a large study, Dougados *et al.*[29] demonstrated that although radiographic improvement was rare, overall clinical improvement at one year follow-up was common. Longer term studies confirmed that radiographic deterioration occurs in one-third to two-thirds of patients, and that radiographic improvement is unusual. A Swedish study documented that among patients with structural change, for example, tibial or femoral sclerosis, the majority experienced radiographic and symptomatic deterioration over 15 years[30,31]. Of those subjects with only osteophyte on baseline radiography, a much smaller proportion suffered deterioration. This is broadly in accord with the American College of Rheumatology Study[32], in which joint space narrowing was judged to be a more important determinant of progression in knee OA than was the presence of osteophyte. However, when variables were considered in combination, this study reported that a score based on joint space narrowing, osteophyte, and sclerosis was reasonably reproducible and a better predictor of progression than any other combination.

Recent British studies have also examined the progression of knee OA, both among subjects attending hospital outpatient departments and in the general population. In an eleven-year follow-up study of 63 subjects who had baseline knee radiographs, the majority of knees did not show a worsening of overall grade of OA, with only 33 per cent deteriorating in Kellgren and Lawrence score over the time period[33]. When a more sensitive global scoring system was used on paired films, the proportion showing a slight deterioration increased to 50 per cent, and 10 per cent showed improvement — the latter estimate is within the limits allowed for by imprecision in radiographic grading. The visual analogue pain scores remained stable over the time period, but it was reported that those with knee pain at baseline had a greater chance of progressing, as did those with existing OA in the contralateral knee. A similar follow-up study was performed in 58

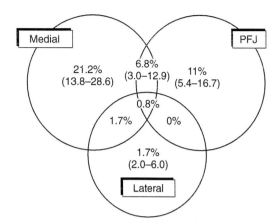

Men: knee pain positive

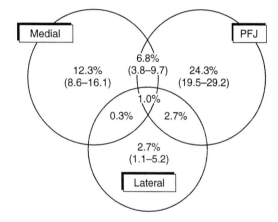

Women: knee pain positive

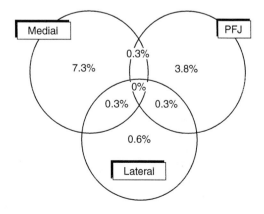

Men and women: knee pain negative

Fig. 8.61 Compartmental involvement of the knee in OA; derived from McAlindon *et al.*[27]

Table 8.10   Studies of the natural history of knee OA

Study		No of subjects	Measure	Follow-up (yrs)	% deteriorated
Hernborg	(1977)[30]	84 knees	C	15	55
			R	15	56
Danielsson	(1970)[31]	106 knees	R	15	33
Massardo	(1989)[35]	31	R	8	62
Dougados	(1992)[29]	353	C	1	28
			R	1	29
Schouten	(1991)[36]	142	R	12	34
Spector	(1992)[33]	63	R	11	33
Spector	(1994)[34]	58	R	2	22
Ledingham	(1995)[37]	350 knees	R	2	72

C = clinical; R = radiographic
Modified from Felson[28]

women aged 45–64, from the general population, in whom unilateral knee OA (Kellgren and Lawrence grade 2 plus) had been assigned at baseline[34]. Follow-up radiographs at 24 months revealed that 34 per cent of the women developed disease in the contralateral knee and that 22 per cent progressed radiologically in the index joint. Despite these studies, several questions remain about the natural history of knee OA. Some studies have excluded from follow-up, subjects whose symptoms were severe enough that they needed surgery. In other studies, many of the patients initially seen were subsequently lost for follow-up. This loss could have occurred because the patients had surgery, or because their knee symptoms had remitted and they felt no need to return.

Hip OA

As with knee OA, it remains uncertain as to whether the anatomically recognized subsets of hip OA represent part of a spectrum or discrete pathophysiological entities. These anatomical subtypes are best classified by the pattern of cartilage loss apparent on hip radiog-

raphy[38]. The most frequent pattern is superolateral, estimated to occur in some 60 per cent of patients with hip OA. The other two patterns are medial and concentric cartilage loss, occurring in 25 and 15 per cent of patients, respectively. The natural history of hip OA is very variable. Many cases that come to surgery have a relatively short history of severe symptoms, suggesting that a progressive phase lasting between three months and three years may often precede the advanced stages of OA.

There are fewer prospective studies of hip OA than of knee OA (Table 8.11). In a Danish follow-up study of 121 hips, over three decades ago, the majority (65 per cent) showed radiographic deterioration over a 10-year follow-up period[39]. Symptomatic improvement in this series was surprisingly common, occurring in the majority of patients. This is at variance with the results of another longitudinal study which documented frequent deterioration in the clinical course of hip OA patients[40]. In a Dutch study of patients identified from the general population who had established OA in one or both hips, 29 per cent of the subjects showed a worsening of their radiographic scores over a 12-year

Table 8.11   Studies of the natural history of hip OA

Study		No. of subjects	Measure	Follow-up (yrs)	% deteriorated
Danielsson	(1964)[39]	121 hips	C	10.0	19
			R	10.0	65
Seifert	(1969)[40]	83 hips	C	5.0	83
Van Saase	(1990)[41]	86	R	12.0	29
Ledingham	(1993)[38]	136	C	2.3	66
			R	2.3	47

C = clinical; R = radiographic
Modified from Felson[28]

follow-up period[41]. Nonetheless, unlike knee OA, a few patients with hip OA can experience clear-cut radiologic and symptomatic recovery[42,43]. This appears to occur most often among patients who have marked osteophytosis and in those with concentric disease. Osteonecrosis is the major complication of hip OA and tends to occur late in the natural history. Rapidly progressive OA can lead to an unusual appearance with extensive bone destruction and a wide interbone distance. This appearance was initially observed among patients who ingested anti-inflammatory drugs and was termed 'analgesic hip[44]'. However, it is now recognized to occur in groups of subjects who ingest few or no such agents[45].

Hand OA

OA principally affects the DIP, PIP, and thumb base in the hand. Detailed studies of the distribution of hand joint involvement have been performed[46] and results are shown in Fig. 8.62. Recent epidemiological data suggest that clinical and radiographic changes in hand OA are concordant in individuals, and that definition is best achieved by a combination of both measures[47]. The evolution of hand OA is usually complete after a period of a few years; it has been studied both clinically and radiographically. The condition usually starts with aching in the affected joints, and tends to have a remit-ting and relapsing course over the initial years. There is often clear evidence of inflammatory phases in which individual joints become warm and tender; bony swelling develops during this phase and cysts may form. After a variable time period, often lasting several years, these flares and the pain tend to subside. The swellings become firm and fixed, and joint movement becomes progressively reduced. The condition then appears to enter a stable phase during the seventh and eighth decades of the life of the subject. Imaging studies show this evolution of change to be accompanied by sequential changes in joint anatomy and physiology.

Kallman *et al.* reported that among men with DIP joint OA, more than 50 per cent experienced progression of radiographic disease over 10 years[25]. The progression was fastest in the DIP joints, and was slower in PIP joints and the thumb base. The presence of narrowing at baseline increased the risk that subjects would develop subsequent osteophytes, and joints with severe radiographic changes at baseline had slower progression rates than joints with milder radiographic changes. The rate of OA progression in individual subjects paralleled the rate of progression hinted at by cross-sectional studies, in which subjects are studied at different ages. Scintigraphic studies have shown that bone activity precedes the radiographic appearances, whether joint space narrowing, sclerosis, or osteophyte[16]. Macroradiographic studies indicate that juxta-articular radiolucencies are an early feature[48].

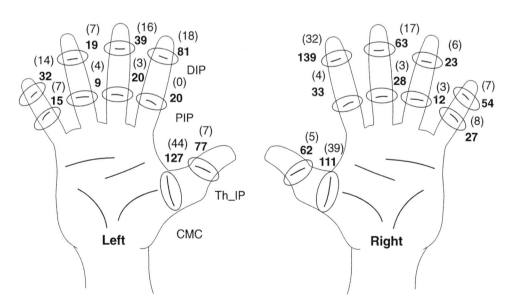

Fig. 8.62 Distribution of hand joint involvement in OA; figures show number of hand joints involved among 967 women age 45–64 years (bold = grade 2+ involvement, parentheses = grade 3+ involvement). Data from Egger *et al.*[46]

Table 8.12   Clustering of hand joint involvement in OA among perimenopausal women

Joint Groups		Radiographic definition of OA	
		Grade 2 + OR (95% CI)	Grade 3+ OR (95% CI)
DIP–DIP	(row)	5.0 (4.2–6.0)	10.0 (7.3–13.7)
PIP–PIP	(row)	3.7 (2.7–5.0)	3.1 (1.4–6.8)
DIP–PIP	(ray)	3.7 (2.2–6.3)	5.9 (0.9–39.4)
CMC–IP		1.4 (1.2–1.6)	1.3 (1.0–1.7)

The odds ratios indicate the hierarchies of association between different joint groups in OA (derived from Egger et al.[46]).
DIP = disted interphalangeal; PIP = proximal interphelangeal; IP = interphelangeal; CMC = carpometacorpal (1st).

The mechanisms implicated in controlling the timing of individual joint involvement remain unknown. However, the pattern of involvement clearly suggests the presence of a polyarticular subset of disease in postmenopausal women[46]. In addition, these studies suggest that symmetry is a more marked feature of the pattern of joint involvement than clustering by row or ray (Table 8.12).

Determinants of progression in OA

Just as the natural history of OA differs at different joint sites, the factors which contribute to disease progression appear to be joint specific. These determinants have been less well studied than the risk factors for prevalent disease. However, Table 8.13 summarizes the known determinants of progression at the knee and hip.

At both sites, multiple joint involvement appears to be a determinant of accelerated disease. For example, in the French study[29], patients who sustained joint space narrowing in the knee over a one-year follow-up period had a larger number of joints throughout the body affected by OA than did those who experienced no joint space narrowing. Spector et al. reported that knee OA progression was more frequent in those with bilateral knee OA than in those with unilateral involvement[34]. This influence of multiple involvement extends from the knee to other joint sites. In a study of 142 subjects with baseline radiographs of the knee, Schouten et al.[49] found that a diagnosis of generalized OA (through the presence of Heberden's nodes) increased the likelihood of progressive cartilage loss in the knee by threefold. This increase in risk persisted after statistical adjustment for age, gender, and body mass index. The coexistence of Heberden's nodes with knee OA, increased the risk of knee deterioration by almost sixfold. Likewise, Doherty et al.[50] found that among patients who had undergone unilateral meniscectomy previously, the presence of radiographic hand OA markedly increased the risk of developing incident knee disease. The explanation for this tendency of generalized OA to increase the rate of progression is not clear — candidates include crystal deposition, and a generalized hormonal or metabolic diathesis. Some studies have suggested that the presence of crystals in association with OA at baseline, increases the risk of progressive disease. Thus, in one study[51], 10 subjects with rapidly progressive OA were, over one year, compared with 84 subjects with more slowly progressive OA. The prevalence of synovial fluid crystals (hydrox-

Table 8.13   Determinants of progression of hip and knee OA

(Risk factor)	Strength of association	
	Knee	Hip
Generalized OA diathesis	++	+
Obesity	++	+
Joint injury	++	+
Crystal deposition	+	
Neuromuscular dysfunction	+	

+ = documented; ++ = strong association

yapatite or calcium pyrophosphate) was substantially higher in those with progressive disease. However, other epidemiological studies[29,49] have failed to document chondrocalcinosis as a risk factor for progression of disease, although the relatively small number of subjects with coexistent knee OA and chondrocalcinosis at baseline has limited the power of these investigations.

Another factor consistently associated with progression of OA is obesity. Several longitudinal studies[29,34,49,52] have reported that obese patients are more likely to experience progressive disease than non-obese patients. The evidence that weight loss slows progression of disease is less clear cut. In the Dutch population study[49], weight loss did not appear to slow progression. These findings contrast with the data from a clinical study of obese patients who underwent rapid weight loss, and an US epidemiological study[53], both of which pointed to an improvement in joint symptoms. Obesity has also been documented as a risk factor for progression in hip OA[41].

Other factors may influence which patients with OA experience progression or not. These include joint injury, which has been most convincingly demonstrated to be a determinant of progression at the knee, muscle weakness, and joint instability[28]. The relationship of growth factors or cytokines to the progression of OA needs further epidemiological and clinical investigation. Studies of insulin-like growth factor 1, a cytokine which might induce increased osteophytes over time, suggest a potential role in modifying progression[54]. Disruption of the neurological input from structures around the joint also appears important in predisposing to accelerated damage. At its most extreme, this leads to the clinical phenomenon termed a 'Charcot joint,' but lesser levels of neurological disruption may lead to accelerated OA in animals.

Conclusions

OA is now firmly established as a public health problem. There have been advances in defining the disorder, measuring its component features clinically, radiographically, and by other investigative techniques. The descriptive epidemiological characteristics of OA, as it affects various joint sites, have been elucidated, and the risk factors for prevalent disease are clearly understood for the knee, hip, and hand. Epidemiological information on the rate of progression of the disorder at these joint sites, and the determinants

of this progression, remains less detailed. However, it is clear that progression is a joint-specific phenomenon and there may be disease subsets at each site in which progression depends on different groups of factors. These factors, though to hasten progression generally, include increasing age, obesity, crystal deposition, the presence of polyarticular OA, joint instability, muscle weakness, and neurogenic dysfunction. The challenge of identifying subjects at risk of rapid progression, through a variety of diagnostic modalities, is currently the subject of intensive research. With the completion of studies examining the efficiency of biochemical markers, scintigraphy, and newer imaging techniques such as magnetic resonance, it is likely that the processes underlying progressive disease will be better understood and developed.

Acknowledgments

This manuscript was prepared by Mrs D. Gould. The authors thank the Medical Research Council, Arthritis and Rheumatism Council, and the Wellcome Trust for research support.

References

1. Felson, D.T. (1988). Epidemiology of hip and knee osteoarthritis. *Epidemiological Reviews*, **10**, 1–28.
2. Rogers, J., Dieppe, P., and Watt, I. (1981). Arthritis in Saxon and medieval skeletons. *British Medical Journal*, **283**, 668–71.
3. Dieppe, T.A. (1994). Osteoarthritis. In *Rheumatology* (ed. J.H. Klippel and P.A. Dieppe), 7.2.1–7.2.6. Mosby Press, London.
4. McAlindon, T. and Dieppe, T. (1989). Osteoarthritis: definitions and criteria. *Annals of the Rheumatic Diseases*, **48**, 531–2.
5. Kellgren, J.K. and Lawrence, J.S. (1957). Radiological assessment of osteoarthritis. *Annals of the Rheumatic Diseases*, **15**, 494–501.
6. Spector, T.D. and Cooper C. (1993). Radiographic assessment of osteoarthritis in population studies: whither Kellgren and Lawrence? *Osteoarthritis and Cartilage*, **1**, 203–6.
7. Spector, T.D., Hart, D.J., Byrne, J., Harris, T.A., Dacre, J.E., and Doyle, D.D. (1993). Definition of osteoarthritis of the knee for epidemiological studies. *Annals of the Rheumatic Diseases*, **52**, 790–4.
8. Croft, P., Cooper, C., Wickham, C., and Coggon, D. (1990). Defining osteoarthritis of the hip for epidemiologic studies. *American Journal of Epidemiology*, **132**, 514–22.

9. Kallman, D.A., Wigley, F.M., Scott, W.W., Hochberg, M., and Tobin, J.D. (1989). New radiographic grading scales of osteoarthritis of the hand. *Arthritis and Rheumatism*, **32**, 1584–91.

10. Dieppe, D.A. (1995). Recommended methodology for assessing the progression of osteoarthritis of the hip and knee joints. *Osteoarthritis and Cartilage*, **3**, 73–7.

11. Cushnaghan, J., Cooper, C., Dieppe, P., Kirwan, J., McAlindon, T., and McCrae, F. (1990). Clinical assessment of osteoarthritis of the knee. *Annals of the Rheumatic Diseases*, **49**, 768–70.

12. Lequesne, M., Mery, C., Sansom, M., and Gerard, D.P. (1987). Indices of severity for osteoarthritis of the hip and knee. *Scandinavian Journal of Rheumatology*. **18** (**supplement 65**), 85–9.

13. Bellamy, N., Buchanan, W.W., and Goldsmith, H. (1988). Validation study of WOMAC: a health status instrument for measuring clinically important patient relevant outcomes to anti-rheumatic therapy in patients with osteoarthritis of the hip or knee. *Journal of Rheumatology*, **15**, 1833–40.

14. McCrae, F., Shoels, J., Dieppe, P., and Watt, I. (1992). Scintigraphic assessment of osteoarthritis of the knee joint. *Annals of the Rheumatic Diseases*, **51**, 938–42.

15. Dieppe, P.A., Cushnaghan, J., Young, P., and Kirwan, J. (1993). Prediction of the progression of joint space narrowing and osteoarthritis of the knee by bone scintigraphy. *Annals of the Rheumatic Diseases*, **52**, 557–63.

16. Hutton, C.W., Higgs, E.R., Jackson, P.C., Watt, I., and Dieppe, D.A. (1986). 99TC-HMDP bone scanning in generalised nodal osteoarthritis. 2. The 4-hour bone scan image predicts radiographic change. *Annals of the Rheumatic Diseases* **45**, 622–6.

17. McAlindon, T.E., Watt, I., McCrae, F.M., Goddard, P., Dieppe, P.A. (1991). Magnetic resonance imaging in osteoarthritis of the knee: correlation with radiographic and scintigraphic findings. *Annals of the Rheumatic Diseases*, **50**, 14–19.

18. Hutton, C.W. and Vennart, W. (1994). Osteoarthritis and magnetic resonance imaging: potential and problems. *Annals of the Rheumatic Diseases*, **54**, 237–43.

19. Lohmander, L.S. (1991). Markers of cartilage metabolism in arthrosis: a review. *Acta Orthopedica Scandinavica*, **62**, 623–32.

20. Thonar, E.J., Shinmei, M., and Lohmander, L.S. (1993). Body fluid markers of articular cartilage changes in osteoarthritis. In Moskowitz R, ed. *Rheumatic disease clinics of North America* (ed. R. Moskowitz), pp. 634–58. W.B. Saunders, Philadelphia.

21. Van Saase, J.L.C.M., Van Romunde, L.K.S., Cats, A. et al. (1989). Epidemiology of osteoarthritis: Zoetermeer Survey. Comparison of radiological osteoarthritis in a Dutch population with that in ten other populations. *Annals of the Rheumatic Diseases*, **48**, 271–80.

22. Felson, D.T., Naimark, A., Anderson, J., et al. (1987). The prevalence of knee osteoarthritis in the elderly. The Framingham osteoarthritis study. *Arthritis and Rheumatism*, **30**, 914–18.

23. Lawrence, J.S. and Sebo, M. (1979). The geography of osteoarthrosis. In Nuki G, ed. *The aetiopathogenesis of osteoarthritis*, (ed. G. Nuki), pp. 155–83. Pitman Medical, London.

24. Wilson, M.G., Michet, C.J., Ilstrup, D.M., and Melton, L.J. (1990). Idiopathic symptomatic osteoarthritis of the hip and knee: a population based incidence study. *Mayo Clinic Proceedings*, **65**, 1214–21.

25. Kallman, D.A., Wigley, F.M., Scott, W.W., Hochberg, M.C., and Tobin, J.D. (1990). The longitudinal course of hand osteoarthritis in a male population. *Arthritis and Rheumatism*, **33**, 1323–32.

26. Oliveria, S.A., Felson, D.T., Reed, J.I., Cirillo, P.A., and Walker, A.M. (1995). Incidence of symptomatic hand, hip and knee osteoarthritis among patients in a health maintenance organisation. *Arthritis and Rheumatism*, **38**, 1134–41.

27. McAlindon, T.E., Snow, S., Cooper, C., and Dieppe, P. (1992). Radiographic patterns of knee osteoarthritis in the community: the importance of the patellofemoral joint. *Annals of the Rheumatic Diseases*, **51**, 844–9.

28. Felson, D.T. (1993). The course of osteoarthritis and factors that affect it. *Rheumatic Disease Clinics of North America*, **19**, 607–15.

29. Dougados, M., Gueguen, A., Nguyen, M., *et al.* (1992). Longitudinal radiologic evaluation of osteoarthritis of the knee. *Journal of Rheumatology*, **19**, 378–83.

30. Hernborg, J.S. and Nilsson, B.E. (1977). The natural course of untreated osteoarthritis of the knee. *Clinical Orthopaedics*, **123**, 130–7.

31. Danielsson, L. and Hernborg, J. (1970). Clinical and roentgenologic study of knee joints with osteophytes. *Clinical Orthopaedics*, **69**, 224–6.

32. Altman, R.D., Fries, J.F., Bloch, D.A., *et al.* (1987). Radiographic assessment of progression in osteoarthritis. *Arthritis and Rheumatism*, **30**, 1214–25.

33. Spector, T.D., Dacre, J.E., Harris, P.A., and Huskisson, E.C. (1992). The radiological progression of osteoarthritis: an eleven-year follow-up study of the knee. *Annals of the Rheumatic Diseases*, **51**, 1107–10.

34. Spector, T.D., Hart, D.J., and Doyle, D.V. (1994). Incidence and progression of osteoarthritis in women with unilateral knee disease in the general population: the effect of obesity. *Annals of the Rheumatic Diseases*, **53**, 565–8.

35. Massardo, L., Watt, I., Cushnaghan, J., *et al.* (1989). Osteoarthritis of the knee joint: an eight year prospective study. *Annals of the Rheumatic Diseases*, **48**, 893–7.

36. Schouten, J. (1991). A twelve-year follow-up study of osteoarthritis of the knee in the general population. PhD Thesis, Erasmus University, The Netherlands.

37. Ledingham, J. Regan, M., Jones, A., and Doherty, M. (1995). Factors affecting radiographic progression of knee osteoarthritis. *Annals of the Rheumatic Diseases*, **54**, 53–8.

38. Ledingham, J.M., Dawson, S., Preston, B., and Doherty, M. (1993). Radiographic progression of hospital referred hip osteoarthritis. *Annals of the Rheumatic Diseases*, **52**, 263–7.

39. Danielsson, L.G. (1964). Incidence and prognosis of coxarthrosis *Acta Orthopedica Scandinavica*, **66** (**supplement**), 1–87.

40. Seifert, M.H., Whiteside, C.G., and Savage, O. (1969). A five-year follow-up of 50 cases of idiopathic

osteoarthritis of the hip (abstract). *Annals of the Rheumatic Diseases*, **28**, 325–6.

41. Van Saase, J.L.C.M. (1990). Osteoarthrosis in the general population: a follow-up study of osteoarthrosis of the hip. Ph.D. Thesis, Leiden State University, Netherlands.

42. Bland, J.H. and Cooper, S.M. (1984). Osteoarthritis: a review of the cell biology involved and evidence for reversibility. *Seminars in Arthritis and Rheumatism*, **14**, 106–33.

43. Perry, G.H., Smith, M.J.G., and Whiteside, C.J. (1979). Spontaneous recovery of the joint space in degenerative hip disease. *Annals of the Rheumatic Diseases*, **31**, 440–8.

44. Newman, N.M. and Ling, R.S.M. (1985). Acetabular bone destruction related to non-steroidal anti-inflammatory drugs. *Lancet*, **2**, 11–14.

45. Rashad, S., Revell, P., Hemingway, A., *et al.* (1989). The effect of non-steroidal anti-inflammatory drugs on the course of osteoarthritis. *Lancet*, **2**, 519–22.

46. Egger, P., Cooper, C., Hart, D.J., Doyle, D.V., Coggon, D., and Spector, T.D. (1995). Patterns of joint involvement in osteoarthritis of the hand: the Chingford study. *Journal of Rheumatology*, **22**, 1509–13.

47. Hart, D.J., Spector, T.D., Egger, P., Coggon, D., and Copper, C. (1994). Defining osteoarthritis of the hand for epidemiologic studies: the Chingford study. *Annals of the Rheumatic Diseases*, **53**, 220–3.

48. Buckland-Wright, J.C., MacFarlane, D.G., Lynch, J.A., and Clark, B. (1990). Quantitative microfocal radiographic assessment of progression in osteoarthritis of the hand. *Arthritis and Rheumatism*, **23**, 57–65.

49. Schouten, J.S.A.G., Van den Ouweland, F.A., and Valkenburg, H.A. (1992). A twelve-year follow-up study in the general population on prognostic factors of cartilage loss in osteoarthritis of the knee. *Annals of the Rheumatic Diseases*, **51**, 932–7.

50. Doherty, M., Watt, I., and Dieppe, P. (1983). Influence of primary generalised osteoarthritis on development of secondary osteoarthritis. *Lancet*, **2**, 8–11.

51. Bardin, T., Bucki, B., Lequesne, M., *et al.* (1985). Crystals in the synovial fluid of osteoarthritic joints are associated with rapid disease progression. *British Journal of Rheumatology*, **27** (**supplement 2**), 94.

52. Felson, D.T., Anderson, J.J., Naimark, A., Walker, A.M., and Meenan, R.F. (1988). Obesity and knee osteoarthritis: the Framingham study. *Annals of Internal Medicine*, **109**, 18–24.

53. Olson, D.T., Zhang, Y., Anthony, J.M., Naimark, A., and Anderson J.J. (1992). Weight loss reduces the risk for symptomatic knee osteoarthritis in women: the Framingham study. *Annals of Internal Medicine*, **116**, 535–9.

54. Schouten, J.S.A.G., Van den Ouweland, F.A., Valkenburg, H.A., and Lamberts, S.W.J. (1993). Insulin like growth factor one: a prognostic factor of knee osteoarthritis. *British Journal of Rheumatology*, **32**, 274–80.

9 | *Management of osteoarthritis*

9.1 Introduction: the comprehensive approach

*Kenneth Brandt, L. Stefan Lohmander, and
Michael Doherty*

The assessment and management of patients with osteoarthritis (OA) is a challenge to the clinical skills and judgment of any health professional. The main problems for which the patient with OA seeks advice are pain and functional impairment. However, the correlation between pain severity, disability, and the extent of structural OA changes is not always strong, and the consequences of pain and impairment on the individual vary greatly, depending on factors such as personality, affect, occupational and recreational aspirations, coexistent disease and disability, and the expectations of available health care delivery. Assessment of the patient with symptomatic OA is, therefore, potentially complex and must occur at at least two levels:

(1) assessment of *the joint* — for example, which joint involved, articular versus periarticular pain, degree of structural damage, instability, inflammation, restriction and disability;

(2) assessment of *the person* — for example, impact and severity of pain, affect, level of distress, handicap, other medical problems, social support, quality of life, and beliefs and knowledge of arthritis.

This requires a global, holistic approach if a successful management plan with realistic goals is to be formulated. Full account must be taken of the individual who is seeking advice, as well as of the severity of OA afflicting their joints.

Management objectives

The principal objectives of management are to:

- educate the patient
- control pain
- optimize function
- reduce handicap.

These clearly interrelate and overlap. To achieve these aims there are a wide variety of interventions from which to choose (Table 9.1). When deciding on the appropriate management strategy for the individual patient, the following general considerations are pertinent:

1. The choice of interventions will, in part, be determined by *the site of OA involvement*, since some treatments are limited in suitability or efficacy to one or a few sites. It follows that data demonstrating success of a treatment at one OA site cannot necessarily be used to justify its use at other OA sites.

2. The order in which different treatments are tried, in sequence or by addition, is also determined by the *individual requirements and characteristics of the patient* (the person and the joint, as above).

3. In general, *simple and safe interventions are tried first*, before more complex, potentially dangerous, treatments.

4. The status and requirements of the patient will change with time, usually slowly but sometimes rapidly. This necessitates *regular review and readjustment of treatment options*, rather than rigid continuation of a single plan.

5. The wide variety of treatment approaches may require the expertise of a number of different health professionals. A *coordinated multidisciplinary team approach* is often required to deliver health care efficiently and to present coherent, rather than contradictory, management advice.

Table 9.1 Available management options for OA

A Non-pharmacological interventions

Patient education, coping
Self-management
Telephone contact
Exercise
Aerobic conditioning
Strengthening, range of motion
Reduction of adverse mechanical factors
Weight loss
Appropriate footwear
'Pacing' of activities
Walking stick
Aids, appliances
Patella taping
Local physical treatments
Heat, cold
Pulsed electrical stimulation

B Local and systemic drug therapies

Topical creams / gels
NSAIDs
Capsaicin
Local injection therapies
Intra-articular and periarticular corticosteroid
Hyaluronan
Oral medications
Simple analgesics, e.g. acetaminophen
Combination analgesics
Oral NSAIDs
Low-dose amitriptyline

C Operative interventions

Invasive physical interventions
Arthroscopic lavage (knee)
Closed tidal irrigation (knee)
Capsular distension (hip)
Surgery
Osteotomy
Joint replacement

The importance of patient education

Central to any management plan is education of the patient and their carers about the nature of OA and its treatments. Knowing about OA helps patients to better manage their condition and to make informed choices between treatment options. Furthermore, provision of access to information and therapist contact can reduce symptoms and disability, as has been shown for monthly 'over-the-telephone' management reviews[1–3] and for educational literature and packages (which may even be impersonal)[4], to improve self-efficacy[5,6].

The cost-effectiveness of such interventions has been well demonstrated[3,6].

OA is often considered a uniformly progressive 'wear and tear' disease, the inevitable consequence of aging, for which there is little effective therapy other than eventual surgical removal. This negative attitude, based on the 'doomsday scenario' of worn-out joints[7], is widespread not only in the community, but among doctors and other health care professionals. In reality, however, OA is not inevitably progressive. Many intervention strategies can reduce symptoms and improve function[7–10]: An optimistic, not fatalistic, approach is, therefore, justified.

Non-pharmacological approaches

Non-pharmacological, non-surgical approaches to management should be considered for every patient, not only because they can be effective[7-10], but because they are safe. Many patients are concerned that continued physical activity may further damage their joints. The musculoskeletal system, however, is designed to move, and reduced activity is detrimental to all its component tissues. Furthermore, poor aerobic fitness, consequent upon reduced activity, is associated with low 'well-being' and more reporting of pain and handicap. Therefore, patients should be encouraged to exercise, using 'small amounts often' to increase general fitness, improve muscle strength and proprioception, and maintain or increase range of movement. For knee OA, there is evidence that supervised fitness walking and exercise[11-13], and quadriceps strengthening[14-16], may reduce symptoms and improve function and gait pattern[13], even in elderly subjects.

Encouraging patients to pace their activities throughout the day may allow them to accomplish more in a given period. The patient may already be utilizing strategies to cope with the consequences of their OA, but such strategies may be improved, or new ones adopted, with the assistance of a therapist[5,6]. Reducing adverse mechanical factors may further help symptoms and improve function. For example, obese patients should be encouraged to lose weight, based on the evidence the weight loss may prevent onset of knee OA symptoms[17]. Weight loss is notoriously difficult to achieve, though slimming regimes may be more effective when combined with exercise. The use of a walking stick[18] is a simple way of reducing symptoms from hip or knee OA. Other mechanical approaches include: wedged insoles for patients with OA and varus deformity[19]; shock-absorbing insoles for hip or knee OA; and taping of the patella for patellofemoral OA[20]. Modification of the patient's home or work environment can further minimise 'external' adverse mechanical factors.

Various local physical therapies are often used for pain relief and to encourage compliance in exercise programs. There is reasonable evidence for some of these modalities, such as pulsed electrical stimulation[21]. Others, however, have empirical rather than evidence-based support. Whether these effects are largely incidental to the clear benefit of therapist contact remains unclear.

Local and systemic drug therapies

The possibility of pharmacological modification of the OA process is considered in Chapter 11. Currently, however, drugs for OA are mainly used for pain relief. Local administration offers the advantage of targeted therapy with low systemic toxicity, and is particularly indicated when one joint or only a few joints are affected. Topical preparations are popular with patients and represent an aspect of therapy that is totally under their control. Rubefacients and counter-irritants are often bought and used by patients, though there are no controlled data to support efficacy. Topical non-steroidal anti-inflammatory drugs (NSAIDs) are certainly safer than oral NSAIDs[22] and, despite a high placebo response data demonstrate, efficacy for some of these agents in OA[23,24]. Topical capsaicin cream has also been demonstrated to be beneficial for OA, as either an adjunct[25] or as monotherapy[26], and its use is increasing, especially for knee and hand OA.

Intra-articular injection of long-acting corticosteroid preparations has long been used, especially for knee OA. This simple procedure may give temporary pain relief[27,28] lasting several weeks or ocasionally several months, and is used particularly to encourage participation in other interventions, such as exercise, or to tide the patient through an important event, such as a holiday. The presence of an effusion has been suggested as a predictor of response[27]. Less widely available injectables include hyaluronan, of various molecular weights, which may give more prolonged symptom control lasting several months [29,30].

Simple oral analgesics, such as acetaminophen, may give effective and safe pain control in OA[31-33]. Stronger analgesics and combination preparations may be more effective[34,35], but this benefit is often countered by frequent troublesome side effects. Oral NSAIDs are effective in OA[32,36,37], but better efficacy than simple analgesics is difficult to show in between-patient comparison (parallel group) study designs[32]. Some studies, however, suggest that certain patients do derive more pain relief from NSAIDs [38,39], though predictors of response are difficult to identify. The main drawback to oral NSAIDs, of course, is the associated morbidity from gastrointestinal bleeding and perforation, and from effects on renal function. Many patients with OA are elderly, have mild renal and cardiac impairment, and are on other medications, making them particularly susceptible to NSAID side effects and drug interactions. In general, therefore, oral NSAIDs are reserved for patients who have failed on simple analgesics and other safe approaches to pain relief. The question of which NSAID to use, and whether co-administration of misoprostol or other 'gastroprotective' agents should be routine, remains a topic of debate. In general, however, low-dose ibuprofen is commonly tried first because of its low gastrointestinal toxicity in comparison to other NSAIDs[40].

A low dose of an antidepressant at night is sometimes given as adjunctive therapy for pain relief, especially in those with poor sleep. The efficacy of this approach in OA, however, has been poorly studied. Overt depression is not uncommon in OA patients, and may justify treatment in its own right. Transcutaneous electrical nerve stimulators and local nerve blocks are used empirically for severe pain that is resistant to other measures.

Operative interventions

Arthroscopic lavage may improve symptoms for some months[41], as may the lesser procedure of closed tidal irrigation[42,43]. Such invasive approaches are predominantly limited to knees and reserved for resistant OA, often as a holding procedure prior to surgical intervention. Capsular distension may be used as an equivalent procedure for the pain of hip OA[44].

Surgery should be considered for patients with persistent, severe pain that is inadequately controlled by other means, particularly when there is associated marked disability. Patients severely incapacitated by hip or knee OA can have their lives transformed by successful joint replacement[45,46]. Osteotomy can be an effective alternative for selected younger patients with isolated medial compartment knee OA[47,48] or, occasionally, hip OA[49]. Surgery, however, is not without its risks. Furthermore, there are no clear guidelines for deciding the timing of surgery or for selecting those who might benefit most. Patients need to be fully informed of the potential benefits, limitations, and dangers of surgery, and the potential influence of any concurrent disease on their outcome. Once they are fully informed, the decision to operate is predominently theirs. As always, a global assessment is paramount, with patients actively involved in determining their own outcome.

Guidelines for effective management of OA

It will be apparent that generic decision trees for management of OA are difficult to formulate, given the variability of OA at different sites and between individuals. Nevertheless, guidelines have been proposed for the management of OA at the knee[10,50] and hip[9,50], these two sites contributing the largest community burden of OA pain, disability, and health care requirement. Such guidelines attempt to offer a framework from which to select appropriate treatments to suit the individual patient. The importance of full patient assessment, education, and support are well emphasised, and non-pharmacological and drug treatments are both presented. The greatest difficulty for such guidelines is ranking treatments in order of OA 'severity', because of the multiple ways in which severity can be defined (for example, X-ray change, pain, disability) and the fact that different assessment measures do not necessarily progress in parallel. Pragmatically, therefore, education, non-pharmacological approaches, and safe drug treatments are given initial, equal priority for all patients, irrespective of severity. Other drug treatments, and more invasive measures, are considered second in order, whilst surgery is reserved for patients with persistent pain and disability, significant to that individual, that are clearly resistant to conservative interventions.

Following chapters discuss the advantages and drawbacks of individual treatment options, and present the evidence for their efficacy in OA at different sites.

References

1. Weinberger, M., Tierny, W.M., Booher, P., and Katz, B.P. (1989). Can the provision of information to patients with osteoarthritis improve functional status? *Arthritis and Rheumatism*, 32, 1577–83.
2. Rene, J., Weinberger, M., Mazzuca, S.A., Brandt, K.D., and Katz, B.P. (1992). Reduction of joint pain in patients with knee osteoarthritis who have received monthly telephone calls from lay personnel and whose medical regimens have remained stable. *Arthritis and Rheumatism*, 35, 511–5.
3. Weinberger, M., Tierney, W.M., Booher, P., and Katz, B.P. (1993). Cost-effectiveness of increased telephone contact for patients with osteoarthritis: a randomised controlled trial. *Arthritis and Rheumatism*, 36, 243–6.

4. Rippey, R.M., Bill, D., Abeles, M., Day, J., Downing, D.S., Pfeiffer, C.A., *et al.* (1987). Computer-based patient education for older persons with osteoarthritis. *Arthritis and Rheumatism*, 30, 932–5.

5. Lorig, K.R., Lubeck, D., Kraines, R.G., Seleznick, M., and Holman, H.R. (1985). Outcomes of self-help education for patients with arthritis. *Arthritis and Rheumatism* 28, 680–5.

6. Lorig, K.R., Mazonson, P.D., and Holman, H.R. (1993). Evidence suggesting that health education for self-management in patients with chronic arthritis has sustained health benefits while reducing health care costs. *Arthritis and Rheumatism*, 36, 439–46.

7. Hurley, M.V. (1995). Conservative management of osteoarthritic knees. *British Journal of Therapeutic Rehabilitation*, 2, 179–83.

8. Puett, D.W. and Griffin, M.R. (1994). Published trials of non-medicinal and non-invasive therapies for hip and knee osteoarthritis. *Annals of Internal Medicine*, 121, 133–40.

9. Hochberg, M.C., Altman, R.D., Brandt, K.D., Clark, B.M., Dieppe, P.A., Griffin, M., *et al.* (1995). Guidelines for the medical management of osteoarthritis. Part I. Osteoarthritis of the hip. *Arthritis and Rheumatism* 38, 1535–40.

10. Hochberg, M.C., Altman, R.D., Brandt, K.D., Clark, B.M., Dieppe, P.A., Griffin, M., *et al.* (1995). Guidelines for the medical management of osteoarthritis. Part II. Osteoarthritis of the knee. *Arthritis and Rheumatism*, 38, 1541–6.

11. Kovar, P.A., Allegrante, J.P., MacKenzie, C.R., Petersen, M.G.E., Gutin, B., and Charlson, M.E. (1992). Supervised fitness walking in patients with osteoarthritis of the knee. *Annals of Internal Medicine*, 116, 529–34.

12. Minor, M.A., Hewett, J.E., Webel, R.R., Anderson, S.K., and Kay, D.R. (1989). Efficacy of physical conditioning exercise in patients with rheumatoid arthritis and osteoarthritis. *Arthritis and Rheumatism*, 32, 1396–1405.

13. Peterson, M.G.E., Kovar, P.A., Otis, J.C., *et al.* (1993). Effect of a walking program on gait characteristics in patients with osteoarthritis. *Arthritis Care and Research*, 6, 11–16.

14. Chamberlain, M.A., Care, G., and Harfield, B. (1982). Physiotherapy in osteoarthrosis of the knees. A controlled trial of hospital versus home exercises. *International Rehabilitation Medicine*, 4, 101–6.

15. Jan, M.H. and Lai, J.S. (1991). The effects of physiotherapy on osteoarthritic knees of females. *Journal of the Formosan Medical Association*, 90, 1008–13.

16. Ettinger, W.F. and Afable, R.F. (1994). Physical disability from knee osteoarthrosis: the role of exercise as an intervention. *Medicine and Science in Sports and Exercise*, 26, 1435–40.

17. Felson, D.T., Zhang, Y., Anthony, J.M., Naimark, A., and Anderson, J.J. (1992). Weight loss reduces the risk for symptomatic knee osteoarthritis in women: the Framingham Study. *Annals of Internal Medicine*, 116, 535–9.

18. Blount, W.P. (1956). Don't throw away the cane. *Journal of Bone and Joint Surgery*, 38A, 695–8.

19. Sasaki, T. and Yasuda, K. (1987). Clinical evaluation of the treatment of osteoarthritic knees using a newly designed wedged insole. *Clinical Orthopedics*, 221, 181–7.

20. Cushnaghan, J., McCarthy, C., and Dieppe, P.A. (1994) Taping the patella medially: a new treatment for osteoarthritis of the knee joint? *British Medical Journal*, 308, 753–5.

21. Zizic, T.M., Hoffman, K.C., Holt, P.A., Hungerford, D.S., O'dell, J.R., Jacobs, M.A., *et al.* (1995). The treatment of osteoarthritis of the knee with pulsed electrical stimulation. *Journal of Rheumatology*, 22, 1757–61.

22. Evans, J.M.M., McMahon, A.D., McGilchrist, M.M., *et al.* (1995). Topical non-steroidal anti-inflammatory drugs and admission to hospital for upper gastrointestinal bleeding and perforation: a record linkage case-control study. *British Medical Journal*, 311, 22–6.

23. Kageyama, T.A. (1987) A double blind placebo controlled multicenter study of piroxicam 0.5% gel in osteoarthritis of the knee. *European Journal of Rheumatology and Inflammation*, 8, 114–15.

24. Rothaker, D., Difigilo, C., and Lee, I. (1994) A clinical trial of topical trolamine salicylate in osteoarthritis. *Current Therapy Research*, 55, 584–97.

25. Deal, C.L., Schnitzer, T.J., Lipstein, E., Seibold, J.R., Posner, M., Stevens, R.M., *et al.* (1991). Treatment of arthritis with topical capsaicin: a double blind trial. *Clinical Therapeutics*, 13, 383–95.

26. Altman, R.D., Aven, A., Holmburg, C.E., Pfeifer, L.M., Sack, M., and Young, G.T. Capsaicin cream 0.025% as monotherapy for osteoarthritis: a double blind study. *Seminars in Arthritis and Rheumatism*, 23 (**supplement** 3); 25–33.

27. Gaffney, K., Ledingham, J., and Perry, J.D. (1995). Intra-articular triamcinolone hexacetonide in knee osteoarthritis: factors influencing the clinical response. *Annals of the Rheumatic Diseases*, 54; 379–81.

28. Jones, A. and Doherty, M. (1996). Intra-articular corticosteroids are effective in osteoarthritis but there are no clinical predictors of response. *Annals of the Rheumatic Diseases*, 55, 829–32.

29. Dougados, M., Nguyen, M., Listrat, V., and Amor, B. (1993). High molecular weight sodium hyaluronate (hyalectin) in osteoarthritis of the knee. A one year placebo-controlled trial. *Osteoarthritis and Cartilage*, 1, 97–103.

30. Jones, A.C., Pattrick, M., Doherty, S., and Doherty, M. (1995). Intra-articular hyaluronic acid compared to intra-articular triamcinolone hexacetonide in inflammatory knee osteoarthritis. *Osteoarthritis and Cartilage*, 3, 269–73.

31. Amadio, P. Jr and Cummings, D.M. (1983). Evaluation of acetaminophen in the management of osteoarthritis of the knee. *Current Therapy Research*, 34, 59–66.

32. Bradley, J.D., Brandt, K.D., Katz, B.P., Kalasinski, L.A., and Ryan, S.I. (1991). Comparison of an anti-inflammatory dose of ibuprofen, an analgesic dose of ibuprofen, and acetaminophen in the treatment of patients with osteoarthritis of the knee. *New England Journal of Medicine*, 325, 87–91.

33. Williams, H.J., Ward, J.R., Egger, M.J., Neuner, R., Brooks, R.H., Clegg D.O., *et al.* (1993). Comparison of

naproxen and acetaminophen in a two-year study of treatment of osteoarthritis of the knee. *Arthritis and Rheumatism*, **36**, 1196–1206.

34. Brooks, P.M., Dougan, M.A., Mugford, S., and Meffin, E. (1982). Comparative effectiveness of five analgesics in patients with rheumatoid arthritis and osteoarthritis. *Journal of Rheumatology*, **9**, 723–6.

35. Kjaersgaard-Anderson, P., Nafei, A., Scov, O., Madsen, F., Andersen, H.M., Kroner, K., *et al.* (1990). Codeine plus paracetamol versus paracetamol in longer-term treatment of chronis pain due to osteoarthritis of the hip. A randomised, double-blind, multi-centre study. *Pain*, **43**, 309–18.

36. Parr, G., Darekar, B., Fletcher, A., and Bulpitt, C.J. (1985). Joint pain and quality of life; results of a randomised trial. *British Journal of Clinical Pharmacology*, **27**, 235–42.

37. Doyle, D.V., Dieppe, P.A., Scott, J., and Huskissen, E.C. (1981). An Articualr index for the assessment of osteoarthritis. *Annals of the Rheumatic Diseases*, **40**, 75–8.

38. March, L., Irwig, L., Schwartz, J., Simpson, J., Chock C., and Brooks, P. (1994). n of 1 trials comparing a non-steroidal anti-inflammatory drug with paracetamol in osteoarthritis. *British Medical Journal*, **309**, 1041–5.

39. Dieppe, P.A., Cushnaghan, J., Jasani, M.K., McCrae, F., and Watt, I. (1993). A two-year, placebo-controlled trial of non-steroidal anti-inflammatory therapy in osteoarthritis of the knee joint. *British Journal of Rheumatology*, **32**, 595–600.

40. Henry, D., Lim, L. L-Y., Garcia Rodriguez, L.A., Gutthann, S.P., Carson, J.L., Griffin, M., *et al.* (1996). Variability in risk of gastrointestinal complications with individual non-steroidal anti-inflammatory drugs; results of a collaborative meta-analysis. *British Medical Journal*, **312**, 1563–6.

41. Livesley, P.J., Doherty, M., Needoff, M., and Moulton, A. (1991). Arthroscopic lavage of osteoarthritic knees. *Journal of Bone and Joint Surgery*, **73-B**, 922–6.

42. Ike, R.W., Arnold, W.J., Rothschild, E.W., and Shaw, H.L. (1992). Tidal irrigation versus conservative medical management in patients with osteoarthritis of the knee: a prospective randomised study. *Journal of Rheumatology*, **19**, 772–9.

43. Chang, R.W., Falconer, J., Stulberg, S.D., Arnold, W.J., Manheim, L.M., and Dyer, A.R. (1993). A randomised, controlled trial of arthroscopic surgery versus closed-needle joint lavage for patients with osteoarthritis of the knee. *Arthritis and Rheumatism*, **36**, 289–96.

44. Egsmose, C., Lund, B., and Anderson, R.B. (1984). Hip joint distension in osteoarthrosis. *Scandinavian Journal of Rheumatology*, **13**, 238–42.

45. Wiklund, I. and Romanus, B. (1991). A comparison of quality of life before and after arthroplasty in patients who had arthrosis of the hip joint. *Journal of Bone and Joint Surgery*, **73-A**, 765–9.

46. Mattsson, E., Brostrom, L-A., and Linnarsson, D. (1990). Changes in walking ability after knee replacement. *International Orthopedics*, **14**, 277–80.

47. Valenti, J.R., Calvo, R., Lopez, R., and Canadell, J. (1990). Long term evaluation of high tibial osteotomy. *International Orthopedics*, **14**, 347–9.

48. Ivarsson, I., Mynerts, R., and Gillquist, J. (1990). High tibial osteotomy for medial osteoarthritis of the knee. *Journal of Bone and Joint Surgery*, **72-B**, 238–44.

49. Werners, R., Vincent, B., and Bulstrode, C. (1990). Osteotomy for osteoarthritis of the hip. *Journal of Bone and Joint Surgery*, **72-B**, 1010–13.

50. Scott, D.L. (1993). Guidelines for the diagnosis, investigation and management of osteoarthritis of the hip and knee. *Journal of the Royal College of Physicians*, **27**, 391–6.

9.2 Why does the patient with osteoarthritis hurt?

Nortin M. Hadler

Nearly three centuries have passed since Thomas Sydenham ushered in the era of scientific medicine. It was his genius that deduced the illness-disease syllogism[1]; symptoms and signs are the illness which is symbolic of some underlying pathoanatomical disorder, a disease. The symbolism of symptoms and signs, a branch of philosophy known as semiotics, was not new with Sydenham; it had been appreciated since antiquity, driving a tradition of treating categories of illness according to the dictates of some abstraction or other. Thanks to Sydenham, forevermore the first

charge to the physician is to define the disease that underlies the category of illness. Then, the physician was to design specific therapy to remediate that disease, with the expectation that the illness would regress as a consequence. Without this conceptual watershed, we might still be diagnosing 'catarrh' instead of curing pneumonias, or 'dropsy' instead of designing therapy specific for each of the causes of the edematous state. The illness-disease syllogism is both the pride and the holy grail of western medicine. It has led to so many triumphs that we seldom question whether it has also left tragedy in its wake. In this chapter, we will explore whether applying the syllogism to regional musculoskeletal illness is such a tragedy.

Every one of us has experienced musculoskeletal discomfort. Sometimes we feel compelled to seek medical care. The moment we describe our morbidity to a physician, we abdicate the station of the person who is trying to cope: we assume the role of the patient. The illness-disease syllogism is joined. What is the cause of this *regional musculoskeletal illness*[2]? For several generations, the usual answer has been 'osteoarthritis.' After all, more often than not, degenerative joint disease is present in the back of the patient with backache, the neck of the patient with neck pain, the knee of the patient with knee pain, and so forth. Medical science was not totally deluded by this coincidence; the age-dependent prevalence of degenerative disease of all regions had been established in necropsy surveys 60 years ago[3].

Everyone will have osteoarthritis, (OA) but not everyone will become a patient with regional joint pain. The mystery that remained was not whether OA was the culprit — that has been generally accepted as the given. The mystery was to define the aspects of OA that afflict the sufferer[4]. I would venture to say that every other chapter in this volume takes this mystery as its starting point. Certainly the 'ACR Criteria for Osteoarthritis', presented in Appendix 1, bears witness to the fashion in which this illness-disease syllogism has commandeered thinking. I am not suggesting that the syllogism is foolish; rather that it falls short as an explanatory model for regional musculoskeletal illness today, and may never serve the vast majority of sufferers at all. To do better, we must reconsider what we mean by 'osteoarthritis', knowing that there are obvious flaws in the illness-disease syllogism with which we are imbued.

Semiotics and OA

The title of this chapter, '*Why does the patient with osteoarthritis hurt?*', is not a rhetorical device; it only seems so. It is a peremptory question. It constrains any response by nature of the implicit tautology; OA is painful, and it is the pain of OA that is somehow responsible for causing the person to choose to be a patient with a regional musculoskeletal illness. Because of this question, the clinician takes recourse in suppressing the discomfort with pharmaceuticals, or trying to extirpate the putatively offending part. It is the question that seduces the pharmaceutical industry to elucidate the mechanisms of joint destruction with the expectation that therein lies the solution to the patient's dilemma.

'*People with osteoarthritis hurt. Why?*' is the question that should drive molecular biology. It is less germane to the clinician, who traditionally is asked to minister to the small fraction of people who hurt and who also choose to be patients. But even this question is not straightforward. As is obvious, from close inspection of Chapter 2, the epidemiology of OA and the epidemiology of regional musculoskeletal discomfort have little in common — not nothing in common, but surprisingly little[5]. Take the example of knee pain, where such an assertion might seem counterintuitive; the relevant data from one survey are presented in Table 9.2. This was a household survey undertaken by the National Center for Health Statistics in the 1970s[6], with follow-up of the patients with OA of the knee a decade later[7]. Clearly, at all ages, more of us suffer knee pain than bear radiographic stigmata of OA of the knee. True, those with more severe radiographic disease are somewhat more likely to experience difficulty with activities requiring mobility[7]. However,

Table 9.2 The % of the US population that recalled having at least one month of daily knee pain in the past year, compared with the prevalence of radiographic arthritis*

	Men		Women	
Age (years)	Symptoms of knee pain (%)	Radiographic arthritis (%)	Symptoms of knee pain (%)	Radiographic arthritis (%)
23–34	5.7	NA	5.2	NA
35–44	7.4	NA	8.1	NA
45–54	12.0	2.3	11.5	3.6
55–64	11.5	4.0	15.0	7.2
65–74	14.9	8.4	19.7	17.9
25–74	9.5	NA	10.9	NA

* Data are from the National Center for Health Statistics.[6]
NA = not available

progression of radiographic OA of the knee is slow, and not predictable, whereas symptoms can exacerbate or regress, regardless of radiographic progression[8]. Clearly, knee pain is the malady, not OA[9].

That insight is central to understanding the semiotics of all the regional musculoskeletal disorders. People — all people — will be forced to cope with musculoskeletal discomfort. Usually, the symptom is exacerbated by usage of the region, and relieved if the region is put to rest. There are some important age-related differences in the distribution of involved regions and even in the quality of some regional symptoms. But that does not take away the fact that each, and every one of us, will 'hurt' in a musculoskeletal region, and do so often and repeatedly. Coping with these predicaments is a fact of life; successfully coping is a prerequisite to healthfulness.

This is not to belittle the fate of so many of our joints. Elegant diarthrodial joints slowly deteriorate. For some joints, such as the apophyseal joints, the process is inexorable and unavoidable. This is the pathoanatomical process we have labeled 'osteoarthritis.' It is not linear over time, nor is it a single process across regions or in a given joint. For example, osteophytes can grow across joints, with little progression in articular dissolution; this is readily demonstrable at the knee, and can be so striking at the spine to warrant the designation 'ankylosing hyperostosis.' However, at no stage in the progression is the clinical consequence predictable. Osteophytes at the knee are more likely to mark a functional joint, than one that has deteriorated[10]. Even people whose joint or joints are ravaged need not be cognizant, or persistently troubled, and certainly need not feel compelled to seek medical attention.

It follows that the clinically relevant question is, '*Why did this person, who may have osteoarthritis, and who is faced with another regional musculoskeletal predicament, choose to be a patient at this time?*' This is the question that should supersede the two above; it is far more consistent with clinical reality. The task for the clinician is to assist the patient in weighing the factors that have compromised their ability to cope. Certainly, the intensity of discomfort, discomfort that is unfamiliar in quality, or compromise in function can be causal. Occasionally, coping can be rendered effete by the magnitude of anatomical distortion consequent to OA. Equally certainly, coping can be confounded by a myriad of psychosocial stresses. Weighing these variables is the art of medicine, rendered all the more challenging because seldom is causation univariate. But, ignoring any of them places the patient at peril.

Focusing on the putative inflammatory nature of OA, or its anatomical stigmata, is to spurn a compelling literature that offers the potential for palliation, if not remediation, of the predicament that caused the person to be a patient in the first place.

Processing regional musculoskeletal symptoms

Most instances of regional musculoskeletal discomfort give us little pause. That is not to say they are trivial. After all, in the course of six weeks, more than 50 per cent of the population of the United States can record, at the end of eight days, that this was a day colored by musculoskeletal discomfort, most often in the axial skeleton[11]. But we cope — most of the time by relying on our common sense and taking recourse in 'over-the-counter' analgesics, home advice, and home remedies. And, most of the time our common sense rewards us with regression of symptoms before our confidence in our personal resources is too shaken. However, common sense is not common; it is not common temporally or geographically, and it is easily perturbed. In fact, in all advanced countries there is an industry committed to perturbing common sense with a cacophony of putatively well-intentioned advice. Osteopathy, the chiropractic, Christian Science, and the entire Pentecostal movement, are the legacy of nineteenth century advice[12]. Today, these practitioners are joined by newer, alternative healers providing recourse to a large segment of the ambulatory ill[13]. No sufferer with a regional musculoskeletal disorder is unaware of these options; all are tempted, and many take advantage. To think otherwise is naive, and to ignore this aspect of a patient's experience of illness creates a barrier to communication that further compromises the marginal benefits of the interventions that are the purview of orthodox medicine.

At some point, some of us suffering with regional musculoskeletal illness will find our personal resources lacking and not adequately supplemented by whatever assistance we obtain from alternative providers. Fig. 9.1 tries to capture the dynamic of coping; choosing to seek professional assistance is indeed a process, always anxiety provoking, never straightforward, and never in a vacuum. For example, each year, 80 per cent of Danes in the suburbs of Copenhagen decide that their personal resources are so inadequate that it makes sense to seek professional care for their backache[14].

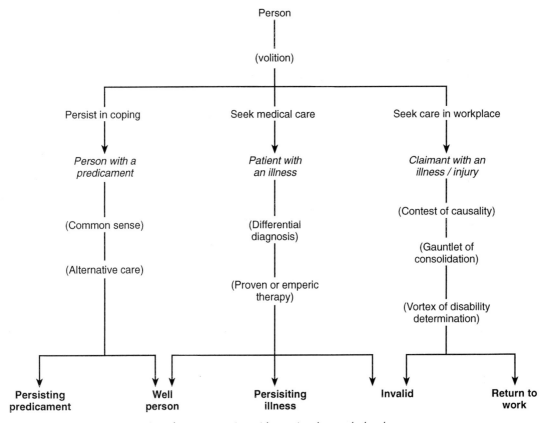

Fig. 9.1 Diagrammatic representation of a person coping with a regional musculosketal symptom.

Americans are far more persistent in coping[11]. Even though low back pain is their chief reason for seeking chiropractic or osteopathic care, and the second most prevalent reason for turning to a physician[15], Americans generally endure their pain for more than two weeks before they conclude that seeking medical care seems sensible[16].

For the past century, the medical care provided in advanced countries has been stratified as to whether the illness is a consequence of an injury that arose out of, and in, the course of employment, or is not work related. The former circumstance entitled one to more comprehensive care and to wage replacement. There have been many experiments with the application of this stratification[17]. However, the most dramatic experiment, and the one most germane to our considerations, was the conceptualization of degenerative joint disease as an injury, if symptoms commenced at work, or even interfered with work. In this fashion, and in this context, backache became 'I injured my back'[18]; degenerative processes of the spine were indemnified under workers' compensation schemes, and processing

of all regional musculoskeletal symptoms would, nevermore, be the same. As is clear in Fig. 9.1, when processing of the symptoms of a regional musculoskeletal disorder results in the decision to seek medical care, there are two alternatives. One can seek the care of a physician outside the industrial context, in which case the illness-disease syllogism is enjoined, focusing on OA. However, if care is sought in the industrial context, and the illness is considered to have arisen in the course of work, 'injury' subjugates OA and the patient assumes the role of workers' compensation insurance claimant. The consequences of traveling these disparate pathways are dramatically different[19]. However, the thesis of this chapter is not the consequences; it is the *reason* for the choice between the three options in Fig. 9.1. Precious little is known about this, but what is known is illuminating.

Choosing to be a patient with knee pain

Nearly every western physician, let alone orthopedic surgeon, is convinced that the secret to evaluating the patient with knee pain is to evaluate the knee. Every medical student is taught, and every orthopedic surgeon never forgets, the signs of meniscal tears, even though we have known for over a decade that their predictive value renders them nearly useless[20]. Imaging the knee defines pathoanatomy, even elegantly, but again the predictive values of these findings are so unimpressive as to render the imaging uninterpretable in the clinical context of the illness-disease syllogism. Yet image we must. Arthroscopy adds little to the definition of pathoanatomy, and arthroscopic surgery is of no demonstrated benefit in the young; in both the young and the elderly, the evidence of its benefit in OA is shortterm, generally anecdotal, and anything but compelling. The upshot is that, try as is our wont, as is our 'standard of care', it is exceptional when we can define the disease that underlies regional knee pain, and truly extraordinary when we can specifically intervene. That is the reason that all interventions are rank empiricisms which, with rare exception, are of no demonstrated value, and probably of little, if any, demonstrable value.

The following chapters detail the limitations of a range of physical, pharmaceutical, and surgical options. These chapters also hold out hope for newer interventions building on the theoretical bases of those currently in use. While efforts to improve diarthrodial joint biology, so as to diminish the likelihood that any one of us will develop biomechanically unsound knees, should be encouraged. It should not be presumed that any such advance will eliminate, or even diminish, our need to cope with intermittent and remittent knee pain and, on occasion, to turn to others for assistance in coping.

The above prediction is based on the results of three separate analyses comparing the influence of psychosocial variables with that of physical measures on the experience of illness in patients with OA, principally of the knee[21-23]. All three used quantification of radiographic OA as the measure of disease, used standard instruments to assess the quantity of pain and disability these patients were experiencing, and assessed the psychological status of the patients by similarly standardized instruments. In all three, the psychological status, particularly disorders in affect, correlated better with the magnitude of pain and dysfunction than the radiographic measures. One could argue that the radiographic scores were insensitive; subtle changes in structure engender significant pain and incapacity, which in turn explains the increased prevalence of depression and other alterations in affect. There is no

incontrovertible counterargument. However, we do know that enthusiastically supervised programs of 'exercise' and social support can impressively alter the patients' perception of their painful and incapacitating knee OA, so that arthroplasty is no longer the only reasonable option[24]. Again, several following chapters will expand on this point.

Choosing to be a claimant with a regional back injury

Although most of this chapter has emphasized the flaws in the illness-disease syllogism as it relates to knee pain, low back pain provides an even more dramatic object lesson. Low back pain was subsumed under the rubric of 'injury' 60 years ago, when 'ruptured disc' was introduced into the clinical lexicon. From then on, particularly in America, any worker who experienced back pain on the job, or whose back pain interfered with function on the job, was potentially eligible for indemnification under the workers' compensation program[17-19]. The choice of the claimant role for back injury (see Fig. 9.1) is seductive, as it offers the promise of all the medical and surgical care money can buy, to put the back injury right, as well as a guarantee of maintenance of wages during the healing phase and, even afterward, should incapacity persist. The consequences of applying the workers' compensation algorithm for redress to regional low back pain include escalation in claims for back injuries, escalation in surgical intervention, escalation in the numbers of workers deemed to suffer permanent partial disabilities, escalation in cost, and the creation of an enormous industry that purports to be helpful. All this can be explained now that we have insight into the processing of the experience of backache that leads a worker to seek care as a 'claimant.'

It is not clear whether any worker performing any task that has been studied, is more likely to experience regional backache than anyone else of similar age and sex. Certainly, if the task he or she is to perform in the workplace is more physically demanding, the challenge to cope is greater. Nonetheless, most do cope, probably because they are fortunate to find themselves in jobs that are accommodating when they are ill. There is a compelling experimental literature that the reason a worker with a backache chooses to be a claimant with an injury, is that the job was not accommodating when he or she was ill, and usually, not accommodating also when he or she was well[25]. Unfortunately, physicians, imbued with the illness-disease syllogism, are still not prepared to pursue the possibility that a complaint of 'my back hurts' is really a complaint that 'my back hurts but I'm here because I can't cope' in the workplace[26]. When resentment, job dissatisfaction, and the like, color the illness, and medical management is constrained by an insurance paradigm that is contentious by design, the process is inherently iatrogenic[19]. It is no surprise that long-term tragedies abound. After all, even if the 'injured worker' returns to work as rapidly as the 'ill' worker with a backache, he or she does so despite the perception of persisting illness[27]. No wonder that workers who have previously claimed back injuries are more likely to claim again, and less likely to enjoy full health in the future.

Conclusion

The thesis of this chapter has been put forth in an unwavering fashion. What if the thesis is incorrect; if the vaunted illness-disease syllogism really does pertain to knee, and hip, and axial pain? Perhaps joint pain can be expunged from the human predicament if we can abrogate OA, or effectively palliate it, or postpone it for decades, so that facet joints and condyles would remain pristine and would articulate harmoniously throughout a lifetime.

It would be far more straightforward to blithely design reductionistic experiments until we honed down on the proximal molecular cause, and then found the remedy for OA. Unfortunately, all attempts to date have fallen so far short. And, whenever we consider the experience of joint pain, we learn that 'osteoarthritis' is a minor variable. If the above thesis is correct, the only way we will serve the joint that hurts, well, is to realize that it is a patient that registered the complaint — we can then explore ways to improve his or her coping[28].

References

1. Foucault, M. (1973). *The birth of the clinic: an archeology of medical perception.* Tavistock Publications, London.
2. Hadler, N.M. (1987). *Clinical concepts in regional musculoskeletal illness.* Grune and Stratton, Orlando.
3. Heine, J. (1926). Über die arthritis deformans. *Virchows Archives.* 260, 521–663.
4. Sokoloff, L. (1969). *The biology of degenerative joint disease.* The University of Chicago Press, Chicago.
5. Hadler, N.M. (1985). Osteoarthritis as a public health problem. *Clinics in the Rheumatic Diseases*, 11, 175–85.
6. National Health and Nutrition Examination Survey (US) (1979). Basic data on arthritis — knee, hip, and sacroiliac joints in adults 25–74 years, United States, 1971–1975. *Vital and Health Statistics Series 11*, No. 213, Publication Number (PHS) 79–1661. Publication Number (PHS)79–1661. National Center for Health Statistics Hyattsville, Maryland.
7. Davis, M.A., Ettinger, W.H., Neuhous, J.M., and Mallon, K.P. (1991) Knee osteoarthritis and physical functioning: evidence from the NHANES I epidemiologic follow-up study. *Journal of Rheumatology*, 18, 591–8.
8. Massardo, L., Watt, I., Cushnaghan, J., and Dieppe, P. (1989). Osteoarthritis of the knee joint: an eight-year prospective study. *Annals of the Rheumatic Diseases*, 48, 893–7.
9. Hadler, N.M. (1992). Knee pain is the malady — not osteoarthritis. *Annals of Internal Medicine*, 116, 598–9.
10. Felson, D.T., Hannan, M.T., Naimark, A., *et al.* (1991). Occupational physical demands, knee bending, and knee osteoarthritis: Results from the Framingham Study. *Journal of Rheumatology* 18, 1587–92.
11. Verbrugge, L.M. and Ascione, F.J. (1987). Exploring the iceberg: common symptoms and how people care for them. *Medical Care*, 12, 264–8.
12. Gevitz, N. (ed.) (1988). *Other healers: unorthodox medicine in America*, pp. 1–302. Johns Hopkins University Press, Baltimore.
13. Murray, R.H. and Rubel, A.J. (1992). Physicians and healers — unwitting partners in health care. *New England Journal of Medicine*, 326, 61–4.
14. Biering-Sorensen, F. (1983). A prospective study of low back pain in a general population. III. Medical service — work consequence. *Scandinavian Journal of Rehabilitation Medicine*, 15, 89–96.
15. Cypress, B.K. (1983). Characteristics of physician visits for back symptoms: a national perspective. *American Journal of Public Health*, 73, 389–95.
16. Deyo, R.A. and Tsue-Wu, Y-J. (1987). Descriptive epidemiology of low-back pain and its related medical care in the United States. *Spine*, 12, 264–8.
17. Hadler, N.M. (1995). The disabling backache. An international perspective. *Spine*, 20, 640–9.
18. Hadler, N.M. (1987). Regional musculoskeletal diseases of the low back. Cumulative trauma versus single incident. *Clinical Orthopaedics*, 221, 33–41.
19. Hadler, N.M. (1993). *Occupational musculoskeletal disorders*, pp. 1–273. Raven Press, New York.
20. Danie, D., Daniels, E., and Aronson, D. (1982). The diagnosis of meniscal pathology. *Clinical Orthopaedics*, 163, 218–24
21. Summers, M.N., Haley, W.E., Reveille, J.D., and Alarcón, G.S. (1988). Radiographic assessment and psychologic variables as predictors of pain and functional impairment in osteoarthritis of the knee or hip. *Arthritis and Rheumatism*, 31, 204–9.
22. Salaffi, F., Cavaliere, F., Nolli, M., and Ferraccioli, G. (1991). Analysis f disability in knee osteoarthritis. Relationship with age and psychological variables but

not with radiographic score. *Journal of Rheumatology*, 18, 1581–6.

23. Dexter, P. and Brandt, K. (1994). Distribution and predictors of depressive symptoms in osteoarthritis. *Journal of Rheumatology*, 21, 279–86.

24. Kovar, P.A., Allegrante, J.P., MacKenzie, R., Peterson, M.G.E., Gutin, B., and Charlson, M.E. (1992). Supervised fitness walking in patients with osteoarthritis of the knee. *Annals of Internal Medicine*, 116, 529–34.

25. Bongers, P.M., de Winter, C.R., Kompier, M.A.J., and Hildebrandt, V.H. (1993). Psychosocial factors at work and musculoskeletal disease. *Scandinavian Journal of Work and Environmental Health*, 19, 297–312.

26. Hadler, N.M. (1994). The injured worker and the internist. *Annals of Internal Medicine*, 120, 163–4.

27. Hadler, N.M., Carey, T.S., and Garrett, J. (1995). The influence of indemnification by workers' compensation insurance on recovery from acute backache. *Spine*, 20, 2710–5.

28. Blalock, S.J., DeVillis, B.M., and Giorgino, K.B. (1995). The relationship between coping and psychological well-being among people with osteoarthritis: a problem-specific approach. *Annals of Behavioural Medicine*, 17, 107–15.

9.3 Nonsteroidal anti-inflammatory drugs*

Marie R. Griffin

Nonsteroidal anti-inflammatory drugs (NSAIDs) are now considered by many to be second line therapy for osteoarthritis (OA)[1,2]. NSAIDs are clearly superior to placebo for pain on movement and at rest, and for morning stiffness associated with OA. Some studies have documented improvement in function as well. However, the efficacy of NSAIDs is modest overall, control of symptoms is rarely complete, and the toxicity of these drugs is substantial, especially in elderly patients using relatively high doses for chronic pain control. This chapter will review the efficacy and toxicity of NSAIDs, and evidence for between-drug differences, and will present an approach to the use of NSAIDs in patients with OA.

Efficacy of NSAIDs

Many trials have addressed the efficacy of short-term administration of NSAIDS, most often compared to placebo or to other NSAIDs. Little information is available on the efficacy of NSAIDs when administered chronically, and almost no information on NSAID dosing schedules other than daily administration. Information on efficacy is summarized as:

• no slowing of disease progression

* Supported in part by the National Institute of Health/National Institute on Aging. 5R01A9 10566

• 10–20 per cent decrease in pain and stiffness with short-term use (1–12 weeks)

• high drop-out rate in longer trials due to side effects and lack of efficacy

• acetaminophen (2–4 g per day) has similar efficacy in many persons.

Appropriate outcome measures in OA

No drug treatment has been shown to delay the progression of disease in humans with OA. *In vitro* and *in vivo* studies in animal models actually suggest that at least some NSAIDs may inhibit cartilage maintenance and or repair mechanisms[2]. Several studies in humans suggest that indomethacin[3–5], and a variety of other NSAIDs[6,7], may accelerate progression of disease in joints. However, these data are controversial and carefully controlled studies are needed to address this issue[2]. Therefore, the aim of NSAID treatment is symptom relief, not cure.

Short-term efficacy of NSAIDs

Many studies have documented the superiority of NSAIDs over placebo[8]. In one double blind study comparing ibuprofen with benoxaprofen[9], patients ranked their overall pain after four weeks of ibuprofen treatment as 34, compared to 55 at baseline, using a

100 mm visual analogue scale (VAS) — a 21 per cent absolute difference. No differences were observed between the effects of ibuprofen and benoxaprofen. These results are similar to those of other studies[10,11] which have reported 10 to 20 per cent differences between NSAID and placebo, and between baseline and active treatment, using similar scales to measure pain and stiffness, with typical baseline values of 40–60 (on a scale of 0 to 100) and post-treatment values of 25–45[12-14].

Other studies have used categorical scales to determine the proportion of patients that may benefit from treatment with an NSAID. In a recent large trial comparing nabumetone to diclofenac, naproxen, ibuprofen, and piroxicam[12], 43 per cent of patients randomized to nabumetone reported improvement after four weeks, 33 per cent reported no change, and 24 per cent had worsening of symptoms. These changes corresponded to a 14 per cent decrease in pain, based on changes in a VAS. Again, there were no significant between-drug differences.

Long-term efficacy of NSAIDs

Most clinical trials of drug efficacy in OA have been relatively short term, usually one to three months. However, many persons with OA take these drugs for years. In a two-year trial, Dieppe *et al.*[15] randomized 89 patients on chronic NSAID therapy for knee OA to 100 mg diclofenac daily or placebo. Patients were permitted to take acetaminophen (paracetamol), up to 4 g daily, as 'rescue' medication. Only 57 per cent completed the two years of the trial. Twenty-seven per cent of those in the placebo group withdrew (primarily in the first three months) due to lack of efficacy, compared to 7 per cent in the diclofenac group (p < 0.01). Approximately 30 per cent of the 38 subjects who did not complete the trial were withdrawn because of side effects, and 15 per cent because of lack of compliance, but there was no appreciable difference between treatment groups in this respect. At the end of two years, among subjects who remained in the trial, 52 per cent of those randomized to diclofenac reported they were better, 16 per cent were the same, and 32 per cent were worse. Outcomes in the placebo group were similar — 45 per cent were improved, 25 per cent were unchanged, and 30 per cent were worse. Placebo recipients consumed an average of 2 g of acetaminophen daily, compared to 1.7 g among those given active drug.

In another two-year study, Williams *et al.*[16] randomized 178 patients with knee OA who had not been on long-term NSAID therapy to naproxen, 750 mg daily, or acetaminophen, 2600 mg daily. Only 35 per cent of these patients completed the two-year trial, 31 per cent of those randomized to acetaminophen and 39 per cent of those assigned to the naproxen group. Withdrawals due to adverse effects were more common among naproxen (23 per cent) than acetaminophen (18 per cent) recipients; however, withdrawals due to lack of efficacy (16 versus 22 per cent) and other reasons (22 versus 30 per cent) were less common among those randomized to naproxen. For those remaining in the trial at two years, improvement was modest and there were few statistically significant differences between treatment groups, although naproxen appeared to be slightly more effective.

Both of these long-term trials[15,16] demonstrate the limited long-term efficacy of both NSAIDs and acetaminophen. These studies suggest that although NSAIDs are clearly superior to placebo overall, they are not clearly superior to acetaminophen, a finding supported also by shorter term studies[17]. The trial by Dieppe *et al.*[15] suggests that a substantial proportion of OA patients receiving chronic NSAID therapy may do as well with withdrawal of their NSAID and use of acetaminophen, 'as-needed'.

Efficacy of differing NSAID regimens

Kvien *et al.*[13] compared a standard fixed dosing regimen of naproxen (500, 750, or 1000 mg daily as determined by patient and physician) to a variable dosing regimen (a maximum of 1000 mg daily, with individual doses and timing determined by the patient) for patients with OA of the hip or knee. There was a decrease in pain on movement as measured on a VAS of about 14 per cent in both groups. However, those assigned to the variable dose regimen consumed 20–30 per cent less naproxen (mean daily dose at eight weeks, 450 mg versus 1335 mg) and had significantly fewer withdrawals due to adverse effects (12 versus 17 per cent). This study suggests that administration of NSAIDs on an as needed basis would be appropriate for many patients.

Studies of NSAID withdrawal in elderly persons[18,19], as well as the two-year studies cited above[15,16], suggest that up to two-thirds of persons who are using NSAIDs chronically may do as well without the NSAID, if other analgesics are available. Periodic attempts at withdrawal and reassessment of NSAID therapy are reasonable. In many clinical trials of NSAIDs, patients have been allowed to take additional analgesics, most often acetaminophen, but cointervention is frequently not evaluated. Seiderman *et al.*[20], in a small, double blind cross-over study of patients with hip OA, found that naproxen plus acetaminophen was more effective than the same dose of naproxen taken alone, and that the effect of naproxen, 500 mg daily, combined with aceta-minophen, 4 g daily, was similar to that of 1000 mg of naproxen alone. Therefore, combination therapy may be preferable to a higher dose of the NSAID, at least for some patients.

Toxicity of NSAIDs

Gastrointestinal tract

NSAIDs have a wide variety of reported adverse effects, the most clinically important of which is their upper gastrointestinal tract toxicity[21]. It has been esti-mated that 15–35 per cent of all peptic ulcer complica-tions are due to these drugs[22–27], and that among the elderly in the United States, 41 000 hospitalizations and 3300 deaths, annually, are attributable to these drugs[21].

Upper gastrointestinal adverse effects of NSAIDs include dyspepsia, ulceration, hemorrhage, perforation, and death[22,23,28–30]. Effects can be summarized as:

• high prevalence of dyspepsia

• doubles usage of H2 receptor antagonists

• increases the risk of ulcer complications four-fold

• ulcer hospitalization rate 1–2 per cent in persons aged 65 and older.

Gastrointestinal symptoms are common, and a fre-quent reason both for withdrawal of NSAIDs and for cotreatment with a 'gastroprotective' drug. In a typical clinical trial, in which patients with known ulcer disease or NSAID intolerance were excluded, 17 per cent of patients randomized to diclofenac reported gas-trointestinal symptoms within four weeks of starting treatment, compared to 0.8 per cent at baseline; 7 per cent withdrew from the trial because of these symptoms[28].

In practice, H2 receptor antagonists, antacids, sucralfate, or misoprostol are often coprescribed to treat such symptoms and / or to prevent ulcer compli-cations. In two population-based studies of older patients, the use of such agents was nearly twice as common in regular NSAID users as in nonusers (11 per cent in nonusers in both studies, and 20 per cent and 26 per cent, respectively, in regular NSAID users)[32,33].

Although dyspepsia is a common symptom that both decreases quality of life[31] and increases the cost of treatment[32,33], it is the more serious gastrointestinal complications that have led to the reconsideration of NSAID therapy as first line treatment for OA[1,2,34,35]. Many studies have now documented that NSAIDs increase the risk of ulcer complications three- to five-fold[29,36,37]. This effect is much more important in older persons because the incidence of ulcer disease increases dramatically with age[25,38]. Hospitalizations for ulcer disease have been reported to be fewer than 1 per 1000 annually, in most populations under age 50[28,39,40]; however, for those 65 years and older, the reported incidence ranges from 2–6 per 1000[27,30,41]. Factors consistently associated with an increased risk of com-plications include:

• increasing age

• increasing NSAID dose[25,30,38,42]

• history of prior ulcer, gastrointestinal hemorrhage, dyspepsia, and/or previous NSAID intolerance[25,38,43]

• use of corticosteroids[25,38,42]

• use of anticoagulants[38,44]

• poor general health[23,42,43]

Older persons are more likely than younger individu-als to use NSAIDs on a regular basis. For an older person, who is a regular NSAID user, the annual rate of hospitalization for ulcer is approximately 16 per 1000 — four-fold higher than for nonusers. Among a cohort of patients with rheumatoid arthritis who were taking NSAIDs, the incidence of hospitalization or death from acute gastrointestinal events was 3 per 1000 person years of NSAID use among those less than 63 years of age, and increased steadily to 42 per 1000 among those older than 75 years of age[42]. In this same cohort, NSAID users with a past history of ulcer disease or gastrointestinal bleeding, serious ulcer com-plications occurred at an annual rate of 40 to 80 per 1000. In-hospital fatality rates associated with peptic ulcer disease are 2–10 per cent,[25,27,38,45] with estimates on the higher end derived from older populations. Therefore, for elderly NSAID users, fatal complications occur at a rate of approximately 1 per 1000 person years of NSAID use, and are higher for those with additional risk factors, such as past history of ulcer disease.

NSAIDs have also been associated with deleterious effects on the small intestine including inflammation associated with loss of blood and protein[46], stricture[47], ulceration, perforation, and diarrhea[48]. Large bowel perforation and hemorrhage are also associated with NSAID use[49]. Although poorly quantitated, clinical consequences of the effects of NSAIDs on the small and large bowel are seen much less frequently than upper gastrointestinal tract problems.

Renal

NSAIDs produce a wide array of undesirable renal effects[50]. Most of these are thought to be due to their ability to inhibit cyclo-ocygenase, a major enzyme in the biosynthesis of prostaglandins. Many studies have shown that a large proportion of patients with conditions that cause a dependence on local production of prostaglandins to maintain renal perfusion (for example, congestive heart failure, dehydration, cirrhosis), will suffer a decline in renal function when exposed to NSAIDs[51,52]. There is some debate over whether all NSAIDs have similar deleterious effects and, specifically, whether sulindac[53] and nabumetone[54] are less likely to cause deterioration in renal function. However, it is clear that all cyclo-oxygenase inhibitors, including sulindac, can decrease renal prostaglandin production and cause a deterioration in renal function if the effective circulating plasma volume is diminished[55–58].

In susceptible patients, NSAIDs can cause a rapid decline in renal function that is usually reversible with discontinuation of the drug. The frequency of this effect may be as high as 13 per cent in frail, elderly nursing home patients[59]. It is much lower in healthier populations. Although most such declines in renal function are transient and clinically insignificant, the decline in renal function may be dramatic, necessitating hospital admission or other acute care. While many case reports suggest a role for NSAIDs in the onset of acute renal failure, few studies have attempted to quantitate the incidence of this effect.

Acute interstitial nephritis has been attributed to most of the NSAIDs, but seems most common with fenoprofen[60–61]. This is an idiosyncratic drug reaction and can occur in patients without any predisposition to renal insufficiency. In contrast to classic, drug-induced allergic nephritis, peripheral blood eosinophilia, fever, and drug rash are uncommon in fenoprofen-induced nephritis[59].

NSAIDs may increase the overall risk for chronic renal failure[62,63], but the contribution of these agents to the development of chronic renal failure, relative to that of acetaminophen, are unknown. However, in two observational studies[64,65], and one clinical trial[17], in which the serum creatinine concentration was measured serially in older patients taking acetaminophen or an NSAID, a decline in renal function was noted among those taking NSAIDs, but not in those taking acetaminophen.

Blood pressure

In experimental studies, the acute administration of a variety of NSAIDs increases both arterial pressure and peripheral resistance[66]. The role of chronic NSAID administration has been less certain. However, more recent data suggest that a variety of NSAIDs interfere with the efficacy of antihypertensive drugs[67–68], raise blood pressure in hypertensive subjects[69], and may result in the initiation of antihypertensive treatment in older persons[70].

Drug interactions

In addition to interference with the efficacy of anti-hypertensive drugs, discussed above, several other drug-drug interactions are fairly frequent and have been shown to produce serious outcomes in population-based studies. Oral corticosteroids, even at the relatively low doses usually used in outpatient care, have been reported to double the rate of serious ulcer disease[25,38,42,71]. The combination of NSAIDs and oral corticosteroids increases the risk of ulcer complication 13 to 15 times that seen in nonusers of either drug, so that older persons using this combination of drugs have an ulcer hospitalization rate of 5 to 6 per cent, per year[25].

In the outpatient setting, anticoagulants increase the risk of upper gastrointestinal bleeding three- to six-fold[38,44]. The combination of NSAIDs and anticoagulants greatly increases the rate of such complications, so that in older persons using this combination, the rate of hospitalization for upper gastrointestinal hemorrhage is about 3 per cent per year[44].

Long-term therapy with angiotensin-converting enzyme (ACE) inhibitors can cause functional renal insufficiency. The presence of factors which decrease renal blood flow will increase the likelihood of renal compromise with these agents. Because NSAIDs interfere with renal hemodynamics, the theoretical potential for problems with this frequently used combination would seem substantial. One population-based study has suggested that renal insufficiency due to this combination may be both serious and relatively common[72].

Other adverse effects

NSAIDs may cause a wide variety of other adverse effects including hepatotoxicity[73], cutaneous toxicity[74], pneumonitis, and neurologic problems including headaches and aseptic meningitis[75].

It has been claimed that NSAIDs may accelerate cartilage damage in OA, either because their analgesic effect results in greater usage of the involved joint, or because some of these agents impair cartilage matrix synthesis by the chondrocyte. There is, however, no evidence from well-controlled clinical trials that NSAIDs accelerate the rate of joint damage in humans with OA (see Chapter 11.5).

Between-drug differences

Efficacy

In a review of nearly 100 comparative trials of NSAIDs in subjects with OA, Hedner[76] found that a daily dose of 2000–4000 mg of aspirin was generally equal to, or less effective in terms of analgesia and function, than 500–700 mg diflunisal, 75–150 mg diclofenac, 100 mg indomethacin, 200–400 mg sulindac, 1200 mg ibuprofen, 400 mg phenylbutazone, and 20 mg piroxicam. In these trials, side effects were generally higher with aspirin than with the comparator NSAIDs. In several trials, ibuprofen, in daily doses of 600– 1200 mg, was less effective than some other NSAIDS. However, in trials using an ibuprofen dose higher than 1200 mg per day, therapeutic efficacy was comparable to that of other NSAIDs. No other consistent between-NSAID differences in efficacy have been found. Bèllamy *et al.* found diclofenac, 75 mg per day, to be less effective for pain and stiffness than meclofenamate, 300 mg per day, but adverse effects with the two treatments were similar[11]. In another study, diclofenac, 150 mg per day, was similar in efficacy to tenoxicam, 20 mg per day, but was associated with significantly more side effects[10]. The between-drug differences in these two trials were not large, but were felt to be clinically significant. However, the results of both studies may be entirely attributable to the doses used, with diclofenac

given at the lower end of the recommended dose in the first study and at the higher end in the second.

Toxicity

Ibuprofen, in doses commonly used in clinical practice, has consistently been associated with a lower risk of serious gastrointestinal complications than other NSAIDs. A recent meta-analysis identified 12 studies of NSAIDs and major upper gastrointestinal tract complications, which included information on individual NSAIDs[36]. Ibuprofen was evaluated in 11 of these 12 studies, and was associated with the lowest risk of complications in 10 of the 11. The increased risk above ibuprofen, for other NSAIDs, varied with the drug: lower than two-fold (fenoprofen, aspirin, dicolfenac), two-fold (sulindac, diflunisal, naproxen, indomethacin), three- to four-fold (piroxicam, ketoprofen, tolmetin), and nine-fold (azapropazone). Although the confidence intervals around many of these estimates were wide, the rank order of drugs within different studies was quite similar, with ibuprofen nearly always associated with the lowest risk, frequently followed by diclofenac. In contrast, piroxicam, ketoprofen, and tolmetin were consistently associated with higher risks. Azapropazone (not available in the United States) was associated with a very high risk in both studies that included this drug.

Fries *et al.*[77] have developed a toxicity index for NSAIDs based on frequency and seriousness of a variety of adverse events: ibuprofen (mean daily dose, 2415 mg), aspirin (2415 mg), and salsalate (2019 mg) had the lowest toxicity scores, whereas ketoprofen (174 mg), meclofenamate (283 mg), tolmetin (1081 mg), and indomethacin (100 mg) had the highest scores. The higher scores for indomethacin and meclofenamate were heavily influenced by central nervous system symptoms and diarrhea, respectively, while the rankings of the other NSAIDs were more influenced by gastrointestinal symptoms and complications.

The lower reported gastrointestinal toxicity of ibuprofen is probably due, at least in part, to a dose phenomenon. There is a clear dose response effect with ibuprofen, as with many other NSAIDs, so that the relative risk reported with higher doses is comparable to that of usual doses of other NSAIDs.

Most large epidemiologic studies of between-NSAID differences did not include non- acetylated salicylates (for example, salsalate) or many of the newer NSAIDs. In short-term clinical trials, salsalate, in doses of 3 to 3.5 g per day, has been associated with lower gastrointestinal blood loss and fewer upper gastrointestinal endoscopic lesions than enteric coated aspirin (2.6 g), naproxen, (750 mg), and piroxicam (20 mg)[78–82]. However, gastrointestinal symptoms were often similar, and overall side effects frequently higher, due to reversible hearing loss and tinnitus reported by about 30 per cent of subjects at these doses[79,81,83]. In the cohort of arthritis patients studied by Fries *et al.*[42], salsalate had a low toxicity score; however, the mean dose used was close to 2 g, and aspirin had a similarly low toxicity index at this dose.

Nabumetone, a relatively new NSAID related to naproxen, is a pro-drug with a long elimination half-life (dosing once daily)[84]. Similar to salsalate, a variety of clinical trials have reported fewer endoscopic lesions with nabumetone (1000 mg daily) than with naproxen (500 mg)[85], ibuprofen (2400 mg)[86], and a variety of other comparison NSAIDs[87]; upper gastrointestinal symptoms are generally slightly less common than with other NSAIDs, whereas the frequency of diarrhea is higher, and overall tolerance appears similar[87,88]. Post-marketing studies of large numbers of subjects suggest a lower rate of clinically significant ulcers than in historical controls; however, direct comparison with other NSAIDs have generally been limited by relatively small numbers of subjects with clinically important ulcers.

An important mechanism of the action of NSAIDs is their ability to inhibit the enzyme cyclo-oxygenase (COX), which controls local prostaglandin production. Of note, two COX molecules, COX-1 and COX-2 have been identified, which are distinct gene product: COX-1, which is present in most tissues, has an important role in maintaining mucosal protection in the gastrointestinal tract; COX-2 is inducible at sites of inflammation[89]. It has been hypothesized that drugs that inhibit COX-2 more selectively than COX-1 will be less likely to cause ulcers, but the ratio of COX-1 to COX-2 inhibition among NSAIDs has been a poor predictor of clinical toxicity[89]. In a study in which gene targeting was used to produce a mouse strain unable to synthesize COX-1, homozygous mutants, surprisingly, showed *less* indomethacin-induced gastric ulceration than wild-type mice, even though their gastric prostaglandin E_2 levels were only about one per cent of those of the wild type[90]. Conversely, in COX-2 knock-out mice, the inflammatory response in several standard models of inflammation was normal[91]. Newer drugs are currently being developed which are much more selective COX-2 inhibitors than those currently available. Whether these drugs will 'spare' the gastrointestinal mucosa is unknown.

There is some evidence that sulindac may not have the deleterious effect on blood pressure reported for other NSAIDs[69,70]; whether it is 'renal-sparing', however, is controversial[54]. Whether significant between-drug differences exist in the frequency of the rarer, serious adverse effects is unknown. Some rare adverse effects have been reported more frequently with specific NSAIDs, for example, hematologic toxicity with phenylbutazone, interstitial nephritis and nephrotic syndrome with fenoprofen, and hepatoxicity with diclofenac. However, most of these adverse effects have been reported with most NSAIDs and it is difficult to determine the relative toxicities of these agents based on these less common side effects[75]. Fries *et al.*[77] have examined more frequent adverse effects and have found patterns similar to those reported by others, for example, an excess of central nervous system symptoms (vertigo, headache, trouble thinking) for indomethacin, an excess of tinnitus for aspirin and salsalate, and an excess of diarrhea for meclofenamate.

Appropriate use of NSAIDs in OA

Population-based studies in the United States[23,92], Canada[25], England[93], and Australia[45] have documented that use of non-aspirin NSAIDs in the elderly is common, and that 10 to 20 per cent have a current or recent NSAID prescription. Use of NSAIDs in the elderly is primarily for symptoms associated with OA and other chronic musculoskeletal conditions. However, the high rate of adverse effects, and the modest efficacy of these agents, suggest that this level of use may not be appropriate. In approaching the patient with symptomatic OA, it is appropriate to consider several options regarding initiation or continuation of NSAID therapy:

(1) try non-pharmacologic measures and topical creams (for example, capsaicin) first;

(2) simple analgesics, such as acetaminophen, are preferable in most patients as first choice for systemic therapy;

(3) consider low-dose ibuprofen as first choice for NSAID;

(4) try 'prn' or intermittent use to limit toxicity;

(5) consider alternatives or misoprostol prophylaxis for those at very high risk of upper gastrointesti-

nal toxicity (for example, the very old, past history of ulcer, high dose NSAID use).

Should an NSAID be used?

Non-medicinal therapies, including behavior modification, (for example, application of joint protection principles), should be considered primary strategies to relieve symptoms and improve function[94]. Simple analgesics, such as acetaminophen, are preferable as an initial choice of systemic medical therapy. NSAIDs should not be continued in patients who do not clearly benefit symptomatically. Even for patients who have had an initial good response to NSAIDs, it is reasonable to try withdrawal periodically. In such patients, a simple analgesic may be prescribed either as needed or on a regular schedule (for example, acetaminophen 1 g, 3–4 times daily).

If an NSAID is used, which one is best?

Although many patients do well with NSAID withdrawal, there are clearly OA patients for whom NSAIDs are superior to acetaminophen for symptomatic relief. For these patients, it is important to minimize the risks of adverse effects. Ibuprofen, especially in doses of less than 1800 mg per day, is a reasonable NSAID of first choice due to its lower gastrointestinal toxicity. Salsalate, and other non-acetylated salicylates, have been less well studied, but may be associated with a lower rate of serious gastrointestinal effects[82]. Lower doses of this drug are often used in practice, in the range of 2 g daily[42]. Furthermore, salsalate has the advantage over ibuprofen of twice daily dosing; higher doses are associated with a high incidence of reversible tinnitus and hearing loss. Further study of nabumetone, and other new NSAIDs, is needed to determine their safety compared to other NSAIDs in comparable doses.

It is reasonable to try to avoid use of those NSAIDs which have consistently ranked higher than others with respect to serious gastrointestinal toxicity (for example, piroxicam, ketoprofen, and tolmetin)[36], especially in patients in whom other risk factors for ulcer disease are present. It is also reasonable to avoid NSAIDs which have other frequent bothersome side effects, such as indomethacin (central nervous system) and meclofenamate (diarrhea). There is much less experience with some of the newer NSAIDs.

What dosing schedule is best?

Although the data are limited, it is reasonable to prescribe NSAIDs on an 'as needed' basis. This type of regimen has been associated with pain control comparable to that of a fixed-dose regimen, but with less toxicity because of the lower amounts of NSAID used[13]. However, NSAIDs which have a long half-life may require several days of repeated dosing before steady-state kinetics and maximum benefits are achieved. Patients with symptoms due to OA may not fit the model for other types of chronic pain, where it has been recommended to give pain medication on a conservative, fixed schedule, rather than as needed[95]. Use of 'as needed' schedules and encouragement of periods of non-use as tolerated, is consistent with encouraging 'self-efficacy' and permitting patients to feel more in control of their symptoms. It also reinforces the principle that these drugs are useful only for symptoms and do not treat the underlying arthritis. Use of other analgesics in combination with NSAIDs, or as 'rescue' analgesia, is also reasonable. Unfortunately, the effects of such chronic analgesic combination on the kidney, in comparison with monotherapy, are unknown.

Is this patient at high risk for an adverse event?

Increasing age and a past history of ulcer disease or dyspepsia are both common in patients with OA. Therefore, older patients, especially those with a history of ulcer disease, should understand that, on average, 2–8 per cent of people treated with an NSAID for one year will be hospitalized with ulcer complications. Other factors that increase the risk include use of anticoagulants and corticosteroids. Anticoagulant therapy and chronic renal failure must be viewed as relative contraindications to the use of NSAIDs. NSAIDs should also be considered as a possible factor in poor blood pressure control, fluid overload, edema, and development of renal insufficiency. An attempt to discontinue the NSAID in response to the appearance of any of these problems is warranted.

Can adverse events be prevented in patients taking NSAIDs?

As noted above, antiulcer drugs are coprescribed for many patients taking NSAIDs. However, while H2 receptor antagonists (the most common class of drugs coprescribed) may relieve symptoms, they have not been shown to prevent NSAID-associated gastric ulcers. Only misoprostol has been demonstrated to prevent clinically important gastric and duodenal ulcers associated with NSAIDs[43]. Recent data suggest that use of high dose H2 blockers or proton pump inhibitors may offer similar protection, but studies of these agents have been limited to ulcers detected during scheduled follow-up endoscopy, rather than symptomatic or clinically important events[96,97].

However, misoprostol is expensive; its efficacy is by no means complete — the estimated decrease in ulcer complications is 40 per cent[43]; adverse effects, predominately diarrhea, are relatively frequent[43,98]; and the drug often does not relieve dyspeptic symptoms. Therefore, the daily quality of life of patients taking misoprostol may be worse than that in those taking an NSAID alone[99]. However, for patients with a high risk of ulcer complications, who receive considerable benefit from an NSAID and not from alternative analgesics, it is reasonable to coprescribe misoprostol. Many patients will not tolerate the recommended dose of 200 μg four times per day, in which case 100 μg four times daily may be used[43]. Misoprostol does not protect, however, against the renal side effects of NSAIDs[100].

Blood pressure and renal function should be monitored in all patients taking an NSAID, especially those concomitantly taking an ACE inhibitor; this combination should be used cautiously. Monitoring of renal function is important also if the patient has other risk factors or events that can lower renal perfusion, such as congestive heart failure or dehydration.

References

1. Sander, J.W.A.S. and Shorvon, S.D. (1988). Non-steroidal anti-inflammatory drugs — prescribe with caution. *Journal of the Royal College of General Practitioners*, **38**, 49–52.
2. Brandt, K.D. (1993). Should osteoarthritis be treated with nonsteroidal anti-inflammatory drugs? *Rheumatic Disease Clinics of North America*, **19**, 697–712.
3. Coke, H. (1967). Long term indomethacin therapy of coxarthrosis. *Annals of the Rheumatic Disease*, **26**, 346–7.
4. Ronningen, H. and Langeland, N. (1977). Indomethacin hips. *Acta Orthopedica Scandinavica*, **48**, 556
5. Rashad, S., Hemingway, A., Rainsford, K., Revell, P., Low, F., and Walker, F. (1989). Effect of non-steroidal anti-inflammatory drugs on the course of osteoarthritis. *Lancet*, **September 2**, (1), 519–22.
6. Solomon, L. (1973). Drug-induced arthropathy and necrosis of the femoral head. *Journal of Bone and Joint Surgery*, **55**, 246–61.
7. Newman, N.M. and Ling, R.S.M. (1985). Acetabular bone destruction related to non-steroidal anti-inflammatory drugs. *Lancet*, **2**, 11–14.
8. Bellamy, N. and Buchanan, W.W. (1984). Outcome measurement in osteoarthritis clinical trials: the case for standardisation. *Clinical Rheumatology*, **3**, 293–303.
9. Tyson, V.C.H. and Glynne, A. (1980). A comparative study of benoxaprofen and ibuprofen in osteoarthritis in general practice. *Journal of Rheumatology*, **7** (supplement 6), 132–8.
10. Bellamy, N., Buchanan, W.W., Chalmers, A., Ford, P.M., Kean, W.F., Kraag, G.R., *et al.* (1993). A multi-center study of tenoxicam and diclofenac in patients with osteoarthritis of the knee. *Journal of Rheumatology*, **20**, 999–1004.
11. Bellamy, N., Kean, W.F., Buchanan, W.W., Gerecz-Simon, E., and Campbell, J. (1992). Double blind randomized controlled trial of sodium meclofenamate (Meclomen) and diclofenac sodium (Voltaren): post validation reapplication of the WOMAC osteoarthritis index. *Journal of Rheumatology*, **19**, 159.
12. Lister, B.J., Poland, M., and DeLapp, R.E. (1993). Efficacy of nabumetone versus diclofenac, naproxen, ibuprofen, and piroxicam in osteoarthritis and rheumatoid arthritis. *American Journal of Medicine* **95**, 2–9.
13. Kvien, T.K., Brors, O., Staff, P.H., Rognstad, S., and Nordby, J. (1991). Improved cost-effectiveness ratio with a patient self-adjusted naproxen dosing regimen in osteoarthritis treatment. *Scandinavian Journal of Rheumatology*, **20**, 280–7.
14. Levinson, D.J. and Rubinstein, H.M. (1983). Double-blind comparison of fenoprofen calcium and ibuprofen in osteoarthritis of large joints. *Current Therapy Research*, **34**, 280–4.
15. Dieppe, P., Cushnaghan, J., Jasani, M.K., McCrae, F., and Watt, I. (1993). A two-year, placebo-controlled trial of non-steroidal anti-inflammatory therapy in osteoarthritis of the knee joint. *British Journal of Rheumatology*, **32**, 595–600.
16. Williams, H.J., Ward, J.R., Egger, M.J., Neuner, R., Brooks, R.H., and Clegg, D.O., *et al.* (1993). Comparison of naproxen and acetaminophen in a two-year study of treatment of osteoarthritis of the knee. *Arthritis and Rheumatism*, **36**, 1196–206.
17. Bradley, J.D., Brandt, K.D., Katz, B.P., Kalasinski, L.A., and Ryan, S. (1991). Comparison of an antiinflammatory dose of ibuprofen, an analgesic dose of ibuprofen, and acetaminophen in the treatment of patients with osteoarthritis of the knee. *New England Journal of Medicine*, **325**, 87–91.
18. Jones, A.C., Berman, P., and Doherty, M. (1992). Non-steroidal anti-inflammatory drug usage and requirement in elderly acute hospital admissions. *British Journal of Rheumatology*, **31**, 45–8.
19. Swift, G.L. and Rhodes, J. (1992). Are non-steroidal anti-inflammatory drugs always necessary? A general practice survey. *British Journal of Clinical Practice*, **46**, 92–4.
20. Seideman, P., Samuelson, P., and Neander, G. (1993). Naproxen and paracetamol compared with naproxen only in coxarthrosis. Increased effect of the combination in 18 patients. *Acta Orthopedica Scandinavica*, **64**, 285–8.

21. Ray, W.A., Griffin, M.R., and Shorr, R.I. (1990). Adverse drug reactions and the elderly. *Health Affairs*, *(Millwood)*, 9, 114–22.

22. Griffin, M.R., Ray, W.A., and Schaffner, W. (1988). Nonsteroidal anti-inflammatory drug use and death from peptic ulcer in elderly persons. *Annals of Internal Medicine*, 109, 359–63.

23. Griffin, M.R., Piper, J.M., Daugherty, J.R., Snowden, M., and Ray, W.A. (1991). Nonsteroidal anti-inflammatory drug use and increased risk for peptic ulcer disease in elderly persons. *Annals of Internal Medicine*, 114, 257–63.

24. Langman, M.J.S., Weil, J., Wainwright, P., Lawson, D.H., Rawlins, M.D., Logan, R.F.A., *et al.* (1994). Risks of bleeding peptic ulcer associated with individual non-steroidal anti-inflammatory drugs. *Lancet*, 343, 1075–8.

25. Gutthann, S.P., Garcia Rodriguez, L.A., and Raiford, D.S. (1994). Individual non-steroidal anti-inflammatory drugs and the risk of hospitalization for upper gastrointestinal bleeding and perforation in Saskatchewan: a nested case-control study. *Pharmacoepidemiology and Drug Safety*, 3, S63.

26. Henry, D., Dobson, A., Turner, C., Hall, P., Forbes, C., and Patey, P. (1991). NSAIDs and risk of upper gastrointestinal bleeding. *Lancet*, 337, 730.

27. Laporte, J., Carné, X., Vidal, X., Moreno, V., and Juan, J. (1991). Upper gastrointestinal bleeding in relation to previous use of analgesics and non-steroidal anti-inflammatory drugs. *Lancet*, 337, 85–9.

28. Garcia Rodriguez, L.A., Walker, A.M., and Gutthann, S.P. (1992). Nonsteroidal antiinflammatory drugs and gastrointestinal hospitalizations in Saskatchewan: a cohort study. *Epidemiology*, 3, 337–42.

29. Gabriel, S.E., Jaakkimainen, L., and Bombardier, C. (1991). Risk for serious gastrointestinal complications related to use of nonsteroidal anti-inflammatory drugs. A meta-analysis. *Annals of Internal Medicine*, 115, 787–96.

30. Smalley, W.E., Ray, W.A., Daugherty, J., and Griffin, M.R. (1995). Nonsteroidal anti-inflammatory drugs and the incidence of hospitalizations for peptic ulcer disease in elderly persons. *American Journal of Epidemiology*, 141, 539–45.

31. Parr, G., Darekar, B., Fletcher, A., and Bulpitt, C.J. (1989). Joint pain and quality of life; results of a randomised trial. *British Journal of Clinical Pharmacology*, 27, 235–42.

32. Smalley, W.E., Griffin, M.R., Fought, R.L., Sullivan, L., and Ray, W.A. (1996). Excess costs for gastrointestinal disease among nonsteroidal anti-inflammatory drug users. *Journal of General Internal Medicine*, 11, 461–9.

33. Hogan, D.B., Campbell, N.R.C., Crutcher, R., Jennett, P., and MacLeod, N. (1994). Prescription of nonsteroidal anti-inflammatory drugs for elderly people in Alberta. *Canadian Medical Association Journal*, 151, 315–22.

34. Dieppe, P.A., Frankel, S.J., and Toth, B. (1993). Is research into the treatment of osteoarthritis with non-steroidal anti-inflammatory drugs misdirected? *Lancet*, 341, 353–4.

35. Liang, M.H. and Fortin, P. (1991). Management of osteoarthritis of the hip and knee. *New England Journal of Medicine*, 325, 125–7.

36. Henry, D., Lim, L. L-Y., Garcia-Rodriguez, L.A., Gutthann, S.P., Carson, J., Griffin, M.R., *et al.* (1996). Variability in risk of major upper gastrointestinal complications with individual NSAIDs. *British Medical Journal*, 312, 1563–6.

37. Bollini, P., Garcia-Rodriguez, L.A., Gutthann, S.P., and Walker, A.M. (1992). The impact of research quality and study design on epidemiologic estimates of the effect of nonsteroidal anti-inflammatory drugs on upper gastrointestinal tract disease. *Archives of Internal Medicine*, 152, 1289–95.

38. Garcia-Rodriguez, L.A. and Jick, H. (1994). Risk of upper gastrointestinal bleeding and perforation associated with individual non-steroidal anti-inflammatory drugs. *Lancet*, 343, 769–72.

39. Steering Committee of the Physicians' Health Study Research Group. (1989). Final report on the aspirin component of the ongoing physicians' health study. *New England Journal of Medicine*, 321, 129–35.

40. Henry, D. and Robertson, J. (1993). Nonsteroidal anti-inflammatory drugs and peptic ulcer hospitalization rates in New South Wales. *Gastroenterology*, 104, 1083–91.

41. Graves, E.J. and Kozak, L.J. (1992). National hospital discharge survey: annual summary, 1990. *Vital Health Statistics*, Series 13. National Center for Health Statistics.

42. Fries, J.F., Williams, C.A., Bloch, D.A., and Michel, B.A. (1991). Nonsteroidal anti-inflammatory drug-associated gastropathy: Incidence and risk factor models. *American Journal of Medicine*, 91, 213–22.

43. Silverstein, F.E., Graham, D.Y., Senior, J.R., Wyn Davies, H., Struthers, B.J., Bittman, R.M., *et al.* (1995). Misoprostol reduces serious gastrointestinal complications in patients with rhematoid arthritis recieving nonsteroidal anti-inflammatory drugs: a randomized, double-blind, placebo-controlled trial. *Annals of Internal Medicine*, 123, 241–9.

44. Shorr, R.I., Ray, W.A., Daugherty, J.R., and Griffin, M.R. (1993). Concurrent use of nonsteroidal anti-inflammatory drugs and oral anticoagulants places elderly persons at high risk for hemorrhagic peptic ulcer disease. *Archives of Internal Medicine*, 153, 1665–70.

45. Savage, R.L., Moller, P.W., Ballantyne, C.L., and Wells, J.E. (1993). Variation in the risk of peptic ulcer complications with nonsteroidal antiinflammatory drug therapy. *Arthritis and Rheumatism*, 36, 84–90.

46. Bjarnason, I., Prouse, P., Smith, T., Gumpel, M.J., Zanelli, G., Smethurst, P., *et al.* (1987). Blood and protein loss via small-intestinal inflammation induced by non-steroidal anti-inflammatory drugs. *Lancet*, September 26, 1, 711–14.

47. Matsuhashi, N., Yamada, A., Hiraishi, M., Konishi, T., Minota, S., Saito, T., *et al.* (1992). Multiple strictures of the small intestine after long-term nonsteroidal anti-inflammatory drug therapy. *American Journal of Gastroenterology*, 87, 1183–6.

48. Kwo, P.Y. and Tremaine, W.J. (1995). Nonsteroidal anti-inflammatory drug-induced enteropathy: case discussion and review of the literature. *Mayo Clinical Proceedings*, **70**, 55–61.

49. Langman, M.J.S., Morgan, L., and Worrall, A. (1985). Use of anti-inflammatory drugs by patients admitted with small or large bowel perforations and haemorrhage. *British Medical Journal*, **290**, 347–9.

50. Clive, D.M. and Stoff, J.S. (1984). Renal syndromes associated with nonsteroidal anti-inflammatory drugs. *New England Journal of Medicine*, **310**, 563–72.

51. Whelton, A., Stout, R.L., Spilman, P.S., and Klassen, D.K. (1990). Renal effects of ibuprofen, piroxicam, and sulindac in patients with asymptomatic renal failure. *Annals of Internal Medicine*, **112**, 568–76.

52. Murray, M.D. and Brater, D.C. (1990). Adverse effects of nonsteroidal anti-inflammatory drugs on renal function. *Annals of Internal Medicine*, **112**, 559–60.

53. Whelton, A. and Hamilton, C.W. (1991). Nonsteroidal anti-inflammatory drugs: effects on kidney function. *Journal of Clinical Pharmacology*, **31**, 588–98.

54. Aronoff, G.R. (1992). Therapeutic implications associated with renal studies of nabumetone. *Journal of Rheumatology*, **19(Supplement 36)**, 25–31.

55. Brater, D.C., Anderson, S.A., Brown-Cartwright, D., and Toto, R.D. (1986). Effects of nonsteroidal anti-inflammatory drugs on renal function in patients with renal insufficiency and in cirrhotics. *American Journal of Kidney Disease*, **5**, 351–5.

56. Brater, D.C. (1988). Clinical aspects of renal prostaglandins and NSAID therapy. *Seminars in Arthritis and Rheumatism*, **17**, 17–22.

57. Kleinknecht, D., Landais, P., and Goldfarb, B. (1986). Analgestic and non-steroidal anti-inflammatory drug-associated acute renal failure: a prospective collaborative study. *Clinical Nephrology*, **25**, 275–81.

58. Stillman, M.T. and Schlesinger, P.A. (1990). Nonsteroidal anti-inflammatory drug nephrotoxicity. Should we be concerned? *Archives of Internal Medicine*, **150**, 568–70.

59. Gurwitz, J.H., Avron, J., Ross-Degnan, D., and Lipsitz, L.A. (1990). Nonsteroidal anti-inflammatory drug-associated azotemia in the very old. *Journal of the American Medical Association*, **264**, 471–5.

60. Cameron, S. (1988). Allergic interstitial nephritis: clinical features and pathogenesis. *Quarterly Journal of Medicine*, **250**, 97–115.

61. Marasco, W.A., Gikas, P.W., Azziz-Baumgartner, R., Hyzy, R., Eldredge, C.J., and Stross, J. (1987). Ibuprofen-associated renal dysfunction. *Archives in Internal Medicine*, **147**, 2107–16.

62. Perneger, T.V., Whelton, P.K., and Klag, M.J., (1994). risk of kidney failure associated with the use of acetaminophen, aspirin, and nonsteroidal antiinflammatory drugs. *New England Journal of Medicine*, **331**, 1675–9.

63. Adams, D.H., Michael, J., Bacon, P.A., Howie, A.J., McConkey, B., and Adu, D. (1986). Non-steroidal anti-inflammatory drugs and renal failure. *Lancet*, **1**, 57–60.

64. Murray, M.D., Brater, D.C., Tierney, W.M., Hui, S.L., McDonald, C.J. (1990). Ibuprofen-associated renal impairment in a large general internal medicine practice. *American Journal of Medicine*, **299**, 222–9.

65. Hale, W.E., May, F.E., Marks, R.G., Moore, M.T., and Stewart, R.B., (1989). Renal effects of nonsteroidal anti-inflammatory drugs in the elderly. *Current Therapy Research*, **46**, 173–9.

66. Smith, M.C. and Dunn, M.J. (1985). The role of prostaglandins in human hypertension. *American Journal of Kidney Disease*, **A32–A39** A32–A39.

67. Chrischilles, E.A. and Wallace, R.B. (1993). Nonsteroidal anti-inflammatory drugs and blood pressure in an elderly population. *Journal of Gerontology*, **48**, M91–M96.

68. Johnson, A.G., Simons, L.A., Simons, J., Friedlander, Y., and McCallum, J. (1993). Non-steroidal anti-inflammatory drugs and hypertension in the elderly: a community-based cross-sectional study. *British Journal of Clinical Pharmacology*, **35**, 455–9.

69. Pope, J.E., Anderson, J.J., and Felson, D.T. (1993). A meta-analysis of the effects of nonsteroidal anti-inflammatory drugs on blood pressure. *Archives in Internal Medicine*, **153**, 477–84.

70. Gurwitz, J.H., Avorn, J., Bohn, R.L., Glynn, R.J., Monane, M., and Mogun, H. (1994). Initiation of anti-hypertensive treatment during nonsteroidal anti-inflammatory drug therapy. *Journal of the American Medical Association*, **272**, 781–6.

71. Piper, J.M., Ray, W.A., Daugherty, J.R., and Griffin, M.R. (1991). Corticosteroid use and peptic ulcer disease: role of nonsteroidal anti-inflammatory drugs. *Annals of Internal Medicine*, **114**, 735–40.

72. Seelig, C.B., Maloley, P.A., and Campbell, J.R. (1990). Nephrotoxicity associated with concomitant ACE inhibitor and NSAID therapy. *Southern Medical Journal*, **83**, 1144–8.

73. Gay, G.R. (1990). Another side effect of NSAIDs. *Journal of the American Medical Association*, **264**, 2677–8.

74. Roujeau, J.C. and Stern, R.S. (1994). Severe adverse cutaneous reactions to drugs. *New England Journal of Medicine*, **331**, 1272–85.

75. Brooks, P.M. and Day, R.O. (1991). Nonsteroidal antiinflammatory drugs — differences and similarities. *New England Journal of Medicine*, **324**, 1716–25.

76. Hedner, T. (1989). Comparative evaluations of NSAIDs and other analgesics in osteoarthrosis. In *Pharmacological treatment of osteoarthritis* (2nd edn.) (ed. National Board of Health and Welfare Drug Information Committee), pp. 173–98. Almqvist and Wiksell, Uppsala.

77. Fries, J.F., Williams, C.A., and Bloch, D.A. (1991). The relative toxicity of nonsteroidal antiinflammatory drugs. *Arthritis and Rheumatism*, **34**, 1353–60.

78. Goldlust, B., Doucette, M., and Verduyn, C. (1991). Developing nonsteroidal anti-inflammatory drugs (NSAIDs) with decreased gastrointestinal (GI) toxicity. *Agents Actions*, **supplement 32**, 27–31.

79. Scheiman, J.M., Behler, E.M., and Berardi, R.R. (1989). Salicylsalicylic acid causes less gastroduodenal mucosal damage than enteric-coated aspirin. An endoscopic comparison. *Digestive Diseases and Sciences*, **34s**, 229–32.

80. Bianchi, P.G., Petrillo, M., and Ardizzone, S. (1989). Salsalate in the treatment of rheumatoid arthritis: a

double-blind clinical and gastroscopic trial versus piroxicam. II. Endoscopic evaluation. *Journal of Internal Medicine Research*, 17, 320–3.

81. Lanza, F., Rack, M.F., Doucette, M., Ekholm, B., Goldlust, B., and Wilson, R. (1989). An endoscopic comparison of the gastroduodenal injury seen with salsalate and naproxen. *Journal of Rheumatology*, 16, 1570–4.

82. Roth, S., Bennett, R., Caldron, P., Hartman, R., Mitchell, C., Doucette, M., *et al.* (1990). Reduced risk of NSAID gastropathy (GI. mucosal toxicity) with nonacetylated salicylate (salsalate): an endoscopic study. *Seminars in Arthritis and Rheumatism*, supplement 2, 11–19.

83. Montrone, F., Caruso, I., and Cazzola, M. (1989). Salsalate in the treatment of rheumatoid arthritis: a double-blind clinical and gastroscopic trial versus piroxicam. I. Clinical trial. *Journal of Internal Medicine Research*, 17, 316–19.

84. Dahl, S.L. (1993). Nabumetone: a 'nonacidic' nonsteroidal antiinflammatory drug. *Annals of Pharmacotherapy*, 27, 456–63.

85. Roth, S.H., Bennett, R., Caldron, P., Mitchell, C., Swenson, C., and Koepp, R. (1994). A longterm endoscopic evaluation of patients with arthritis treated with nabumetone vs naproxen. *Journal of Rheumatology*, 21, 1118–23.

86. Roth, S.H., Tindall, E.A., Jain, A.K., McMahon, F.G., April, P.A., and Bockow, B.I. (1993). A controlled study comparing the effects of nabumetone, ibuprofen, and ibuprofen plus misoprostol on the upper gastrointestinal tract mucosa. *Archives of Internal Medicine*, 153, 2565–71.

87. Eversmeyer, W., Poland, M., DeLapp, R.E., and Jensen, C.P. (1993). Safety experience with nabumetone versus diclofenac, naproxen, ibuprofen, and piroxicam in osteoarthritis and rheumatoid arthritis. *American Journal of Medicine*, 95, 10S–18S.

88. Morgan, G.J., Poland, M., and DeLapp, R.E. (1993). Efficacy and safety of nabumetone versus diclofenac, naproxen, ibuprofen, and piroxicam in the elderly. *American Journal of Medicine*, 95, 19S–27S.

89. Hayllar, J. and Bjarnason, I. (1995). NSAIDs, Cox-2 inhibitors and the gut. *Lancet*, 346, 521–2.

90. Langenbach, R., Morham, S.G., Tiano, H.F., Loftin, C.D., Chanayem, B.I., Chulada, P.C., *et al.* (1995). Prostaglandin synthetase 1 gene disruption in mice reduces arachidonic acid-induced inflammation and indomethacin-induced gastric ulceration. *Cell*, 83, 483–92.

91. Dinchuk, J.E., Car, B.D., Focht, R.J., Johnston, J.J., Jaffee, B.D., Covington, M.B., *et al.* (1995). Renal abnormalities and an altered inflammatory response in mice lacking cyclooxygenase II. *Nature*, 378, 406–9.

92. Chrischilles, E.A., Lemke, J.H., Wallace, R.B., and Drube, G.A. (1990). Prevalence and characteristics of multiple analgesic drug use in an elderly study group. *Journal of the American Geriatric Society*, 38, 979–84.

93. Somerville, K., Faulkner, G., and Langmen, M. (1986). Non-steroidal anti-inflammatory drugs and bleeding peptic ulcer. *Lancet*, 1, 462–4.

94. Griffin, M.R., Brandt, K.D., Liang, M.H., Pincus, T. Ray and W.A. (1995). Practical management of osteoarthritis: integration of pharmacologic and nonpharmacologic measures. *Archives of Family Medicine*, 4, 1049–55.

95. Fordyce, W.E. (1978). Evaluating and managing chronic pain. *Geriatrics*, 33, 59–62.

96. Ekstrom, P., Carling, L., Wetterhus, S., Wingren, P.E., Ankerhansen, O., Lundegardh, G. *et al.* (1996). Prevention of peptic ulcer and dyspeptic symptoms with omeprazole in patients receiving continuous nonsteroidal anti-inflammatory drug therapy — a Nordic multicentre study. *Scandinavian Journal of Gastroenterology*, 31, 753–8.

97. Taha, A.S., Hudson, N., Hawkey, C.J., Swannell, A.J., Trye, P.N., Cottrell, J., *et al.* (1996). Famotidine for the prevention of gastric and duodenal ulcers caused by nonsteroidal antiinflammatory drugs. *New England Journal of Medicine*, 334, 1435–9.

98. Raskin, J.B., White, R.H., Jackson, J.E., Weaver, A.L., Tindall, E.A., Lies, R.B., *et al.* (1995). Misoprostol dosage in the prevention of nonsteroidal antiinflammatory drug-induced gastric and duodenal ulcers: a comparison of three regimens. *Annals of Internal Medicine*, 123, 344–50.

99. Gabriel, S.E., Campion, M.E., and O'Fallon, M. (1993). Patient preferences for nonsteroidal antiinflammatory drug related gastrointestinal complications and their prophylaxis. *Journal of Rheumatology*, 20, 358–61.

100. Rudy, D.W., Rudy, A.C., Black, P.K., Ciu, Y., Hamman, M., and Brater D.C. (1995). Influence of misoprostol on the adverse renal effects and stereospecific pharmacokinetics of ibuprofen in chronic renal insufficiency. *American Journal of Therapeutics*, 2, 864–74.

9.4   Systemic analgesics

John D. Bradley and Kenneth D. Brandt

Joint pain is the complaint which most frequently brings the patient with osteoarthritis (OA) to the physician and is a major determinant of disability in this disease. While treatment of the underlying cause of the joint pain is desirable, treatment of the pain itself is incumbent on the physician. For many patients with OA this treatment frequently begins and ends with nonsteroidal anti-inflammatory drugs (NSAIDs). These have been the mainstay of therapy for this disease for over 50 years. While aspirin has been supplanted by newer, 'safer' NSAIDs, these drugs are frequently prescribed for patients with OA, at the upper ends of their dose range, with the intent of suppressing inflammation as well as providing pain relief[1].

This practice has been called into question, however, by studies demonstrating that, in many patients with OA, the efficacy of simple analgesics (drugs devoid of clinically significant anti-inflammatory effects) is comparable to that of NSAIDs. For example, in a short-term randomized clinical trial by Bradley *et al.*[2], acetaminophen, 4000 mg per day, was as effective as either an analgesic dose (1200 mg per day) or anti-inflammatory dose (2400 mg per day) of ibuprofen in subjects with knee OA. Similarly, no significant difference with regard to relief of joint pain was found in a comparative clinical trial in which patients with knee OA were treated with either the NSAID, flurbiprofen, or the analgesic, nefopam[3]. Indeed, these results could have been anticipated; previous evidence indicated that ibuprofen, in a daily dose of only 1200 mg, which has only minimal anti-inflammatory effect[4], was as effective as several other NSAIDs, including phenylbutazone, in relieving joint pain in patients with OA — even when the other NSAIDs were given in anti-inflammatory doses[5,6]. Similarly, a long-term comparison of acetaminophen, 2600 mg per day, and naproxen, 750 mg per day, showed no difference in outcome between the two treatment groups with respect to pain relief[7]. Furthermore, the risks of NSAID therapy, particularly in the elderly, are receiving increasing attention (see Chapter 9.3).

Origins of joint pain in OA

Articular cartilage, the tissue that generally exhibits the most striking pathologic changes in OA, is aneural. OA pain, therefore, must originate in other articular and periarticular tissues. Candidates include the synovium and joint capsule, which are richly innervated by neurons with nociceptor and mechanoreceptor functions[8]. Synovial inflammation in OA may be induced by proteoglycans[9] or cartilage fragments[10] released from the damaged articular surface, or by calcium-containing crystals, which result in the release of proinflammatory mediators, for example, bradykinin and prostaglandins, which sensitize the nociceptor. Other potential sites of origin of OA pain include[11]:

- synovium
- periosteum
- subchondral bone
- joint capsule
- intra- and para-articular ligaments
- para-articular tendons and associated muscles.

Joint inflammation in OA may not be persistent or even clinically apparent. Common clinical features of OA which suggest the presence of joint inflammation include soft tissue swelling and joint tenderness. Morning stiffness is usually of only brief duration (less than 20 minutes). Erythema and warmth over the joint are uncommon. In the short-term clinical trial cited above[2], improvement in knee tenderness and swelling occurred as frequently when acetaminophen was given in a dose of 4000 mg per day, as with an anti-inflammatory dose of ibuprofen[12]. In patients with knee OA who had a synovial effusion, Schumacher *et al.* found that ibuprofen, 2400 mg per day, was superior to a lower dose of acetaminophen, 2600 mg per day, and noted a positive correlation between the synovial fluid leukocyte count and pain relief, with the anti-inflammatory therapy[13]. Perhaps a subset of patients with OA responds preferentially to anti-inflammatory therapy but, in general, evidence that NSAIDs are superior to a simple analgesic for symptomatic treatment of OA is lacking.

Concerns have been expressed about possible acceleration of joint damage by analgesic therapy in patients with OA. It has been suggested that use of analgesics will impair protective muscle reflexes that are triggered by joint pain, with a resultant increase in usage of the damaged joint. Schnitzer *et al.*[14] recently demonstrated an increase in joint loading in subjects with medial compartment knee OA treated with the NSAID, piroxicam. Although most subjects experienced considerable reduction in joint pain during treatment, this was associated with significant increases in knee adductor moment, and maximum quadriceps moment, that is, an increase in loading of the arthritic knee, as determined by computerized analysis of gait. Whether the increase in loading occurred as a result of the analgesic effect of the NSAID is not entirely clear, but is likely because treatment with acetaminophen resulted in similar loading changes at the knee[15]. Additional studies are required to determine whether the increase in loading is relevant to the question raised above, that is, whether analgesics might accelerate the progression of OA.

In addition to the possibility that the analgesic effects of NSAIDs may increase joint damage as a result of increased joint trauma, aspirin and several other (although not all) NSAIDs inhibit the synthesis of proteoglycans by chondrocytes *in vitro* in a concentration-dependent fashion[16]. Furthermore, cartilage loss in animal models of OA has been accelerated by administration of aspirin[17,18]. Rashad *et al.*[19] reported an increase in the rate of joint space narrowing (implying loss of articular cartilage) in radiographs of patients with hip OA who were treated with the cyclo-oxygenase (COX)-inhibiting NSAID, indomethacin, in comparison with those who received the weak COX inhibitor, azapropazone. However, that study had several limitations: for example, baseline pain scores were higher in the azapropazone group than in the indomethacin group; the timing of hip replacement surgery, which was based on clinical features such as joint pain and functional limitation, was determined by a physician who was not blinded to the treatment group; and, even though azapropazone-treated patients had higher post-treatment pain scores, they were determined to be surgical candidates later in their course of treatment than the indomethacin group.

In a more recent study, Huskisson *et al.*[20] concluded that indomethacin use was related to acceleration of joint breakdown in patients with knee OA. In a double-blind parallel study in which 376 patients with knee OA completed at least one year of treatment with indomethacin (75 mg per day), tiaprofenic acid (600 mg per day), or placebo, more than twice as many patients in the indomethacin group showed narrowing of the joint space in serial radiography of the OA knee, as those in the placebo group. However, a number of concerns exist relative to the design of that study, as enumerated by Doherty and Jones[21]. In summary, the data supporting the association of indomethacin use with acceleration of joint breakdown in OA remain far from convincing at this time; it is, furthermore, worth noting that in a recent study of practice variations among various medical specialties[22] only 1.2 per cent of 397 patients with knee OA, cared for by either primary care physicians or rheumatologists in Indiana, were taking indomethacin.

At present, the choice of an analgesic for the patient with OA is dictated largely by effectiveness, convenience, tolerability, cost, and risks of injury to organ systems other than the musculoskeletal system.

Acetaminophen

The classification of analgesics based upon a 'peripheral' or 'central' site of action is misleading and outmoded. For example, although acetaminophen has been called a 'peripheral' analgesic, it readily penetrates the central nervous system (CNS) at therapeutic doses, and clearly has central activity. Its central action may be mediated through activation of the diffuse noxious inhibitory control pathway[23]. Acetaminophen has minimal effect on the activity of COX, regardless of whether the constitutive or inducible isoform of the enzyme is tested. Although COX is present in the CNS, particularly in the glial cells, there is no evidence that COX in the CNS is more sensitive to inhibition by acetaminophen than COX at peripheral sites[24]. Furthermore, even if prostaglandins are administered centrally during treatment with acetaminophen, an analgesic effect is evident[25].

Because it is readily available, inexpensive, well tolerated, and effective, acetaminophen deserves a place at the top of the list of initial drug therapies for OA. Acetaminophen remains the sole agent in the class of simple non-narcotic analgesics available in the United States; others, such as nefopam and dipyrone, are available elsewhere. Like aspirin, acetaminophen shows a nearly linear dose-response curve for analgesia which reaches a plateau at about 1000 mg[26]. The maximum recommended daily dose is 1000 mg four times daily. For those with underlying renal or liver disease, lower doses may be appropriate.

Like its predecessor, phenacetin, acetaminophen can cause chronic interstitial nephritis when consumed in large quantities over a long period of time[27]. The mechanisms and specific metabolites responsible for chronic interstitial nephritis due to acetaminophen are not well characterized. Acute overdoses of acetaminophen, usually greater than 6 g, can occasionally cause acute renal tubular necrosis[28].

In patients with alcoholic liver disease, doses of acetaminophen as small as 3 g per day have been associated with hepatic necrosis[29]. Ethanol induces the hepatic cytochrome P-450 enzymes responsible for the metabolism of acetaminophen, enhancing production of the toxic metabolite, N-acetyl-benzoquinoneimine[30]. This metabolite, which is normally inactivated by conjugation with glutathione, becomes problematic when glutathione stores are depleted, either as a result of a pre-existing condition (for example, alcoholism) or the acetaminophen overload itself. Hepatotoxicity can be prevented by timely administration of N-acetylcysteine, which repletes intracellular glutathione.

NSAIDs

Although NSAIDs have been classified as peripherally-acting analgesics, they have substantial effects in the spinal cord and brain. The ability of NSAIDs to penetrate the CNS is variable, and is dependent largely on their pKa and lipophilicity. Those NSAIDs which penetrate the CNS (for example, indomethacin, ketoproten, diclofenac) may inhibit COX centrally. However, the effectiveness of NSAIDs as analgesics correlates poorly with their potency as COX inhibitors[31]. Some NSAIDs (particularly propionic acid derivatives) are racemic mixtures of R- and L-stereoisomers. The L-form inhibits COX and has analgesic and anti-inflammatory activity, while the R-form is essentially devoid of biologic effects. The R-forms of some NSAIDs, for example, ibuprofen, are readily converted *in vivo* to the S-form. However, even though R-flurbiprofen does

not undergo bioconversion in humans, its analgesic potency has been found to be comparable to that of S-flurbiprofen[32]. In patients with hip or knee OA, only a weak correlation was noted between the magnitude of pain relief and the serum concentration of either total ibuprofen or the S-enantiomer[33].

The effectiveness of some NSAIDs as analgesics may be attributable to mechanisms unrelated to inhibition of COX, for example, inhibition of central hyperalgesia induced by glutamate and substance P[34]. Interestingly, the analgesic effect of some NSAIDs is inhibited by naloxone, implying a mechanism involving opioid receptors[35]. Because prostaglandins can inhibit the pain-suppressing influences of spinal noradrenergic synapses, NSAIDs may reduce pain by eliminating prostaglandin-mediated disinhibition of pain messages[36].

The role of lipoxygenase inhibition in NSAID-induced analgesia is unclear. While 8,15-diHETE, a leukotriene produced by stimulated neutrophils, induces hyperalgesia by sensitization of the primary afferent nociceptor[37], most NSAIDs have little effect on production of 8, 15-diHETE.

All NSAIDs provide essentially comparable relief of OA pain. There is no demonstrated analgesic superiority of those NSAIDs which are marketed as analgesics, for example, ibuprofen, naproxen. To sustain the analgesic effect, NSAIDS with a short half-life must be dosed more frequently than those with a long half-life. The latter require more time to reach steady state concentrations, and their peak effect, therefore, may be delayed. Relief of OA pain by NSAIDs is often apparent within a few days of initiation of therapy[38], and tends to increase over four or more weeks of continued therapy[39] — an observation unexplained by their pharmacokinetics. Some NSAIDs, especially propionic acid derivatives, produce maximal analgesia at doses much lower than those needed for their optimal anti-inflammatory effect. Although non-acetylated salicylates (for example, salsalate, choline magnesium trisalicylate) are only weak COX inhibitors, they are as effective as aspirin (a more powerful, irreversible COX inhibitor) in relieving OA pain[40] and inflammation[41].

Aspirin is the least expensive analgesic, but the direct cost of treatment with this agent, as is the case for most NSAIDs (see Chapter 9.5), is compounded by the cost of treatment of its complications. The incidence of dyspepsia, upper gastrointestinal ulcers and bleeding can be reduced by use of more expensive enteric-coated preparations of aspirin, and by keeping the total daily dose low (less than 2600 mg) or administering a non-acetylated salicylate[42–44]. Some older patients, particularly those with pre-existing hearing loss, experience annoying tinnitus, even with a low dose of salicylate. Bruising may also be evident at a low dose, particularly with aspirin, and hyperuricemia may be induced or exacerbated by analgesic doses of salicylates.

Ibuprofen, which is available 'over-the-counter', is relatively safe and effective in low doses (less than 1600 mg per day). Considering overall costs of treatment, and the lower incidence of dyspepsia, it is preferable to aspirin if an NSAID is required for analgesia in patients with OA pain (see Chapter 9.5). Naproxen, which recently became available 'over-the-counter' in the United States, offers the advantage of less frequent dosing (two times daily, compared to 3–4 times daily for ibuprofen). While the optimum dose has not been defined, naproxen is effective in treating OA pain in the range of 500–750 mg per day. Chapter 9.3 reviews in detail the adverse effects associated with NSAID use.

Other generic and proprietary NSAIDs are comparably effective for treatment of OA symptoms. Some have more favorable side effect profiles, and some are more convenient, permitting once-daily dosing, but are more expensive; some patients prefer one of these agents over the others, and the difference in cost may be justified.

Patients frequently experience an initial response to an NSAID which then 'wears off', resulting in serial prescription of multiple other NSAIDs. It is not clear whether this loss of effectiveness is due to a change in pharmacodynamics or attenuation of a placebo effect. In any event, because of either this limited duration of efficacy, or side effects, only 5–20 per cent of patients with OA who are started on an NSAID are still using the same NSAID one year later[45].

Opioids

Opioids are often referred to as 'centrally acting' analgesics, but have been shown to be effective when administered intra-articularly (that is, peripherally) in low doses[46]. Indeed, the primary afferent nociceptor cell body synthesizes opioid receptors and transports them centrally and peripherally[47]. Opioids inhibit the sensitization of nociceptors by inflammatory mediators, for example, prostaglandins and leukotrienes, and by elevation of the activation threshold via G protein activation and subsequent inhibition of adenyl cyclase[48]. The above consequences of activation of μ-opioid receptors are complemented by the activation of δ and κ opioid receptors, which not only produces analgesia, but alters sympathetic nerves to prevent release of nociceptor-

sensitizing agents, such as prostanoids[49]. Activation of μ and δ opioid receptors can inhibit release of substance P from peripheral afferent nociceptors[50].

In general, commercially available opioid analgesics interact predominantly with μ-receptors, as does the predominant pain-modulating endogenous opioid, β-endorphin. Other endogenous opioids, for example, enkephalins and dynorphins, interact chiefly with δ and κ opioid receptors, respectively. High concentrations of these opioid receptors are found along the central neural pathways involved in nociception, for example, the dorsal horn of the spinal cord, periaqueductal gray matter, and thalamus.

β-endorphin is generated in the hypothalamus and pituitary gland as a cleavage product during release of adrenocorticotrophic hormone[51]. Production of β-endorphin in the pituitary gland permits systemic release, whereas β-endorphin synthesized in the hypothalamus remains confined to the central nervous system. β-endorphin concentrations in serum and spinal fluid are decreased in many chronic pain conditions, including OA and several other arthritides[52], and may be 'normalized' by successful therapy, such as hypnotherapy and acupuncture[53,54]. Exercise can induce release of β-endorphin, but the exertion must be sustained for at least 10–20 minutes, at about 70 per cent of maximum heart rate — a level which relatively few patients with arthritis can achieve.

While a body of evidence supports the role of β-endorphin in modulation of acute pain[55], its role in regulation of *chronic arthritis pain* is questionable. We evaluated the effect of naloxone, a μ-receptor antagonist, on the relief of joint pain in subjects with knee OA. Analgesia, induced by either ketorolac or placebo, was unaffected by naloxone in both placebo responders and non-responders, implying that production of analgesia by placebo and by this NSAID did not involve the μ-receptor[56]. Overall, because of the relatively high density of opioid receptors in the central nervous system, and the permeability of that region to exogenous opioids, central mechanisms probably predominate over peripheral effects when exogenous opioids are administered systemically.

Propoxyphene is a relatively weak opioid analgesic which generally causes minimal effects on mood and mentation and, therefore, has low abuse potential. However, propoxyphene tablets may be pulverized, suspended in a vehicle, and injected intravenously by narcotic abusers.

The effectiveness of propoxyphene as an analgesic is enhanced by combination with acetaminophen[57]. Such combinations usually contain propoxyphene napsylate (100 mg), or propoxyphene hydrochloride (65 mg) and acetaminophen (650 mg), as a single tablet which may be taken as often as every 4–6 hours, as needed. In a four-week randomized comparison of slow-release diclofenac (100 mg per day) versus dextropropoxyphene (180 mg per day)/acetaminophen (1.95 g per day), in subjects with joint pain (not necessary due to OA), improvement in joint pain and mobility were significantly greater in the diclofenac group, and a higher proportion of those in the propoxyphene/acetaminophen group developed problems with their job of work and lost time from work, than those treated with diclofenac[58]. Like all opioid analgesics, propoxyphene is most effective when used short-term for acute pain or intermittently for exacerbations of chronic pain. Chronic use may result in development of tolerance[59].

Codeine is also a more effective analgesic when combined with acetaminophen. A recent study showed that the analgesic effectiveness of codeine, 30 mg/acetaminophen, 325 mg, dosed 1–2 tablets every 4–6 hours, as needed, was comparable to that of propoxyphene/acetaminophen, but intolerable side effects (for example, nausea, constipation, dizziness, dysphoria, and sedation) were relatively more common with the codeine combination[60]. Although a long-term study showed sustained efficacy of codeine/acetaminophen, adverse effects severely limited its usefulness[61]. Tolerance may develop to the analgesic effects of codeine, but not to many of the adverse effects of this agent, including constipation and respiratory suppression.

The effectiveness and adverse effects of hydrocodone/acetaminophen combinations are similar to those for codeine/acetaminophen at comparable doses (hydrocodone, 2.5 mg, approximates codeine, 30 mg). Use of propoxyphene and of codeine has been associated with an increased risk of hip fracture in the elderly, particularly during the period of initial use and when these agents are taken in combination with other psychoactive agents, for example, antidepressants[62].

Tramadol is an analgesic with both μ-opioid receptor agonist activity, and serotonin and norepinephrine reuptake inhibitory activity, both of which contribute to its analgesic effects[63]. Administered in a dose of 50–100 mg up to four times a day, as needed, it provides pain relief comparable to that of one or two tablets of acetaminophen, 325 mg/codeine, 30 mg, taken up to four times a day (up to 240 mg codeine)[64].

The adverse event profile of tramadol is similar to that of propoxyphene. Nausea and vomiting can be minimized by phasing in the full dose of tramadol over 4–7 days. Interestingly, tolerance to the analgesic effects of tramadol has not been demonstrated, and its abuse and addiction potential levels are reported to be very low. Because of its inhibition of norepinephrine reuptake, tramadol should not be given to patients receiving a monoamine oxidase inhibitor[65].

Pentazocine has been marketed in various formulations, for example, as a single agent, in combination with acetaminophen, and in combination with naloxone. Because the orally non-absorbable naloxone is fully available if the preparation is injected parenterally, and antagonizes the pentazocine and any other opioid present, the latter formulation minimizes the intravenous abuse potential of pentazocine. However, the abuse potential of pentazocine, even without addition of naloxone, is relatively low, perhaps because it does not produce euphoria but rather frequently causes dysphoria[66]. The recommended dosing schedule is 50–100 mg as often as every four hours, as needed.

Higher potency *opioid analgesics* including oxycodone, meperidine, and morphine analogs, are more likely to lead to tolerance, dependency, and abuse than propoxyphene, codeine, pentazocine, or tramadol; and may cause undesirable changes in mood, affect, and behavior, in addition to the adverse effects listed above for the weaker opioids. Many produce a rapid onset of analgesia but have a duration of effect of less than four hours, making them unsuitable as mainstays of treatment for chronic severe pain.

A large proportion of rheumatologists and primary care physicians prescribe narcotic analgesics for patients with arthritis[67]. Many patients with OA pain, who require high potency opioid analgesics, are candidates for total joint arthroplasty. Certainly, other pharmacologic and non-pharmacologic modalities should be considered before high potency opioids are prescribed for OA pain. However, in some patients with OA, specific circumstances may limit the options of the physician in management of the disease, and necessitate the use of opioid analgesics. The effectiveness of narcotic analgesics may be improved, and the dose therefore minimized, by combination with acetaminophen, an NSAID, or an antidepressant[68].

The physician can be somewhat reassured by the evidence that dependency and addiction are relatively infrequent with these agents.

Antidepressants

Although no antidepressant is approved by the United States Food and Drug Administration for treatment of pain, antidepressants are often prescribed for management of chronic pain syndromes. Their efficacy is best documented in treatment of neuropathic pain, for example, diabetic peripheral neuropathy, post-herpetic neuralgia, post-stroke pain. Few antidepressants have been formally tested in patients with arthritis pain, in general, or OA pain, in particular. Thus, any recommendation regarding their use in management of OA pain is supported by few data. Pain threshold and pain tolerance are increased by these agents[69].

While mechanisms of pain in various chronic pain syndromes may differ, some antidepressants exhibit multiple mechanisms of action. Obviously, depressed patients may benefit from the antidepressant effect of the drug, regardless of the neurochemical specificities of the agent used. Chronic pain and depression frequently coexist (see Chapter 9.13), and may share neurochemical mechanisms[70]. In such patients, improvement in depressive symptoms correlates with reduction in pain, and both may correlate with the serum concentration of the antidepressant and its active metabolites[71]. Furthermore, antidepressants may be useful therapeutic adjuncts in non-depressed patients who have chronic pain. Several observations suggest that the analgesic and antidepressant effects of these agents are separable:

1. The dose required for pain relief is often substantially lower than that needed to treat the depression.

2. The time course of the analgesic usually precedes the antidepressant effect, sometimes by weeks. In a study in which the onset of pain reduction was rapid, the peak analgesic effect with imipramine occurred after serum concentrations of the drug had begun to decline[72], supporting the concept that distribution of the drug to the central nervous system (which is delayed) is essential for the analgesic activity.

3. Some effective antidepressants are relatively poor analgesics. The newer, selective serotonin (5-hydroxytryptamine, 5-HT)-reuptake inhibitors (for example, fluoxetine, sertraline, paroxetine) may be less effective in managing chronic pain than older agents which inhibit reuptake of both norepinephrine and serotonin, for example, imipramine, amitriptyline, and nortriptyline[73].

Several studies have helped clarify the sites of action and mechanisms underlying the analgesia produced by antidepressants: levels of 5-HT, in particular, but also of norepinephrine, are relatively depleted in chronic pain conditions[74,75]. Receptors for 5-HT are enriched in the diffuse noxious inhibitory control pathway in the brainstem[76]. Stimulation of these 5-HT receptors may induce release of endogenous opioids, which may exert local or distant analgesic effects[77]. Agents inhibiting reuptake of 5-HT (and, perhaps, of norepinephrine) potentiate morphine-induced analgesia[75]. Inhibition of reuptake results in persistence of the neurotransmitter in the synaptic cleft, leading initially to increased signal transmission. However, if the high concentration of neurotransmitter is sustained, receptor expression may be down-regulated, resulting in a decrease in the number of receptors and re-establishment of equilibrium at a lower level of reuptake (that is, fewer receptors). This does not appear to result in a loss of effect, however[71].

The most extensively tested and widely utilized antidepressants for management of chronic arthritis pain are amitriptyline[78] and imipramine[79], both of which are tricyclic heterocyclic antidepressants. Low doses, that is, 10–25 mg, may be administered up to three times daily, with a similar or larger dose at bedtime, especially if sleep is disturbed by pain. The analgesic effect should be apparent within 2–4 weeks, following which the dose may be adjusted accordingly. Imipramine is less sedating than amitriptyline, but both cause anticholinergic side effects, such as dry mouth, constipation, difficulty initiating urination, and slowed urine stream[80]. Serious concerns, including ileus, urinary retention, cardiac conduction block, arrhythmia, and lowering of the seizure threshold, are much more problematic with overdoses than with therapeutic doses.

Other antidepressants that have been shown to be effective in treatment of chronic arthritis pain include trimipramine[81], dothiepin, and dibenzepine. These drugs have been tested in patients with rheumatoid arthritis, and in mixed arthritis populations, which often included patients with concomitant depressive symptoms who were receiving other antirheumatic / analgesic therapy.

The antidepressant, S-adenosyl methionine (SAM), is a physiologic intermediary of metabolism which is essential in transmethylation and transulfuration reactions. In pharmacologic doses, SAM induces a modest increase in the spinal fluid concentration of monoamines[82].

SAM is well absorbed after oral administration but undergoes extensive first-pass metabolism in the liver, reducing the systemic bioavailability of the drug to less than 10 per cent[83]. In a large study of patients with OA, in which oral SAM treatment (1200 mg perday) was compared with naproxen (750 mg per day), efficacy of the two agents after four weeks was comparable but, in contrast to naproxen, no effect of SAM was evident prior to that time[84]. Intravenous loading, however, followed by oral maintenance doses of 600 mg per day, accelerated onset of the SAM effect in subjects with knee OA, which in some cases was evident within 14 days after initiation of intravenous treatment[85]. Notably, subjects in that study were not depressed, and improvement of joint pain was not associated with a change in depression or mood scale scores. SAM has no significant effect on prostaglandins, and no significant anticholinergic (for example, dry eyes, dry mouth, constipation) or antidopaminergic (for example, dystonia, tardive dyskinesia) side effects, which are common with the older heterocyclic antidepressants. However, hypomania or mania may develop in about 10 per cent of patients with bipolar affective disorder who are treated with parenteral SAM.

SAM is not available in the United States but is marketed in Europe and South America, with an indication for the treatment of OA. The minimum effective dose is probably 200 mg three times daily[72]; 1200 mg per day may be optimal[84]. SAM is unstable when exposed to oxygen, light, and heat, and has a limited storage life, all of which lead to high costs of manufacturing, packaging, and distribution. Furthermore, although SAM causes essentially no serious adverse effects (other than mania in predisposed patients), it frequently produces nausea and dyspepsia[85]. These limitations may be overcome with further advances in manufacturing and changes in formulation.

Conclusion

The future will undoubtedly witness the availability of new classes of analgesics. Development of analgesic NSAIDs which are free of undesirable anti-prostaglandin effects in the gastrointestinal tract or kidney appear to be feasible[86]. Selective COX-2 inhibitors (that is, NSAIDs which inhibit only the

inducible, inflammation-associated COX-2 enzyme and not the constitutive COX-1 enzyme) may have analgesic and anti-inflammatory activity, without the adverse effects on the gastric mucosa and kidney exhibited by currently available NSAIDs and largely attributable to inhibition of COX-1[87]. However, as discussed in Chapter 9.3, the relationship between COX selectivity and the clinical gastroprotective or, for that matter, anti-inflammatory effect of an NSAID is not fully understood. Opioids may be improved by development of agents which bind selectively to μ_1 receptors (inducing analgesia) and not to μ_2 sites (causing respiratory depression)[88]. Inhibitors of specific neural receptors, for example, the N-methyl D-aspartate (NMDA) and NK-1 receptor, and agonists of other receptors, for example, the gamma amino butric acid (GABA) receptor, may provide effective analgesia without the side effects of opioids. NMDA and NK-1 receptors are found on pain-responsive neurons in the dorsal horn of the spinal cord, and respond primarily to glutamate and substance-P, respectively, released from the axon terminal of the primary afferent neuron (PAN)[50]. These are prominent, if not predominant, pathways of pain signal transmission[89]. GABA and the endogenous opioids are pain-inhibitory, and are involved in segmental spinal pain control mechanisms[90].

In summary, pain control is the primary objective of the currently available systemically-acting phramacologic agents used to treat patients with OA. Function and quality of life can be enhanced by adequate control of joint pain, but impaired by the side effects of many of the currently available analgesics; this is especially true of the elderly — the population at greatest risk for OA. Because of marked inter-individual variations in efficacy and side effects, the choice of an analgesic agent must be individualized. Finally, it should be emphasized that while the above discussion highlights concepts relevant to systemic analgesic therapy for OA pain and dosing guidelines, it cannot rigidly define a treatment regimen or provide strict treatment guidelines. The treatment of OA pain today is driven to a large extent by the art, rather than the science, of medicine.

References

1. Mazzuca, S.A., Brandt, K.D., Katz, B.P., Stewart, K.D., and Li, W. (1993). Therapeutic strategies distinguish community-based primary care physicians from rheumatologists in the management of osteoarthritis. *J Rheumatol*, **20**, 80–6.

2. Bradley, J.D., Brandt, K.D., Katz, B.P., Kalasinski, L.A., and Ryan, S.I. (1991). Comparison of an anti-inflammatory dose of ibuprofen, an analgesic dose of ibuprofen and acetaminophen in the treatment of patients with osteoarthritis of the knee. *N Engl J Med*, **325**, 87–91.

3. Stamp, J., Rhind, V., and Haslock, I. (1989). A comparison of nefopam and flurbiprofen in the treatment of osteoarthritis. *Br J Clin Prac*, **43**, 24–6.

4. Huskisson, E.C., Hart, F.D., and Shenfield, G.M., *et al.* (1971). Ibuprofen: a review. *Practitioner*, **207**, 639–43.

5. Cimmino, M.A., Cutolo, M., Samanta, E., *et al.* (1982). Short-term treatment of osteoarthritis: a comparison of sodium meclofenamate and ibuprofen. *J Int Med Res*, **10**, 46–52.

6. Moxley, T.E., Royer, G.L., Hearron, M.S., *et al.*. (1975). Ibuprofen versus buffered phenylbutazone in the treatment of osteoarthritis: Double-blind trial. *J Am Geriatr Soc*, **23**, 343–9.

7. Williams, H.J., Ward, J.R., Egger, M.J., Neuner, R., Brooks, R.H., Clegg, D.O., *et al.* (1993). Comparison of naproxen and acetaminophen in a two-year study of treatment of osteoarthritis of the knee. *Arthritis Rheum*, **36**, 1196–1206.

8. Kidd, B.L., Mapp, P.I., Blake, D.R., Gibson, S.J., and Polak, J.M. (1990). Neurogenic influences in arthritis. *Ann Rheum Dis*, **49**, 649–52.

9. Boniface, R.J., Cain, P.R., and Evans, C.H. (1988). Articular responses to purified cartilage proteoglycans. *Arthritis Rheum*, **31**, 258–66.

10. Evans, C.H., Mears, D.C., and Stanitski, C.L. (1982). Ferrographic analysis of wear in human joints: evaluation by comparison with arthroscopy of symptomatic knees. *J Bone Joint Surg*, **64B**, 572–8.

11. Altman, R. and Dean, D. (1989). Introduction and overview: pain in osteoarthritis. *Semin Arthritis Rheum*, **18 (Suppl 2)**, 1–3.

12. Bradley, J.D., Brandt, K.D., Katz, B.P., Kalasinski, L.A., and Ryan, S.I. (1992). Treatment of knee osteoarthritis: relationship of clinical features of joint inflammation to the response to a nonsteroidal anti-inflammatory drug or pure analgesic. *J Rheumatol*, **19**, 1950–4.

13. Schumacher, H.R. Jr, Stineman, M., Rahman, M., Magee, S., and Huppert, A. (1990). The relationship between clinical and synovial fluid findings and treatment response in osteoarthritis (OA) of the knee. (Abstract) *Arthritis Rheum*, **33**, S92.

14. Schnitzer, T.J., Popovich, J.M., Andersson, G.B.J., and Andriacchi, T.P. (1993). Effect of piroxicam on gait in patients with osteoarthritis of the knee. *Arthritis Rheum*, **36**, 1207–13.

15. Schnitzer, T.J., Andriacchi, T.P., Feddor, D., and Lindeman, M. (1990). Effect of NSAIDs on knee loading in patients with osteoarthritis (OA). *Arthritis Rheum*, **33**, 592.

16. Palmoski, M. and Brandt, K.D. (1979). Effect of salicylate on proteoglycan metabolism in normal canine articular cartilage *in vitro*. *Arthritis Rheum*, **22**, 746–54.

17. Palmoski, M. and Brandt, K.D. (1983). *In vivo* effect of aspirin on canine osteoarthritic cartilage. *Arthritis Rheum*, **26**, 994–1001.

18. Wilhelmi, V.J. (1978). Fordende and hemmende Einflusse von Tribenosid and Acetylsalicylsaure auf die spontane Arthrose der Maus. *Arzniemittelforschung*, **28**, 1724.

19. Rashad, S., Revell, P., Hemmingway, A., Low, F., Rainsford, K., and Walker, F. (1989). Effect of nonsteroidal anti-inflammatory drugs on the course of osteoarthritis. *Lancet*, **2**, 519–22.

20. Huskisson, E.C., Berry, H., Gishen, P., Jubb, R.W., and Whitehead, J. (1995). Effects of antiinflammatory drugs on the progression of osteoarthritis of the knee. *J Rheumatol*, **22**, 1941–6.

21. Doherty, M. and Jones, A. (1995). Indomethacin hastens large joint osteoarthritis in humans — how strong is the evidence? *J Rheumatol*, **22**, 2013–16.

22. Mazzuca, S.A., Brandt, K.D., Katz, B.P., Freund, D.A., Dittus, R.S., Lubitz, R.M., *et al.* (1995). Risk of iatrogenic gastropathy from drugs prescribed by family physicians general internists and rheumatologists for osteoarthritis of the knee. *Arthritis Rheum*, **38 (suppl 9)**, S227.

23. Tjolson, A., Lund, A., and Hole, K. (1991). Antinociceptive effect of paracetamol in rats is partly dependent on spinal serotonergic systems. *Eur J Pharmacol*, **193**, 193–201.

24. Bruchhausen, F.V. and Baumann, J. (1982). Inhibitory actions of desacetylation products of phenacetin and paracetamol on prostaglandin synthetases in neuronal and glial cell lines and rat renal medulla. *Life Sci*, **30**, 1783–91.

25. Piletta, P., Porchet, H.C., and Dayer, P. (1991). Central analgesic effect of acetaminophen but not of aspirin. *Clin Pharmacol Ther*, **49**, 350–4.

26. Cooper, S.A. (1981). Comparative analgesic efficacies of aspirin and acetaminophen. *Arch Intern Med*, **141**, 282–5.

27. Sandler, D.P., Smith, J.C., Weinberg, C.R., Buckalew, V.M. Jr, Dennis, V.W., Blythe, W.B., *et al.* (1989). Analgesic use and chronic renal disease. *N Engl J Med*, **320**, 1238–43.

28. Prescott, L.F. (1983). Paracetamol overdosage. Pharmacological considerations and clinical management. *Drugs*, **25**, 290–314.

29. Denison, H., Kaczynski, J., and Wallerstedt, S. (1987). Paracetamol medication and alcohol abuse: a dangerous combination for the liver and the kidney. *Scand J Gastroenterol*, **22**, 701–4.

30. Licht, H., Seeff, L.B., and Zimmerman, H.J. (1980). Apparent potentiation of acetaminophen hepatotoxicity by alcohol. *Ann Intern Med*, **92**, 511.

31. McCormack, K. and Brune, K. (1991). Dissociation between the antinociceptive and antiinflammatory effects of the nonsteroidal anti-inflammatory drugs. A survey of their analgesic efficacy. *Drugs*, **41**, 533–47.

32. Brune, K., Beck, W.S., Geisslinger, G., Menzel-Soglewek, S., Peskar, B.M., and Peskar, B.A. (1991). Aspirin-like drugs may block pain independently of prostaglandin synthesis inhibition. *Experientia*, **47**, 258–61.

33. Bradley, J.D., Rudy, A.C., Katz, B.P., Ryan, S.I., Kalasinski, L.A., Brater, D.C., *et al.* (1992). Correlation of serum concentrations of ibuprofen stereoisomers with clinical response in the treatment of hip and knee osteoarthritis. *J Rheumatol*, **19**, 130–4.

34. Urquhart, E. (1993). Central analgesic activity of nonsteroidal anti-inflammatory drugs in animal and human pain models. *Semin Arthritis Rheum*, **23**, 198–205.

35. Björkman, R., Hedner, J., Hedner, T., and Henning, M. (1990). Central, naloxone-reversible antinociception by diclofenac in the rat. *Nauyn-Schmiedeberg's Arch Pharmacol*, **342**, 171–6.

36. Taiwo, Y.O. and Levine, J.D. (1988). Prostaglandins inhibit endogenous pain control mechanisms by blocking transmission of spinal nonadrenergic synapses. *J Neurosci*, **8**, 1346–9.

37. White, D.M., Basbaum, A.I., Goetzl, E.J., and Levine, J.D. (1990). The 15-lipoxygenase product, 8R, 15-diHETE, stereospecifically sensitizes C-fiber mechanoheat nociceptors in hairy skin of rat. *J Neurophysiol*, **63**, 966–70.

38. Altman, R.D. and Hochberg, A.C. (1983). Degenerative joint disease. *Clin Rheum Dis*, **9**, 681–93.

39. Bellamy, N., Buchanan, W.W., and Grace, E.E. (1986). Double-blind randomized controlled trial of isoxicam *vs* piroxicam in elderly patients with osteoarthritis of the hip and knee. *Br J Clin Pharmac*, **22**, 149S–155S.

40. Liyange, S.P. and Tambar, P.K. (1978). Comparative study of salsalate and aspirin in osteoarthritis of the hip or knee. *Curr Ther Res Opin*, **5**, 450–3.

41. Preston, S.J., Arnold, M.H., Beller, F.M., Brooks, P.M., and Buchanan, U.W. (1989). Comparative analgesic and anti-inflammatory properties of sodium salicylate and acetylsalicylic acid (aspirin) in rheumatoid arthritis. *Br J Clin Pharmac*, **27**, 607–11.

42. Lanza, F.L., Royer, G.L., and Nelson, R.S. (1980). Endoscopic evaluation of the effects of aspirin, buffered aspirin, and enteric-coated aspirin on gastric and duodenal mucosa. *N Engl J Med*, **303**, 136–8.

43. Mielants, H., Veys, E.M., Verbruggen, G., and Schelstraete, K. (1981). Comparison of serum salicylate levels and gastrointestinal blood loss between salsalate (Disalcid) and other forms of salicylates. *Scand J Rheumatol*, **10**, 169–73.

44. Scheiman, J.M. and Elta, G.H. (1990). Gastroduodenal mucosal damage with salsalate versus aspirin: results of experimental models and endoscopic studies in humans. *Semin Arthritis Rheum*, **20**, 121–17.

45. Scholes, D., Stergachis, A., Penna, P.M., Normand, E.H., and Hansten, P.D. (1995). Nonsteroidal antiinflammatory drug discontinuation in patients with osteoarthritis. *J Rheumatol*, **22**, 708–12.

46. Stein, C., Comisel, K., Haimerl, E., Yassouridis, A., Lehrberger, K., Herz, A. *et al.* (1991). Analgesic effect of intra-articular morphine after arthroscopic knee surgery. *N Engl J Med*, **325**, 1123–6.

47. Basbaum, A.I. and Levine, J.D. (1991). Opiate analgesia: how central is a peripheral target? *N Engl J Med*, **325**, 1168–9.

48. Levine, J.D. and Taiwo, Yo. (1989). Involvement of the mu-opiate receptor in peripheral analgesia. *Neuroscience*, **32**, 571–5.

49. Taiwo, Y.O. and Levine, J.D. (1991). K- and Δ-opioids block sympathetically dependent hyperalgesia. *J Neurosci*, **11**, 928–32.

50. Levine, J.D., Fields, A.L., and Basbaum, A.I. (1993). Peptides and the primary afferent nociceptor. *J Neurosci*, **13**, 2273–86.

51. Millan, M.J. and Herz, A. (1985). The endocrinology of the opioids. *Int Rev Neurobiol*, **26**, 1–83.

52. Denko, C.W., Aponte, J., Gabriel, P., and Petricevic, M. (1982). Serum beta-endorphin in rheumatic disorders. *J Rheumatol*, **9**, 827–33.

53. Domangue, B.B., Margolis, C.G., Leiberman, D., and Kaji, H. (1985). Biochemical correlates of hypoanalgesia in arthritic pain patients. *J Clin Psychiatry*, **46**, 235–8.

54. He, L.F. (1987). Involvement of the endogenous opioid peptides in acupuncture anesthesia. *Pain*, **31**, 99–121.

55. Levine, J.D., Gordon, N.C., Junes, R.T., and Fields, H.L. (1978). The narcotic antagonist naloxone enhances clinical pain. *Nature*, **272**, 826–7.

56. Bradley, J.D. Unpublished observations

57. Beaver, W.T. (1981). Aspirin and acetaminophen as constituents of analgesic combination. *Arch Intern Med*, **141**, 293–300.

58. Parr, G., Darekar, B., Fletcher, A., and Bulpitt, C.J. (1989). Joint pain and quality of life; results of a randomized trial. *Br J Clin Pharmac*, **27**, 235–42.

59. Jaffe, J.H. and Martin, W.R. (1990). Opioid analgesics and antagonists. In *The Pharmacological basis of therapeutics* (8th edn) (ed. A.G. Gilman, T.W. Rall, A.S. Nies, P. Taylor), pp. 485–521. MacMillan Publishing Company, New York.

60. Boissier, C., Perpoint, B., Laporte-Simitsidis, P., Hocquart, J., Gayel, J.L., Rambaud, C., *et al.* (1992). Acceptability and efficacy of two associations of paracetamol with a central analgesic (dextropropoxyphene or codeine): comparison in osteoarthritis. *J Clin Pharmacol*, **32**, 990–5.

61. Kjaersgaard-Andersen, P., Nafei, A., Skov, O., Madsen, F., Andersen, H.M., Krøner, K., *et al.* (1990). Codeine plus paracetamol versus paracetamol in longer-term treatment of chronic pain due to osteoarthritis of the hip. A randomized, double-blind multicentre study. *Pain*, **43**, 309–18.

62. Schorr, R.I., Griffin, M.R., Daughtery, J.R., and Ray, W.A. (1992). Opioid analgesics and the risk of hip fracture in the elderly: codeine and propoxyphene. *J Gerontol*, **47**, M111–M115.

63. Raffa, R.B., Friderichs, E., Reimann, W., Shank, R.P., Codd, E.E., and Vaught, J.L. (1992). Opioid and non-opioid components independently contribute to the mechanism of action of tramadol, an 'atypical' opioid analgesic. *J Pharmacol Exp Ther*, **260**, 275–85.

64. Rauck, R.L., Rouff, G.E., and McMillen, J.I. (1994). Comparison of tramadol and acetaminophen with codeine for long-term pain management in elderly patients. *Curr Ther Res*, **55**, 1417–31.

65. Lee, C.R., McTavish, D., and Sorkin, E.M. (1993). Tramadol: a preliminary review of its pharmacodynamic and pharmacokinetic properties, and therapeutic potential in acute and chronic pain states. *Drugs*, **46**, 313–40.

66. Kantor, T.G. (1986). Pentazocine: clinical analgesic studies. In *Advances in pain research and therapy*,

Vol. 8, (ed. K.M. Foley and C.E. Inaturrisi), pp. 241–5. Raven Press, New York.

67. Turk, D.C., Brody, M.C., and Okifuji, E.A. (1994). Physicians' attitudes and practices regarding the long-term prescribing of opioids for non-cancer pain. *Pain*, **59**, 201–8.

68. Sunshine, A., Slafta, J., and Gruber, C. Jr (1978). A comparative study: propoxyphene, fenoprofen, the combination of propoxyphene and fenoprofen, aspirin and placebo. *J Clin Pharmacol*, **18**, 11–16.

69. Poulsen, L., Arendt-Nielsen, L., Brøsen, K., Nielsen, K.K., Gram, L.F., and Sindrup, S.H. (1995). The hypoalgesic effect of impramine in different human experimental pain models. *Pain*, **60**, 287–93.

70. Feinmann, C. (1985). Pain relief by antidepressants: possible modes of action. *Pain*, **23**, 1–8.

71. Magni, G. (1993). The use of antidepressants in the treatment of chronic pain. A review of the current evidence. *Drugs*, **42**, 730–48.

72. Sindrup, S.H., Gram, L.F., Skjold, T., Frøland, A., and Beck-Nielsen, H. (1990). Concentration-response relationship to imipramine treatment of diabetic neuropathy symptoms. *Clin Pharmacol Ther*, **47**, 509–15.

73. Max, M.B., Lynch, S.A., Muir, J., Shoaf, S.E., Smoller, B., and Dubner, R. (1992). Effects of desipramine, amitriptyline, and fluoxetine on pain in diabetic neuropathy. *N Engl J Med*, **326**, 1250–6.

74. Messing, R.B. and Lytle, L.D. (1977). Serotonin containing neurons: their possible role in pain and analgesia. *Pain*, **4**, 1–21.

75. Kuraishi, Y., Harada, Y., Aratani, S., Satoh, M., and Takagi, H. (1983). Separate involvement of the spinal noradrenergic and serotonergic systems in morphine analgesia: the differences in mechanical and thermal algesic tests. *Brain Res*, **273**, 245–52.

76. Andersen, E. and Dafny, N. (1983). An ascending serotonergic pain modulation pathway from the dorsal raphe nucleus to the parafascicularis nucleus of the thalamus. *Brain Res*, **269**, 57–67.

77. Sacerdote, P., Boni, A., Mantegazza, P., and Panerai, A.E. (1987). A role for serotonin and beta endorphin in the analgesia induced by some tricyclic antidepressant drugs. *Pharmacol Biochem Behav*, **26**, 153–8.

78. Frank, R.G., Kashani, J.H., Parker, J.C., Beck, N.C., Brownlee-Duffeck, M., Elliott, T.R., *et al.* (1988). Antidepressant analgesia in rheumatoid arthritis. *J Rheumatol*, **15**, 1632–8.

79. Gringas, M. (1976). A clinical trial of Tofranil in rheumatic pain in general practice. *J Int Med Res*, **4(suppl 2)**, 41–9.

80. Egbunike, I.G. and Chaffee, B.J. (1990). Antidepressants in the management of chronic pain syndromes. *Pharmacotherapy*, **10**, 262–70.

81. Macfarlane, G.J., Jalali, S., Grace, E.M. (1986). Trimipramine in rheumatoid arthritis: a randomized double-blind trial in relieving pain and joint tenderness. *Curr Med Res Opin*, **10**, 89–93.

82. Baldessarini, R. (1987). Neuropharmacology of S-adenocele-L-methionine. *Am J Med*, **83(supple 5A)**, 95–103.

83. Stramentinoli, G. (1987). Pharmacologic aspects of S-adenosyl-methionine. Pharmacokinetics and pharmacodynamics. *Am J Med*, **83(Suppl 5A)**, 35–42.

84. Caruso, I. and PietroGrande, V. (1987). Italian double-blind multicenter study comparing S-adenasylmethionine, naproxen, and placebo in the treatment of degenerative joint disease. *Am J Med*, **83(suppl 5A)**, 66–71.

85. Bradley, J., Flusser, D., Katz, B., Schumacher, H.R. Jr, Brandt, K., Chambers, M., *et al.* (1994). A randomized double-blind, placebo-controlled trial of intravenous loading with S-adenosylmethionine (SAM) followed by oral SAM therapy in patients with knee osteoarthritis. *J Rheumatol*, **21**, 905–11.

86. Brune, K., Geisslinger, G., and Menzel-Soglowek, S. (1992). Pure enantiomers of 2-arylpropionic acids: Tools in pain research and improved drugs in rheumatology. *J Clin Pharmacol*, **32**, 944–52.

87. Mitchell, J.A., Akarasereenont, P., Thiemermann, C., Flower, R.J., and Vane, J.R. (1994). Selectivity of nonsteroidal anti-inflammatory drugs as inhibitors of constitutive and inducible cyclooxygenase. *Pharmacology*, **90**, 11693–7.

88. Ling, G.S.F., Spiegel, K., Nishimura, S.L., and Pasternak, G.W. (1983). Dissociation of morphine's analgesic and respiratory depressant actions. *Eur J Pharmacol*, **86**, 487–8.

89. Konttinen, Y.T., Kemppinen, P., Segerberg, M., Hukkanen, M., Rees, R., Santavirta, S. *et al.* (1994). Peripheral and spinal neural mechanisms in arthritis, with particular reference to treatment of inflammation and pain. *Arthritis Rheum*, **37**, 965–82.

90. Bannwarth, B., Demotes-Mainard, F., Schaeverbeke, T., and Dehais, J. (1993). Where are peripheral analgesics acting? *Ann Rheum Dis*, **52**, 1–4.

9.5   Economic considerations in the use of nonsteroidal anti-inflammatory drugs

Wayne A. Ray

NSAIDs are today among the most widely used medications. Aspirin, the best known NSAID, has been available and widely used since 1899[1]. The first prescription NSAID, phenylbutazone, was approved for use by the Food and Drug Administration (FDA) in 1952[2], but the use of prescription NSAIDs became common only after the marketing of ibuprofen in 1974[3]. In 1973, only four drugs were marketed and drug stores dispensed close to 30 million prescriptions per year[3–5]. By 1991, patients received 70 million prescriptions (3.8 per cent of all prescriptions) at a cost of about 2.2 billion dollars[6]. In addition, a growing number of NSAIDs have become available without a prescription; thus, this value is an underestimation, as it excludes expenditure on such 'over-the-counter' agents. Use of NSAIDs increases with the age of the subject, so that at any given time an estimated 10 to 15 per cent of persons 65 years and over are taking prescription NSAIDs[7–9].

Although there are three major FDA-approved indications for NSAIDs — arthritis and related conditions, pain, and dysmenorrhea — over 50 per cent of use of these drugs is associated with arthritis or other musculoskeletal conditions. Of physician visits in 1987 for arthritis, sprains and strains, and dysmenorrhea, it has been estimated that 59, 31, and 68 per cent, respectively, resulted in the prescription of an NSAID[4].

This wide use of NSAIDs has been controversial[10,11]. The costs of NSAID therapy and of its complications have caused several economic issues to be raised, which are the focus of this review. Four broad topics are considered: (1) the rationale underlying growing interest in economic evaluation of pharmacotherapy; (2) terminology and methods of economic analysis of therapeutic interventions; (3) direct drug costs for individual NSAIDs; and (4) the costs associated with the gastrointestinal toxicity of NSAIDs, their most common serious adverse effect.

Rationale for economic analysis of pharmaceuticals

Economic analysis plays a growing role in therapeutics. Two trends have led to the increasing contempory focus on cost as an important outcome. The first is the growing availability of therapeutic alternatives, which leads to the natural question as to how both clinical and economic outcomes vary for the several available options. The second is the realization that the seemingly unconstrained growth in expenditures for health care in the past cannot continue indefinitely.

Recently, increased economic scrutiny has been applied to the use of pharmaceuticals throughout the world[12]. In the US, growing recognition of the economic consequences of suboptimal pharmacotherapy[13–15] has led to an increase in efforts to improve the quality and economy of prescribing, including voluntary physician education programs[16], mandated drug utilization review for Medicaid[17–19], wide use of restrictive access policies (formularies, service limitations, prior approval requirements, and generic and therapeutic substitution requirements)[20], and direct federal regulation of prescribing indications[21]. In Australia, Medicare, the national health insurance plan[22,23], now uses economic analysis in deciding whether or not to approve new drugs for reimbursement and in determining the rate of reimbursement. Similar guidelines have been implemented in the Canadian province of Ontario. The National Health Service (NHS) in England and Wales has scrutinized the £3.6 billion annual expenditures for drugs prescribed by general practitioners in 1992–1993[24]. An audit commission concluded that £425 million (11.8 per cent) could be saved annually by reducing overprescribing (£275 million); reducing prescribing drugs of little clinical value (£45 million); substitution of cheaper alternative drugs (£25 million); more appropriate use of expensive preparations (£30 million).

Because drugs are generally much less expensive than many other therapeutic interventions (such as hospitalizations or surgery)[25], the growth in scrutiny of medicine costs may seem somewhat perplexing. Clearly, it is not the relative magnitude of expenditures for pharmaceuticals that drives the current focus on economic evaluation. In my judgment, there are several underlying factors. First, although a relatively small component of overall health care expenditures, the expenditures for pharmaceuticals often are large in absolute terms (for example, about $70 billion in the US at present). Second, for pharmaceuticals, there often are clearly identifiable alternatives with substantially different prices; for example, there are at least 14 currently available non-salicylate NSAIDs[26] with a 12–to–1 range of costs at the pharmacy[27]. Thus, consumers — particularly third-party payers — naturally consider whether or not expenditures for the more expensive NSAIDs are justified. Third, in the US, the proportion of costs paid for 'out of pocket' by patients for medicines is greater than that for other health services, such as hospital stays. This increased visibility focuses attention on drugs. Fourth, introduction of pharmaceutials is regulated already by governments; thus, to add economic requirements to those already present for efficacy and safety is a relatively modest step. Finally, all sectors of health care are receiving intense price scrutiny and pharmaceuticals cannot expect to be exempt from this trend. Indeed, the movement of payers to greater consideration of total health care costs — thinking in terms of total payments per subscriber — may result in greater use of pharmaceuticals, which often are low cost relative to other therapeutic interventions.

Terminology and methods of economic evaluation

The objective of this section is to provide a brief overview of terminology and methods used in economic evaluations. The reader interested in further detail is referred to the very readable introductory text by Drummond[28] and to articles by Detsky[29], Eisenberg[30], Bloom[23], and Drummond[22].

A full economic analysis of a health care intervention requires two components: appraisal of both the clinical (benefits and adverse effects) and economic (costs) outcomes of the intervention, and comparison with one or more alternatives. Other types of analyses, such as cost-identification studies that quantify the costs associated with a particular treatment, are useful, but in themselves do not assist in the choice between competing alternatives.

There are four basic types of economic analyses: cost-minimization, cost-effectiveness, cost-utility, and cost-benefit. A *cost-minimization* analysis assumes each of the interventions compared has equivalent benefits; thus, the objective of the economic analysis is to identify the least expensive. A variant is *cost-analysis*, which simply describes the costs of two alternatives, with no attempt to evaluate clinical benefits.

However, competing treatments or health programs infrequently have precisely equivalent benefits. Thus, *cost-effectiveness* analysis calculates the cost per unit of clinical outcome, such as adverse events averted, deaths prevented, or years of life gained. Detsky[29] provides a simple example of this type of analysis. Assume that there are two treatments for a serious disease, such as therapy for lung cancer. Assume treatment A has costs of $20 000 and provides a life expectancy of 4.5 years, and treatment B, costs of $10 000 and life expectancy of 3.5 years. In this example, treatment A, when compared to treatment B, provides an additional year of life expectancy at a cost of $10 000. Thus, the marginal cost-effectiveness of treatment A is $10 000 per additional year of life gained.

Cost-effectiveness analysis assumes that all differences between the treatments can be expressed in terms of the chosen unit of effectiveness, such as years of life. However, interventions may differ in other ways. For example, anti-hypertensive drugs may be equally effective in reducing blood pressure, but may have different side effect profiles[31]. Patients quite naturally prefer treatments with fewer side effects. *Cost-utility* analysis attempts to place a subjective value on the clinical outcome, such as years of life, by weighting by the subjective utilities. Results often are expressed in terms of quality adjusted life years (QALYs). This method can adjust for the effects of severe disability or frequent, painful side effects on the quality of life.

Drummond notes that cost-utility analysis is appropriate if: (1) quality of life is a primary objective of treatment (as in osteoarthritis (OA)); (2) when a treatment affects multiple health states and it is desired to have a summary measure of impact; or (3) when comparing diverse treatments. The controversial aspect of cost-utility analysis is obtaining the utilities — a value for each possible health state that reflects its relative desirability. These generally are obtained either from patients, other members of the population, or health care professionals. Drummond[28] notes that for some health states, different panels provide generally consistent utilities. However, if there is a well-defined, more narrow instrument that measures quality of life in a particular clinical situation, such as the Sickness Impact Profile[32] in arthritis, or measures of mood in studies of antihypertensives[31], its use is preferable.

When economic methods first were applied to evaluation of health treatments, *cost-benefit* analyses were most commonly used, where all benefits were valued in monetary terms[33]. Cost-benefit analyses were initially applied to evaluate the benefits of dams and other public works projects. These analyses usually defined all benefits in terms of wages gained or lost (the human capital method). However, the difficulty of equating health states to dollars has led to the virtual abandonment of this method in health economics.

NSAIDs would appear to be excellent candidates for economic analyses. There are multiple drugs in this class, with a wide range of costs. Furthermore, there are both pharmacologic and non-pharmacologic alternatives to NSAIDs in the management of OA. However, there are at least three major problems with economic analysis of OA therapies.

First, the therapeutic effect of NSAIDs and other drugs is reduction of symptoms. There is no evidence that NSAIDs retard progression of OA or prolong life[34,35]. Thus, it is not possible to use a straightforward cost-effectiveness analysis which would compare therapies with regard to adverse events prevented (such as joint replacements), or to years of life saved.

Second, extant data are inadequate to perform comparative, comprehensive economic analyses with regard to pain and function. These types of analyses would require data that precisely quantified the relative efficacy and safety of therapeutic alternatives for OA with regard to these endpoints. The primary source of such data would be the controlled clinical trials. However, such trials generally compare a very limited number of agents (such as active drug versus placebo, or two active drugs). Thus, comprehensive economic analysis would require combining data from multiple trials. However, the heterogeneity of patient populations, therapeutic regimens, instruments for measure of pain and function, and follow-up procedures, would make this exercise futile. Furthermore, the available data are even more limited for biomechanical and other non-medicinal approaches, which ultimately may become important components of OA management[36].

Third, to fairly assess both the benefits and costs of NSAID therapy, long-term follow-up of large populations would be required. However, clinical trials have tended to encompass small numbers of subjects followed for relatively short periods of time.

Thus, the objectives of this review are more modest. The first objective is to describe present data on the direct drug cost component of NSAID therapy. A key issue will be whether or not there is evidence supporting the proposition that the wide cost disparity in NSAIDs is readily justified by differences in efficacy or safety. The second objective is to review data on the costs associated with the gastrointestinal toxicity of NSAIDs, their most common serious adverse effect. This will include a brief review of the controversy regarding the economic analyses of misoprostol.

Direct drug costs for individual NSAIDs

The clinician wishing to treat a patient with an NSAID has a broad spectrum of choices. In 1991, the *Medical Letter* listed 14 available non-salicylate drugs[26]. Individual NSAID prices differ substantially, with the more expensive agents having a cost as much as 12 times that of generic ibuprofen[27]. Ibuprofen, one of the least expensive drugs, had an average wholesale cost of $12.83[26] for 30 days of treatment; whereas flurbiprofen, one of the most expensive of these agents, had an average monthly cost of $81.30[26]. In the US, market survey data show that the majority of NSAIDs prescribed are the more expensive drugs[3].

Given these data, an obvious means of cost cutting would be encouraging use of less expensive NSAIDs. The utility of this strategy depends upon whether or not there are systematic differences in efficacy and safety between different individual NSAIDs. This topic is one of considerable controversy. Some analyses have focused on the limited data suggesting different pharmacokinetic and pharmacodynamic properties for individual NSAIDs, and different patient responsiveness to individual drugs. However, a more balanced view suggests that although patient responsiveness to individual

NSAIDs may vary, for as yet poorly understood reasons, there is limited evidence of systematic differences in efficacy[34]. Indeed, ibuprofen[37] compares very favorably with flurbiprofen[38].

Safety of individual NSAIDs is another controversial topic. Ibuprofen is consistently associated with lower rates of upper gastrointestinal bleeding (see Chapter 9.3)[39], the most common serious NSAID side effect. For other NSAIDs, there are differences in the perceived frequency of less common adverse reactions[40], such as excess case reports of hepatotoxicity for diclofenac, increased dermatologic reactions with piroxicam, increased central nervous system side effects with indomethacin, and a greater frequency of interstitial nephritis with fenoprofen. However, without epidemiologic data from well-controlled studies, the differences between individual drugs with regard to these uncommon adverse reactions cannot be quantified, which underlines the need to collect better data on the relative safety of pharmaceuticals with the same therapeutic indication[10].

We evaluated a 'natural experiment' in which there was a sudden shift from expensive non-generic to less expensive generic NSAIDs[41]. In October of 1989, the Tennessee Medicaid program implemented a prior authorization requirement for non-generic drugs. We evaluated the effects of this policy on clinical and economic outcomes of NSAID therapy using a longitudinal Medicaid database[42]. Our objectives were to quantify the effects of the program on use of prescribed NSAIDs, and to determine if there were unanticipated increases in use of other medications or medical services. Such increases could offset savings from reduced NSAID prescription costs, and could indicate deterioration of clinical outcomes. We compared monthly Medicaid expenditures for medical care potentially affected by the policy change, for the year preceding, and two years following its implementation on 1 October 1989.

In the baseline year, Medicaid paid $22.41 (95% confidence interval = $21.19 to $23.62) for NSAID prescriptions for each person year of enrollment. Following the implementation of the prior authorization program, there was an abrupt drop in expenditure rates (Fig. 9.2).

An interrupted time-series analysis estimated a decrease (Δ) of $14.63 million or 65 per cent (60 to 71 per cent) in NSAID expenditures immediately following the policy change. This resulted from both a shift from non-generic to generic NSAIDs (Fig. 9.2(a)) and a 26 per cent (21 to 31 per cent) reduction in overall days of NSAID use (Fig. 9.2(b)). When the two years following prior authorization are compared with the baseline year in the entire Medicaid population, there was an $11.78 million reduction (53 per cent (48 to 57 per cent)) in mean annualized NSAID expenditures. During the two years following prior authorization, the policy change led to a $12.8 million reduction in NSAID expenditures.

There was no evidence that utilization of other services increased following the policy change. Expenditures for other analgesic and anti-inflammatory drugs did not increase, nor did those for outpatient services for management of pain and inflammation. Regular users of non-generic NSAIDs (most affected by the policy change) had a similar reduction in NSAID expenditures and use, with no increase in expenditures for other study medical care. Cost savings were greatest among persons over 65 years of age.

Given its low administrative costs (less than $100 000), the program was highly effective in terms of its intended effect on NSAID expenditures. Although we were initially concerned that the program could lead to a corresponding increase in equally expensive, but potentially less desirable drugs, such as opioid analgesics, or oral corticosteroids, this did not occur. Furthermore, expenditures for outpatient or inpatient services for management of musculoskeletal disorders did not increase. These data provide further evidence that less costly generic NSAIDs are an appropriate alternative to expensive generic drugs for many patients, and that encouragement of generic use can achieve substantial cost savings. If the findings of this study can be extrapolated to the US, they suggest that preferential use of less expensive NSAIDs could result in savings of up to $1 billion annually.

Evaluation of the costs of NSAIDs must also consider the costs of alternative medicinal and non-medicinal therapies. The low correlation between the degree of synovial inflammation in OA and response to NSAID therapy[43] suggest that the therapeutic effects of NSAIDs in OA result primarily from their analgesic, rather than anti-inflammatory properties[44,45]. Thus, other simple analgesics may be considered as pharmacotherapy. Acetaminophen, a safe[46] and inexpensive drug, is an attractive alternative to NSAIDs, for OA[45,47–50]. Its analgesic efficacy compares favorably to that of aspirin and other NSAIDs[47,48]. The clinical trial of Bradley *et al.*[51], in patients with OA of the knee, demonstrated that acetaminophen at 4 g per day was comparable to 1200 or 2400 mg of ibuprofen. In most patients taking acetaminophen, there is a substantially

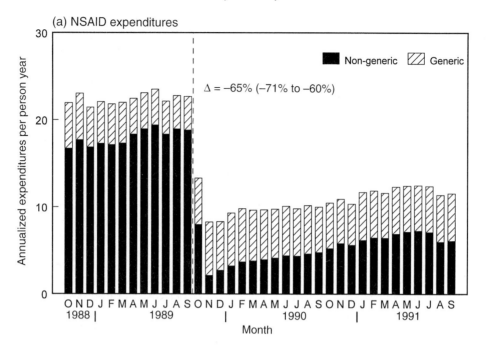

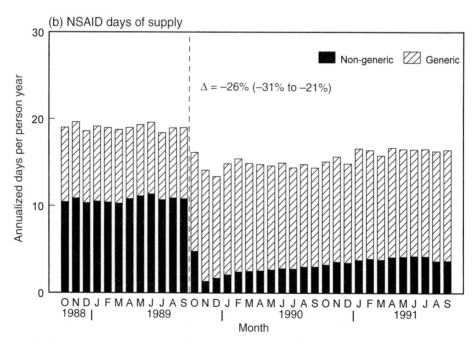

Fig. 9.2 Annualized rates of NSAID expenditures (a) and prescribed days of supply (b) among all Tennessee Medicaid enrollees, before and after implementation of the prior authorization program. The solid bars denote non-generic drugs; the hatched bars, generic drugs; the dashed line indicates the date of program implementation; Δ indicates the immediate effect of the program, as estimated from the interrupted time-series analysis; the values in parentheses, the 95 per cent confidence interval. From reference 41.

lower incidence of serious toxicities — hepatotoxicity and renal failure — than NSAID-associated gastrointestinal bleeding[52–55].

Puett and Griffin recently reviewed published trials of non-medicinal and non-invasive therapies for hip and knee OA[36]. These included superficial and deep heat, cold, exercise, weight loss, acupuncture, transcutaneous electrical nerve stimulation, low-energy laser, vibration, topically applied creams, pulsed electromagnetic fields, and orthotic devices. They concluded that exercise reduced pain and improved function in knee OA, and that some evidence suggested topical capsaicin and laser treatments reduced pain in knee OA. Thus, these therapies should be considered in an economic analysis. However, current data on the efficacy of, and costs for, these therapies are inadequate to support direct economic comparisons with NSAIDs.

Costs of NSAID-associated gastrointestinal bleeding

It is now widely recognized that NSAIDs have frequent and serious upper gastrointestinal adverse effects in elderly patients, which include gastrointestinal symptoms, ulceration, hemorrhage, and death[7,9,14,56–62]. The incidence of serious peptic ulcer disease is greatest in elderly NSAID users[63]. In a large study of elderly Tennessee Medicaid enrollees, we found that for current NSAID users, the annual rate of hospitalization was 16 per 1000, a four-fold greater rate than that for non-users of NSAIDs[14]. Risk increased with dose: the annual rate of hospitalization increased from 4 per 1000 for persons who were non-users of NSAIDs, to more than 40 per 1000 for persons receiving the largest doses. Data from this and other[7,9] studies suggest that among persons 65 or older, 20 to 30 per cent of all peptic ulcer hospitalizations or deaths are attributable to NSAID use. Among elderly NSAID users, nearly two-thirds of ulcer-related hospitalizations or deaths are due to the NSAID. Thus, in the US, as many as 41 000 excess hospitalizations and 3300 deaths occur, each year, among elderly NSAID users[64].

Because the gastrointestinal side effects of NSAIDs are so frequent, quantification of medical care resource utilization for these disorders is central to economic evaluation of NSAIDs. However, despite the importance of this topic, it is not well studied. Prior economic analyses of the adverse gastrointestinal effects of NSAIDs have had a more narrow scope, focusing on

the cost effectiveness of misoprostol prophylaxis for prevention of gastric ulcers[65]. Furthermore, most of these studies have not directly ascertained costs, but have estimated them by various indirect methods[63,65–69].

To obtain more accurate data, we conducted a large retrospective cohort study among Tennessee Medicaid enrollees of the costs for gastrointestinal disease attributable to NSAID use[70]. The cohort consisted of all enrollees of Tennessee Medicaid, 65 years of age or older on 1 January 1989, who were enrolled in Medicaid throughout 1988, the baseline year. Each cohort member was classified according to NSAID use in the baseline year as *non-users* (no NSAID use), *occasional users* (fewer than 75 per cent of days with NSAID use), and *regular users* (75 per cent or more of days with NSAID use). Study outcomes were the utilization and cost of medical care, provided during up to one year of follow-up, for the diagnosis and treatment of gastrointestinal disorders potentially related to the use of NSAIDs. The three components of medical care studied were hospital admissions, outpatient visits, and medication prescriptions. We defined costs as the total amounts paid by Medicaid and Medicare for qualifying medical care. The analysis estimated annual mean utilization of, and payments for, medical care for study gastrointestinal disorders within each NSAID use group, adjusted for baseline differences in demographics and other medical care utilization.

The study cohort included 75,350 Medicaid enrollees, 65 years of age or older, with 67,593 person-years of follow-up. There were 29,555 (39 per cent) persons in the cohort who had one or more NSAID prescriptions in the baseline year, 24,633 (33 per cent) were occasional users; and 4922 (6 per cent) were regular users. Among non-users of NSAIDs, adjusted mean annual payments for all types of medical care for study gastrointestinal disorders were $132. This increased to $182 among occasional users, an excess of $50 (p < 0.001); and to $246 among regular users, an excess of $114 (p < 0.001; comparison with both non-users and occasional users). Among regular NSAID users, Medicare and Medicaid payments increased with NSAID dose. Medication prescriptions (mostly histamine-2 receptor antagonists) and hospital admissions were the largest component of excess costs.

The frequency and severity of NSAID-associated gastrointestinal bleeding has led to the development and marketing of misoprostol (a synthetic prostaglandin E_1 analogue), that in clinical trials has been shown to prevent gastric ulceration associated with NSAID use[71,72]. Because the complications of gastric ulcer are expensive, misoprostol may have economic as well as clinical benefits. Conversely, misoprostol is an expensive medication (more than $1000 per year for 200 mg, four times per day); thus, the cost of providing prophylaxis to patients not at high risk of NSAID-associated ulcers may be unacceptably high.

Economic analyses of the cost-effectiveness of misoprostol prophylaxis for prevention of gastric ulcers have had widely divergent results[63,65-69,73]. The analysis of Hillman and Bloom[66] reported that prophylaxis of patients with OA and abdominal pain was cost-saving. In contrast, the analysis of Edelson et al.[63] reported that the costs of prophylaxis, per year of life saved, were $667 400 for all NSAID users, $186 700 for users 60 years or older, and $95 600 for users with rheumatoid arthritis (although these estimates were revised downward in subsequent correspondence). The primary factor underlying these differences are the estimates of the incidence of, and costs for, NSAID-associated gastric ulcers[73]. Our data, as well as a preliminary cost analysis[74] of data from the MUCOSA[72] study, suggest that misoprostol therapy would almost never be cost- saving. In a specific patient population, the cost-effectiveness of misoprostol will be determined by the underlying risk of gastric ulcer complications. In a preliminary economic analysis of data from the MUCOSA[74] study, Levine estimated that in patients in that trial with no risk factors, the cost per complication prevented was $276 916. In contrast, for patients with four risk factors, the comparable cost was $12 486.

Conclusion

Unfortunately, the quantitative data on the relative efficacy, safety, and costs of the numerous therapies for OA are presently inadequate to support a full economic analysis. However, the available data do lead one to several useful practical conclusions. Interestingly, for OA, economic considerations seem to reinforce those based on clinical grounds alone. The following conclusions can be supported:

1. NSAIDs are widely used drugs and much of this use is of expensive agents.

2. There are no data to support systematic differences in efficacy between the individual NSAIDs; thus, although for idiosyncratic reasons some patients may ultimately require the more expensive drugs, less expensive agents should be tried first.

Ibuprofen, presently one of the least expensive drugs, also appears to have the advantage of lower gastrointestinal toxicity, which leads to further cost savings.

3. Gastrointestinal bleeding is an expensive complication of NSAID therapy, particularly in older patients. Misoprostol may have clinical benefits; however, except in a very small subgroup of extremely high risk patients, this drug is unlikely to be cost-saving.

4. Economic as well as clinical[11] considerations suggest that acetaminophen should be a primary therapy in OA. Acetaminophen is both less expensive than non-generic NSAIDs and it does not have expensive gastrointestinal bleeding complications.

5. Non-medicinal non-invasive therapies should be considered further on clinical grounds; however, data presently are insufficient to conduct comparative economic analysis of these modalities.

Acknowledgments

Supported in part by a grant from the Agency for Health Care Policy Research (HS07768) and a cooperative agreement with the Food and Drug Administration (FD-U-0000073).

References

1. Mills, J.A. (1991). Aspirin, the ageless remedy? N Engl J Med, 325, 1303-4.

2. Baum, C., Kennedy, D.L., and Forbes, M.B. (1985). Utilization of nonsteroidal anti-inflammatory drugs. Arthritis Rheum, 28, 686-92.

3. Tomita, D.K., Baum, C., Kennedy, D.L., Knapp, D.E., and Perry, Z.A. (1988). Drug utilization in the United States: 1987, ninth annual review. Dept. of Health and Human Services, Washington DC.

4. Tomita, D.K., Kennedy, D.L., Baum, C., Knapp, D.E., and Anello, C. (1989). Drug utilization in the United States: 1988, tenth annual review. Dept. of Health and Human Services, Washington DC.

5. Burke, L.B., Baum, C., Jolson, H.M., and Kennedy, K.D. (1991). Drug utilization in the United States: 1989, eleventh annual review. Dept. of Health and Human Services, Washington DC.

6. Anti-arthritic medication usage: 1991. Statistical Bulletin 1992, 73, 25-34.

7. Griffin, M.R., Ray, W.A., and Schaffner, W. (1988). Nonsteroidal anti-inflammatory drug use and death

from peptic ulcer in elderly persons. *Ann Intern Med*, **109**, 359–63.

8. Griffin, M.R., Piper, J.M., Daugherty, J.R., Snowden, M., and Ray, W.A. (1991). Nonsteroidal anti-inflammatory drug use and increased risk for peptic ulcer disease in elderly persons. *Ann Intern Med*, **114**, 257–63.

9. Somerville, K., Faulkner, G., and Langmen, M. (1986). Non-steroidal anti-inflammatory drugs and bleeding peptic ulcer. *Lancet*, **1**, 462–4.

10. Ray, W.A., Griffin., M.R., and Avorn, J. (1993). Evaluating drugs after their approval for clinical use. *N Engl J Med*, **329**, 2029–32.

11. Griffin, M.R., Brandt, K.D., Liang, M.H., Pincus, T., and Ray, W.A. (1995). Practical management of osteoarthritis: integration of pharmacologic and non-pharmacologic measures. *Arch Fam Med*, **4**, 1049–55.

12. US Congress Oo. (1993). *Pharmaceutical R and D: costs, risks and rewards, OTA-H-522.* US Government Printing Office, Washington DC.

13. Ray, W.A., Griffin, M.R., Schaffner, W., Baugh, D.K., and Melton, L.J. (1987). Psychotropic drug use and the risk of hip fracture. *N Engl J Med*, **316**, 363–9.

14. Shalat, L., True, L.D., Fleming, L.E., and Pace, P. (1989). Kidney cancer in utility workers exposed to polychlorinated biphenyls (PCBs). *Br J Ind Med*, **46**, 823–4.

15. Schondelmeyer, S.W. and Thomas, J. III. (1990). Data watch: trends in retail prescription expenditures. *Health Aff (Millwood)*, **9**, 131–45.

16. Soumerai, S.B. and Avorn, J. (1990). Principles of educational outreach ('academic detailing') to improve clinical decision making. *JAMA*, **263**, 549–56.

17. Avorn, J. and Soumerai, S.B. (1983). Improving drug-therapy decisions through educational outreach. A randomized controlled trial of academically based 'detailing'. *N Engl J Med*, **308**, 1457–74.

18. Schaffner, W., Ray, W.A., Federspiel, C.F., and Miller, W.O. (1983). Improving antibiotic prescribing in office practice: a controlled trial of three educational methods. *JAMA*, **250**, 1728–32.

19. Feinberg, J.L. (1991). OBRA '90: remnants of the Medicaid Prudent Pharmaceutical Purchasing Act become law. *The Consultant Pharmacist*, **6**, 6–11.

20. Soumerai, S.B. and Ross-Degnan, D. (1990). Experience of state drug benefit programs. *Health Aff (Millwood)*, **9**, 36–54.

21. Winograd, C.H. and Pawlson, L.G. (1991). OBRA 87 – a commentary. *J Am Geriatr Soc*, **39**, 724–6.

22. Drummond, M.F. (1992). Basing prescription drug payment on economic analysis: the case of Australia. *Health Aff (Millwood)*, **11**, 191–6.

23. Bloom, B.S. (1992). Issues in mandatory economic assessment of pharmaceuticals. *Health Aff (Millwood)*, **11**, 197–201.

24. Ramsey, S. (1994). UK prescription for change. *Lancet*, **343**, 663.

25. Sonnefeld, S.T., Waldo, D.R., Lemieux, J.A., and McKusick, D.R. (1991). Projections of national health expenditures through the year 2000. *Health Care Financing Review*, **13**(1), 1–27.

26. (1991). Drugs for rheumatoid arthritis. In *The Medical Letter on drugs and therapeutics* (33th edn) (ed. M. Abramowicz), pp. 65–70. The Medical Letter Inc., New York.

27. (1992). Facts and Comparisons. Drug Facts and Comparisons. St Louis: Facts and Comparisons.

28. Drummond, M.F., Stoddart, G.L., and Torrance, G.W. (1993). *Methods for the economic evaluation of health care programmes.* Oxford University Press, Oxford.

29. Detsky, A.S. and Naglie, I.G. (1990). A clinician's guide to cost-effectiveness analysis. *Ann Intern Med*, **113**, 147–54.

30. Eisenberg, J.M. (1989). Clinical economics: a guide to the economic analysis of clinical practices. *JAMA*, **262**, 2879–86.

31. Croog, S.H., Levine, S., Testa, M.A., Brown, B., Bulpitt, C.J., Jenkins, C.D, et al. (1986). The effects of antihypertensive therapy on the quality of life. *N Engl J Med*, **314**, 1657–64.

32. Bergner, M., Bobbitt, R.A., Carter, W.B., and Gilson, B.S. (1981). The sickness impact profile: development and final revision of a health status measure. *Med Care*, **XIX**, 787–805.

33. Luce, B.R. (1993). Cost-effectiveness analysis. Obstacles to standardisation and its use in regulating pharmaceuticals. *Pharmaco Economics 3*, **1**, 1–9.

34. Brooks, P.M. and Day, R.O. (1991). Nonsteroidal antiinflammatory drugs — differences and similarities. *N Engl J Med*, **324**, 1716–25.

35. Rashad, S., Hemingway, A., Rainsford, K., Revell, P., Low, F., and Walker, F. (1989). Effect of non-steroidal anti-inflammatory drugs on the course of osteoarthritis. *Lancet*, **2**, 1149.

36. Puett, D.W. and Griffin, M.R. (1994). Published trials of nonmedicinal and noninvasive therapies for hip and knee osteoarthritis. *Ann Intern Med*, **121**, 133–40.

37. Gall, E.P., Caperton, E.M., McComb, J.E., Messner, R., Multz, C.V., O'Hanlan, M., et al. (1982). Clinical comparison of ibuprofen, fenoprofen, calcium, naproxen and tolmetin sodium in rheumatoid arthritis. *J Rheumatol*, **9**, 402–7.

38. (1989). Flurbiprofen. In *The Medical Letter on drugs and therapeutics* (31th edn) (ed. M. Abramowicz), pp. 31–4. The Medical Letter Inc., New York.

39. Langman, M.J.S., Weil, J., Wainwright, P., Lawson, D.H., Rawlins, M.D., Logan, R.F.A. et al. (1994). Risks of bleeding peptic ulcer associated with individual nonsteroidal anti-inflammatory drugs. *Lancet*, **343**, 1075–8.

40. Brooks, P.M. and Day, R.O. (1991). Drug therapy. *N Engl J Med*, **324**, 1716–25.

41. Smalley, W.E., Griffin, M.R., Fought, R.L., Sullivan, L., and Ray, W.A. (1995). Effect of a prior-authorization requirement on the use of nonsteroidal antiinflammatory drugs by Medicaid patients. *N Engl J Med*, **332**, 1612–17.

42. Ray, W.A. and Griffin, M.R. (1989). Use of Medicaid data for pharmacoepidemiology. *Am J Epidemiol*, **129**, 837–49.

43. Hugenberg, S.T., Myers, S.L., Brandt, K.D., and Ryan, S. (1991). Synovitis does not predict response to nonsteroidal antiinflammatory drug therapy in knee osteoarthritis. *Arthritis Rheum*, **34** (**suppl**), S84.

44. Dieppe, P.A., Frankel, S.J., and Toth, B. (1993). Is research into the treatment of osteoarthritis with nonsteroidal anti-inflammatory drugs misdirected? *Lancet*, **341**, 353–4.

45. Pinals, R.S. (1992). Pharmacologic treatment of osteoarthritis. *Clin Ther*, **14**, 336–46.

46. Jackson, C.H., MacDonald, N.C., and Cornett, J.W.D. (1984). Acetaminophen: a practical pharmacologic overview. *Can Med Assoc J*, **131**, 25–32.

47. Amadio, P. Jr and Cummings, D.M. (1983). Evaluation of acetaminophen in the management of osteoarthritis of the knee. *Curr Ther Res*, **34**, 59–66.

48. Calin, A. (1984). Pain and inflammation. *Am J Med*, **77** (3A), 9–15.

49. Steele, K., Mills, K.A., Gilliland, A.E.W., Irwin, W.G., and Taggart, A. (1987). Repeat prescribing of nonsteroidal anti-inflammatory drugs excluding aspirin: how careful are we? *Br Med J*, **295**, 962–4.

50. Quinet, R.J. (1986). Osteoarthritis: increasing mobility and reducing disability. *Geriatrics*, **41**, 36–50.

51. Bradley, J.D., Brandt, K.D., Katz, B.P., Kalasinski, L.A., and Ryan, S. (1991). Comparison of an antiinflammatory dose of ibuprofen, an analgesic dose of ibuprofen, and acetaminophen in the treatment of patients with osteoarthritis of the knee. *N Engl J Med*, **325**, 87–91.

52. Denison, H., Kaczynski, J., and Wallerstedt, S. (1987). Paracetamol medication and alcohol abuse: a dangerous combination for the liver and the kidney. *Scand J Gastroenterol*, **22**, 701–4.

53. Whitcomb, D.A. and Block, G.D. (1994). Association of acetaminophen hepatotoxicity with fasting and ethanol use. *JAMA*, **272**, 1845–50.

54. Sandler, D.P., Smith, J.C., Weinberg, C.R., Buckalew, V.M. Jr, Dennis, V.W., Blythe, W.B., *et al.* (1989). Analgesic use and chronic renal disease. *N Engl J Med*, **320**, 1238–43.

55. Perneger, T.V., Whelton, P.K., and Klag, M.J. (1994). Risk of kidney failure associated with the use of acetaminophen, aspirin, and nonsteroidal antiinflammatory drugs. *N Engl J Med*, **331**, 1675–9.

56. Collier, D.S. and Pain, J.A. (1985). Non-steroidal antiinflammatory drugs and peptic ulcer perforation. *Gut*, **26**, 359–63.

57. McIntosh, J.H., Byth, K., and Piper, D.W. (1985). Environmental factors in aetiology of chronic gastric ulcer: a case control study of exposure variables before the first symptoms. *Gut*, **28**, 789–98.

58. McIntosh, J.H., Fung, C.S., Berry, C., and Piper, D.W. (1988). Smoking, nonsteroidal anti-inflammatory drugs, and acetaminophen in gastric ulcer. A study of associations and of the effects of previous diagnosis on exposure patterns. *Am J Epidemiol*, **128**, 761–70.

59. Duggan, J.M., Dobson, A.J., Johnson, H., and Fahey, P. (1986). Peptic ulcer and non-steroidal anti-inflammatory agents. *Gut*, **27**, 929–33.

60. Clinch, D., Banerjee, A.K., Levy, D.W., Ostick, G., and Faragher, E.B. (1987). Nonsteroidal anti-inflammatory drugs and peptic ulceration. *J R Coll Physicians Lond*, **21**, 183–7.

61. Armstrong, C.P. and Blower, A.L. (1987). Non-steroidal anti-inflammatory drugs, and life threatening complications of peptic ulceration. *Gut*, **28**, 527–32.

62. Guess, H.A., West, R., Strand, L.M., Helston, D., Lydick, E.G., Bergman, U., *et al.* (1988). Fatal upper gastrointestinal hemorrhage or perforation among users and non-users of non-steroidal anti-inflammatory drugs in Saskatchewan, Canada 1983. *J Clin Epidemiol*, **41**, 35–45.

63. Edelson, J.T., Tosteson, A.N.A., and Sax, P. (1990). Cost-effectiveness of misoprostol for prophylaxis against nonsteroidal anti-inflammatory drug-induced gastrointestinal tract bleeding. *JAMA*, **264**, 41–7.

64. Ray, W.A., Griffin, M.R., and Shorr, R.I. (1990). Adverse drug reactions and the elderly. *Health Aff (Millwood)*, **9**, 114–22.

65. Gabriel, S.E., Jaakimainen, R.L., and Bombardier, C. (1993). The cost-effectiveness of misoprostol for nonsteroidal antiinflammatory drug-associated adverse gastrointestinal events. *Arthritis Rheum*, **36**(4), 447–59.

66. Hillman, A.L. and Bloom, B.S. (1989). Economic effects of prophylactic use of misoprostol to prevent gastric ulcer in patients taking nonsteroidal anti-inflammatory drugs. *Arch Intern Med*, **149**, 2061–5.

67. Knill-Jones, R., Drummond, M., Kohli, H., and Davies, L. (1990). Economic evaluation of gastric ulcer prophylaxis in patients with arthritis receiving nonsteroidal anti-inflammatory drugs. *Postgrad Med J*, **66**, 639–46.

68. Carrin, G.J. and Torfs, K.E. (1990). Economic evaluation of prophylactic treatment with misoprostol in osteoarthritic patients treated with NSAIDs. The case of Belgium. *Rev Epidemiol Sante Publique*, **38**, 187–99.

69. de Pouvourville, G. (1992). The economic consequences of NSAID-induced gastropathy: the French context. *Scand J Rheumatol*, **suppl. 96**, 49–53.

70. Smalley, W.E., Griffin, M.R., Fought, R.L., and Ray, W.A. (1996). Excess costs for gastrointestinal disease among nonsteroidal anti-inflammatory drug users. *J Gen Intern Med*, **11**, 461–69.

71. Graham, D.Y., Agrawal, N.M., and Roth, S.H. (1988). Prevention of NSAID-induced gastric ulcer with misoprostol: multicentre, double-blind, placebo-controlled trial. *Lancet*, **2**, 1277–80.

72. Silverstein, F.E., Graham, D.Y., Senior, J.R., Wyn Davies, H., Struthers, B.J., Bittman, R.M., *et al.* (1995). Misoprostol reduces serious gastrointestinal complications in patients with rhematoid arthritis recieving nonsteroidal anti-inflammatory drugs: a randomized, double-blind, placebo-controlled trial. *Ann Intern Med*, **123**, 241–9.

73. Stuki, G., Johannesson, M., and Liang, M.H. (1995). Is misoprostol cost-effective in the prevention of nonsteroidal anti-inflammatory drug-induced gastropathy in patients with chronic arthritis? *Arch Intern Med*, **154**, 2020–5.

74. Levine, J.S. (1995). Misoprostol and nonsteroidal anti-inflammatory drugs: a tale of effects, outcomes, and costs. *Ann Intern Med*, **123**, 309–10.

9.6   Topical NSAIDs

Michael Doherty and Adrian Jones

Introduction

Topical delivery of salicylate and, subsequently, the newer nonsteroidal anti-inflammatory drugs (NSAIDs) has been investigated for over 60 years[1]. It is claimed that this method of delivery is effective in relieving locomotor pain but avoids the serious side effects associated with oral NSAIDs. Although topical products are popular with patients, most physicians remain sceptical of such efficacy and safety claims, largely due to the paucity of published controlled trials, the high associated placebo response, and cost[2].

Nevertheless, an increasing number of topical NSAIDs have been promoted and they now form a significant proportion of total NSAID sales. In some countries this represents over 50 per cent of all antirheumatic agents, and they are often available 'over the counter', without prescription. Available topical NSAIDs include salicylate, benzydamine, diclofenac, felbinac, flurbiprofen, ibuprofen, indomethacin, ketoprofen, and piroxicam. All have oral equivalents except benzydamine. Felbinac (biphenylacetic acid) is the active form of the prodrug fenbufen. As for oral NSAIDs, the major market is for regional soft tissue pain. Few studies relate to osteoarthritis (OA), and only a minority of topical NSAIDs are licensed for use in OA. Once available, however, usage is often extended to OA and other forms of arthritis.

In this chapter we review the potential advantages and disadvantages of topical NSAIDs and examine data relating to their use in OA.

Theoretical suitability of topical NSAID delivery

At first sight, there seem several potential advantages to topical compared to oral NSAIDs (Table 9.3). For patients with only one, or a few, painful joints — the usual situation with OA — it seems appropriate to target the site where analgesia is required, thereby avoiding unnecessary systemic exposure. Topical products are generally well tolerated and popular with patients; applying a safe, soothing treatment where it is needed, makes sense, and compliance is usually high. Such popularity may partly relate to self-efficacy — the patient participating in and controlling their own treat-

Table 9.3   Theoretical advantages and disadvantages of topical application of NSAIDs

Advantages
- makes sense for single regional pain syndromes
- very popular with patients
- well tolerated
- good compliance
- self-efficacy; shift of locus of control to patient
- possible concomitant benefit from massage
- lower serum levels — therefore safer.

Disadvantages
- inappropriate for multiple regional pain syndromes
- may be difficult, or messy, to apply
- possible local skin reactions
- systemic (especially hypersensitivity) reactions may still occur, despite low serum levels
- may not achieve adequate tissue levels
- cost
- may be no better than cheaper rubefacients.

ment. The massage required to rub in topical creams or gels may itself alleviate pain. Importantly, compared to oral delivery, topical NSAIDs result in lower blood levels. Since the risk of major adverse events, especially gastrointestinal (GI), are dose and blood level related, topical NSAIDs should be safer.

Local application, however, may have its problems. It may be less suitable than oral delivery for multiple regional pain; relatively inaccesible sites such as the spine; or pain arising from deep structures such as the hip or glenohumeral joint. Patients with compromised hand function may have difficulty applying topical agents, and some products are messy and stain clothing. Side effects may still occur — local reactions to the NSAID or carrier, for example, reddening, itching, photosensitivity; more widespread hypersensitivity reactions, such as bronchoconstriction or extensive skin/mucous membrane reactions; or even severe renal adverse reactions, for example, interstitial nephritis and renal failure following excessive[3] or normal[4] application. Whether topical agents penetrate locally and achieve adequate periarticular and joint tissue levels has also been questioned. Furthermore, many topical NSAIDs cost more per day than the equivalent oral drug. Whether they are better or safer than cheaper 'over the counter' rubefacients or embrocations (themselves not formally tested in OA) remains unknown.

Given these various considerations, what is the evidence for efficacy and safety in man?

Pharmacokinetics and mode of action

The skin presents a barrier through which only a limited amount of active substance from a given preparation will penetrate, for example, approximately 25 per cent for ibuprofen. Several factors, such as dose, fat solubility, and ionised state of the drug determine penetration into the stratum corneum, with lipid soluble, unionised drugs penetrating best. Diffusion through skin is accelerated by occlusive dressings and local hyperemia. Some additives induce hyperemia and, thus, influence absorption as well as exerting possible effects from hyperemia *per se*. Topical NSAIDs come as creams, gels, foams, patches, or sprays. Premedicated patches offer standard doses of NSAID, but all other modalities give variable self-administered dosing which presents special problems for efficacy and costing studies.

For many drugs that penetrate skin, rapid clearance via skin capillaries prevents local accumulation; this explains the systemic efficacy of transdermal nitrates and estrogen. However, this may not be inevitable and there are limited data from animal and human studies to support high local tissue levels of salicylate and certain NSAIDs, with minor uptake into the systemic circulation, after topical delivery. For example, in dogs, topical salicylate achieves higher concentrations than oral aspirin in cartilage, fascia, ligament, muscle, and tendon, despite much lower blood levels[5]. In one study of felbinac applied to human knees six hours prior to orthopedic surgery[6], drug concentrations in skin, subcutaneous fat, muscle, synovium, synovial fluid, and serum were in descending approximate ratios of 750: 230: 220: 100: 3: 1. Similarly, topical ibuprofen and piroxicam may reach several hundred-fold higher concentrations in periarticular tissues compared to plasma[7-9]. However, not all data support such high tissue concentrations from topical delivery. One study, in orthopedic patients[10], found oral fenbufen gave higher concentrations in periarticular tissues and synovial fluid than topical felbinac; all tissue concentrations were lower than those previously reported[6]. Meticulous technique is required to avoid contamination during sampling of contiguous periarticular/articular tissues, and methodological differences may account for the disparity in these studies[10].

Understandably, there are more data on synovial fluid and plasma levels than periarticular tissues. All studies concur in showing low plasma levels after topical salicylate or NSAID — in the order of 20–100 times less than following oral administration of identical or equivalent drugs at recommended doses[5-11]. With few exceptions[11], drug concentrations in synovial fluid after topical application are lower than those following oral administration[5,6,9,10]. When it has been examined, for example, for diclofenac[12], fenbufen[13], and piroxicam[9], similar synovial fluid concentrations occur in topically treated and contralateral untreated knees of the same patient, suggesting that NSAID absorption is mainly into the plasma, with secondary reperfusion into synovium. However, topical salicylate may achieve synovial fluid levels 60 per cent of those following oral aspirin, but with plasma levels several hundred-fold lower[5], supporting local penetration as well as blood-borne delivery.

The balance of evidence, therefore, confirms low plasma levels following topical delivery, but questions whether adequate levels are achieved in target tissues. Such inconclusive pharmacokinetic evidence of efficacy fuels the scepticism on topical NSAIDs[2]. However, the issue is clouded since:

1. 'Adequate' therapeutic levels of NSAIDs in peri-articular and joint tissue sites are not established.

2. Much pharmacokinetic data on topical NSAIDs is unpublished, as 'data on file', in pharmaceutical houses.

3. Synovial fluid data are only available for the knee — extrapolation to smaller, more superficial joints, for example, finger interphalangeal joints, is problematic.

Of course, 'adequate' synovial fluid levels may not be required for symptom benefit in OA. Mechanisms of pain production in OA are complex and much OA pain may be periarticular rather than intracapsular in origin[14]. Furthermore, effects on afferent nociceptor fibers in skin might influence spinal cord handling of afferents from adjacent joints[15], and neurovascular interactions between skin and underlying deep structures might modulate pain[16]. Wider investigation of possible effects of topical NSAIDs, therefore, seems warranted.

Data on clinical efficacy in OA

Most clinical data on topical NSAIDs relate to studies of soft-tissue lesions. A number of problems exist for most such studies:

(1) poor definition of acute regional pain syndrome, often with pooling of different conditions;

(2) short observation period (mainly 7–14 days);

(3) self-limiting nature of many lesions;

(4) questionable assessments of pain, function, or clinical signs;

(5) marked placebo response in all studies (up to 40–70 per cent).

Few studies appear in peer-reviewed journals. Despite these caveats, there are randomized placebo-controlled studies that attest to the efficacy of topical NSAIDs, including piroxicam[17], diclofenac[18], indomethacin[19], flurbiprofen[20], and felbinac[21], in acute and chronic soft tissue injury.

Relatively fewer, particularly placebo-controlled, studies relate to OA. Again, many of these have problems such as definitions of 'OA'; short-term observation (usually 14 days); very high placebo response (averaging about 60–70 per cent); and inappropriate primary and secondary outcome measures. Such paucity of data has led in the UK, for example, to only two topical agents, piroxicam and diclofenac, being licensed for use in OA.

Placebo-controlled studies in OA

There are limited data for hand and knee OA. In a double-blind cross-over study of 50 patients with hand OA[22], topical trolamine salicylate gave better relief of pain and stiffness than placebo cream; this benefit largely went within two hours of application. The placebo had no counterirritant action, and benefit from massage alone probably lasted approximately 30 minutes.

A randomized double-blind study of piroxicam versus placebo gel, applied three or four times daily to the most symptomatic knee of 246 OA patients, demonstrated greater efficacy with piroxicam at two weeks[23]. Global patient opinion showed improvement in 80 versus 68 per cent of patients, with marked-moderate improvement in 51 versus 33 per cent. Interestingly, improvement in the contralateral OA knee occurred to a lesser, but equal extent, in piroxicam (31 per cent) and placebo (36 per cent) patients, suggesting no clinical benefit at distant sites following single joint treatment.

Comparative studies

Several studies report similar efficacy when the topical is compared to the parent or alternative oral NSAID. For example, in a double-blind double-dummy study of 275 patients with mild-moderate knee OA, felbinac was as effective over a two-week period as oral fenbufen, with a similar low incidence of side effects[24]. Parity was also demonstrated in a similarly designed study of 235 patients with mild knee OA, comparing thrice daily piroxicam gel and oral ibuprofen (1200 mg per day) over a four-week period[25]. In three smaller (40–50 patient) double-blind double-dummy studies of patients with various diagnoses, including OA, equal efficacy, after one week, was found with salicylate cream or oral aspirin (2600 mg daily) at various peripheral and axial sites[26,27]. Topical salicylate, however, had advantages of faster pain relief and fewer side effects.

The ability to substitute topical for oral NSAID has been demonstrated in one open UK study[28]. One hundred and ninety-one elderly subjects on oral NSAID for OA (mainly knee) were randomized to continue their NSAID for four weeks, or to use piroxicam gel, plus half their oral NSAID dose, for two weeks and then gel alone for a further two weeks. Both groups improved from baseline, but the gel group showed greater improvements in joint tenderness and movement, and in AIMS (Arthritis Impact Measurement Scale) scores.

When topical NSAIDs have been directly compared in OA, there are little or no differences in efficacy between products. The design of such studies, however, is often questionable[29,30], with a strong likelihood of type II error.

Safety and economic considerations

Short-term studies in OA all report a very low incidence of side effects from topical NSAIDs, similar to[22–25,28], or lower [26,27] than, oral NSAIDs. Large surveillance studies in general practice appear to confirm their safety. For example, in 23,590 patients given felbinac for two weeks for locomotor pain (22 per cent for OA or arthritis), only 1.5 per cent developed adverse events, mainly local reactions[31]. However, six adverse events relating to the upper GI tract were attributed to felbinac. Other case reports of upper GI events in patients using topical NSAIDs suggest that the risk from these products, although low, may not be negligible.

A recent case-control study evaluated the risk of a major upper GI event associated with topical NSAID use[32]. Using a record-linkage database, 1103 patients, hospitalized for upper GI bleeding or perforation, were each compared to matched community and hospital controls (eight controls per case) for prior drug exposures. After adjusting for the confounding effect of concomitant exposure to oral NSAIDs and ulcer-healing drugs, no association between topical NSAIDs and upper GI events was discerned.

A number of studies have estimated the economic benefits of topical versus oral NSAIDs using various models of comparative efficacy, GI ulcer rates, and clinical decision making. Although generally considered an expensive alternative to oral NSAIDs[2], two studies, at least, suggest that topical piroxicam should be more

cost effective than oral ibuprofen for treatment of mild OA [33], as would felbinac compared to a combination product containing diclofenac and misoprostol[34].

Conclusions

Several observations support positioning of topical NSAIDs above oral NSAIDs in the preference order of symptomatic agents for OA:

1. Topical NSAIDs achieve only low blood levels and appear very safe in comparison to oral NSAIDs.

2. Several placebo-controlled studies attest to the clinical efficacy of topical NSAIDs for knee, and possibly hand OA.

3. Comparative studies suggest equal efficacy of topical NSAIDs to oral NSAIDs.

4. Topical NSAIDs may prove more cost effective than oral NSAIDs.

There are, however, relatively few published studies in this area. There is, therefore, a need for further well-designed studies with good definition of OA; appropriate pain and functional assessments; adequate power; and many, rather than just a few, weeks' duration; in order to:

(1) confirm clinical efficacy at common OA sites, and;

(2) clarify the mechanisms of action of topical NSAIDs.

References

1. Nothmann, M. and Wolff, M. (1933). The absorption of salicylic acid by human skin. *Klin Wochscht*, **12**, 345–6.
2. Anonymous. (1989). Topical NSAIDs: a gimmick or a godsend? *Lancet*, **2**, 779–80.
3. O'Callaghan, C.A., Andrews, P.A., and Ogg, C.S. (1994). Renal disease and use of topical non-steroidal anti-inflammatory drugs. *Br Med J*, **308**, 110–11.
4. Fernando, A.H.N., Thomas, S., Temple, R.M., and Lee, H.A. (1994). Renal failure after topical use of NSAIDs. *Br Med J*, **308**, 533.
5. Rabinowitz, J.L., Feldman, E.S., Weinberger, A., and Schumacher, H.R. (1982). Comparative tissue absorption of oral 14 C-aspirin and topical triethanolamine 14

C-salicylate in human and canine knee joints. *J Clin Pharmacol*, **22**, 42–8.

6. Sugawara, Y. (1985). Percutaneous absorption and tissue absorption of L-141 topical agent. *Jpn Med Pharmacol*, **13**, 183–94.

7. Peters, H., Chlud, K., Berner, G., et al. (1987). Percutaneous kinetics of ibuprofen. *Akt Rheumatol*, **12**, 208–11.

8. Kanazawa, M., Ito, H., Shimooka, K., and Mase, K. (1987). The pharmacokinetics of 0.5% piroxicam gel in humans. *Eur J Rheumatol Inflamm*, **8**, 117.

9. Sugawara, S., Ohno, H., Ueda, R., et al. (1984). Studies of percutaneous absorption and tissue distribution of piroxicam gel. *Jpn Med Pharmacol Sci*, **12**, 1233–8.

10. Bolten, W., Salzman, G., Goldmann, R., and Miehlke, K. (1989). Plasma and tissue concentrations of biphenylacetic acid following one week oral fenbufen medication and topical administration of felbinac gel on the knee joint. *J Rheumatol*, **48**, 317–22.

11. Riess, W., Schmid, K., Botta, L., et al. (1986). Percutaneous absorption of diclofenac. *Arzneimittel Forschung Drug Research*, **36**, 1092–6.

12. Radermacher, J., Jentsch, D., Scholl, M.A., Lustinetz, T., and Frolich, J.C. (1991). Diclofenac concentrations in synovial fluid and plasma after cutaneous application in inflammatory and degenerative joint disease. *Br J Clin Pharmacol*, **31**, 537–41.

13. Dawson, M., McGee, C.M., Vine, J.H., et al. (1988). The disposition of biphenylacetic acid following topical application. *Eur J Clin Pharmacol*, **33**, 639–42.

14. Jones, A. and Doherty, M. (1992). The treatment of osteoarthritis. *Rheumatology Review*, **1**, 205–16.

15. Woolf, C.J. and Wall, P.D. (1986). Relative effectiveness of C primary fibres of different origins in evoking a prolonged facilitation of the flexor reflex in the rat. *J Neuroscience*, **6**, 1433–42.

16. Kidd, B.L., Mapp, P.I., Blake, D.R., Gibson, S.J., and Polak, J.M. (1990). Neurogenic influences in arthritis. *Ann Rheum Dis*, **49**, 649–52.

17. Russell, A.L. (1991). Piroxicam 0.5% topical gel compared to placebo in the treatment of soft tissue injuries: a double blind study comparing efficacy and safety. *Clin Invest Med*, **14**, 35–43.

18. Schapira, D., Linn, S., and Scharf, Y. (1991). A placebo-controlled evaluation of diclofenac diethylamine salt in the treatment of lateral epicondylitis of the elbow. *Curr Ther Res*, **49**, 162–8.

19. Ginsburgh, F. and Famaey, J–P. (1991). Double-blind, randomised cross-over study of the percutaneous efficacy and tolerability of a topical indomethacin spray versus placebo in the treatment of tendinitis. *J Int Med Res*, **19**, 131–6.

20. Poul, J., West, J., Buchanan, N., and Grahame, R. (1993). Local action transcutaneous flurbiprofen in the treatment of soft tissue rheumatism. *Br J Rheumatol*, **32**, 1000–3.

21. Hosie, G. and Bird, H. (1994). The topical NSAID felbinac versus oral NSAIDs: a critical review. *Eur J Rheum atol Inflamm*, **14**, 21–8.

22. Rothacker, D., Difigilo, C., and Lee, I. (1994). A clinical trial of topical 10% trolamine salicylate in osteoarthritis. *Curr Ther Res*, **55**, 584–97.

23. Kageyama, T. (1987). A double blind placebo controlled multicenter study of piroxicam 0.5% gel in osteoarthritis of the knee. *Eur J Rheumatol Inflamm*, **8**, 114–15.

24. Tsuyama, N., Kurokawa, T., Nihei, T., Nagano, A., Tachibana, N., and Hanaoka, K. (1985). Clinical evaluation of L-141 topical agent on osteoarthrosis deformans of the knees. *Clin Med*, **1**, 697–729.

25. Dickson, D.J. (1991). A double-blind evaluation of topical piroxicam gel with oral ibuprofen in osteoarthritis of the knee. *Curr Ther Res*, **49**, 199–207.

26. Shamszad, M., Perkal, M., Golden, F.L., and Marlin, R. (1986). Two double-blind comparisons of a topically applied salicylate cream and orally ingested aspirin in the relief of chronic musculoskeletal pain. *Curr Ther Res*, **39**, 470–9.

27. Golden, E.L. (1978). A double-blind comparison of orally ingested aspirin and a topically applied salicylate cream in the relief of rheumatic pain. *Curr Ther Res*, **24**, 524–9.

28. Browning, R.C. and Johnson, K. (1994). Reducing the dose of oral NSAIDs by use of feldene gel: an open study in elderly patients with osteoarthritis. *Adv Ther*, **11**, 198–207.

29. Giacovazzo, M. (1992). Clinical evaluation of a new NSAID applied topically (BPAA gel) versus diclofenac emulgel in elderly osteoarthritic patients. *Drugs Exptl Clin Res*, **18**, 201–3.

30. Rau, R. and Hockel, S. (1989). Piroxicam gel versus diclofenac gel in activated gonarthrosis. *Fortschr Med*, **22**, 485–8.

31. Newbery, R., Shuttleworth, P., and Rapier, C. (1992). A multicentre post marketing surveillance study to evaluate the safety and efficacy of felbinac 3% gel in the treatment of musculoskeletal disorders in general practice. *Eur J Clin Res*, **3**, 139–50.

32. Evans, J.M.M., McMahon, A.D., McGilchrist, M.M., et al. (1995). Topical non-steroidal anti-inflammatory drugs and admission to hospital for upper gastrointestinal bleeding and perforation: a record linkage case-control study. *Br Med J*, **311**, 22–6.

33. McKell, D. and Stewart, A. (1994). A cost-minimisation analysis comparing topical versus systemic NSAIDs in the treatment of mild osteoarthritis of the superficial joints. *Br J Med Econ*, **7**, 137–46.

34. Peacock, M. and Rapier, C. (1993). The topical NSAID felbinac is a cost effective alternative to oral NSAIDs for the treatment of rheumatic conditions. *Br J Med Econ*, **6**, 135–42.

9.7   Topical capsaicin cream

Kenneth D. Brandt and John D. Bradley

Capsaicin (trans-8-methly-n-vanillyl-6-nonenamide) is an alkaloid derived from the seeds and membranes of the Nightshade family of plants, which includes the common pepper plant[1] (Fig. 9.3). It is the active ingredient in tabasco sauce.

Capsaicin has received attention recently as a topical analgesic agent. Initially, it was believed that capsaicin worked by a 'counterirritant' mechanism[2], that is by stimulation of faster conducting nonciceptors which activated the descending diffuse noxious inhibitory control system which, in turn, inhibited the more slowly conducting pain signals transmitted along small diameter unmyelinated fibers in the spinal cord. (This 'gate control' concept may be relevant also to the mechanism of action of transcutaneous electrical nerve stimulation (TENS) and acupuncture)[3].

Subsequently, however, it was shown that capsaicin, when applied topically, stimulates the release of the neuropeptide, substance P, from peripheral nerves and prevents its reaccumulation from cell bodies and nerve terminals in both the central and peripheral nervous system. Substance P is an important chemical mediator responsible for transmission of pain from the periphery to the central nervous system.

Capsaicin has been used in treatment of a variety of painful disorders, including postherpetic neuralgia, cluster headaches, diabetic neuropathy, phantom limb pain, and postmastectomy pain[4-7]. Local application of capsaicin results in depletion of substance P from the entire neuron, so that branches from the peripheral nerves to deeper structures, such as the joint, are effectively depleted[1,8]. Initially, external transport of substance P is blocked; with continued treatment, synthesis of substance P is reduced.

Although articular cartilage has no nerve supply and, therefore, cannot be a source of pain, histologic studies of joint innervation have shown that the joint capsule, tendons, ligaments, and periosteum are extensively innervated[9,10]. Nerve fibers are also present in the subchondral bone[11]. Small diameter nerve fibers in the synovium[12] and subchondral plate[13] have been shown to stain immunohistochemically for substance P, as has sclerotic bone[14] and areas of bony eburnation[15] and of fibrillated cartilage[15] in OA joints. Synovial concentrations of substance P are increased in patients with OA[16,17].

There is some evidence that, in addition to modulating pain, substance P may mediate inflammation within the joint. Intra-articular infusion of substance P in rats with adjuvant arthritis increased the severity of joint inflammation, and this effect could be blocked by infusion of a substance P antagonist[18]. Intra-articular injection of substance P increases blood flow to the joint, transudation of plasma proteins, and release of lysosomal enzymes[19]. In addition, substance P is a chemoattractant for neutrophils and monocytes[19], and stimulates synovial cells to produce prostaglandins and collagenase, mediators associated with joint damage[18,20]. Although the importance of substance P in the pathogenesis of joint inflammation in OA is not clear, and mediators other than substance P are undoubtedly involved, substance P may play an important role in mediating joint pain in OA and pharmacologic inhibition of substance P may be useful in symptomatic management of OA.

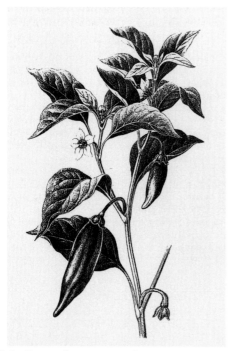

Fig. 9.3   Pepper plant, a source of capsaicin.

In 1991, Deal *et al.*[21] reported the results of a randomized, double-blind, placebo-controlled multi-center trial involving patients with moderate to very severe pain due to knee OA. Patients in the active treatment group applied either 0.025 per cent capsaicin cream, or the vehicle, four times daily to anterior, posterior, and lateral aspects of the most severely affected knee. Thirty-six patients received the active agent and 34, the placebo. Patients were evaluated after one, two and four weeks of treatment (Table 9.4).

Improvement in joint pain was significantly greater (p = 0.02) in subjects who received capsaicin than in the placebo group. After four weeks of treatment, the evaluation of the physician and the pain score of the patient both showed a mean reduction of 22 per cent (p = 0.05) for those using the active cream, but of only 14 per cent (p = 0.05) and 10 per cent (p = 0.06), respectively, for those using the placebo cream.

A local burning sensation was noted by 44 per cent of patients using the capsaicin preparation and by one patient in the placebo group. However, burning diminished with continuation of treatment, and 94 per cent of patients in the active treatment group and 88 per cent of those in the placebo group completed the study. Although the burning, which occurred at the site of application, obviously affected blinding of the study, and may have favored a positive response to the capsaicin, the authors attempted to take this into account by comparing the results in patients treated with capsaicin who experienced burning, with those in capsaicin-treated patients who did not have this side effect. No difference in drug response was apparent between the two groups.

In 1992, McCarthy and McCarty reported similar beneficial effects from topical application of a more potent formulation of capsaicin (0.075 per cent) in a placebo-controlled, four-week, double-blind randomized trial involving 14 subjects with painful OA of the distal or proximal interphalangeal joints or first carpometacarpal joint[22]. By week four, topical application of capsaicin had reduced joint pain by nearly 60 per cent and joint tenderness by approximately 40 per cent, in comparison with the baseline values, while improvement in these parameters in patients treated with topical application of the vehicle alone was only about 20 and 10 per cent, respectively. No changes were noted, however, with respect to grip strength, joint swelling, duration of morning stiffness, or joint function. As in the study by Deal *et al.*[21], all patients who received capsaicin reported a burning sensation in the skin. However, none discontinued treatment because of this side effect, and the local discomfort diminished over the first week and became increasingly tolerable with continued treatment (Table 9.4).

In both of the above studies, patients were permitted to continue their usual treatment with NSAIDs or analgesics; capsaicin was used as an adjunct to the usual therapy. In contrast, Altman *et al.* recently reported a clinical trial of 0.025 per cent capsaicin cream as *monotherapy* for OA[23]. In this double-blind study, NSAIDs and other medications which the patients were receiving for treatment of OA were discontinued before entry into the study. Use of acetaminophen was permitted during the study but was restricted to three days per month, and patients were given only 12 tablets of

Table 9.4 Results of placebo-controlled trials of capsaicin cream in patients with OA

Study	OA joint site	Capsaicin strength	Duration of study	Number of subjects treated	Decrease in joint pain at end of study	
					Capsaicin	Placebo
Deal *et al.*[21]	Knee	0.025%	4 weeks	36 capsaicin 34 placebo	22%	14%
McCarthy and McCarty[22]	DIP, PIP, MCP	0.075%	4 weeks	7 capsaicin 7 placebo	60%	20%
Altman *et al.*[23]	Various (70% knee)	0.025%	12 weeks	57 capsaicin 56 placebo	53%	27%
Schnitzer *et al.*[24]	Various (approx. 80% knee)	0.25%	4 weeks	32 capsaicin 32 placebo	74%	65%

DIP = distal interphalangeal
PIP = proximal interphalangeal
MCP = metacarpophalangeal

acetaminophen per month, to be used for non-arthritic pain or fever. Patients were evaluated for 12 weeks, that is, considerably longer than in either of the two trials cited above. Although subjects had OA at a variety of joint sites, 70 per cent of those treated with capsaicin and 79 per cent of those treated with the vehicle had knee OA. Among the 113 patients included in the study, 57 received capsaicin and 56 were treated with the vehicle.

Baseline pain scores in the two groups, measured on a visual analogue scale, were comparable (57 mm for capsaicin, 56 mm for vehicle). Based on global evaluation of the patients, those who received capsaicin reported significantly greater reduction of pain at weeks 4, 8, and 12, than the controls. At week 12, a mean improvement of 52.9 per cent was noted in the capsaicin group but of only 27.4 per cent in the placebo-treated group (p = 0.02). Global assessment by the physician also revealed a difference between groups at week 12 (Table 9.4).

This study is important insofar as it shows that improvement in joint pain can occur with capsaicin as the *sole* analgesic therapy and can be sustained. Indeed, pain relief was as great after 12 weeks of treatment as after only four weeks. Furthermore, the magnitude of improvement in joint pain was as great as that seen with NSAIDs.

In a recent single-blind study of patients with OA at a variety of joint sites[24], a high strength (0.25 per cent) capsaicin cream (not currently available in the United States), applied only twice a day, provided greater pain relief, with a more rapid onset of action, than 0.025 per cent capsaicin cream applied four times daily. It is unclear, however, whether the fact that the dosing regimens were not comparable may have affected outcomes in the two treatment groups. As in the study by Altman *et al.*[23], medications that might have interfered with the efficacy evaluation (for example, NSAIDs, systemic analgesics) were withdrawn prior to randomization. Furthermore, only one patient in the high-strength capsaicin treatment group discontinued therapy because of a sensation of burning at the site of application. Although the incidence of burning was initially greater with the high-strength formulation, by day seven, and subsequently for the remainder of this 28-day study, the number of patients who reported burning was no greater in the high-strength capsaicin group than in the 0.025 per cent capsaicin group (Table 9.4).

Topical capsaicin therapy appears to be safe and effective, and warrants initial consideration in management of OA pain. Patients should apply the medication in a thin film to all sides of the involved joint and should be instructed to wash their hands immediately after application of the cream, and to avoid contact with eyes and mucus membranes, and broken or inflamed skin. In all of the studies cited above, the topical burning sensation caused by capsaicin generally subsided with continued treatment and seldom resulted in discontinuation of treatment. Intolerance may also be managed by temporarily switching to a lower strength preparation (if the 0.025 per cent formulation is not the initial choice). A higher potency cream may then be used, if necessary, after tolerance to the skin irritating effect of the lower strength preparation has developed.

References

1. Virus, R.M. and Gebhart, G.F. (1979). Pharmacologic actions of capsaicin: apparent involvement of substance P and serotonin. *Life Science*, **25**, 1273–84.

2. Kantor, T. (1989). Concepts in pain control. *Semin Arthritis Rheum*, **18**, 94–9.

3. Gunn, C.C. (1978). Transcutaneous neural stimulation, acupuncture, and the current of injury. *Am J Acupuncture*, **6**, 191–6.

4. Bernstein, J.E., Korman, N.J., Bickers, D.R., Dahl, M.V., and Millikan, L.E. (1989). Topical capsaicin treatment of chronic postherpetic neuralgia. *J Am Acad Dermatol*, **21**, 265–70.

5. Sicuteri, F., Fusco, B., Marabini, S., and Fanciullacci, M. (1988). Capsaicin as a potential medication for cluster headache. *Med Sci Res*, **16**, 1079–80.

6. Ross, D.R. and Varipapa, R.J. (1989). Treatment of painful diabetic neuropathy with topical capsaicin. *N Engl J Med*, **321**, 474–5.

7. Raynor, H.C., Atkins, R.L., and Westerman, R.A. (1989). Relief of local stump pain by capsaicin cream. *Lancet* **2**, 1276–7.

8. Fitzgerald, M. (1983). Capsaicin and sensory neurones — a review. *Pain*, **15**, 109–30.

9. Samuel, E.P. (1952). The autonomic and somatic innervation of the articular capsule. *Anat Rec*, **113**, 84–93.

10. Ralson, H.J., Miller, M.R., and Kasahara, M. (1960). Nerve endings in human fasciae, tendons, ligaments, periosteum and joint synovial membrane. *Anat Rec*, **136**, 137–47.

11. Milgram, J.W. and Robison, R.A. (1965). An electron microscopic demonstration of unmyelinated nerves in the Haversian canels of the adult dog. *Bull Johns Hopkins Hosp*, **117**, 163–73.

12. Kidd, B.L., Mapp, P.I., Blake, D.R., Gibson, S.J., and Polak, J.M. (1990). Neurogenic influences in arthritis *Ann Rheum Dis*, **49**, 649–52.

13. Nixon, A.J. and Cummings, J.F. (1994). Substance P immunohistochemical study of the sensory innervation

of normal subchondral bone in the equine metacarpophalangeal joints. *Am J Vet Res*, 55, 28–33.

14. Badalamente, M.A. and Cherney, S.B. (1989). Periosteal and vascular innervation of the human patella in degenerative joint disease. *Semin Arthritis Rheum*, 18, 61–6.

15. Wojtys, E.M., Beaman, D.N., Glover, R.A., and Janda, D. (1990). Innervation of the human knee joint by substance-P fibers. *Arthroscopy: J Arth Rel Surg*, 6, 254–63.

16. Menkes, C.J., Mauborgne, A., Loussadi, S., *et al.*: (1991). Substance P (SP) levels in synovial tissue and synovial fluid from rheumatoid arthritis (RA) and osteoarthritis (OA) patients. In *Scientific Abstracts of the 54th annual meeting of the American College of Rheumatology, Seattle, WA, October 27 — November 1.*

17. Marshall, K.W., Chiu, B., and Inman, R.D. (1990). Substance P and arthritis: analysis of plasma and synovial fluid levels. *Arthritis Rheum*, 33, 87–90.

18. Levine, J.D., Clark, R., Devor, M., Helms, C., Moskowitz, M.A., and Basbaum, A.I. (1984). Intra-neuronal substance P contributes to the severity of experimental arthritis. *Science*, 226, 547–9.

19. Kimball, E.S. (1990). Substance P, cytokines and arthritis. *Ann NY Acad Sci*, 594, 293–308.

20. Lotz, M., Carson, D.A., and Vaughan, J.H. (1987). Substance P activation of rheumatoid synoviocytes: Neural pathway in pathogenesis of arthritis. *Science*, 235, 893–5.

21. Deal, C.L., Schnitzer, T.J., Lipstein, E., *et al.* (1991). Treatment of arthritis with topical capsaicin: a double-blind trial. *Clin. Ther*, 13, 383.

22. McCarthy, G.M. and McCarty, D.J. (1992). Effect of topical capsaicin in the therapy of painful osteoarthritis of the hands. *J Rheumatol*, 19, 604.

23. Altman, R.D., Aven, A., Holmburg, C.E., *et al.* (1994). Capsaicin cream 0.025% as monotherapy for osteoarthritis: a double-blind study. *Semin Arthritis Rheum*, 23, 25–33.

24. Schnitzer, T., Posner, M., and Lawrence, I. (1995). High strength capsaicin cream for osteoarthritis pain: rapid onset of action and improved efficacy with twice daily dosing. *J Clin Rheumatol*, 1, 268–73.

9.8   Intra-articular therapies in osteoarthritis

Adrian Jones and Michael Doherty

Introduction

Although systemic factors are discussed in relation to its etiopathogenesis, osteoarthritis (OA) is essentially a disease that is localized to the joint when it comes to symptomatology. It seems logical, therefore, to attempt to minimize potential adverse effects of therapy by using local measures. Fortunately, many of the symptomatic joints of OA — knee, hip, hand — are accessible to the suitably trained practitioner, and much is to be potentially gained by the use of intra- or periarticular approaches. In this chapter, we shall first present a brief historical overview of intra-articular therapies, and then concentrate on the evidence for the efficacy and safety of the different agents that may be used. Since corticosteroids are the most widely used drugs in this context, the focus of this chapter will be on them, but other agents will also be discussed.

Historical considerations

The history of intra-articular therapy in OA is surprisingly long. Following on from observations in the 1930s that synovial fluid in OA joints develops an alkaline pH, and the resulting hypothesis that acidity may stimulate joint repair, some workers attempted to treat OA by intra-articular injection of various acids, including lactic acid[1] and phosphoric acid[2]. Although encouraging results were reported from large series of patients[3], the studies were largely uncontrolled and the practice slowly faded. It was not really until the discovery of the power of factor F (adrenal extract) to ameliorate the effect of rheumatoid arthritis that interest in intra-articular agents was rekindled. Thorn is generally credited with the first use of intra-articular factor F, but it was Hollander who reported the first large series involving OA joints[4]. These showed promising efficacy, and subsequent controlled trials in OA have demonstrated efficacy, albeit of short duration. However, the use of corticosteroids in uncomplicated OA remains controversial, as will be discussed later.

The increasing use of arthroscopy and arthrography in the diagnostic evaluation of OA led to uncontrolled reports of symptomatic benefit following these procedures. Uncontrolled series of patients treated by these methods followed. However, only a few methodologically sound studies demonstrate clear benefit.

Just as synovial fluid in OA is alkaline, so too does it have reduced viscosity, principally as a result of degradation of complex proteoglycans. Using the logic that this decreased viscosity would impair lubrication of the joint and hence movement, various agents have been used to attempt to restore viscosity. Initial reports concerned mineral oils such as silicone. Results were disappointing[5], and a marked chemical synovitis can occur as a result of this 'inert' agent. More recently though, work on 'viscosupplementation' with high molecular weight hyaluronans has been reported, with some promising results. The mechanism of these actions is, however, not as a result of direct 'viscosupplementation' but a result of the effect of these complex molecules on the biochemistry of the joint. Indeed, a greater appreciation of the biology of OA has led to speculation concerning several potential mechanisms for altering cartilage biochemistry favorably. Many of these agents will need to be administered intra-articularly.

Corticosteroids

Efficacy

Although the history of intra-articular corticosteroid use in OA now extends over 30 years, there are surprisingly little controlled data to support either its use or the choice of the optimal agent. Early reports, using hydrocortisone (factor F) in an open fashion, suggested an effect in OA, although this was generally transient, lasting only a few days. When subjected to controlled clinical trial, no significant therapeutic effect of hydrocortisone acetate could be demonstrated[6]. The synovial membrane is readily permeable to hydrophilic molecules such as hydrocortisone acetate and such rapid loss from the site of action probably explains much of the inefficacy. Studies on more hydrophobic agents have, therefore, been undertaken, although these are surprisingly few in number, given the widespread use of this agent.

In a comparison of hydrocortisone actetate, hydrocortisone tertiary butylacetate, and placebo, in a randomized cross-over study of 38 OA knees in 25 patients, a greater improvement was seen with the longer acting hydrocortisone tertiary butlyacetate than either of the other two preparations[7].

In a parallel group, double-blind comparison of 20 mg triamcinolone hexacetonide versus carrier in 34 patients, symptomatic benefit was demonstrated in the steroid group, but only at one week post-injection, the difference being lost at four weeks[8].

Dieppe *et al.* conducted two related studies of 20 mg triamcinolone in OA of the knee[9]. In the first, 12 patients with bilateral symptomatic OA of the knee received, in an observer-blind fashion, 20 mg triamcinolone in one knee and, simultaneously, 1 ml saline in the opposite knee. In the second, 16 patients with 24 symptomatic knees received, in an observer-blind one-week cross-over study, 20 mg triamcinolone or saline in randomized order. Both studies demonstrated short-term benefit of triamcinolone over saline placebo, with clear patient preference for the steroid. Benefit could not be related to any disease characteristics, although numbers were small. An order effect was noted with greater benefit resulting from the first injection, perhaps reflecting the marked placebo effect of any intra-articular procedure.

In a parallel-group, observer-blind comparison of 20 mg triamcinolone hexacetonide versus 6 mg betamethasone, the former was more effective at reducing pain[10]. In a parallel-group, double-blind, placebo-controlled study in 84 patients with painful knee OA, 20 mg triamcinolone hexacetonide produced significant improvements in pain and walking distance in one minute, compared to placebo[11]. This effect was still apparent at six weeks.

Although there is some evidence for efficacy at the knee, the use of intra-articular injection at other sites is largely unproven. Thumb-base injection for OA has been asserted to be of long-lasting efficacy but controlled data to support this are lacking. Injection into other small joints in the hands and feet are anecdotally often successful, but again, this is on the basis of clinical impression. In addition, the dose of corticosteroid in relation to the size of the joint has been raised as a concern, since this may be associated with increased cartilage and bone loss. At the hip, intra-articular steroids have been used but little controlled data are available. In a small double-blind study comparing 10 ml (0.5 per cent) bupivicaine and triamcinolone, versus 10 ml (0.5 per cent) bupivicaine alone, or 10 ml N saline, the group receiving triamcinolone fared worse in terms of a deterioration of symptoms than either of the other two groups. Furthermore, there are concerns regarding safety; injections around the hip have been suggested to be linked to increased progression of cartilage loss[12].

Perhaps an equally controversial area concerns the use of corticosteroid injections for 'OA' of the spine. Although spinal OA is well recognized both radiographically and pathologically, it is perhaps the site where it is the most difficult to link symptoms with structural change. Whilst a large number of paraspinal steroid injections have been, and continue to be given, perhaps the only situation in which one is using them specifically for OA is when injecting facet joints. Although proponents describe good efficacy at this site, there are no appropriately controlled data to support its use. Within-patient comparisons, using injections of local anesthetic or placebo into the region of the facet joint, can demonstrate that symptoms may be abolished by a suitable agent, but whether corticosteroids have any additional role in this is a moot point.

The temporomandibular joint is a site in which corticosteroid injections have also been widely used, although generally this is outside the realm of the rheumatologist and in the remit of dental services. Good symptomatic benefit is claimed for this procedure, but again controlled data are lacking. In addition, although temporomandibular pain and dysfunction may be associated with OA change, there are a number of other structures, including the joint meniscus, which may be the source of symptoms.

In summary, the data regarding the efficacy of corticosteroid injections in OA is surprisingly sparse, given that they are widely used. At the knee, however, there is some evidence that long-acting corticosteroids, and in particular triamcinolone hexacetonide, are effective, although the duration of action is typically short, at approximately three weeks. Decisions regarding more widespread use of this approach must, therefore, be based on considerations of safety and individual patient response.

Adverse effects

The adverse effects of corticosteroid injections are generally relatively minor but some, such as skin atrophy, may result in costly litigation. Sepsis is, of course, the most feared complication, since it may result in severe morbidity and significant mortality. Finally, there are also, as yet, unresolved issues regarding possible effects of corticosteroids on bone and cartilage metabolism.

Local reactions to corticosteroid injection

Two principle reactions will be considered here; post-injection flares and corticosteroid induced atrophy. Although corticosteroids are anti-inflammatory, most clinicians will have experienced patients who have a flare of synovitis following corticosteroid injection. The

incidence of such a reaction is unclear, as is the specificity for steroid injections. Post-injection flares following saline and other pharmaceutical agents are reported in a number of studies[8,10]. In the study by Gaffney *et al.*, 4 of 42 (10 per cent) patients receiving saline placebo, and none of the triamcinolone group, reported a deterioration of symptoms[11]. Our own study of triamcinolone hexacetonide versus hyaluronic acid was associated with a post-injection flare in 3 of 32 (10 per cent) of patients receiving triamcinolone. Other studies have reported incidences of the order of 12–24 per cent[8,13,14]. In a direct comparison of two corticosteroids, 4 of 21 patients receiving triamcinolone hexacetonide experienced flares, compared to 1 of 21 receiving betamethasone.

The incidence of corticosteroid-induced tissue atrophy is less clear cut. Two types of atrophy are particularly important: skin and subcutaneous fat, and tendon. Damage to both may be an important cause of patient harm and possible litigation. Atrophy of subcutaneous fat and skin produces a depressed, atrophic area which is often made more noticeable by associated hypopigmentation. Factors associated with development of atrophy include poor localization of the injection, particularly when superficial structures are being injected or potent fluorinated steroids used. It is, therefore, prudent to specifically warn patients of this possibility when injecting superficial sites, for example, acromioclavicular joints and small joints of the hands, and to record this fact in the notes. In addition, fluorinated steroids should be avoided at these sites. Similar considerations apply to tendon injury. Injections under pressure should be avoided, and we would advise against paratendinous injection.

Systemic effects of corticosteroid injection

Temporary deterioration in diabetic control might be expected due to systemic absorption of corticosteroid; significant problems with this are not common[13], although it is best to warn patients of the possibility. Facial flushing, presumably due to altered vascular tone, occurs in some patients after intra-articular corticosteroid injection. Its incidence is unclear, but one prospective study has suggested that it may be as much as 40 per cent, although only severe in 12 per cent[15]; it seems prudent to warn patients of the possibility. Changing to a different corticosteroid may reduce the risk of subsequent flushing[15]. Anaphylaxis has also been reported after corticosteroid injection but is fortunately rare[16].

Sepsis following corticosteroid injection

A major fear in the use of intra-articular injection is the risk of introducing infection. Not only is this simply as a result of intra-articular puncture, but it is felt that the risk is greater in the presence of corticosteroids. In fact, the true risk of infection following corticosteroid injection is unknown. Most estimates are derived from retrospective records and these are of the order of 1 : 15 000–50 000 injections. In a retrospective study of septic arthritis, over a ten-year period in Nottingham (population 600 000), only three cases of septic arthritis possibly related to intra-articular steroid were identified. As in most studies of this type, the denominator is unknown and the presence of infection prior to injection not excluded. The risk of infection would seem slight.

Cartilage and bone

Corticosteroids have the theoretical and experimental potential to affect the OA process or to produce avascular necrosis. Animal experiments on this point are inconclusive and depend on the species used and the dose of corticosteroid employed. Little data about humans are available. An early analysis of radiographs of patients receiving intra-articular hydrocortisone acetate and hydrocortisone tertiary butylacetate for rheumatoid arthritis, was thought to show a rapid deterioration in radiographic appearance[17]. In children with juvenile chronic arthritis, receiving multiple triamcinolone injections, little deterioration in the joints was observed over a prolonged period of follow-up, with the possible exception of the hip[12]. In this series, one case of avascular necrosis of the femoral head was observed. Further suggestion that corticosteroid injection at the hip may be detrimental arises from a small case-control study in patients awaiting total hip replacement which demonstrated a more rapid deterioration in symptoms in the group given steroid injection[18]. Further work is required to confirm this, but it would seem prudent to be cautious about the use of intra-articular steroids at the hip.

The number of injections per joint or per person that should be undertaken is unclear, as there is little direct evidence on which to base the decision. Extrapolating from animal models suggests that in small joints, such as those of the hand, the number of injections should perhaps be limited to one or two per lifetime, whereas in larger joints, such as the knee, three-monthly injec-

tions may be safe. At present, the validity of these figures remains a matter of opinion.

Accuracy

There has been debate about the need for accurate joint injections as it has been suggested that provided the corticosteroid is placed in the vicinity of the joint, benefit will accrue. There are, thus, two issues to consider:

(1)   how accurate is the placement of joint injections, and

(2)   does this matter?

It would appear that injections are often inaccurate, and that this does indeed matter. In a study of unselected patients receiving intra-articular steroid injections into a variety of joints and for a variety of rheumatological diagnoses, injections were shown, by contrast radiography, to be extra-articular in 30 per cent of cases[19]. This varied to some extent by joint site but was still inaccurate in as many as 30 per cent of the knees injected. Aspiration of joint fluid was associated with improved accuracy. This would obviously not matter if accuracy did not affect efficacy but, unfortunately, the same study suggested that inaccurate injections produced a smaller benefit in terms of inflammation of the joint. Whether accuracy can be improved is unclear, but if an injection is ineffectual then it is reasonable to assume that this may be due to inaccuracy, and worth repeating.

Indications

Several studies have failed to demonstrate any clear-cut predictors of response to corticosteroids apart, possibly, from the presence of effusion[11]. The latter, however, may be acting as a surrogate for injection accuracy[19], although in an earlier study, prior aspiration of fluid did not predict response[8]. All this does mean is that, although many authors suggest that corticosteroids should be reserved for acute synovitis in OA, there is little direct experimental support for this view. Decisions regarding the more widespread adoption of corticosteroid injections have, therefore, to be made on the basis of cost and safety. It would seem reasonable to consider using corticosteroid injections in patients who have failed to respond to other conservative therapies and who are unwilling, or unable, to have surgery.

Para-articular injection

Although it has been suggested that, in general, accurate joint injection is associated with improved efficacy, it is also true that in many patients with OA, pain may arise from para-articular structures. In 1939, Kellgren described many of the possible para-articular pain sources in the knee, but their role and prevalence remains unclear[20]. At least one study has demonstrated that peripatellar injection at the knee may be as efficacious as intra-articular injection[21]. The role of a placebo effect in this study cannot be excluded.

Nerve blocks

An alternative to intra-articular injection is to attempt to reduce pain from a joint by blocking afferent nerves with either local anesthetics or neurodestructive agents. The techniques have been particularly applied at the hip and shoulder, and for a variety of pathologies including OA. Pain relief from such procedures can be good and of prolonged benefit, and may be of importance when surgical or other options have failed or are inappropriate. The only concern is that such nerve blocks may be detrimental to the OA process, a view that is suggested by animal experiments involving denervation of joints[22].

Radiosynovectomy

Clinical and histological data supports a role for synovial hypertrophy and inflammation in OA. Accordingly, radiation synovectomy has been proposed as a means of controlling local synovitis in OA. In a comparison of external beam radiotherapy (800 radiographs over four weeks) versus short-wave diathermy and physiotherapy in 46 evaluated patients, no convincing difference in benefit was observed between the two groups[23].

In a study of pyrophosphate arthropathy, 5 mCi of ^{90}Y and 20 mg triamcinolone was more effective in relieving pain at six months than 20 mg triamcinolone and saline[24]. Our own experience of radiosynovectomy in OA is also disappointing, and there are concerns, of course, with the long-term safety of radiosynovectomy both on the joint itself and due to a possible increased risk of carcinogenesis — a risk presently unquantified, and probably negligible. At present, we would be reluctant to recommend radiosynovectomy for the OA patient except in exceptional circumstances.

Novel therapies

Other agents which may be of benefit in OA may be given intra-articularly. Some are older agents which are being re-evaluated, others are novel agents which may have effects on the OA process itself.

Anesthetic agents

Local anesthetics can be used as a component of intra-articular steroid or may be used on their own for nerve blocks. It is not clear, however, whether they would have an effect on the OA joint itself. At the hip, bupivicaine alone may be as effective as triamcinolone, and both may be less effective than saline alone[18]. Some preliminary data from Creamer *et al.* suggests that lignocaine is more effective than placebo in knee OA, and may have an equivalent duration of action[25].

Joint distension

It has been suggested that simple joint injection with saline may improve OA symptoms. It has further been suggested that distension of the joint may have an additive effect. However, in a double-blind, placebo-controlled study in 38 patients with hip OA, joint distension with radiographic contrast was not more effective in reducing symptoms than para-articular injection with saline[26].

Nonsteroidal anti-inflammatory drugs (NSAIDs)

Since OA is essentially a local disease, it would seem at face value that direct administration of NSAIDs into the joint would bypass some of the potential problems of systemic administration. To date, only a few studies of this approach have been published. In a comparison of hip joint distension with and without indoprofen, no additional benefit was conferred by the addition of the

NSAID[27]. Further evaluation of a possible role for intra-articular NSAIDs is necessary.

Hyaluronic acid

Hyaluronic acid is a normal component of synovial fluid, being a high molecular weight glycosaminoglycan. In OA, it is degraded into small molecular weight complexes. Initially, it was argued that injecting high molecular weight hyaluronans into an affected joint would restore synovial fluid viscosity and, hence, joint function. It would thus act in a manner as proposed for silicone oils. In fact, hyaluronans have now been demonstrated to have a multiplicity of biological actions which may underpin any possible beneficial role on the OA process[28].

There is a difference, however, between understanding possible mechanisms and demonstrating symptomatic benefit. Several double-blind controlled studies on the benefit of hyaluronic acid preparations have been performed; several general comments should be made. Firstly, hyaluronic acids are highly viscous, making blinding of the injector difficult. For this reason, studies in which the investigator and injector are the same, need to be considered with caution. Secondly, hyaluronic acid preparations differ widely in their molecular weight and, hence, properties. Extrapolation from one preparation to the other is, thus, difficult. The following is a summary of some of the more major controlled studies.

Studies of Hyalgan, a 750 kD hyaluronan, have produced varying results. In a double-blind, placebo-controlled study of three weekly injections of Hyalgan versus an equivalent number of phosphate buffer injections in 40 knee joints in 34 patients, Hyalgan produced bigger reductions in visual analogue pain scores than placebo[29]. This difference persisted for sixty days. Similar results were seen in a larger study of longer duration (23 weeks) involving up to 11 injections[30]. A one-year, single-blind study of five hyaluronic acid injections versus placebo in 110 patients failed to demonstrate any significant differences between the two treatments, except when analyzed by a single-tailed t-test[31]. Similarly, in a double-blind, placebo-controlled study in 91 patients, no significant differences were seen in the active as compared to the placebo group during the initial five-week treatment period[32]. In a double-blind, placebo-controlled study of Hyalgan against 20 mg triamcinolone hexacetonide, similar efficacy for the two agents was seen in the

initial five-week injection period[33]. All these studies tantalizingly suggest a possible long-term effect of the agent, but because of drop-out during the study, statistically this fails to reach significance.

In a observer-blind study of 209 patients using a 600–12 000 kD hyaluronan manufactured by the Seikagaku Corporation, a significant difference between the two groups was demonstrated after five weeks, lasting up to the end of the study at 14 weeks[34]. However, in a double-blind, placebo-controlled study of the same agent in 52 patients with arthroscopic cartilage damage, no significant symptomatic benefit was seen over that of the placebo, even up to one year[35].

In an observer-blind comparison of seven injections of hyaluronic acid (500–730 kD) versus mucopolysaccharide polysulfuric acid ester, the former was more effective in symptom relief[36]. Hylan G-F 20 is a preparation of hyaluronic acid in the form of a gel. Some studies have demonstrated efficacy, but a note of caution has been sounded due to a relatively high incidence of local reactions in clinical use. One study of 22 patients, who received a total of 88 injections into 28 knees, has suggested an incidence of post-injection 'flares' in 27 per cent of patients and 11 per cent of injections[37]. What is not clear is how this compares to other hyaluronic acid preparations, as well as to that occurring after corticosteroids or, indeed, simple needling of a joint.

Overall, the place of hyaluronic acid injections in OA is unclear. The injections are currently expensive and the frequency of the injection protocols, usually 3–5 weekly injections, may make their use unpopular with health purchasers and patients alike.

Orgotein

Orgotein is a preparation of bovine Cu-Zn super-oxide dismutase that has been subject to a number of clinical trials. The rationale of its use is unclear, but it is assumed that the drug will inhibit the phagocytic response to hydroxyapatite crystals and inhibit any hypoxic reperfusion cycle. Notwithstanding the mechanism, symptomatic benefit has been demonstrated. In a 24-week, double-blind, placebo-controlled trial of 45 patients with inflammatory OA of the knee, 12 fortnightly injections of 2 mg orgotein was compared to placebo[38]. Although the precise details of the evaluation may be criticized, a decrease in pain and an increase in function in the orgotein group was observed, compared to placebo. These effects took

8–14 weeks to develop. Six of the 29 patients receiving orgotein experienced a post-injection flare, attributed by the authors to residual endotoxin in the preparation; it may, of course, been due to the effect of joint needling, as discussed above.

In a randomized double-blind comparison of 40 mg methylprednisolone and either 8 mg or 16 mg orgotein, no statistically significant differences were seen between the groups except at 24 weeks, when 16 mg orgotein was more efficacious[14]. Due to the small size of the study, both type I and II statistical errors may be important.

A comparison of three doses of orgotein (8 mg × 3, 16 mg × 2, or 32 mg × 1) with three placebo injections, at weekly intervals, was performed in a double-blind fashion in 139 patients with knee OA[39]. The major outcome measures in this study were that there were more withdrawals due to inefficacy in the placebo group and higher efficacy ratings for all three doses of orgotein, compared to placebo. Convincing differences between the orgotein dosing regimes were not demonstrated.

In another study, 419 patients with knee OA were randomized to receive either 4 mg or 8 mg orgotein or betamethasone[40]. A faster onset of action with the steroid was observed, but after seven weeks efficacy was comparable: there was no difference between the patients receiving different doses of the orgotein. There are a number of important caveats to the study. Firstly, only the dose of orgotein was blinded; patients and physicians were not blinded as to whether the patients received steroid. Secondly, the injection schedule of the orgotein groups was different to that of the steroid groups; one-to-three, compared to single injections. Thus, as with hyaluronic acid, orgotein may be of symptomatic benefit in OA but at the expense of the need for multiple injections. The onset of action may be slower compared to corticosteroids, but the duration of action may be more prolonged. Local adverse effects, especially pruritus and skin eruptions, are not uncommon.

Glycosaminoglycan polysulphate

Glycosaminoglycan polysulphate (GAGPS) is a macromolecule related to heparin which has multiple biochemical actions including inhibition of cartilage degradation, and promotion of proteoglycan and collagen synthesis. Therapeutically, it is normally given intramuscularly, but it may be administered intra-articularly. In a one-year, double-blind, placebo-controlled study comparing GAGPS to saline, no statistically significant benefit of the active agent could be demonstrated[41].

Summary

1. Several intra-articular agents have been used in the treatment of OA but few, as yet, have stood up to the test of randomized double-blind controlled studies.

2. Intra-articular long-acting corticosteroids have, however, been shown to be effective in OA, and with few serious side effects, but their duration of action is short lived.

3. There are no predictors of clinical response except that accuracy of injection is probably important.

References

1. Waugh, W.G. (1938). Treatment of certain joint lesions by injection of lactic acid. *Lancet*, i, 487–9.
2. Crowe, H.W. (1944). Treatment of arthritis with acid potassium phosphate. *Lancet*, i, 563–4.
3. Waugh, W.G. (1945). Mono-articular osteo-arthritis of the hip. *Br Med J*, i, 873–4.
4. Hollander, J.L., Brown, E.M., and Jessar, R.A. (1951). Hydrocortisone and cortisone injected into arthritic joints. *JAMA*, 147, 1629–35.
5. Wright, V., Haslock, D.I., Dowson, D., Seller, P.C., and Reeves, B. (1971). Evaluation of silicone as an artificial lubricant in osteoarthrotic joints. *Br Med J*, 2, 370–3.
6. Miller, J.H., White, J., and Norton, T.H. (1958). The value of intra-articular injections in osteoarthritis of the knee. *J Bone Jt Surg (Br)*, 40-B, 636–43.
7. Wright, V., Chandler, G.N., Monson, R.A.H., and Hartfall, S.J. (1960). Intra-articular therapy in osteoarthritis. *Ann Rheum Dis*, 19, 257–61.
8. Friedman, D.M. and Moore, M.E. (1980). The efficacy of intraarticular steroids in osteoarthritis: a double-blind study. *J Rheumatol*, 7, 850–6.
9. Dieppe, P.A., Sathapatayavongs, B., Jones, H.E., Bacon, P.A., and Ring, E.F.J. (1980). Intra-articular steroids in osteoarthritis. *Rheumatol Rehabil*, 19, 212–17.
10. Valtonen, E.J. (1981). Clinical comparison of triamcinolone hexacetonide and betamethasone in the treatment of osteoarthrosis of the knee joint. *Scan J Rheumatol*, **suppl S41**, 1–7.
11. Gaffney, K., Ledingham, J., and Perry, J.D. (1995). Intra-articular triamcinolone hexacetonide in knee osteoarthritis: factors influencing the clinical response. *Ann Rheum Dis*, 54, 379–81.
12. Sparling, M., Malleson, P., Wood, B., and Petty, R. (1990). Radiographic followup of joints injected with

triamcinolone hexacetonide for the management of childhood arthritis. *Arthritis Rheum*, **33**, 821–6.

13. Clemmesen, S. (1971). Triamcinolone hexacetonide for intraarticular and intramuscular therapy. *Acta Rheum Scand*, **17**, 273–8.

14. Gammer, W. and Brobäck, L-G. (1984). Clinical comparisons of orgotein and methylprednisolone acetate in the treatment of osteoarthrosis of the knee joint. *Scand J Rheumatol*, **13**, 108–12.

15. Pattrick, M. and Doherty, M. (1987). Facial flushing after intra-articular injection of steroid. *Br Med J*, **295**, 1380.

16. Hopper, J.M. and Carter, S.R. (1993). Anaphylaxis after intra-articular injection of bupivicaine and methylprednisolone. *J Bone Jt Surg (Br)*, **75-B**, 505–6.

17. Chandler, G.N. and Wright, V. (1958). Deleterious effect of intra-articular hydrocortisone. *Lancet*, **ii**, 661–3.

18. Flanagan, J., Thomas, T.L., Casale, F.F., and Desai, K.B. (1988). Intra-articular injection for pain relief in patients awaiting hip replacement. *Ann Royal Coll Surg Eng*, **70**, 156–7.

19. Jones, A., Regan, M., Ledingham, J., Pattrick, M., Manhire, A., and Doherty, M. (1993). Importance of placement of intra-articular steroid injections. *Br Med J*, **307**, 1329–30.

20. Kellgren, J.H. (1939). Some painful joint conditions and their relation to osteoarthritis. *Clin Sci*, **4**, 193–201.

21. Sambrook, P.N., Champion, G.D., Browne, C.D., Cairns, D., Cohen, M.L., Day, R.O., *et al.* (1989). Corticosteroid injection for ostreoarthritis of the knee: peripatellar compared to intra-articular route. *Clin Exp Rheumatol*, **7**, 609–13.

22. O'Connor, B.L. and Brandt, K.D. (1992). Neurogenic acceleration of osteoarthrosis. *J Bone Jt Surg (Am)*, **74-A**, 367–76.

23. Gibson, T., Winter, P.J., and Grahame, R. (1973). Radiotherapy in the treatment of osteoarthrosis of the knee. *Rheumatol Rehabil*, **12**, 42–6.

24. Doherty, M. and Dieppe, P.A. (1981). Effect of intra-articular yttrium-90 on chronic pyrophosphate arthropathy of the knee. *Lancet*, **ii**, 1243–6.

25. Creamer, P., Hunt, M., and Dieppe, P. (1995). Pain mechanisms in osteoarthritis of the knee: effect of intra-articular anaesthetic. *Br J Rheumatol*, **34 (suppl 2)**, 45.

26. Høilund-Carlsen, P.F., Meinicke, J., Christiansen, B., Karle, A.K., Stage, P., and Uhrenholdt, A. (1985). Joint distension arthrography for disabling hip pain. *Scand J Rheumatol*, **14**, 179–83.

27. Egsmose, C., Lund, B., and Andersen, R.B. (1984). Hip joint distension in osteoarthrosis. A triple-blind controlled study comparing the effect of intra-articular indoprofen with placebo. *Scand J Rheumatol*, **13**, 238–42.

28. Strachan, R.K., Smith, P., and Gardner, D.L. (1990). Hyaluronate in rheumatology and orthopaedics: is there a role? *Ann Rheum Dis*, **49**, 949–52.

29. Grecomoro, G., Martorana, U., and Di Marco, C. (1987). Intra-articular treatment with sodium hyaluronate in gonarthrosis: a controlled clinical trial versus placebo. *Pharmatherapeutica*, **5**, 137–41.

30. Dixon, A.S.J., Jacoby, R.K., Berry, H., and Hamilton, E.B.D. (1988). Clinical trial of intra-articular injection of sodium hyaluronate in patients with osteoarthritis of the knee. *Curr Med Res Opinion*, **11**, 205–13.

31. Dougados, M., Nguyen, M., Listrat, V., and Amor, B. (1993). High molecular weight sodium hyaluronate (hyalectin) in osteoarthritis of the knee: a 1 year placebo-controlled trial. *Osteoarthritis and Cartilage*, **1**, 97–103.

32. Henderson, E.B., Smith, E.C., Pegley, F., and Blake, D.R. (1994). Intra-articular injections of 750 kD hyaluronan in the treatment of osteoarthritis: a randomised single centre double-blind placebo-controlled trial of 91 patients demonstrating lack of efficacy. *Ann Rheum Dis*, **53**, 529–34.

33. Jones, A.C., Pattrick, M., Doherty, S., and Doherty, M. (1995). Intra-articular hyaluronic acid versus intra-articular triamcinolone hexacetonide in knee osteoarthritis. *Osteoarthritis and Cartilage*, **3**, 269–73.

34. Puhl, W., Bernau, A., Greiling, H., Köpcke, W., Pförringer, W., Steck, K.J., *et al.* (1993). Intra-articular sodium hyaluronate in osteoarthritis of the knee: a multicenter, double-blind study. *Osteoarthritis and Cartilage*, **1**, 233–41.

35. Dahlberg, L., Lohmander, S., and Ryd, L. (1994). Intraarticular injections of hyaluronan in patients with cartilage abnormalities and knee pain. *Arthritis Rheum*, **37**, 521–8.

36. Graf, J., Neusel, E., Schneider, E., and Niethard, F.U. (1993). Intra-articular treatment with hyaluronic acid in osteoarthritis of the knee joint: a controlled clinical trial versus mucopolysaccharide polysulfuric acid ester. *Clin Exp Rheumatol*, **11**, 367–72.

37. Puttick, M.P.E., Wade, J.P., Chalmers, A., Connell, D.G., and Rangno, K.K. (1995). Acute local reactions after intraarticular Hylan for osteoarthritis of the knee. *J Rheumatol*, **22**, 1311–14.

38. Lund-Oleson, K. and Menander-Huber, K.B. (1983). Intra-articular orgotein therapy in osteoarthritis of the knee. *Arzneim Forsch*, **33**, 1199–203.

39. McIlwain, H., Silverfield, J.C., Cheatum, D.E., Poiley, J., Taborn, J., Ignaczak, T. *et al.* (1989). Intra-articular orgotein in osteoarthritis of the knee: a placebo-controlled efficacy, safety, and dosage comparison. *Am J Med*, **87**, 295–300.

40. Mazieres, B., Masquelier, A-M., and Capron, M-H. (1991). A French controlled multicenter study of intraarticular orgotein versus intraarticular corticosteroids in the treatment of knee osteoarthritis: a one-year followup. *J Rheumatol*, **18 (suppl 27)**, 134–7.

41. Pavelka, K., Sedlćková, M., Gatterová, J., Becv!ar, R., and Pavelka, K. (1995). Glycosaminoglycan polysulfuric acid (GAGPS) in osteoarthritis of the knee. *Osteoarthritis and Cartilage*, **3**, 15–23.

9.9 Physical therapy

Janet Cushnaghan and Susan Forster

Introduction

Physical therapy plays an important part in the complete management of osteoarthritis (OA), because it can equip the patient with the knowledge, skills, and attitudes to take control of their own disease and its treatment. There are almost no side effects to physical treatments used, an important consideration as the majority of patients will be in the older age group where the side effects of drug treatment may be considerable. Developments in the physiotherapy profession over the last 50 years have been marked; there are now highly skilled and specialized therapists delivering high quality care to patients with OA. Research into the efficacy of physical therapy is growing steadily and is essential in the present cost conscious health market. Many treatments are still given empirically, without evidence of efficacy, and this situation must be rectified. It has been shown, however, that patients with OA demonstrate an improvement after physiotherapeutic intervention[1].

Assessment

The key to successful therapy is accurate assessment, leading to a problem list and treatment plan, which will include treatment goals for both the therapist and the patient. These goals are usually to control pain and other symptoms, reduce disability, and educate the patient and their carers about the disease and its therapy. Assessment of the patient should reveal the following information:

(1) the stage of the disease;

(2) joints involved;

(3) influence of biomechanical alterations;

(4) pain threshold;

(5) causes of pain, either biomechanical or active inflammation;

(6) lifestyle and aspirations of the patient, and how these are affected by the disease;

(7) understanding by the patient of the condition;

(8) medications they are using;

(9) other medical problems.

Time spent initially on thorough and accurate assessment will result in an appropriate and, ultimately, more successful treatment plan being designed. Assessment tools to measure pain, dysfunction, and disability must be valid, reliable, easy to use, quantifiable, sensitive to change, and useful.

Pain

Although a subjective phenomenon, pain can be measured objectively by a variety of means. It is important to know the nature or type of pain being measured — overall, night, at rest, on use, or pain in a specific joint. The time and duration over which the pain has been present is important, for example, in the last 24 hours, over the last week, or since the patient was last seen. The exact level of pain or the degree of change in pain can be assessed.

Stiffness

Joint stiffness is another symptom of OA requiring assessment. It is usually worse after a period of inactivity such as sitting for a length of time or standing in one position, though early morning stiffness is commonly short lived. Actual measurements of the range of motion at individual joints, using a goniometer, will reveal where problems lie and where treatment is necessary[2]. Evaluation of joint deformities can also be made using a goniometer, for example, the extent of varus or valgus deformity at the knee.

Muscle strength

It is becoming increasingly accepted that muscle strength plays a major role in determining disability in OA. This being the case, it is important to assess the muscle strength of individuals, over various joints, to plan a treatment program that will strengthen the appropriate muscles, leading to improved joint function and, therefore, reduced disability. A variety of methods to measure muscle strength are available (see Chapter 7.6). For the quadriceps, for example, the best of three isometric torque values, obtained on the same occasion, may confidently be used to monitor a disease process, guide physical rehabilitation programs, and help to design and evaluate the efficacy of innovative therapeutic interventions[3].

Joint stability

Biomechanical assessments are gaining popularity and technological advances have been made enabling complex assessment of joints during activities such as ambulation. Gait analysis laboratories are increasing in number but such facilities would not routinely be available to physiotherapists in hospital or community settings. Ligament laxity does occur in OA, leading to instability of joints; measures should be taken to strengthen surrounding musculature in order to compensate for the instability, or a suitable orthosis should be provided to support the unstable joint.

Functional assessment

How OA impacts on a patient will be decided by many factors including age, gender, employment, hobbies, aspirations, and other personal factors. It is important to individualize the goals of treatment and make them relevant to each patient. Assessment also has to be individualized to reveal the limitations of each patient. Many standardized questionnaires exist to assess functional disability and this is part of a more general health status measure in some cases (see Chapter 10).

Therapeutic techniques

General goals to rehabilitate patients with OA are: (1) to increase function; (2) to maintain current function; (3) to prevent dysfunction or preserve normal function. The aims are thus *restoration*, *maintenance*, and *prevention*. These goals are achieved by relieving pain and maintaining muscle strength and range of movement; preservation of energy and provision of supportive measures are also important. Additionally, assistance in coping with a changing condition and functional status is vital. There are many therapeutic modalities that can be employed to achieve both the general and the more specific goals of rehabilitation.

Exercise

The benefits of exercise therapy are beginning to be evaluated. Most attention has been paid to the quadriceps mechanism, but the data may be extrapolated to other muscle groups. Marks[4a], in a case study, reports improvements in quadriceps torque, clinical status, and pain with walking after isometric exercise training. The exercises were carried out three times a week for six weeks, with the knee at an angle of 60°. In a review of quadriceps training[4b], Marks states that despite many studies, there is still no consensus on dosage, mode of administration, or frequency of treatment. There is also a need to establish the reliability, validity, and sensitivity of outcome measures designed to measure functional change in trials of treatment for OA. This information would assist in establishing whether reported significant changes hold clinical significance. Most of the trials reviewed reported an improvement in function and a reduction in pain after quadriceps exercises, but design problems prevented conclusions being made as to whether the exercises are any more effective than rest or placebo for improving function in this population. General exercise programs have also been found to be beneficial in OA. Kovar *et al.*[5] assessed the value of an eight-week supervised fitness walking program in 102 patients with knee OA and found the exercise group improved significantly, compared with the controls.

Biomechanical manoeuvres

Appliances that can alter the biomechanics of a joint may be helpful. Cushnaghan *et al.*[6]. showed that taping the patella medially was effective in reducing knee pain in patients with patellofemoral OA. In a randomized, single-blind, cross-over trial with 14 subjects, medial taping was better than lateral or neutral taping for pain scores, symptom change, and patient preference. McConnell[7] recommends taping followed by quadriceps exercises for the treatment of chondromalacia patellae in young people. Further studies are needed to establish the combination of taping and exercise needed to treat OA, and produce lasting relief of pain and permanent alteration of abnormal biomechanics. Appliances such as medial or lateral wedged insoles can be fitted to the shoe to alter varus or valgus deformities at the knee joint and, thereby, reduce pain[8]. Knee bracing may be necessary for painful, unstable joints, but unfortunately may promote atrophy of the quadriceps.

Assistive devices

Mobility is one of the most important goals for patients with OA. Walking aids can unload affected joints, resulting in less pain, improved balance, and greater confidence for the user in a crowded situation. A walking aid should be used in the opposite hand to the joint affected to enable an even gait pattern and maintain good posture. Aids include a simple walking stick, a stick with a moulded handle for those with hand problems, elbow crutches, and walking frames.

Education

Patient education can improve knowledge, skills, and attitudes; armed with information, patients can take control of their disease and use self-help techniques to manage their symptoms. Improved coping skills will reduce the need for patients to consult with their physician or physiotherapist. It has been shown that regular telephone contact results in improvements in pain and functional status, and is cost effective[9]. (See Chapter 9.12).

Hydrotherapy

The use of hydrotherapy can assist the therapist to achieve the goals of rehabilitation; physiological effects can be summarized as:

- rise in body temperature
- increased sweating
- superficial vasodilatation
- increase in peripheral circulation
- heart and respiratory rates increased
- fall in blood pressure after immersion
- increased metabolism
- sedative effect on sensory nerve endings
- muscle relaxation
- fatigue.

The pool can be used to induce muscle relaxation and, thereby, assist in the mobilization of joints. The buoyancy of the water helps to assist or resist muscle work and enable partial weight bearing exercises to be performed. Pain may be relieved due to the temperature of the water and the muscle relaxation achieved; water temperature should be 34–37 °C, with the pool area kept at 23–24 °C. Contraindications to hydrotherapy are skin infections or lesions, cardiovascular disorders, and respiratory distress[10]. One study of hydrotherapy and home exercises, compared to home exercises alone, in OA of the hip, found no significant difference between the two groups. The authors do, however, state that compliance with the exercise regime was high due to frequent follow-up, and diary cards being monitored closely[11].

Electrical and physical measures

There are numerous electrical and physical modalities which can be used to achieve the goals of rehabilitation. Table 9.5 gives an overview of equipment using electromagnetic or mechanical energy. The most widely owned and frequently used electrotherapeutic modalities in the UK are ultrasound, pulsed short-wave diathermy, and interferential; transcutaneous electrical neuromuscular stimulation (TENS) and flowtron show high use[12]. There is a general trend to athermal techniques[13], though this change in emphasis is not necessarily reflected in studies abroad[14,15].

Table 9.5   Therapeutic energy forms

	Electromagnetic energy
Radio frequency	
Very low frequency < 30 kHz	Faradism: 30–100 Hz, pulse duration 0.1–1 ms
	TENS: 50–100 Hz, pulse duration 0–0.5 ms
	Interferential: 4 kHz continuous. Two interfering signals, 10–130 Hz resultant
High frequency 3–30 MHz	SWD: 27.12 MHz continuous
	PSWD: 27.12 MHz, pulse duration 25–400 μs, PRF 15–800/s
Very high frequency 30–300 MHz	None
Ultra high frequency 300–3000 MHz	Microwave: 433.9, 915, 2450 MHz continuous
Infra red	Infra red lamp
Light	
Laser	915–660 nM
	Mechanical energy
Ultrasound	0.5–5 MHz, continuous or pulsed with variable duty cycle

TENS = Transcutaneous electrical nerve stimulations; SWD = Short wave diathermy; PSWD = Pulsed short wave diathermy; PRF = Pulsed repetition frequency.

Heat

Most tissues demonstrate a therapeutic response to heat at temperatures of 41–45 °C[16]. Heat can be applied superficially, transferred to the skin by conduction, radiation, or deep heating (where one form of energy, for example, electromagnetic or mechanical, is converted to heat in the tissue). It is worth noting that even superficially applied heat increases the intraarticular temperature[17]. Before any therapeutic heat is used, thermal sensation of the subject must be checked to safeguard against tissue injury.

The therapeutic effects of heating include reduction of pain and muscle spasm, acceleration of healing, and increased range of joint movement. Pain relieving effects are thought to be achieved by afferent nerve stimulation, possibly having an analgesic effect by acting on the pain gate control mechanism, with the resulting increased blood flow 'washing out' some pain-provoking metabolites resulting from tissue injury[18]. A reduction in muscle spasm is a secondary effect of pain reduction. Heating the secondary afferent muscle spindle nerve endings and golgi tendon endings could lead to this muscle spasm reduction[19]. Physiologically, heating collagen tissue increases its extensibility[20], but this only occurs with simultaneous stretching and near the maximum therapeutically acceptable range of 40–45 °C. This effect, along with heat-induced pain relief, and the reduction in tissue viscosity leading to a reduction in joint stiffness[21], all contribute to an improved range of joint motion.

Heat should not be regarded as a complete treatment but as a precursor to another regimen, for example, exercise, mobilization, or traction. Indeed, the use of heat should be used with caution as joint damage *may* be enhanced[22].

Superficial heating

The benefit of superficial heating (temperature application 40–44 °C) is that it can be carried out, after careful instruction, by the patient at home using a towel-wrapped hot water bottle, gel-filled (hydrocollator) hot pack, or thermostatically controlled electric heated pad. Other methods of applying superficial heat include paraffin wax baths, infra red radiation, and hydrotherapy.

Paraffin wax baths are generally used for hands, wrists, feet, and ankles. A 2–3 mm coating of wax is built up by immersing the area into molten wax, six to twelve times. The body part is then wrapped in plastic and a towel to retain the heat, for 15 minutes, until the wax solidifies sufficiently to remove but remains adequately malleable for exercising the treated part.

Hydrocollator packs are traditionally filled with 'Fullers earth', though gel-filled packs are now available. The packs are heated in hot water to 75–80 °C, wrapped in four to eight layers of towel, and applied to the area to be treated. This increases the skin temperature to the therapeutically acceptable 40–44 °C.

Deep heat

The three modalities used to create deep heat are shortwave diathermy, continuous therapeutic ultrasound, and microwave.

Shortwave diathermy (SWD) is an electromagnetic radiation of 27.12 MHz frequency and 11.062 M wavelength. The field is delivered via two electrodes or an inductothermy cable for approximately 20 minutes. Therapeutic effects are considered to be related to the increase in skin, intramuscular, and intraarticular temperature, increasing blood flow and pain threshold. The pain threshold appears to return to normal after 15–30 minutes of cessation of treatment[23].

Patients with OA treated with continuous SWD, in combination with exercise, may demonstrate significant pain relief[24] and improvement in the overall clinical condition[25]. However, although historically a popular modality in the treatment of OA, careful thought should be exercised before use. SWD may exacerbate the condition, possibly due to heat-induced proliferation of collagenous tissue and the development of adhesions, leading to limitation of movement[26]. SWD may also encourage enzymatic reactions within damaged joints, leading to cartilage breakdown[22]. Possibly a low thermal dose would be an acceptable option if SWD is selected as a form of pre-exercise heating.

Pulsed shortwave diathermy (PSWD) was first introduced in the early 1950s and has become popular over the last 20 years. It is the application of pulsed modulated electromagnetic energy. A 27.12 MHz carrier is amplitude modulated with pulse lengths of 25–400 μs, with a repetition frequency of 15–800 per second[27]. It is postulated that the alternating field excites the speed of phagocytic and enzymatic activity, and transport across membranes is increased[28]; it may also alter cell membrane potential, repolarising damaged cell membranes[29].

A recent concept is 'frequency windows' or 'amplitude windows', whereby a cellular activity is provoked or enhanced by absorbed energy at a particular narrow range of frequencies or amplitudes[30,31]. There is some controversy regarding PSWD and its heating effect; though it seems that the term 'athermic' is inappropriate, the heating being below the subjective detectable threshold[32].

PSWD has been demonstrated to improve pain, functional performance, and joint tenderness[33,34]. It may be more effective than SWD in chronic conditions[35] and, given that heat from continuous SWD may be damaging to an OA joint, PSWD could be a more effective modality due to the exciting effect of an alternating field, rather than the heating effect. For the greatest pain relief, a pulse width of 65 μs and a 200–300 pulse repetition rate for 20 minutes has been suggested[29]. Latest clinical evidence suggests chronic conditions appear to require a mean power of more than 5W to achieve a reasonable tissue response.

Studies in PSWD and OA are sparse and call for further clinical investigation[36]. Of the studies carried out, they usually include an exercise element, making it difficult to establish which part of the treatment is effective.

Therapeutic ultrasound (TUS) has been used therapeutically for over 40 years. TUS is a 0.5–5 MHz mechanical vibration generated by a transducer supplied by an electronic circuit converting electrical energy into mechanical energy. The therapeutic mechanisms of TUS are both thermal and mechanical. Ultrasound is absorbed and creates heat in structures with a high protein content. The heat is dissipated rapidly in vascular tissue such as muscle, creating only a small temperature rise. However, less vascular, dense connective tissue for example, tendons and ligaments, may experience greater temperature increase[27]. The physiological effects of local tissue heating, discussed above, include temporary extensibility of fibrous tissue structures, increase in pain threshold, reduction of muscle spasm, and promotion of the healing process.

The mechanical or non-thermal effects include 'microstreaming' — small fluid movements around cells which may affect cell membrane permeability, promote collagen synthesis, and alter electrical activity in nerves involved in pain relief[37]. The absorption of TUS by nociceptive fibers may also block pain transmission[38]. TUS is administered as continuous or pulsed — continuous TUS has both thermal and mechanical effects; with pulsed TUS, the mechanical effects dominate, as there is time for the heat created by each ultrasound pulse to be dissipated.

TUS is used in the management of OA for pain relief, reduction in muscle spasm, and improved extensibility of fibrous tissue, prior to an exercise regimen aimed to improve range of joint movement and functional ability. Again, there is little documented evidence of the effectiveness of TUS, leaving uncertainty as to the most effective dosage for this condition. With the poor calibration demonstrated in some ultrasound machines[39], even with a documented treatment protocol, ineffective doses could be administered. However, TUS is a non-invasive technique that is quick and easy to administer.

Microwave is used rarely now[12]. This reflects the trend to athermal techniques, but also in the last 20 years there has been concern as to its safety. Microwave is an electromagnetic radiation. Therapeutically in the UK three frequencies are used — 2450, 915, and 433.9 MHz. Doses are given for approximately 20 minutes, usually with the patient setting the intensity at the level of heat required.

The main therapeutic benefits are thought to be from the heat created. However, low dose or pulsed treatments, giving barely or imperceptible heating, are not necessarily ineffective. Unlike SWD, where heat can be created in deep tissue, microwave heats the superficial tissue and is, therefore, only used in treating superficial muscle and joints, for example, anterior knee pain.

Cold therapy

This is another popular treatment that can be easily self-administered at home, promoting a self-management regimen for coping with OA. As with therapeutic heat, skin sensation must be tested before cold application. Methods of application include:-

(1) *cold pack*, consisting of a damp towelling bag filled with ice chips, gel hydropack, or simple bag of frozen peas, separated from the skin by layers of towel to prevent burning, and applied for 10–20 minutes;

(2) *cold immersion* of a limb into ice water for one minute repeated periods;

(3) *ice cube massage*, applied for 5–10 minutes;

(4) *evaporating sprays* of volatile fluids.

Cold application reduces tissue metabolic rate, peripheral nerve conduction velocity, synapse transmission, and blood flow, due to vasoconstriction and increased blood viscosity. However, cutaneously, the vasoconstriction alters to vasodilatation after a few minutes, and then oscillates between the two states.

Cold therapy is used before exercise in the treatment of OA to reduce pain and muscle spasm, and to assist in muscle strengthening. Pain reduction is due to reduced conduction velocity of peripheral nerves, notably A delta fibers, reduced synaptic transmission and, possibly, by effects on the pain gate mechanism. Ice therapy has been shown to improve pain and joint stiffness in OA[40], and there is evidence that the pain relief lasts longer than the application period[41]. Muscle spasm reduction is enhanced by the pain relief. Probably most interesting is the improved muscle strength after short periods of cryotherapy, which is also retained for longer than the application time[42].

Interferential therapy

Interferential therapy (IF) was first introduced in the early 1950s. Two medium frequency (approximately 4 kHz) alternating currents, which differ slightly in frequency, are passed through tissue. The resultant low frequency, therapeutic current, whose frequency is the difference between the two original frequencies, is used. In treating OA, the current is applied via two- or four-plate electrodes, using damp 'spontex' or lint to make effective contact with the skin, or electrodes held within suction cups. The intensity of the current creates a prickling sensation but is just short of a muscle contraction. It is applied for 10–20 minutes, for up to 12 treatments, preferably daily, but no less than twice a week.

It has been shown to produce significant reduction in pain intensity during treatment, but does not affect pain threshold[43]. Different frequencies are thought to activate different pain relieving mechanisms: 90–150 Hz triggers the pain gate mechanism with some speculation that specifically 130 Hz is the optimum; it is thought that over 50 Hz temporarily blocks finely or non-myelinated nociceptive fibres; and a low 10–25 Hz activates A delta and C fibers, thereby releasing encephalin and endorphin. Lower frequencies of 1–5 Hz can be used to activate the opioid mechanism. Finally, fluid movements created by mild muscle contractions assist removal of chemical irritants affecting pain nerve endings[27].

For the treatment of OA hip, four electrodes are 'cross fired' and seven minutes of a constant sedative frequency of 100 or 130 Hz, followed by seven minutes of 10–100 Hz sweep, are recommended. The same frequencies can be used for spondylosis, but for 10 minutes on each. For OA knee, two or four electrodes can be used and set on a sedative dose for 15 minutes[44].

Transcutaneous electrical neuromuscular stimulation

Transcutaneous electrical nerve stimulation (TENS) is a battery driven, short pulse width (50–250 μs), low frequency (2–150 Hz) therapy used specifically for pain relief. The intensity, like IF, should give a mild prickling sensation and not be painful or produce a muscle contraction. Different size carbon-rubber electrodes are used, with a coupling gel for good contact; self-adhesive electrodes are also available. The recommendations on duration of use vary from 30–60 minutes, once to twice daily[45], to continuous use for 8–24 hours[46]. TENS can be delivered in three modes — conventional, burst, and acupuncture-like. It is possible to utilize both the pain gate and opioid mechanisms by setting the frequency at 130 Hz and using the 'burst' mode at 2–5 per second. Its popularity can be partly attributed to the fact that it can be self-administered at home, as part of a self-management program. It is relatively inexpensive, non-invasive, and portable.

Pain relief mechanisms of TENS are much the same as those of IF. Active TENS produces a significant increase in pain threshold, but not in pain intensity[43]. It has been demonstrated to assist in improving pain, joint stiffness, and range of movement in treatment of OA knees, with a significant, lasting reduction in joint stiffness after treatment[47]. Pain relief is also shown to extend beyond the treatment period[48].

For the treatment of OA, no set protocol has been established. Perhaps no ideal settings have been defined because, as some researchers believe, individual patient preference for TENS pulse parameters maximize the analgesic effects of TENS[49].

Faradism

This is a low frequency (30–100 Hz), short duration (0.1–1 ms) muscle stimulating electrical current. Pulses with a slow rise time are applied via two metal electrodes, separated from the skin by layers of damp lint. One electrode is generally sited over the nerve trunk supplying the group of muscle to be treated, and the other is placed over the motor point of the muscle to be stimulated.

Among the physiological effects of faradism are the stimulation of sensory and motor nerves, facilitating a muscle contraction. In the management of OA, it is this effect that is utilised to re-educate a muscle action. It is not proposed as an alternative to active exercise[50], but to initiate a muscle contraction in a wasted muscle or when a voluntary contraction is inhibited due to pain[51]. The patient contracts the muscle along with the electrical stimulation. Studies have shown an average gain in muscle strength due to electrical stimulation, over a one-month period, to be 20 per cent with, interestingly, an increase in muscle strength on the untreated contralateral muscles[52].

Laser

This is a relative newcomer to the physiotherapy armamentarium. Laser is an acronym for light amplification by stimulated emission of radiation. The equipment produces a coherent, essentially parallel, beam of light at a fixed frequency. Most apparatus generate light at 630–1300 nM wavelength, mean power of 1–100 mW; applications are measured in Joules/cm^2, that is energy density. Therapeutically, a 1–500 mW intensity laser is used for tissue healing and pain control. It is applied by a single head 'wand' probe with a beam of 1–7 mm width, or a multi-head cluster probe consisting of a number of laser diodes producing different wavelengths of energy. The treatment head is held in firm contact with the area to be treated. Protective eye goggles must be worn by everyone present. Short treatment times are used, as the radiation is focused and a large amount of energy is delivered to a small region with each application. Output can be pulsed or continuous.

OA has been found to benefit from laser therapy[53]. However, no specific dosages are established for OA treatment; an energy density of 12 J cm^2, twice weekly, is suggested for chronic musculoskeletal pain. This differs from the suggestion of a therapeutic 'window' for laser dosage of 0.5–4 J cm^{2,54}.

Summary

In conclusion, in managing OA, electrotherapy and other physical techniques appear to have their place, but primarily as a precursor to exercise for pain relief, reduction in muscle spasm, increase of muscle strength, and extensibility of fibrous tissue structures — all of which lead to improved joint mobility and restoration of function. It would be naïve not to mention the placebo effect of these physical modalities. However, it is also recognized that physical measures assist in pain relief in OA. The modalities may continue to be used to complement the manual skills of the therapists, and as part of a self-care package in the management of OA, along with exercise regimens and joint protection advice.

References

1. Dobson, C. (1995). A study of the quality and effectiveness of the treatment of knee conditions. *Physiotherapy*, **81**, 217–21.

2. Wright, V. (1979). Conference on measurement of joint movement. *Rheumatol Rehabil*, **18**, 261.

3. Oldham, J.A. and Howe, T.E. (1995). Reliability of isometric quadriceps muscle strength testing in young subjects and elderly osteo-arthritic subjects. *Physiotherapy*, **81**(7), 399–404.

4a. Marks, R. (1993). Quadriceps strength training for osteoarthritis of the knee: a literature review and analysis. *Physiotherapy*, **79**(1), 13–18.

4b. Marks, R. (1993). The effect of isometric quadriceps strength training in mid-range for osteoarthritis of the knee. *Arth Care Res*, **6**(1), 52–6.

5. Kovar, P.A., Allegrante, J.P., MacKenzie, C.R., Peterson, M.G.E., Gutin, B., and Charlson, M.E. (1992). Supervised fitness walking in patients with osteoarthritis of the knee: A randomized, controlled trial. *Ann Intern Med*, **116**, 529–33.

6. Cushnaghan, J., McCarthy, C., and Dieppe, P. (1994). Taping the patella medially: a new treatment for osteoarthritis of the knee joint? *Brit Med J*, **308**, 753–5.

7. McConnell, J.S. (1986). The management of chondromalacia patellae: a long term solution. *Austr J Physiotherapy*, **32**, 215–23.

8. Sasaki, T. and Yasuda, K. (1987). Clinical evaluation of the treatment of the osteoarthritic knee with a wedged insole. *Clin Orthop Rel Research*, **221**, 181–7.

9. Weinberger, M., Tierney, W.M., Booher, P., and Katz, B.P. (1989). Can the provision of information to patients with osteoarthritis improve functional status? A randomized, controlled trial. *Arth Rheum*, **32**, 1577–83.

10. Lee, J.M. (1978). *Aids to physiotherapy* (ed. J.M. Lee), pp. 12–13. Churchill Livingstone, Edinburgh.

11. Green, J., McKenna, F., Redfern, E.J., and Chamberlain, M.A. (1993). Home exercises are as effective as outpatient hydrotherapy for osteoarthritis of the hip. *Brit J Rheum*, **32**(9), 812–15.

12. Pope, G.D., Mockett, S.P., and Wright, J.P. (1995). A survey of electrotherapeutic modalities, ownership and use in the N.H.S. in England. *Physiotherapy*, **81**, 82–91.

13. ter Haar, G., Dyson, M., and Oakley, S. (1987). The use of ultrasound by physiotherapists in Britain. *Ultrasound in Medicine and Biology*, **13**, 659–64.

14. Lindsey, D., Dearness, J., Richardson, C., Chapman, A., and Cuskelly, G. (1990). A survey of electromodality usage in private physiotherapy practices. *Austr J Physiotherapy*, **36**, 249–56.

15. Lambrechtsen, J., Sorensen, H.G., Frankeld, S., and Raismussen, G. (1992). Use of thermotherapy, ultrasound and laser by practising physiotherapists: physiotherapists choice of treatment. *Ugeskrift for Laeger*, **154**(21), 1478–81.

16. Delpizzo, V. and Joyner, K.H. (1987). On the safe use of microwave and shortwave diathermy units. *Austr J Physiotherapy*, **33**(3), 157–61.

17. Oosterveld, F.G., Rasker, J.J., Jacobs, J.W., and Overmars, H.J. (1992). The effect of local heat and cold therapy on the intraarticular and skin surface temperature of the knee. *Arth Rheum*, **35**(2), 146–51.

18. Wadsworth, H. and Chanmugan, A.P.P. (1980). In *Electrophysical agents in physiotherapy*. Cited in: *Electrotherapy explained, principles and practice*. Eds. Low, J.L., Reed, A. (1995). Butterworth Heinemann, Oxford.

19. Lehmann, J.F. and de Lateur, B.J. (1982). Therapeutic heat. In *Therapeutic heat and cold* (ed. J.F. Lehmann), pp. 404–562. Williams and Wilkins, Baltimore.

20. Lehmann, J.F., Mascock, A.J., Warren, C.G., *et al.* (1970). Effect of therapeutic temperatures on tendon extensibility. *Arch Phys Med Rehab*, **51**, 481–7.

21. Wright, V. and Johns, R.J. (1961). Quantitative and qualitative analysis of joint stiffness in normal subjects and in patients with connective tissue disease. *Ann Rheum Dis*, **20**, 36–46.

22. Van Laranta, H. (1982). Shortwave diathermy effects on 35-S-sulphate uptake and glycosamine concentration in rabbit knee tissue. *Arch Phys Med Rehab*, **63**, 25–8.

23. Benson, T.B. and Copp, E.P. (1974). The effect of therapeutic foms of heat and ice on the pain threshold of the normal shoulder. *Rheumatol Rehabil*, **13**, 101–4.

24. Sylvester, K.L. (1990). Investigation of the effect of hydrotherapy in the treatment of osteoarthritic hips. *Clinical Rehabil*, **4**, 223–8.

25. Quirk, A., Newman, R., and Newman, K. (1985). An evaluation of interferential therapy, shortwave diathermy and exercise in the treatment of osteoarthrosis of the knee. *Physiotherapy*, **71**(2), 55–7.

26. Van Laranta, H. (1982). Effect of shortwave diathermy on mobility and radiological stage of the knee in the development of experimental osteo-arthritis. *Am J Phys Med*, **61**(2), 59–65.

27. Kitchen, S., Partridge, C. (1992). Review of shortwave diathermy continuous and pulsed patterns. Physiotherapy, **78**(4), 243–52.

28. Evans, A. (1980). The healing process at cellular level: a review. *Physiotherapy*, **66**, 256–8.

29. Hayne, C.R. (1984). Pulsed high frequency energy — its place in physiotherapy. *Physiotherapy*, **70**(12), 459–66.

30. Tsong, T.Y. (1989). Deciphering the language of cells. *Trends Biol Sci*, **14**, 92.

31. Charman, R.A. (1990). Exogenous currents and fields — experimental and clinical application. *Physiotherapy*, **76**(12), 743–50.

32. Low, J. (1995). Dosage of some pulsed shortwave clinical trials. *Physiotherapy*, **81**(10), 611–16.

33. Trock, D.H., Bollet, A.J., Dyer, R.H. Jr, Fielding, L.P., Miner, W.K., and Markoll, K. (1993). A double blind

trial of the clinical effects of pulsed electromagnetic fields in osteoarthritis. *J Rheumatol*, 20(3), 456–60.

34. Trock, D.H., Bollet, A.J., and Markoll, R. (1994). The effects of pulsed electromagnetic fields in the treatment of osteoarthritis of the knee and cervical spine: report of randomized, double blind, placebo trials. *J Rheumatol*, 21(10), 1903–11.

35. Wagstaff, P., Wagstaff, S., and Downey, M. (1986). A pilot study to compare the efficacy of continuous and pulsed magnetic energy (shortwave diathermy) on the relief of low back pain. *Physiotherapy*, 72, 563–6.

36. Puett, D.W. and Griffin, M.R. (1994). Published trials of nonmedicinal and noninvasive therapies for hip and knee osteoarthritis. *Ann Intern Med*, 121(2), 133–40.

37. Dyson, M. (1987). Mechanisms involved in therapeutic ultrasound. *Physiotherapy*, 73, 116–20.

38. Mardiman, S., Wessel, J., and Fisher, B. (1995). The effects of ultrasound on the mechanical pain threshold of healthy subjects. *Physiotherapy*, 81(12), 718–23.

39. Pye, S. (1996). Ultrasound therapy equipment: does it perform? *Physiotherapy*, 82(1), 39–44.

40. Clarke, G.R., Willis, L.A., Stenner, L., and Nichols, P.J. (1974). Evaluation of physiotherapy in the treatment of osteoarthritis of the knee. *Rheumatol Rehabil*, 13, 190.

41. Lee, J., Warren, M., and Mason, S. (1978). Effects of ice on nerve conduction velocity. *Physiotherapy*, 64, 2–6.

42. Rajadhyaksha, V., Dastoor, D., and Shahani, M. (1982). Influence of cooling of anterior aspect of thigh on maximal isometric tension of quadriceps muscle. In *Proceedings of the IXth International Congress of World Confederation for Physical Therapy*, pp. 494–8. Stockholm,

43. Salisbury, L. and Johnson, M. (1995). The analgesic effects of interferential therapy compared with TENS on experimental cold induced pain in normal subjects. *Physiotherapy*, 81(12), 741.

44. Savage, B. (1984). *Interferential therapy*, pp. 78–80. Faber and Faber, London.

45. Klein, J. and Pariser, D. (1987). Transcutaneous electrical nerve stimulation. In *Clinical electrotherapy* (ed. R. Nelson and P. Curner), pp. 209–30. Appleton and Lange, Norwalk, Conneticut.

46. Frampton, V. (1988). Transcutaneous electrical nerve stimulation and chronic pain. In *Pain: management and control in physiotherapy* (ed. P. Wells, V. Frampton, and D. Bowsher), pp. 89–112. Heinemann Medical Books, London.

47. Grimmer, K. (1992). A controlled double blind study comparing the effects of strong burst mode TENS and high rate TENS on painful osteoarthritic knees. *Austr J Physiotherapy*, 38, 49–56.

48. Jensen, H., Zesler, T., and Christensen, T. (1991). Transcutaneous electrical stimulation TNS for painful osteoarthrosis of the knee. *Int J Rehabil Res*, 14, 356–8.

49. Johnson, M.I., Ashton, C.H., and Thompson, J.W. (1991). An in depth study of long term users of transcutaneous electrical stimulation: implications for clinical use of TENS. *Pain*, 44, 221–9.

50. Lloyd, T., DeDomenico, G., Strauss, G.R. *et al.* (1986). A review of the use of the electro-motor stimulation in human muscle. *Aust J Physiotherapy*, 32, 18–30.

51. Eriksson, E. and Haggmark, T. (1979). Comparison of isometric muscle training and electrical stimulation supplementing isometric muscle training in the recovery after major knee ligament surgery. *Am J Sports Med*, 17, 169.

52. Balogun, J.A., Onilari, O.O., Akeju, O.A., and Marzouk, D.K. (1993). High voltage electrical stimulation in the augmentation of muscle strength: effects of pulse frequency. *Arch Phys Med Rehab*, 74, 910–16.

53. Seitz, L.M. and Kleinkort, J.A. (1986). Low power laser: its application in physical therapy. In *Thermal agents in rehabilitation*, (ed. S.L. Michlovitz), pp. 217–37. F.A. Davies, Philadelphia.

54. Laakso, L., Richardson, C., and Cramond, T. (1993). Factors affecting low level laser therapy. *Austr J Physiotherapy*, 39, 95–9.

9.10   The role of occupational therapy

Rebecca Barton and Judy Feinberg

This chapter discusses the role of the occupational therapist in treatment of the patient with osteoarthritis (OA), and specific evaluation and treatment techniques employed by occupational therapists for this population of patients. It is important first, however, to define the role of occupational therapy in management of the general patient population.

General function of the occupational therapist

The occupational therapist is an integral member of the health care team of today. The primary goal of this specialist is to identify, in collaboration with the patient and other team members, those areas of daily tasks of the patient which are impaired or affected by the disease or disability. Daily tasks, which vary depending upon the roles the patient fulfills in life, are referred to as activities of daily living (ADL). They include self-care tasks, home management tasks, work tasks, and avocational activities. Once the impairments in ADL have been identified, the primary goal of the therapist is to improve the ability of the patient to perform the relevant ADL more independently or more effectively. This may be accomplished through use of compensatory strategies or restoration of function.

The occupational therapist is trained to evaluate and assess various components of function, such as range of motion, muscle strength, endurance, coordination, sensation, and psychosocial skills, and to assess how limitations in these areas affect the ability of the patient to perform ADL. Treatment should address the components which have been found to be impaired; treatment techniques may include use of therapeutic exercise or activity to improve mobility and strength, fabrication of splints or other assistive devices to improve function, training to compensate for dysfunction in performance of ADL, or retraining to improve function. For example, the occupational therapist may teach a patient who has OA of the hand to utilize joint protection principles or adaptive equipment in the performance of daily tasks. At the same time, the therapist may work toward rehabilitation of the affected joints through appropriate exercise or activity to improve or restore function.

It is essential for members of the health care team to understand and delineate the roles of each discipline, and for team members to work together to provide comprehensive care. This occurs through frequent communication and coordination of services among team members. It has been found that integrated interdisciplinary 'team care' may be more effective than isolated provision of treatment by specialists in the care of patients with a chronic disease, such as arthritis[1]. An integrated team approach to patient care can improve compliance and patient attitudes, and decrease conflict between treatment goals of various team members[2]. A comprehensive team includes those professionals needed to adequately treat the patient population it must serve. A typical 'arthritis team' might include the physician, nurse, educator, occupational therapist, physical therapist, and social worker, as described by Gross et al.[2].

Patients with OA frequently have difficulty in performance of ADL because of joint pain or stiffness.

In addition, patients and their families often experience difficulty coping emotionally with the pain and functional limitations which result from the disease process. It is the role of the occupational therapist to help the patient cope with the physical and emotional demands of the disease.

Evaluating the patient with OA

The occupational therapist must evaluate the impact of the disease or disability upon the ability of the patient to perform their normal daily activities. A face-to-face interview is a good way to establish rapport with the patient and permits direct communication regarding what the patient perceives as his or her major deficits. Some therapists supplement the interview assessment with a questionnaire which is completed by the patient. Direct observation of skills may be used to validate information obtained through the interview or questionnaire.

Articular involvement

Elucidating sites of current and previous articular involvement will help the therapist and the patient ascertain which areas of function are, or may become, affected. For example, knowing that a patient has shoulder involvement will direct attention to functional activities requiring shoulder mobility (for example, reaching to comb the hair, or to put on a shirt); a person with thumb-base involvement may have difficulty gripping a pen or turning a doorknob; hip involvement may impair the ability of the patient to put on and take off shoes and stockings.

Pain

Visual analogue scales are useful in quantifying the level of joint pain[3]. These are linear scales which range from one extreme to the other; the patient indicates pain intensity somewhere along the scale. One can ask: 'On a scale from 0 to 10, with 10 being the most severe pain you've ever had, and zero being no pain, how would you quantify your pain today (or over the past two days, or the past week)?'

Feinberg and Brandt[4] have suggested the use of the terms mild, moderate, and severe to quantify level of pain. They defined severe pain as pain present at rest, with no joint movement or pressure; moderate pain as pain that is present with minimal exertion or routine movement; and mild pain as pain that occurs only with strenuous exercise or activity. This categorization of pain focuses on the effect of pain on function, rather than on the severity of the pain itself.

In OA, joint pain is seen with joint motion or loading, and diminishes with rest[5]. Many subjects with OA who have significant changes in joint structure, as noted by physical examination or radiography, do not have significant joint pain[6]. Nonetheless, quantification of pain is important to establish a baseline from which improvement or worsening of symptoms can be measured. The level of pain will have implications for assessing the efficacy of pharmacologic therapy and non-pharmacologic interventions, such as splinting or exercise, and measuring the ability of the patient to perform ADL.

Joint stiffness

Stiffness, which is experienced as a feeling of resistance to movement, may involve the whole body or may be isolated to certain joints. It is important to have patients describe their stiffness and document its duration (in minutes or hours). It is also important to ascertain what time of day, or during which activities, stiffness is most prominent, because this may guide therapeutic interventions to assist the patient in completion of ADL tasks. For example, to avoid the onset of stiffness for a patient with hip OA employed in a sedentary job, the occupational therapist may recommend breaks, alternating periods of sitting with periods of activity requiring lower extremity movement.

Endurance, strength, and fatigue

Fatigue is a symptom of many chronic diseases. It is often more apparent in rheumatoid arthritis than in OA, but can be seen in any patient who experiences chronic pain. Many individuals with OA cite fatigue as a factor limiting completion of their normal activities. Activities which produce fatigue should be identified and modified, or eliminated, if possible. For example, if the patient finds that playing 18 holes of golf is tiring, a suggestion might be to reduce the game to nine holes: the activity is modified but not eliminated.

Muscle strength can be reduced by the disuse engendered by joint pain. A manual muscle test can be performed to assess the strength of individual muscles or groups of muscles; the grading scale in Table 9.6 can be used to assess strength objectively[7]. When performing manual muscle testing, care should be taken to avoid exacerbating pain and damaging joints by application of excessive resistance by the therapist. In lieu of formal testing, muscle strength can be assessed as it relates to the ability to complete functional tasks.

To measure isolated strength in the digits and thumb, grip and pinch strength can be assessed. A dynamometer can be used to measure grip strength, and a pinchometer to measure different types of prehensile pinch strength (Fig. 9.4). Lateral pinch strength should be assessed routinely in patients with OA of the first carpometacarpal joint, insofar as many common activities require use of lateral pinch (for example, turning a key in the ignition of a car or the knob on a stove or washing machine). An adapted sphygmomanometer can serve as an alternative to the standard dynamometer for measurement of grip strength, and is less stressful to the hand and wrist[6] (Fig. 9.4). It should be emphasized that measurement of grip and pinch strength in the patient with arthritis reflects not only actual strength, but provides a measure of pain. The more pain that is present, the less likely that the subject will be able to exert maximum force, either with a metered instrument or against manual resistance.

Table 9.6 Manual muscle test grading scale[*]

Grade	Results of evaluation
5 or Normal	Full range of motion (ROM) against gravity, with maximum resistance
4 or Good	Full ROM against gravity, with minimal to moderate resistance
3 or Fair	Full ROM against gravity, with no resistance
2 or Poor	Full ROM in a gravity eliminated plane, with either minimal or no resistance; P- would indicate only partial ROM in a gravity eliminated plane
1 or Trace	No movement noted, however, a muscle contraction is felt
0	No muscular contraction palpable

* From reference 7

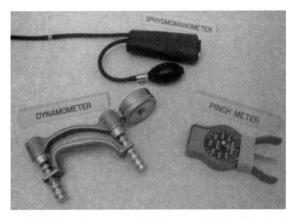

Fig. 9.4 Tools for evaluating grip and pinch strength. (Reprinted from the ARHP Arthritis Teaching Slide Collection. Used with permission of the American College of Rheumatology).

Joint mobility or range of motion

Range of motion can be limited in patients with OA by capsular fibrosis or osteophytes[5]. Therefore, it is important to quantify the mobility of each joint so that a baseline can be established from which improvement or deterioration of function can be documented over time. A goniometer may be used to quantify joint motion.

The therapist should note whether the recorded measurements represent active or passive motion of the joint. In assessing passive movement of a joint, care should be taken not to aggravate joint pain by application of excessive manual force.

Hand function

In evaluating hand function, it is important to assess the ability of the patient to perform tasks which require both prehensile and non-prehensile grip[6]. Prehensile tasks involve pinch or grip of the hand and thumb around, or on to, an object; non-prehensile tasks involve use of the hand in a static manner (for example, tucking in clothing, cleaning a window)[6]. Functional tests may include assessment of gross and fine coordination and sensation. Performance can be scored with respect to the time needed to complete the task, the proportion of the task which can be completed, subjective complaints generated during completion of the task, and the agility or dexterity of hand use during the test[8]. The 'Box and Block' Test[9], the Jebsen–Taylor Hand Function Test[10], and the 'Nine Hole Peg' Test[11] are examples of standardized tests

which may be used in patients with OA to quantify hand function.

Deformities of the hand and wrist

The presence of osteophytes, such as Heberden's nodes at the distal interphalangeal joints (DIP) and Bouchard's nodes at the proximal interphalangeal joints (PIP), should be noted. Although these usually develop slowly, in some patients the onset of nodal OA is acute and accompanied by pain and inflammation which interfere with hand function[5]. Patients with nodal OA may experience tenderness with external pressure on the nodes during certain prehensile activities, such as gripping a pencil.

OA of the first carpometacarpal (CMC) joint can impair hand function during activities requiring grip or lateral pinch (for example, opening a jar, turning a key in a lock). In such cases, the first CMC joint is often tender and has a squared appearance secondary to partial subluxation and osteophyte formation[5].

Primary OA of the wrist or elbow is uncommon. However, patients with OA of the CMC joint may experience pain at the wrist or the elbow as a result of tendinitis or tenosynovitis, caused by an alteration of mechanics as they try to minimize pain during use of the involved joint[6]. The presence of coexisting lateral or medial epicondylitis at the elbow, or DeQuervain's tenosynovitis at the thumb and wrist, should be noted. The assessment should differentiate pain due to arthritis from that due to soft tissue rheumatism.

Activities of daily living

Each area of ADL should be addressed with the patient; deficits should be identified and recorded. It is important to ascertain which tasks the patient is able to complete independently, and in which he or she is limited, partially or completely. The patient with arthritis is often independent in the performance of many tasks but may place excessive mechanical stress on joints during the performance of those tasks. The type of questions that can be asked to ascertain functional ability, joint stress, and the support systems available to assist the patient with task completion include:

1. What can you do?

2. What can you not do?

3. What things are difficult or painful for you to do?

4. Who helps with those activities?

5. How do you feel about them helping?

6. How do you feel about having to have help?

7. What do you want to be able to do that you cannot do now?

These questions can also help the therapist identify areas which the patient has prioritized as being important.

The occupational therapist is trained to analyze how the patient utilizes the joints in self-care tasks, at work, and in other ADL. The spectrum of **self-care tasks** is extensive and includes every aspect of daily self-care chores such as toileting, bathing, dressing, grooming, and self-feeding. **Home management tasks** include the ability to perform various household chores such as cleaning, cooking, and lawn maintenance. In this context, it is important to evaluate architectural barriers within the home. **Work tasks** should be analyzed and the patient should identify areas of deficit or mechanical stress. Assessment of the ability of the patient to perform **avocational tasks or enjoy leisure skills** is also important with respect to maintenance of a balanced lifestyle and psychological well-being.

General functional mobility should be addressed, including the ability to ambulate with or without assistive devices, use a toilet or bathtub, and safely navigate stairs; it is extremely useful to observe the patient performing these tasks. Many standardized ADL evaluations are available, including the Functional Independence Measure[12] and Revised Kenny Self-Care Evaluation[13]. The Rancho Los Amigos Hospital's 'Arthritis Hand Assessment' includes a checklist for observation of various functional tasks[14].

Psychosocial needs

It is important to assess the emotional status of the patient and the support systems available. Family involvement should be noted, including the availability of relatives to assist the patient with areas of impairment; in some cases, the patient may be needed to take care of the family. This, too, should be noted because it represents a component of the ADL tasks of the patient and it may influence compliance with treatment recommendations. Dealing with changing functional ability and the impact of having a chronic disease can be emotionally stressful and may affect how well the patient is able to cope with the disease and the recommended

therapeutic interventions. This area is addressed in more detail in Chapter 9.14.

Treatment considerations

Joint protection and energy conservation

Instruction of patients in adapting their lifestyle and daily activities to the changes imposed by the disease is an important component of treatment for OA[15]. Learning to protect the involved joint by use of joint protection principles is important in reducing joint stress and pain. The occupational therapist is trained in analysis of activity and can teach the patient how to protect the involved joint by changing the ways in which ADLs are performed.

The several principles of joint protection are[15]:

(1) distribute stress evenly over joints;

(2) place stress on larger joints or over surface area that is not a joint;

(3) use joints in their most mechanically effective position;

(4) avoid static positions for extended periods of time;

(5) eliminate excess weight when lifting objects, or completely avoid lifting;

(6) use adaptive equipment as a form of joint protection;

(7) avoid twisting type movements with the hand, wrist, and thumb;

(8) raise seating heights to eliminate stress to lower extremity joints;

(9) avoid repetitive activities.

In general, these principles involve the redistribution of stress from smaller joints to larger joints, utilization of the most mechanically efficient joint to perform stressful movements or tasks, avoidance of positions which will promote deformity, and avoidance of static positions. Specific examples might include use of both hands, rather than one, to lift heavy objects; use of lever-type handles to open doors and to turn faucets, thereby eliminating the need to twist the fingers and wrist; and use of utensils with thick handles to avoid the stressful tight grip needed for standard size imple-

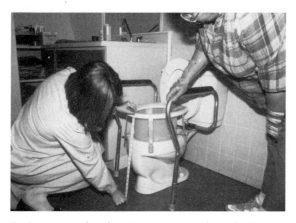

Fig. 9.5 Principles of joint protection: an elevated toilet seat to protect the hip and knee. (Reprinted from the ARHP Arthritis Teaching Slide Collection. Used with permission of the American College of Rheumatology).

ments. These modifications can reduce the stresses placed on the proximal interphalangeal joints, distal interphalangeal joints, and thumb base. Joint protection may be accomplished also by modifying household equipment, such as switching from use of heavy pottery dishes to lighter weight dinnerware. Use of specially designed equipment such as a jar opener, elevated toilet seat, or a long-handled hair brush, may protect hand joints, knees, and shoulder, respectively (Fig. 9.5).

The occupational therapist may need to modify the work site of the patient to reduce stress on the arthritic joint during performance of work tasks. In some cases, it may be desirable for the occupational therapist to visit the job site and make recommendations for appropriate modifications. An example of a simple adaptation for a patient who is a grade school teacher with nodal OA, is the use of an enlarged pen grip to assist in grading papers; a laboratory technician with OA of the first CMC joint may need to wear a thumb support or splint to assist with pipetting.

The patient should be educated with respect to the use of energy conservation techniques. Although fatigue is often not a major problem for patients with OA, learning to balance rest and activity can improve activity tolerance when limited endurance is a problem. The several principles of energy conservation are:

(1) learn to set priorities and do those tasks that are most important or necessary;

(2) distribute tasks over a period of time, instead of trying to complete them in one short period;

(3) take frequent rest periods, several times a day;

(4) sit to work, instead of standing;

(5) utilize relaxation techniques;

(6) balance rest with activity;

(7) continue to lead a balanced lifestyle, taking time for leisure and spiritual enrichment;

(8) work more slowly to save energy, instead of rushing through task performance;

(9) pace yourself;

(10) instead of eliminating activity, do a portion of the activity desired.

The occupational therapist can assist patients in learning how to apply these principles during performance of their daily routines.

Exercise and activity

The occupational therapist can prescribe exercises or therapeutic activities specific for the joints or muscle groups which require treatment. The general goals of exercise are to maintain or gradually increase mobility, flexibility, and strength[16]. It is important to avoid overly aggressive exercise, or excessive resistance or weights, which may increase pain or joint stress. Range of motion exercises should be performed independently by the patient, if possible, to avoid exacerbation of pain from passive force. Use of water as a medium in which to perform exercise is often recommended, because it provides buoyancy and facilitates greater mobility[17]. Aerobic exercise under water can improve cardiovascular conditioning while still protecting the joints. Aerobic exercise, once thought to be contraindicated in patients with arthritis, has been shown to facilitate better outcomes with respect to overall cardiovascular and musculoskeletal function, occupational status, and physical parameters, when performed in conjunction with a range of motion exercises that incorporate use of joint protection principles to decrease joint stress[18–21].

Thermal modalities may be used as an adjunct to exercise. Heat is beneficial in reducing stiffness and preparing the joint for exercise[22]. Principles of exercise and thermal modalities are described in more detail in Chapter 9.9.

Isolated digital flexion and extension, and composite flexion and extension (for example, making a fist) should be emphasized to maintain mobility of metacarpophalangeal (MCP), DIP, and PIP joints. Thumb opposition, flexion, and extension, and radial and palmar abduction, can be achieved via appropriate exercises — this will help to maintain the ability of the patient to pinch and grasp. Exercises for the wrist should encompass flexion, extension, and ulnar and radial deviation and circumduction. The goal is to teach the patient how to regulate his or her exercise program and to recognize signs of mechanical stress resulting from exercise or activity. If joint pain is exacerbated by the exercise regimen, the patient should decrease the number of repetitions or the amount of exercise.

Positioning and splinting

The provision or fabrication of specifically designed splints or positional aids may help decrease pain and joint stress, and improve function[23] (Fig. 9.6). A splint may be fabricated out of a thermoplastic (for example, Orthoplast™) that can be molded by the therapist to fit each patient individually. These materials, which are soft and malleable when heated, become rigid as they cool and assume the shape that is fashioned by the therapist. Many commercially available splints are available, fabricated out of leather, neoprene, or other more flexible materials. Upon request from the physician, the type of splint most appropriate for the symptoms of the patient can be selected by the therapist. Whether it is prefabricated or custom-made, the splint should fit properly; care should be taken to avoid creating pressure points. The patient should be able to apply and remove the splint independently, unless assistance with application and removal is readily available.

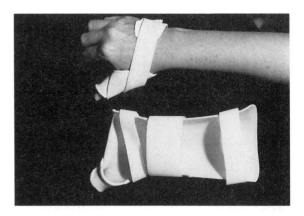

Fig. 9.7 Thumb post splint.

The splint most commonly utilized for hand OA is the thumb post splint (Fig. 9.7) which supports the first CMC and first MCP joints. It is used to stabilize these joints, and reduce pain and joint stress. Because of the support it provides, this splint is also helpful in improving hand function. A longer version, the thumb spica splint, provides support for the wrist, as well as the thumb base, and can be useful if the patient has wrist pain or DeQuervain's tenosynovitis (Fig. 9.8). Individual gutter splints can be molded to support a painful or inflamed interphalangeal joint. The full resting splint, which is more often prescribed for patients with rheumatoid arthritis than OA, supports the entire hand and wrist; it may be useful for the occasional patient with OA who has pain in the hand, wrist, and thumb.

Adaptive equipment

The occupational therapist is trained to design and fabricate adaptive devices to improve the independence of

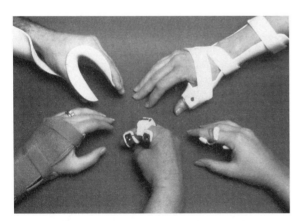

Fig. 9.6 Hand splints. (Reprinted from the ARHP Arthritis Teaching Slide Collection. Used with permission of the American College of Rheumatology).

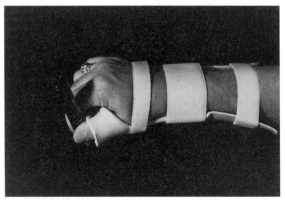

Fig. 9.8 Thumb spica splint.

the patient in the performance of their daily activities, and to instruct patients in the use of such devices. Many of these items are commercially available. The therapist can recommend which items would be most beneficial, based upon the needs of the patient and specific joint involvement. Adaptive equipment for individuals with arthritis serves also as a means of joint protection; because patients may be reluctant to use such equipment, perhaps feeling it connotes a loss of independence, the joint protective aspect of the equipment should be stressed. Only equipment which is necessary should be recommended. Examples of adaptive equipment include long-handled items to assist in performance of self-care tasks requiring reaching or bending (for example, a long-handled sponge for bathing, a reacher or dressing stick to assist with putting on trousers). These are helpful for the patient with shoulder, hip, or knee involvement. Various items of adaptive safety equipment are available for the bathroom, such as elevated toilet seats, bathtub seats, and shower safety rails, all of which should be considered for the individual with lower extremity involvement (Fig. 9.5, Fig. 9.9). Adaptive devices are also available for the individual with hand, wrist, or thumb OA, to assist with turning keys, opening jars, or holding a book or pen. Use of a bookstand will decrease stress to

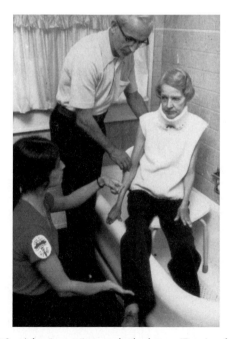

Fig. 9.9 Adaptive equipment: bathtub seat. (Reprinted from the ARHP Arthritis Teaching Slide Collection. Used with permission of the American College of Rheumatology).

the cervical spine; the patient with stiff or painful Heberden's or Bouchard's nodes which interfere with the fine dexterity needed for manipulation of buttons or zippers, can use an adapted button hook and zipper pull, or Velcro™ fasteners, to replace buttons.

The Arthritis Foundation publishes a Self Help Manual which serves as an excellent resource book for the patient with OA (Arthritis Foundation, 1314 Spring St. NW, Atlanta GA 30309).

The role of the occupational therapist in care of the patient who has had joint replacement surgery

The occupational therapist is often involved in the rehabilitation of patients who have recently undergone total knee or hip replacement. The role of the therapist, in the management of these individuals, is to educate them about precautions related to the prosthetic joint and how these precautions apply to their ADL[24]. Adaptive equipment is frequently prescribed in such cases to permit the patient to maintain independence in self-care tasks while complying with these precautions. For example, an elevated toilet seat may be helpful for the patient who has undergone total hip replacement; long-handled sponges for bathing, adapted stocking aids, dressing sticks and reachers can be helpful for patients who have had a hip or knee replacement. The occupational therapist can provide the necessary equipment and educational material, and can teach the patient how to use the prescribed devices and perform requisite daily tasks as independently and safely as possible, with or without the equipment.

The occupational therapist may also be involved with the rehabilitation of individuals after cervical spine surgery for OA. Postoperative patient education should be performed in the same manner as with rehabilitation of patients who have undergone total joint replacement surgery, with instruction in precautions related to ADL performance and provision of equipment, as needed, to improve independence and safety.

After surgical intervention for OA of the hand, wrist, and thumb, treatment by the occupational therapist should focus on control of edema, protective splinting, wound care and scar management, and initiation of appropriate exercise and activity, as indicated by the treatment protocol of the surgeon. Function in the areas of self-care, work tasks, and home maintenance should be evaluated. Instruction should be provided, as needed, to increase independence through use of compensatory techniques, joint protection principles, and adaptive equipment.

Edema control includes instruction of the patient in elevation of the hand and wrist above the level of the heart, use of elastic compressive dressings, and active exercise of those joints in which postoperative movement is permitted[25]. Splints are used to immobilize the surgical site and adjacent joints to promote healing. (The splint designs discussed earlier are also used post-operatively.) The type of splint used depends on the specific surgical procedure performed and the joints requiring immobilization. For example, a thumb spica splint immobilizing the wrist, first CMC, and first MCP joints would be utilized for the patient with OA who underwent surgical fusion of the joints of the thumb base.

Scar management focuses on decreasing the stresses placed on healing tissue; techniques include early active and passive motion (as permitted), scar massage to reduce postsurgical adhesions, and compressive techniques, such as the compressive wraps described above. A scar pad, molded directly over the healed incision and secured with a compressive wrap, may also be utilized to provide continuous, even compression over the scar, thereby assisting with remodeling of the scar[25].

Exercise and activity after surgery is initiated according to the protocol of the surgeon. Selection of specific exercises depends upon the type of surgical procedure performed and the joints involved. Principles of joint protection should be stressed postoperatively in the exercise regimen.

ADL intervention includes retraining the hand and wrist for use during normal activities, and provision of adaptive equipment to assist with ADL performance. This is accomplished during the immediate post-operative immobilization, when the patient needs to learn to compensate for lack of use of the immobilized hand, and, subsequently, in the postoperative rehabilitation period.

References

1. Feinberg, J. and Brandt, K. (1984). Allied health team management of rheumatoid arthritis patients. *Am J Occup Ther*, **38**, 613–20.
2. Gross, M., Brandt, K., Feinberg, J., Korba, E., Rankin, M., and Roche, V. (1982). Team care for patients with chronic rheumatic disease. *J Allied Health*, **11**, 239–47.
3. Huskisson, E.C., Jones, J., and Scot, P.J. (1976). Application of visual analog scales to the measurement of functional capacity. *Rheumatol Rehab*, **15**, 185–7.
4. Feinberg, J. and Brandt, K.D. (1981). Use of resting splints by patients with rheumatoid arthritis. *Am J Occup Ther*, **19**, 285–94.
5. Feinberg, J. and Trombly, C. (1995). Arthritis. In *Occupational therapy for physical dysfunction* (4th edn) (ed. C. Trombly), pp. 815–30. Williams and Wilkins, Baltimore.
6. Melvin, J. (1989). Rheumatic diseases in the adult and child. In *Occupational therapy and rehabilitation* (3rd edn) (ed. J. Melvin), pp. 49–61. F.A. Davis, Philadelphia.
7. Trombly, C. (1995). Evaluation of biomechanical and physiological aspects of motor performance. In *Occupational therapy for physical dysfunction*, (4th edn) (ed. C. Trombly), pp. 73–156. Williams and Wilkins, Baltimore.
8. Apfel, E. (1990). Preliminary development of a standardized hand function test. *J Hand Ther*, **3**, 191–4.
9. Mathiowetz, V., *et al.* (1985). Adult norms for the Box and Block Test of manual dexterity. *Am J Occup Ther*, **39**, 386–91.
10. Jebsen, R.W., *et al.* (1969). An objective and standardized test of hand function. *Arch Phys Med*, **50**, 311–19.
11. Mathiowetz, V., *et al.* (1985). Adult norms for the nine hole peg test of finger dexterity. *Occup Ther J Res*, **5**, 24–38.
12. Uniform Data System for Medical Rehabilitation. Guide for use of the uniform data set for medical rehabilitation. (1993) (Booklet, obtainable from Project Office, Department of Rehabilitation Medicine, State University of New York at Buffalo, Buffalo General Hospital, 100 High St., Buffalo, New York.)
13. Iversen, I.A., Silberberg, N.E., Stever, R.C., and Schoening, H.A. (1973). *The revised Kenny self care evaluation*. Publication No. 722. Sister Kenny Institute Abbott-Northwestern Hospital, Minneapolis.
14. Professional Staff Association of the Rancho Los Amigos Hospital. (1979). *Upper extremity surgeries for patients with arthritis: a pre- and post-operative treatment guide*. Obtainable through Rancho Los Amigos Hospital, Downey CA.
15. Cordery, J. (1965). Joint protection: a responsibility of the occupational therapist. *Am J Occup Ther*, **19**, 285–94.
16. Banwell, B. (1988). Exercise for arthritis. In *Physical therapy management of arthritis*, (ed. B. Banwell and V. Gall), pp. 67–76. Churchill Livingstone, New York.
17. Jetter, J. and Kadlec, N. (1985). *The arthritis book of water exercise*, pp. 8–20. Holt, Rinehart, and Winston, New York.
18. Ekblom, B., *et al.* (1974). Physical performance in patients with rheumatoid arthritis. *Scand J Rheumatol*, **3**, 121–5.
19. Ekblom, B., *et al.* (1985). Effect of short-term physical training on patients with rheumatoid arthritis. *Scand J Rheumatol*, **4**, 80–6.
20. Ekblom, B., *et al.* (1975). Effect of short-term physical training on patients with rheumatoid arthritis. *Scand J Rheumatol*, **4**, 87–91.
21. Nordemar, R. (1981). Physical training in rheumatoid arthritis: a controlled long-term study, II: functional

capacity and general attitudes. *Scand J Rheumatol*, **10**, 25–30.

22. Haralson, K. (1988). Physical modalities. In *physical therapy management of arthritis* (ed. B. Banwell and V. Gall), pp. 77–106. Churchill Livingston, New York.

23. Schultz-Johnson, K. (1992). Splinting: a problem solving approach. In *Concepts in hand rehabilitation* (ed. B. Stanley and S. Tribuzi), pp. 239–71. F.A. Davis, Philadelphia.

24. Daniel, M. and Strickland, L.R. (1992). Surgical conditions. In *Occupational therapy protocol management in adult physical dysfunction*, pp. 139–49. Aspen Publishers, Gaithersburg.

25. Walsh, M. and Muntzer, E. (1992). Wound management. In *Concepts in hand rehabilitation*, (ed. B. Stanley and S. Tribuzi), pp. 152–77. F.A. Davis, Philadelphia.

9.11 Patient education

Kate Lorig

There are several features of osteoarthritis (OA) which set it apart from other health problems. First, it is chronic, often spanning a third or more of the total lifetime of the patient. Second, its major feature, from the point of view of the patient, is pain. Third, medical and surgical interventions are, at best, only partially ameliorative. Finally, both physicians and patients often believe that little can be done for OA. Patients are often told, 'You will have to learn to live with it.' They are seldom taught 'how to live with it.' The operative word, however, is 'learn'. Patient education is an important treatment for all people with OA and, for many, it is the most important intervention.

This chapter will discuss OA patient education from three perspectives: (1) what the patient wants and needs; (2) what is known about the effectiveness of various forms of patient education; (3) how physicians can integrate patient education into clinical practice.

OA perspective of the patient

The usual role of the physician is to diagnose and then, based on scientific knowledge of anatomy, physiology, pharmacology, and so on, suggest a treatment plan. The unique role of the physician is as holder and applier of scientific knowledge.

Many patients, on the other hand, are not particularly interested in scientific knowledge, except as it applies to helping them get on with their lives. For them, a disease is just that: a 'dis — ease' or a disruption. Unfortunately, the patients are often educated as though they were health professionals. They are taught about the physiological causes of their disease and instructed to follow prescribed medical or exercise routines. These instructions sometimes have little to do with the disease as seen by the patient.

In a large qualitative study, Corbin and Strauss[1] interviewed patients with chronic conditions. They identified three major ways in which the lives of patients were disrupted. First, patients had to conform to a new set of medical issues. That is, they had to take medicine, exercise in new ways, visit physicians, and carry out other activities necessitated by their illness. Second, they had to accommodate changes in their life roles. For example, they had to change the patterns of their work, family, social, and recreational lives. Sometimes, these accommodations were small, such as asking for help in opening jars, and, sometimes, very large, such as moving to be closer to relatives.

Finally, people with chronic conditions have an altered and often uncertain future. This realization often causes emotional problems such as depression, frustration, or anger. The findings of Corbin and Strauss have been verified in studies of people with OA. For example, it has been estimated that 20 to 40 per cent of people with arthritis are clinically depressed, and that depression is similar in OA and RA patients[2].

Community samples of OA patients identified pain, activity problems, and depression as their major concerns. When rheumatologists were asked about the concerns of patients, they gave similar responses, but rated them to be less important than did patients[3]. Table 9.7 suggests some ways in which patients and health care providers differ in how they view OA.

Other studies have found that the beliefs of arthritis patients and their physicians differ. For example,

Table 9.7 How views of patients and providers differ

Views of the provider	Views of the patient
— Anatomy and physiology	— Why do I feel bad?
— Behaviors to maintain or improve health	— Behaviors to solve problems
— Facts about disease	— Beliefs about disease
— Skills to perform health behaviors	— Skills to maintain a 'normal' life
— Frustration about non-compliance	— Frustration about living with disease
— Fear of malpractice	— Fear about the future

physicians believe that their patients are much more compliant than they actually are[4]. They also believe that their patients know less about their disease and use non-traditional therapies more than is the reality[3]. A final set of studies has shown that patients find physicians their most credible source of information[5]. Unfortunately, many physicians do not feel that they are effective in educating their patients.

In summary, patients and their physicians have similar, but not concordant, concerns and beliefs. To the extent that concerns and beliefs are similar, communication and education are possible. One of the first rules in establishing good patient/physician communication is for the physician to solicit, and then act on, the concerns of the patient. Specific techniques for doing this are discussed later. Pain and disability are the two greatest concerns of OA patients — concerns that should be addressed by patient education programs. Dekker *et al.* wrote an excellent review of the biobehavioral mechanisms of these symptoms in OA patients[6]. They concluded that 'pain and disability are associated with degeneration of cartilage and bone (articular level) with muscle weakness, limitation in joint motion (kinesiological level), limitation with anxiety coping styles, attention focus on symptoms and possibly depression (psychological level).'

What we know about OA patient education

There are now more than 150 published arthritis patient education studies[7,8]. Of these, approximately 25 per cent involve people with OA. The literature, although limited, suggests that OA patient education can increase the practice of healthy behaviors, improve health status, and decrease health care utilization.

Before discussing specific programs and their outcomes, some definitions are necessary. 'Patient education' is any set of planned educational activities designed to help patients change behaviors, health

status, or health care utilization. While it is true that most patient education programs also alter the knowledge that patients have, this is not the ultimate aim. Changes in knowledge are necessary, but not sufficient, to bring about changes in behaviors or health status; if all that was necessary was having the correct knowledge, there would be few overweight patients and most would exercise appropriately and be compliant with medication taking. In short, good patient education combines the giving of knowledge with skills development, problem solving, and motivational activities.

'Patients' are people with diagnosed disease. When health professionals see these people in a clinical setting, they are patients. Most of the time, however, they are people living in the community who happen to have OA.

'Health status', for the purpose of this chapter, refers to health from the perspective of the patient. For OA, this means disability, pain, depression, and fatigue. Health status does not refer to X-ray findings or joint space. While these physiological states of the disease may relate to patient symptoms, these states by themselves are usually not important to patients.

Two other terms which merit discussion are 'coping' and 'self-management'. These terms are often incorrectly used as synonyms. Coping is the response to a negative stimulus and is usually short-term; self-management, on the other hand, entails a wide range of skills such as planning, problem-solving, and using consultants, and is long-term. Consider, for example, that businesses advertise for managers, not copers. For patients with long-term chronic conditions such as OA, self-management becomes the key ingredient in successful patient education.

Having examined some of the important concepts, we will now turn to what is known about OA patient education. Many of the studies have focused on determining the effectiveness of a specific therapy modality such as weight management, cognitive pain management, or exercise. Templeton *et al.*[9] held a 17-week group intervention focusing on weight loss; the eight participants reached their expectations for weight loss (5–20 pounds). While it is widely accepted that excess weight is a risk factor in OA, this small study is the only example the author has found of OA patient education aimed at weight loss.

Relaxation or cognitive pain management is widely thought to be helpful for people with arthritis. One of the most popular cognitive techniques is progressive muscle relaxation, which teaches patients to tense and relax muscles in a systematic manner[10]. Other cognitive techniques include visualization or guided day dreams, distraction or thinking of something other than pain, and various forms of meditation. For a short overview of cognitive pain management techniques see *The arthritis helpbook*[11]. While there have been a number of studies evaluating these modalities with non-OA patients, there have been few parallel studies focusing on OA. Investigators have demonstrated that cognitive pain management techniques are useful in decreasing pain, and, sometimes, depression, for RA and fibro-myalgia patients[12,13,14,15,16,17]. The results of studies using relaxation with OA patients have been somewhat mixed. Laborde and Powers randomized 160 people with OA into five groups[18]. Group one received an informational brochure, group two received instructions in joint protection, group three received relaxation training plus the brochure, group four received all three interventions, and group five received no interventions. Subjects receiving relaxation training (when compared to controls) demonstrated significant reduction in pain ($p < 0.05$).

In a study of 222 hip and knee surgery patients (73 per cent OA), Daltroy *et al.* used four interventions: informational classes, Benson's relaxation training, both of these interventions combined, and no intervention. They found no main effects for length of hospital stay, postoperative pain, anxiety, or medication usage[19].

Calfas *et al.* studied 40 OA patients[20]. The intervention subjects were taught cognitive pain management techniques, while control subjects received lectures from health professionals. As in the Daltroy study, there were no main effects, although both groups demonstrated decreases in depression and improvements in physical functioning.

Several conclusions can be drawn from these few studies. First, for some OA patients, cognitive pain management techniques may be useful. However, when used as the only behavioral modality, or when combined only with didactic material, these techniques do not appear to be very powerful. The work of Bill-Harvey *et al.* suggests one reason for this lack of response. They found that in a program which taught several behaviors — use of assistive devices, relaxation, and exercise — only 3 per cent of the population continued relaxation exercises[21]. While this percentage is probably low, it does point out that cognitive techniques are usually new to patients; like all other new behaviors, these techniques need practising before effects can occur. If used, emphasis should be placed on long-term practice.

Another behavior taught in most arthritis patient education programs is exercise. In the past, it was believed that arthritis patients needed to be careful when exercising; the fear was that they would 'wear out their joints'. In the past dozen years, we have learned the importance of a full conditioning program for people with OA. Minor *et al.* have conducted a series of important studies on this subject. Twenty-four OA and RA patients were randomized to a physical conditioning program including aerobic exercise (walking or swimming) or a range of motion exercise program. The aerobic group, as compared to the range of motion group, demonstrated improvements in walking time, morning stiffness, pain, and grip strength[22].

In a second study by Minor *et al.*, 40 RA and 80 OA patients were randomized to an aerobic walking group program, a group aerobic aquatic program, or a range of motion group. The aerobic groups, compared to the range of motion group, improved significantly in aerobic capacity, endurance, physical activity, anxiety, and depression[23].

Kovar *et al.* randomized 102 OA patients with knee involvement to an eight-week group walking program or weekly phone calls about activities of daily living[24]. The walking subjects significantly decreased their disability and increased their six-minute walk distance; no changes in joint involvement were seen, suggesting that there were no adverse effects from the walking program.

The above discussion of patient education interventions aimed at specific strategies suggests that patient education can be helpful in lessening weight, pain, and disability. Next, we will examine patient education programs which combine the teaching of several behavioral strategies. All of these programs have several common elements:

(1) the education takes place in small groups;

(2) the education is carried out over several weeks;

(3) the education is highly participatory, with structured practice and feedback;

(4) the education is geared to the concerns of the patients.

Lorig *et al.* have carried out a series of studies on the six-week Arthritis Self-Management Program (ASMP). This program is taught in the community by teams of trained lay leaders who conducted two-hour weekly group sessions with 10 to 15 people (75 per cent with OA). The following are the major findings:

1. In four-month randomized trials, ASMP participants, when compared to wait list controls, experienced increased physical activity, increased use of cognitive pain management techniques, and decreased pain[25].

2. Reinforcement after one year did not add to the effect; both reinforced and non-reinforced groups retained most of the initial gains two years after the original course[26].

3. Subjects that were followed for four years continued to demonstrate decreased pain; they also decreased their arthritis-related visits to physicians[27].

4. The mechanisms by which the ASMP affects pain appear to be much more psychological than behavioral. The program enhances self-efficacy of participants, increasing their confidence that they can do something about specific disease-related problems. The changes in self-efficacy are significantly associated with changes in pain. There are no significant associations between changes in pain and changes in behaviors (exercise and the use of cognitive pain management techniques)[28].

The ASMP is now sponsored by national voluntary arthritis organizations (Arthritis Foundation, Arthritis Society, Arthritis Care) in the United States, Australia, Canada, and Great Britain.

Another series of studies was conducted by Goeppinger *et al.* with 450 subjects (72 per cent OA) living in rural areas. Subjects were randomized to a small group self-management program similar to the ASMP, a home-study program with the same content, or a wait list control group[29]. At four months, both intervention groups demonstrated improvements in knowledge, self-care behaviors, perceived helplessness and pain, when compared to controls; these improve-

ments were sustained for one year[30]. There were no significant changes in depression or function, nor were there differences between the two intervention groups — both interventions had high (82 per cent) retention rates and high acceptability to the participants. When the control group subjects were allowed to choose, half chose the small group and half chose the home-study interventions[31].

Bill-Harvey *et al.* utilized a quasi-experimental pre-test–post-test design to study 76 inner-city (mostly African–American) subjects who attended a 10-hour group intervention[21]; all subjects had OA. Classes were taught by trained lay leaders. Results included an increase in knowledge and exercise, and improved attitude ($p < 0.05$ function); the use of assistive devices also increased.

These studies of psychoeducational group interventions emphasizing multiple behaviors and individualized programs based on problems as perceived by the patients, suggest that these interventions can positively affect quality of life. The interventions were all community based and utilized non-health professionals as instructors; they appeared useful for a wide strata of people with OA — urban and rural people with little education, university graduates, and people of different races. Two studies have investigated the use of lay instructors compared to instruction given by health professionals[32,33]. In both studies, outcomes for participants taught by professionals were the same as those taught by lay people.

Several studies have examined other patient education delivery systems. Nineteen women, age 50 and above, with OA in the knee, were randomized to individualized 15–30 minute sessions or a small group one-hour session[34]. Both were taught by a nurse–physician team. There were no differences in outcomes between groups; both groups improved in knee flexion and extension, and pain. There were no changes in weight, mobility, physical activity, anxiety, or depression. The failure of this study to change behaviors suggests the need for education to be carried out in several sessions over time.

Goeppinger *et al.* conducted a dissemination study of a home-study arthritis education program combined with the availability of a community advisor. Subjects improved in behaviors, helplessness, pain, and depression[35]. When this study was repeated without advisors, no beneficial effects were noted (personal communication).

The importance of personalization was also demonstrated by Weinberger *et al.*[36]. Four hundred and thirty-nine OA patients in a general medicine practice were randomized to receive monthly phone calls, attend the clinic, or receive both monthly phone calls and attend the clinic. There were no significant clinic-by-phone interactions. Those contacted by phone had less disability and pain than those not receiving phone calls; disability and follow-up were significantly worse for the clinic only group compared to the phone groups.

Finally, two studies have utilized computers for patient education. Seventy-two OA patients from small-town senior centers used a computer to access eight OA lessons, totaling less than three hours. Significant pre–post increases were reported in knowledge, exercise, rest, and use of heat; no differences were reported in locus of control or pain[37].

OA patients belonging to a large health maintenance organization (HMO) filled out questionnaires about their arthritis[38]. Utilizing a computer program, the questionnaires were analyzed, and participants received highly personalized letter responses with self-management suggestions; they also received a book about arthritis self-management and an audio relaxation tape. Every three months, they repeated the questionnaire and received a response showing progress or problems since the previous questionnaire. At six months, study subjects who completed the program, when compared to controls, reported less pain, greater mobility, and greater sense of control over their symptoms; there were also trends towards less health care utilization.

Several conclusions can tentatively be drawn from the reviewed studies:

1. Patient education is most effective when several behaviors are taught.

2. Patient education should be based on the concerns and problems of the patient.

3. Patient education should be interactive and personalized.

4. If teachers are well trained, professional qualifications do not appear to give any advantage.

5. Many methods of patient education are effective: small group, proactive telephone, home-study, and computerized.

6. The most effective programs are carried out over time.

7. Focusing on self-management skills and behaviors appears to be more effective than focusing on the acquisition of knowledge or compliance to a set of prescribed behaviors.

Patient education in clinical practice

The following are suggestions of how patient education can be integrated into clinical practice; most of these suggestions require little or no extra time:

1. Frame teaching to match the concerns and expectations of the patient. For example, if patients are concerned about pain, suggest that exercise will help reduce pain by strengthening muscles. Also, reassure patients that they will not 'wear out' their joints and that they will not make their arthritis worse by exercising: in reality, the reverse is true. Tell them that they will make their arthritis worse by not exercising.

2. Be specific — Do not just suggest that a patient walk more. Find out what they can do now and suggest that they do this, four times a week, adding to it 10 per cent a week until they can exercise for 20–30 minutes.

3. Tell patients what you want them to do. If you do not tell a patient to walk, practise relaxation, or loose weight, they will not do it. Many times patients tell us that they are not doing things because their doctor never told them to.

4. Inform patients of the purposes and expected effects of medications. Also, tell them when to expect effects. Patients usually think that they are taking medications, so they will feel better. They should be told that sometimes medications do not make them better — they prevent symptoms from becoming worse, or they slow the progression of the disease.

   Another patient expectation is that medications will make them feel better in a short period of time, usually hours or, at most, a day. When this does not happen they stop taking the medication. By knowing what to expect, and when to expect it, there is a greater compliance with medication taking[39].

5. It is probably easier for patients to add new behaviors than to eliminate established ones. For

example, starting an exercise program is easier for most patients than changing eating habits[40].

6. Ask patients to tell you how they are going to integrate your suggestions into their lives. For example, ask them when they are going to take their medicine or do their exercises. Do not let them repeat your exact words; rather, get them to think about how they will do things. In this way, you can often discuss problems before they occur.

7. Use a combination of educational strategies; this can be done in any setting. Have literature for your patients, tell them what you want them to do, maybe have video tapes of exercise programs that they can borrow, teach your office staff to reinforce what is taught — in this way your patients will not get mixed messages.

8. Involve your office staff — patients learn a great deal from the receptionist and other staff in the office. Be sure that everyone is giving the same messages to patients.

9. Refer — in a short visit you cannot possibly do all the necessary teaching. Many patients will never find their way to patient education courses, exercises classes, or voluntary arthritis organizations, without your suggestion. Most patients, especially new patients and those not previously referred, should not leave your office without some sort of a referral. To make referrals easier, have referral prescription pads made up at any copy shop. They should contain the names of books, tapes, and organizations which you have found helpful. In addition, they should contain phone numbers. All you have to do is to check off what you want the patient to do.

    Another time-saving way of doing referrals is to have a bulletin board in the waiting area; across the top it can say 'Things your doctor suggests'. Have someone on your staff assigned to keep the board updated with information about classes, support groups, new literature and tapes, and local arthritis organizations.

10. Monitor progress — note what you asked patients to do so that next time you see them you can ask about the arthritis class, or exercise program, or whatever. This personalizes the visit and shows the patient you are truly interested; it also gives you direct feedback on the programs to which you are referring.

In summary, patient education can be one of the most important interventions for OA. It is true that this is a disease that patients 'have to learn to live with': the operative word is 'learn'. The job of good clinical practice is to assist patients with this learning.

References

1. Corbin, J.M. and Strauss, A. (1988). *Unending work and care: managing chronic illness at home*. Jossey-Bass Publishers, San Francisco.
2. Hawley, D.J. and Wolfe, F. (1993). Depression is not more common in rheumatoid Arthritis: A 10-year longitudinal study of 6153 patients with rheumatic disease. *Journal of Rheumatology*, 20, 2025–31.
3. Lorig, K., Cox, T., Cuevas, Y., Kraines, R.G., and Britton, M.C. (1984). Converging and diverging beliefs about arthritis: Caucasian patients, spanish-speaking patients and physicians. *Journal of Rheumatology*, 11(1), 76–9.
4. Allegrante, J.P., Peterson, M.G.E., Kovar, P.A., and Gordon, K.A. (1990). Beliefs held by physicians and patients regarding compliance with treatment and educational needs in arthritis and musculoskeletal diseases. In *25th Annual Meeting: Arthritis Health Professions Association in Seattle, WA*, S204.
5. Hanumappa, S., Murphy, B.B., and Schumacher, H.R. (1988). Patient sources of information about treatment of arthritis. In *23rd Annual Meeting: Arthritis Health Professions Association in Houston, TX*, S162.
6. Dekker, J., Boot, B., Van der Woude, L.H.V., and Bijlsma, J.W.J. (1992). Pain and disability in osteoarthritis: A review of biobehavioral mechanisms. *Journal of Behavioral Medicine*, 15(2), 189–213.
7. Hirano, P.C., Laurent, D.D., and Lorig, K.R. (1994). Arthritis patient education studies, 1987–1991: a review of the literature. *Patient Education Counsel*, 24, 9–54.
8. Lorig, K., Konkol, L., and Gonzalez, V. (1987). Arthritis patient education: a review of the literature. *Patient Education Counsel*, 10, 207–52.
9. Templeton, C.L., Petty, B.J., and Harter, J.L. (1978). Weight control — a group approach for arthritis clients. *Journal of Nutritional Education*, 10, 33–5.
10. Jacobson, E. (1938). *Progressive relaxation*. University of Chicago Press, Chicago.
11. Lorig, K. and Fries, J. (1995). *The arthritis helpbook*, pp. 191–206. Addison-Wesley, Reading.
12. Basler, H.D. and Rehfisch, H.P. (1991). Cognitive-behavioral therapy in patients with ankylosing spondylitis in a German self-help organization. *Journal of Psychosomatic Research*, 35, 345–54.
13. Bruce, J., Parker, S., Wellman, F., Kunce, J., and Meyer, A. (1984). Pain management in rheumatoid arthritis: cognitive behavior modification and transcutaneous neural stimulation. 1–3. Paper presented at the 19th Annual Meeting of the Arthritis Health Professionals Association in Minneapolis, MN.
14. Goldenberg, D.L., Kaplan, K.H., and Nadeau, M.G. (1991). The impact of cognitive-behavioral therapy

(CBT) on fibromyalgia. In *American College of Rheumatology 55th Annual Meeting in Boston, MA*, S190.

15. Randich, S.R. (1982). Evaluation of pain management program for rheumatoid arthritis patients. *Arthritis and Rheumatism*, (suppl) 25, S11.

16. Shearn, M.A. and Fireman, B. (1985). Stress management and mutual support groups in rheumatoid arthritis (RA): a controlled study. *American Journal of Medicine*, 78, 771–5.

17. Spilberg, F. and Gilner, F.H. (1985). A pain management program for rheumatoid arthritis patients. *Arthritis and Rheumatism*, (suppl) 28, S139.

18. Laborde, J.M. and Powers, M.J. (1983). Evaluation of educational interventions for osteoarthritis. *Multiple Linear Regression Viewpoints*, 12, 12–37.

19. Daltroy, L., Morlino, C., and Liang, M. (1989). Preoperative education for total hip and knee replacement patients. In *24th Annual Meeting: Arthritis Health Professions Association in Cincinnati, OH*, S193.

20. Calfas, K.J., Kaplan, R.M., and Ingram, R.E. (1992). One-year evaluation of cognitive-behavioral intervention in osteoarthritis. *Arthritis Care Research*, 5(4), 202–9.

21. Bill-Harvey, D., Rippy, R., Abeles, M., Donald, M.J., Dawning, D., Ingemito, F., *et al.* (1989). Outcome of an osteoarthritis education program for low-literacy patients taught by indigenous instructors. *Patient Education Counsel*, 13, 133–42.

22. Minor, M.A., Hewett, J.E., and Kay, D.R. (1986). Monitoring for harmful effects of physical conditioning exercise (PCE) with arthritis patients. *Arthritis and Rheumatism*, (suppl) 29, S144.

23. Minor, M.A., Hewettm, J.E., Webel, R.R., Anderson, S.K., and Kay, D.R. (1989). Efficacy of physical conditioning exercise in patients with rheumatoid arthritis and osteoarthritis. *Arthritis and Rheumatism*, 23(11), 1396–405.

24. Kovar, P.A., Allegrante, J.P., MacKenzie, C.R., Peterson, M.G.E., and Gutin, B. (1992). Supervised fitness walking in patients with osteoarthritis of the knee: A randomized, controlled trail. *Annals of Internal Medicine*, 116, 529–34.

25. Lorig, K., Kraines, R.G., and Holman, H.R. (1981). A randomized prospective controlled study of the effects of health education for people with arthritis. *Arthritis and Rheumatism*, 24 (4, Suppl.), S90.

26. Lorig, K. and Holman, H. (1989). Long-term outcomes of an arthritis self-management study: effects of reinforcement efforts. *Social Science Medicine*, 29, 221–4.

27. Lorig, K., Mazonson, P., and Holman, H. (1993). Evidence suggesting that health education for self-management in patients with chronic arthritis has sus-tained health benefits while reducing health care costs. *Arthritis and Rheumatism*, 36(4), 439–46.

28. Lorig, K., Seleznick, M., Lubeck, D., Ung, E., Chastain, R., and Holman, H.R. (1989). The beneficial outcomes of the arthritis self-management course are inadequately explained by behavior change. *Arthritis and Rheumatism*, 32(1), 91–5.

29. Goeppinger, J., Brunk, S.E., Athur, M.W., and Reidesel, S. (1987). The effectiveness of community-based arthritis self-care programs. *Arthritis and Rheumatism*, 30, S194.

30. Goeppinger, J., Arthur, M.W., Baglioni, A.J., Brunk, S.E., and Hawdon, J.E. (1988). Effectiveness of arthritis self-care education: a longitudinal perspective. In *23rd Annual Meeting: Arthritis Health Professions Association in Houston, TX*, S155.

31. Goeppinger, J., Arthur, M.W., Baglioni, A.J., Brank, S.E., and Brunner, C.M. (1989). A re-examination of the effectiveness of self-care education for persons with arthritis. *Arthritis and Rheumatism*, 32, 706–16.

32. Lorig, K., Feigenbaum, P., Regan, C., Ung, E., and Holman, H.R. (1986). A comparison of lay-taught and professional-taught arthritis self-management courses. *Journal of Rheumatology*, 13(4), 763–7.

33. Cohen, J.L., Sauter, R., DeVellis, R.F. and DeVellis, B.M. (1986). Evaluation of arthritis self-management courses led by lay persons and by professionals. *Arthritis and Rheumatism*, 29, 388–93.

34. Doyle, T.H. and Granda, J.L. (1982). Influence of two management approaches on the health status of women with osteoarthritis. *Arthritis and Rheumatism*, suppl 25, S153.

35. Goeppinger, J., Macnee, C., Anderson, M.K., Boutaugh, M., and Stewart, K. (1995). From research to practice: the effects of jointly sponsored dissemination of an arthritis self-care nursing intervention. *Applied Nursing Research*, 8(3), 106–13.

36. Weinberger, M., Tierney, W.M., Booker, P., and Katz, B. (1989). Can the provision of information to patients with oseoarthritis improve functional status. *Arthritis and Rheumatism*, 23(12), 1577–83.

37. Rippey, R.M., Bill, D., Abels, M., Day, J., Downing, D.S., Pfeiffer, C.A., *et al.* (1987). Computer-based patient education for older persons with osteoarthritis. *Arthritis and Rheumatism*, 30(8), 932–5.

38. Gale, F.M., Kirk, J.C., and Davis, R. (1994). Patient education and self-management: randomized study of effects on health status of a mail-delivered program. *Arthritis and Rheumatism*, 37(9), S197.

39. Daltroy, L.H., Katz, J.N., and Liang, M.H. (1992). Doctor-patient communications and adherence to arthritis treatments. *Arthritis Care Research*, 5, S19.

40. Mullen, P.D., Simons-Morton, D.G., Ramirez, G., *et al.* (1993). A meta-analysis of studies evaluating patient education for three groups of preventive behaviors. In *Prevention '93 in St. Louis, MO*.

9.12 Social support

Steven A. Mazzuca and Morris Weinberger

The relationship between pathophysiology in osteoarthritis (OA) and clinical outcomes of pain and related dysfunction is complex[1]. Only 30–40 per cent of subjects with evidence of OA apparent by radiography report significant joint pain[2,3]. While pain and function are related to the presence and radiographic severity of OA, persons with similar degrees of radiographic changes experience markedly different levels of joint pain and dysfunction[4,5]. Obviously, many factors may mediate or moderate the effects of cartilage destruction on clinical outcomes of OA. In this chapter, we will describe the phenomenon of social support as a potential mediator of joint pain and dysfunction from OA; we will summarize research evidence concerning the capacity of social support to enhance the effectiveness of therapeutic interventions in OA; and finally, we will offer some guidelines and cautions for assessing and utilizing social support in practice.

Overview of social support

For decades, social scientists have hypothesized that persons who are exposed to stressful life events (for example, death of a loved one, divorce, marriage, childbirth, the diagnosis of a chronic illness) experience worse health outcomes than persons who avoid major stressors. However, the strength of the observed correlations between exposure to stressful life events and health parameters is only modest. This consistent finding has led social scientists to explore factors that may mediate the stress–health relationship, thereby accounting for the modest correlations. One factor that has been examined as a potential mediator of the relationship between stress and well-being is social support.

What is social support?

Social support is generally defined as the gratification of basic social needs through interactions with others[6]. Within the context of health, social support refers to processes by which interpersonal relationships promote physical, social, and emotional well-being[7]. Like many terms used by social scientists, social support has come to be used commonly in other research disciplines and by the general public: this is a double-edged sword. While common usage of the term assures a broad appreciation of its meaning, the popularity of the term also makes communication of precise operational definitions of social support and, therefore, implications of research findings, more difficult.

Two theoretical approaches to social support are popular today among social scientists. The *social network approach* emphasizes the quantifiable, structural characteristics of support systems[8,9]. This approach assumes that factors such as the size of a social network and the frequency with which members contact one another are critical. All social ties which an individual possesses are assumed to be both accessible and supportive. An alternative conceptualization represents a *functional approach* to understanding support systems[10,11]. This approach requires an individual to identify a person or person who fulfill basic social needs. As such, this approach makes qualitative distinctions between the types of support from which a person may benefit. For patients with chronic medical conditions, supportive functions include:

(1) *emotional support* to promote feelings of belonging and being valued;

(2) *informational support* to assure understanding of the medical condition, treatment options, and prognosis;

(3) *tangible support* in the form of financial and other assistive services to individuals (for example, help with transportation and other activities of daily living).

These two approaches are not antithetical. Pearlin argues that they provide different, but complementary, information[12]. Social networks reflect support that is potentially available (that is, the totality of the social resources from which persons may draw), while functionally-defined support better represents the resources that one actually uses when dealing with specific stressors.

How does social support operate to maintain health?

Two causal models are used currently by social science researchers attempting to explain how social support influences health (Fig. 9.10). The *buffering model* states that social support influences health only when a stressor is present[13,14]. Thus, when individuals are exposed to stressors, the existence of social support protects them from negative health-related sequelae. However, in the absence of stress, social support does not affect health. The *additive* or *main-effects model* posits that social support is beneficial, regardless of the stress level of a person[15-17]. It has been hypothesized that social support, by providing individuals with an overall sense of well-being, a sense of stability in their life, and a recognition of self-worth, prevents the occurrence, or reduces the severity, of stressors — thereby, protecting individuals from poor health outcomes.

Who can provide social support?

Regardless of how social support is defined (structurally or functionally) or how it operates to maintain health (as a buffer or as prophylaxis against stress), a further distinction between the sources of social support is important.

Social scientists differentiate between primary and secondary social groups. *Primary social groups* are composed of persons involved in personal, intimate, and non-specialized relationships (for example, families). While primary group members often develop close, intimate, and enduring relationships with each other, primary relationships are not always loving or supportive. Primary group members need not live in close physical proximity, but periodic interaction is necessary to maintain primary group status. In contrast, members of *secondary social groups* relate to one other in the context of limited, specific roles (for example, as coworkers). In secondary groups, members have few emotional bonds, and ties are impersonal; relationships are task-oriented, and members associate to achieve specific, practical goals; interactions are more superficial and utilitarian than in primary groups.

Adapting these definitions, potential *primary sources of social support* are generally considered to be the family of the patient and close friends. Persons capable of functioning as primary sources of social support usually comprise a limited group of individuals with whom the patient shares deeply personal, often intimate, relationships. The support offered by primary sources is non-specialized; that is, primary sources can perform a variety of emotional, informational, and tangible functions. In contrast, *secondary sources of social support* are usually a larger group of less intimate acquaintances who can offer context-specific, but nevertheless valuable, support (for example, health care professionals, members of peer-support groups). Notably, through repeated contact over time, secondary sources of social support can evolve into primary sources.

Research on social support in arthritis

To date, research on the effects of social support on outcomes in arthritis has been dominated by investiga-

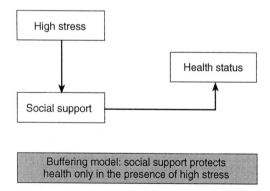

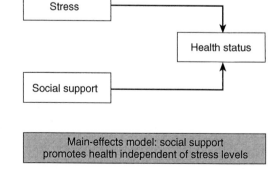

Fig. 9.10   Theoretical models of the effects of social support on health status.

tions of patients with rheumatoid arthritis (RA). Even though patients with RA and OA differ with respect to clinical, therapeutic, and demographic characteristics — to the extent that patients with either disease must cope with stressful life events, joint pain, and the prospect of progressive dysfunction — several conclusions about social support and RA may generalize to patients with OA:

1. In numerous observational studies (both cross-sectional and longitudinal) comparing patients with differing levels of measurable social support, patients with higher levels of support also reported more effective coping strategies[18], greater psychological adjustment to illness[19], greater self-esteem[20], fewer depressive symptoms[21–23], and higher levels of life satisfaction[24].

2. The participation of family and friends (primary sources of social support) in cognitive-behavioral therapy for arthritis patients can enhance the capacity of such interventions to reduce the psychological impact of arthritis[25] and prolong initial therapeutic response to treatment[26].

3. Instruction of patients on how to communicate their needs for support to family members can increase compliance[27] and a sense of control over pain[28].

4. The beneficial effects of social support are more consistently seen in psychological and behavioral outcomes than in pain and dysfunction[7].

A limited number of studies of social support in OA have been published — the results of which are consistent with several of the above generalizations from studies of RA. Summers *et al.*[29] demonstrated that psychological variables are stronger correlates of joint pain in patients with hip and knee OA than are objective (radiographic) indicators of disease severity. While social support was not among the psychological variables included in that study, the variables that were included (that is, depression, anxiety, and coping style) are all related to social support. However, observational studies of social support and OA outcomes are rare. In a longitudinal study of 193 patients with OA, Weinberger *et al.*[30] found functional indicators of social support to be better correlated with the subjective appraisal of the patient of satisfaction with social support, than were structural indicators. However, neither aspect of social support was found to buffer the effects of stressors on health over six months. This

investigation was followed by a larger study (n = 439) of the direct benefits of social support in OA[31]. In this study, low self-esteem was associated with joint pain, physical disability, and psychological disability. In addition, physical disability was related to a lack of tangible support, and the absence of a sense of belonging among OA patients was inversely related to psychological health. These relationships were independent of the effects of stress, that is, the data were consistent with a direct main effect (rather than a buffering effect) of social support on health.

Prospective intervention studies targeted at patients with OA indicate a clearly positive role for social support. In two studies, social support was shown to be a mediating factor in the long-term response of OA patients to treatment. Calfas *et al.*[32] evaluated a cognitive-behavioral modification intervention designed to teach patients to reconceptualize their pain; to monitor the interrelatedness of their thoughts, beliefs, and actions as they relate to pain; to believe they can cope effectively; and to adapt their behaviors to improve functioning. While only immediate post-intervention improvements in quality of life could be attributed to the intervention, baseline social support and mobility were the only significant (inverse) predictors of depressive symptoms 12 months after intervention.

Using a different form of non-pharmacologic treatment for arthritis, Minor *et al.*[33] have shown that aerobic walking and aquatic exercise programs (three 60–minute sessions per week, for 12 weeks) can have significant positive effects on physical and emotional function in patients with OA or RA. In a secondary analysis of self-directed maintenance of the exercise routines by the original subjects, the investigators determined that the perceived support of friends for continued exercise was a significant predictor of exercise behavior nine months after completion of the study intervention[34]; by 18 months, social support was no longer a direct predictor of self-directed behavior. However, at that point, prior exercise behavior (to which social support had contributed) became a significant determinant.

The literature contains several controlled evaluations of educational interventions for patients with OA in which elements of the design of the intervention were intended to facilitate support of patients by family members, friends, or peers. While the discrete effects of such elements cannot be teased out of the overall results, their support-engendering potential are noteworthy, nevertheless.

The most widely documented model for arthritis patient education is the intervention first named the Arthritis Self-Management Program (ASMP) by Lorig and other investigators at Stanford University[35,36]. Now disseminated in the United States, Canada, Australia, and New Zealand, the basic paradigm for the ASMP is a series of six two-hour sessions that combine conventional topics of patient education (for example, disease processes, exercise, side effects of drugs) with cognitive-behavioral techniques (visualization, contracting for behavioral change, and so on). Participation of family members is encouraged, but the discrete effects of such participation have not been documented. As in the RA study by DeVellis et al.[27], participants are led through a communication exercise in which they learn to elicit supportiveness from family and friends. Most notable is the fact that the ASMP is designed to be led by an autonomous lay person who is also an arthritis patient. Formative evaluation data from early trials of the ASMP showed greater knowledge gains among participants in sessions led by health professionals, but greater implementation of self-care behaviors (for example, relaxation techniques) in sessions with lay leaders[37].

Kovar et al.[38] published a trial in which the intervention (supervised walking and patient education for patients with symptomatic knee OA) included social support from secondary sources. The authors designed the eight-week intervention (three 90–minute sessions per week) to include both supportive encouragement by the intervention facilitator (a physical therapist) and peer interactions during educational and walking sessions[39]. In comparison with subjects in an attention-control group, patients participating in the walking / education program exhibited significant improvements in walking capacity, functional status, and joint pain[38].

More direct evidence for the beneficial effects of social support from secondary sources can be found in a series of reports by Weinberger et al.[40-42]. In an early study of social support in OA, subjects (193 patients with knee and / or hip OA) were telephoned bi-weekly for six months by a research assistant, to document current stressors, social support, and arthritis outcomes with standardized research instruments[30]. An uncontrolled (and unexpected) observation in the study was that social support and functional status parameters both improved significantly over the six months[40]. This observation led to the hypothesis that periodic communication between lay personnel and patients, about the status of their OA, could serve a beneficial, supportive function.

The hypothesis was tested directly in a randomized controlled trial of various strategies for achieving periodic communication between trained lay personnel and OA patients for the purpose of reviewing the health of the subject[41]. Contacts were structured to assure a uniform set of inquiries: medications (compliance, adequacy of supply), joint pain, presence of gastrointestinal symptoms, status of acute symptoms for comorbid conditions (for example, hypertension, diabetes, heart or pulmonary disease), recall of next scheduled outpatient visit, barriers to keeping clinic appointments, and recall of an 'after-hours' telephone number at which healthcare providers could be reached. Two formats for delivery of the intervention were studied: by monthly telephone call and in clinic, immediately prior to seeing a physician for a scheduled appointment. Subjects were 439 patients with OA who were assigned at random to one of four treatment conditions: telephone intervention, in-clinic intervention, both telephone and in-clinic intervention, or neither (that is, a pure control group).

After one year of contacts and informational support under their assigned conditions, subjects in the groups receiving monthly telephone calls exhibited significant improvements in joint pain and physical function. In contrast, the in-clinic (only) intervention was not beneficial and, in fact, had an adverse effect on physical health[41]. Several possible explanations may be offered for this observation. Perhaps most importantly, the clinic may be a poor setting in which to deliver such interventions. When patients have an appointment with their physician, the busy clinical environment and thoughts about the primary purpose of the visit may undermine efforts to provide support. In contrast, telephone calls were made at times convenient for the patient — if the patient was busy or feeling ill, interviewers were instructed to call back at a more convenient time.

It is especially noteworthy that the effects of the telephone intervention not only were apparent, but also were strongest, among those patients who were maintained on a stable medical regimen throughout the study[42]. The magnitude of experimental effects on pain and physical function (65 and 53 per cent of the respective pooled standard deviations) for this subsample of subjects was more than twice that found in the study as a whole. Effects of this size compare favorably to the results of open-label trials of nonsteroidal anti-inflammatory drugs[43]. This is striking evidence that periodic, supportive communication with patients about their health status should be considered adjunctive therapy for patients with OA.

Social support in clinical practice

Assessment of social support

To our knowledge, currently available instruments for the measurement of quantitative and functional aspects of social support have not been validated for 'real-world' clinical use. Nevertheless, the basic definitions and causal assumptions about the interrelatedness of social support and well-being provide an adequate framework within which social support can be assessed briefly, as a part of the patient history, by asking the following questions:

1. Are you married?

2. Are there other family members or friends with whom you keep close contact?

3. To whom do you talk when something is bothering you?

4. On whom do you count when you need help with doing something?

5. Whose advice do you trust for information about your health?

Structural issues of social support include the marital status of the patient and the number and roles of persons other than a spouse (for example, friends, and other family members) with whom the patient maintains close or frequent contact. Membership in a church congregation or in social organizations may be suggestive of the types of supportive environments and activities available to the patient. As an added measure, questions about specific supportive functions (that is, emotional, tangible, informational) may identify areas of need that are currently unmet.

Enhancement of social support in care of the patient with OA

With the exception of the social support intervention designed by Weinberger *et al.* and delivered by trained lay persons[41], specific protocols or guidelines for addressing social support in clinical practice have not been subjected to controlled evaluation among patients with OA. Nevertheless, published evidence of a mediating role of social support in OA care[30–32,34], and general social support dynamics implicit in previous intervention studies in both RA[25–28] and OA[37,38], offer a firm basis for a systematic approach to addressing social support in clinical practice. Elements of that approach can be listed as follows:

(1) include the support-giver in discussions regarding prognosis, self-care recommendations, and drug effects and side effects;

(2) have the support-giver accompany the patient to self-care education programs;

(3) monitor, prospectively, the continued functionality of the relationship between patient and support-giver;

(4) make sure the support-giver maintains social ties outside the relationship / marriage;

(5) be alert to the need for peer support or a mental health professional for the support-giver during times of high stress;

(6) consider specific functional requirements of the patient for community service organizations regarding transportation, nutrition, and so on;

(7) initiate interim (telephone) contacts with patients to monitor health status and effects and side effects of therapy, and to reinforce self-care.

When the social history of a patient reveals a primary relationship with an individual who is committed to the general well-being of that patient, every effort should be made to permit that individual to fulfill his or her role as a primary support-giver. With the permission of the patient, the person primarily entrusted with a supportive role should be present during any discussions between physician and patient in which disclosure of information occurs regarding prognosis, self-care recommendations, and drug effects and side effects. To the extent that the primary support-giver is able to participate in the clinical encounter, the information that is shared will enable him or her to anticipate the stresses the patient will endure and to adapt existing support schemes to accommodate the new demands of drug therapy, exercise regimens, and observance of principles of joint protection. Most free-standing programs of arthritis self-care education (for example, the ASMP) permit, but do not require, attendance of 'significant others'. Patients enrolling in such programs should be encouraged to attend with their primary support-giver.

Research on the interrelationships among patients with RA and their family members has revealed several pitfalls to the mustering of social support which, on face value, bear mention in the context of care for OA. Either by their own limitations, or because of temporary and uncontrollable circumstances, primary support-givers cannot always be counted upon to be unfailing sources of help and encouragement. Among the real or perceived behaviors of family and friends that can, at times, be detrimental to the well-being of the patient are the trivialization of symptoms, pessimistic comments, and over-solicitousness[19]. For some patients, social support is helpful only as a buffer against stress (for example, a flare of disease activity); as the stress subsides, the otherwise supportive actions of others can be perceived as threats to the sense of autonomy and self-esteem of the patient[44]. The clinician should assess, periodically, the status of relationships between OA patients and family members in order to detect early any dysfunction due to the fallibility of supportive relationships.

The clinician who utilizes social support in practice must recognize that support-givers pay an emotional cost to fulfill their roles. This is a particular concern when support-givers are elderly and have their own array of medical conditions, or when children of elderly adults with OA have obligations to their own families. In such cases, the support-givers themselves are subject to stress. Interviewing the spouses of RA patients, Revenson and Majerovitz[45] found that support-givers often feel burdened and are hesitant to reveal the stress of their role to their spouse (that is, the patient). Many support-givers find they can be more helpful to their spouse if they maintain and nurture social ties outside the marriage. Also, about a third of the spouses of RA patients learn to cope with the prolonged burden of their roles with the help of support groups or mental health professionals[45].

The physician and his or her staff should consider themselves the chief source of *informational support* for all patients (and their support-givers) coping with OA. This responsibility extends beyond the disclosure of essential information during routine office visits to enable patients to make informed choices about their treatment. As demonstrated by Weinberger *et al.*[41], periodic contact by telephone for the purpose of assessing the health status of the patient and reinforcing self-care can have dramatic, beneficial effects on the physical and psychological well-being of patients with OA — over and above routine clinical contact.

The responsibility of the clinician also entails making patients and their care-givers aware of community service organizations specializing in *tangible support*, in the forms of transportation, nutrition, personal

hygiene, and other domestic needs of the elderly and infirmed. Finally, while health care professionals strive to provide a degree of *emotional support* to all patients, this need may be greatest for elderly OA patients who, because of widowhood or the death of close friends, may have no primary source of social support. Older OA patients have support-givers who are themselves elderly or burdened by other commitments (for example, the child of a patient may also be a parent). In such cases, clinicians can facilitate access to secondary sources of support (for example, patient support groups, social and religious organizations) which may, in time, develop into primary sources of support.

In summary, among the psychosocial variables that have been studied in patients with OA, social support is noteworthy because it serves both as an indicator of the psychological response of the patient to pain and dysfunction and as a target for intervention by clinicians. Important structural and functional aspects of social support are readily discernible in the social history of the patient. Involvement of key individuals (primary sources of social support) who have insight into the stresses faced by the patient and a willingness to buffer their detrimental effects may, with a modest investment of effort on the part of the clinician, pay large dividends in terms of the ability of the patient to cope effectively with chronic pain and dysfunction. Clinicians (physicians and staff) should recognize that they too are important, albeit secondary, sources of social support. Research evidence supports the proposition that provision of informational support and interim monitoring of patient progress (for example, by telephone) results in improved patient outcomes.

References

1. Hadler, N.M. (1992). Knee pain is the malady — not osteoarthritis. *Annals of Internal Medicine*, **116**, 598–9.
2. Lawrence, J.S., Bremner, J.M., and Bier, F. (1966). Osteoarthrosis, prevalence in the population and relationship between symptoms and X-ray changes. *Annals of the Rheumatic Diseases*, **25**, 1–24.
3. Cobbs, S., Merchant, W.R., and Rubin, T. (1957). The relationship of symptoms to osteoarthritis. *Journal of Chronic Diseases*, **5**, 197–204.
4. Davis, M.A., Ettinger, W.H., Neuhaus, J.M., and Mallon, K.P. (1991). Knee osteoarthritis and physical functioning: evidence from the NHANES I Epidemiologic Followup Study. *Journal of Rheumatology*, **18**, 591–8.

5. Davis, M.A., Ettinger, W.H., Neuhaus, J.M., Barclay, J.D., and Segal, M.R. (1992). Correlates of knee pain among US adults with and without radiographic knee osteoarthritis. *Journal of Rheumatology*, **19**, 1943–9.

6. Kaplan, B.H., Cassel, J.C., and Gore, S. (1977). Social support and health. *Medical Care*, **15**, 47–58.

7. Lanza, A.F. and Revenson T.A. (1993). Social support interventions for rheumatoid arthritis patients: the cart before the horse? *Health Education Quarterly*, **20**, 97–117.

8. Berkman, L.F. and Syme, L. (1979). Social networks, host resistance, and mortality: a nine-year follow-up study of Alameda County residents. *American Journal of Epidemiology*, **109**, 186–204.

9. Mitchell, R.E. and Trickett, E.J. (1980). Social networks as mediators of social support: an analysis of the effects and determinants of social networks. *Community Mental Health Journal*, **16**, 27–44.

10. Sarason, I.G., Levine, H.M., Basham, R.B., and Sarason, B.R. (1983). Assessing social support: the social support questionnaire. *Journal of Personality and Social Psychology*, **44**, 127–39.

11. Porritt, D. (1979). Social support in crisis: quantity or quality. *Social Science and Medicine*, **13A**, 715–21.

12. Pearlin, L.I. (1989). The sociological study of stress. *Journal of Health and Social Behavior*, **30**, 241–56.

13. Dean, A. and Lin, N. (1977). The stress-buffering role of social support: problems and prospects for systematic investigation. *Journal of Nerve and Mental Disorders*, **165**, 403–17.

14. Dohrenwend, B.S. and Dohrenwend, B.P. (1978). Some issues in research on stressful life events. *Journal of Nerve and Mental Disorders*, **168**, 7–15.

15. Blazer, D. (1982). Social support and mortality in an elderly community population. *American Journal of Epidemiology*, **115**, 684–94.

16. Norris, F.H. and Murrell, S.A. (1984). Protective function of resources related to life events, global stress, and depression in older adults. *Journal of Health and Social Behavior*, **25**, 424–37.

17. Williams, A.W., Ware, J.E., and Donald, C.A. (1981). A model of mental health, life events, and social support applicable to general populations. *Journal of Health and Social Behavior*, **22**, 324–36.

18. Manne, S.L. and Zautra, A.J. (1989). Spouse criticism and support: their association with coping and psychological adjustment among women with rheumatoid arthritis. *Journal of Personality and Social Psychology*, **56**, 608–17.

19. Affleck, G., Pfeiffer, C., Tennen, H., and Fifield, J. (1988). Social support and psychological adjustment to rheumatoid arthritis. *Social Science and Medicine*, **27**, 71–7.

20. Fitzpatrick, R., Newman, S., Lamb, R., and Shipley, M. (1988). Social relationships and psychological well-being in rheumatoid arthritis. *Social Science and Medicine*, **27**, 399–403.

21. Brown, G.K., Wallston, K.A., and Nicassio, P.M. (1989). Social support and depression in rheumatoid arthritis: a one-year prospective study. *Journal of Applied Social Psychology*, **19**, 1164–81.

22. Fitzpatrick, R., Newman, S., Archer, R., and Shipley, M. (1991). Social support, disability and depression: a longitudinal study of rheumatoid arthritis. *Social Science and Medicine*, **33**, 605–11.

23. Goodenow, C., Reisine, S.T., and Grady, K.E. (1990). Quality of social support and associated social and psychological functioning in women with rheumatoid arthritis. *Health Psychology*, **9**, 266–84.

24. Smith, C.A., Dobbins, C.J., and Wallston, K.A. (1991). The mediational role of perceived competence in psychological adjustment to rheumatoid arthritis. *Journal of Applied Social Psychology*, **21**, 1218–47.

25. Bradley, L.A., Young, L.D., Anderson, K.O., Turner, R.A., Agudelo, C., McDaniel, L.K., *et al.* (1987). Effects of psychological therapy on pain behavior of rheumatoid arthritis patients. *Arthritis and Rheumatism*, **30**, 1105–14.

26. Radojevic, V., Nicassio, P.M., and Weisman, M.H. (1992). Behavioral intervention with and without family support for rheumatoid arthritis. *Behavior Therapy*, **23**, 13–30.

27. DeVellis, B.M., Blalock, S.J., Hahn, P.M., DeVellis, R.F., and Hochbaum, G.M. (1988). Evaluation of a problem-solving intervention for patients with arthritis. *Patient Education and Counseling*, **11**, 29–42.

28. Parker, J.C., Frank, R.G., Beck, N.C., Smarr, K.L., Buesher, K.L., Philips, L.R., *et al.* (1988). Pain management in rheumatoid arthritis patients: a cognitive-behavioral approach. *Arthritis and Rheumatism*, **31**, 593–601.

29. Summers, M.N., Haley, W.E., Reveille, J.D., and Alarcon, G.S. (1988). Radiographic assessment and psychological variables as predictors of pain and function in osteoarthritis of the knee or hip. *Arthritis and Rheumatism*, **31**, 204–9.

30. Weinberger, M., Hiner, S.L., Tierney, W.M. (1987). Assessing social support in elderly adults. *Social Science and Medicine*, **25**, 1049–55.

31. Weinberger, M., Tierney, W.M., Booher, P., and Hiner, S.L. (1990). Social support, stress and functional status in patients with osteoarthritis. *Social Science and Medicine*, **30**, 503–8.

32. Calfas, K.J., Kaplan, R.M., and Ingram, R.E. (1992). One-year evaluation of cognitive-behavioral intervention in osteoarthritis. *Arthritis Care and Research*, **5**, 202–9.

33. Minor, M.A., Hewett, J.E., Webel, R.R., Anderson, S.K., Kay, D.R. (1989). Efficacy of physical conditioning exercise in patients with rheumatoid arthritis or osteoarthritis. *Arthritis and Rheumatism*, **32**, 1396–1405.

34. Minor, M.A. and Brown, J.D. (1993). Exercise maintenance of persons with arthritis after participation in a class experience. *Health Education Quarterly*, **20**, 83–95.

35. Lorig, K., Lubeck, D., Kraines, R.G., Seleznick, M., and Holman, H.R. (1985). Outcomes of self-help education for patients with arthritis. *Arthritis and Rheumatism*, **28**, 680–5.

36. Lorig, K. and Holman, H.R. (1989). Long-term outcomes of an arthritis self-management study: effects of

reinforcement efforts. *Social Science and Medicine*, 29, 221–4.

37. Lorig, K., Feigenbaum, P., Regan, C., Ung, E., Chastain, R.L., and Holman, H.R. (1986). Comparison of lay-taught and professional-taught arthritis self-management courses. *Journal of Rheumatology*, 13, 763–7.

38. Kovar, P.A., Allegrante, J.P., MacKenzie, C.R., Peterson, M.G.E., Gutin, B., and Charlson, M.E. (1992). Supervised fitness walking in patients with osteoarthritis of the knee. *Annals of Internal Medicine*, 116, 529–34.

39. Allegrante, J.P., Kovar, P.A., MacKenzie, C.R., Peterson, M.G.E., and Gutin, B. (1993). A walking education program for patients with osteoarthritis of the knee: theory and intervention strategies. *Health Education Quarterly*, 20, 63–81.

40. Weinberger, M., Hiner, S.L., and Tierney, W.M. (1986). Improving functional status in osteoarthritis: the effect of social support. *Social Science and Medicine*, 23, 899–904.

41. Weinberger, M., Tierney, W.M., Booher, P., and Katz, B.P. (1989). Can provision of information to patients with osteoarthritis improve functional status? A randomized, controlled trial. *Arthritis and Rheumatism*, 32, 1577–83.

42. René, J., Weinberger, M., Mazzuca, S.A., Brandt, K.D., and Katz, B.P. (1992). Monthly telephone contacts with lay personnel reduce join pain in patients with knee osteoarthritis maintained on stable medical management. *Arthritis and Rheumatism*, 35, 511–15.

43. Anderson, J.J., Firschein, H.E., and Meenan, R.F. (1989). Sensitivity of a health status measure to short-term clinical changes in arthritis. *Arthritis and Rheumatism*, 32, 844–50.

44. Cohen, S. (1988). Psychological models of the role of social support in the etiology of physical disease. *Health Psychology*, 7, 269–97.

45. Revenson, T.A. and Majerovitz, S.D. (1990). Spouse's support provision to chronically ill patients. *Journal of Social and Personal Relationships*, 7, 575–86.

9.13   Depression in osteoarthritis

Phyllis A. Dexter and John R. Hayes

Perhaps no health problem better illustrates the biopsychosocial model of health[1] than osteoarthritis (OA). The complex interactions among the OA symptoms of joint pain and disability, psychological characteristics of the patient, social support, aging, activity, sleep, obesity, and other factors, in this mostly elderly population, require a holistic approach to care. This chapter will discuss some of the ways in which a common psychological problem — depression — can interact with many of these factors in the context of OA. Depression can interfere with clinical assessment of the patient with OA, cost-effective care delivery, and disease outcomes. Depression is debilitating and costly, but treatable, and should always be diagnosed and treated. When depression occurs in patients with a complex illness, such as OA, its recognition and treatment are particularly important for good outcomes.

Several introductory comments are in order. First, because costly longitudinal research studies with initially healthy subjects are needed to establish precise cause-and-effect relationships, it is not surprising that our current knowledge of depression in arthritis is based mostly on statistical correlations and cross-sectional studies. Such studies, while often very suggestive, can address causality only indirectly. For example, the extent to which depression leads to pain and disability versus the extent to which pain and disability lead to depression is unknown; however, for clinicians treating depressed OA patients, such problems are more of academic than practical importance.

Second, whereas the effects of many of the individual factors discussed in this chapter are, by themselves, limited, their potential cumulative effects on OA outcomes may be considerable. That multiple factors interact to affect joint pain and disability in patients with OA is a central thesis.

Third, most studies of depression in arthritis have been conducted on patients with rheumatoid arthritis (RA). Fortunately, in the few studies that have included both RA and OA patients, no important response differences have been identified that would seem to preclude extrapolating findings from RA studies to OA. Discussion of such studies, therefore, is included in this chapter.

Finally, although anxiety differs conceptually from depression, in practice it is difficult to separate the two and there is a large amount of overlap in symptoms[2].

Anxiety will not be treated separately in this chapter, but it is assumed that anxiety and depression occur together much, or even most, of the time.

Epidemiology

Prevalence

Major depression, as defined by the Diagnostic and Statistical Manual of Mental Disorders, 4th edition (DSM-IV)[3] is thought to be relatively infrequent among those in the general population who are over the age of 65, that is, the group most likely to have OA. The prevalence rate in persons of this age group who live in the community is probably less than 2 per cent[4]. On the other hand, even low-level chronic depression in the OA patient may interfere with treatment outcomes, and the rate for substantial depressive symptoms (as opposed to major depression) in the elderly is much higher — 10 to 20 per cent[4–6].

Because depression is highly correlated with functional disability[5], chronic pain[7], and health care utilization[8], it is not surprising that the rate of depression among persons who seek treatment for arthritis is higher than that for the general population. Approximately 17 per cent of clinic patients with hip or knee OA were found to be 'probably' depressed and an additional 16 per cent 'possibly' depressed[9]. Depression rates in OA and RA do not differ significantly from each other or from those in other chronic diseases[9,10].

Recognition

In 1988, because of accumulating evidence that depression in the United States was greatly under-recognized, misdiagnosed, and/or under-treated by physicians, an educational initiative was launched by the National Institute of Mental Health (NIMH)[11]. Depending on study design and sample, estimates of the percentage of depression cases missed by physicians in non-psychiatric outpatient settings have ranged from 25 to 90 per cent[12]. Considering that the great majority of patients with depression are seen in such settings[11], this lack of recognition is a serious problem. Furthermore, even when physicians recognize the condition, they may not properly treat it; one large multi-site study found that only about 10 per cent of depressed patients were receiving appropriate treatment[13]. Reasons for this lack of recognition and treatment may include lack of skill or confidence among primary care physicians in making the diagnosis of depression, discomfort of the physician with discussing the possibility of depression with patients, and preoccupation of the physician with other medical problems[14].

The elderly, especially, underutilize mental health services[15]. Although physicians may be relatively less likely to refer elderly patients for mental health treatment[16], this underutilization may relate more to prevailing attitudes and lack of knowledge in this age group. Older persons have strongly negative attitudes toward mental health problems and mental health professionals, and overwhelmingly prefer a general physician for treatment of such problems[17]. It has been estimated that perhaps only one in five elderly persons with severe mental health problems recognizes or admits that they need help[6].

Risk factors

Physicians are accustomed to thinking in terms of sociodemographic risk factors for diseases, and such factors, indeed, have been identified for depression. In the general population, these include female sex, low education and income, and lack of social support[5,6,18]. However, one of the strongest and most consistent predictors of depression in all age groups is poor physical health and/or functional disability[5,19]. Although the causal relationships are uncertain — how, and to what extent, does poor health or disability lead to depression, and vice versa? — evidence suggests both physiological and psychosocial influences, as well as some reciprocal effects between these factors over time, especially in the elderly[19].

Studies of depression in arthritis have found that education, economic resources, social support, and coping abilities attenuate the association between disease-related factors and depression[20–23]. In a study of persons with hip or knee OA, 40–50 per cent of depressive symptoms were explained by three factors: education, self-reported disease impact, and age[24]. Specifically, low education, severe disease, and being under age 75 (perhaps because severe OA is relatively more disruptive to the more active lives of the 'young old') were strong risk factors for depression. Importantly, these associations were interactive rather than additive; even at high disability levels, older and better educated individuals were relatively much less likely to be depressed.

Links between depression and OA

Utilization/somatization

It has long been recognized in the general population that, controlling for objective physical health status, depressed persons are disproportionately high users of health care services[8,25]; this pattern also has been found in elderly populations[26] and among persons with arthritis[21,24]. We recently found that, for all except those at the highest educational level, depression was a better predictor of who would be under the care of a physician for OA than pain and disability[24].

Perhaps the most important explanation for the observed association between depression and utilization of health services is the phenomenon of somatization, that is, the tendency to express psychological stress through physical symptoms and to seek medical help for these symptoms[27]. Many depressed persons will not only selectively focus on the somatic symptoms associated with their depression and seek care accordingly but also, for whatever reasons, will minimize or deny the affective symptoms[25]. Hypochondriacal tendencies are much better predictors of OA pain than the rating by the physician of disease severity[28].

Most physicians easily recognize the possibility of psychological influences in patients who have an array of vague symptoms that are medically unexplained, who 'doctor shop', and who have a history of repeated and extensive negative medical workups. However, it is much more difficult to identify those patients who may be amplifying the symptoms of an existing medical condition and/or whose depressive symptoms overlap with those that could result from the medical condition. Nevertheless, in addition to being a great waste of medical resources, the unnecessary testing and inappropriate treatments and medications often prescribed for these patients put them at risk for iatrogenic harm.

Physicians treating OA may not recognize depression for several reasons. First, most OA patients are elderly women, and there is some evidence that this group is especially predisposed to somatization when depressed[29]. Second, there is considerable overlap between somatic symptoms of depression, such as fatigue and restless sleep, and symptoms that can be associated with OA. Finally, although pain and disability, independent of objective measures of disease severity, are strongly associated with depression[5,7] and somatization[25,27], they are also important symptoms of OA. Despite these diagnostic problems, a physician who does not routinely screen for depression in OA patients, or who automatically assumes that any depression must be secondary to the OA and, therefore, only offers symptomatic treatment, frequently will not provide optimal care.

Pain and disability

Much has been written in the context of arthritis about the associations between disease factors, disability, and pain. Although the methodologies and findings of various studies differ considerably and can be confusing in their specifics, researchers have established, not surprisingly, that objective indicators of disease activity or severity, such as radiographs, joint count, and erythrocyte sedimentation rates do not fully explain variability in the two most important clinical outcomes of all types of arthritis: pain and functional disability. Because of this discrepancy, much interest exists in determining what other potentially modifiable factors — including depression — may contribute to these outcomes.

Although the exact amount varies depending on the measures used, most studies have been able to predict, at best, only about 20 per cent of total pain variability and 15 per cent of disability using objective disease measures of arthritis alone[28,30–32]. However, by adding depression, and sometimes anxiety, to the prediction equation, close to 50 per cent of both pain and disability has been explained[30–32]. Conversely, other researchers have examined the extent to which pain and disability, as opposed to objective disease factors, can explain depression. They have usually found that disease parameters alone are very poor predictors[21,23,33], but have been able to predict as much as 30 per cent of depression variability with measures of pain and disability[33].

'Predict' or 'explain', as used in the research context, is obviously different from 'cause', and the above, mostly cross-sectional, studies did not clarify causal relationships. Several recent longitudinal studies, however, have provided this type of evidence in relation to pain. For example, in a sample of 600 metal industry workers, Leino and Magni[34] found that, controlling for the level of baseline pain, depression significantly predicted chronic musculoskeletal pain five years later. A smaller study found support for the causal impact of arthritis pain on depression over a 12-month period[35]. And a third study, using a population sample of 2000 adults, found evidence of both effects[36]. Among subjects who did not have pain at baseline, those who were depressed were more than twice as likely to have chronic musculoskeletal pain eight years later as those who were not depressed at baseline. Similarly, among subjects who were not depressed at baseline, those who had pain at baseline were almost three times more likely to be depressed after eight years than those without pain at baseline.

Whether arthritis pain is the primary problem or is, to some extent, caused or amplified by depression is not as important as the fact that, when screening and adequate treatment for depression are achieved, somatic symptoms can improve[25]. Two recent reviews[37,38] concluded that antidepressants can be beneficial in the treatment of chronic pain, although the mode of action is not entirely clear and much more research is needed to determine which drugs are most effective for which types of pain.

Devins *et al.*[39] postulated that the burden of illness in arthritis — including pain, disability, treatment regimens, and, perhaps, economic problems — leads to illness-induced lifestyle disruptions which, in turn, can lead to depression; this model has empirical support[39–41]. A central point is that different patients may perceive a given level of OA symptoms as being more or less burdensome in their lives and these differential perceptions are dependent on particular psychosocial characteristics of the patient. The following sections describe two of these mediating characteristics: coping resources and social support.

Personal coping resources

Particular coping responses are independently related to depression and other disease outcomes in the context of chronic disease, disability, and arthritis. Perceptions of personal control and competence seem to be very important for avoiding depression. Feelings of low 'personal mastery'[42], 'helplessness'[43,44], and inability to cope[22] have all been associated with depression.

Coping strategies can be categorized as passive or active. In arthritis, active strategies include attempts to control the pain or to keep active despite limitations; passive strategies might involve dependency on others or limiting social activities. Not surprisingly, the use of passive coping strategies has been linked to depression[45].

Particularly maladaptive coping strategies in relation to pain, function, and depression in arthritis include cognitive distortions such as personalizing, over-generalizing, self-blame, 'catastrophizing', and avoiding reality[46–50]. On the other hand, active efforts, such as

information seeking[46,49] and restructuring goals[48] have been associated with less depression and better functional status. The fact that formal education is related to the use of more effective coping strategies[51] may help explain why education is independently associated with better arthritis outcomes[52].

The individual effects of each of the above factors on OA outcomes tend to be modest, although collectively these effects may be significant. However, the cost-effectiveness of including interventions in routine OA care aimed at strengthening self-efficacy and coping resources, or decreasing negative thought patterns, has not been determined. The limited evidence to date suggests that some of these 'cognitive-behavioral' interventions can reduce pain, disability, and/or depression in some patients[53]. It will be important to determine which types of psychological interventions might be most cost-effective as adjuncts to standard OA therapies.

Social support

Social integration and perceived social support are significant predictors of depression in the general elderly population[18], among the disabled elderly[42], and in persons with arthritis[22,23,54]. Importantly, the perceived quality of social support appears to be of greatest importance to persons with arthritis, as opposed to merely the number of social contacts[20]. Fitzpatrick found that maintenance of friendships was a particular problem in arthritis and that the absence of such relationships was strongly associated with depression[54]. Weinberger *et al.* showed that monthly telephone calls by trained non-medical personnel, offering information and support to OA clinic patients, were related to significant improvements in physical health and pain, and marginal improvements in psychological health[55]. Taken together, these studies suggest that arthritis patients who lack satisfying social relationships may be at special risk for depression and other negative disease outcomes and, therefore, that attention to this area by health and social services professionals is important.

Sleep, exercise, obesity

Three other factors may interact with depression in clinically relevant ways in OA: sleep, exercise, and obesity. Sleep disturbance is a symptom of depression[3] and also is common in chronic pain and arthritis[56,57]. However, the nature and direction of the causal relationships here are important in terms of treatment; two recent studies are helpful in this regard. In a two-year longitudinal study, baseline pain predicted subsequent sleep disruption, and the interaction of severe pain with sleep problems predicted subsequent depression[57]. That is, pain apparently caused problems with sleeping, which then led to depression over time. Supporting this sequence, Devins *et al.*[56] found evidence that the extent to which arthritis was seen as interfering with quality of life mediated the relationship between restless sleep and depression. This suggests that restless sleep may lead to fatigue and lessened involvement in valued activities during the day which, in turn, lead to depression.

Strengthening and stretching exercises[58], as well as fitness walking[59], are beneficial in OA, and depression has the potential to interact in several ways with such exercise. Depression has been associated with physical inactivity in the general population[60] and with 'dropping out' of arthritis[61] and other[62] exercise programs. Arthritis patients are often markedly impaired in exercise tolerance, flexibility, and biomechanical efficiency, and inactivity, as opposed to disease-related factors, appears to be the major cause of this impairment[63]. Perhaps of relevance to this, repetitive motor activity can raise brain serotonin levels, and low levels of serotonin are associated with depression[64].

The correlation between depression and disability in a sample of persons with OA of the hip or knee was found to be significantly higher in patients with weak periarticular muscles[65]. The authors speculated that depression may promote a vicious cycle of avoidance of activity, muscle weakness, instability of joints, and disability.

Finally, because obesity is a risk factor for OA, (at least of the knees[66], any relationship between depression and obesity is of clinical interest. There is minimal evidence of an overall positive association in the general population between obesity and depression[67]. In fact, depressed older persons generally tend to lose weight over time[68]. However, the onset of depression in persons who are already dieting may lead to increased eating[69]. Furthermore, a subgroup of obese persons may become depressed when placed on a diet[70]. For these reasons, the clinician is wise to monitor depression when trying to help the OA patient lose weight.

Diagnosis of depression

As discussed above (p.00), the diagnosis of depression in OA patients is complicated by the fact that many of the symptoms of the illness itself mimic depression. The diagnostic criteria from the fourth edition of the *Diagnostic and statistical manual* of the American Psychiatric Association (DSM-IV)[3] are listed in Table 9.8. Experiencing any five of the nine symptoms for a period exceeding two weeks, as long as this represents a change from previous levels of functioning and at least one of the symptoms is either depressed mood or loss of interest or pleasure, qualifies a patient for the diagnosis of major depression[3].

Notably, whether or not they are depressed, many OA patients may suffer some sleep disturbance, weight change, low energy, inability to concentrate, and decreased psychomotor activity related to their joint pain and disability and/or to their treatment. This leaves only depressed mood, diminished pleasure in life, feelings of worthlessness or guilt, and recurrent thoughts of death or suicide as clear symptoms of major depression. Even if these four factors are present, if the other symptoms were all ascribed to OA the diagnosis could not be made cleanly, given the requirement for five symptoms not otherwise explained.

Psychiatrists who deal with patients with medical and surgical illnesses have always struggled with this diagnostic problem[71]. Consequently, there are continuing attempts to refine the diagnosis of depression in patients who come to the offices of physicians with other complaints. A number of screening instruments are available to detect depressive symptoms in patients with OA or other medical disorders[72]; most of these are useful for screening in medical settings. However, all such instruments suffer from the same tendency to confuse the symptoms of other underlying illness with the somatic symptoms of depression[73]. Furthermore, even though relatively high levels of depressive symptomatology have been identified in all medically ill groups, including OA, recent studies in large primary care populations suggest that simply identifying depressed patients at a higher rate does not guarantee improved outcomes because many patients in primary care settings have vague, and often self-limited, depressive complaints[74]. This makes it even more important for clinicians caring for OA patients to understand how they can best sort out those patients who are truly in

Table 9.8   Criteria for major depressive episode

Five (or more) of the following symptoms have been present during the same two-week period and represent a change from previous functioning; at least one of the symptoms is either (1) depressed mood or (2) loss of interest or pleasure:

(1) depressed mood most of the day, nearly every day, as indicated by either subjective report (e.g. feels sad or empty) or observation made by others (e.g. appears tearful);

(2) markedly diminished interest or pleasure in all, or almost all, activities most of the day, nearly every day (as indicated by either subjective account or observation made by others);

(3) significant weight loss when not dieting or weight gain (e.g. a change of more than 5% of body weight in a month), or decrease or increase in appetite nearly every day;

(4) insomnia or hypersomnia nearly every day;

(5) psychomotor agitation or retardation nearly every day (observable by others, not merely subjective feelings of restlessness or being slowed down);

(6   fatigue or loss of energy nearly every day;

(7) feelings of worthlessness, or excessive or inappropriate guilt (which may be delusional), nearly every day (not merely self-reproach or guilt about being sick);

(8) diminished ability to think or concentrate, or indecisiveness, nearly every day (either by subjective account or as observed by others);

(9) recurrent thoughts of death (not just fear of dying), recurrent suicidal ideation without a specific plan, or a suicide attempt or a specific plan for committing suicide;

The symptoms cause clinically significant distress or impairment in social, occupational, or other important areas of functioning.

The symptoms are not due to the direct physiological effects of a substance (e.g. a drug of abuse, a medication condition such as hypothyroidism).

In the case of the loss of a loved one, symptoms which persist for longer than two months or are characterized by marked functional impairment, morbid preoccupation with worthlessness, suicidal ideation, psychotic symptoms, or psychomotor retardation may represent major depressive episode, but in less severe or prolonged cases, the symptom may simply be bereavement.

---

need of treatment for depression, to help their overall condition.

Researchers have studied medically ill patients with various screening instruments for depression and with interviews by expert psychiatric diagnosticians familiar with medical patients[75-79]. These approaches have resulted in very similar sets of weighted criteria for depression in medically ill patients. This technique for modifying the DSM-IV criteria has been used most often for cancer patients, but can be applied to OA patients. Endicott[78] has suggested substitution of psychological and social symptoms for the somatic symptoms that commonly lead to false positive diagnoses (Table 9.9). Comparing her substitutive criteria with the standard DSM-IV criteria makes the diagnostic dilemma clear, and defines the correct diagnostic approach.

These efforts to formulate clear diagnostic criteria for medically ill patients or to develop screening instru-ments for use in this population have been fruitful. However, the most important diagnostic tools of the clinician remain empathy and a high index of suspi-cion; there is no technical substitute for asking patients about their feelings. The psychological (as opposed to somatic) symptoms are crucial to making the diagnosis of depression in the OA patient. It is these issues of guilt, depressed mood, inability to experience pleasure or enjoyment in usually enjoyable things (anhedonia), and preoccupation with worthlessness or feeling like a burden to family and friends, that are most important to uncover. It is essential to remember that even though 10–30 per cent of OA patients are depressed, the remaining 70–90 per cent are *not* feeling that way; being depressed is not the norm for OA patients. Rather, it is an abnormal added burden for the OA patient for which treatment is very likely to improve quality of life at any level of illness and disability.

Table 9.9 Suggested criteria for major depressive syndrome for use with medical patients

A	Dysphoric mood or loss of interest or pleasure in all, or almost all, usual activities and pastimes. The dysphoric mood is characterized by symptoms such as the following: depressed, sad, blue, hopeless, low, down in the dumps, irritable. The mood disturbance must be prominent and relatively persistent, but not necessarily the most dominant symptom, and does not include momentary shifts from one dysphoric mood to another dysphoric mood, e.g. anxiety to depression to anger, such as are seen in states of acute psychotic turmoil.
B	At least four of the following symptoms have each been present nearly every day for a period of at least two weeks. If the medical condition is likely to affect the specific symptom, do not score it — use the substitute symptoms indicated in the footnotes.

1 Poor appetite or significant weight loss (when not dieting), or increased appetite or significant weight gain[1]
2 Insomnia or hypersomnia[2]
3 Psychomotor agitation or retardation (but not merely subjective feelings of restlessness or being slowed down)
4 Loss of interest or pleasure in usual activities, or decrease in sexual drive not limited to a period when delusional or hallucinating
5 Loss of energy, fatigue[3]
6 Feelings of worthlessness, self-reproach, or excessive or inappropriate guilt (either may be delusional)
7 Evidence of diminished ability to think or concentrate, such as slowed thinking, or indecisiveness not associated with marked loosening of association or incoherences[4]
8 Recurrent thoughts of death, suicidal ideation, wishes to be dead, or suicide attempt

C	Neither of the following dominate the clinical picture when an affective syndrome is absent, i.e. symptoms in criteria A and B above.

1 Preoccupation with a mood-incongruent delusion or hallucination
2 Bizarre behavior

D	Not superimposed on either schizophrenia, schizophreniform disorder, or a paranoid disorder.
E	Not due to any organic mental disorder or uncomplicated bereavement.

[1]Fearfulness or depressed appearance in face or body posture
[2]Social withdrawal or decreased talkativeness
[3]Brooding, self-pity, or pessimism
[4]Cannot be cheered up, does not smile, no response to good news or funny situations
Adapted from Endicott[78]

'Subthreshold' diagnosis

What about the troublesome, but very common, patient who complains about depressive symptoms that are either too few or too mild to reach the threshold for a diagnosis of major depression? As discussed earlier, even such mild or 'subthreshold' depression may have an impact on the abilities of patients to maximize their functioning. We are not speaking of patients with simply mild and transient feelings of sadness, but of patients who chronically exhibit, suffer from, and complain about depressive symptoms, but never fully fulfill the diagnostic criteria.

The best approach for such patients remains controversial, but the advent of antidepressant drugs with few side effects now allows the physician to make a pharmacotherapy decision for these people whose depression is apparent, but not severe enough to meet criteria for major depressive episode.

In the past, the side effects of antidepressant medications created a need for clinicians to be very sure of potential benefit before exposing patients to the risks of added treatment. However, as discussed below, the safety and ease of use of medications now available make it possible, perhaps advisable, for the clinician to err on the side of a treatment trial whenever chronic depressive complaints seem to play a part in failure of an OA patient to achieve maximal functioning.

Clinical management

An integrated treatment approach for the depressed OA patient is likely to be of greatest help. At the very least, a psychoeducational and supportive approach by the primary medical physician will allow patients to understand how depression fits into their disease management and promote compliance with treatment recommendations. Studies that have attempted to compare psychotherapeutic approaches with psychopharmacologic approaches, in general, often have come to the conclusion that using both together is better than either alone, but the approach should be cognitive and behavioral, not psychoanalytic. At its very best, such psychotherapy may help patients to rearrange life priorities, come to grips with losses, and regain self-esteem, even in the face of disability.

The question of when to refer to a psychotherapist or psychiatrist is best addressed by simply saying that the majority of depressed OA patients can be treated with supportive and explanatory discussions by their primary physician, in conjunction with antidepressant drug therapy prescribed by that same physician. Only when an adequate course of such treatment has not yielded results, when the patient is severely ill (for example, delusional or suicidal), or when there are obvious situational or personality issues which exist apart from the depression, would referral usually be indicated. When such conditions do lead to referral, it should be to a mental health professional with whom the primary care physician can easily communicate and coordinate a comprehensive treatment plan.

As noted above, attention to the multiple psychological and social issues that are likely to be active in the life of the OA patient may have a positive effect on depressive symptoms and clinical outcomes. Importantly, however, such effects are likely to be modest in those patients who qualify for a diagnosis of major depression, unless the physician utilizes concomitant psychopharmacologic therapy. Historically, the most widely used psychopharmacologic treatments for all depressed patients have been tricyclic antidepressant medications. These have been used especially for patients with pain problems because they have been shown to produce improvement not only in the depression, but also in the pain itself[80].

There has been considerable conjecture about whether such improvement is an artifact of reducing depression (and the self-absorption that accompanies it and magnifies perceptions of pain and discomfort), or whether there are direct analgesic effects of tricyclics. The best current theories are that modification of serotonin levels in the brain is useful in attenuation of pain, as well as relief of depression, and that both may be primary pharmacologic effects[80]. Given that opinion, the notion that serotoninergic tricyclics are the drugs of choice for depressed patients with painful OA may be modified to a belief that any antidepressant that favorably influences serotonin levels should be useful in this population.

This may seem a minor or specialized consideration for the non-psychiatric clinician caring for OA patients. However, this pharmacologic inference translates clinically into a recommendation that, for the vast majority of depressed, elderly patients with OA, the newer selective serotonin reuptake inhibitors (SSRIs) (Table 9.10) are the first-line drugs of choice. The anticholinergic side effects and orthostatic hypotension that plague many elderly patients taking tricyclics are, in general, not a problem with the SSRIs (Table 9.11). Furthermore, with several SSRIs, once-a-day dosing is possible. Given the great difficulties for OA patients (and elderly patients in general) of taking multiple medicines on multiple schedules, these SSRIs offer a distinct advantage in treating depression for such patients.

It should be noted that, even though trazadone, and its newer relative, nefazadone, are seratonin agonists and have some utility in treating patients with chronic pain, sedation and orthostatic hypotension can still be a problem, especially in elderly patients. Bupropion has a favorable side-effects profile but does not act through serotonin pathways directly, and its usefulness in pain patients is less clear.

For those few patients (15–20 per cent) who develop bothersome side effects from SSRIs, perseverance for five to ten days may suffice to eliminate these side effects or make them tolerable. Four to five per cent of patients may not be able to take an SSRI because of side effects such as agitation and 'jitteriness', or gastrointestinal distress. In these cases, rather than switching to another newer antidepressant, as might be done for a young patient with uncomplicated depression, the clinician should consider using the older tricyclic drug, nortriptyline. Although nortriptyline has all the usual tricyclic side effects, they occur to a lesser degree than with other tricyclic drugs. In very small starting doses, and with slow increases to an average dose, in most cases it may be used to advantage in an elderly patient with chronic pain from OA without limiting side effects, and provides an alternative to SSRIs.

By offering care that addresses the emotional as well as the medical needs of our OA patients, we can often provide them with a much better quality of life, regardless of the degree of limitation due to their arthritis. All OA patients have to live with some degree of chronic

Table 9.10   Pharmacology of antidepressant medications

Drug	Therapeutic dosage range (mg/d)	Average (range) elimination half-life[*] (hours)	Potentially fatal drug interactions
Tricyclics			
Amitriptyline (Elavil, Endep)	75–300	24 (16–46)	Antiarrhythmics, MAOIs
Clomipramine (Anafranil)	75–300	24 (20–40)	Antiarrhythmics, MAOIs
Desipramine (Norpramin, Pertofrane)	75–300	18 (12–50)	Antiarrhythmics, MAOIs
Doxepin (Adapin, Sinequan)	75–300	17 (10–47)	Antiarrhythmics, MAOIs
Imipramine (Janimine, Tofranil)	75–300	22 (12–34)	Antiarrhythmics, MAOIs
Nortriptyline (Aventyl, Pamelor)	40–200	26 (18–88)	Antiarrhythmics, MAOIs
Protriptyline (Vivactil)	20–60	76 (54–124)	Antiarrhythmics, MAOIs
Trimipramine (Surmontil)	75–300	12 (8–30)	Antiarrhythmics, MAOIs
Heterocyclics			
Amoxapine (Asendin)	100–600	10 (8–14)	MAOIs
Bupropion (Wellbutrin)	225–450	14 (8–24)	MAOIs (possibly)
Maprotiline (Ludiomil)	100–225	43 (27–58)	MAOIs
Trazodone (Desyrel)	150–600	8 (4–14)	—
Selective serotonin reuptake inhibitors (SSRIs)			
Fluoxetine (Prozac)	10–40	168 (72–360)[†]	MAOIs
Paroxetine (Paxil)	20–50	24 (3–65)	MAOIs[‡]
Sertraline (Zoloft)	50–150	24 (10–30)	MAOIs[‡]
Monoamine Oxidase Inhibitors (MAOIs)[§]			
Isocarboxazid (Marplan)	30–50	Unknown	For all 3 MAOIs:
Phenelzine (Nardil)	45–90	2 (1.5–4.0)	vasoconstrictors", decongestants",
Tranylcypromine (Parnate)	20–60	2 (1.5–3.0)	meperidine, and possibly other narcotics

[*]Half-lives are affected by age, sex, race, concurrent medications, and length of drug exposure
[†] Includes both fluoxetine and norfluoxetine
[‡] By extrapolation from fluoxetine data
[§] MAO inhibition lasts longer (7 days) than drug half-life
" Including pseudoephedrine, phenylephrine, phenylpropanolamine, epinephrine, norepinephrine, and others
Adapted from Depression Guideline Panel. (1993). *Depression in primary care: volume 2. Treatment of major depression. Clinical practice guideline, no. 5* p. 59. US Department of Health and Human Services, Public Health Service, Agency for Health Care Policy and Research. AHCPR pub, no 93–0551.

medical trouble, but when that translates into exhaustion, depression, despair, and hopelessness, the primary care physician can help a great deal more than is often recognized.

References

1. Engel, G.L. (1977). The need for a new medical model: a challenge for biomedicine. *Science*, **96**, 129–36.
2. Stavrakaki, C. and Vargo, B. (1986). The relationship of anxiety and depression: a review of the literature. *Br J Psychiatry*, **149**, 7–16.
3. (1994). *Diagnostic and statistical manual of mental disorders* (4th edn), p. 327. American Psychiatric Association, Washington DC.
4. Blazer, D. (1989). Current concepts: depression in the elderly. *N Engl J Med*, **320**, 164–6.
5. Berkman, L.F., Berkman, C.S., Kasl, S., Freeman, D.H., Leo, L. Ostfeld, A.M., *et al.* (1986). Depressive symptoms in relation to physical health and functioning in the elderly. *Am J Epidemiol*, **124**, 372–88.
6. Murrell, S.A., Himmelfarb, S., and Wright, K. (1983). Prevalence of depression and its correlates in older adults. *Am J Epidemiol*, **117**, 173–85.
7. Sternbach, R.A. (1974). *Pain and depression, patients, traits and treatment.* Academic Press, New York.
8. Tessler, R., Mechanic, D., and Dimond, M. (1976). The effect of psychological distress on physician utilization: a prospective study. *J Health Soc Behav*, **17**, 353–64.
9. Hawley, D.J. and Wolfe, F. (1993). Depression is not more common in rheumatoid arthritis: a 10-year longitudinal study of 6,153 patients with rheumatic disease. *J Rheumatol*, **20**, 2025–31.
10. Cassileth, B.R., Lusk, E.J., Strouse, T.B., Miller, D.S., Brown, L.L., Cross, P.A., *et al.* (1984). Psychosocial status in chronic illness: a comparative analysis of six diagnostic groups. *N Engl J Med*, **311**, 506–11.

Table 9.11 Side-effect profiles of antidepressant medications

	Anticholinergic[*]	Drowsiness	Insomnia/ agitation	Orthostatic hypotension	Cardiac arrhythmia	Gastrointestinal distress	Weight gain (> 6 kg)
Amitriptyline	4+	4+	0	4+	3+	0	4+
Desipramine	1+	1+	1+	2+	2+	0	1+
Doxepin	3+	4+	0	2+	2+	0	3+
Imipramine	3+	3+	1+	4+	3+	1+	3+
Nortriptyline	1+	1+	0	2+	2+	0	1+
Protriptyline	2+	1+	1+	2+	2+	0	0
Trimipramine	1+	4+	0	2+	2+	0	3+
Amoxapine	2+	2+	2+	2+	3+	0	1+
Maprotiline	2+	4+	0	0	1+	0	2+
Trazodone	0	4+	0	1+	1+	1+	1+
Bupropion	0	0	2+	0	1+	1+	0
Fluoxetine	0	0	2+	0	0	3+	0
Paroxetine	0	0	2+	0	0	3+	0
Sertraline	0	0	2+	0	0	3+	0
Monoamine oxidase inhibitors (MAOIs)	1+	1+	2+	2+	0	1+	2+

0–4+ = Relative frequency, with 0 indicating absent or rare and 4+ indicating relatively common occurrence.
[*] Dry mouth, blurred vision, urinary hesitancy, constipation
Adapted from Depression Guideline Panel. (1993). *Depression in primary care: volume 2. Treatment of major depression. Clinical practice Guideline, No. 5*, p. 56 US Department of Health and Human Services, Public Health Service, Agency for Health Care Policy and Research. AHCPR pub. no. 93–0551.

11. Regier, D.A., Hirschfeld, R.M.A., Goodwin, F.K., Burke, J.D., Lazar, J.B., Judd, L.L. (1988). The NIMH Depression Awareness, Recognition, and Treatment Program: structure, aims, and scientific basis. *Am J Psychiatry*, **145**, 1351–7.

12. Prestidge, B.R. and Lake, C.R. (1987). Prevalence and recognition of depression among primary care outpatients. *J Fam Pract*, **25**, 67–72.

13. Keller, M.B., Klerman, G.L., Lavori, P.W., Fawcett, J.A., Coryell, W., and Endicott, J. (1982). Treatment received by depressed patients. *JAMA*, **248**, 1848–55.

14. Zung, W.W.K., Magill, M., Moore, J.T., and George, D.T. (1983). Recognition and treatment of depression in a family medicine practice. *J Clin Psychiatry*, **44**, 3–6.

15. Redick, R.W. and Taube, C.A. (1980). *Demography and mental health care of the aged: handbook of mental health and aging* (ed. J.E. Birren and R.B. Sloane). Prentice-Hall, Englewood Cliffs, NJ.

16. Kucharski, L.T., White, R.M., and Schratz, M. (1979). Age bias, referral for psychological assistance, and the private physician. *J Gerontol*, **34**, 423–8.

17. Waxman, H.M., Carner, E., and Blum, A. (1983). Depressive symptoms and health service utilization among the community elderly. *J Am Geriatr Soc*, **31**, 417–20.

18. Phifer, J.F. and Murrell, S.A. (1986). Etiologic factors in the onset of depressive symptoms in older adults. *J Abnorm Psychol*, **95**, 282–91.

19. Aneshensel, C.S., Frerichs, R.R., and Huba, G.J. (1984). Depression and physical illness: a multiwave, non-recursive causal model. *J Health Soc Behav*, **25**, 350–71.

20. Goodenow, C., Reisine, S.T., and Grady, K.E. (1990). Quality of social support and associated social and psychological functioning in women with rheumatoid arthritis. *Health Psychol*, **9**, 266–84.

21. Hawley, D.J. and Wolfe, F. (1988). Anxiety and depression in patients with rheumatoid arthritis: a prospective study of 400 patients. *J Rheumatol*, **15**, 932–41.

22. Hurwicz, M. and Berkanovic, E. (1993). The stress process in rheumatoid arthritis. *J Rheumatol*, **20**, 1836–44.

23. Newman, S.P., Fitzpatrick, R., Lamb, R., and Shipley, M. (1989). The origins of depressed mood in rheumatoid arthritis. *J Rheumatol*, **16**, 740–4.

24. Dexter, P. and Brandt, K. (1994). Distribution and predictors of depressive symptoms in osteoarthritis. *J Rheumatol*, **21**, 279–86.

25. Katon, W. (1987). The epidemiology of depression in medical care. *Int J Psychiatry Med*, **17**, 93–112.

26. Waxman, H.M., Carner, E.A., and Klein, M. (1984). Underutilization of mental health professionals by community elderly. *Gerontologist*, **24**, 23–30.

27. Lipowski, Z.J. (1988). Somatization: the concept and its clinical application. *Am J Psychiatry*, **145**, 1358–68.

28. Lichtenberg, P.A., Skehan, M.W., and Swenson, C.H. (1984). The role of personality, recent life stress and arthritic severity in predicting pain. *J Psychosom Res*, **28**, 231–6.

29. Berry, J.M., Storandt, M., and Coyne, A. (1984). Age and sex differences in somatic complaints associated with depression. *J Gerontol*, **39**, 465–67.

30. Hagglund, K.J., Haley, W.E., Reveille, J.D., and Alarcon, G.S. (1989). Predicting individual differences in pain and functional impairment among patients with rheumatoid arthritis. *Arthritis Rheum*, **32**, 851–8.

31. Salaffi, F., Cavalieri, F., Nolli, M., and Ferraccioli, G. (1991). Analysis of disability in knee osteoarthritis: rela-

tionship with age and psychological variables but not with radiographic score. *J Rheumatol*, **18**, 1581–6.

32. Summers, M.N., Haley, W.E., Reveille, J.D., and Alarcon, G.S. (1988). Radiographic assessment and psychologic variables as predictors of pain and functional impairment in osteoarthritis of the knee or hip. *Arthritis Rheum*, **31**, 204–9.

33. Wolfe, F. and Hawley, D.J. (1993). The relationship between clinical activity and depression in rheumatoid arthritis. *J Rheumatol*, **20**, 2032–7.

34. Leino, P. and Magni, G. (1993). Depressive and distress symptoms as predictors of low back pain, neck-shoulder pain, and other musculoskeletal morbidity: a 10-year follow-up of metal industry employees. *Pain*, **53**, 89–94.

35. Brown, G.K. (1990). A causal analysis of chronic pain and depression. *J Abnorm Psychol*, **99**, 127–37.

36. Magni, G., Moreschi, C., Rigatti-Luchini, S., and Merskey, H. (1994). Prospective study on the relationship between depressive symptoms and chronic musculoskeletal pain. *Pain*, **56**, 289–97.

37. Magni, G. (1991). The use of antidepressants in the treatment of chronic pain: a review of the current evidence. *Drugs*, **42**, 730–48.

38. Onghena, P. and Van Houdenhove, B. (1992). Antidepressant-induced analgesia in chronic non-malignant pain: a meta-analysis of 39 placebo-controlled studies. *Pain*, **49**, 205–19.

39. Devins, G.M., Edworthy, S.M., Guthrie, N.G., and Martin, L. (1992). Illness intrusiveness in rheumatoid arthritis: differential impact on depressive symptoms over the adult lifespan. *J Rheumatol*, **19**, 709–15.

40. Rudy, T.E., Kerns, R.D., and Turk, D.C. (1988). Chronic pain and depression: toward a cognitive-behavioral mediation model. *Pain*, **35**, 129–40.

41. Katz, P.P. and Yelin, E.H. (1994). Life activities of persons with rheumatoid arthritis with and without depressive symptoms. *Arthritis Care Res*, **7**, 69–77.

42. Turner, R.J. and Noh, S. (1988). Physical disability and depression: a longitudinal analysis. *J Health Soc Behav*, **29**, 23–37.

43. Nicassio, P.M., Wallston, K.A., Callahan, L.F., Herbert, M., and Pincus, T. (1985). The measurement of helplessness in rheumatoid arthritis: the development of the Arthritis Helplessness Index. *J Rheumatol*, **12**, 462–7.

44. Stein, M.J., Wallston, K.A., and Nicassio, P.M. (1988). Factor structure of the Arthritis Helplessness Index. *J Rheumatol*, **15**, 427–32.

45. Brown, G.K., Nicassio, P.M., and Wallston, K.A. (1989). Pain coping strategies and depression in rheumatoid arthritis. *J Consult Clin Psychol*, **57**, 652–7.

46. Felton, B.J. and Revenson, T.A. (1984). Coping with chronic illness: a study of illness controllability and the influence of coping strategies on psychological adjustment. *J Consult Clin Psychol*, **52**, 343–53.

47. Lefebvre, M.F. (1981). Cognitive distortion and cognitive errors in depressed psychiatric and low back pain patients. *J Consult Clin Psychol*, **49**, 517–25.

48. Parker, J., McRae, C., Smarr, K., Beck, N., Frank, R., Anderson, S., *et al.* (1988). Coping strategies in rheumatoid arthritis. *J Rheumatol*, **15**, 1376–83.

49. Revenson, T.A. and Felton, B.J. (1989). Disability and coping as predictors of psychological adjustment to rheumatoid arthritis. *J Consult Clin Psychol*, **57**, 344–8.

50. Smith, T.W., Peck, J.R., Milano, R.A., and Ward, J.R. (1988). Cognitive distortion in rheumatoid arthritis: relation to depression and disability. *J Consult Clin Psychol*, **56**, 412–16.

51. McLeod, J.D. and Kessler, R.C. (1990). Socioeconomic status differences in vulnerability to undesirable life events. *J Health Soc Behav*, **31**, 162–72.

52. Pincus, T. (1988). Formal educational level — a marker for the importance of behavioral variables in the pathogenesis, morbidity, and mortality of most diseases? (editorial). *J Rheumatol*, **15**, 1457–60.

53. Young, L.D. (1992). Psychological factors in rheumatoid arthritis. *J Consult Clin Psychol*, **60**, 619–27.

54. Fitzpatrick, R., Newman, S., Archer, R., and Shipley, M. (1991). Social support, disability and depression: a longitudinal study of rheumatoid arthritis. *Soc Sci Med*, **33**, 605–11.

55. Weinberger, M., Tierney, W.M., Booher, P., and Katz, B.P. (1989). Can the provision of information to patients with osteoarthritis improve functional status? *Arthritis Rheum*, **32**, 1577–83.

56. Devins, G.M., Edworthy, S.M., Paul, L.C., Mandin, H., Seland, T.P., Klein, G., *et al.* (1993). Restless sleep, illness intrusiveness, and depressive symptoms in three chronic illness conditions: rheumatoid arthritis, end-stage renal disease, and multiple sclerosis. *J Psychosom Res*, **37**, 163–70.

57. Nicassio, P.M. and Wallston, K.A. (1992). Longitudinal relationships among pain, sleep problems, and depression in rheumatoid arthritis. *J Abnorm Psychol*, **101**, 514–20.

58. Brandt, K.D. (1997). Management of osteoarthritis. In *Textbook of rheumatology*, (5th edn) (ed. W.N. Kelley, E.D. Harris, S. Ruddy, and C. Sledge), pp. 1394–403. W.B. Saunders, Philadelphia.

59. Kovar, P.A., Allegrante, J.P., MacKenzie, C.R., Peterson, M.G.E., Gutin, B., and Charlson, M.E. (1992). Supervised fitness walking in patients with osteoarthritis of the knee. *Ann Intern Med*, **116**, 529–34.

60. Ross, C.E. and Hayes, D. (1988). Exercise and psychologic well-being in the community. *Am J Epidemiol*, **127**, 762–71.

61. Minor, M.A. and Brown, J.D. (1993). Exercise maintenance of persons with arthritis after participation in a class experience. *Health Educ Q*, **20**, 83–95.

62. Dishman, R.K., Sallis, J.F., and Orenstein, D.R. (1985). The determinants of physical activity and exercise. *Pub Health Rep*, **100**, 158–71.

63. Minor, M.A., Hewett, J.E., Webel, R.R., Dreisinger, T.E., and Kay, D.R. (1988). Exercise tolerance and disease related measures in patients with rheumatoid arthritis and osteoarthritis. *J Rheumatol*, **15**, 905–11.

64. Jacobs, B.L. (1991). Serotonin and behavior: emphasis on motor control. *J Clin Psychiatry*, **52**[12, **suppl**], 17–23.

65. Dekker, J., Tola, P., Aufdemkampe, G., and Winckers, M. (1993). Negative affect, pain and disability in

osteoarthritis patients: the mediating role of muscle weakness. *Behav Res Ther*, **31**, 203–6.

66. Felson, D.T., Anderson, J.J., Naimark, A., Walker, A.M., and Meenan, R.F. (1988). Obesity and knee osteoarthritis: the Framingham study. *Ann Intern Med*, **109**, 18–24.

67. Istvan, J., Zavela, K., and Weidner, G. (1992). Body weight and psychological distress in NHANES I. *Int J Obes*, **16**, 999–1003.

68. DiPietro, L., Anda, R.F., Williamson, D.F., and Stunkard, A.J. (1992). Depressive symptoms and weight change in a national cohort of adults. *Int J Obes*, **16**, 745–53.

69. Baucom, D.H. and Aiken, P.A. (1981). Effect of depressed mood on eating among obese and nonobese dieting and nondieting persons. *J Pers Soc Psychol*, **41**, 577–85.

70. Nutzinger, D.O., Cayiroglu, S., Sachs, G., and Zapotoczky, H.G. (1985). Emotional problems during weight reduction: advantages of a combined behavior therapy and antidepressive drug therapy for obesity. *J Behav Ther Exp Psychiatry*, **16**, 217–21.

71. Robinson, R.G. (1989). Introduction to depression and chronic medical illness. In *Depression and coexisting disease*, (ed. R.G. Robinson and P.V. Rabins), pp. 1–9. Igaku-Shoin, New York.

72. Mulrow, C.D., Williams, J.W. Jr, Gerety, M.B., Ramirez, G., Montiel, O.M., and Kerber, C. (1995).

73. Callahan, L.F., Kaplan, M.R., and Pincus, T. (1991). The Beck Depression Inventory, Center for Epidemiological Studies Depression Scale (CES-D), and General Well-Being Schedule Depression Subscale in Rheumatoid Arthritis: criterion contamination of responses. *Arthritis Care Res*, **4**, 3–11.

74. Simon, G.E. and VonKorff, M. (1995). Recognition, management, and outcomes of depression in primary care. *Arch Fam Med*, **4**, 99–105.

75. Cavanaugh, S.V. (1983). The prevalence of emotional and cognitive dysfunction in a general medical population using the MMSE, GHQ, and BDI. *Gen Hosp Psych*, **5**, 15–24.

76. Cavanaugh, S., Clark, D.C., and Gibbons, R.D. (1983). Diagnosing depression in the hospitalized medically ill. *Psychosomatics*, **24**, 809–15.

77. Clark, D.C., Cavanaugh, S.V., and Gibbons, R.D. (1983). The core symptoms of depression in medical and psychiatric patients. *J Nerv Ment Dis*, **171**, 705–13.

78. Endicott, J. (1984). Measurement of depression in patients with cancer. *Cancer*, **53**, 2243–9.

79. Noyes, R. and Kathol, R.G. (1986). Depression and cancer. *Psychiatric Dev*, **4**, 77–100.

80. Institute of Medicine. (1987). Psychiatric aspects of chronic pain. In *Pain and disability*, (ed. M. Osterweis, A. Kleinman and D. Mechanic), pp. 165–85. National Academy Press, Washington DC.

Casefinding instruments for depression in primary care settings. *Ann Intern Med*, **122**, 913–21.

9.14   Coping strategies for the patient with osteoarthritis

Francis J. Keefe, Susmita Kashikar-Zuck, and David S. Caldwell

Patients with osteoarthritis (OA) vary greatly in their abilities to cope with the disease[1]. Consider two patients, both of whom have very similar levels of OA of the hips. The first patient, a 70-year-old man, reports having severe hip pain, is discouraged, spends most of his time in a wheelchair, and is increasingly dependent upon his family. The second patient, a 72-year-old woman, reports having minimal to moderate pain, is optimistic about the future, walks daily, and is very active socially. In order to explain such variations in adjustment, biobehavioral scientists are increasingly turning their attention to coping processes in patients with OA. Over the past 10 years, a number of research studies have examined coping in OA patients and investigated whether training in coping skills can reduce pain and psychological disability.

This chapter provides an overview of recent studies in the OA coping literature. The chapter is divided into four sections: the first section presents a biopsychosocial model of coping in OA and contrasts it with the more traditional biomedical models of OA; the second section focuses on methods for assessing coping in OA; the third section describes coping skills training and arthritis education interventions used to enhance coping efforts of OA patients; the fourth section highlights a number of important future directions for work in this area.

Conceptual background

OA is typically assessed and treated on the basis of a biomedical or disease model. This model, depicted in Fig. 9.11, focuses on impairment as the primary cause of pain and disability. Impairment in the form of cartilage destruction and changes in bone surfaces can range from minimal to severe. According to the biomedical model, patients with severe impairment can be expected to have more severe pain and higher levels of disability than patients with minimal impairment. Treatments based on this model are designed to correct or minimize the effects of underlying impairments. Thus, a surgical joint replacement might be used to treat a patient with very advanced disease. Alternatively, medical treatments in the form of nonsteroidal anti-inflammatory agents might be used to treat a patient with moderate disease and significant swelling.

The biomedical model (Fig. 9.11) has several problems. First, the relationship between the degree of impairment and the amount of pain and disability is not uniform; some patients with advanced disease report less pain than patients with minimal disease. Second, patients who receive the same medical or surgical treatment often show very different outcomes. For example, two patients with very similar demographic and medical profiles may show quite different outcomes following knee replacement surgery.

The biopsychosocial model of OA is depicted in Fig. 9.12. The major tenet of this model is that to understand pain and disability in OA, one needs to not only be concerned about impairment, but also about psychological and social factors. This model differs in several ways from the biomedical model. First, it highlights the important role that coping and appraisal play in determining adjustment to OA. Coping refers to the efforts that patients make to deal with or minimize the effects of their disease. Coping strategies might include, for example, relaxing, pacing activities, or intentionally calming oneself when upset or feeling pain. Coping strategies that are adopted and used over a long time period can have a significant impact on pain and disability. Appraisal refers to the way in which a patient views their situation and their own ability to cope effectively with it. The second difference is that the biopsychosocial model takes a broader view of disability and considers not only pain and disability, but also psychological disability due to depression, anger, frustration, or guilt. Finally, this model considers the social context of OA; patients who receive support from a spouse or family members may show much better coping and adjustment to OA.

Assessing coping in OA patients

Researchers have taken two basic approaches to the assessment of coping in OA patients. The first

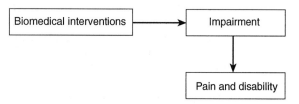

Fig. 9.11   The biomedical model.

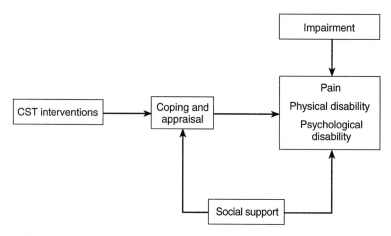

Fig. 9.12   The biopsychosocial model.

approach involves assessing general coping skills, and the second involves assessing pain-specific coping skills.

Assessing general coping skills

Conceptual background

Lazarus and Folkman[2] proposed a general model of stress and coping that has been used to analyze coping in many medical conditions, including OA. According to this model, the relationship between a stressful event (for example, having arthritis) and health outcomes (for example, pain and disability) is mediated by two factors: coping strategies and appraisal. Coping strategies are the efforts of a person to reduce, manage, or deal with stress; appraisal refers to their perceptions of their situation as being potentially threatening/harmful (primary appraisal) and about their own ability to cope effectively (secondary appraisal).

A major tenet of the stress and coping model of Lazarus and Folkman[2] is that the particular coping strategies used by the person are likely to have important consequences for their adjustment. For example, an individual with OA who uses planful problem-solving as a coping strategy (for example, seeking out educational information about their disease in an active fashion) is very likely to have less pain and disability than a patient who uses escape-avoidance strategies to deal with their disease (for example, simply wishing their condition would go away). According to this model, how an individual appraises their arthritis is a very important determinant of adjustment. The OA patient who anticipates a high level of pain and dysfunction, and doubts their own ability to cope, may become much more disabled by their disease.

To measure general coping efforts used by OA patients, researchers have used three questionnaire instruments. These instruments are somewhat similar in that they are based on the same general coping model, but also have notable differences.

1. The ways of coping scale (WOC)

The WOC[3] is the most general measure of coping that has been used to assess coping in OA patients. This is a 66-item questionnaire that asks respondents to describe the most stressful event they have experienced in the past month, and then to indicate on a four-point scale (0 = not used, 3 = used a great deal) how often they have used different strategies to cope with the event. The WOC has eight subscales, each of which assesses a distinct coping strategy. These strategies include confrontive coping, distancing, self-control, seeking social support, accepting responsibility, escape-avoidance, problem-solving, and positive reappraisal. Sample items for each of the WOC subscales are presented in Table 9.12. Research has shown that the WOC is internally reliable, and alpha coefficients for the subscales generally fall in the moderately high range (that is, from 0.61–0.79)[3].

A recent study by Burke and Flaherty[4] used the WOC to assess coping in a sample of elderly women with OA. The study found that the most frequently employed strategy was self-control, for example, keeping feelings to oneself; other commonly used strategies included positive reappraisal and distancing. Correlational analyses revealed that there was a significant negative relationship between the use of escape-avoidance strategies and health status. That is, women who reported that they cope with arthritis by engaging in wishful thinking and hoping were much more likely to have poor physical health and psychological functioning.

The WOC has the advantages of being theoretically based, having wide applicability, and good reliability. It was initially developed for use in stress research, and has only recently been extended to arthritis populations. Further research is needed to determine whether this very general coping instrument is likely to be useful in understanding pain and disability in OA patients.

Table 9.12 Subscales of the WOC, and sample items

Subscale	Sample item
Confrontive coping	Stood my ground and fought for what I wanted
Distancing	Made light of the situation; refused to think too much about it
Self-controlling	I tried to keep my feelings to myself
Seeking social support	Talked to someone to find out more about the situation
Accepting responsibility	Criticized or lectured myself
Escape-avoidance	Wished that the situation would go away or somehow be over
Planful problem-solving	I knew what had to be done, so I doubled my efforts to make it work
Positive reappraisal	Changed or grew as a person in a good way

2. *The Jalowiec Coping Scale (JCS)*

The JCS[5] is also based on the Folkman and Lazarus model of stress and coping, but was specifically designed to be applicable to medical populations. The JCS is a self-report instrument that consists of 40 items designed to measure coping strategies derived from the Folkman and Lazarus model. Patients are asked to rate each item on a 5-point scale (1 = never, to 5 = almost always) to indicate how often they use that strategy.

Jalowiec[5] conducted a study to identify the underlying factor structure of the JCS; subjects included patients having a variety of medical conditions (for example, cardiac patients, arthritis patients, pulmonary patients, and cancer patients) as well as non-patients (for example, relatives of patients, nurses, and graduate students.) A factor analysis of the responses of the patients on the JCS identified three factors that accounted for a significant proportion of variance in questionnaire responses. The three factors were: (1) confrontive coping (for example, thinking through solutions); (2) palliative coping (for example, accepting the situation); and (3) emotive coping (for example, getting nervous / angry). The factors were found to be highly reliable, showing evidence of good internal consistency (alphas ranging from 0.70–0.85) and test-retest reliability (test-retest coefficients ranging from 0.78–0.91).

Downe-Wambolt[6] used the JCS to study coping in a sample of women having OA. This study found that the most frequently used coping strategies were palliative strategies such as accepting the situation and being resigned to one's fate. The next most frequently used coping strategies were confrontive strategies, such as thinking through solutions and maintaining control over the situation. Data analysis revealed that the overall level of coping, as assessed by total scores on the JCS, was related to life satisfaction. Women who reported high levels of coping were found to have much higher levels of life satisfaction than those reporting low levels of coping[7].

The JCS appears to be a reliable instrument that has the advantage of being specifically designed for use with medical populations. Available evidence suggests that there is a relationship between the frequency of coping, as assessed by the JCS, and life satisfaction in OA patients.

3. *The Arthritis Appraisal and Ways of Coping Scale (AAWOC)*

The AAWOC is an arthritis-specific coping questionnaire based on the Lazarus and Folkman model of stress and coping[8]. In developing the AAWOC, Regan *et al.*[8] modified items from the WOC to make them more relevant to arthritis patients. For example, two WOC items ('changed something so that things would turn out all right' and 'bargained or compromised to get something positive from the situation') were changed because in these patients, having arthritis is a given fact that cannot be changed, bargained, or compromised with. These two items, thus, were combined to form the AAWOC item 'modified my plans or activity to get something positive from the situation'. The AAWOC also included items from the Catastrophizing subscale from the Coping Strategies Questionnaire[9] — a pain-specific coping measure we will discuss below. The AAWOC differs from the WOC and JCS in that it not only assesses coping strategies, but also appraisal. On the AAWOC, there are items that assess primary appraisal (threat / harm / loss) and secondary appraisal (self-efficacy).

Regan *et al.*[8] carried out a factor analysis of the AAWOC and identified five coping factors: dependency; adapting; distancing; anger-withdrawal; and expanding thoughts and actions. Table 9.13 lists sample items for each of the factors. The AAWOC has been found to have acceptable reliability; test-retest reliability for each of the factors ranged from 0.45–0.82 and internal consistency reliabilities ranged from 0.64–0.81. The internal consistency estimate for

Table 9.13   Coping subscales of the AAWOC and sample items

Subscale	Sample item
Dependency	Talked to someone who could do something
Adapting	Did something to help myself relax
Anger-withdrawal	Took it out on other people
Distancing	Refused to think about it too much
Expanding thought and action	Thought about a person I admire and used that as a role model

the items measuring appraisal was also found to be good (primary appraisal scale, $\alpha = 0.83$) as were the estimates for internal consistency for the secondary appraisal items ($\alpha = 0.75$–0.90).

Regan *et al.*[8] have presented evidence supporting the validity of the AAWOC. Arthritis patients scoring high on items measuring fear of harm or threat (primary appraisal), and low on items measuring perceived self-efficacy (secondary appraisal), had higher levels of pain and depression. The scores of patients on the coping factors were also found to relate to adjustment. Individuals who scored high on the dependency factor had higher levels of pain and depression, and lower activity levels. Individuals scoring high on the anger-withdrawal factor had higher levels of depression and lower activity levels.

To summarize, the AAWOC is a theoretically based instrument that shows reasonably good psychometric properties. In addition, it has the advantage of being specifically applicable to arthritis patients. Scores on the AAWOC have been shown to be related to pain, depression, and activity level in OA patients.

Comment

The general measures of coping in OA research are based on the Lazarus and Folkman model of stress. The AAWOC was specifically developed for use with arthritis populations and research has provided support for its reliability and validity. Of the general coping measures currently available, the AAWOC appears to be the instrument of choice for use with OA patients.

Assessing pain-specific coping strategies

Conceptual background

OA patients consider pain to be the most common and difficult problem they have to contend with[10]. Not

suprisingly, a major focus in coping research has been on understanding the use of strategies patients specifically employ to cope with pain. Pain coping strategies have been defined as the cognitive and behavioral methods patients use to tolerate, deal with, or minimize their pain[9]. These strategies might include distraction, calming self-statements, or changing activity level. In a chronic disease such as OA, these strategies can have a substantial impact on pain and function. Patients who develop and apply adaptive strategies over long time periods may have much less pain and lower levels of disability. Those patients, however, who develop and apply maladaptive strategies may be much more disabled by their pain.

Assessment of pain coping strategies

The most commonly used method of assessing pain coping strategies in arthritis patients is the Coping Strategies Questionnaire[9] (CSQ). This 44-item instrument measures the frequency of use and perceived effectiveness of a variety of cognitive-behavioral pain coping strategies. The CSQ contains seven subscales, each of which measures a different cognitive or behavioral strategy. Table 9.14 lists the subscales along with sample items. Questionnaire respondents rate each item, indicating how frequently they use that strategy when they feel pain; the item ratings are made using a seven-point scale on which, for example 0 = never, 3 = sometimes, and 6 = always. The last two items of the questionnaire ask subjects to provide two ratings of the overall effectiveness of the pain coping strategies: (1) how much their strategies allow them to control pain (for example, 0 = no control, 3 = some control, and 6 = complete control); (2) how much their strategies allow them to decrease pain (for example, 0 = cannot decrease it at all, 3 = can decrease it somewhat, and 6 = can decrease it completely).

Table 9.15 summarizes data for each of the CSQ subscales gathered from a sample of 51 patients having

Table 9.14   Coping Strategy Questionnaire: subscales and sample items

Subscale	Sample item
Diverting attention	I try to think of something pleasant
Reinterpreting pain sensations	I don't think of it as pain but rather as a dull or warm feeling
Coping self-statements	I tell myself I can overcome the pain
Ignoring pain sensations	I don't think about the pain
Catastrophizing	It's terrible and I feel it's never going to get any better
Praying and hoping	I pray to God it won't last long.
Increasing activity level	I leave the house and do something, such as going to the movies or shopping

Table 9.15   Coping Strategies Questionnaire statistical data

Subscale	α^a	Item rating M	SD	Factor loading 1	2
		Factor 1: Coping Attempts			
Diverting attention	0.84	2.55	1.56	0.83	−0.05
Reinterpreting pain sensations	0.89	1.18	1.50	0.78	0.15
Coping self-statements	0.82	4.06	1.36	0.75	0.03
Ignoring pain sensations	0.78	2.40	1.41	0.70	0.34
Praying and hoping	0.80	3.41	1.52	0.67	−0.44
Increasing activity level	0.78	2.89	1.45	0.79	−0.08
		Factor 2: Self-control and Rational Thinking			
Catastrophizing	0.74	1.29	1.15	0.37	−0.63
Ability to control pain	–	3.56	1.13	0.30	0.71
Ability to decrease pain	–	2.96	1.12	0.06	0.76

*Cronbach's (1970) alpha. Alpha coefficients were based on n = 52 (including 1 subject who was missing data on other measures).
Reprinted from reference 1. This table is reprinted from p. 210 in Keefe, F., Keefe, F.J., Caldwell, D.S., Queen, K.T., Gil, K.M., Martinez, S., Crisson, J.E., Ogden, W. and Nunley, J. (1987). Pain coping strategies in osteoarthritis patients. *Journal of Consulting and Clinical Psychology*, 55, 208–12. © 1987, by the American Psychological Association, Reprinted with permission.

OA of the knees[1]. As can be seen, these patients varied in the frequency of coping strategies; patients reported frequent use of coping self-statements and praying and hoping, and rarely reported the use of catastrophizing and reinterpreting pain strategies. Patients rated the perceived effectiveness of their pain coping strategies in controlling and decreasing pain in the moderate range (2.96 to 3.56).

To assess the internal reliability of the CSQ, Cronbach alpha coefficients were computed for each subscale. As displayed in Table 9.15, these coefficients were in the 0.78 to 0.89 range, indicating that this measure has a good degree of internal consistency.

Factor analysis of CSQ responses revealed two factors accounting for 60 per cent of the variance in questionnaire responses — the subscales and factor loadings for each of these are shown in Table 9.15. Patients scoring high on the first factor, Coping Attempts, are active copers, in that they report frequent use of a wide variety of strategies including diverting attention, reinterpreting pain, coping self-statements, ignoring pain sensations, praying and hoping, and increasing activity level. Patients scoring high on the second factor, Pain Control and Rational Thinking, report they are effective in decreasing and controlling pain, and also avoid overly negative thinking (catastrophizing) when having pain. Interestingly, these same two factors, with nearly identical factor loadings, have been identified by Parker *et al.*[11] in a study of pain coping strategies used by rheumatoid arthritis patients.

We have conducted several studies of pain coping in patients having OA of the knees. Our initial study[1], for example, found that patients scoring high on the Pain Control and Rational Thinking factor had significantly lower levels of pain, physical disability, psychological disability, and overall psychological distress than patients scoring low on this factor. In a second study[12], we found that high scores on Pain Control and Rational Thinking also were related to functional impairment; patients scoring high on this factor took less time to make transfers from standing to sitting, and standing to reclining position. They also walked a five-meter course more rapidly and reported on the Arthritis Impact Measurement Scales that they had higher levels of dexterity, mobility, and household activities. These findings, regarding coping, are particularly impressive because they were obtained after controlling for demographic variables (age, sex) and medical status variables (X-ray evidence of disease, obesity status, financial disability workers compensation status) believed to explain pain and disability in this population.

Further evidence for the validity of pain coping strategies in understanding pain and disability has come from treatment outcome studies. For example, we have found that changes in scores on the Pain Control and Rational Thinking factor of the CSQ are related to short- and long-term outcomes of pain coping skills training in OA patients[13,14]. Patients who showed increases on the Pain Control and Rational

Thinking factor were more likely to show immediate improvements in physical disability[13]; patients who showed increases on this factor during treatment, also were found to have lower levels of pain, physical disability, and pain behavior at six months follow-up[14].

Comment

Research suggests that a focus on specific pain coping strategies may be useful in understanding pain and functional disability in OA patients. The CSQ has been used in a number of studies we have conducted and is now being used in several ongoing studies by other investigators. Available evidence provides support for the reliability and validity of this instrument in assessing pain-specific coping strategies in OA patients.

Coping skills training for OA patients

Over the past 10 years, behavioral researchers have developed and refined protocols that teach arthritis patients how to cope with their disease[13,15]. To illustrate the methods used in these protocols, we will describe a pain coping skills training intervention for OA that we have developed[13]. In this chapter, we provide a brief description of this intervention; readers interested in a more detailed description are referred to a recent chapter by Keefe *et al.*[16]. The present description includes a discussion of the general treatment format, treatment rationale, and specific coping skills training methods. We will then examine research studies that have tested the efficacy of coping skills interventions for OA patients.

General format

The pain coping skills training intervention we have developed is carried out in group sessions consisting of six to nine patients. The sessions are held weekly, for 10 weeks, and last 90 minutes. Two therapists serve as group leaders: a psychologist, having a background in cognitive-behavioral approaches to pain management; and a nurse, having experience in educational interventions. Each session involves the presentation of didactic material on pain coping, followed by a discussion of the material and guided practice with the skills learned.

The small group format is an ideal one for training in pain coping skills. It provides patients with exposure to other individuals who have similar problems and concerns about their arthritis. The group setting is also small enough that each patient has an opportunity to talk and to get individual attention from the therapists. Finally, the group setting provides opportunities for patients to learn from each other; patients who are experiencing success in the use of newly learned pain coping skills often serve as effective models for other patients in the group.

Treatment rationale

The treatment rationale is introduced early in the group sessions and is designed to help patients reconceptualize their pain and to understand that they have a role to play in coping with their disease. The rationale has three basic elements: (1) presentation of an adaptational model; (2) discussion of the gate control theory; and (3) description of skills training.

The adaptational model used in the treatment rationale focuses on the adjustment of patients to their disease. Patients are asked to identify changes in their life that have occurred as a result of having OA and pain symptoms. Specifically, they are asked about changes in three areas of adjustment: (1) daily activities (for example, ability to work, carry out household chores, participate in recreational activities); (2) thoughts (for example, thoughts about self, others, and the future); and (3) feelings (for example, anxiety, anger, or depression). Several points are highlighted in the discussion including: the fact that: (1) the changes identified are common and shared by most of the patients; (2) the patterns of adjustment have usually developed gradually over the course of time; and (3) the changes in adjustment can, in turn, influence arthritis pain (for example, feeling discouraged is often associated with increased pain). Patients are told that training in coping skills can provide a new and more effective alternative to learned patterns of adjustment.

The second element of the rationale consists of a simplified presentation of the gate control theory of pain[17]. The discussion begins with a brief description of traditional pain theories that highlights some of the problems of these theories, such as the failure to explain the absence of pain following injury (for example, in battlefield and sports injuries), the poor correlation between amount of tissue damage and amount of perceived pain, and the failure to account for psychological and behavioral factors that can influence pain. The gate control theory is then presented as an alternative to traditional pain theories. It stresses the fact that pain is a complex experience and that the cognitive and behavioral responses of the patients themselves can influence pain. Patients are asked to identify specific thoughts, feelings, and behaviors that they have found influence their own pain. Coping skills are then introduced as techniques for altering cognitive and behavioral responses to pain and, thereby, enhance pain control.

The third component of the rationale is designed to help patients understand that learning how to cope with arthritis is a skill; like any skill, practice is important. Patients are given the opportunity to practise each coping skill in the group setting, and the therapists provide feedback and guidance on performance. At the end of each session, the patients are also given explicit instructions about how to practice at home, and their compliance with these instructions is monitored at the start of the next group session. Obstacles to regular practice are pinpointed in the group sessions and problem-solving is used to identify innovative ways to overcome these obstacles.

Specific skills training

The coping skills training protocol is designed to increase sense of control over pain by the patient and to reduce the use of catastrophizing — variables that we have found are related to pain in OA patients.

Controlling pain through attention diversion

To help patients control and decrease pain more effectively, they are provided with systematic training in three attention diversion techniques: progressive relaxation training; imagery; and distraction methods. Progressive relaxation training[18] consists of slowly tensing and relaxing major muscle groups, starting with those in the feet and legs, and progressing to those in the face, scalp, and neck. The therapists initially demonstrate the relaxation exercises and then use a relaxation tape to guide patients through the relaxation process; patients are asked to listen to the relaxation tape at least twice daily. Imagery is introduced as a way to heighten relaxation and enhance pain control. Patients are asked to focus on a pleasant image (for example, relaxing at the beach or by a mountain lake or stream) and to try to involve each of their senses in the imagery. They are encouraged to use pleasant imagery at the end of each relaxation session and whenever they are feeling increased pain. The distraction techniques help patients alter thought patterns during episodes of increased pain. One distraction method involves counting backwards slowly from 100 to 1; another technique involves focusing on distracting features of the physical environment such as a pleasant picture on the wall or a photograph of a loved one. To help patients become more aware of the pain reducing effects of distraction, they are asked to record their pain level before and after practice, and note any differences in pain that occur.

Controlling pain by changing activity patterns

Patients are trained in two activity-based coping skills for controlling pain: activity–rest cycling and pleasant activity scheduling. Activity–rest cycling is designed to help patients better pace their activities over the day.[19] Many OA patients overdo daily activities such as shopping or gardening, and push themselves until they reach the point of pain tolerance before stopping and allowing themselves to rest. In activity–rest cycling, patients learn to break up activities that they tend to overdo into periods of moderate activity, followed by limited rest. A patient who reports having severe knee pain after hours of gardening, for example, might be taught to break up the yardwork into 30 minute periods of work, followed by 10 minutes of rest. The activity–rest cycle works best when it is repeated frequently. To encourage repetition of the cycle, patients are asked to keep track of the number of activity–rest cycles they complete each week. as patients become accustomed to the cycle, the amount of time spent in the activity phase of the cycle can be increased, and the amount of time spent in the rest phase decreased.

Pleasant activity scheduling[20] is a second activity-based coping skill that helps patients better manage pain. Many patients with moderate or severe arthritis pain have reduced their involvement in pleasant activities and tend to live very restricted and unrewarding lifestyles. As a result, they have few distractions from pain and often feel discouraged and depressed. To counter this behavioral pattern, patients are encouraged to identify a range of pleasant activities they might enjoy doing. A list of 20 to 30 activities is typically developed and patients are asked to select activity goals from this list on a weekly basis; different goals are set each week and attainment by the patients of these goals is systematically monitored in the group. Many patients report reductions in pain and improvements in mood when they are involved in pleasant activities.

Research on coping skills interventions for OA patients

We have carried out a controlled study testing the efficacy of coping skills training for OA patients[13,14]. In our study, we randomly assigned 99 patients having OA of the knees to one of three interventions: pain coping skills training: arthritis education: or a standard care control condition. Patients in the pain coping skills training condition received an intervention identical to that described above, that is, 10 weekly, 90-minute sessions focused on enhancing pain coping skills; patients in the arthritis education intervention attended 10 weekly, 90-minute group sessions that used a lecture — discussion format to present basic information on the diagnosis and treatment of OA; patients in the standard care condition continued with their routine care. Data analysis revealed that patients in the pain coping skills training condition had significantly lower levels of pain and psychological disability than patients in the arthritis education or standard care condition. At six months follow-up, patients in the pain coping skills training condition had significantly lower levels of psychological disability and physical disability than patients in the arthritis education condition, and marginally lower levels of psychological and physical disability than patients in the standard care condition. Correlational analyses showed that changes in coping were related to treatment outcome. Patients in the pain coping skills training condition, who showed increases in scores on the Pain Control and Rational Thinking (PCRT) factor of the Coping Strategies Questionnaire, had significantly lower levels of pain, physical disability, psychological disability, and pain behavior at long-term follow-up.

Calfas et al.[21] have also conducted a study comparing the efficacy of a cognitive-behavioral coping skills training intervention and a traditional educational intervention for patients having OA. This study found that both the coping skills training group and the educational group had significant improvements in depression, and short-term (six months) improvements in physical and psychological functioning. There was a borderline ($p < 0.07$) tendency for the coping skills training group to show improvement relative to the education group when comparing outcomes before and after treatment. At one year follow-up, however, these group differences were not apparent. These findings suggest that both educational and coping skills training interventions may have benefits for OA patients, but that patients may have difficulty maintaining their treatment gains.

One approach to enhancing the short- and long-term effects of a coping skills training intervention is to combine it with an educational program designed to increase the knowledge of patients about their disease. Lorig et al.[22] were the first to investigate the efficacy of a combined coping skills training-arthritis education intervention for OA patients. Their protocol, called the Arthritis Self-Management Program, systematically taught patients about their disease and also provided training in relaxation, exercise, and a variety of cognitive self-management strategies. Training was carried out in group sessions of 10 to 15 patients who met weekly for two hours, for six weeks; each group was led by two lay leaders who had been trained in the program. Outcome data have demonstrated that this program was effective in reducing pain and improving knowledge about arthritis in a heterogeneous population of arthritis patients, 75 per cent of whom had OA[22,23]. A four-year follow-up of the Arthritis Self-Management Program has shown that patients were able to maintain their gains in pain relief, with a highly significant reduction in physician office visits[24]. The program appears to be cost-effective, in that the savings in terms of medical care substantially outweigh the costs of the program. In fact, Lorig et al.[24] estimated that if only 1 per cent of individuals with OA in the USA participated in the program, the net savings over four years would be $14.5 million.

Taken together, the results of recent treatment outcome studies suggest that coping skills training, or combined coping skills training and arthritis education interventions, can reduce pain and improve the psychological functioning of patients with OA.

Future directions

As we have seen, recent studies suggest that a focus on coping is important in understanding pain and disability in patients having OA. The results of these studies potentially have important implications for future assessment and treatment efforts.

In terms of assessment, clinicians working with populations of OA patients need to be more aware of how individual patients cope with their disease. Patients who report their coping strategies are ineffective, and who tend to worry and focus excessively on the negative aspects of pain, may be at risk for increased pain and disability. To identify these patients, clinicians may wish to gather baseline data on coping using questionnaire instruments such as the Coping Strategies Questionnaire or AAWOC. Individuals who are having difficulty coping could be referred for coping skills training interventions that may prevent the development of maladaptive behavioral and cognitive responses to OA. Periodic assessments of coping may also be useful in tracking the progress of patients over the course of treatment. Our clinical observations suggest that patients who have a good response to medical or surgical treatments for OA, for example, often show an increase in the use and perceived effectiveness of their own cognitive and behavioral coping skills.

In terms of treatment, there a number of important future directions. First, coping skills training and related educational interventions need to be more fully integrated into the management of OA. One obstacle has been the costs involved in having psychologists or highly skilled mental health professionals conduct such treatments. Studies by Lorig *et al.*,[22,23] however, suggest that nurse educators and lay individuals can deliver these interventions in a cost-effective manner. Innovative computer-based formats for coping skills training are also being developed and evaluated[25] and are likely to significantly reduce the costs of this intervention.

Second, methods for enhancing the long-term efficacy of coping skills training interventions need to be developed. The relapse prevention model developed by Marlatt and Gordon[26] can serve as a theoretical foundation to guide therapists interested in enhancing the maintenance of coping skills training interventions in arthritis patients[27]. This model maintains that relapse is a process, and that patients can learn to analyze and to cope with specific episodes of relapse. Arthritis patients, for example, can be trained to recognize early warning signs of setback or relapse and then to apply coping skills in a timely fashion. Through behavioral rehearsal, arthritis patients can also learn strategies for dealing with major setbacks or relapse episodes. Finally, by training arthritis patients in self-monitoring and self-reinforcement skills, one can potentially maintain a much more frequent use of coping skills.

As indicated in the biopsychosocial model presented earlier, coping occurs in a social context. Adaptations to OA by patients affect individuals in their social environment, and the responses of these individuals to the patient can, in turn, affect coping and adaptation. There is a need to explore whether involving family members, friends, or companions in treatment can improve the outcome of coping skills training. We are currently conducting a study of spouse-assisted coping skills training for patients having OA of the knee. Preliminary results suggest that the spouse-assisted training is more effective than an arthritis education — spousal support control condition in reducing pain and psychological disability.

Conclusions

The coping perspective has much to offer clinicians working with OA patients. Research findings gathered over the past 15 years suggest that an analysis of coping not only can help in understanding pain and disability, but that it can also be useful in symptom management. By extending the coping perspective even more fully into clinical practice, one may be able to significantly reduce the pain and suffering experienced by OA patients.

References

1. Keefe, F.J., Caldwell, D.S., Queen, K.T., Gil, K.M., Martinez, S., Crisson, J.E., *et al.* (1987a). Pain coping strategies in osteoarthritis patients. *Journal of Consulting and Clinical Psychology*, 55, 208–12.

2. Lazarus, R.S. and Folkman, S. (1984). *Stress, appraisal and coping*. Springer, New York.

3. Folkman, S., Lazarus, R.S., Dunkel-Schetter, C., DeLongis, A., and Gruen, R. (1986). The dynamics of a stressful encounter: cognitive appraisal, coping and encounter outcomes. *Journal of Personality and Social Psychology*, 50, 992–1003.

4. Burke, M. and Flaherty, M.J. (1993). Coping strategies and health status of elderly arthritic women. *Journal of Advanced Nursing*, 18, 7–13.

5. Jalowiec, A. (1988). Confirmatory factor analysis of the Jalowiec Coping Scale. In *The measurement of nursing outcomes, vol 1: measuring client outcome* (ed. C.F. Waltz and O.L. Strickland), pp. 287–308. Springer, New York.

6. Downe-Wambolt, B. (1991a). Stress, emotions and coping: a study of elderly women with OA. *Health Care Women International*, 12, 85–98.

7. Downe-Wambolt, B. (1991b). Coping and life satisfaction in elderly women with OA. *Journal of Advanced Nursing*, 16, 1328–35.

8. Regan, C.A., Lorig, K., and Thorensen, C.E. (1988). Arthritis appraisal and ways of coping: scale development. *Arthritis Care and Research*, 1, 139–50.

9. Rosenstiel, A.R. and Keefe, F.J. (1983). The use of coping strategies in chronic low back pain patients: Relationship to patient characteristics and current adjustment. *Pain*, 17, 33–40.

10. Kazis, L.E., Meenan, R.F., and Anderson, J. (1983). Pain in the rheumatic diseases: investigations of a key health status component. *Arthritis and Rheumatism*, (**No 4 suppl. 2**), 10–13.

11. Parker, J.C., Frank, R.G., Beck, N.C., *et al.* (1988). Pain management in rheumatoid arthritis patients: a cognitive-behavioral approach. *Arthritis and Rheumatism*, **29**, 1456–66.

12. Keefe, F.J., Caldwell, D.S., Queen K.T., Gil, K.M., Martinez, S., Crisson, J.E., *et al.* (1987b). Osteoarthritic knee pain: a behavioral analysis. *Pain*, **28**, 309–21.

13. Keefe, F.J., Caldwell, D.S., Williams, DA., Gil, K.M., Mitchell, D., Robertson, D., *et al.* (1990a). Pain coping skills training in the management of osteoarthritic knee pain: a comparative study. *Behavior Therapy*, **21**, 49–62.

14. Keefe, F.J., Caldwell, D.S., Williams, D.A., Gil, K.M., Mitchell, D., Robertson, C., *et al.* (1990b). Pain coping skills training in the management of osteoarthritic knee pain: follow-up results. *Behavior Therapy*, **21**, 435–48.

15. Bradley, L.A., Young, L.D., Anderson, K.O., *et al.* (1987). Effects of psychological therapy on pain behavior of rheumatoid arthritis patients: treatment outcome and six-month follow-up. *Arthritis and Rheumatism*, **30**, 1105–14.

16. Keefe, F.J., Beaupre, P.M., and Gil, K.M. (in press). Group therapy for patients with chronic pain. *Psychological treatments for pain; a practitioner's handbook* (ed. D.C. Turk and R.J. Gatchel), pp. 259–82. Guilford Press, New York.

17. Melzack, R. and Wall, P. (1965). Pain mechanisms: a new theory. *Science*, **50**, 971–9.

18. Bernstein, D.A. and Borkovec, T.D. (1973). *Progressive relaxation training; a manual for the helping professions*. Research Press, Champaign, Illinois.

19. Gil, K.M., Ross, S.L., and Keefe, F.J. (1988). Behavioral treatment of chronic pain: four pain management protocols. In *Chronic pain* (ed. R.D. France and K.R. Krishnan), pp. 376–413. American Psychiatric Press, New York.

20. Lewinsohn, P.M. (1975). The behavioral study and treatment of depression. In *Progress in behavior modification: volume 1* (ed. M. Hersen, R.M. Eisler and P.M. Miller), pp. 19–65. Academic Press, New York.

21. Calfas, K.J., Kaplan, R.M., and Ingram, R. (1992). One-year evaluation of cognitive-behavioral intervention in osteoarthritis. *Arthritis Care and Research*, **5**, 202–9.

22. Lorig, K., Laurin, J., and Holman, H.R. (1984). Arthritis self-management: a study of the effectiveness of patient education in the elderly. *The Gerontologist*, **24**, 455.

23. Lorig, K., Lubeck, D.P., Kraines, R.G., Seleznick, M., and Holman, H.R. (1985). Outcomes of self-help education for patients with arthritis. *Arthritis and Rheumatism*, **28**, 680–5.

24. Lorig, K.R., Mazonson, P.D., and Holman, H.R. (1993). Evidence suggesting that health education for self-management in patients with chronic arthritis has sustained health benefits while reducing health care costs. *Arthritis and Rheumatism*, **36**, 439–46.

25. Gale, F.M., Kirk, J.C., and Davis, R. (1994). Patient education and self-management: randomized study of effects on health status of a mail delivered program. *Arthritis and Rheumatism*, **37**, S197 (abstract).

26. Marlatt, G.A. and Gordon, J.R. (1985). *Relapse prevention*. Guilford Press, New York.

27. Keefe, F.J. and Van Horn, Y. (1993). Cognitive-behavioral treatment of rheumatoid arthritis pain: maintaining treatment gains. *Arthritis Care and Research*, **6**, 213–22.

9.15 Joint lavage

Robert W. Ike

Introduction

Therapeutic arthrocentesis of an osteoarthritic joint is usually followed by delivery of corticosteroids. However, measures that remove additional material have drawn interest for decades[1]. American College of Rheumatology guidelines for management of knee osteoarthritis (OA)[2] recommend that referral for joint lavage be considered for patients who have not responded to medical therapy.

The effect of passing fluid through a joint was first noted in Burnam's 1934 accounts[3] of clinical arthroscopy: 'It was in this group of arthritic cases that we had the pleasant surprise of seeing a marked improvement of the joint following arthroscopy'. One patient — arthroscoped to rule out tuberculosis and to judge whether synovectomy or arthrodesis should be performed — had such a good result that '... he begged us to do the same for the other knee', and they did, speculating that improvement was '... due to the withdrawal of the synovial effusion and to the distention and thorough irrigation of the joint'[3]. Capabilities of arthroscopy have grown considerably since then, as have indications for arthroscopy in the arthritic knee. Discussions[4,5] from both ends of the two-decade 'arthroscopy revolution' cite joint lavage as an important component of arthritis arthroscopy that can confound assessment of surgical interventions. Less costly alternatives to conventional arthroscopy now include small diameter 'needle-scopes' for use with local anesthesia and mild systemic sedation, to lavage the joint and assess intra-articular anatomy[6], and other simple techniques for office-based joint lavage. Regardless of lavage method, evidence for clinical efficacy in OA has accumulated, although reasons for the observed effects remain elusive.

Clinical effects of joint lavage in knee OA

Open studies

The first reports to quantify outcome following joint lavage in knee OA were three open trials of arthroscopic lavage[7-10] in each of which OA patients constituted one of several subgroups (Table 9.16). In each report, half or more of the OA patients derived some benefit, coupled with objective improvements as highlighted in a short-term prospective analysis from Moscow[10]. Reviewing 207 arthroscopies showing tibiofemoral articular cartilage defects consistent with OA, Canadian orthopedists[11] found that initial benefits were similar whether knees had been lavaged or subjected to resective procedures, but were maintained in a larger fraction for the latter group. Two open studies analyzed lavage using needle arthroscopy. In his report of 100 needle arthroscopy cases, Wei[12] included 43 patients with knee OA whose visual analogue scale (VAS) pain improved substantially one week and one month afterwards, but drifted toward pretreatment levels by six months. A preliminary report[13] of a study correlating outcome with lavage effluent characteristics found VAS pain significantly reduced one week following needle arthroscopy in 10 patients.

Eight open studies examined joint lavage performed *without* arthroscopy. Watanabe's 'articular pumping' differs from modern techniques by recirculating lavage effluent after withdrawal rather than discarding it; about the same fraction of OA patients were relieved by this procedure as that of an arthroscoped group[7,8].

Eriksson and Häggmark[14] described 10 middle-aged runners whose symptomatic knee OA resolved following arthroscopic lavage. When pain and effusion returned within four months to a year, lavage with a large-bore needle effected relief, and was repeated at regular intervals in some. Arnold[15] reintroduced the concept of closed joint lavage to American rheumatologists at their 1985 national meeting, presenting results with 20 OA knees in 17 patients: half the knees were deemed improved for one to nine months after the procedure. Advanced radiographic OA seldom got better. A larger retrospective review[16] two years later calculated probabilities of maintaining a good result and found the 26 knees with milder OA much more likely to respond (6 months: 42 per cent; 12 and 18 months: 34 per cent) than the more severely affected knees. Intra-articular steroids seemed not to influence outcome. Jungmichel et al.[17] subjected knees to 'joint washing' as follows: local anesthesia, arthrocentesis, lactated Ringer's instillation (40–60 mL), repeated flexion and extension for 10 minutes, then complete evacuation lavage fluid; of patients who underwent an average of five 'washings', twice a week, nearly all considered themselves better, with concomitant improvements in several objective measures. A review of tidal irrigation from the Cleveland Clinic[18] found that 75 per cent of those with knee OA obtained some relief, which lasted longer than six months in 61 per cent. Edelson et al.[19] lavaged 29 knees in 23 patients using a two-cannula system whereby the knee was inflated by inflow through one cannula, then drained by turning a stopcock on the other, repeated until three liters of hypertonic lactated Ringer's instillation had passed through. Most subjects improved on a variety of subjective and objective measures collected over two years, although radiographic stage of OA did not correlate with results. Hyaluronic acid, randomly injected to half following lavage, had no effect. In 17 older patients, Espósito[20] found that tidal irrigation significantly reduced pain one month after treatment and eliminated crepitus in all but two.

Controlled studies

Prospective, controlled evaluations of the effects of joint lavage comprise six reports (Table 9.17). Two trials[21,22] examined joint lavage performed without arthroscopy. Knee lavage performed by British rheumatologists[21] differed from the 'tidal irrigation' method Arnold had devised, using separate cannulas to instill and evacuate the joint, and avoiding intra-articular

Table 9.16 Summary of open studies examining clinical effects of joint lavage inpatients with OA of the knee

Ref	Patients (Knees)	Demographics	X-ray Severity of OA	Lavage Technique	Volume	Study Design	Outcome Measures	Total Dur'n	Time Points	Results Subjective	Objective	Overall Assessment
7,8	76	Not stated	Not stated	Arthroscopic (N = 12); 'Articular pumping' (N = 64)	Not stated; >1L	Retrospective Open	Pain, Dull feeling, Stiffness, Swelling	Not stated		Arthroscopic lavage: 3/12 (25%): 'excellent'; 7/12 (58.3%): 'good'; 0/12 (0%): 'fair'; 2/12 (16.7%): 'unimproved'. 'Articular pumping': 45/64 (70.3%): 'excellent'; 13/64 (20.3%): 'good'; 3/64 (4.7%): 'fair'; 3/64 (4/7%): 'unimproved'	Not stated	Not stated
9	2	Not stated	Not stated	Arthroscopic	≥1L	Prospective Open	Thermographic index, Subjective improvement	4 wks	2 hr, 8 d, 4 wks	1: better; 1: no change	No change	Not stated
14	10	Mean age, 55.8 yrs	'Mild,' 6 'Moderate,' 4	Arthroscopic, followed by large-bore needle lavage q 4–12 mos	Not stated	Retrospective Open	Pain, Effusion	2–4 yrs		Pain improved after initial and repeat lavage	Effusions resolved after initial and repeat lavage	All resumed running
10	44	Age 21–39 yrs: N = 25; Age 40–59 yrs: N = 19; 12m, 32f	K&L grade / N: 0-I 28; II-III 16	Arthroscopic	3–4L	Prospective Open	Pain, Joint circumference, Range of motion, Thermography	7–8 d		Improvement in joint pain — K&L grade / Much / Some / None / Worse: 0-I: 2, 19, 6, 1; II-III: –, 12, 4, –; Overall: 2, 31, 10, 1	Change in knee circumference — K&L grade / ↓0.5–1 cm / None / ↑: 0-I: 12, 15, 1; II-III: 6, 9, 1; Overall: 18, 24, 2. Change in ROM — K&L grade / ↑0.5–1 cm / None / ↑: 0-I: 19, 6, 1; II-III: 12, 4, –; Overall: 31, 10, 1. Change in temp — K&L grade / ↓0.5–1° / ↓<0.5° / None: 0-I: 2, 6, 2; II-III: 1, 4, 2; Overall: 3, 10, 4	Not stated
15	17 (20)	Mean age, 68 yrs; 2m, 15f	K&L grade / N: I 3; II 3; III 4; IV 10	TI (with IA anesthesia)	1L	Retrospective Open	Subjective clinical outcome score	Mean, 5.3 mos		Good/excellent — K&L grade: I-III 8/10; II-III 2/10; Overall 10/20	Not stated	Not stated

5/10 with fair/poor outcome went on to surgery (arthroscopy, total joint arthroplasty)

Table 9.16 *Continued*

Ref	Patients (Knees)	Demographics	X-ray Severity of OA	Lavage — Technique	Lavage — Volume	Study Design	Outcome Measures	Follow-up — Total Dur'n	Follow-up — Time Points	Results — Subjective	Results — Objective	Overall Assessment
11	207	Mean age, 47.8 yrs	Not stated (OA diagnosed by arthroscopy)	Arthroscopic lavage (69 knees) or Arthroscopic debridement, (138 knees) Chondral (C): 72 Meniscal (M): 15 C + M: 51	Not stated	Retrospective Open	Recall of any improvement	Mean, 39.6 mos		% with improvement — at any time / at end of f/u: Lavage 80% / 45%; Debridement C 85% / 65%; M 87% / 67%; C + M 88% / 68%	Not stated	Not stated
16	36 (48)	Mean age, 66.8 yrs; 9m, 27f	K&L grade / N: I 9; II 17; III 4; IV 18	TI (with IA anesthesia), followed by IA corticosteroid injection in 32/48	1L	Retrospective Open	Life table analysis based on patient's subjective outcome, recalled at specified time intervals to provide cumulative probability of 'good or excellent result' (CPGER)	Mean, 8 mos	2 wks 6 mos 12 mos 18 mos	CPGER — K&L grade / 2 wks / 6 mo / 12 mo / 18 mo: I-II 75% 42% 34% 34%; III-IV 55% 14% 0% 0%; Overall 62% 29% 23% 13%	Not stated	Not stated
17	45 (Follow-up reports on only 33)	Mean age, 40.3 yrs; 33m, 27f	'II&III'	'Joint washing' (40–60 mL) 2x/wk; avg 5 washings/patient		Prospective Open	Walking distance, kM ROM Swelling Effusion Pain (rest, exertion) Subjective outcome	6 mos		Before / After: Pain, rest 17/33 / ↓ in 15/17; Pain, exertion 33/33 / ↓ in 18/33	Before / After: Walking, kM: 2.9 / 4.9; Swelling: 29/33 / 12/33; Effusion: 26/33 / ↓ or absent in 4/26	Asymptomatic: 7/33 Improved: 23/33 Unchanged: 3/33
18	47 (52)	Mean age, 68.1 yrs 24m, 23f	Available on 27/42 pts, but results not discussed	TI (with IA anesthesia)	Not stated	Prospective Open (later retrospective f/u)	Pain (VAS): assessed by pt, assessed by physician 50' walk time 4-stair climb Telephone contact (41 pts) Pain relief (now, ever) Surgery Some relief	32 wks (max)	1 wk 4 wks q4 wks, thereafter	Sig ↓ in pain c/w baseline Patient assessment at 1,4,8,16 wks Physician assessment at 1,4,8,12,16,28 wk	↓ 50' walk time at 4,8,12,16,28 wks ↓ 4-stair climb time at 8,12,16,28 wks; Both reductions sig, c/w baseline	Some pain relief: 30/41 Relief lasting > 6 mos: 25/41
12	43	Not stated	Not stated	Needle arthroscopy	Not stated	Prospective Open	Pain (VAS)	6 mos	1 wk 1 mos 6 mos	Mean VAS pain: Baseline 8.4; 1 wk 2.8; 1 mos 4.0; 6 mos 6.7	Not stated	Not stated

Table 9.16 *Continued*

Ref	Patients (Knees)	Demographics	X-ray Severity of OA	Lavage Technique	Lavage Volume	Study Design	Outcome Measures	Follow-up Total Dur'n	Follow-up Time Points	Results Subjective	Results Objective	Overall Assessment
19	23 (29)	Mean age, 58 yrs 20m, 3f	K&L grade N I 11 II 13 III 5 IV 0	2 cannulas; inflow: lateral outflow: medial; (no IA anesthesia)	3L	Prospective Open	VAS pain: at rest, after exertion, rising from chair 10M, 100M, 1 kM walk Running or sports Knee scales (HSS, KS) Knee ROM Effusion	2 yrs	2 wks 6 wks 3 mos 6 mos 9 mos 1 yr 2 yrs	VAS pain (rest, rise, walk) sig ↓ at 1 yr and 2 yrs, c/w baseline HSS/KS pain/function scales 1 yr 2 yrs 'Excellent' 12 9 'Good' 13 8 'Fair' 2 2 'Poor' 2 6 Lost to f/u 4	Mean effusion ↓ at 1 yr; (P < 0.05 c/w baseline) ROM unchanged	At 1 yr: 15 'greatly improved' 7 'somewhat improved' 1 'same' 1 'worse'
20	17	All < 65 yrs (m/f not stated)	'Non end-stage' OA; 4 with chondro-calcinosis	TI (with IA anesthesia)	Not stated	Prospective Open	Pain (VAS) Rest pain Activity pain Pain on passive Tenderness Knee circumference Maximum flexion Crepitus Effusion Walk time (100 M)	1 mo	1 wk 1 mo	Base-line 1 wk 1 mo VAS (cm) 6.1 2.4 1.0 Rest pain 17/17 6/17 1/17 Activity pain 17/17 8/17 6/17 Motion pain 17/17 2/17 0/17 Tenderness 17/17 5/17 2/17 (For all reductions, P < 0.05 c/w baseline)	Base-line 1 wk 1 mo Circumference, cm 37.7 36 36 Max flexion, degrees 95 107 107 Crepitus 17/17 2/17 2/17 Effusion 13/17 0/17 0/17 Walk time, sec 7.35 4.05 4.05 (For all reductions, P < 0.05 c/w baseline)	Not stated
13	10	Not stated	Not stated	Needle arthroscopy	Mean, 1.7L, 'until clear'	Prospective Open	Pain (VAS) ROM Weight of debris obtained	1 wk		Mean VAS pain Baseline 4.3 ± 0.7 1 wk 2.6 ± 0.6 (P < 0.001)	ROM unchanged	Not stated

Abbreviations: pts, patients; (Knees), number of knees studied is not equal to number of patients in study); Ref, reference; L, liter; c/o, complaint of; TI, tidal irrigation; IA, intraarticular; avg, average; ROM, range of motion; kM, kilometers; VAS, visual analogue scale; c/w, compared with; HSS, Hospital for Special Surgery; KS, Knee Society; f/u, follow-up; M, meters; ↓ = decrease; ↑ = increase; K&L, Kellgren and Lawrence; m, male; f, female; OA, osteoarthritis; max, maximum; sec, seconds; hr, hour; d, day; wks, weeks; yrs, years; mos, months; N, number of subjects; q, every; sig, significant(ly).

Table 9.17 Summary of prospective controlled studies comparing joint lavage to other modalities in patients with knee OA.

Ref	N	Study Design	Demographics	X-ray Severity of OA	Lavage Technique, volume, L	Comparison Treatment, (Other)	Outcome Measures	Total Dur'n	Time Points	Results Subjective	Results Objective	Overall assessment
21	20	Prosp, rand	Lavage (N = 10) mean age, 57.7 yrs; 6m, 4f Other (N = 10) mean age, 63.3 yrs; 2m, 8f	Scale not defined (range = 1–3) Lavage Score = 1.9 Other Score = 2.0	2 cannulae; outflow medial; inflow lateral; 2L, no IA anesthesia	Aspiration and injection of 10 ml of saline	Pain: rest, walking, night Sleep Δ, % with Stiffness: AM, immobility ROM Circumference Quadriceps bulk	12 wks	1 wks 4 wks 12 wks	Lavage and Other ↓ Pain ↓ AM stiffness ↓ % with sleep Δ	Other ↑ Knee flexion ↓ Walk time	Not stated
22	57	Prosp, rand	Lavage (N = 29) mean age, 66.3 yrs; 15m, 14f Other (N = 28) mean age, 67.4 yrs; 11m, 17f	K&L grade N I 4 II 8 III 17 K&L grade N I 0 II 10 III 18	TI, 1 L, with IA anesthesia	'Conservative medical management': PT instruction, Counseling, Adjustment of NSAIDs and analgesics	Pain: prev day, after walk, stairs Days of AM stiffness Frequency of gelling ROM Warmth Swelling Tenderness Inflammation 50' walk time 4-stair climb Patient global Physician global	12 wks	1 wks 2 wks 4 wks 8 wks 12 wks	Sig improvement, Lavage c/w Other ↓ Pain: rest, walking, night ↓ Stiffness: AM, after rest ↓ Tenderness	No differences between Lavage and Other	Lavage sig more effective than Other, based on patient global and physician global
23	61	Prosp, not rand	Lavage (N = 37) mean age, 60.7 yrs; 25m, 12f Other (N = 24) mean age, 61.0 yrs;	'Modified Thomas score' Lavage 5.3 ± 2.6 Other 5.3 ± 2.7	Arthroscopic, 2L, followed by PT	Physical therapy	Pain: rest, activity, night Stiffness: AM, after rest Sleep Δ Perceived swelling Walking difficulty ROM Effusion Tenderness Warmth Stress pain Wasting Crepitus Patient global	12 mos	1 mo 3 mos 6 mos 12 mos	Lavage Sig improvement, cf Baseline ↓ Rest pain 2 mos ↓ Activity pain 2 mos ↓ Night pain 2 mos ↓ AM stiffness 3 mos ↓ Sleep Δ 2 mos ↓ Swelling 6 mos ↓ Tenderness 2 mos Other Sig improvement, cf Baseline ↓ Rest pain 6 mos ↓ Activity pain 6 mos ↓ Night pain 6 mos ↓ Sleep Δ 2 mos ↓ Tenderness 3 mos	Lavage Sig improvement, cf Baseline ↓ Warmth 2 mos ↓ Effusion 2 mos ↓ Stress pain 2 mos Other ↓ Warmth 3 mos ↓ Stress pain 2 mos	Lavage group improved to 12 mos; Other group improved to 6 mos; Difference between groups, favoring Lavage, was sig only at 3 mos 14/37 knees in Lavage group had 'severe' x-ray changes and did not improve

Table 9.17 Continued

Ref	N	Study Design	Demographics	X-ray Severity of OA	Lavage Technique, volume, L	Comparison Treatment, (Other)	Outcome Measures	Follow-up Total Dur'n	Follow-up Time Points	Results Subjective	Results Objective	Overall assessment
24	20	Prosp, rand	Lavage (N = 10) age, 38–68 yrs 6m, 4f; Other (N = 10) age, 45–69 yrs 8m, 2f	Not stated	Arthroscopic, 3L	Arthroscopic debridement	BOA scale for symptoms; Muscle torque: quadriceps and hamstrings; Muscle biopsy; Weight of debris removed	12 wks	6 wks, 12 wks	No change in either treatment group	Lavage ↑Iskoinetic torque Debris weight: 0.9 ± 0.8 gm; Other ↑Diameter of type II fibers Debris weight: 2.4 ± 1.9 gm	Not stated
25	32	Prosp, rand	Lavage (N = 14) mean age, 65 yrs; 4m, 10f; Other (N = 18) mean age, 61 yrs; 5m, 14f	K&L grade N: I 4, II 8, III 17; K&L grade N: I 0, II 10, III 18	TI, 1 L, with IA anesthesia	Arthroscopic debridement	AIMS; Active/passive ROM; Swelling; Tenderness; 50' walk time; Patient global; Physician global	12 mos	3 mos, 12 mos	Lavage ↓Pain; Other ↓Pain ↓Physical activity ↓Tenderness	Other ↓Swelling	Patient global and physician global improved in both groups
26	52	Prosp, rand	Lavage, major (N = 22) mean age, 62.9 yrs; 10m, 12f; Lavage, minimal (N = 30) mean age, 57.7 yrs; 11m, 19f	K&L grade, sum of 3 compartments (max = 12) mean for both treatment groups, 4.1	Lavage, major Arthroscopic, needle, 3 L	Lavage, minimal Arthroscopic, needle, <250 mL (minimum volume necessary for visualization)	Physician global; WOMAC	3 mos	1 mos, 3 mos	WOMAC: both groups sig improved c/w baseline; improvement more substantial after major lavage c/w minimal lavage (p < 0.05)	Not stated	Physician global improved in both groups, c/w baseline; improvement greater after major lavage c/w minimal lavage (p < 0.01)

Abbreviations: Ref, reference cited; L, liter; N, number of subjects; Dur'n, duration; Pros, prospective; rand, randomized; mL, milliter; ROM, range of motion; TI, tidal irrigation (see text); m, male; f, female; NSAIDs, non-steroidal anti-inflammatory drugs; sig, significant(ly); BOA, British Orthopaedic Association; AIMS, Arthritis Impact Measurement Scale; WOMAC, Western Ontario and MacMaster University Osteoarthritis Index; K&L, Kellgren and Lawrence; c/w, in comparison with; IA, intraarticular; wks, weeks; mos, months; yrs, years.

anesthesia; 10 OA patients fared no differently that 10 others given a saline injection, although pain and stiffness were reduced in both groups. A cadre of rheumatologists[22] prospectively compared tidal irrigation to comprehensive medical management in randomized patients for whom previous treatment — which had included intra-articular steroids in several, and NSAIDs in all — had been unsatisfactory. Overall outcome for the lavaged knees was judged by patients and by physicians, blinded to treatment, as superior throughout the 12-week study.

Two prospective studies[23,24] of arthroscopic lavage yielded conflicting results. Differing orthopedic practice styles in Nottingham permitted comparison of arthroscopic lavage (performed when referrals came to one office) to formal physiotherapy (undertaken when referrals came to the other office)[23]. Followed for 12 months, the lavaged patients tended to do better, especially regarding pain and overall assessment, but both groups had similar objective changes. For 20 patients with knee OA randomized to arthroscopic lavage or arthroscopic debridement, there were no differences in outcome, and no significant clinical improvements in either group[24], although the multi-item outcome scale used may have masked small changes.

In a landmark study, Chang et al.[25] offered tidal irrigation as an alternative to arthroscopic surgery for knee OA. Less than half the patients evaluated remained symptomatically eligible after a period of observation and physiotherapy instruction. Clinical parameters improved similarly for both groups (Table 9.18), although some of the arthroscoped patients with certain patterns of intra-articular pathology (that is, lateral meniscal abnormalities) seemed to do better than the rest. While failing to provide strong support for arthroscopic surgery in knee OA, these data suggest that lavage by tidal irrigation might be considered as a nearly equivalent, and far less costly, alternative. Further, an evaluation for patterns of intra-articular pathology might help classify subsets of knee OA patients. Interim three-month follow-up results[26] from a prospective trial comparing outcomes following needle arthroscopy, in which either large volume (3 liter) lavage or minimal lavage necessary for visualization (less than 250 mL) was used, indicated that lavage helped both groups, but to a significantly greater degree when a large volume was delivered. A 12-month follow-up was planned, as was further patient enrollment and correlation of intra-articular features with outcome.

Knee joint lavage in crystalline arthropathies

Although the phlogistic agents in crystalline arthropathies are known and easily identified, their removal by lavage is hardly an established part of the therapeutic armamentarium, despite some promising observations (Table 9.19). With crystals implicated in the pathogenesis of OA, an overview of joint lavage in conditions defined primarily by presence of crystals is germane to any discussion of joint lavage in OA.

O'Connor[27] reported a large series of patients with crystals or macroscopic collections of bright, white material identified as 'calcinosis' at arthroscopy. No surgery was performed, although several patients went on to open procedures because of the intra-articular pathology identified. Excluding the operated patients, and reorganizing data for those remaining, four distinct groups emerge: acute synovitis (gout or pseudogout) responded well to lavage; only half the patients with non-inflammatory CPPD and a normal X-ray got completely better following arthroscopy; less than half of the patients with non-inflammatory CPPD and radiographic OA, without chondrocalcinosis, had 'complete relief'; in contrast, all five knees with radiographic OA and chondrocalcinosis got complete relief, although one patient requested a second lavage.

Bennett et al.[28] sought to duplicate this effect with closed needle techniques, using calcium chelating solutes (EDTA or $MgSO_4$). In four patients with CPPD and prior recurrent pseudogout episodes (quiescent at time of the procedure), lavage precipitated a severe pseudogout attack within 24 hours, in all four.

Nevertheless, two subsequent arthroscopy series[9,12] included patients with crystal-associated arthropathies who felt better after the procedure. Observations[29] that meniscal pathology may be common in patients with CPPD and OA imply that lavage by needle arthroscopy might be preferred, identifying intra-articular pathology which could influence further management.

Lavage of other joints

The shoulder

Several interventions described to treat certain painful shoulder conditions resemble those used to lavage the knee. However, OA has seldom been a major component of the conditions discussed. For the 'frozen

Table 9.18 Comparison of outcomes after lavage or arthroscopic surgery in patients with knee OA*

Outcome measure	Clinical, functional, and global outcomes						Between-Group Comparisons	
	Lavage (N = 14)			Arthroscopy (N = 18)			Improvement	Statistically Significant Difference
	Baseline	3 mos	12 mos	Baseline	3 mos	12 mos		
Active ROM (degrees)	111.0	112.0	115.0	114.0	115.0	116.0	Neither group	—
% with knee tenderness improved	—	38.0	31.0	—	47.0†	47.0†	Both groups	No
% with knee swelling improved	—	14.0	14.0	—	35.0	35.0	Both groups	No††
AIMS pain**	6.1	5.4†	5.0†	6.5	5.0†	5.3†	Both groups	—
AIMS physical activity**	5.3	6.3	6.2	6.9	5.0†	4.8†	Arthroscopy	No
AIMS physical function**	1.7	2.0	2.0	2.3	1.5	1.7	Arthroscopy	No
AIMS social activity**	4.7	4.7	4.3	4.7	4.3	4.6	Neither group	—
AIMS depression**	2.6	2.5	2.6	2.6	2.7	1.8	Neither group	—
AIMS anxiety**	3.9	3.9	3.5	3.9	3.8	3.2	Neither group	—
50-ft walk time (seconds)	15.0	15.0	14.1	14.9	14.2	13.9	Neither group	—
Physician's global assessment (% of pts improved)	—	46.0	23.0	—	47.0	41.0	Both groups	No††
Patient's global assessment (% improved)**	4.6	3.6	3.4	4.6	3.4†	4.1	Both groups	No

*Data from reference 25

Abbreviations: ROM, range of motion; AIMS, Arthritis Impact Measurement Scale; pts, patients; mos, months; N, number of subjects

** AIMS categories, on 10-cm visual analogue scale; from 0 (best) to 10 (worst)

†significant improvement over baseline

††comparison of proportions improved, by group, is significant at $P < 0.05$ by chi-square [but results are suspect because of missing observations (Chang, R.W., personal communication)]

368

Table 9.19 Summary of studies examining clinical effects of joint lavage in crystal-associated arthropathies

Ref	Patients (Knees)	Demographics	Clinical Presentation	Lavage Technique	Lavage Volume	Calcinosis	Meniscal Abnormality	Cartilage Degeneration	Follow-up	Outcome	Knees	Comments
27	7, 7	Mean age, 37.9 yrs; 7m	Acute synovitis; CPPD in 6, gout in 1	Arthroscopic	≥ 4L	6/7	0/7	2/7	8.5±1.1 mos (4–13 mos)	Complete relief / Relief, relapse	6 / 1	Relapsed case relieved by 2nd lavage
	4, 5	Mean age, 41.8 yrs; 3m, 1f	Pain/normal X-ray	Arthroscopic	≥ 4L	2/5	1/5	1/5	10.3±3.0 mos (5–18 mo)	Complete relief / Partial relief	3 / 2	2nd lavage performed in one 'partial relief' knee
	9, 10	Mean age, 53.5 yrs; 6m, 3f	Pain/OA X-ray	Arthroscopic	≥ 4L	3/10	5/10	10/10	8.1±1.0 mos (5–18 mos)	Complete relief / Partial relief / No relief	4 / 5 / 1	Complete relief more likely in knees with calcinosis on arthroscopy (3/3 vs 1/7; $P < 0.05$)
	4, 5	Mean age, 47.8 yrs; 4m	Pain/OA + chondrocalcinosis	Arthroscopic	≥ 4L	5/5	2/5	5/5	10.8±1.7mos (7–15 mos)	Complete relief	5	One knee required repeat lavage
28	4, 4	Mean age, 63.8 yrs; 1m, 3f	Pain/OA + chondrocalcinosis (history of recurrent pseudogout in all)	Lavage through 17 gauge intracath (no IA anesthesia)	20–705 mL.	Not applicable	Not applicable	Not applicable	18 mos	Acute pseudogout within 24 hours / Lavage not completed because of pain	4 / 1	Lavage with EDTA (20 mM), 3 knees; magnesium sulfate (20 mM), 1 knee
9	4, 4	Not stated	Pain/chondrocalcinosis	Arthroscopic	≥ 1L	Not stated	Not stated	Not stated	4 wks	3/4 'much better', 1/4 'better'		
12	10, 10	Not stated	Pain/effusion (crystal diagnosis first established at arthroscopy in 5/10)	Needle arthroscopy	Not stated	Not stated	Not stated	Not stated	6 mos	Mean VAS pain / Baseline 8.0 / 1 wk 4.7 / 1 mo 2.9 / 6 mo 5.1		

Abbreviations: Ref, reference; L, liter; mL, milliliter; IA, intraarticular; mM, millimolar; VAS, visual analogue scale; yrs, years; m, male; f, female; mos, months; wks, week; cm, centimeter

shoulder', arthrography is sometimes performed with anticipation of a therapeutic effect from the bolus of dye and fluid administered[30]. Joint distention, sufficient to rupture the capsule, may be required to achieve relief[31], while the effect of added corticosteroids remains unsettled[32,33] This 'brisement' with repeated large-volume shoulder injections[34], whether done after arthrography or in the clinic, resembles lavage in which removal of instilled fluid is neglected. With arthroscopic distention proposed for treatment of the frozen shoulder[35,36] consideration to other methods of joint lavage seems warranted.

Calcific tendinitis can be treated by instilling fluid through a large needle inserted into the shoulder region, affected to break up and remove the calcific deposits[37]. This intervention has not been compared to modern arthroscopic approaches, which usually resect tissues[38], but might be considered as an alternative.

Lavage in the treatment of severe secondary shoulder OA with effusion has been described[39]; for two patients, the pain and effusion of 'Milwaukee shoulder' syndrome was palliated by sequential tidal irrigations done three to four months apart, with remission lasting nearly a year, and relapse in one patient treated successfully with another lavage.

The hip

Hip arthrography, which delineates a small joint space and thick capsule in some cases of OA, has been used for treatment[40,41]. In an open trial of distention arthrography, Spector[40] found two-thirds of his patients reporting good to excellent results lasting three months. Whether indoprofen or saline was instilled, hip distention palliated symptoms in a prospective trial[41], with about 50 per cent sustaining relief for three months, but only two remaining asymptomatic. Joint distention did not, predictably, relieve hip pain and restricted motion in a prospective trial[42] comparing pump-directed infusion of saline (20 ml, plus whatever volume raised intracapsular pressure to 1600 mm Hg) with a sham periarticular injection of saline (20 ml), as no treatment-related differences in outcome for 38 patients (including 22 with normal X-rays) were detected after three months; however, not all patients had capsular constriction (the component expected to respond to joint distention), since the median injected volume was 20 ml — similar to that of the normal hip[43]. Pain in otherwise normal hips, with a constricted joint capsule at arthrography, has been relieved

by forceful reexpansion followed by corticosteroid instillation[44].

Arthroscopy of the hip joint is a technically difficult procedure with limited indications[45]. Arthroscopic techniques have been applied to hip OA, with joint lavage cited[46] as one component contributing to symptom relief. However, outcome following arthroscopy of hip OA performed without 'debridement' cannot be discerned from published accounts.

Theoretical questions regarding joint lavage

How might lavage work in OA?

Features in OA that could be altered by joint lavage are as follows:

(1) removal of cartilage debris ('wear particles', macromolecules);
    (a) present in OA synovium
    (b) correlate with articular cartilage lesions
    (c) induce release of destructive compounds *in vitro*
    (d) produce OA-like lesions in animal models;

(2) removal of crystals;

(3) temporary changes
    (a) cooling
    (b) dilution of degradative compounds;

(4) disruption of intra-articular adhesions, capsular fibrosis;

(5) placebo effect.

Some interruption of the interaction between synovium and disintegrating articular cartilage seems the most likely mechanism; several lines of indirect evidence delineate this interaction.

OA joint fluid commonly contains cartilage fragments[47–49] — or 'wear particles'[50–52] — of sizes and shapes correlating with articular cartilage lesions[53–57]. Meniscal lesions generate long strands lacking cellular detail, whereas irregular fragments with chondrocyte nuclei arise from disrupted hyaline cartilage, the area and depth of damage proportionate to their size and number[56]. Ferrography, a technique for analyzing lubricating fluids to detect machine wear, has been used to study joint wear by examining particles from joint lavage resuspended in magnetizing solution and pumped across a microscope slide in a strong magnetic field[50]. This technique has detected 'microdamage' not seen by arthroscopy[57]. However, gross inspection of synovial fluid is usually adequate to detect wear particles (Fig. 9.13)[54].

The relationship between cartilage components and synovium was elegantly described by Hultén and Gellerstedt[58] in 1940, and the basic precepts of their model endure. Examining operative and autopsy material from knee joints with various degrees of cartilage degeneration, they surmised that fragments of disrupted articular cartilage passed off to 'quiet nooks and corners of the joint' — usually the suprapatellar recess and peripatellar areas — to become embedded in synovium and, eventually, transformed. Further, the synovial reaction followed a characteristic pattern, with hyperemia, histiocytosis, and an increase in synovial connective tissue gradually producing a fibroplastic synovitis. The structure of embedded fragments was altered beyond recognition within a few days, often leaving no traces of cartilage debris in later stages.

Horwitz[59] described five cases of early tabetic arthropathy diagnosed or substantiated by finding cartilage and bone shards in synovium, a feature of all established neuropathic joints surveyed but of only a few, far advanced OA cases. In surgical specimens from severe hip OA, Lloyd-Roberts[60] found cartilage shards surrounded by fibrotic synovium in 23 of 25 patients. Knee synovium from autopsy contained cartilage shards in 11 out of 30 individuals with advanced OA by inspection, with synovitis in all 30[61]. However, cartilage shards were not found in synovium from arthroscopy in 'early' OA (minimally abnormal radiographs and short duration symptoms), despite deep cartilage ulcers in some cases and synovitis in many[62].

Nevertheless, the phlogistic properties of cartilage fragments have been demonstrated in several systems. *In vitro* exposure to cartilage fragments induces release of neutral proteases from cultured monocytes and synoviocytes[63], and generates kinin-like activity from platelet-deficient plasma[64]. The range of synovial and cartilage pathology in knees of experimental animals injected with variously prepared cartilage derivatives approximates that of naturally-occurring human OA. Hultén and Gellerstedt[58] found mild transient synovitis after single injections of hyaline cartilage homogenate, whereas marked synovitis with thickening of the joint capsule and atrophy of adjacent muscles followed injections repeated once or twice a month for six to seven months. More than 20 years later, Chrisman *et al.*[65] induced synovitis in dogs by repeatedly injecting homogenates of autologous costal cartilage. Knees receiving weekly injections for six months or less were grossly indistinguishable from saline-injected controls, but developed chronic synovitis with some fibrosis.

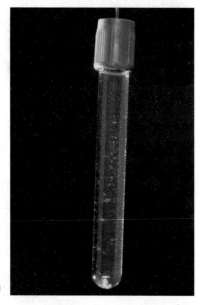

(a)

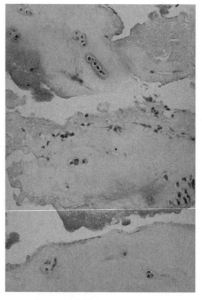

(b)

Fig. 9.13 (a), (b)   Cartilaginous debris from patients with knee OA: (a) debris-laden synovial fluid; (b) sediment from effluent collected during tidal irrigation; note irregularly shaped fragments with 'brood clusters' of proliferated chondrocyte nuclei. (H and E x200. Courtesy of W.J. Arnold, MD)

Injections given for 9 to 12 months led to restricted joint motion, more extensive synovial fibrosis, and marginal ridges and exostoses on X-rays and gross inspection. Thrice-weekly injections of allogenic cartilage homogenates produced remarkably consistent time-dependent changes in rabbit knee joints[66]. After one month, a joint effusion, mild histologic features of synovitis, and slightly raised degradative enzyme activity in *ex vivo* explants of synovium were detectable. By two months, joint inflammation was clinically detectable, synovitis was worse, and activity of neutral proteases and acid hydrolases elaborated by cultured synovium was markedly elevated. Hyaline cartilage showed histologic changes at three months, and fissuring of deeper layers, along with surface pitting and gross discoloration, at five months. Despite the vigorous local inflammatory response, no systemic humoral or cellular immune response to the injected particles occurred.

Certain macromolecular components of cartilage can induce a synovial reaction. Dogs, receiving weekly intra-articular injections of either autologous dermal collagen or a chondromucoprotein from calf nasal cartilage, developed synovitis with the latter preparation after two to four months[67]. Rabbits, given 10 to 15 weekly intra-articular injections of protein-free cartilage extracts, developed more pronounced synovitis when the source contained proteoglycans typical of 'aging' cartilage (keratan sulfate and chondroitin sulfate-C from shark cartilage, compared with chondroitin sulfate-A rich bovine nasal cartilage)[67]. Twenty years later, Evans[68] found similar consequences of intra-articular proteoglycan injections in rabbits, whether the source was adult rabbit cartilage extract or highly purified monomers from bovine nasal cartilage: synovial hypertrophy and inflammation, erosion of articulating surfaces, and loss of cartilage metachromasia. If comparable mechanisms operate in clinical human OA, synovium could become inflamed in response to components of degenerating articular cartilage, yet not contain identifiable cartilage particles.

Other components found in OA joint fluid might provoke a synovial reaction. It has been proposed that crystals[61] — found in OA far more frequently than polarized light microscopy would estimate[69] — contribute to OA synovitis; thus, their removal could ameliorate inflammation. CPPD crystals were found in the lavage effluent from 7 out of 10 knees undergoing arthroscopy for knee OA[70], although only one knee had chondrocalcinosis on X-ray. Furthermore, for all but one knee, crystals were more abundant after the

two or three liters had passed through the joint. Red blood cells can evoke a synovial reaction[71], and chronic destructive synovitis can follow repeated intra-articular bleeding, as in the hemophiliac patient[72]. While frank hemarthrosis is uncommon in knee OA[73], some red blood cells are always present in OA synovial fluid and would be among the elements removed by lavage.

Thus, the synovitis of OA almost certainly develops in response to several different factors (Fig. 9.14). Although most of these factors would be altered by joint lavage, the specific changes that predict clinical response have yet to be identified. The decrement in pain reported by 10 patients with knee OA, one week after arthroscopic lavage, correlated with the amount of debris removed[13], — a finding that could be used to predict response if confirmed in larger cohorts.

Other temporary changes in the joint milieu following joint lavage — including cooling and reduction in concentration of degradative enzymes and cytokines — could have a short-term effect on symptoms, although longer term effects are uncertain. Changes in the joint capsule which reduce joint compliance have been described[74,75] in some patients with knee OA, and could sensitize the capsule to pain and enhance reflex muscle inhibition[76] produced by a joint effusion. Joint overdistention, to disrupt intra-articular adhesions and capsular fibrosis, has been used to treat pain in hip OA[40,41]. In a multicenter trial[22] comparing joint lavage with medical management of knee OA, many investigators noted that the volume accepted by some knees increased as the lavage progressed.

Whether joint lavage exerts its effect, at least in part, by a placebo mechanism cannot be satisfactorily determined by studies performed to date. The placebo effect of any intervention involving puncture of a symptomatic knee[77] can never be completely discounted. Blinding subjects to treatment in any studies that would compare joint lavage to a sham procedure might be difficult, as a subject informed of the distention–irrigation mechanics involved could probably distinguish any sham procedure from 'true' joint lavage.

Could lavage harm the joint?

During joint lavage, cartilage and synovium are exposed to fluids with different physiochemical properties than normal synovial fluid. Studies of what occurs when these tissues are bathed in various irrigating solutions show potential for harm. Radiolabeled sulfate incorporation by bovine cartilage samples *in vitro* — an assessment of metabolic activity — was almost com-

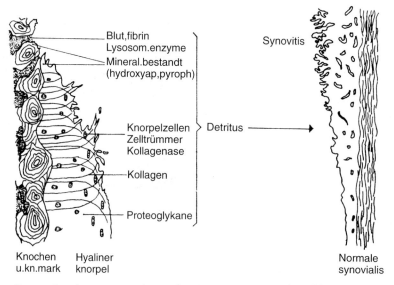

Fig. 9.14 Schematic of interactions between synovium and various components released from disintegrating joint surface in OA, as envisioned by Jungmichel *et al.*[17]. (German– English translations: *blut*, blood; *mineral. bestandt.*, mineral composition; *knorpelzellen*, chondrocyte; *zelltrümmer*, debris; *knochen u. kn. mark*; bone and bone marrow; *hyaliner knorpel*, hyaline cartilage.)

pletely suppressed by normal saline, but progressed nearly as well in lactated Ringer's as in tissue culture medium[78]. However, similar assays on explants of rabbit cartilage taken from knees continuously irrigated for two hours were unaffected by agents used (saline, Ringer's, or water)[79]. Scanning electron microscopy demonstrated irrigant-induced damage in non-weight bearing cartilage exposed to one of five irrigating solutions during arthroscopy. Changes were worst after water irrigation, but barely detectable after 1.5 percent glycine or 2.6 percent glycerol, with alterations from Ringer's lactate worse than those from saline[80]. Extraction of matrix proteoglycan can alter cartilage structure. More proteoglycan was eluted from samples of bovine articular cartilage by ionic media (saline, Ringer's) than by non-ionic media (mannitol, sorbitol, glycerol, Dextran, or glycine); the difference between elution rates was more pronounced when intact rat femoral heads were used[81]. Cartilage ultrastructure (and, in a similar comparison study[82], cartilage firmness) was altered only after exposure to ionic media.

Contrary to these *in vitro* findings, articular cartilage in lavaged knees of intact living animals seems remarkably resilient. Cartilage from rabbit knees irrigated through indwelling catheters for 1–14 days was depleted of matrix proportionate to irrigation time. However, animals allowed to run freely for six months

after irrigation lost no knee cartilage matrix when compared to controls[83]. Cartilage and synovium from rabbit knees irrigated for 20 minutes with saline, water, or one of several non-ionic solutions showed subtle changes by electron microscopy, but were indistinguishable from controls 3–4 weeks after irrigation[84]. Further investigations will be needed to determine whether human articular cartilage, especially in OA, is adversely affected by the solutions used for lavage, and whether differential effects occur according to type of solution used.

Practical matters regarding joint lavage

Technique

The clinical studies reviewed describe several methods for joint lavage, with main differences derived from: (1) whether arthroscopy is done; (2) whether single or multiple entry sites are used; and (3) characteristics of lavaging fluid.

Conventional arthroscopy, done in a sterile operating room, minimizes infection risk and provides lavage quicker than other available techniques, as fluids flow through large-bore cannulae, often assisted by mechanical pumps. Using smaller bore ('needle') arthroscopes, it is feasible to inspect and lavage a knee, at a lower cost, in a procedure room or office setting; lavage proceeds slower and often uses less fluid, as 250–1000 mL is usually sufficient to provide clear viewing. Because lavage fluid flows in through the arthroscope, the tibiofemoral compartments are thoroughly irrigated. Pressure gradients carry any debris to the suprapatellar space to be evacuated through an outflow cannula; lavage techniques that use only a single cannula in the suprapatellar pouch probably do not achieve this. Arthroscopically directed interventions that might be used to alter intra-articular pathology are not as readily available to the needle arthroscopist, although these capabilities are expanding[85,86].

Techniques devised to lavage the knee joint without arthroscopy can be mastered by any practitioner who is competent at arthrocentesis; 'Tidal irrigation' is among the simplest of these, and has received the most attention[15,16,18,20,22,25,39]. After skin preparation and draping, an entry site at the superolateral border of the patella is palpated, then instilled with lidocaine to anesthetize skin, subcutaneaous tissue, and joint capsule; arthrocentesis follows, and 30–50 mL of longer acting anesthetic (for example, bupivicaine) is instilled. A larger bore irrigating needle is placed into the joint through the anesthetized tract (this author uses an 11 g Vere's needle, which has a sharp removable trochar and an on-off valve on the proximal end of the cannula), then attached to an appropriate closed system (Fig. 9.15) to evacuate the joint and reinstill irrigating fluid. The instilled fluid is then withdrawn and the process repeated until the desired volume of fluid has been used. The entire procedure takes 30–45 minutes for a one liter lavage, and the patient is permitted to ambulate immediately afterward. Two-cannula techniques have been described[1,19,21] for more rapid and higher volume lavage.

Commonly available physiologic fluids are usually chosen for lavage, with lactated Ringer's and normal saline predominating while aforementioned studies on the effects of various fluids on articular cartilage await clinical confirmation. Necessary volume for optimal effect is currently being tested in a prospective trial[26]. Although it has been proposed[87] that joint distention with cooler fluid exerts superior effects for some conditions, most practitioners use fluids at room temperature.

Complications

The rates for various complications that might follow joint lavage for knee OA have not been extensively

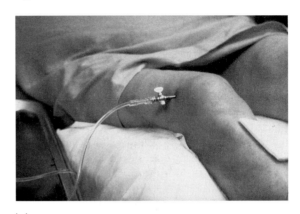

(a)

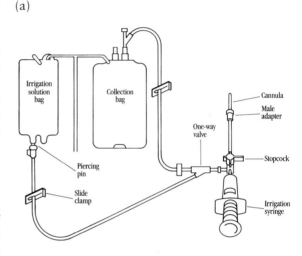

(b)

Fig. 9.15 Joint lavage by tidal knee irrigation. (a) Patient's right knee penetrated with sterile 11 gauge Vere's needle after skin preparation, local anesthetic to skin and subcutaneous tissues to capsule, and distention of knee with long-acting anesthetic (bupivicaine); Vere's needle connected to closed system for delivery of saline and collection of effluent. (b) Schematic of tidal irrigation kit (Abbott Laboratories, Abbott Park, IL, USA); no longer commercially available, but can be duplicated using conventional intravenous fluid management supplies.

documented. In the reports of arthroscopic lavage reviewed previously, no major complications were mentioned. The large surveys[88–91] of complication rates for knee arthroscopy have focused mainly on surgical procedures and have not analyzed subgroups in which lavage might have been the only intervention. Thus, the occurrence and incidence of recognized complications — hemarthrosis, joint infection, venous thrombosis, reflex sympathetic dystrophy, nerve palsies, ligament damage, and joint rupture — cannot be extrapolated to lavage of the OA knee done by conventional arthroscopy.

Overall rate of complications following needle arthroscopy was 1.7 per cent in a mail survey[92] of 16 physicians recounting 582 cases, and 11.5 per cent in a retrospective review[93] of four year's experience at two centers. Minor complications included cellulitis, hemarthrosis, other effusions requiring arthrocentesis, vasovagal reactions, flare of crystal arthropathy, fluid extravasation, allergic reactions to skin preparation, and synovial sinus formation; most events occurred once or twice in each series. Intra-articular corticosteroids and non-compliance with postarthroscopy directions probably contributed to the sole major complication: culture-negative septic arthritis occurring two weeks after arthroscopy for severe knee OA[93].

Some local discomfort following knee arthroscopy is expected. Of 84 patients with knee OA who completed a questionnaire two weeks after needle arthroscopy with lavage, some (25 per cent) had no pain, but 71 per cent had sufficient pain to hamper their daily activities, often for a few days (less than one day, 44 per cent; less than two days, 55 per cent; less than one week, 79 per cent); nevertheless, 90 per cent of the patients tolerated the procedure well, and 82 per cent considered their joint symptoms improved[94].

The complications of joint lavage done without arthroscopy have not been delineated by formal survey, but reports of clinical use have not mentioned any. Problems related to joint puncture with a large-bore instrument (pain at puncture site, sinus tract formation, cellulitis) and joint distention with fluid under pressure (vasovagal reaction, fluid extravasation, joint rupture) might be expected, but in 10 years of clinical use at this author's institution, these complications have been rare, and some (infection, sinus formation) have never occurred. Because joint proprioception is impaired by intra-articular anesthesia, patients are discouraged from driving for six hours after lavage.

Regardless of lavage technique used, the most common technical problem involves removing all instilled fluid. The synovium absorbs fluid at a rate measured as 1.1–7.1 mL per minute (mean = 4.1 mL per min.) in a study of 35 young men[95]. Fluid can extravasate into soft tissues along puncture tracts, and can be forced into a popliteal cyst when a patent connection exists. The intra-articular pressure prompting these events rises when the knee approaches 90° flexion[96], a common position when the patient is seated while undergoing arthroscopy. Unless the system used

for lavage provides a route for spontaneous escape of fluid under pressure, the volume of fluid in the joint should be reduced when moved from a position of maximal compliance (20–30° flexion) to full extension or to greater flexion, lest spontaneous joint rupture occur. Removal of fluid can be impeded when the outflow cannula becomes clogged with tissue or debris, or comes to rest in a position where tissue can collapse around it, such as the uppermost reaches of the suprapatellar pouch or under a synovial plica. Although lavage effluent volume rarely matches the total infused into the joint, the retained fluid seldom causes more than a temporary cosmetic problem, even when extruded into a popliteal cyst, as physiologic solutions such as saline are not phlogistic and are usually reabsorbed within a few days.

Summary and conclusions

Palliation of knee OA symptoms by joint lavage — whether delivered by arthroscopy or closed needle techniques — has been observed by several generations of arthroscopists and documented in a number of uncontrolled trials. Prospective controlled investigations suggest the 'lavage effect' is real and worth considering for non-end stage knee OA that has not responded to comprehensive conventional medical management, possibly delivered by lower-cost office-based alternatives to conventional arthroscopy, such as 'needle' arthroscopy and tidal irrigation. Other conditions of the hip and shoulder have occasionally been approached with lavage-like interventions that might be adaptable to office practice. Therapeutic effects of lavage on the OA joint could derive from several mechanisms — most likely, removing potentially phlogistic cartilage detritus of various forms. Promising preliminary reports from several ongoing prospective trials designed to determine the clinical, microscopic, and biochemical correlates of therapeutic outcome following joint lavage have recently appeared. In addition, two large clinical trials involving tidal irrigation are ongoing, compared with sham lavage in one study (Bradley, personal communication), and to arthroscopic surgery, as well as lavage by needle arthroscopy, in the other (Chang, personal communication). Results from these studies should shed light both on proper patient selection for joint lavage and on mechanisms of pain production and relief in OA.

References

1. Ayral, X. and Dougados, M. (1995). Joint lavage. *Revue du Rhumatisme (English Edition)*, **62**, 281–7.
2. Hochberg, M.C., Altman, R.D., Brandt, K.D., *et al.* (1995). Guidelines for the medical management of osteoarthritis. Part II: osteoarthritis of the knee. *Arthritis and Rheumatism*, **38**, 1541–6.
3. Burman, M.S., Finkelstein, F.H., and Mayer, L. (1934). Arthroscopy of the knee joint. *Journal of Bone and Joint Surgery*, **16**, 255–68.
4. Jackson, R.W. and Abe I. (1972). The role of arthroscopy in the management of disorders of the knee joint. *Journal of Bone and Joint Surgery (British)*, **54B**, 310–22.
5. Burks, R.T. (1990). Arthroscopy and degenerative arthritis of the knee: a review of the literature. *Arthroscopy*, **6**, 43–7.
6. O'Rourke, K.S. and Ike, R.W. (1994). Diagnostic arthroscopy in the arthritis patient. *Rheumatic Disease Clinics of North America*, **20**, 321–42.
7. Watanabe, M. (1949). Articular pumping. *Journal of the Japanese Orthopedic Surgical Society*, **24**, 30–2.
8. Watanabe, M., Takeda, S., and Ikeuchi, H. (1979). Therapeutic value of arthroscopic procedure. In *Atlas of arthroscopy* (3rd edn), pp. 52–5. Igaku-Shoiu Ltd, Tokyo.
9. Bird, H.A. and Ring, E.F.J. (1978). Therapeutic value of arthroscopy. *Annals of the Rheumatic Diseases*, **37**, 78–9.
10. Luchikhina, L.V. (1981). (Irrigation of the knee joint during arthroscopy as a method of treating of patients with rheumatoid arthritis and osteoarthritis deformans). Irrigatsiia kolennogo sustava pri artroskopii kak metod lechebnogo vozdeistviia u bol'nykh revmatoidnym artritom i deformiruiushchim osteoartrozom. *Terapevticheskii Arkhiv*, **53**, (7), 99–103.
11. Jackson, R.W., Silver, R., and Marans, H. (1986). Arthroscopic treatment of degenerative joint disease. *Arthroscopy*, **2**, 114.
12. Wei, N., Delauter, S.K., and Erlichman, M.S. (1993). Office knee arthroscopy: the first 100 cases. *Rheumatology Review*, **2**, 151–8.
13. Rangiwala, M.A., Michalska, M., and Block, J.A. (1995). Pain inprovement and quantity of articular debris after arthroscopy for osteoarthritis of the knee. *Arthritis and Rheumatism*, **38**, 9(suppl), S240.
14. Eriksson, E. and Häggmark, T. (1980). Knee pain in the middle-aged runner. In *Symposium on the foot and leg in running sports*, pp. 106–8. American Academy of Orthopedic Surgeons, Park Ridge, IL.
15. Arnold, W.J., Mather, S.E., Mostello, N., and Tongue, J. (1985). Tidal knee lavage in patients with chronic pain due to osteoarthritis of the knee. *Arthritis and Rheumatism*, **28** (suppl), S66.
16. Ike, R.W., Arnold, W.J., Simon, C., and Eisenberg, G.M. (1987). Tidal knee irrigation as an intervention for chronic pain due to osteoarthritis of the knee. *Arthritis and Rheumatism*, **30**, 1(suppl), S17.
17. Jungmichel, D., Weber, H., and Gatzsche, L. (1988). (Joint washing — a treatment possibility in active arthritis). Gelenkwaschung — eine behandlungsmoglichkeit bei aktivierter arthrose. *Beitrage zur Orthopadie und Traumatologie*, **35**, 512–17.
18. Mohr, B.W., Danao, T., Gragg, L.A., and Segal, A.M. (1991). Tidal knee lavage for osteoarthritis and rheumatoid arthritis: long-term results. *Arthritis and Rheumatism*, **34**, 9(suppl), S85.
19. Edelson, R., Burks, R.T., and Bloebaum, R.D. (1995). Short-term effects of knee washout for osteoarthritis. *American Journal of Sports Medicine*, **23**, 345–9.
20. Espósito, P., Rodriguez-Albán, M., Barbero, N., and Rodríguez-de la Serna, A. (1995). Tidal irrigation in old patients with osteoarthritis of the knee. *Rheumatology in Europe*, **24**, (suppl 3), 195.
21. Dawes, P.T., Kirlew, C., and Haslock, I. (1987). Saline washout for knee osteoarthritis: results of a controlled study. *Clinical Rheumatology*, **6**, 61–3.
22. Ike, R.W., Arnold, W.J., Rothschild, E.W., Shaw, H.L., and the Tidal Irrigation Cooperating Group. (1992). Tidal irrigation versus conservative medical management in patients with osteoarthritis of the knee: a prospective randomized study. *Journal of Rheumatology*, **19**, 772–9.
23. Livesley, P.J., Doherty, M., Needhoff, M., and Moulton, A. (1991). Arthroscopic lavage of osteoarthritic knees. *Journal of Bone and Joint Surgery (British)*, **73B**, 922–6.
24. Alistair Gibson, J.N., White, M.D., Chapman, V.M., and Strachan, R.K. (1992). Arthroscopic lavage and debridement for osteoarthritis of the knee. *Journal of Bone and Joint Surgery (British)*, **74B**, 534–7.
25. Chang, R.W., Falconer, J., Stulberg, S.D., Arnold, W.J., Mannheim, L.M., and Dyer, A.R. (1993). A randomized controlled trial of arthroscopic surgery versus closed-needle joint lavage for patients with osteoarthritis of the knee. *Arthritis and Rheumatism*, **36**, 289–96.
26. Kalunian, K., Klashman, D., Singh, R., *et al.* (1995). Office-based arthroscopy in early osteoarthritis of the knee: preliminary results of a multi-center study of the effects of visually guided irrigation on outcome. *Arthritis and Rheumatism*, **38**, 9(suppl), S240.
27. O'Connor, R.L. (1973). The arthroscope in the management of crystal-induced synovitis of the knee. *Journal of Bone and Joint Surgery (American)*, **55A**, 1443–9.
28. Bennett, R.M., Lehr, J.R., and McCarty, D.J. (1976). Crystal shedding and acute pseudogout. A hypothesis based on a therapeutic failure. *Arthritis and Rheumatism*, **19**, 93–7.
29. Ike, R.W. (1993). The role of arthroscopy in the differential diagnosis of osteoarthritis of the knee. *Rheumatic Disease Clinics of North America*, **19**, 673–96.
30. Rizk, T.E. and Pinals, R.S. (1982). Frozen shoulder. *Seminars in Arthritis and Rheumatism*, **11**, 440–52.
31. Rizk, T.E., Gavant, M.L., and Pinals, R.S. (1994). Treatment of adhesive capsulitis (frozen shoulder) with arthrographic capsular distension and rupture. *Archives of Physical Medicine and Rehabilitation*, **75**, 803–7.

32. Jacobs, L.G., Barton, M.A., Wallace, W.A., Ferrousis, J., Dunn, N.A., and Bossingham, D.H. (1991). Intra-articular distension and steroids in the management of capsulitis of the shoulder. *British Medical Journal*, **302**, 1498–501.

33. Rizk, T.E., Pinals, R.S., and Talaiver, A.S. (1991). Corticosteroid injections in adhesive capsulitis: investigation of their value and site. *Archives of Physical Medicine and Rehabilitation*, **72**, 20–2.

34. Simon, W.H. (1975). Soft tissue disorders of the shoulder. Frozen shoulder, calcific tendinitis, and bicepital tendinitis. *Orthopedic Clinics of North America*, **6**, 521–9.

35. Hsu, S.Y. and Chan, K.M. (1991). Arthroscopic distension in the management of frozen shoulder. *International Orthopedics*, **15**, 79–83.

36. Pollock, R.G., Duralde, X.A., Flatow, E.I., and Bigliani, L.U. (1994). The use of arthroscopy in the treatment of resistant frozen shoulder. *Clinical Orthopedics and Related Research*, **304**, 30–6.

37. Comfort, T.H. and Arafiles, R.P. (1978). Barbotage of the shoulder with image-intensified fluoroscopic control of needle placement for calcific tendinitis. *Clinical Orthopedics and Related Research*, **135**, 171–8.

38. Ark, J.W., Flock, T.J., Flatow, E.L., and Bigliani, L.U. (1992). Arthroscopic treatment of calcific tendinitis of the shoulder. *Arthroscopy*, **8**, 183–8.

39. Caporali, R., Rossi, S., and Montecucco, C. (1994). Tidal irrigation in Milwaukee shoulder syndrome. *Journal of Rheumatology*, **21**, 1781–2.

40. Spector, G.W. (1973). Joint distension arthrography: alternate method of treatment of osteoarthritis of the hip. *Missouri Medicine*, **70**, 605–10.

41. Egsmose, C., Birger, L., and Andersen, R.B. (1984). Hip joint distension in osteoarthrosis: a triple-blind controlled study comparing the effect of intra-articular indoprofen with placebo. *Scandinavian Journal of Rheumatology*, **13**, 238–42.

42. Hoilund-Carlsen, P.F., Meinicke, J., Christiansen, B., Karle, A.K., Stage, P., and Uhrenholdt, A. (1985). Joint distension arthrography for disabling hip pain. A controlled clinical trial. *Scandinavian Journal of Rheumatology*, **14**, 179–83.

43. Razzano, C.D., Nelson, C.L., and Wilde, A.H. (1974). Arthrography of the adult hip. *Clinical Orthopedics and Related Research*, **99**, 86–94.

44. Keroack, B.J., Lunquist, C., and Ike, R.W. (1992). Idiopathic capsular constriction of the hip, an under appreciated cause of hip pain. *Arthritis and Rheumatism*, **35**, 5(suppl), S123.

45. Villar, R. (1995). Hip arthroscopy. *Journal of Bone and Joint Surgery (British)*, **77B**, 517–18.

46. Eriksson, E., Arvidsson, I., and Arvidsson, H. (1986). Diagnostic and operative arthroscopy of the hip. *Orthopedics*, **9**, (2), 169–76.

47. Hollander, J.L. (1960). The most neglected differential diagnostic test in arthritis. *Arthritis and Rheumatism*, **3**, 364–7.

48. Kitridou, R., McCarty, D.J., Prockop, D.J., and Hummler, K. (1969). Identification of collagen in synovial fluid. *Arthritis and Rheumatism*, **12**, 580–8.

49. Cheung, H.S., Ryan, L.M., Kozin, F., and McCarty, D.J. (1980). Identification of collagen subtypes in synovial fluid segments from arthritic patients. *American Journal of Medicine*, **68**, 73–9.

50. Mears, D.C., Hanley, E.N., Rutkowski, R., *et al.* (1978). Ferrography: its application to the study of human joint wear. *Wear*, **50**, 115–25.

51. Evans, C.H. and Mears, D.C. (1981). The wear particles of human synovial fluid: their ferrographic analysis and pathophysiological significance. *Bulletin of Prosthetics Research*, **10**, (36), 13–28.

52. Evans, C.H., Mears, D.C., and McKnight, J.L. (1981). A preliminary ferrographic analysis of the wear particles in human synovial fluid. *Arthritis and Rheumatism*, **24**, 912–18.

53. Mori, Y. (1979). Debris observed by arthroscopy of the knee. *Orthopedic Clinics of North America*, **10**, 559–63.

54. Sedgwick, W.G., Gilula, L.A., Lesker, P.A., and Whiteside, L.A. (1980). Wear particles: their value in knee arthrography. *Radiology*, **136**, 11–14.

55. Tew, W.P. and Hackett, R.P. (1981). Identification of cartilage wear fragments in synovial fluid from equine joints. *Arthritis and Rheumatism*, **24**, 1419–24.

56. Hotchkiss, R.N., Tew, W.P., and Hungerford, D.S. (1982). Cartilaginous debris in the injured human knee. Correlation with arthroscopic findings. *Clinical Orthopedics and Related Research*, **168**, 144–56.

57. Evans, C.H., Mears, D.C., and Stanititski, C.L. (1982). Ferrographic analysis of wear in human joints. Evaluation by comparison with arthroscopic examination of symptomatic knees. *Journal of Bone and Joint Surgery (British)*, **64B**, 572–8.

58. Hultén, O. and Gellerstedt, N. (1940). (Products of use in joints and their resorbtion in synovitis detritica.) Uber abnutzungsprodukte in gelenken und ihre resorption unter dem bilde einer synovitis detritica. *Acta Chirurgica Scandinavica*, **84**, 1–29.

59. Horwitz, T. (1948). Bone and cartilage debris in the synovial membrane. *Journal of Bone and Joint Surgery (American)*, **30A**, 579–88.

60. Lloyd-Roberts, G.C. (1953). The role of capsular changes in osteoarthritis of the hip joint. *Journal of Bone and Joint Surgery (British)*, **35B**, 627–42.

61. Schumacher, H.R., Gorgon, G., Paul, H., *et al.* (1981). Osteoarthritis, crystal deposition, and inflammation. *Seminars in Arthritis and Rheumatism*, **11**, (suppl), 116–22.

62. Myers, S.L., Flusser, D., Brandt, K.D., and Heck, D.A. (1992). Prevalence of cartilage shards in synovium and their association with synovitis in early and endstage osteoarthritis. *Journal of Rheumatology*, **19**, 1247–51.

63. Evans, C.H., Mears, D.C., and Cosgrove, J.L. (1981). Release of neutral proteinases from mononuclear phagocytes and synovial cells in response to cartilagenous wear particles *in vitro*. *Biochemica Biophysica Acta*, **677**, 287–94.

64. Moskowitz, R.W., Schwartz, H.J., Michel, B., Ratnoff, O.D., and Astrup, T (1970). Generation of kinin-like agents by chondroitin sulfate, heparin, chitin sulfate, and human articular cartilage: possible pathophysio-

logic implications. *Journal of Laboratory and Clinical Medicine*, 76, 790–8.

65. Chrisman, O.D., Fessel, J.M., and Southwick, W.O. (1965). Experimental production of synovitis and marginal articular exostoses in the knee joints of dogs. *Yale Journal of Biology and Medicine*, 37, 409–12.

66. Evans, C.H., Mazzocchi, R.A., Nelson, D.D., and Rubash, H.E. (1984). Experimental arthritis induced by intraarticular injection of allogenic cartilagenous particles into rabbit knees. *Arthritis and Rheumatism*, 27, 200–7.

67. George, R.C. and Chrisman, O.D. The role of cartilage proteoglycans in osteoarthritis. *Clinical Orthopedics and Related Research*, 57, 259–66.

68. Boniface, R.J., Cain, P.R., and Evans, C.H. Articular responses to purified cartilage proteoglycans. *Arthritis and Rheumatism*, 31, 258–66.

69. Swan, A., Chapman, B., Heap, P., Seward, H., and Dieppe, P. (1994). Submicroscopic crystals in osteoarthritic synovial fluids. *Annals of the Rheumatic Diseases*, 53, 467–70.

70. Klashman, D.J., Moreland, L.W., Ike, R.W., and Kalunian, K.C. (1994). Occult presence of CPPD crystals in patients undergoing arthroscopic knee irrigation for refractory pain related to OA. *Arthritis and Rheumatism*, 37, 9(suppl), S240.

71. Tate, G., Schumacher, H.R. Jr, Reginato, A., and Clayburne, G. (1988). Inflammation after blood injection into a synovial-like space is a result of the cellular component rather than the plasma. *Journal of Rheumatology*, 15, 1686–92.

72. Madhok, R., York, J., and Sturrock, R.D. (1991). Haemophilic arthritis. *Annals of the Rheumatic Diseases*, 50, 588–91.

73. Kawamura, H., Ogata, K., Miura, H., Arizono, T., and Sugioka, Y. (1994). Spontaneous hemarthrosis of the knee in the elderly: etiology and treatment. *Arthroscopy*, 10, 171–5.

74. Caughey, D.E. and Bywaters, E.G.L. (1963). Joint fluid pressure in chronic knee effusions. *Annals of the Rheumatic Diseases*, 22, 106–9.

75. Myers, D.B. and Palmer, D.G. (1972). Capsular compliance and pressure-volume relationships in normal and arthritic knees. *Journal of Bone and Joint Surgery (British)*, 54B, 710–16.

76. deAndrade, J.R., Grant, C., and Dixon, A.St.J. (1965). Joint distension and reflex muscle inhibition in the knee. *Journal of Bone and Joint Surgery (American)*, 47A, 313–22.

77. Miller, J.H., White, J., and Norton, T.H. (1958). The value of intra-articular injections in osteoarthritis of the knee. *Journal of Bone and Joint Surgery [British]*, 40B, 636–43.

78. Reagan, B.F., McInerny, V.K., Treadwell, B.V., Zaris, B., and Mankin, H.J. (1983). Irrigating solutions for arthroscopy: A metabolic study. *Journal of Bone and Joint Surgery (American)*, 65, 629–31.

79. Arciero, R.A., Little, J.S., Liebenberg, S.P., and Parr, T.J. (1986). Irrigating solutions used in arthrosocopy and their effect on articlar cartilage. *Orthopedics*, 9, 1511–15.

80. Bert, J.M., Posalaky, Z., Snyder, S., McGinley, D., and Chock, C. (1990). Effect of various irrigating fluids on the ultrastructure of articular cartilage. *Arthroscopy*, 6, 104–11.

81. Gradinger, R., Träger, J., and Klauser, R.J. (1995). Influence of various irrigation fluids on articular cartilage. *Arthroscopy*, 11, 263–9.

82. Jurvelin, J.S., Jurvelin, J.A., Kiviranta, I., and Klauser, R.J. (1994). Effects of different irrigation liquids and times on articular cartilage: an experimental, biomechanical study. *Arthroscopy*, 10, 667–72.

83. Johnson, R.G., Herbert, M.A., Wright, S., *et al.* (1983). The response of articular cartilage to the *in vivo* replacement of synovial fluid with saline. *Clinical Orthopedics and Related Research*, 174, 285–92.

84. Maarshall, G.J., Kirchen, M.E., Sweeney, J.R., and Snyder, S. (1988). Synoviosol as an irrigant for electrosurgery of joints. *Arthroscopy*, 4, 187–92.

85. Small, N.C., Glogau, A.I., Berezin, M.A., and Farless, B.L. (1994). Office operative arthroscopy of the knee: technical considerations and a preliminary analysis of the first 100 patients. *Arthroscopy*, 10, 534–9.

86. Wei, N., Delauter, S.K., and Erlichman, M.S. (1995). Office based arthroscopy. Evolution of the procedure: the next 100 cases. *Journal of Clinical Rheumatology*, 1, 219–27.

87. Chen, S.C., Helal, B., Revell, P.A., Brocklehurst, R., and Currey, H.L. (1986). Experimental cryo-irrigation of the knee joint. *Annals of the Rheumatic Diseases*, 45, 865–72.

88. Sherman, O.H., Fox, J.M., Snyder, S.J., *et al.* (1986). Arthroscopy — 'no-problem surgery'. An analysis of complications in two thousand six hundred and forty cases. *Journal of Bone and Joint Surgery (American)*, 68A, 256–65.

89. Committee on Complications of the Arthroscopy Association of North America. (1986). Complications in arthroscopy: the knee and other joints. *Arthroscopy*, 2, 253–8.

90. Small, N.C. (1988). Complications in arthroscopic surgery performed by experienced arthroscopists. *Arthroscopy*, 4, 215–21.

91. Bamford, D.J., Paul, A.S., Noble, J., and Davies, D.R. (1993). Avoidable complications of arthroscopic surgery. *Journal of the Royal College of Surgeons of Edinburgh*, 38, 92–5.

92. Huff, J.P., Segueira, W., Harris, C.A., Blackburn, W.D., and Moreland, L.W. (1992). Survey of physicians doing office-based arthroscopy. *Arthritis and Rheumatism*, 35, 9(suppl), S292.

93. Szachnowski, P., Wei, N., Arnold, W.J., and Cohen, L.M. (1995). Complications of office based arthroscopy of the knee. *Journal of Rheumatology*, 22, 1722–5.

94. Ayral, X., Dougados, M., Listrat, V., *et al.* (1993). Chondroscopy: a new method for scoring chondropathy. *Seminars in Arthritis and Rheumatism*, 22, 289–97.

95. Visuri, T. and Kiviluoto, O. (1986). Arthroscopic volume of the knee joint in young male adults. *Scandinavian Journal of Rheumatology*, 15, 251–4.

96. Funk, D.A., Noyes, F.R., Grood, E.S., and Hoffman, S.D. (1991). Effect of flexion angle on the pressure-volume of the human knee. *Arthroscopy*, 7, 86–90.

9.16   Surgical approaches to preserving and restoring articular cartilage[*]

Joseph A. Buckwalter and L. Stefan Lohmander

Most patients, and many physicians, consider joint replacement as the only surgical option for the treatment of osteoarthritic joints, yet procedures that preserve or restore articular cartilage, instead of resecting and replacing it with synthetic materials, make up an important part of the spectrum of treatments available to patients with degenerative joints. These procedures can decrease pain and improve joint function for selected patients, including younger patients with localized loss or early articular cartilage degeneration[1,2]. For these individuals, maintaining or restoring synovial joint structure and function may make possible a high level of physical activity, and delay or eliminate the need for joint replacement or fusion. Improvements in methods of preserving and restoring articular cartilage may expand the role of these operations to include treatment of older individuals with early degenerative disease, and possibly individuals with advanced joint degeneration.

Procedures performed with the intent of preserving or restoring articular cartilage surfaces include joint debridement — shaving fibrillated cartilage, perforation of subchondral bone to stimulate formation of a new articular surface, osteotomies, resection arthroplasty, and resection of localized regions of degenerated articular cartilage. Such a procedure may be followed by implantation of periosteal, perichondrial, and osteochondral autografts and allografts to create a new articular surface[1–3]. Surgeons have used joint debridement, and resection or penetration of subchondral bone, most commonly for treatment of degenerative disease of the knee and, less frequently, for the elbow, shoulder, hip, ankle, and other joints. Osteotomies have been used most frequently for treatment of degenerative disease of the knee and hip, while resection arthroplasties appear to be most effective for treatment of osteoarthritis (OA) involving the first metatarsal phalangeal joint, the carpalmetacarpal joint of the thumb, and, less commonly, other joints.

Periosteal, perichondrial, and osteochondral grafts have been used in a variety of joints including the knee, hip, and hand joints.

Experimental procedures being developed to preserve or restore articular surfaces include implantation of growth factors, chondrocytes, and mesenchymal stem cells, and synthetic matrices or combinations of growth factors, cells, and matrices[1,3]. Although the effectiveness of these procedures has not yet been demonstrated in treating OA joints, experimental studies suggest they have potential to improve current procedures performed with the intent of restoring articular cartilage.

Joint debridement

Joint debridement usually includes joint irrigation, resecting cartilage flaps, and removing loose cartilaginous, osteochondral, and meniscal fragments: in some instances it includes shaving regions of severely degenerated meniscal and articular cartilage surfaces, resecting synovium, and removing osteophytes (cheilectomy)[4,5]. Although surgeons have debrided OA joints for more than 50 years, by arthrotomy[21,22] or by arthroscopy[3–20], the efficacy of debridement in altering the course of OA, relieving pain, or improving joint function has not been established by prospective long-term randomized studies.

The lack of these studies makes critical evaluation of the effects of different procedures involved in joint debridement especially important in making treatment decisions for individual patients. Removal of chondral flaps and free cartilage, osteochondral and meniscal fragments causing mechanical disturbances of joint function, improves function and decreases symptoms[15,23]. In addition, since intra-articular osteochondral fragments can cause synovitis and excoriation of articular cartilage[24], removing free tissue fragments may slow progression of joint degeneration. The potential benefits of other debridement procedures are less clear.

[*] Many of the observations presented in this chapter were included in a previously published review[1].

Despite widespread clinical use, shaving or debriding fibrillated articular cartilage and menisci remains controversial. Although careful removal of fibrillated tissue can leave a smoother articular surface, published reports of animal experiments and clinical studies do not demonstrate beneficial effects of this procedure. Shaving normal animal articular cartilage did not stimulate regeneration of an articular surface[25,26], and in one experiment, the remaining cartilage degenerated following shaving[25]. Fibrillated human OA cartilage may respond differently to debridement, but clinical studies indicate that shaving is not likely to restore an articular surface[27-30].

Despite the lack of evidence for beneficial effects of debridement on joint structure and function — other than correcting mechanical disturbances of joint function due to free or displaced tissue fragments, and questions concerning its clinical efficacy[31], — many clinical series indicate that joint debridement decreases pain[1]. The symptomatic improvement could result from a placebo effect[17] or from a decrease in the stimulus for joint pain. Observations from experimental studies[32,33], combined with the clinical observation that joint irrigation may temporarily decrease pain in OA joints[17,31,34], suggest that removal of tissue debris and joint irrigation could improve symptoms by decreasing a source of synovial irritation.

Penetration of subchondral bone

Some surgeons combine debridement of a degenerated joint with penetration of subchondral bone to stimulate formation of a new articular surface. In regions with full thickness loss or advanced degeneration of articular cartilage, penetration of the exposed subchondral bone disrupts subchondral blood vessels, leading to formation of a fibrin clot over the bone surface[3,35,36]. If the surface is protected from excessive loading, undifferentiated mesenchymal cells migrate into the clot, proliferate, and differentiate into cells with the morphologic features of chondrocytes[37]. In many instances, they form a fibrocartilaginous repair tissue over the bone surface[38,39].

Currently, it is not clear which method of penetrating subchondral bone produces the best new articular surface, and differences in patient selection and technique among surgeons using the same method may be responsible for variations in results, making it difficult to compare techniques[1]. However, comparison of bone abrasion with subchondral drilling for treatment of an experimental chondral defect in rabbits showed that while neither treatment predictably restored the articular surface, drilling appeared to produce better long-term results than abrasion[40]. This observation fits well with previous experimental work showing that tissue that grows up through multiple drill holes that pass from the articular surface into vascularized bone will spread over exposed subchondral bone between holes and form a fibrocartilaginous articular surface[41].

Examination of joint surfaces following arthroscopic abrasion has shown that in many individuals it results in formation of fibrocartilaginous articular surface that varies in composition from dense fibrous tissue, with little or no type II collagen, to hyaline cartilage-like tissue with predominantly type II collagen[38,39]. In some patients, this tissue persists for years. Some of the variability in the clinical results of this procedure may result from the variability in the extent or quality of the repair tissue. However, no studies have documented a relationship between the extent and type of repair tissue, and symptomatic or functional results.

Prospective randomized controlled trials of arthroscopic abrasion treatment of OA joints have not been reported, but several authors have reviewed series of patients and found that some 60–85 per cent those treated with arthroscopic debridement and abrasion of subchondral bone reported improvement[7,11,15,19,21,22,38,39,42-46]. However, the probability of a satisfactory clinical result decreased with increasing severity of the joint disease[11]. Other studies have reported less favorable outcome of this procedure, for example, only 12 per cent of the patients in one series had no symptoms at two years following treatment[38,39], and another study reported up to 50 per cent failures[7].

Although an increase in radiographic joint space following subchondral abrasion presumably indicates formation of a new articular surface[38,39], the development of this new surface does not necessarily result in symptomatic improvement. Bert and Maschka[8,9] found that about half of 59 patients treated with abrasion arthroplasty had evidence of increased radiographic joint space two years after treatment, but one out of three of these individuals either had no symptomatic improvement or more severe symptoms at follow-up.

These observations suggest that formation of a new articular surface following penetration of subchondral bone does not necessarily relieve pain. This lack of predictable benefit may result from variability among patients in the severity of the changes, joint alignment, patterns of joint use, age, perception of pain, preoperative expectations, or other factors. It may also result from the inability of the newly formed tissue to replicate the properties of articular cartilage. Examination of the tissue that forms over the articular surface following penetration of subchondral bone shows that it lacks the structure, composition, mechanical properties, and, in most instances, the durability of articular cartilage[3,35,36,41]. For these reasons, even though it covers the subchondral bone, it may fail to distribute loads across the articular surface in a way that avoids pain with joint loading and further degeneration of the joint[1,3]. We are also reminded of the fact the specific sources of pain in OA are usually unknown, and may well vary between different patients, different joints, and different disease stages.

Despite the evidence that penetration of subchondral bone stimulates formation of fibrocartilaginous repair tissue, and reports of symptomatic improvement in several series of patients[19,39,45], the clinical value of this approach remains uncertain. One investigator has concluded that while joint debridement can improve symptoms in many patients, abrasion or drilling of subchondral bone do not benefit patients with OA of the knee, and may increase symptoms[8]. The short periods of follow-up, lack of well-defined evaluations of outcomes, lack of randomized controlled trials, and the possibility for a significant placebo effect[17] or an improvement in symptoms due to joint irrigation alone[31,34] make it difficult to define the indications for penetration of subchondral bone to stimulate formation of a new articular surface.

Osteotomies

Treatment of an OA joint, with an osteotomy, consists of cutting the bone adjacent to the involved joint and then stabilizing the cut bone surfaces in a new position, thereby changing the alignment of the joint (Fig. 9.16 a and b). In general, the osteotomy procedure aims to decrease loads on the most severely degenerated regions of the joint surface, bring regions of the joint surface that have remaining articular cartilage into opposition with regions that lack articular cartilage, or correct joint malalignment that may be contributing to symptoms and joint dysfunction. Most hip and knee osteotomies performed to treat OA alter joint alignment in the coronal plane (varus and valgus osteotomies). However, surgeons design some hip osteotomies to change joint alignment in the sagittal plane (flexion and extension osteotomies) or alter the relationship of the joint surfaces by rotation of the

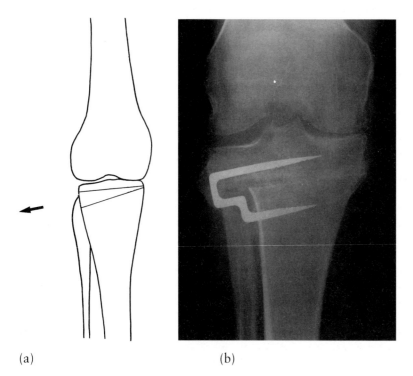

(a)   (b)

Fig. 9.16 Tibial valgus osteotomy for OA of the medial compartment of the knee: (a) schematic drawing, showing resection of bone wedge; (b) postoperative radiograph showing closed osteotomy.

femoral head relative to the acetabulum (rotational osteotomies). Clinical experience shows that osteotomies of the hip and knee can decrease symptoms and stimulate formation of a new articular surface[1]. The mechanisms of symptomatic improvement and formation of new articular surfaces remain poorly understood. The decreased pain may result from decreasing stresses on regions of the articular surface with the most advanced cartilage degeneration, decreasing intraosseous pressure or formation of a new articular surface[1].

Most clinical studies have shown that osteotomies lead to improvement in the radiographic signs of joint degeneration including resolution of subchondral cysts or lucencies, decreased subchondral bone density, and increased radiographic joint space. This latter change may result either from the altered relationship between the articular surfaces or from the formation of a new articular surface. That is, osteotomies may alter joint alignment to separate previously opposed joint surfaces, or they may rotate a cartilage-covered articular surface into opposition with a surface consisting of exposed bone, thus creating a radiographically visible joint space where, prior to the osteotomy, bone, opposed bone. In one series of 757 osteotomies performed to treat OA of the hip, the radiographic joint space increased immediately following the procedure in approximately one-third of the patients[47]. In these patients, the increased joint space presumably resulted from alterations in the relationships between the joint surfaces. In another third of the patients, the radiographic joint space increased during the next 18 months, and these individuals had better clinical results. This result suggests that these patients developed a new articular surface in some areas of the joint as a result of the altered loading. Evidence that hip osteotomies stimulate formation of fibrocartilaginous tissue over articular surfaces that previously consisted of exposed bone supports this suggestion[48,49].

Reports of the treatment of OA of the knee with osteotomies also describe increased radiographic joint space accompanied by decreased subchondral sclerosis, and, in some patients, formation of a new fibrocartilaginous articular surface[1,50,51]. However, no correlation was found between the formation of a new fibrocartilaginous articular surface, radiographic appearance, postoperative varus–valgus angle, and clinical outcome[50,51].

Long-term follow-up of patients treated with osteotomies for hip and knee OA shows that the clinical results deteriorate with time[47,52]. At one year following surgery, 70 per cent of 103 hips treated by intertrochanteric osteotomy had a good result; at five years, 51 per cent had a good result; and, at ten years, only 30 per cent of the hips still showed a beneficial effect of the osteotomy[53]. Studies of patients treated with tibial osteotomies have reported that the proportion of patients with good or excellent results declined from some 90 per cent at two-year follow-up, to 50–85 per cent at three to five years, and that only 15–57 per cent of the knees were pain free nine years or more following surgery[52,54,55]. Variables that appear to adversely affect the results of knee osteotomies include advanced patient age, obesity, severe joint degeneration, joint instability, limited joint motion, operative over correction or under correction, and postoperative loss of correction[52,54,55,56]. However, many patients who appear to be optimal candidates for osteotomy and who have a good initial surgical outcome, tend to develop recurrent pain and evidence of advancing OA with time.

Several studies indicate that the results of osteotomies could be improved through advances in technique and patient selection[57,58]. Evaluation of preoperative joint mechanics may also lead to improved results. Surgeons generally use radiographs that demonstrate joint alignment, subchondral bone density, and cartilage space to plan osteotomies that will redistribute articular surface loading. They base this practice on the assumption that static joint alignment can be used to predict loading in different regions of a joint. One group of investigators showed that dynamic joint loading also should be considered[59,60]. They studied patients with varus gonarthrosis, using gait analysis, and found that the patients could be separated into two groups: those with high adduction moments at the knee, and those with low adduction moments. The two groups did not differ in preoperative knee score, initial knee alignment, postoperative knee alignment, age, or weight; but those with high preoperative adduction moments had only 50 per cent good or excellent results at an average of 3.2 years following osteotomy, compared with 100 per cent good or excellent results for patients with low preoperative adduction moments[59]. With increasing time, the results for both groups deteriorated, but the patients with low preoperative adduction moments maintained better clinical results[60].

At present, the overall clinical results of hip and knee osteotomies vary more than those of joint replacement, and the relationships among the degree of alteration of joint loading, type of osteotomy, quality and extent of articular surface repair, radiographic changes, and clinical outcome remain unclear. Given the available information, identifying the patients most likely to benefit from osteotomy, planning the optimal osteotomy for a specific joint, and predicting the outcome of the procedure for an individual patient are difficult. However, recent investigations by Odenbring suggest that advances in osteotomies through improved selection of patients, preoperative planning, and surgical techniques have the potential to provide better and, possibly, longer lasting results than arthroplasties, in young physically active patients[57,58,61].

Resection arthroplasty

Resection of an OA joint surface, followed by joint motion, results in the formation of fibrocartilaginous tissue over the surfaces of the resected bone[1,3,35]. When the degenerated articular surfaces are resected along with some of the underlying bone, the space between the bone surfaces fills with a fibrin clot and, then, granulation tissue. With motion, a firm fibrocartilaginous tissue may replace the soft vascular granulation tissue. In many instances, the fibrocartilaginous tissue covering the opposing bone ends assumes the appearance of an articular surface. In addition to motion, some distraction, or at least limited loading of the new joint facilitates formation of fibrocartilaginous articular surfaces; whereas, immobilization and compression may lead to bony or fibrous union. The articulations that result from resection arthroplasty lack stability and may be painful, but in selected patients and joints they provide acceptable function.

Resection arthroplasty may be most successful in joints that do not require a high degree of stability, and where shortening due to resection of bone does not prevent near normal function. One of the most commonly performed resection arthroplasties — the Keller arthroplasty (performed to treat hallux valgus deformity and degenerative disease of the first metatarsalphalangeal joint) — consists of resecting degenerated articular cartilage, along with 30 to 50 per cent of the proximal portion of the proximal phalanx of the great toe[62,63]. The reasons for the relatively good clinical outcomes of this procedure have not been fully explored. Possibly, the limited loading and early motion at the resection site allows formation of an articular surface. The limited loading of the newly formed articular

surface may also prevent degeneration of this tissue and decrease the probability of pain from motion.

Fibrous or fibrocartilaginous articular surfaces also form after resection arthroplasty of the hip or knee. Surgeons most commonly perform these procedures in an attempt to save some joint function following a failed total joint arthroplasty, or to treat joint infections that cannot be controlled by other means. Generally, the instability of the joint and, in some instances, limb shortening and pain, compromise function. However, some investigators have found relatively good results of resection arthroplasty treatment of infected total knee arthroplasties[64,65].

Soft tissue grafts

Treatment of OA joints by soft tissue grafts usually involves debriding the joint and interposing soft tissue grafts consisting of fascia, muscle, tendon, periosteum, or perichondrium between debrided or resected articular surfaces[3]. The potential benefits of soft tissue grafts relative to resection arthroplasty or penetration of subchondral bone include introduction of a new cell population along with an organic matrix, a decrease in the probability of ankylosis before a new articular surface can form, and some protection of the graft or host cells from excessive loading. The success of soft tissue arthroplasty depends not only on the severity of the joint abnormalities and the type of graft, but on postoperative motion to facilitate generation of a new articular surface.

Soft tissue interposition arthroplasties have been used most frequently to treat degenerative joints of the upper extremity; in particular, tendon or fascial arthroplasty treatment of OA of the thumb carpometacarpal joint[66]. The surgeon debrides the joint and usually resects a portion of the articular surface, along with subchondral bone, to allow interposition of tendon or fascia. The joint is temporarily stabilized, followed by controlled motion. This procedure has been found to provide acceptable relief of symptoms in a high proportion of the patients and to allow retention of some joint motion.

Fascial arthroplasty has been used for other joints of the upper extremity including the elbow. In selected young patients with post-traumatic degenerative disease of the elbow, some surgeons have used soft tissue interposition arthroplasty as an alternative to total joint arthroplasty, with variable functional results. The investigators have concluded that in selected patients, fascial arthroplasty can provide a functional range of motion with little pain, but that it is not indicated in patients requiring a strong stable extremity[67,68].

Animal experiments and clinical experience show that perichondral and periosteal grafts can replace lost or degenerated regions of articular cartilage[15]. These grafts have the potential advantage of containing cells with the capacity to differentiate into chondrocytes and synthesize a cartilaginous matrix. Engkvist and Johansson treated 26 patients, with painful stiff small joints, with rib perichondral arthroplasty[69]. Some individuals had improved motion and decreased pain, but a roughly equal number were not improved. Seradge *et al.* studied the results of rib perichondrial arthroplasties in 16 metacarpophalangeal joint and 20 proximal interphalangeal joints at a minimum of three years following surgery[70]: patient age was directly related to the results. In metacarpophalangeal joint arthroplasties, 100 per cent of the patients in their twenties and 75 per cent of the patients in their thirties had good results; in proximal interphalangeal joint arthroplasties, 75 percent of the patients in their teens and 66 per cent of the patients in their twenties had good results; None of the patients older than 40 years had a good result with either type of arthroplasty. The authors concluded that perichondrial arthroplasty could be used for treatment of post-traumatic OA of the metacarpophalangeal joint and proximal interphalangeal joints of the hand in young patients.

Perichondrial grafts have also been used to replace lost or damaged cartilage in the knee[71]. The knee function improved significantly and arthroscopic examination showed that 28 of the 30 chondral defects had filled, almost completely, with a tissue resembling articular cartilage in 25 patients with an average age of 31 years.

The clinical observation that perichondrial grafts produced the best results in younger patients[70] agrees with the concept that age may adversely affect the ability of undifferentiated cells or chondrocytes to form an articular surface, or that, with age, the population of cells that can form an articular surface declines[72]. The age-related differences in the ability of cells to form a new articular surface may also help explain some of the variability in the results of other procedures including osteotomies or procedures that penetrate subchondral bone — that is, younger people

may have greater potential to produce a more effective articular surface when all other factors are equal.

Cartilage grafts

Compared with soft tissue grafts, cartilage or meniscal grafts have the advantage of more closely resembling the structure and composition of articular cartilage, and they have the potential for transplantation of viable chondrocytes. Experimental work using meniscal[73] and sternal cartilage[74] autografts have shown promising results. Because of the limited sources of autogenous cartilage, it is rarely used, but osteochondral patellar autografts used to replace portions of the tibial articular surface, healed and provided satisfactory joint function[75]. With their greater availability, and because they can be prepared in any size, osteochondral allografts are more frequently used to replace damaged segments of articular surfaces.

Clinical experience with fresh and frozen allografts shows that they can heal to the host tissue and restore an articular surface. Several studies have thus shown that osteochondral allografts can provide at least temporary improvement in symptoms and function for selected patients with isolated regions of degenerated articular cartilage[76-79]. They suggest that the grafts may delay or even prevent the development of degenerative changes in the joint surfaces opposing the grafts, although more long-term follow-up studies are needed to determine if this suggestion is correct. The limited sources of acceptable osteochondral grafts prevents extensive use of this treatment, but the results of these grafts indicate that in selected patients, restoring localized regions of an articular surface can improve joint function.

Experimental treatments

Experimental surgical methods of restoring articular cartilage include implantation of growth factors, cells, and artificial matrices. In animal experiments, these approaches have resulted in formation of new articular surfaces following creation of an acute cartilage, or cartilage and subchondral bone, defect in normal joints[1]. In interpreting these studies, it is important to recognize that methods which stimulate articular cartilage formation in a normal animal joint will not necessarily lead to similar success in an OA human joint.

Growth factors influence a variety of cell activities including cell proliferation, migration, matrix synthesis, and differentiation. Many of these factors have been shown to affect chondrocyte metabolism and chondrogenesis[1]. Bone matrix contains a variety of these molecules including transforming growth factor (TGF), insulin-like growth factors, bone morphogenic proteins, platelet-derived growth factors, and others. In addition, mesenchymal cells, endothelial cells, and platelets produce many of these factors. Thus, osteochondral injuries and exposure of bone due to loss of articular cartilage may release these agents that affect the formation of cartilage repair tissue, and they probably have an important role in the formation of new articular surfaces after currently used surgical procedures including resection arthroplasty, penetration of subchondral bone, soft tissue grafts, and, possibly, osteotomies.

Local treatment of chondral or osteochondral defects with these factors has the potential to stimulate restoration of an articular surface superior to that formed after penetration of subchondral bone alone, especially in joints with normal alignment and range of motion and with limited regions of cartilage damage. A recent experimental study of the treatment of partial thickness cartilage defects with timed release of TGF-showed that this growth factor can stimulate cartilage repair[80]. Despite the promise of this approach, the wide variety of growth factors, their multiple effects, the interactions among them, the possibility that the responsiveness of cells to growth factors may decline with age[72,81] and the limited understanding of their effects in OA joints make it difficult to develop a simple strategy for using these agents to treat patients with OA. However, development of growth factor based treatments for early cartilage degenerative changes in younger people appears promising.

The limited ability of host cells to restore articular surfaces[3] has led investigators to seek methods of transplanting cells that can form cartilage into chondral and osteochondral defects. Experimental work has shown that both chondrocytes and undifferentiated mesenchymal stem cells, placed in articular cartilage defects, survive and produce a new cartilage matrix, in animal experiments[72,82–86].

In addition to these animal experiments with cell transplants, a group of investigators has reported using autologous chondrocyte transplants for treatment of localized cartilage defects of the femoral condyle or patella in 23 patients[87]. The investigators harvested chondrocytes from the patients, cultured the cells for 14 to 21 days, and then injected them into the area of the defect and covered them with a flap of periosteum. At two or more years following chondrocyte transplantation, 14 of 16 patients with condylar defects, and two of seven patients with patellar defects, had good or excellent clinical results. Biopsies of the defect sites showed hyaline-like cartilage in 11 of 15 femoral, and one of seven patellar defects. These results indicate that chondrocyte transplantation, combined with a periosteal graft, can promote restoration of an articular surface in humans, but much more work is needed to assess the function and durability of the new tissue and to determine if it improves joint function and delays or prevents joint degeneration, and if this approach will be beneficial in OA joints.

Treatment of chondral defects with growth factors or cell transplants requires a method of delivering and, in most instances, at least temporarily stabilizing the growth factors or cells in the defect. For these reasons, the success of these approaches often depends on an artificial matrix. In addition, artificial matrices may allow, and in some cases stimulate ingrowth of host cells, matrix formation, and binding of new cells and matrix to host tissue; combined with materials currently used to fabricate artificial joints, they have the potential to improve the fixation of the artificial joints. Implants formed from a variety of biologic and non-biologic materials including treated cartilage and bone matrices, collagens, collagens and hyaluronan, fibrin, carbon fiber, hydroxyapatite, porous polylactic acid, polytetrafluoroethylene, polyester and other synthetic polymers can facilitate restoration of an articular surface[72]. Lack of studies that directly compare different types of artificial matrices makes it difficult to evaluate their relative merits, but the available reports show that this approach can contribute to restoration of an articular surface. For example, in animal experiments, collagen gels have proven to be an effective way of implanting chondrocytes and mesenchymal stem cells[1], and fibrin has been used to implant and allow timed release of a growth factor[80]. Treatment of osteochondral defects in rats and rabbits, with carbon fiber pads, resulted in restoration of a smooth articular surface consisting of firm fibrous tissue that filled the pads[88]. Use of the same approach to treat osteochondral defects of the knee in humans produced a satisfactory result in 36 of 47 patients evaluated clinically and arthroscopically three years after surgery[88].

Conclusions

Current surgical treatments that attempt to preserve or restore articular cartilage include joint debridement, penetration of subchondral bone, osteotomies, and replacement of lost or damaged articular cartilage with soft tissue or cartilage grafts. Unfortunately, the efficacy of these procedures has not been demonstrated by prospective, controlled randomized studies, and the basic mechanisms by which they may relieve pain and improve function remain poorly understood. Generally, these procedures produce less predictable results than joint replacement, and their efficacy, as measured by relief of symptoms and improved function, varies among joints, among patients, and among procedures.

Debridement of OA joints may provide symptomatic relief in some patients, but prospective randomized controlled clinical studies are needed to define the indications and optimal techniques for this approach; the same is true of the multiple methods of stimulating formation of a new articular surface by penetration of subchondral bone. In selected patients, osteotomies decrease pain, but more work is needed to refine the indications for osteotomies and improve the techniques. In particular, we need to learn more about how altering loads on the articular surfaces and subchondral bone affects joint pain and regeneration or preservation of articular cartilage, and to develop better methods of assessing the static and dynamic loads on articular surfaces and determining how osteotomies alter these loads. Resection arthroplasties and soft tissue interposition arthroplasties can be effective in a limited number of joints, but the resulting instability, shortening, and, in some instances, pain, make these procedures inappropriate for many joints and patients. Osteochondral allografts can replace limited regions of articular degenerated cartilage, but they have less value in joints with more extensive changes, they may expose the patients to risk of disease transmission, and the supply of grafts is restricted. Promising experimental methods of stimulating formation of a new joint surface include growth factors, cell transplants, and artificial matrices. Thus far, none of these approaches has been shown to regenerate tissue that duplicates the structure, composition, mechanical properties, and durability of articular cartilage; nor have these methods been compared in clinical trails to other approaches to stimulating formation of a new articular surface in localized chondral defects, including penetration of subchondral bone and perichondral grafts.

It is unlikely any single one of these methodologies will be generally successful in the treatment of OA. Instead, the available clinical and experimental evidence indicates that future optimal surgical methods of preserving and restoring articular surfaces will begin with a detailed analysis of the structural and functional abnormalities of the involved joint, and the expectations of the patient for future joint use. Based on this analysis, the surgeon will develop a treatment plan that potentially combines correction of mechanical abnormalities (including malalignment, instability, and intra-articular causes of mechanical dysfunction), debridement (that may nor may not include limited penetration of subchondral bone and applications of growth factors or implants that may comprise a synthetic matrix that incorporates cells or growth factors), followed by a post-operative course of controlled loading and motion.

References

1. Buckwalter, J.A. and Lohmander, S. (1994). Operative treatment of osteoarthrosis: Current practice and future development. *J Bone Joint Surg*, **76A**, 1405–18.
2. Buckwalter, J.A., Mow, V.C., and Ratcliffe, A. (1994). Restoration of injured or degenerated articular surfaces. *J Am Acad Orthop Surg*, **2**, 192–201.
3. Buckwalter, J.A. and Mow, V.C. (1992). Cartilage repair in osteoarthritis. In *Osteoarthritis: diagnosis and medical/surgical management* (ed. R.W. Moskowitz *et al.*), pp. 71–107. Saunders, Philadelphia.
4. Geldwert, J.J., Rock, G.D., McGrath, M.P., and Mancuso, J.E. (1992). Cheilectomy: still a useful technique for grade I and grade II hallux limitus/rigidus. *J Foot Surg*, **31**, 154–9.
5. Mann, R.A. and Clanton, T.O. (1988). Hallux rigidus: treatment by cheilectomy. *J Bone Joint Surg*, **70A**, 400–6.
6. Aichroth, P.M., Patel, D.V., and Moyes, S.T. (1991). A prospective review of arthroscopic debridement for degenerative joint disease of the knee. *Int Orthop*, **15**, 351–5.
7. Baumgaertner, M.R., Cannon, W.D., Vittori, J.M., Schmidt, E.S., and Maurer, R.C. (1990). Arthroscopic debridement of the arthritic knee. *Clin Orthop*, **253**, 197–202.
8. Bert, J.M. (1993). Role of abrasion arthroplasty and debridement in the management of osteoarthritis of the knee. *Rheum Dis Clinics North America*, **19**(3), 725–39.
9. Bert, J.M. and Maschka, K. (1989). The arthroscopic treatment of unicompartmental gonarthrosis. *J Arthroscopy*, **5**, 25.
10. Dandy, D.J. (1991). Arthroscopic debridement of the knee for osteoarthritis. *J Bone Joint Surg*, **73B**, 877–8.

11. Ewing, J.W. (1990). Arthroscopic treatment of degenerative meniscal lesions and early degenerative arthritis of the knee. In *Articular cartilage and knee joint function: basic science and arthroscopy* (ed. J.W. Ewing), pp. 137–45. Raven Press, New York.

12. Ha'eri, G.B. and Wiley, A.M. (1980). High tibial osteotomy combined with joint debridement: a long-term study of results. *Clin Orthop*, **151**, 153–9.

13. Hawkins, R.B. (1988). Arthroscopic treatment of sports-related osteophytes in the ankle. *Foot Ankle*, **9**, 87–90.

14. Jackson, R.W., Silver, R., and Marans, R. (1986). The arthroscopic treatment of degenerative joint disease. *J Arthroscopy*, **2**, 114.

15. Johnson, L.L. (1980). *Diagnostic and surgical arthroscopy*. C.V. Mosby, St. Louis.

16. Morrey, B.F. (1992). Primary degenerative arthritis of the elbow. Treatment by ulnohumeral arthroplasty. *J Bone Joint Surg*, **74B**, 409–13.

17. Moseley, J.B., Wray, N.P., Kuykendall, D., Willis, K., Landon, G.C. (1996). Arthroscopic treatment of osteoarthritis of the knee: a prospective, randomized, placebo-controlled trial: results of a pilot study. *American Journal of Sports Medicine*, **24**(1), 28–34.

18. Rand, J.A. (1991). Role of arthroscopy in osteoarthritis of the knee. *J Arthroscopy*, **7**, 358.

19. Sprague, N.F. (1981). Arthroscopic debridement for degenerative knee joint disease. *Clin Orthop*, **160**, 118–23.

20. Tsuge, K. and Mizuseki, T. (1994). Debridement arthroplasty for advanced primary osteoarthritis of the elbow. Results of a new technique in 29 elbows. *J Bone Joint Surg*, **76B**, 641–6.

21. Haggart, G.E. (1940). The surgical treatment of degenerative arthritis of the knee joint. *J Bone Joint Surg*, **22**, 717–29.

22. Magnuson, P.B. (1941). Joint debridement: surgical treatment of degenerative arthritis. *Surg Gynecol Obstet*, **73**, 1–9.

23. Hubbard, M.J.S. (1987). Arthroscopic surgery for chondral flaps in the knee. *J Bone Joint Surg*, **69B**, 794–6.

24. Huber, M.J., Schmotzer, W.B., Riebold, T.W., Watrous, B.J., Synder, S.P., and Scott, E.A. (1992). Fate and effect of autogenous osteochondral fragments implanted in the middle carpal joint of horses. *Am J Vet Res*, **53**, 1579–88.

25. Kim, H.K.W., Moran, M.E., and Salter, R.B. (1991). The potential for regeneration of articular cartilage in defects created by chondral shaving and subchondral abrasion. *J Bone Joint Surg*, **73A**, 1301–15.

26. Mitchell, N. and Shepard, N. (1987). Effect of patellar shaving in the rabbit. *J Orthop Res*, **5**, 388–92.

27. Bentley, G. (1980). Chondromalacia patellae. *J Bone Joint Surg*, **52A**, 221–32.

28. Bentley, G. and Dowd, G. (1984). Current concepts of etiology and treatment of chondromalacia patellae. *Clin Orthop*, **189**, 209–28.

29. Milgram, J.W. (1985). Injury to articular cartilage joint surfaces. I. chondral injury produced by patellar shaving: a histopathologic study of human tissue specimens. *Clin Orthop*, **192**, 168–73.

30. Schmid, A. and Schmid, F. (1987). Results after cartilage shaving studied by electron microscopy. *Am J Sports Med*, **15**, 386–7.

31. Gibson, J.N.A., White, M.D., Chapman, V.M., and Strachan, R.K. (1992). Arthroscopic lavage and debridement for osteoarthritis of the knee. *J Bone Joint Surg*, **74B**, 534–7.

32. Boniface, R.J., Cain, P.R., and Evans, C.H. (1988). Articular response to purified cartilage proteoglycans. *Arthritis Rheum*, **31**, 258–66.

33. Evans, C.H., Mazzocchi, R.A., Nelson, D.D., and Rubash, H.E. (1984). Experimental arthritis induced by intra-articular injection of allogenic cartilagenous particules into rabbit knees. *Arthritis Rheum*, **27**, 200–15.

34. Livesley, P.J., Doherty, M., Needoff, M., and Moulton, A. (1991). Arthroscopic lavage of osteoarthritic knees. *J Bone Joint Surg*, **73B**, 922–6.

35. Buckwalter, J.A., Einhorn, T.A., Bolander, M.E., and Cruess, R.L. (1996). Healing of the musculoskeletal tissues. In *Fractures*, fourth edition (ed. D.P. Green, R.W. Bucholz, and J.D. Heckman), pp. 261–304. Lippincott, Philadelphia. (Based on a chapter published in 1991.)

36. Buckwalter, J.A., Rosenberg, L.C., and Hunziker, E.B. (1990). Articular cartilage: composition structure, response to injury and methods of facilitating repair. In *Articular cartilage and knee joint function: basic science and arthroscopy* (ed. J. W. Ewing), pp. 19–56. Raven Press, New York.

37. Shapiro, F., Koide, S., and Glimcher, M.J. (1993). Cell origin and differentiation in the repair of full-thickness defects of articular cartilage. *J Bone Joint Surg*, **75A**, 532–53.

38. Johnson, L.L. (1986). Arthroscopic abrasion arthroplasty. Historical and pathologic perspective: present status. *Arthroscopy*, **2**, 54–9.

39. Johnson, L.L. (1990). The sclerotic lesion: pathology and the clinical response to arthroscopic abrasion arthroplasty. In *Articular cartilage and knee joint function: basic science and arthroscopy* (ed. J.W. Ewing), pp. 319–33. Raven Press, New York.

40. Fenkel, S.R., Menche, D.S., Blair, B., Watnik, N.F., Toolan, B.C., and Pitman, M.I. (1994). A comparison of abrasion burr arthroplasty and subchondral drilling in the treatment of full-thickness cartilage lesions in the rabbit. *Trans Orthop Res Soc*, **19**, 483.

41. Mitchell, N. and Shepard, N. (1976). The resurfacing of adult rabbit articular cartilage by multiple perforations through the subchondral bone. *J Bone Joint Surg*, **58A**, 230–3.

42. Bentley, G. (1978). The surgical treatment of chondromalacia patellae. *J Bone Joint Surg*, **60B**, 74–81.

43. Childers, J.C. and Ellwood, S.C. (1979). Partial chondrectomy and subchondral bone drilling for chondromalacia. *Clin Orthop*, **144**, 114–20.

44. Ficat, R.P., Ficat, C., Gedeon, P.K., and Toussaint, J.B. (1979). Spongialization: a new treatment for diseased patellae. *Clin Orthop*, **144**, 74–83.

45. Friedman, M.J., Berasi, D.O., Fox, J.M., Pizzo, W.D., Snyder, S.J., and Ferkel, R.D. (1994). Preliminary results with abrasion arthroplasty in the osteoarthritic knee. *Clin Orthop*, **182**, 200–5.

46. Insall, J. (1974). The Pridie debridement operation for osteoarthritis of the knee. *Clin Orthop*, **101**, 61–7.

47. Weisl, H. (1980). Intertrochanteric osteotomy for osteoarthritis. A long-term follow-up. *J Bone Joint Surg*, **62B**, 37–42.

48. Beyers, P.D. (1974). The effect of high femoral osteotomy on osteoarthritis of the hip. *J Bone Joint Surg*, **56B**, 279–90.

49. Itoman, M., Yamamoto, M., Yonemoto, K., Sekiguchi, M., and Kai, H. (1992). Histological examination of surface repair tissue after successful osteotomy for osteoarthritis of the hip. *Int Orthop (Germany)*, **16**, 118–21.

50. Bergenudd, H., Johnell, O., Redlund-Johnell, I., and Lohmander, L.S. (1992). The articular cartilage after osteotomy for medial gonarthrosis: biopsies after 2 years in 19 cases. *Acta Orthop Scand*, **63**, 413–16.

51. Odenbring, S., Egund, N., Lindstrand, A., Lohmander, L.S., and Wilén, H. (1992). Cartilage regeneration after proximal tibial osteotomy for medial gonarthrosis. *Clin Orthop*, **277**, 210–16.

52. Insall, J.N., Joseph, D.M., and Msika, C. (1984). High tibial osteotomy for varus gonarthrosis. A long-term follow-up study. *J Bone Joint Surg*, **66A**, 1040–8.

53. Reigstad, A. and Gronmark, T. (1984). Osteoarthritis of the hip treated by intertrochanteric osteotomy. A long-term follow up. *J Bone Joint Surg*, **66A**, 1–6.

54. Berman, A.T., Bosco, S.J., Kirshner, S., and Avolio, A. (1991). Factors influencing long-term results in high tibial osteotomy. *Clin Orthop*, **272**, 192–8.

55. Matthews, L.S., Goldstein, S.A., Malvitz, T.A., Katz, B.P., and Kaufer, H. (1988). Proximal tibial osteotomy. Factors that influence the duration of satisfactory function. *Clin Orthop*, **229**, 193–200.

56. Coventry, M.B., Ilstrup, D.M., and Wallrichs, S.L. (1993). Proximal tibial osteotomy. A critical longterm study of eighty-seven cases. *J Bone Joint Surg*, **75A**, 196–201.

57. Odenbring, S., Egund, N., Knutson, K., Lindstrand, A., and Larsen, S.T. (1990). Revision after osteotomy for gonarthrosis. A 10–19 year follow-up of 314 cases. *Acta Orthop Scand*, **61**, 128–30.

58. Odenbring, S., Egund, N., Lindstrand, A., and Tjörnstrand, B. (1989). A guide instrument for high tibial osteotomy. *Acta Orthop Scand*, **60**, 449–51.

59. Prodromos, C.C., Andriacchi, T.P., and Galante, J.O. (1985). A relationship between gait and clinical changes following high tibial osteotomy. *J Bone Joint Surg*, **67A**, 1188–94.

60. Wang, J-W., Kuo, K.N., Andriacchi, T.P., and Galante, J.O. (1990). The influence of walking mechanics and time on the results of proximal tibial osteotomy. *J Bone Joint Surg*, **72A**, 905–9.

61. Odenbring, S., Tjörnstrand, B., Egund, N., Hagstedt, B., Hovelius, L., Lindstrand, A., *et al.* (1989). Function after tibial osteotomy for medial gonarthrosis below aged 50 years. *Acta Orthop Scand*, **60**, 527–31.

62. Richardson, E.G. (1987). The foot in adolescents and adults. In *Campbell's operative orthopedics* (ed. A.H. Crenshaw), pp. 829–988. C.V. Mosby, St Louis.

63. Sherman, K.P., Douglas, D.L., and Benson, D.A. (1984). Keller's arthroplasty: is distraction useful? *J Bone Joint Surg*, **66B**, 765–9.

64. Falahee, M.H., Matthews, L.S., and Kaufer, H. (1987). Resection arthroplasty as a salvage procedure for a knee with infection after a total arthroplasty. *J Bone Joint Surg*, **69A**, 1013–21.

65. Lettin, A.W.F., Neil, N.J., Citron, N.D., and August, A. (1990). Excision arthroplasty for infected constrained total knee replacements. *J Bone and Joint Surg*, **72B**, 220–4.

66. Dell, P.C. and Muniz, R.B. (1987). Interposition arthroplasty of the trapeziometacarpal joint for osteoarthritis. *Clin Orthop*, **220**, 27–34.

67. Knight, R.A. and Zandt, I.L.V. (1952). Arthroplasty of the elbow. *J Bone Joint Surg*, **34A**, 610–18.

68. Shahriaree, H., Sajadi, K., Silver, C.M., and Sheikholeslamzadeh, S. (1987). Excisional arthroplasty of the elbow. *J Bone Joint Surg*, **61A**, 922–7.

69. Engkvist, O. and Johansson, S.H. (1980). Perichondrial arthroplasty: a clinical study in twenty-six patients. *Scand J Plast Reconstr Surg*, **14**, 71–87.

70. Seradge, H., Kutz, J.A., Kleinert, H.E., Lister, G.D., Wolff, T.W., and Atasoy, E. (1984). Perichondrial resurfacing arthroplasty in the hand. *J Hand Surg*, **9A**, 880–6.

71. Homminga, G.N., Bulstra, S.K., Bouwmeester, P.M., and Linden, A.J.V.D. (1990). Perichondrial grafting for cartilage lesions of the knee. *J Bone Joint Surg*, **72B**, 1003–7.

72. Buckwalter, J.A., Woo, S. L-Y., Goldberg, V.M., Hadley, E.C., Booth, F., Oegema, T. R., *et al.* (1994). Soft tissue aging and musculoskeletal function. *J Bone Joint Surg*, **75A**, 1533–48.

73. Kusayama, T., Tomatsu, T., Akasaka, O., and Imai, N. (1991). Autogenous meniscus grafts in articular cartilage defects — an experimental study. *Tokai J Exp Clin Med*, **16**, 145–51.

74. Vachon, A.M., Mcllwraith, C.W., Powers, B.E., McFadden, P.R., and Amiel, D. (1992). Morphologic and biochemical study of sternal cartilage autografts for resurfacing induced osteochondral defects in horses. *Am J Vet Res*, **53**, 1038–47.

75. Jacobs, J.E. (1965). Follow-up notes on articles previously published in the journal: patellar graft for severely depressed comminuted fractures of the lateral tibial condyle. *J Bone Joint Surg*, **47A**, 842–7.

76. Flynn, J.M., Springfield, D.S., and Mankin, H.J. (1994). Osteoarticular allografts to treat distal femoral osteonecrosis. *Clin Orthop*, **303**, 38–43.

77. Gross, A.E., Beaver, R.J., and Mohammed, M.N. (1992). Fresh small fragment osteochondral allografts used for posttraumatic defects in the knee joint. In *Biology and biomechanics of the traumatized synovial joint: the knee as a model* (ed. G.A.M. Finerman and F.R. Noyes), pp. 123–41. American Academy of Orthopedic Surgeons, Rosemont, IL.

78. Locht, R.C., Gross, A.E., and Langer, F. (1984). Late osteochondral allograft resurfacing for tibial plateau fractures. *J Bone Joint Surg*, **66A**, 328–35.

79. Meyers, M.H., Akeson, W., and Convery, F.R. (1989). Resurfacing the knee with fresh osteochondral allograft. *J Bone Joint Surg*, **71A**, 704–13.

80. Hunziker, E.B. and Rosenberg, R. (1994). Induction of repair partial thickness articular cartilage lesions by timed release of TGF-Beta. *Trans Orthop Res Soc*, **19**, 236.

81. Pfeilschifter, J., Diel, I., Brunotte, K., Naumann, A., and Ziegler, R. (1993). Mitogenic responsiveness of human bone cells *in vitro* to hormones and growth factors decreases with age. *J Bone Min Res*, **8**, 707–17.

82. Itay, S., Abramovici, A., Ysipovitch, Z., and Nevo, Z. (1988). Correction of defects in articular cartilage by implants of cultures of embryonic chondrocytes. *Trans Orthop Res Soc*, **13**, 112.

83. Noguchi, T., Oka, M., Fujino, M., Neo, M., and Yamamuro, T. (1994). Repair of osteochondral defects with grafts of cultured chondrocytes. Comparison of allografts and isografts. *Clin Orthop*, **302**, 251–8.

84. Robinson, D., Halperin, N., and Nevo, Z. (1990). Regenerating hyaline cartilage in articular defects of old chickens using implants of embryonal chick chondro-cytes embedded in a new natural delivery substance. *Calcif Tissue Int*, **46**, 246–53.

85. Wakitani, S., Goto, T., Mansour, J.M., Goldberg, V.M., and Caplan, A.I. (1994). Mesenchymal stem cell-based repair of a large articular cartilage and bone defect. *Trans Orthop Res Soc*, **19**, 481.

86. Wakitani, S., Kimura, T., Hirooka, A., Ochi, T., Yoneda, M., Natsuo, N., *et al.* (1989). Repair of rabbit articular surfaces with allograft chondrocytes embedded in collagen gel. *J Bone Joint Surg*, **71B**, 74–80.

87. Brittberg, M., Lindahl, A., Nilsson, A., Ohlsson, C., Isaksson, O., and Peterson, L. (1994). Treatment of deep cartilage defects in the knee with autologous chondrocyte transplantation. *New Eng J Med*, **331**, 889–95.

88. Muckle, D.S. and Minns, R.J. (1990). Biological response to woven carbon fiber pads in the knee: a clinical and experimental study. *J Bone and Joint Surg*, **72B**, 60–2.

??. Beltran, J.E. (1987). Resection arthroplasty of the patella. *J Bone Joint Surg*, **69B**, 603–7.

9.17 Arthroplasty and its complications

Kaj Knutson

Arthroplasty is the reconstruction, by natural modification or artificial replacement, of a diseased, damaged, or ankylosed joint. This chapter deals with endoprosthetic joint replacement arthroplasty.

Clinical picture

Joint degeneration in osteoarthritis (OA) is slow and gradual. The OA joint may be painful on weight-bearing and incapacitating as soon as radiographs show only a reduced thickness of the joint cartilage in the load-bearing areas. However, some patients have an asymptomatic joint degeneration like that found on postmortem examinations. The degenerative process goes on to complete loss of cartilage and attrition of the subchondral bone. Finally, the joint is painful even at rest. The time from the onset of OA on radiographs to the onset of pain or to the complete loss of cartilage varies considerably between patients and between joints.

In hinge-like joints, such as the knee, one part of the joint often takes more load than the other with an asymmetric progress of the degeneration. As a result, a varus or valgus malalignment follows which increases the uneven load distribution. The end result is a severely malaligned joint, with subluxation of the condyles. However, pain reduces joint mobility which, together with sclerosis of the loaded parts of the condyles, osteophytes, and fibrosis of the joint capsule, stops the process at some advanced level. Sometimes, the joint spontaneously ankyloses.

The radiographic prevalence of OA of the hip has been shown to be three per cent in the Swedish population aged over 55, and it increases with age. The sex distribution is uniform, and bilateral involvement occurs in 40 per cent. The prevalence has not changed in two decades. Similar studies from Denmark have shown a slightly higher prevalence, especially in women. Studies on risk factors show that overweight, high occupational joint load, and strenuous high-level sports activities are risk factors.

The prevalence of OA of the knee varies with the definitions used. Radiographic changes are seen in one third of the population aged over 65, but only half of them have symptoms; symptomatic OA is twice as common in women; symptoms may disappear, but are more usual with more advanced radiographic changes;

it is not clear whether the prevalence increases in the population over age 70; progression is commoner in advanced cases, but is not inevitable; the risk factors are the same as for the hip.

Historical review

One hundred years ago, attempts were made to treat diseased joints with endoprosthetic replacement. Péan designed a rubber ball to replace the humeral head and Gluck, an ivory hinge for the knee, that were implanted in patients with tuberculous joints. The initial failures were due to unsuitable materials and surgical technique, as well as to a lack of antisepsis and proper indications. A search for implant materials for fracture treatment and joint replacement continued, and by the middle of the century, stainless steel, cobalt-chromium alloy, and acrylics were found to be suitable. The first successes came with a stainless steel reinforced acrylic hinged knee prosthesis introduced by Walldius in 1953. The Walldius knee was further developed into a cobalt-chromium hinge that was universally accepted; it relied on fibrous encapsulation of its stems in the femoral and tibial shafts. Young and Shiers independently made similar designs.

Parallel with this development, attempts were made to treat arthritic joints with materials interposed between the joint surfaces. The idea was to prevent the degenerated surfaces from making direct contact, thus reducing pain and the progression of attrition and malalignment. Autogenous materials, such as fascia lata and split-thickness skin grafts, were used, but also pig-bladder and synthetic materials have been tried. In weight-bearing joints, the materials were too soft, or they evoked a serious foreign-body reaction. However, autogenous materials in the joints of the upper extremity still have their use in modern orthopedic surgery in rheumatoid patients. In the 1950s, inert metal alloys were successfully introduced as hemiprostheses, replacing one of a pair of degenerated articular surfaces, for example, the Smith–Petersen hip cup, the MacIntosh and McKeever tibial inlays. Femoral head-replacing prostheses were also introduced by Judet, Moore, and Thomson.

An important breakthrough came with the work of Charnley[26]. He realized that a hip hemiarthroplasty would never achieve the low friction of a normal joint when a metallic head articulated against subchondral bone in the acetabulum; high friction caused the implants to loosen by putting stress on the boundaries between the bone and the implant. Others, such as McKee, had tried metal-against-metal hip implants with screw fixation, but Charnley found that the friction was too high and the fixation inadequate. From a chemist in the field of dental surgery, Charnley had learnt about self-curing acrylic resin that could be used for implant fixation — a powder of polymethyl methacrylate was mixed with fluid methyl methacrylate, giving a doughy cement that could be used to fill the gap between the stem of a hip prosthesis and the femoral shaft. The cement cured in 15 minutes, with some heat generation. Once cured, the substance was inert and strong enough to keep the femoral component fixed to the bone. Charnley also looked for other materials to use as an articulating surface against the Moore prosthesis. Low friction was first achieved with an acetabular cup of polytetrafluoroethylene (PTFE) and was improved by gradual reduction of the head diameter from 42 to 22 mm. Despite low friction, the PTFE wore rapidly, and the wear particles evoked a strong foreign-body reaction — another cup material was needed. High-density polyethylene (HDPE) combined inertness with low friction and low wear rate. In 1962, Charnley's low friction arthroplasty (LFA) was finalized with a set of orthopedic instruments and a strict surgical routine for the procedure. Although the procedure was a success, Charnley continued to refine the operation. The components were redesigned to improve cement pressurization during insertion, which also improved cement interlocking with the intramedullary cancellous bone. He also introduced drill holes in acetabulum, lavage systems and brushes for cleaning the cancellous surfaces, and the technique of plugging the distal femoral canal with a bone-block to further improve fixation.

Another important step in making the LFA a safe procedure was the development of an ultraclean environment for the operation. Charnley assumed that the seven per cent deep infection rate in the early years was due to intraoperative contamination. Operating in a small tent-like enclosure in the operating room, with a vertical flow of filtered air, reduced the number of infective particles to two per cent. Further reduction was achieved with body gowns of new impermeable materials, a helmet with glass visor, body exhaust systems, and double gloves. After ten years' development, the infection rate was less than one tenth of the original rate.

Once the usefulness of the LFA became obvious, the implant and technique were copied and modified by others: Buchholz in Hamburg added antibiotics to the bone cement to reduce the infection rate; Müller made an implant with curved stem and a larger head to reduce the risk of dislocation; in the United States, new bone cements with lower viscosity were introduced in an attempt to get better penetration into cancellous bone surfaces — it had to be applied with a cartridge and a cement gun. Eventually, hundreds of modifications of the original LFA were marketed.

Evolution of hip prostheses

In hip arthroplasty, the load of the implant is carried to the bone through shearing forces in the cement. This load is high, and methods have been employed to increase the strength of the cement and, thus, prevent it from deforming and cracking. The traditional mixing of cement in a bowl led to air entrapment causing a porous and weakened cement. Low viscosity cement was easier to mix, and centrifugation after mixing reduced the number of large voids, while microporosity was the same. Mixing in thin air (so-called partial vacuum) has been shown to improve further the fatigue properties of cement, and is nowadays commonly used.

The bone cement monomer is toxic, the curing process generates high temperatures with a potential risk of bone necrosis, and the cement is brittle, and more so with age. Once the cement is loose, it wears down and generates cement particles that can induce an inflammatory process which increases bone resorption and promotes further loosening of the implant. Concern about heat necrosis during the cement-curing process has led to the development of new types of cement with lower heat generation. However, *in vivo* measurements of interfacial temperatures have not supported the validity of this concern in arthroplasty. At least one of the new low-heat generating cements had to be withdrawn because of poor mechanical properties[16]. As an alternative, biological fixation methods, with direct bone-to-implant contact, were investigated. Initial macroscopic fixation was a prerequisite for microscopic fixation, with bone growing on to the surface of the implant.

The polyethylene cup was reinforced with a metal outer shell in an attempt to better redistribute the load and to minimize deformation through creep of the plastic material. The metallic shell was supplied with an outer thread to allow cementless fixation by screwing the cup into the acetabular cavity. However, the screw cup had only the inadequate area of the edge of the threads in contact with bone, and results were infe-

rior. Instead, a layer of porous coating was added to the metal shell to combine instant macrolocking with later microlocking through bone ingrowth[28]. Concern was expressed that the cup failed to make bone contact centrally, thus preventing bone ingrowth which cannot span millimetre-wide gaps. Conventional screws inserted through holes in the metal shell were introduced. The thickness of the metal shell had to be increased to harbour the screw heads, thus reducing the thickness of the plastic parts to an unsafe level, with increased plastic deformation and wear as a result. Because of the screw holes, only a fraction of the plastic shell was actually supported by the metal shell. The latest step has been a solid metal shell with a smooth inner surface that makes full contact with the plastic part. These porous-coated cups rely on under-reamed acetabulae and a peripheral pressfit for fixation. The latter type of acetabular implant has proved to be as reliable as cemented HDPE cups.

Porous coating for biological fixation is also used in the femoral shaft[20]. The technique requires a large number of sizes to allow optimal filling of the medullary cavity for an initial, stable pressfit. In animal experiments porous coating along all of the stem induced proximal bone atrophy through stress shielding; has been abandoned for proximal porous coating alone. Initial stability is essential to bone ingrowth and as little as 150 μ of micromotion has been found to prevent bone ingrowth. The natural variability in the shape of the proximal femur makes it impossible to obtain more than isolated areas with good bone-to-prosthesis contact.

In later years, great interest has been focused on bioactive coatings to create an active bond between the implant and the bone bed. The coating most often used is made of hydroxyapatite. The bioactive coating improves early fixation, but does not replace the need for porous coating or pressfit design. Its effect is probably short lasting, and the coating may resorb or become yet another source of particles that may interfere with the articulation, thus creating more wear.

The shafts of uncemented femoral components are considerably stiffer than the femoral cortex. This has been pointed out as a possible explanation of the common problem of mid-thigh pain during the first postoperative year. Attempts have been made to improve the elasticity match of the femoral component by weakening the distal end. This can be done with slots or hollow implants, a thinner stem with an outer sleeve, and by using titanium alloy components. However, more flexible implants have more interfacial motion and less ingrowth in porous surfaces. Again, the solution to one problem causes another[9].

Concern about wear has led to improvement in the surface quality of the femoral heads and the use of ceramic heads. Ceramic cups have been designed for the same reason. A renewed interest in metal-against-metal articulation has also started. Modern production techniques make it possible to produce perfectly matching pairs with minimal wear. Modern metal-to-plastic implants have a wear rate of 0.1–0.2 mm per year; ceramic and all metal articulations are more than ten times better. The friction in all metal articulations are the same as in the LFA, and the high friction found by Charnley has since been ascribed to his having evaluated a poorly designed copy of the McKee–Farrar prosthesis.

Evolution of knee prostheses

It was soon realised that the low-friction technique, with HDPE-against-metal components fixed with bone cement, was also the solution for knee arthroplasty. The interposition implants were developed into surface replacements, with a HDPE tibial component and a metal runner on the femoral condyle, as in the polycentric knee developed by Gunston, the Marmor knee, and the St. Georg sled designed by Buchholz. These implants were suitable for single-compartment degeneration. For generalized degeneration, it was easier to use interconnected surface replacement parts (Geomedic) or true bicondylar implants, for example, the Freeman–Swanson knee. Later, the patellar articulation was included and the implants became tricompartmental or 'total knees', for example, the total condylar knee by Insall, the Townley knee, and the ICLH knee by Freeman and Swanson. Hinged implants were more anatomically redesigned, as in the French GUEPAR prosthesis, and soon included HDPE bearings to avoid direct metal-to-metal connections as in the St. Georg hinged prosthesis. Hybrid solutions were created, either as rotating hinges or stabilized prostheses with more than single-axis mobility. The latter had loose interference connections between the tibial and femoral parts, restricting varus and valgus mobility, and a forced rollback of the femoral component on the tibia through a cam axis or similar design. Most of these implants were fixed with bone cement.

The initial clinical experience of knee arthroplasty was rewarding, with good mobility, stability, and pain relief. However, the failure rate was higher than for contemporary hip arthroplasties. Large implants were easy to use because they replaced both the degenerated joint surfaces and the accompanying stabilizing structures. The positioning of the implants relative to the bony parts was simplified by using long intramedullary stems. Despite the rigid fixation, these implants had a high failure rate because of loosening and deep infection[12]. During the 1980s, the larger implants were replaced by smaller ones, as more was learned about soft tissue techniques with ligament release procedures to correct deformities. The surface replacement prostheses were supplied with increasingly complex guide instruments to ensure proper alignment of the leg, position of the implant, and soft tissue balance. Surface replacement prostheses rely on the support of the condylar cancellous bone for fixation, and cement injection techniques were developed, using a cement gun and low viscosity cement.

Further attempts were made to improve prosthetic fixation. In particular, the tibial component constituted a problem because of its basically flat design; the first polyethylene tibial components covered only a part of the resected tibial condyle. They were anchored to the cement and bone bed by a textured surface or by small dovetail-shaped pegs. Development of better fixation was a gradual process, starting with better coverage by using more sizes, short intracondylar stems, integrated metal reinforcement, or a metal base plate with stems, pegs, or screws. Parallel to this, attempts were made to reduce the stresses transmitted through the tibial component. Initially, the femoral and tibial parts were highly congruent, allowing only single-axis rotation. Thus, the rotation of the lower leg around its longitudinal axis was restricted by the implant, with high stresses on the tibial component anchorage. By redesigning the articulate surfaces into a flat tibial contact area, these stresses were instead transmitted through the soft tissues. However, in solving one problem, that is, the overload of the tibial component fixation, other problems were created. Articulating a curved femoral component on a flat tibial component meant a very high stress level at the point of contact, with an increased wear rate as a result.

Biological fixation methods with direct bone-to-implant contact have also been investigated in knee arthroplasty. Initial macroscopic fixation is a prerequisite for microscopic fixation, with bone growing on to the surface of the implant. The former was achieved through a pressfit design, with additional screw fixation, and the latter through a porous coating of the implant. The first design to be clinically used was the

PCA total knee by Hungerford and Kenna — it had a porous layer of chrome-cobalt beads sintered to the metal parts. Others followed, with titanium alloy components having a porous wire mesh fixed to the substrate by diffusion bonding, that is, a low-temperature, high-pressure sintering technique. Porous titanium surfaces were also created by plasma-spraying metal on to a cold metal substrate. Again, it seemed that a problem was solved, but instead, new problems were created. The sintering process changed the properties of the substrate metal, making it more vulnerable to metal fatigue; beads came off and tibial trays broke. Furthermore, the porous structure greatly enlarged the surface, with increased risk of metal ion leakage into the surrounding tissues. Although the alloys were inert, the isolated ions were not.

In animal models of the hip and knee, it was demonstrated that with porous stems, the load was transmitted from the implant to the bone at the tip of the stem. The condylar regions were thus stress-shielded, and responded with severe bone atrophy. This phenomenon is not so obvious in human knees, probably because little, if any, bone ingrowth occurs. These have been the findings at the examination of postmortem retrieved tibial components.

Micromotion

Computer-assisted radiostereometric analysis (RSA) of tibial component migration can detect very small changes in the prosthetic position over time[22]. Collected data have indicated that most implants migrate for up to one year after insertion, but then they stabilize[21]; A small subset migrated more, and continued to migrate. Cases that eventually were revised for loosening of the implant, all belonged to the continuously migrating group. Thus, the loosening process was gradual and started shortly after implantation. The pattern was the same, whether the interface material was bone cement, polyethylene, or metal. Less migration was seen when a water-cooled saw-blade was used to cut bone, instead of cutting with a conventional heat-generating blade[24]. Proper alignment of the leg also reduced migration.

RSA has also been used to record the inducible displacement of the tibial component when the replaced knee is physiologically loaded. The observed micromotion occurs at a level that inhibits bone ingrowth in porous surfaces. However, stems and screws have a stabilizing effect, with reduced interfacial motion.

RSA indicates that the early findings govern the final outcome of the arthroplasty, and they are influenced by prosthetic design, surgical technique, fixation and position of implants, alignment, and bone quality. The interface in stable implants has been shown to be mainly dense fibrocartilage. Unstable implants have a softer, fibrous tissue encapsulation that is permeable to polyethylene wear particles. These, and other wear particles, induce an inflammatory reaction capable of inducing bone resorption: this makes failure more likely[4].

Scandinavian national arthroplasty registers

In 1975, the Swedish Orthopaedic Society initiated a prospective nationwide study of knee arthroplasty[15]. It was followed by a national hip arthroplasty study in 1979[17]. The former is organized as a prospective study of primary operations, while the latter, due to the much larger number of procedures, focused on revisions, using estimates of the number of primary operations. The Norwegian and Finnish counterparts have started similar registers[3,6–8]. The registers use the unique social security numbers to keep track of all patients. Individual patient mortality has been checked against national census registers. Data are regularly analyzed by actuarial methods, since there are many censored observations. The multicenter design gives large samples that are used to calculate the cumulated risk of revision for various groups of patients, implants, and surgical techniques. The results provide a better calculation of risks than reports from highly specialized units and are part of an ongoing quality control of joint replacement procedures. The registers have shown some underperforming designs, but also that the modern conventional cemented implants have been a safe choice. On the other hand, the constant change in designs, and the complexity of implants with modularity and optional combinations, have made analysis increasingly difficult.

The registers focus on revision, but not all revisions are equal. An implant with a higher rate of simple revisions may be a better choice than an implant with fewer, but devastating, failures. The second problem is that results are so good that differences become obvious only after prolonged observation times, when the implants have already been replaced by newer models. Another problem is that clinical performance is not taken into account; a slightly higher failure rate may be offset by a better clinical outcome in the vast majority of successful cases. Nonetheless, these large-scale studies have given information that could not have been collected in any other way, and they have never been meant to replace detailed studies in smaller units. Selected data from the registers have also been used to analyze uncommon conditions (for example, osteonecrosis of the knee), complications (for example, deep infection), and techniques (arthrodesis for knee failure).

Hip arthroplasty

In Scandinavian countries, the usual procedure is a cemented total hip replacement with a cobalt-chromium-molybdenum or stainless steel femoral component articulating against a UHMWPE acetabular cup (Fig. 9.17). The four commonest types in Sweden, in 1991, were Charnley, Lubinus SP, Exeter polished, and Scan Hip. Head sizes varied between 22 and 32 mm. Use of a cement-restricting plug, lavage, cleaning of the bone bed, and cement pressurization of vacuum-mixed cement with a gun was standard practice and affected the revision rate, according to the Swedish Total Hip Arthroplasty Register[17]. The same source shows a cumulative revision rate of 0.6 per cent for infection at ten years. This infection rate was influenced by the use of ultraclean air filtration and of gentamicin-containing bone cement, but not by the use of body-exhaust gowns. The ten-year revision rate for loosening was just above ten per cent; it was higher in men and in younger patients. Modern implants differed little. The limited experience of uncemented implants did not encourage its continued use. These findings have been supported by the Norwegian Arthroplasty Register in which uncemented implants had twice as high a risk of revision as the cemented, and even more among younger patients[7].

Knee arthroplasty

Early single-compartment OA of the knee can be treated with unicondylar implants. The commonly used Richards' modular knee and Endo sled are femoral onlay implants with pegs for fixation. On the tibial side, they have UHMWPE parts with a flat top. They can be used with or without a metal backing, and they

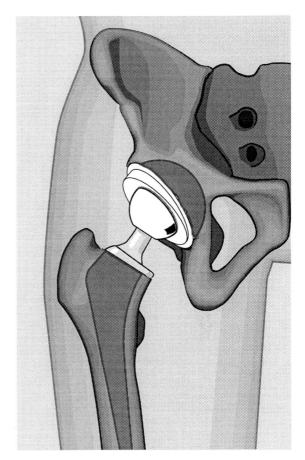

Fig. 9.17 Conventional hip prostheses have a cobalt-chromium stem fixed with bone cemented to the femoral shaft. The head is modular and fixed to the neck with a taper lock. The polyethylene cup is fixed with bone cement in the acetabular cavity.

rely on bone cement for fixation. Additional implants have been introduced recently. They differ in having femoral components that are fixed to the femoral condyle after resection of the distal and posterior parts of the femoral condyle. The tibial part is often metal backed, sometimes with screw fixation. These implants are available with or without porous coating, for cemented or uncemented fixation. The fraction of knee arthroplasties for OA performed with unicondylar implants varies from country to country. In Sweden, it is approximately one third[15].

Advanced or generalized OA of the knee is, nowadays, treated with tricompartmental (total) knee prostheses (Fig. 9.18). Most of them are cobaltchromium-molybdenum alloy implants with an anatomically-shaped femoral component. Both smooth

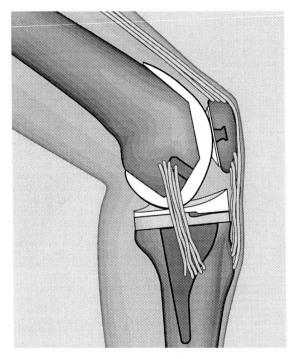

Fig. 9.18 A side view of the knee shows the extent of a tricompartmental knee prosthesis. The femoral part is fixed, with or without bone cement, to the resected femoral condyle covering all joint surfaces. The tibial part is a metal tray with pegs or stem fixed with bone cement to the resected surface of upper tibia. A polyethylene component of appropriate thickness is fitted in the tray. Despite the completely incongruent contact, the design is stable through the action of the ligaments and muscles. A small polyethylene button may be fixed on the resected joint surface of the patella. Unicompartmental prostheses cover only one of the femorotibial articulations.

and porous-coated femoral implants are used, and uncemented fixation is regarded as safe. The tibial component is usually modular, with a cemented metal tray that gains additional stability from a short central stem or from pegs. The UHMWPE part is usually fixed to the tray with a snap-fit. Modularity is increasingly popular, and several implants can be fitted with stem extension and wedges to fill the gap between the implant and the worn-down tibial condyle. Attempts are being made to reduce the high contact stresses inherent in a knee prosthesis with a flat tibial component and a rounded femoral component. By changing the tibial component to a more 'dished' shape, a higher degree of congruence is achieved with larger contact area. The most radical design has a fully congruent polyethylene component, which has a second articulation on its lower surface against the flat and polished top of the metal tray. By separating the articulation for flexion from that of axial rotation, these discal knees combine a large contact area with low shear forces and wear.

In total knees, a polyethylene patellar component can be fitted. It usually has the shape of a small button and is cemented against the resected joint surface of the patella. Metal backing is avoided because of the thin implant that may wear through causing metal to scratch against metal. The need for patellar replacement is debated[19].

Stabilized implants with a forced roll-back of femur on tibia have limited use in primary knee arthroplasty[15] — the exception being patellectomized knees, and knees with severe insufficiency of the posterior cruciate ligament.

Ankle arthroplasty

OA of the ankle is rare and often secondary to deformity, joint instability, ankle fractures, or vascular necrosis of the talus. The condition is painful; cartilage reduction and osteophyte formation lead to early loss of motion. The commonest surgical treatment is ankle fusion through an anterior approach or lateral with malleolar osteotomy; fixation is achieved with oblique screws inserted through the joint.

In sedentary OA patients aged over 60, without instability, deformity, or neuropathic disorders, but with normal vascular status, a joint replacement arthroplasty may be considered. A variety of implants have been designed, most of them having a metal talar dome and an UHMWPE tibial insert, with more or less constrained articulation. Cement fixation is commonly used, but at least one porous-coated design intended for biological fixation has been introduced. This implant is discal, with a lower conventional talar articulation and an upper flat tibial articulation that eliminates shear forces.

Ankle replacement arthroplasty is still being investigated. It has a low success rate that deteriorates with time, and reports are few and short term[10].

Foot arthroplasties

OA of the subtalar joints and the first metatarsophalangeal joints has been experimentally treated with joint replacement arthroplasty. The most extensive attempt has used silicone rubber interposition in the first metatarsophalangeal joint. Safe alternative methods, such as arthrodesis, osteotomy, and resection arthroplasty, have completely replaced these experimental methods[1].

Shoulder arthroplasty

OA of the shoulder follows the same pattern as OA of other joints: the cartilage is reduced in the loaded areas, and the periphery of the humeral head and glenoid is enlarged with osteophytes; usually the rotator cuff remains intact or mildly degenerated; Fibrosis of the joint capsule restricts mobility, but this restriction is compensated by the thoracoscapular mobility. OA of the shoulder is not the main indication for shoulder arthroplasty, a procedure constituting one per cent of all large joint arthroplasties. The implants used today are all similar unconstrained designs derived from the original Neer design, but with a modular, anatomically-sized head fixed with a taper to a humeral stem (Fig. 9.19); an UHMWPE glenoid surface replacement component is optional. (Resection of the head is a necessary part of the procedure if the glenoid is to be replaced.) The approach is anterior, through the deltopectoral groove. Only the subscapularis tendon must be divided and the joint dislocated to obtain access. At closure, the tendon can be lengthened to improve joint mobility, (since this tendon is often shortened in OA). Prosthetic components are pressfit or cemented. A simple metal cup fixed to the surface of the head has been designed for hemiarthroplasty — its usefulness in OA has not been established.

Little has been reported concerning the clinical outcome of shoulder hemiarthroplasty — pain relief is incomplete, and mobility depends on the condition of the rotator cuff and the shoulder muscles. A glenoid component seems to increase pain relief, at least for as long as it remains fixed. Failure of this component, however, is quite common.

Elbow arthroplasty

The elbow is a hinge-like joint and the first attempts to replace it were performed using hinged prostheses. Because of the high failure rate, with loosening due to overload of the bone-cement interface, the hinge was abandoned. Today, constrained surface replacement implants with short stems, such as the capitello-

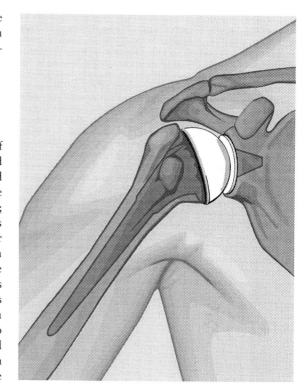

Fig. 9.19 A shoulder prosthesis is a design with a cemented or uncemented stem, a modular head, and an optional, rather flat, glenoid component. As in the normal shoulder, the joint is stable through the tension of the joint capsule and muscles.

condylar and Kudo implants, are used when possible (Fig. 9.20). In severely destroyed joints, 'sloppy' hinged prostheses may be used; they allow some axial rotation along the shafts, which reduces the interfacial stress. The approach is either posterior through the triceps tendon or lateral, with detachment of the radial collateral ligament. OA of the elbow is a rare condition and more than 95 per cent of all elbow arthroplasties are performed for other indications.

Arthroplasties of the hand

OA of the fingers affects both the proximal and distal joints. The initially painful arthritis and joint degeneration eventually cause stiff, slightly deformed but stable joints that need not be treated with implants, although these are available for rheumatoid arthritis.

The commonest OA affliction of the hand is found in the saddle-shaped trapeziometacarpal (TMC) joint of the thumb. Every fourth woman will have some joint

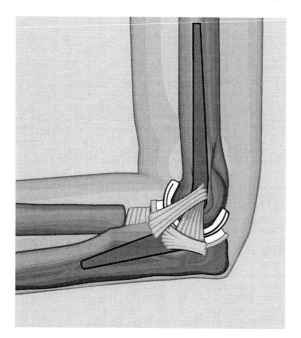

Fig. 9.20 A constrained elbow surface replacement has a metal humeral joint surface with a thin intramedullary stem. The ulnar component usually consists of a short-stemmed, metal-backed component with a congruent polyethylene part against the humeral component. Joint stability is achieved by the tension of the ligaments.

degeneration and as many as one in twenty will be a candidate for surgery[2]. The OA loss of cartilage is combined in many cases with subluxation of the TMC joint, and the end-stage is pantrapezial OA with fixed adduction contracture.

Surgical treatment of TMC OA includes partial or total excision of the trapezium with ligament reconstruction and interposition of tendinous structures or a silicone rubber implant. The implant can be designed to replace the base of the first metacarpal or the trapezium. Cemented ball-and-socket prostheses, like miniature hip prostheses, are also being evaluated in the TMC joint[2].

Primary OA of the wrist is rare and in many cases unilateral. Although silicone rubber interposition devices and cemented or porous-coated ball-and-socket prostheses have been designed for use in rheumatoid arthritis, they are seldom used in OA. Arthrodesis of the wrist permanently relieves pain and improves finger function, but at the expense of motion — This affects daily living activities. Partial wrist fusion and proximal row carpectomy are alternatives in localized, often secondary, OA of the wrist joints[27].

Arthroplasty complications

General complications

The prevalence of symptomatic OA increases with the age of the patient, as also do the risks of general complications due to major surgery. Improvements in risk assessment and anesthesiological technique have made it possible to offer arthroplasty even to the very old. Early reports on hip arthroplasty have dealt mainly with surgical risk aspects and early clinical outcome. These reports indicate that the immediate mortality rate was 0.5—2 per cent, mainly because of cardiac problems and pulmonary embolism. One type of pulmonary embolism was seen during pressurization of cement in the femoral shaft. It has been suggested that thromboplastic products are pushed out into the venous circulation in the cancellous bone by the cement. Changes in surgical technique with the introduction of lavage, brushing, and retrograde cement-filling of the shaft have eliminated this risk of intraoperative mors subita. With modern hip arthroplasty technique and hypotensive epidural anesthesia, Sharrock et al.[23] have reported a 0.1 per cent mortality at the Hospital for Special Surgery in New York.

The risk of deep vein thrombosis has been reported to be 10–70 per cent, and pulmonary embolism 1–4 per cent. Half of the thrombi were proximal and sometimes asymptomatic, and these were associated with pulmonary embolism. Deep-vein thrombosis, even when treated, is associated with later deep-venous insufficiency. Many methods have been introduced to reduce these figures: by using epidural instead of general anesthesia, the risk was reduced to less than half; Mechanical methods, such as leg elevation, graduated elastic compression stockings, foot compression pumps, and early ambulation all contribute. The main improvement came with pharmacologic prophylaxis. Dextran, heparin, dihydroergotamine, antithrombin III, and warfarin/dicumarol have been successfully used. Today, the low molecular weight heparins are favoured because of simple administration (once daily), and good prophylactic effect with negligible pulmonary embolism and few bleeding complications. Similarly good results, that is, 11 per cent deep-vein thrombosis and 1 per cent pulmonary embolism, have been reported using hypotensive epidural anesthesia combined with aspirin[23].

Urinary retention is a common problem seen in one third of the patients undergoing hip arthroplasty. Indwelling catheters are used to prevent retention and to monitor kidney function, but they increase the risk of urinary tract infection.

Rare general complications include paralytic intestinal obstruction, gastrointestinal bleeding, kidney dysfunction, cardiac failure, arrhythmia and infarction, pulmonary infection, stroke, and postoperative confusion and psychosis. The best prevention against these complications is a properly selected, well-informed, well-nourished, well-monitored patient, with blood loss replaced and pain-free. The importance of being pain-free has recently led to changes in the postoperative routines, including continued epidural analgesia, personally adjusted doses, and even self-administration of morphine.

Local complications in hip arthroplasty

The surgical procedure of hip arthroplasty is quite safe, but some intraoperative complications remain. The hip is close to both vessels and nerves; accidental damage to these structures has been reported (neural damage in 0 to 3 per cent[25]). Especially when arthroplasty is combined with lengthening of the hip, distension of the sciatic nerve may cause injury.

The preparation of the bone beds has been reported to cause fractures of the greater trochanter, the shaft, and acetabulum, particularly when uncemented pressfit prostheses are used (shaft fractures in 2 to 20 per cent[11]); if not dislocated, they usually heal uneventfully. The orientation of the implants must be reasonably correct to allow a normal range of motion and stability. Malpositioned components may cause impingement, early loosening, and dislocation. The reason for malposition can be altered anatomical landmarks, combined with an unstable position of the patient on the operating table. Failure to anchor the components properly may result in the patient having a prosthesis that is loose from the beginning. One serious intraoperative complication is bacterial contamination of the joint.

Early local postoperative complications include delayed wound-healing, deep infection, dislocation, avulsion of the greater trochanter, or pseudarthrosis of a trochanteric osteotomy. Dislocation has been reported in 0.5–5 per cent. The joint can usually be reduced and the problem may resolve as a pseudocapsule develops around it. Dislocation is associated with prior surgery of the hip, use of a posterior approach, and malaligned components, but not with head-size, leg or neck length, or nursing instructions[18]. Trochanteric problems are reported with the same frequency and to these should be added the formation of heterotopic bone seen in every other patient. When pronounced, it may seriously reduce mobility.

Late local complications include deep infection, loosening of implants, osteolysis, periprosthetic fractures, implant wear, and breakage. Wear has so far been unavoidable, but it causes no problems during the first ten postoperative years. Severe wear of the cup may result in instability and dislocation of the joint. More serious is the bone loss caused by osteolysis triggered by wear particles; this asymptomatically reduces the bone stock later needed for revision.

Low virulent infection may develop as a late complication, or the joint may be hematogenously seeded from some other focus, that is, urinary tract, gall bladder, lungs, or dental abscess. The overall infection rate today is below one per cent and less than half is believed to be hematogenous.

Loosening of components is the indication for 80 per cent of the hip revisions; using survival statistics, the risk is approximately 10 per cent at 10 years and is higher in men and in younger patients (Fig. 9.21). Modern cemented implants differ little from one another. Most steps in modern cementation technique have an impact on prosthetic survival. In half of the revisions, both components are exchanged and, overall, more stems than cups. Standard revision usually means the recementation of new, sometimes larger components. Components designed for revision, with a prolonged stem to create anchorage below the previous implant, are used in cases with severe bone loss. Various oddly shaped acetabular cups have been designed to fit and fill various defects.

An alternative method to compensate for severe bone loss is to fill the femoral shaft with morselized cancellous bone grafts from donors. Donated bone consists of heads from previous hip arthroplasties, temporarily stored in a bone bank at −80°C until tests show that it is safe to use for reconstruction. A cavity is created centrally in the shaft with impaction instruments and a conventional implant is cemented into the cavity. Cortical defects are covered with stainless steel mesh, fixed with wires. After some years, the impaction-grafted shafts show a normalized cortex, but the central core of dead donor bone remains dead. Early results are promising, but long-term results are lacking. Acetabular bone defects can be treated in the same manner.

Deep infection is a serious complication. Three types are encountered: early and delayed postoperative, and late hematogenous. The former are regarded as intra-

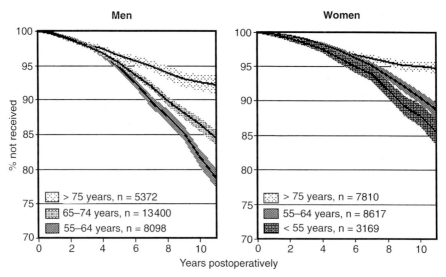

Fig. 9.21 On the basis of findings in 92 000 hip arthroplasties performed in Sweden between 1978–1990, Malchau *et al.*[17] derived the following prosthetic survival rates, that is, the percentage not revised for men and women of various ages with OA. (Published by permission of *Acta Orthopaedica Scandinavica*, **64**, 501. (1993).)

operative contaminations. Typically, the patient is not pain-free, the erythrocyte sedimentation rate remains elevated, and, sometimes, low-grade fever is noted. Wound healing may be disturbed or a fistula may develop. Radiographic examination usually shows rapid loosening of the components that is indistinguishable from aseptic loosening. Osteolysis and perforation of the cortex are subsequently seen. The clinical condition can range from no signs of infection to life-threatening septic shock.

A broad spectrum of micro-organisms has been isolated from infected hip arthroplaties; staphylococci are seen in half of the cases, with more *S. epidermidis* than *S. aureus* infections. The latter was the commonest infective organism in the early days of hip arthroplasty, and the change in bacteriologic findings may be due to modern antimicrobial prophylaxis. Some bacteria are glycocalyx-forming, and this protects them from the effects of antibiotics and body defence mechanisms.

Surgical treatment of deep infection, without removal of the implants, can occasionally be effective in cases with well-fixed components. Antibiotics alone can only slow down the destructive process, but this may be the only alternative in elderly persons with medical contraindications to surgery. For the majority, the only safe method is removal of the implant, other foreign material, and all infected tissue; multiple tissue biopsies for cultures; and prolonged antibiotic treatment according to results of the cultures. In many cases, cultures from joint fluid aspirate are negative and

cultures from sinus tracts show non-specific organisms. A controversial question is whether and if so, when to reimplant a new prosthesis. Leaving the patient without a hip joint — the Girdlestone procedure — causes leg shortening, severe limp, and often pain and is, therefore, usually avoided. Buchholz has a long experience of one-stage revision, with immediate reimplantation of a new prosthesis using bone cement loaded with gentamicin or other appropriate antibiotics. Other investigators have waited months to years before reimplantation, that is, a two-stage revision. Modern two-stage techniques include extraction of the prosthesis, a 4- to 6-week period with chains of gentamicin-containing cement beads inserted in the bone defects and antibiotic treatment on the basis of the cultures, and then reimplantation of a new prosthesis. Attempts have been made to select treatment in conformity with bacterial virulence and proven sensitivity to nontoxic antibiotics — the overall success rate is in the range of 75 to 95 per cent.

Local complications in knee arthroplasty

Knee arthroplasty is associated with some problems. The knee is more superficial than the hip; it is also a hinge-like joint having considerable mobility combined with stability in the opposite direction. Very high forces are transmitted through the joint and the extensor mechanism, especially in the loaded flexed knee.

The knee may have undergone surgery before arthroplasty. This increases the risk of conflicting skin incisions with healing disturbances. Overdistension of the capsular sutures, due to oversized implants, may cause capsular dehiscence. The end result may be wound rupture and skin necrosis, with a high risk of deep infection. Intraoperative contamination of the joint is related to problems with wound healing. An exposed implant must be promptly covered and a gastrocnemic muscle-flap can be turned over the anterior part of the joint to save the patient from serious consequences. Wound-healing problems are commoner and more often associated with deep infection when large and complex implants are used. Over distension of the patellar ligament may lead to its rupture or necrosis, a complication that cannot be safely treated.

Correct articulation of patella is a prerequisite for knee function. Medial capsular dehiscence, a tight lateral patellar retinaculum, malposition of components, unbalanced ligaments, and deformed patella are some reasons for patellar subluxation and dislocation which make the knee weak and unreliable. All of the causes of patellar dislocation can be corrected, but the results of revision are unpredictable. Postoperative patellar pain is not uncommon but it usually resolves, with time, in patients with an unresurfaced patella. Resurfacing the patella is not without problems — The component is thin and wears quickly because of a small contact area; deformation of the component causes loosening; and the anchoring holes make the patella weaker, with an increased risk of fatigue fracture. Lateral release to improve patellar tracking may render the patella avascular, with flattening or fragmentation. Overall, six per cent of all revisions are made for patellar problems including secondary resurfacing of the patella.

During total knee arthroplasty, the mechanical axis is restored, that is, the knee is so aligned that it is placed on the axis joining the hip with the ankle. Specially designed instruments are used to achieve correct bone cuts; soft tissues around the knee then must be released to balance ligament tensions. Failure to do so may cause instability and even complete dislocation of the joint. Seven per cent of all revisions are due to instability and 15 per cent to other mechanical reasons[15]. For revision of unstable knees, implants with more or less inherent stability are available. Some reports indicate that unbalanced tension may accelerate loosening of the implant, and the same is found when the mechanical axis is not corrected. Ligament insufficiency is a minor problem. If muscle control is good, or if the knee is protected in a brace, the ligament spontaneously adapts within a few months.

Periprosthetic fractures, in combination with a loose prosthesis, can be treated with exchange arthroplasty, using long-stem components. Treatment of a fracture is the indication in one per cent of all revisions. With a fixed prosthesis, treatment is dictated by the degree of malalignment. Intramedullary supracondylar rods or angulated plates are used if alignment cannot be controlled by conservative means.

Loosening of components, mainly the tibial, is the indication in half of all revisions. In total knee arthroplasty, the cumulative risk of revision for loosening is three per cent at 10 years (Fig. 9.22). This risk has constantly been reduced by improvements in instrumentation, prosthetic design, and cementation technique; the risk in unicondylar implants is twice as high, with less improvement over time (Fig. 9.22). The best results are achieved if a new total knee implant is used and if all components are exchanged. If bone loss is minor, a primary type of implant is used, or else a thicker long-stem revision type is advocated. Modular systems are marketed, with various spacers that can be fitted on any of the bone-prosthesis contact areas. Central bone defects, after loose stems, can be reconstructed with bank bone in the same way as hips, but experience of this is limited.

Deep infection occurs after intraoperative contamination, at secondary procedures, and in the form of hematogenous seeding from distant foci, most commonly leg ulcers. Early septic arthritis can be treated with conventional therapy, that is, debridement and lavage. If intramedullary guide instruments have been used during the index operation, medullitis must be suspected and the implants, must be removed. Late infection from intraoperative contamination may occur as chronic arthritis, with fibrosis and joint contracture. Eventually the implants become loose. Late infection can also present as an abscess or a fistula. Usually, the bone–cement interface is also infected, and revision is needed. Hematogenous infections may start as septic arthritis. If the implants show fibrous encapsulation, seen as a radiolucent zone on the radiographs, this is also infected. The infection may occasionally be necrotizing, toxic, and life-threatening; in such a case, prompt removal of the implant or even amputation may be necessary.

The cumulative risk of revision for deep infection is below 1 per cent at 10 years. Half of the revisions are performed as one- or two-stage exchange arthroplasties, and the remainder as knee fusions. The eradication rate after exchange arthroplasty is 75 to 85 per cent, regardless of the staging technique. However, the clinical success rate is lower; residual pain and restricted

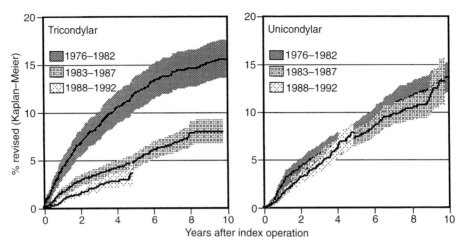

Fig. 9.22   Based on the findings in 30 000 knee arthroplasties for OA performed in Sweden between 1976–1992, Knutson *et al.*[15] derived the following prosthetic revision rates in men and women, various age groups, and unicompartmental/tricompartmental prostheses used during three periods. (Published by permission of *Acta Orthopaedica Scandinavica*, **65**, 375–86 (1994).)

mobility are common. An attempt to preserve leg length by use of a cement spacer in the void after the removed implant, during the interim period with a two-stage method, is an attractive possibility, but it has not been shown to improve mobility. Deep infection in combination with large implants, severe bone loss, a disrupted extensor mechanism, or soft tissue damage is not suitable for exchange arthroplasty. Attempts have been made using resection arthroplasty, that is, leaving the joint empty; the results have been discouraging with instability, pain, and persistent deep infection. More reliable results have been achieved with knee fusion; a modified two-stage technique is used. The empty knee is fixed with a stable external fixator, plates, or an intramedullary rod and gentamicin-containing cement beads are inserted and combined with appropriate antibiotic therapy according to intra-operative tissue cultures. After six weeks, the beads are removed and, at the same time, an autogenous cancellous bone graft is placed around the joint. Healing can be expected in 90 per cent, but it may take four to eight months; failed fusion can be treated with another attempt.

Local complications in ankle arthroplasty

The complication rate after ankle arthroplasty is high. Delayed wound healing has been reported in 40 per cent and deep infection in three to five per cent. In one report, radiolucent zones were seen in 88 per cent after one year, and loosening of almost all components after six years. More typical results show that one fourth of

the components become loose at five years; the talar component is most often involved. Impingement, malleolar fracture, subluxation, and dislocation are also reported.

Local complications in shoulder arthroplasty

Complications occurred in 11 per cent of a mixed material, using the Neer prosthesis; other similar designs produced the same complication rate. The most frequent complication, one third of patients, is impingement with the acromion, rotator cuff tears, and tuberosity problems, followed by instability. The loosening, seen in a few per cent, mainly affects the glenoid component. In a compilation of 13 reports with various durations of follow-up, half of the glenoid components had a radiolucent zone, and two to ten per cent a shift in position, indicating that loosening might be imminent or underestimated. In one six-year follow-up of Neer arthroplasties, many of the humeral components showed a shift in position, although the clinical results continued to be excellent.

Other rare complications include intra- or post-operative periprosthetic fractures, intraoperative nerve injury, notably of the axillary nerve, and deep infection. Pain is sometimes reported in otherwise successful shoulder arthroplasties; one reason for this is OA pain from the acromioclavicular joint.

Loose glenoid components can be exchanged, if bone stock so permits, by temporarily removing the modular humeral head. In half the revisions, the glenoid component is permanently removed and a bone graft is placed in the defect. Instability can be treated with a new larger head or soft-tissue repair; infection is treated with component removal. In hemiarthroplasty, glenoid attrition and medialization of the head weaken the joint and make it painful. Secondary glenoid replacement is sometimes possible, but a similar effect can be achieved by replacing the head by a bipolar type, where the inside of the outer head articulates against a smaller humeral head.

Local complications in elbow arthroplasty

Most reports on elbow arthroplasty are based on materials with a majority of rheumatoid cases. The commonest complications with modern surface replacements are ulnar nerve palsy in 20 to 40 per cent and instability or dislocation in 10 per cent. Wound-healing disturbances are not uncommon and deep infection is seen in a few per cent; implant loosening is a less common problem than infection. The overall revision rate is estimated as 5 per cent at five years with the best designs; hinged prostheses with a 'sloppy' or similar rotation are used for revision. Infected cases are, as a rule, treated with resection arthroplasty; fusion is not an alternative, because of the limited usefulness of a stiff elbow.

Local complications in silicone rubber arthroplasties

Silicone rubber has been used extensively as an interpositional implant, with good early results. Some loss of motion is common when the implant bridges from one shaft, over the joint, to the next cortical shaft. Although the material is soft and pliable, fatigue fracture of the implant is a common finding after some years. The fracture may pass unnoticed, but may lead to malalignment, instability, and dislocation. The implant may also fret against the hard cortical shafts causing the production of wear particles. These are not so biocompatible as the bulk material, and severe synovitis and cyst formation have been noted in the adjacent bones. Concern regarding this reaction has limited the use of silicone implants in joints where other options are available.

References

1. Campbell II, D.C. (1991). Arthroplasty of the metatarsophalangeal joint. In *Joint replacement arthroplasty* (ed. B.M. Morrey), pp. 1183–92. Churchill Livingstone, Rochester.

2. Cooney, W.P. (1991). Arthroplasty of the thumb axis. In *Joint replacement arthroplasty* (ed. B.M. Morrey), pp. 173–94. Churchill Livingstone, Rochester.

3. Espehaug, B., Havelin, L.I., Engesæter, L.B., Vollset, S.E., and Langeland, N. (1995). Early revision among 12,179 hip prostheses. A comparison of 10 different brands reported to the Norwegian Arthroplasty Register, 1987–1993. *Acta Orthopaedica Scandinavica*, **66**, 487–93.

4. Goodman, S. and Lidgren, L. (1992). Polyethylene wear in knee arthroplasty. *Acta Orthopaedica Scandinavica*, **63**, 358–64.

5. Grelsamer, R.P. (1995). Current concepts review. Unicompartmental osteoarthrosis of the knee. *Journal of Bone and Joint Surgery (American)*, **77-A**, 278–92.

6. Havelin, L.I., Espehaug, B., Vollset, S.E., Engesæter, L.B., and Langeland, N. (1993). The Norwegian arthroplasty register: a survey of 17,444 hip replacements 1987–1990. *Acta Orthopaedica Scandinavica*, **64**, 245–51.

7. Havelin, L.I., Espehaug, B., Vollset, S.E., and Engesæter, L.B. (1994). Early failures among 14,009 cemented and 1,326 uncemented prostheses for primary coxarthrosis: the Norwegian Arthroplasty Register, 1987–1992. *Acta Orthopaedica Scandinavica*, **65**, 1–6.

8. Havelin, L.I., Vollset, S.E., and Engesæter, L.B. (1995). Revision for aseptic loosening of uncemented cups in 4352 primary total hip prostheses: a report from the Arthroplasty Register. *Acta Orthopaedica Scandinavica*, **66**, 494–500.

9. Huiskes, R. (1993). Failed innovation in total hip replacement. Diagnosis and proposals for a cure. *Acta Orthopaedica Scandinavica*, **64**, 699–716.

10. Johnson, K.A. (1991). Ankle replacement arthroplasty. In *Joint replacement arthroplasty* (ed. B.M. Morrey), pp. 1173–82. Churchill Livingstone, Rochester.

11. Kavanagh, B.F. (1992). Femoral shaft fractures associated with total hip arthroplasty. *Orthopedic Clinics of North America*, **23**, 249–457.

12. Knutson, K., Lindstrand, L., and Lidgren, L. (1986). Survival of knee arthroplasties. A nation-wide multicentre investigation of 8000 cases. *Journal of Bone and Joint Surgery (British)*, **68-B**, 795–803.

15. Knutson, K., Lewold, S., Robertsson, O., and Lidgren, L. (1994). The Swedish knee arthroplasty register. A nation-wide study of 30,003 knees 1976–1992. *Acta Orthopaedica Scandinavica*, **65**, 375–86.

16. Linder, L. (1995). Boneloc® — the Christiansen experience revisited. *Acta Orthopaedica Scandinavica*, **66**, 205–6.

17. Malchau, H., Herberts, P., and Ahnfelt, L. (1993). Prognosis of total hip replacement in Sweden: follow-up of 92,675 operations performed 1978–1990. *Acta Orthopaedica Scandinavica*, **64**, 497–506.

18. Morrey, B.F. (1992). Instability after total hip arthroplasty. *The Orthopedic Clinics of North America*, **23**, 237–48.

19. Rand, J.A. (1994). Current concepts review. The patellofemoral joint in total knee arthroplasty. *Journal of Bone and Joint Surgery (American)*, **76-A**, 612–20.

20. Rothman, R.C. and Cohn, J.C. (1990). Cemented versus cementless total hip arthroplasty: a critical review.

Clinical Orthopaedics and Related Research, **254**, 153–69.

21. Ryd, L., Albrektsson, B.E.J., Carlsson, L., Dansgård, F., Herberts, P., Lindstrand, A., et al. (1995). Roentgen stereophotogrammetric analysis as a predictor of mechanical loosening of knee prostheses. *Journal of Bone and Joint Surgery (British)*, **77**, 377–83.

22. Selvik, G. (1974). Roentgen stereophotogrammetry. A method for the study of kinematics of the skeletal system. (Thesis, University of Lund, Sweden). Reprinted 1989 in *Acta Orthopaedica Scandinavica*, **60** (**supplementum 232**).

23. Sharrock, N.E., Cazan, M.G., Hargett M.J.L., Williams-Russo, P., and Wilson Jr, P. D. (1995). Changes in mortality after hip and knee arthroplasty over a ten-year period. *Anesthesia and Analgesia*, **80**, 242–8.

24. Toksvig-Larsen, S., Ryd, L., and Lindstrand, A. (1990). An internally cooled saw-blade for bone cuts: lower temperatures in 30 knee arthroplasties. *Acta Orthopaedica Scandinavica*, **61**, 321–3.

25. Wasielewski, R.C., Crossett, L.S., and Rubash, H.E. (1992). Neural and vascular injury in total hip arthroplasty. *Orthopedic Clinics of North America*, **23**, 219–35.

26. Waugh, W. (1990). *John Charnley. The man and the hip*. Springer-Verlag, London.

27. Wood, M.B. (1991). Alternative reconstructive procedures. In *Joint replacement arthroplasty* (ed. B.M. Morrey), pp. 217–35. Churchill Livingstone, Rochester.

28. Yahiro, M.A., Gantenberg, J.B., Nelson, R., Lu, H.T.C., and Mishra, N.K. (1995). Comparison of the results of cemented, porous-ingrowth, and threaded acetabular cup fixation. A meta-analysis of the orthopaedic literature. *Journal of Arthroplasty*, **10**, 339–50.

Evaluating outcome in osteoarthritis for research and clinical practice

Charles Rivest and Matthew H. Liang

Introduction

The basic goals in managing osteoarthritis (OA) are to reduce symptoms (stiffness, pain, instability), and to maintain and improve function. To this end, one needs to assess whether the patient is getting better or worse, in a disease where early on, the symptoms are subtle and unfold over years. In advanced disease, where significant structural damage has occurred, the assessment of pain in weight-bearing joints is confounded by the fact that patients adapt to pain by giving up activities to spare themselves of symptoms. These self-imposed limitations may further aggravate the problem by accelerating physical deconditioning.

Definitions

Impairment, disability, and *handicap* refer to the major impacts of illness on individuals[1]. *Impairment* is an 'objective' loss or abnormality of psychological, physiological, or anatomical structure or function, and signifies a pathological state. In OA, measures of impairment include radiographic assessment of cartilage thickness and standard assessment of joint deformation, circumference, and range of motion by physical examination.

Impairment can result in *disability* or restricted ability, or inability to perform normal activities. *Disability* can affect behavior, communication, personal care, locomotion, dexterity, and activities of daily living. *Disability*, or function, cannot be captured by a single standard measure because, at any given time, it is the result of three factors: capacity, will, and need. Capacity is the physical and mental potential to do something; will includes personality factors, such as drive and motivation, and the need of the person to function. In clinical practice, function is improved or maintained by manipulating or enhancing capacity, will, or need.

Handicap is the disadvantage for an individual that limits fulfillment of normal functions. Handicaps include work ability, social integration, and economic self-sufficiency. Questionnaires developed to evaluate the health status or quality of life measure a multi-attribute state that includes physical, emotional, and social functioning.

Symptoms of OA and reported functional difficulties should be considered within the experience of the patient. There is a view that the report of the patient is subjective and less important or, less objective, than hard clinical findings. However, in the last three decades, advances in clinical research have produced a number of sophisticated questionnaires with excellent psychometric properties to measure pain, well-being, and functional limitations (physical, emotional, or social).

Validity, reliability, and *sensitivity* to change are the basic attributes used to judge the quality of questionnaires and other quantitative measures. The *validity* of an assessment method refers to its capacity to measure what it intends to measure. There are four types of *validity: face, content, construct*, and *criterion*. An instrument has *face validity* when in the eyes of experienced individuals, it appears to measure the domain of interest (for instance, joint pain). *Content validity* refers to the extent to which a measure is able to comprehensively evaluate the domain of interest (for example, all joint symptoms). *Construct validity* is demonstrated when measures obtained with an instrument are consistent with hypothetical constructs (or concepts) related to the domain of interest (for example, physical disability resulting from rheumatic diseases). *Criterion validity* is assessed by comparing the instrument to a '*gold standard*' (such as, a pathognomonic finding or a biopsy). However, such irrefutable standards are generally not available for the measure of health status.

Reliability (reproducibility) is assessed by comparing the results obtained with an instrument administered to the same individuals at different times, and under the same experimental conditions. The instrument is considered reliable if the measurements show little random error. *Sensitivity* of a measure refers to its capacity to detect any changes. *Responsiveness* is the ability to detect a clinically meaningful change.

Studies have shown that patient-derived data are *valid*, *reliable*, and as *sensitive*, or more *sensitive* to change than traditional radiographic measures or physical findings. We review these assessment methods and indicate how they can be practically incorporated in patient care.

Patient self-assessment

Patient self-assessment techniques have generated considerable interest because of their low cost, simplicity, and acceptability by patients. The information relies exclusively on the information provided by the patient, generally collected by questionnaires, either self-administered or administered by interviewers. Rateable domains include joint symptoms, and emotional, physical, and social functioning.

Pain rating

Pain scales

The major tools used to evaluate pain include verbal transition scales (VTS), verbal rating scales (VRS) or Likert scales, numerical rating scales (NRS), and visual analogue scales (VAS). The VTS (Fig. 10.1(a)) has the respondent estimate whether the pain has been stable or has changed over a period of time, (better or worse). With the VRS (Fig. 10.1(b)), the respondent is asked to quantify his or her pain ranging, for example, from total absence (no pain) to extreme pain, with a number of intermediate levels (mild, moderate, severe). The NRS (Fig. 10.1(c)(i) and 10.1 (c)(ii)), has the respondent assign a number from an ordinal scale, usually ranging from 0 (no pain) to 10 (extreme pain), or from 0 (no pain) to 100 (extreme pain), rather than endorsing an adjective. The VAS is typically a 10 cm line marked '*least*' at one end '*most*' at the other end on which the patient marks a point representing his level of pain (Fig. 10.1(d)); and the distance from this point to the origin of the line is recorded. All of these techniques show changes when an intervention is effective.

As a general principle, more reproducible information is obtained by framing the question in a specific and consistent manner, such as specifying the period of time of interest and whether one is interested in the worst pain or average pain during that period[2]. Irrespective of the period covered by the questions, however, people seem to weigh and / or remember their current discomfort.

Verbal transition, verbal rating, and numerical rating scales are the most practical, and most patients find them easy to use. The VRS and NRS are summarized by a number; the VAS[3] offers the theoretical advantages of a continuous pain score. However, some patients cannot complete the visual analogue scale or numerical scales because of functional illiteracy or limited cognitive function. The addition of adjectives (mild, moderate, severe) along the line can improve comprehension but individuals may circle or check these anchors, instead of marking the line. This phenomenon, which is more frequent when a vertical scale is used, technically converts the VAS into a verbal rating scale equivalent, and results in significant loss in sensitivity[4].

Pain scales which require that the respondent endorse a facial expression (Fig. 10.1(e)) that corresponds to their affective state, are useful in evaluating pain in children[5] and mood in patients with rheumatoid arthritis[6]. These faces scales can also be used in illiterate populations or across different languages. However, faces scales cannot be completed over the telephone and their validity in OA has not yet been studied.

Pain questionnaires

Pain questionnaires emerged from efforts to describe pain as a multidimensional process with sensory, emotional, social, and behavioral inputs. The McGill pain questionnaire[7], based on an inventory of 78 adjectives, is often considered to be the '*gold standard*' for this type of instrument. A shorter version exists[8] but it has received only limited application in OA research.

The Knee Pain Scale, a self-administered 12-item questionnaire, was developed in an OA population to evaluate the intensity and frequency of knee pain in transfer and ambulation[9]. This valid and reliable scale, if it proves to be responsive, may become a valuable tool for pain assessment in clinical trials.

Stiffness

Joint stiffness (early morning, after awakening, or after a period of inactivity) is frequently reported in clinical

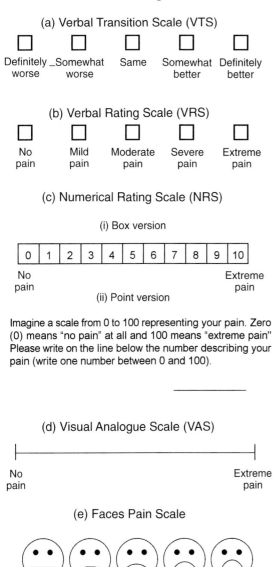

Fig. 10.1 Pain rating scales.

trials. The duration of morning stiffness is a reliable measure when assessed by experienced interviewers[10], particularly after standardization of the question[11]. In clinical trials, morning stiffness, measured either by VRS or VAS, is generally responsive to active therapy[12].

Health status or quality of life instruments

A variety of self-administered or interviewer-assisted instruments have been applied to the study of

rheumatic diseases. Measures developed for general populations are referred to as *generic*, while others, distinguished as *disease-specific* or *organ-specific*, refer to specific pathologic processes or involved structures and or organs.

Generic instruments

Generic health status questionnaires which have been applied to OA populations include the Sickness Impact Profile[13] (SIP), the Nottingham Health Profile[14,15] (NHP), and the Medical Outcome Study (MOS) Short Form-36[16] (SF-36). All have excellent psychometric properties in general populations and have been tested for reliability and validity, at least to some extent, in orthopedic surgery patients or populations with OA[15,17,18].

The SIP[13] is composed of 138 yes–no questions; it takes approximately 30 minutes to complete as a self-reported or an interviewer-administered survey. Individual items are weighted and aggregated to provide scores for seven dimensions: physical (ambulation, mobility, body care, and movement), psychological (communication, social interaction, emotional behavior, alertness behavior), sleep and rest, eating, work, home management, and recreational activities. The SIP is one of the most responsive instruments in the evaluation of joint arthroplasty[19–21]. In a longitudinal study of hip and knee OA[22], the performance of the SIP was similar to the Arthritis Impact Measurement Scale[23] (AIMS), an arthritis-specific health status instrument (p. 00).

The NHP[24] is a 38-item self-administered questionnaire which can be completed in approximately 10 minutes. It was designed for population surveys to measure mobility, pain, emotion, energy level, sleep, and social isolation. The instrument has been validated in OA[15] and used in a study of total hip arthroplasty[25]. The NHP may not be sensitive enough, however, to assess small improvements in individuals with mild or very severe OA.

The SF-36[16], the most widely used health status measure, is a self-administered questionnaire which takes less than 10 minutes to complete. It has excellent psychometric properties and has been validated and tested for reliability in OA[18]. A shorter version (SF-12) is available from the originators of the SF-36, but its psychometric properties have not yet been reported. In evaluating outcome of hip joint arthroplasty[26], the SF-36 performs as well as the SIP and a short version of the AIMS[27].

Arthritis-specific instruments

The term *arthritis-specific* describes instruments developed to quantify health status and functional impact in populations with rheumatic diseases. *Joint-specific* instruments focus on one joint (for example, the knee) or a set of joints (for example, the hips and knees). Instruments developed to assess the impact of a particular disease, such as OA, in specific joints are described as *disease-and-joint-specific*.

Most *arthritis-specific* instruments were developed to study rheumatoid arthritis. The two most popular are the AIMS[23] and the Health Assessment Questionnaire (HAQ)[28]. The HAQ is a 24-item questionnaire rating self-assessed performance in activities of daily living (ADL), with emphasis on mobility, personal care, need for equipment or physical assistance, drug side effects, and pain; about 8–10 minutes are needed to complete the instrument. The disability and pain subscale scores of the HAQ have been extensively used in RA and many other rheumatic conditions, with or without modifications[29]. The HAQ is included in the US National Health and Nutrition Survey (NHANES). A modified shorter version of the HAQ is available (MHAQ)[30].

The AIMS[23] is a self-administered questionnaire, with 45 items, taking about 15–20 minutes to complete; nine subscales measure pain, mobility, physical activity, dexterity, social role, social activity, depression, well being, and anxiety. AIMS2 includes new scales for arm function, work, and social support, and new sections to evaluate satisfaction with function, attribution of problem to arthritis, and self-designation of priority areas for improvement[31]. The new version takes 20–25 minutes to complete. Reliability and validity are excellent for both the AIMS[23] and AIMS2[31], but the sensitivity to change of the AIMS2 is yet to be tested.

Compared to the AIMS, the HAQ is simpler and shorter. However, in a comparative study, the HAQ was considerably less efficient than the AIMS to judge changes in pain and mobility in subjects undergoing total joint arthroplasty[19].

Joint-specific instruments

Instruments to rate single joints have been developed to evaluate outcomes of joint surgery[32,33]. Until recently, these instruments were unstandardized, untested for reliability and validity, and based on arbitrary anthropometric criteria or on the assessment of the surgeon.

The Hip Rating Questionnaire (HRQ), developed to assess total hip replacement, is one of the few instruments that has been tested for validity, reliability, and responsiveness[34,35]. The 15 questions, probing the overall impact of the arthritis, walking ability, and performance in daily life activities, can be answered in approximately 10 minutes.

The Total Hip Arthroplasty Outcome Evaluation Questionnaire (THAOEQ) is based on a consensus recommendation of the American Academy of Orthopedic Surgeons (AAOS), the HIP Society, and the Société Internationale de Chirurgie Orthopédique et de Traumatologie (SICOT)[36]. The baseline form (15 questions) and postoperative form (13 questions) include items on pain, level of activity, ADL, walking capacity, gait, patient satisfaction, expectations, and reasons for choosing the operation. The instrument is valid and reliable, but its responsiveness has not been assessed[36].

Disease- and joint-specific instruments

The Lequesne Indices of Severity for Osteoarthritis of the Hip and the Knee[37] and the Western Ontario and McMaster Universities Osteoarthritis Index (WOMAC)[38] were designed for OA patients. The Lequesne Indices consist of one 10-item scale for the knee and one 10-item scale for the hip; these can be administered by trained individuals in 5–10 minutes. Both scales rate pain or discomfort, stiffness, performance on activities of daily living, and need for assistive devices in maximum walking capacity. In the hip scale, an additional question addresses arthritis-related sexual dysfunction in sexually active women. The knee and the hip indices are reliable[37,39] and responsive in clinical trials[37,40].

The WOMAC Osteoarthritis Index[38] is a 24-item questionnaire focusing on pain, stiffness, and functional limitations related to knee and/or hip OA. The WOMAC is available in two equivalent versions, one using verbal rating scales and another using visual analogue scales; both versions are self-reported and can be completed in less than five minutes. The WOMAC has been extensively tested for validity, reliability, and responsiveness[38]; It has been translated into several different languages and used as the main outcome in evaluations of pharmacologic[41], surgical[20,42], and acupuncture therapy trials[43].

The Lequesne Indices had similar sensitivity to change as the Doyle[44] and the WOMAC indices in a trial comparing meclofenate to diclofenac sodium for OA of the knee[45]. Both instruments are recommended for long-term OA research studies[46]. However, the Lequesne Indices have disadvantages compared to the WOMAC; some of the items are not clearly described; the time period covered is not stated; there is no clear 'breakpoint' within categories of 'walking distance'; and interviewer training is required.

Semiobjective assessments

Semiobjective assessments combine patient-report and the assessment by the physician of the subject's report. These include the measures of medication consumption, joint counts, and performance testing.

Consumption of medications

Having patients to collaborate in methods evaluating their consumption of medications is a typical example of semiobjective assessment. Quantification of the use of analgesics and NSAIDs for OA could reflect how much discomfort a patient experiences, but this approach has limitations. Many patients with OA reduce their level of medication use after a few years, even if symptoms persist[47]. Potential explanations for this observation include the natural evolution of the disease (the maximal aggravations of OA symptoms generally occurring in the first few years[48]), limitation of joint use to reduce symptoms, adaptation to pain, and, possibly, drug side effects.

Physical examination

Few physical examination findings of OA have been tested for their reliability and sensitivity to change over time[10,49].

Joint count

The Doyle Index[44] was adapted for OA populations from the Ritchie Index[50], which is used in rheumatoid arthritis. It is a standardized examination protocol of 48 OA target joints. The examiner records the number of joints in which pain or tenderness is produced under firm digital pressure or movement. Each joint is scored on a 4-point scale (0 = no tenderness, 1 = patient complained of pain, 2 = patient complained of pain and winced, 3 = patient complained of pain, winced, and withdrew the joint). The index has been tested for reliability and validity[44], and has been used in OA

trials[45,51]: sensitivity to change has been demonstrated[44]. A joint count is recommended for the long-term evaluation of a drug with disease modification properties in OA[46].

Performance testing methods

Timed walking capacity

Timed walking capacity measures lower-limb function[52]. The measure is obtained by calculating the time a patient needs to walk a predetermined distance (for example, 20 or 50 meters) as fast as possible. The validity of timed walking capacity in OA has been demonstrated[53]. In trials evaluating pharmacological, rehabilitation, and surgical interventions for knee OA, timed walked capacity showed improvement[34,54–58]. Therefore, walking time is part of the recommendations for long-term OA trials[46].

Muscle strength

The applicability of muscle strength in assessing OA has received limited attention[58–60], but these measures are reliable, valid, and responsive. In an elderly population, muscle strength of the lower limb was a better predictor of walking velocity than joint pain[61]; quadriceps muscle strength was a stronger predictor of functional impairment than the radiologic severity of knee OA[62].

Objective methods

Objective measures include physical findings (that do not rely on self-report) and direct or indirect evaluation of joint damage. In this section, we will limit our discussion to objective physical examination methods. Other objective methods, such as arthroscopy, standard radiographs, microradiographs, sonography, magnetic resonance imaging, scintigraphy, and biological markers of cartilage damages are covered in detail elsewhere in this book.

Physical examination

In a comparison of swelling, crepitus, tenderness, and instability, only bony tenderness and tibiofemoral crepitus showed moderate to good intrarater and interrater reliability[49] in subjects with OA of the knee. Not surprisingly, the reproducibility of joint count, range of motion measures, and bony swelling assessment can be improved by training and standardization of the procedures[11].

Joint circumference

Measurement of joint circumference or bony *swelling* or *enlargement* is one of the most reliable physical signs of OA[49], as confirmed in a cross-sectional study[63]. The validity of this method for cross-sectional studies is, however, questionable because of variation in joint shape and size. Joint circumference may be suitable for longitudinal assessment, but the rate of change is not known and it is likely to be insensitive.

Range of movement

The techniques for the measurement of joint range of motion that have been tested for inter and intra rater reliability have shown important variations[64]. The general findings can be summarized as follows: (1) measurements of passive motion are generally greater than those for active motion; (2) intrarater reliability is better than interrater reliability; (3) reliability can be substantially improved with proper training and standardization of the examination[11]; (4) warming-up exercises, before measurements, may affect the results[65]; and (5) responsiveness for these measures has not been documented in OA.

Summary and methodologic considerations

Many factors influence the report of the patient on function and health status including the time of the day when the questions are asked[66], the season[67,68], the learning effect from previous experience with a questionnaire, and, possibly, the effects of warming up[65]. Informing patients of their previous answers may influence their response and affect sensitivity and reliability of the results; such an effect may also be condition specific. When a pain VAS was used in patients with painful rheumatic conditions, a majority of patients, not informed of their previous answers, overestimated their previous pain score two weeks later[69]. However, Bellamy *et al.*[70] were not able to reduce response variation when the baseline WOMAC was given to patients before a follow-up WOMAC was completed, in a trial of NSAIDs for hip and knee OA.

Aggregated versus signal measurement strategy?

Results of health assessment questionnaires are generally reported as aggregates or summations of the weighted or unweighted items. In contrast, a signal measurement strategy identifies one or more 'target' joints or symptoms from an inventory which the patient identifies as areas in which potential improvement would have personal importance. This customizes the evaluation process to the individual and improves the efficiency of the measure by concentrating on items with the highest potential for response. In patients with OA, undergoing total hip or knee joint replacement surgery[71], and in a clinical trial comparing two NSAIDs[72], such a strategy reduced response variation.

The signal measurement strategy may be problematic, however, because different individuals may chose different signals, and the stability of patient choices has not been demonstrated over time. Others problems include the possibility of overlooking relevant or clinically important changes in items not chosen as signals, the tendency of patients to choose the functional items which are most severely affected and, possibly, less responsive, and the added time needed to negotiate preferences.

Floor and ceiling effects

Health status instruments are sometimes insensitive to change in individuals who score near the extreme values for a scale. The *floor effect* refers to an inability to measure improvement in individuals already at the minimal allowable disability score, and the *ceiling effect* refers to the inability to measure deterioration in individuals at the worst possible score[73].

Which instrument to choose?

All the questionnaires described in this chapter have been tested for validity and reliability. The decision of which instrument to use depends on which joints are under study (some instruments being joint-specific), the purpose of the study, the responsiveness of the instrument, and practical considerations, such as the need for an interviewer and the time required to complete the questionnaire.

Because of their narrow focus, joint-or disease-specific instruments may be more pertinent and more sensitive to change in studies assessing specific joints. However, because of their broader perspective, generic instruments may detect complications or side effects in areas which are not specific to the disease under investigation. Generic instruments are also particularly valuable in studies of resource allocation or health policy because they permit comparison of the impact of the disease or therapy across a variety of medical conditions[18].

Quantitative approaches from clinical research applied to the practice setting

An international task force has proposed guidelines for the long-term clinical trials evaluating potential disease modifying drugs in OA[46] (Table 10.1). Restrictions in time and available resources limit the application of these guidelines to the practice setting. However, they provide a framework for a practical approach to long-term clinical follow-up of patients with OA.

Table 10.2 summarizes the components of a comprehensive and practical assessment of OA which takes into account the constraints of routine office care. The approach follows a step-wise progression, starting with traditional, open-ended screening questions, using basic principles of good questionnaire construction. These questions rapidly establish the priorities of the patient and assess whether the condition has changed. If deterioration has occurred, the questions progress to more detailed inquiry and systematic review, especially in the complicated elderly, reticent, stoic, or unreliable historian. Observation of the gait of the patient and ability to transfer from a chair to the examination table, will help to confirm reported problems and anchor the assessment of the clinician to those of other patients with the same impairments.

For the reliable patient who is stable and doing well, the examination adds little. When there has been a change in reported problems, additional history, particularly details of medication use and changes in activ-

Table 10.1 Recommended outcome assessment for evaluating therapy for OA[46]

Symptomatic slow-acting drugs*		Disease-modifying drugs[¶]
Measures:	(5 to 8 of the following)	(One of the following)
	1 Pain scale	Assessment of the cartilage status
	2 Algofunctional indices:	and rate of change by serial:
	(a) Lequesne Index	1 Radiography (joint space narrowing)
	or	2 Fiberoptic arthroscopy
	(b) WOMAC	3 Other techniques:
	3 Medication consumption:	(a) CT-scan
	(a) Analgesics	(b) MRI
	(b) NSAIDs	(c) Ultrasonography
	4 Number of articular flares:	
	(with and without effusion, particularly	
	those necessitating articular tap)	
	5 Physical examination:	
	(a) Doyle Index (original or adaptations)	
	(b) Articular mobility	
	6 Timed performances:	
	(a) Walk 20 or 50 meters	
	(b) Go up and down a standard flight of stairs[†]	
	7 Global judgment of effectiveness:	
	(a) From the patient	
	(b) From the physician	
	8 Quality of life scale	
Duration:	3–12 months	Therapeutic trial[‡] — 2–4 years
		Prophylactic trial[§] — many years
		(allow a sufficient time interval
		between trauma or exposure)

*Drugs that are neither rapidly acting analgesics nor nonsteroidal anti-inflammatory agents nor chondroprotective, but have a slow onset of action and are alleged to improve OA symptoms.
[¶] Drugs that may prevent, retard, or reverse cartilage lesions in humans.
[†] Standard has not been defined.
[‡] Aimed at slowing or reversing the OA articular changes.
[§] Aimed at preventing the development of OA change (in selected high-risk populations).

Table 10.2   Clinical assessment of OA Patients[†]

Variables	Assessment
Global rating	Verbal transition scale (VRS)
	Are you better, same, or worse?
Pain	Numerical rating scale (NRS)
	Over the last month, how much discomfort have you had on a scale of 1–5 (5 = the most)?
	Have you had:
	1) Pain at rest?
	2) Pain with any weight bearing?
	3) Pain at night?
Function	*What is the most difficult thing for you to do on a regular day?*
Flares	Number of exacerbations or joint effusions[‡]
Examination	Range of motion and effect of mobilization on pain
	Functional testing, if necessary (see Table 10.3)
Therapy	Analgesics
	NSAIDs
	Joint aspirations[§]
	Intra-articular steroids

[†] Should be done initially, and every 6 months
[‡] Joint effusion = accumulation of joint fluid, documented by a physician
[§] Joint aspiration = evacuation of joint fluid with the use of a syringe and a bored needle
NRS = numeric rating scale; VRS = verbal rating scale;
NSAIDs = nonsteroidal anti-inflammatory drugs

ity, will provide insight into potential management strategies. When severe discomfort is reported, knowing what critical functions are disturbed, such as sleep or weight bearing, grades the pain even more finely.

The physical examination will identify coexisting periarticular soft tissue rheumatism (for example, trochanteric, iliopsoas, or anserine bursitis; supraspinatus, epitrochlear, DeQuervain's, or Achilles tendinitis, nerve entrapments such as carpal, Guyon's, or tarsal tunnel syndromes) which may respond to local therapy. Biomechanical factors such as flexion, recurvatum, valgus or varus deformities which may cause ligament strain, can be approached with orthotic compensation or correction. Finally, whether mobilizing the joint induces discomfort may be used as a clue for unreported functional limitation. For the unreliable historian, simple performance tests (p. 412) may quickly identify potential functional problems and the joints that may be involved.

With the current state of therapy, radiographic imaging is important for confirmation of the diagnosis but has little value in the routine monitoring of patients because of its poor correlation with symptoms and function. Radiographies are useful when surgery is contemplated, when there has been a major change in symptoms or physical findings, or when another diagnosis is under consideration. Monitoring should include global rating from the care giver and the

patient, a pain assessment, a check on the number of flare-ups, a functional diagnosis (p. 00), a focused examination, and selective performance testing.

General principles

The development of valid, reliable, patient-centered questionnaires have taught us how to pose more useful and quantitative questions for the day-to-day monitoring of the patient with OA. The minimal history should include questions which are:

(1) comprehensible-stated in the simplest language;

(2) consistent-framed or asked in a way to insure reproducible replies, by having the same anchors, time of reference, response categories;

(3) mutually exclusive-minimal overlap with one another;

(4) sensitive to change-respond to the range of severity.

Patient and physician global rating

We ask people to rate their symptoms over a defined period of time (for example, a week or a month or since their last visit) using verbal, numerical, or verbal transition rating scales.

Pain rating

Global pain rating can be accomplished with a NRS. Intuitively, pain may be rated lower than expected for patients with a high threshold or for those taking pain medication, or rated higher than expected for patients with low thresholds or nonorganic pain. Pain perception can be substantiated by examination and observed behavior. Spontaneous attempts by the patient to avoid a painful activity or painful examination, and facial expressions of discomfort can be used to develop a clinical grading where 0 = spontaneous complaint; 1 = spontaneous complaint; 2 = wincing only with movement; 3 = wincing and withdrawal with movement; and 4 = wincing with activity, and the presence of night pain.

Count of flares

Episodic deteriorations (flares) are frequently reported by OA patients. During these episodes, patients may experience exacerbation of their pain, with or without joint inflammation signs (that is, joint warmth, joint swelling, or effusions). The number of such events, if closely monitored over a period of time, may provide guidance in the adjustment of the therapeutic regimen.

Functional diagnosis

It is important to recognize that there is a natural trajectory of functional decline, which is hastened by chronic and acute illnesses in patients with OA. Many individuals decline slowly, accommodate the decline in function, and accept it. Unfortunately, by the time function has declined, effective intervention may be difficult. Regular functional evaluation may be particularly useful in this regard; function is an important end point to be measured in a standardized, quantitative manner. Two approaches are useful to evaluate function: (1) the one-second drill asks the patient what single function is the most difficult for him or her to perform during the day, and how difficult it is on a scale of 1 to 5; (2) the 10-second drill permits patients to express how they are affected by the condition, communicate which activity is the most difficult, compare

their condition to baseline, and determine their priority for treatment. Questioning in the 10-second drill might take the following course:

1. How does your condition affect you?
2. What is the most: a) difficult thing for you to do in an average day? b) important thing for us to work on?
3. What can you not do: a) that you were able to do? b) that you need or would like to do?
4. Are you able to sleep through the night?

In patients with polyarticular OA, or when the patient is a poor observer or cognitively impaired, a systematic inventory of activities of daily living (ADL) such as ambulation, dressing, eating, personal hygiene, transfers, and toileting should be obtained (ADEPTT is a mnemonic). Disease-specific[38] or joint-specific[34] instruments might be administered while the patient is waiting to be seen. To be most helpful, the physician should incorporate these ratings into his assessment to obtain additional details on the problem areas.

Functional testing

A useful method of evaluating function in elderly, sick, cognitively impaired, or unreliable subjects is performance testing[74]. One performance test that can be done rapidly in the office, to screen for potential problems, has the patient imitate the assessor in maneuvers that test musculoskeletal areas (Table 10.3). If there is asymmetry between sides, or if the patient is unable to perform these maneuvers because of pain or mechanical restrictions, limitations in certain self-care areas probably exist.

In following functional ability, adoption of a single-signal function can help the evaluator and the physician to focus on relevant problems. However, because function is multideterminant, interrelated factors (emotion, social and economical environments, education, and vocational status) should be explored for potential deleterious contributions. Activity is frequently inversely proportional to the level of pain. When function is not proportional to objective evidence, psychosocial factors should be considered.

Table 10.3 Screening for functional disability in patients with OA

Task	Musculoskeletal areas tested	Function
Touch fingers to palmar crease†	Finger small joints(F)	Grip
Touch index finger pad to thumb pad	Thumb (AB, O) and thumb opponens muscle (S)	Grip and pinch
Place palm of hand to contralateral trochanter	Wrist (F) and shoulder (AD)	Hygiene (perineal and back care)
Touch 1st MCP joint to top of head	Shoulder (AB, F, ER) and elbow (F)	Hygiene (face, neck, hair, oral), feeding, and dressing
Touch waist in back	Shoulder (IR)	Dressing and low back care
Touch tip of shoe	Back, hip, and knee (F) and elbow (E)	Dressing of lower extremities
Arise from chair without using hands‡	Hip girdle and quadriceps rectus femoris (S)	Transfer ability
Stand unassisted	Hip, knee, and ankle (F, E) and quadriceps femoris muscle (S)	Standing
Step over a 6-inch block	Hip, knee, and ankle (F, E) and Hip girdle (S)	Stairs
Gait	Hip, knee, ankle, and small joints of feet (F, E), hip girdle and quadriceps femoris muscle (S)	Walking

AB = abduction ER = external rotation F = flexion E = extension
AD = adduction IR = Internal rotation O = opposition S = strength
† If abnormal, test grip strength; lateral pinch strength is the last to diminish
‡ If abnormal, test ability to get up from bed
(Adapted from Liang *et al.*[74], with permission.)

References

1. Liang, M.H. and Jette, A.M. (1981). Measuring functional ability in chronic arthritis: a critical review. *Arthritis Rheum*, **24**, 80–6.
2. Williams, R.C. (1988). Toward a set of reliable and valid measures for chronic pain assessment and outcome research. *Pain*, **35**, 239–51.
3. Huskisson, E.C. (1974). Measurement of pain. *Lancet*, **2**, 1127–31.
4. Scott, J. and Huskisson, E.C. (1976). Graphic representation of pain. *Pain*, **2**, 175–84.
5. Bieri, D., Reeve, R.A., Champion, G.D., Addicoat, L., and Ziegler, J.B. (1990). The Faces Pain Scale for the self-assessment of the severity of pain experienced by children: development, initial validation, and preliminary investigation for ratio scale properties. *Pain*, **41**, 139–50.
6. Lorish, C.D. and Maisiak, R. (1986). The Face Scale: a brief, nonverbal method for assessing patient mood. *Arthritis Rheum*, **29**, 906–9.
7. Melzack, R. (1975). The McGill pain questionnaire: major properties and scoring methods. *Pain*, **1**, 277–99.
8. Melzack, R. (1987). The short-form McGill Pain Questionnaire. *Pain*, **30**, 191–7.
9. Rejeski, W.J., Ettinger, W.H. Jr, Shumaker, S., Heuser, M.D., James, P., Monu, J., *et al.* (1995). The evaluation of pain in patients with knee osteoarthritis: the knee pain scale. *J Rheumatol*, **22**, 1124–9.
10. Jones, A., Hopkinson, N., Pattrick, M., Berman, P., and Doherty, M. (1992). Evaluation of a method for clinically assessing osteoarthritis of the knee. *Ann Rheum Dis*, **51**, 243–5.
11. Bellamy, N., Carette, S., Ford, P.M., Kean, W.F., le Riche, N.G., Lussier, A., *et al.* (1992). Osteoarthritis antirheumatic drug trials. I: Effects of standardization procedures on observer dependent outcome measures. *J Rheumatol*, **19**, 436–43.
12. Bellamy, N. and Buchanan, W.W. (1984). Outcome measurement in osteoarthritis clinical trials: the case for standardization. *Clin Rheumatol*, **3**, 293–303.
13. Bergner, M., Bobbitt, R.A., Pollard, W.E., Martin, D.P., and Gilson, B.S. (1976). The Sickness Impact Profile: validation of a health status measure. *Med Care*, **14**, 57–67.
14. McDowell, I.W., Martini, C.J., and Waugh, W. (1978). A method for self-assessment of disability before and after hip replacement operations. *Br Med J*, **2**, 857–9.
15. Hunt, S.M., McKenna, S.P., and Williams, J. (1981). Reliability of a population survey tool for measuring perceived health problems: a study of patients with osteoarthrosis. *J Epidemiol Community Health*, **35**, 297–300.
16. Ware, J.E. Jr and Sherbourne, C.D. (1992). The MOS 36-item short-form health survey (SF-36). A conceptual framework and item selection. *Med Care*, **30**, 473–83.
17. Summers, M.N., Haley, W.E., Reveille, J.D., and Alarcon, G.S. (1988). Radiographic assessment and psychologic variables as predictors of pain and functional impairment in osteoarthritis of the knee or hip. *Arthritis Rheum*, **31**, 204–9.
18. Bombardier, C., Melfi, C.A., Paul, J., Green, R., Hawker, G., Wright, J., *et al.* (1995). Comparison of a

generic and a disease-specific measure of pain and physical function after knee replacement surgery. *Med Care*, 33, AS131–44.

19. Liang, M.H., Larson, M.G., Cullen, K.E., and Schwartz, J.A. (1985). Comparative measurement efficiency and sensitivity of five health status instruments for arthritis research. *Arthritis Rheum*, 28, 542–7.

20. Laupacis, A., Bourne, R., Rorabeck, C., Feeny, D., Wong, C., Tugwell, P., *et al*. (1993). The effect of elective total hip replacement on health-related quality of life. *J Bone Joint Surg (Am)*, 75–A, 1619–26.

21. Liang, M.H., Fossel, A.H., and Larson, M.G. (1990). Comparisons of five health status instruments for orthopedic evaluation. *Med Care*, 28, 632–42.

22. Weinberger, M., Samsa, G.P., Tierney, W.M., Belyea, M.J., and Hiner, S.L. (1992). Generic versus disease specific health status measures: comparing the sickness impact profile and the arthritis impact measurement scales. *J Rheumatol*, 19, 543–6.

23. Meenan, R.F., Gertman, P.M., and Mason, J.H. (1980). Measuring health status in arthritis. The arthritis impact measurement scales. *Arthritis Rheum*, 23, 146–52.

24. Hunt, S.M. and McEwen, J. (1980). The development of a subjective health indicator. *Soc Health Illn*, 2, 231–46.

25. Wiklund, I. and Romanus, B. (1991). A comparison of quality of life before and after arthroplasty in patients who had arthrosis of the hip joint. *J Bone Joint Surg (Am)*, 73–A, 765–9.

26. Katz, J.N., Larson, M.G., Phillips, C.B., Fossel, A.H., and Liang, M.H. (1992). Comparative measurement sensitivity of short and longer health status instruments. *Med Care*, 30, 917–25.

27. Wallston, K.A., Brown, G.K., Stein, M.J., and Dobbins, C.J. (1989). Comparing the short and long versions of the Arthritis Impact Measurement Scales. *J Rheumatol*, 16, 1105–9.

28. Fries, J.F., Spitz, P.W., and Young, D.Y. (1982). The dimensions of health outcomes: the health assessment questionnaire, disability and pain scales. *J Rheumatol*, 9, 789–93.

29. Daltroy, L.H., Larson, M.G., Roberts, N.W., and Liang, M.H. (1990). A modification of the Health Assessment Questionnaire for the spondyloarthropathies. *J Rheumatol*, 17, 946–50.

30. Pincus, T., Summey, J.A., Soraci, S.A. Jr, Wallston, K.A., and Hummon, N.P. (1983). Assessment of patient satisfaction in activities of daily living using a modified Stanford Health Assessment Questionnaire. *Arthritis Rheum*, 26, 1346–53.

31. Meenan, R.F., Mason, J.H., Anderson, J.J., Guccione, A.A., and Kazis, L.E. (1992). AIMS2. The content and properties of a revised and expanded Arthritis Impact Measurement Scales Health Status Questionnaire. *Arthritis Rheum*, 35, 1–10.

32. Larson, C. (1963). Rating scale for hip disabilities. *Clin Orthop*, 31, 85–93.

33. Harris, W.H. (1969). Traumatic arthritis of the hip after dislocation and acetabular fractures: treatment by mold arthroplasty. An end result study using a new method of result evaluation. *J Bone Joint Surg (Am)*, 51–A, 737–55.

34. Johanson, N.A., Charlson, M.E., Szatrowski, T.P., and Ranawat, C.S. (1992). A self-administered hip-rating questionnaire for the assessment of outcome after total hip replacement. *J Bone Joint Surg (Am)*, 74–A, 587–97.

35. Mancuso, C.A. and Charlson, M.E. (1995). Does recollection error threaten the validity of cross-sectional studies of effectiveness? *Med Care*, 33, AS77–88.

36. Katz, J.N., Phillips, C.B., Poss, R., Harrast, J.J., Fossel, A.H., Liang, M.H., *et al*. (1995). The validity and reliability of a total hip arthroplasty outcome evaluation questionnaire. *J Bone Joint Surg*, 77A, 1528–34.

37. Lequesne, M., Mery, C., Samson, M., and Gerard, P. (1987). Indexes of severity for osteoarthritis of the hip and knee. Validation — value in comparison with other assessment tests. *Scand J Rheumatol*, Suppl 65, 85–9.

38. Bellamy, N., Buchanan, W.W., Goldsmith, C.H., Campbell, J., and Stitt, L.W. (1988). Validation study of WOMAC: a health status instrument for measuring clinically important patient relevant outcomes to antirheumatic drug therapy in patients with osteoarthritis of the hip or knee. *J Rheumatol*, 15, 1833–40.

39. Pavelka, K., Gatterova, J., Pelitskova, Z., Svarcova, Z., Fencl, F., Urbanova, Z., *et al*. (1992). Correlation between knee roentgenogram changes and clinical symptoms in osteoarthritis. *Rev Rhum Mal Osteoartic*, 59, 553–9.

40. Mazieres, B., Masquelier, A.M., and Capron, M.H. (1991). A French controlled multicenter study of intraarticular orgotein versus intraarticular corticosteroids in the treatment of knee osteoarthritis: a one-year follow up. *J Rheumatol*, suppl 27, 134–7.

41. Bellamy, N., Bensen, W.G., Ford, P.M., Huang, S.H., and Lang, J.Y. (1992). Double-blind randomized controlled trial of flurbiprofen-SR (ANSAID-SR) and diclofenac sodium-SR (Voltaren-SR) in the treatment of osteoarthritis. *Clin Invest Med*, 15, 427–33.

42. Bellamy, N., Buchanan, W.W., Goldsmith, C.H., Campbell, J., and Stitt, L. (1988). Validation study of WOMAC: a health status instrument for measuring clinically important patient relevant outcomes following total hip or knee arthroplasty in osteoarthritis. *J Orthop Rheumatol*, 1, 95–108.

43. Takeda, W. and Wessel, J. (1994). Acupuncture for the treatment of pain of osteoarthritic knees. *Arthritis Care Res*, 7, 118–22.

44. Doyle, D.V., Dieppe, P.A., Scott, J., and Huskisson, E.C. (1981). An articular index for the assessment of osteoarthritis. *Ann Rheum Dis*, 40, 75–8.

45. Bellamy, N., Kean, W.F., Buchanan, W.W., Gerecz-Simon, E., and Campbell, J. (1992). Double blind randomized controlled trial of sodium meclofenamate (Meclomen) and diclofenac sodium (Voltaren): post validation reapplication of the WOMAC Osteoarthritis Index. *J Rheumatol*, 19, 153–9.

46. Lequesne, M., Brandt, K.D., Bellamy, N., Moskowitz, R., Menkes, C.J., Pelletier, J.P., *et al*. (1994). Guidelines for testing slow acting drugs in osteoarthritis. *J Rheumatol*, 21 (suppl 41), 65–71.

47. Lequesne, M., Dougados, M., Abiteboul, M., Bontoux, D., Bouvenot, G., Dreiser, R.L., *et al.* (1990). How to evaluate the long-term course of osteoarthritis. Tests for trials of fundamental treatments (spine excluded). *Rev Rheum Mal Osteoartic*, **57**, 24S–31S.

48. Auquier, L., Paolaggi, J.B., Cohen de Lara, A., Siaud, J.R., Limon, J., Emery, J.P., *et al.* (1979). Long term evolution of pain in a series of 273 coxarthrosis patients. *Rev Rheum Mal Osteoartic*, **46**, 153–62.

49. Cushnaghan, J., Cooper, C., Dieppe, P., Kirwan, J., McAlindon, T., and McCrae, F. (1990). Clinical assessment of osteoarthritis of the knee. *Ann Rheum Dis*, **49**, 768–70.

50. Ritchie, D.M., Boyle, J.A., Mclnnes, J.M., Jasani, M.K., Dalakos, T.G., Grieveson, P., *et al.* (1968). Clinical studies with an articular index for the assessment of joint tenderness in patients with rheumatoid arthritis. *Q J Med*, **37**, 393–406.

51. Buckland-Wright, J.C., Macfarlane, D.G., Lynch, J.A., and Jasani, M.K. (1995). Quantitative microfocal radiography detects changes in OA knee joint space width in patients in placebo controlled trial of NSAID therapy. *J Rheumatol*, **22**, 937–43.

52. Spiegel, J.S., Paulus, H.E., Ward, N.B., Spiegel, T.M., Leake, B., and Kane, R.L. (1987). What are we measuring? An examination of walk time and grip strength. *J Rheumatol*, **14**, 80–6.

53. Marks, R. (1994). Reliability and validity of self-paced walking time measures for knee Osteoarthritis. *Arthritis Care Res*, **7**, 50–3.

54. Minor, M.A., Hewett, J.E., Webel, R.R., Anderson, S.K., and Kay, D.R. (1989). Efficacy of physical conditioning exercise in patients with rheumatoid arthritis and osteoarthritis. *Arthritis Rheum*, **32**, 1396–405.

55. Kovar, P.A., Allegrante, J.P., MacKenzie, C.R., Peterson, M.G., Gutin, B., and Charlson, M.E. (1992). Supervised fitness walking in patients with osteoarthritis of the knee. A randomized, controlled trial. *Ann Intern Med*, **116**, 529–34.

56. Chang, R.W., Falconer, J., Stulberg, S.D., Arnold, W.J., Manheim, L.M., and Dyer, A.R. (1993). A randomized, controlled trial of arthroscopic surgery versus closed-needle joint lavage for patients with osteoarthritis of the knee. *Arthritis Rheum*, **36**, 289–96.

57. Williams, H.J., Ward, J.R., Egger, M.J., Neuner, R., Brooks, R.H., Clegg, D.O., *et al.* (1993). Comparison of naproxen and acetaminophen in a two-year study of treatment of osteoarthritis of the knee. *Arthritis Rheum*, **36**, 1196–206.

58. Fisher, N.M., Gresham, G.E., Abrams, M., Hicks, J., Horrigan, D., and Pendergast, D.R. (1993). Quantitative effects of physical therapy on muscular and functional performance in subjects with osteoarthritis of the knees. *Arch Phys Med Rehabil*, **74**, 840–7.

59. Fisher, N.M., Gresham, G.E., and Pendergast, D.R. (1993). Effects of a quantitative progressive rehabilitation program applied unilaterally to the osteoarthritic knee. *Arch Phys Med Rehabil*, **74**, 1319–26.

60. Hochberg, M.C., Lethbridge-Cejku, M., Plato, C.C., Wigley, F.M., and Tobin, J.D. (1991). Factors associated with osteoarthritis of the hand in males: data from the Baltimore Longitudinal Study of Aging. *Am J Epidemiol*, **134**, 1121–7.

61. Chang, R.W., Dunlop, D., Gibbs, J., and Hughes, S. (1995). The determinants of walking velocity in the elderly. An evaluation using regression trees. *Arthritis Rheum*, **38**, 343–50.

62. McAlindon, T.E., Cooper, C., Kirwan, J.R., and Dieppe, P.A. (1993). Determinants of disability in osteoarthritis of the knee. *Ann Rheum Dis*, **52**, 258–62.

63. Theiler, R., Stucki, G., Schütz, R., Hofer, H., Seifert, B., Tyndall, A., *et al.* (1996). Parametric and nonparametric measures in the assessment of knee and hip osteoarthritis: interobserver reliability and correlation with radiology. *Osteoarthritis and Cartilage*, **4**, 35–42.

64. Bellamy, N. (1993). Mechanical and electromechanical devices. In *Musculoskeletal clinical metrology*, pp. 117–34. Kluwer Academic Publishers, Dordrech.

65. Roberts, W.N., Liang, M.H., Pallozzi, L.M., and Daltroy, L.H. (1988). Effects of warming up on reliability of anthropometric techniques in ankylosing spondylitis. *Arthritis Rheum*, **31**, 549–52.

66. Bellamy, N., Sothern, R.B., and Campbell, J. (1990). Rhythmic variations in pain perception in osteoarthritis of the knee. *J Rheumatol*, **17**, 364–72.

67. Hawley, D.J. and Wolfe, F. (1994). Effect of light and season on pain and depression in subjects with rheumatic disorders. *Pain*, **59**, 227–34.

68. Harris, C.M. (1984). Seasonal variations in depression and osteoarthritis. *J R Coll Gen Pract*, **34**, 436–9.

69. Scott, J. and Huskisson, E.C. (1979). Accuracy of subjective measurements made with or without previous scores: an important source of error in serial measurement of subjective states. *Ann Rheum Dis*, **38**, 558–9.

70. Bellamy, N., Goldsmith, C.H., Buchanan, W.W., Campbell, J., and Duku, E. (1991). Prior score availability: observations using the WOMAC osteoarthritis index. *Br J Rheumatol*, **30**, 150–1.

71. Bellamy, N., Buchanan, W.W., Goldsmith, C.H., Campbell, J., and Duku, E. (1990). Signal measurement strategies: are they feasible and do they offer any advantage in outcome measurement in osteoarthritis? *Arthritis Rheum*, **33**, 739–45.

72. Barr, S., Bellamy, N., Buchanan, W.W., Chalmers, A., Ford, P.M., Kean, W.F., *et al.* (1994). A comparative study of signal versus aggregate methods of outcome measurement based on the WOMAC Osteoarthritis Index. *J Rheumatol*, **21**, 2106–12.

73. Stucki, G., Stucki, S., Bruhlmann, P., and Michel, B.A. (1995). Ceiling effects of the Health Assessment Questionnaire and its modified version in some ambulatory rheumatoid arthritis patients. *Ann Rheum Dis*, **54**, 461–5.

74. Liang, M.H., Gall, V., Partridge, A.J., and Eaton, H. (1983). Management of functional disability in homebound patients. *J Fam Practice*, **17**, 429–35.

11 Prospects for pharmacological modification of joint breakdown in osteoarthritis

11.1 Introduction

Kenneth Brandt, L. Stefan Lohmander, and Michael Doherty

Because of the limitations of current therapy of osteoarthritis (OA), interest has arisen in pharmacologic agents which are not principally analgesic, but whose fundamental actions result in the alteration of pathogenetic mechanisms within the OA joint, that is, disease-modifying drugs[1]. Claims have been made — often based on *in vitro* effects on chondrocytes or on cartilage slices — that a variety of agents are 'chondroprotective', although no drug has yet been shown to modify the pathologic changes of OA in a well-designed placebo-controlled clinical trial in humans. Nonetheless, hopes are spurred by recent studies which show that pharmacologic modification of joint damage in animal models of OA is feasible.

In considering guidelines for testing new drugs, a Committee of the International League of Associations for Rheumatology recommended recently that the term, disease-modifying drug for osteoarthritis (DMOAD), be reserved for agents which prevent, retard the progression of, or reverse *morphologic changes* of OA[1]; an effect only on the biochemistry or metabolism of cartilage matrix molecules or on the concentration in body fluids of molecules derived from cartilage or bone in the diseased joint ('osteoarthritis marker' molecules) was considered to be insufficient to qualify an agent as a DMOAD. Furthermore, because *all* of the structures of the joint, and not only the cartilage, are involved in OA, it is conceivable that a drug that acts primarily on bone or other tissues of the joint may prove to be as effective in protecting against OA as an agent whose primary target lies within the cartilage. For this reason, in particular, OA mavins now

consider that the designation, DMOAD, more accurately describes agents in this class than the label, 'chondroprotective drug'.

In animal models, several agents have met the above criterion for a DMOAD. They range from empirical compounds, for example, tissue extracts, to site-specific inhibitors designed to fit precisely into the catalytic site of collagenase, and include tribenoside, tamoxifen, diacerhein, chloroquine, hyaluronic acid, glucocorticoids, and tranexamic acid. Excellent reviews of these agents have been published recently[2–4]. Chapter 11.2 brings the discussion up to date, and Chapters 11.3 and 11.4 discuss the advantages and limitations of the use of animal models for the development of DMOADs.

Previous reports which suggested that the pathologic changes of OA advance very slowly are, to a large extent, responsible for the fact that this is a field which, until recently, moved very slowly; it was assumed that vast numbers of subjects and many years of treatment would be required to demonstrate a DMOAD effect in humans. This view deterred efforts by the pharmaceutical industry to develop DMOADs. However, as discussed in Chapter 11.5, the mean rate of articular cartilage loss in OA, as judged by the reduction of joint space width in a standard radiograph, is much more rapid than previously believed[1,5]. Standardization of radioanatomic positioning of the knee can reduce the variability in measurements of joint space to only 1–2 per cent[6] and computerized analysis of the digitized radiograph will reduce the variability inherent in manual measurements of the radiographic image, further reducing the number of subjects required to demonstrate a true drug effect.

Epidemiologic data suggest that a clinical trial of a DMOAD can be facilitated by focusing on a joint at high risk for OA; for example, 50 per cent of middle-aged, obese women with radiographic evidence of uni-lateral knee OA will develop OA in the contralateral knee within the next two years[7]. Several strategies can be applied to maximize retention of subjects in a long-term clinical trial and compliance with the dosing regimen[8], as exemplified by the 82 per cent retention rate in a 48-week trial of minocycline in patients with rheumatoid arthritis[9]. A 'faintness-of-heart' test[10], to eliminate non-compliers prior to randomization into treatment groups, and use of computerized medicine caps to permit study personnel to direct their efforts to enhance compliance toward those subjects who can best benefit from such efforts, may further increase retention of the subject in a long-term trial. With use of these techniques, the logistics of a clinical trial of a DMOAD need not be daunting; efficacy of a DMOAD might be demonstrated in a controlled clinical trial with only 2–2½ years of treatment and enrollment of fewer than 500 subjects. Appendix 4 contains guidelines for the conduct of clinical studies of DMOADs published recently by the Osteoarthritis Research Society[11].

A need exists now for clinical researchers with an interest in OA, members of the pharmaceutical industry, and representatives of regulatory authorities to agree upon appropriate outcome measures and assessment tools for evaluation of DMOADs. Once a drug with DMOAD activity in humans has been identified, it will be possible to determine whether reduction in the rate of cartilage loss is accompanied by reductions in joint pain, the frequency of joint arthroplasty, and the rate of disability.

Finally, the possibility exists that some drugs, rather than having a beneficial effect, may accelerate or exacerbate the pathologic changes of OA. For example, in animal models, salicylate administration has been shown to lead to more severe changes in the arthritic joint than those seen in untreated animals[12,13]. Several investigators have suggested that indomethacin, in particular, has an adverse effect on the OA joint. Although these reports have been based largely on anecdotal evidence, a recent randomized controlled trial in humans[14], albeit limited by problems in the experimental design and interpretation of the data[15], also has sug-

gested that this nonsteroidal anti-inflammatory drug (NSAID) has a detrimental effect on the OA joint. The issue is far from settled.

References

1. Lequesne, M., Brandt, K., Bellamy, N., Moskowitz, R., Menkes, C.J., Pelletier, J.P., *et al.* (1994). Guidelines for testing slow-acting and disease-modifying drugs in osteoarthritis. *J Rheumatol*, **21**,suppl 41,(9), 65–71.
2. Burkhart, D. and Ghosh, P. (1987). Laboratory evaluation of antirheumatic drugs as potential chondroprotective agents. *Semin Arth Rheum*, **17**, 3–34.
3. Howell, D.S., Altman, R.D., Pelletier, J-P., Martel-Pelletier, J., and Dean, D.D. (1995). Disease modifying anti-rheumatic drugs: current status of their application in animal models of osteoarthritis. In *New horizons in osteoarthritis* (ed. K. Kuettner and V. Goldberg), pp. 365–77. American Academy of Orthopedic Surgeons, Chicago.
4. Di Pasquale, G. (1993). Pharmacologic control of cartilage degeneration in osteoarthritis. In *joint cartilage degradation: basic and clinical aspects* (ed. J.F. Woessner and D.S. Howell), pp. 475–501. Marcel Dekker; New York.
5. Dougados, M., Guegen, A., Nguyen, M., Thiesce, A., Listrat, V., Jacob, L., *et al.* (1992). Longitudinal radiologic evaluation of osteoarthritis of the knee. *J Rheumatol*, **19**, 378–84.
6. Buckland-Wright, J.C. and MacFarlane, D.G. (1995). Radio-anatomic assessment of therapeutic outcome in osteoarthritis. In *Osteoarthritic disorders* (ed. K. Kuettner and V. Goldberg), pp. 51–65. American Academy of Orthopedic Surgeons, Rosemont, IL.
7. Spector, T.D., Hart, D.J., and Doyle, D.V. (1994). Incidence and progression of osteoarthritis in women with unilateral knee disease in the general population: the effect of obesity. *Ann Rheum Dis*, **53**, 565–8.
8. Haynes, R.B., Wang, E., and Da Mota Gomes, M. (1987). A critical review of interventions to improve compliance with prescribed medications. *Pt Educ Couns*, **10**, 155–66.
9. Tilley, B., Alarcon, G., Heyse, S., Trentham, D., Neuner, R., Caplan, D.A., *et al.* (1995). Minocycline in rheumatoid arthritis. A 48-week, double-blind, placebo-controlled trial: the MIRA trial group. *Ann Intern Med*, **122**(2), 81–9.
10. Lang, J.M. (1990). The use of a run-in to enhance compliance. *Statistics in Med*, **9**, 87–95.
11. Altman, R., Brandt, K., Hochberg, M., Moskowitz, R., Bellamy, N., Bloch, DA., *et al.* (1996). Design and conduct of clinical trial in patients with osteoarthritis. *Osteoarthritis and Cartilage*, **4**, 217–43.
12. Palmoski, M.J., Colyer, R., and Brandt, K.D. (1980). Marked suppression by salicylate of the augmented proteoglycan synthesis in osteoarthritic cartilage. *Arthritis Rheum*, **23**, 83–91.

13. Wilhelmi, V.J. (1978). Fordende and hemmende einflusse von tribenosid and acetylsalicylsaure auf die spontane arthrose der maus. *Arzniemittelforschung*, **28**, 1724–6.

14. Huskisson, E.C., Berry, H., Gishen, P., Jubb, R.W., and Whitehead, J. (1995). Effects of antiinflammatory drugs

on the progression of osteoarthritis of the knee. *J Rheumatol*, **22**, 1941–6.

15. Doherty, M. and Jones, A. (1995). Indomethacin hastens large joint osteoarthritis in humans — how strong is the evidence? *J Rheumatol*, **22**, 2013–16.

11.2 Disease-modifying osteoarthritis drugs

Roy D. Altman and David S. Howell

Introduction

Osteoarthritis (OA) is no longer considered a 'degenerative' or 'wear-and-tear' disease but is now recognized to involve dynamic biological and biochemical processes[1]. Many of the changes in the OA joint represent active remodeling. Furthermore, although articular cartilage continues to be at the center of change, OA is increasingly viewed as a disease which affects all of the tissues of the joint and, therefore, represents the failure of the joint as an organ[2]. This appreciation has opened new avenues of research; efforts directed toward the development of better symptomatic therapy for OA are now complemented by approaches that address the fundamental biological, biochemical, and biomechanical alterations. Conceptually, OA may be modified by surgical or pharmacologic measures or a combination of such approaches[3].

For lack of a better term, pharmacologic agents with reparative properties have been called disease-modifying OA drugs (DMOADs)[4] (also called structure modifying drugs for OA; Appendix 4). Specifically, the term, DMOAD, is used to describe an agent that arrests or retards the progression of OA and/or enhances normal reparative processes in the diseased joint. The effects of a DMOAD on tissue injury or repair may be distinct from its effect on symptoms, which may be direct or indirect. The long-term goal of DMOAD therapy is to diminish the need for joint replacement; it may augment other non-invasive or minimally invasive (for example, arthroscopic) treatment. Because OA is a disease of the entire joint, and not only of the articular cartilage, the adjective used previously to describe DMOAD effects — 'chon-

droprotective' — is inappropriate: for example, a drug could, hypothetically, exert a DMOAD effect via an action on the remodeling of subchondral bone, rather than directly on the articular cartilage. Although several agents are currently being evaluated for DMOAD properties, none has yet been identified as an effective DMOAD in humans.

As discussed below, combinations of surgical and pharmacologic methods seem promising in the treatment of OA, for example, local arthroscopically-directed application of medication supplemented with passive motion of the joint. Agents can be applied directly to the developing OA lesion, or upon (or within) surgically implanted cartilage explants or cell-matrix constructs. The immediate goals are to fill in defects in the cartilage surface, improve the biomechanical properties of the cartilage, and strengthen host-graft interfaces.

Table 11.1 lists some of the agents that have been tested for DMOAD properties. The potential value of surgical application of such agents is of great interest but has not yet been adequately tested.

Animal models in the evaluation of DMOADs

Only the most promising DMOADs will be tested in clinical trials in humans. For this reason, a wide variety of animal models have been developed which have characteristics mimicking various aspects of human OA and facilitate the testing of potential DMOADs[5–7]. Animal models of OA hold promise for demonstration of both surgical and pharmacologic disease-modifying

Table 11.1 Disease-modifying osteoarthritis drugs (DMOADs)

Sulfated glycosaminoglycans
    Glycosaminoglycan-peptide (GAG-peptide)
    Glycosaminoglycan polysulfuric acid (GAGPS)
    Pentosan polysulfate
    Chondroitin sulfate
    Glucosamine sulfate
Non-sulfated glycosaminoglycans
    Hyaluronic acid
Agents acting on bone
    Bisphosphonates
        Etidronate
    Calcitonin
Anti-inflammatory agents
    Nonsteroidal anti-inflammatory drugs
    Glucocorticoids
        Oral
        Intra-articular
    Anthroquinones
        Diacerhein
    Lipids
Enzyme inhibitors
    Tetracyclines
        Doxycycline
        Chemically-modified tetracyclines
    Specific stromelysin inhibitors
    Specific collagenase inhibitors
Cytokines / growth factors
    Growth hormone
    Insulin-like growth factor-1 (IGF-1)
    Transforming growth factor-beta (TGF-β)
    Interleukin-1 receptor antagonist (IL-1ra)

effects. Insofar as OA in humans comprises a spectrum of disorders, no single animal model can fully reflect human OA. Although virtually all vertebrates develop, or can be induced to develop, OA, among the best characterized and most commonly used models are the canine cruciate deficiency model, the lapine partial meniscectomy model, and the ovine meniscectomy model[5–7]. The morphologic, biochemical, and metabolic changes in articular cartilage in all of these animal models mimic those of human OA. Notably, all three of these models are based on joint instability, changes in joint mechanics, and/or irregularity of intra-articular surfaces, and, therefore, represent secondary (that is, post-traumatic) OA. The relatively slow progression of OA in the canine cruciate deficiency model may be accelerated by interruption of sensory input from the unstable limb[8] or by a strenuous exercise program, as provided by treadmill running.

Surgical approaches to cartilage repair

Because the capacity of the host chondrocytes to restore the articular surface is limited[9,10], investigators have sought methods of transplanting cells or using explants to fill chondral and osteochondral defects. The objective of such studies has been to stimulate formation of a new articular surface after the development of a superficial or deep defect in the cartilage, with or without an associated subchondral bony defect[11]. Such studies are based on the fact that damaged cartilage, because it has no blood supply, heals poorly. It is believed that coating of the fibrillar matrix of the articular cartilage with proteoglycans, (particularly dermatan sulfate proteoglycans), prevents blood vessels and repair cells from entering the site of injury[12]. Thus, undifferentiated stem cells from the underlying bone marrow have little chance of participating in repair of the cartilage defect without surgical manipulation to deliver them to the site of damage.

Some examples of surgical strategies aimed at the production of repair cartilage include the following:

- arthroscopic cartilage abrasion

- chondral auto- or allografts

- osteochondral auto- or allografts

- periosteal inversion.

Use of an abrasion burr to expose subchondral bone permits vascular invasion from the underlying marrow, leading to resorption of the damaged hyaline cartilage and replacement with fibrocartilage. A chondral or osteochondral auto- or allograft is secured in a cartilage defect with an inverted periosteal flap from which progenitor cells may differentiate into chondrocytes[11]. This may lead to formation of new tissue, filling the defects in both bone and cartilage.

These surgical techniques have been augmented with the use of passive motion of the joint to increase lymphatic flow and the delivery of nutrients to the host and graft cartilages[13]. It should be noted that studies of the repair tissue produced in the canine cruciate-deficiency model of OA by mechanical abrasion of the joint surface have shown ineffective articular cartilage repair, with eventual enlargement of the defect, suggesting that stabilization may be required for the abrasion technique to be of value[10].

In osteochondral grafts, the bony portion of the graft usually heals uneventfully, while the cartilage often remains viable but seldom bonds to the surrounding host cartilage, giving the graft an 'osteochondritis dissecans-like' appearance. Attempts to fuse the grafted cartilaginous surface to the host cartilage by the use of chemical agents, such as glycosaminoglycan polysulfate (GAGPS) or chondroitinase AC, have been unsuccessful (Altman, R.D., Molinin, T., and Lavernia, C. — unpublished). Proper placement of the graft is critical. Failure of the graft is seen when the surface between the residual cartilage and the graft is uneven: traumatic injury of the graft will occur if the graft is too high relative to the residual surrounding cartilage surface, while the graft will atrophy if it is too low relative to the residual surrounding cartilage surface.

Pharmacologic approaches to modification of OA

As shown in Table 11.1, a variety of pharmacologic agents have been investigated for potential DMOAD effects; some are described in more detail below. The agent may be delivered orally or by intramuscular or intra-articular injection. Alternative delivery systems, for example, liposomes, hyaluronate beads, retroviral constructs — which may provide a longer duration of action within the joint — are being explored. These new techniques may be of particular value for administration of growth factors and cytokine inhibitors[14].

Repair of partial thickness articular cartilage lesions by the timed release of TGF-β encapsulated in liposomes has been attempted in an animal model[15]. Following treatment, the defects exhibited an increase in cellularity due to infiltration of mesenchymal cells from the synovial membrane. The repair tissue resembled normal hyaline cartilage and persisted for as long as one year after surgery.

Gene therapy of OA may also become a reality in the future[16]. For example, the regulation of genes for tissue inhibitor of metalloproteinases (TIMP) and for the metalloproteinases (MMPs), themselves, may provide an opportunity to modulate the disease.

Combinations of surgical and pharmacologic therapies

In the future, better results may be achieved by the use of osteochondral grafts. Implantation of chondrocytes into isolated cartilage defects is possible in humans[11], and the differentiation of stem cells into bone and cartilage after their implantation into an osteochondral defect has been observed in a rabbit model[17]. If these procedures become practical, they may radically alter the management of OA.

In addition to the frequent failure of the explant or graft to firmly anneal to the existing cartilage, a major limitation of surgical approaches to restoration of the articular surface has been the failure to establish space-filling cell matrix constituents that do not deteriorate. The combination of open surgical or arthroscopic techniques and local application of a DMOAD has great appeal. New attempts in this direction have been made using growth factors in conjunction with enzymatic degradation of the host-graft interface with trypsin or chondroitinase ABC. Attempts have also been made to fill the defect with cultured chondrocytes or other cells to promote synthesis of a collagen network[15].

Other approaches under investigation include the implantation of mesenchymal cells or chondrocytes, with or without synthetic matrices[11,17,18], the local application of paracrine or endocrine factors which stimulate chondrogenesis[19], and stimulation with pulsed electrical fields[20].

Recently studied DMOADs

Clinical investigators have only recently focused on the numerous issues involved in establishing guidelines for clinical evaluation of DMOADs[21]. The lack of such guidelines and the continued emphasis on development of drugs that are directed primarily at symptomatic relief (joint pain), rather than at modification of the underlying pathologic processes, has resulted in a dearth of published clinical trials of agents with potential DMOAD activity.

However, a number of pharmacologic agents with DMOAD potential are now under study. As a group, these agents prevent and / or reduce breakdown of cartilage components. As shown in Table 11.1, DMOADs range from empirical compounds, for example, tissue extracts, to highly specific inhibitors of the catalytic site of a matrix-degrading protease. Nonsteroidal anti-inflammatory drugs, antimalarials, hormones, and cytokines have been examined for DMOAD activity and are described in detail in excellent recent reviews of the subject[22-24]; some are discussed below.

Heparinoids

Originally used in the form of crude extracts of animal cartilage and other tissues, these agents contain highly sulfated glycosaminoglycans (GAGs). Reports on the use of heparinoids in therapy of OA have accumulated over the last three decades, but only recently has information become available concerning the basis for their therapeutic effect.

GAG-peptide

Glycosaminoglycan (GAG)-peptide complex (Rumalon®) has perhaps been the most extensively

studied and is, historically, the most important of the heparinoids[22]. GAG-peptide is an aqueous extract of bovine cartilage and bone marrow, containing approximately 1.8 mg per ml of GAGs (mainly chondroitin-4 sulfate and chondroitin-6 sulfate) and 0.7 mg per ml of peptides. GAG-peptide has the capacity to stimulate cartilage matrix synthesis. In the partial meniscectomy lapine model, both prophylactic and therapeutic administration of GAG-peptide retarded the evolution of OA[25,26]. Gross and microscopic changes in the articular cartilage, levels of proteinase activity, cartilage concentrations of proteoglycan, and of tissue inhibitor of metalloproteinase (TIMP)[25] all showed improvement, in comparison with untreated OA controls. Studies in humans with OA to whom GAG-peptide was administered intramuscularly twice weekly for three to six weeks, every six months, patients with hip OA (treated for up to 10 years) and knee OA (treated for five years) showed improvement in several clinical parameters[27]. The results of a recent five-year prospective trial of GAG-peptide in patients with hip or knee OA are currently being analyzed (Pavelka, K. and Altman, R.D., unpublished). Although it contains bovine peptides, GAG-peptide has been well tolerated and adverse events are uncommon.

GAGPS

Glycosaminoglycan polysulfate (GAGPS) (Arteparon®; Adequan®), an aqueous extract of bovine tracheal and bronchial cartilages which contains synthetically over-sulfated chondroitin-4 sulfate and chondroitin-6 sulfate, ranges in molecular weight from 2000–16000 daltons and possesses some heparin-like properties[22]. GAGPS stimulates cartilage matrix synthesis and is a pan-protease inhibitor. Although GAGPS is rapidly removed from extracellular fluids and visceral organs after administration, biochemical analysis and autoradiography of labeled GAGPS have shown that it is retained in articular cartilage, at levels sufficient to inhibit proteases, for as long as three weeks after injection[28,29].

Weekly intra-articular injections of GAGPS, for four weeks, were shown to have a prophylactic effect in reducing cartilage damage in the canine cruciate deficiency model of OA[30]. Hydroxyproline and uronic acid concentrations in cartilage of GAGPS-treated dogs were higher, and levels of active and latent stromelysin in extracts of the OA cartilage, significantly lower than those in untreated OA control dogs. GAGPS therapy also reduced the swelling of OA cartilage following immersion *ex vivo* in 0.9 per cent saline, suggesting that it preserved the integrity of the collagen network of the tissue.

Notably, GAGPS retarded development of OA in the cruciate deficiency canine model, even when treatment did not commence until four weeks after ligament transection[31]. A four-week therapeutic trial of GAGPS resulted in a normalization of the gross and histologic appearance of the cartilage, reduced cartilage swelling and levels of latent and active collagenase, and increased the proteoglycan content of the cartilage. Preliminary studies of the prophylactic and therapeutic administration of GAGPS in a lapine partial meniscectomy model have shown reduction in the severity of joint pathology and in levels of proteoglycan-degrading enzymes[32].

When GAGPS was given prophylactically by intramuscular injection, twice weekly, in a dose of 2.5 to 5.0 mg per kg, to Labrador retrievers which were predisposed to hip dysplasia, the severity of joint damage was reduced in comparison with that in untreated control dogs[33]. In addition, the volume of synovial fluid was diminished and fibronectin levels in cartilage of the GAGPS-treated animals were lower than those in the untreated controls. This important observation, made over an eight-month period of treatment, strongly suggests that this agent has important DMOAD activity.

In a five-year trial in humans with OA of the knee, GAGPS treatment was reported to improve a variety of outcome measurements, including the frequency of surgical intervention and amount of time lost from work[27]. Although GAGPS remains available for equine use, concern about hypersensitivity reactions and heparin-like effects have sharply limited its use in humans.

Pentosan

Pentosan polysulfate (Cartrofen®, SP 50), a polysaccharide sulfate ester derived from beechwood hemicellulose, is a potent inhibitor of many proteases, including leukocyte elastase, hyaluronidase, and matrix metalloproteases[22,34]. Like GAG-peptide, pentosan has been shown by both autoradiography and biochemical analyses to remain undegraded in articular cartilage and intervertebral disc for a prolonged period of time after administration[35].

Like GAGPS, this strongly anionic compound disappears from extracellular fluid and visceral organs within two to three days after administration, but is selectively bound in collagenous tissues, including intervertebral disc and articular cartilage. Since proteoglycans are anionic, it is surprising that pentosan, a highly polyanionic compound, has an affinity for cartilage. The theoretical basis for penetration of pentosan into cartilage includes the following: (1) the low molecular weight of the agent (6000 daltons); (2) facilitated diffusion of linear polyelectrolytes through cartilage[36]; and (3) binding to non-proteoglycan proteins, such as thrombospondin (Ghosh P *et al*, — unpublished). As shown by circular dichroism, pentosan inhibits leukocyte elastase by binding near its catalytic site[37].

Pentosan polysulfate and heparin down-regulate phorbol-induced cancer cell proliferation by interfering with the binding of transcription factor to gene promoter AP1 sites[38]. This group of agents may have an analogous effect on down-regulation of metalloproteinase transcription.

In the ovine medial meniscectomy model, in which severe OA develops after 16 weeks of exercise, pentosan polysulfate, hyaluronan, and a combination of the two had significant effects on joint pathology, gait analysis, and cartilage histomorphometry; hyaluronan, alone, showed less impressive cartilage conservation than the combination. In the lapine partial meniscectomy model of OA, prophylactic treatment with pentosan polysulfate preserved proteoglycan content and structure, and reduced the severity of gross and histologic changes in the articular cartilage[39]. Pentosan also provided partial cartilage protection in the canine cruciate deficiency model of OA, particularly when used in combination with intra-articular injection of IGF-1[40]. Although sodium pentosan must be given by intramuscular or intra-articular injection, calcium pentosan has shown good bioavailability after oral administration[41] and protection against cartilage damage in lapine models of inflammatory arthritis[42].

Chondroitin sulfate

An orally administered formulation of chondroitin sulfate is currently marketed in several countries for therapy of hip and knee OA. In a double-blind, placebo-controlled study which included a three-month treatment phase followed by a two-month observation period[43] in which the major outcome parameter was the level of consumption of a nonsteroidal antiinflammatory drug (NSAID), those who received chondroitin sulfate consumed less NSAID than the controls, both at the end of treatment and during the subsequent observation period.

Chondroitin sulfate is available as a food supplement. There is little information concerning the effective absorption of this agent. Its mechanism of action is unknown, as is its DMOAD potential. It is possible, however, that chondroitin sulfate is the major active component in GAG-peptide, described above (p. 420).

Glucosamine sulfate

Glucosamine sulfate (Dona®), an intermediate in glycosaminoglycan biosynthesis, has been used orally and intramuscularly in symptomatic treatment of OA. When given intramuscularly, 400 mg twice weekly, for six weeks, in comparison with placebo, glucosamine sulfate reduced the severity of OA symptoms, as judged by the Lequesne Algofunctional Index[44,45].

Glucosamine is available as a food supplement. Although the above clinical findings are interesting, inadequate information exists concerning the pharmacology of this agent. Whether glucosamine sulfate has DMOAD activity is unknown.

Non-sulfated glycosaminoglycans

Synthetic and naturally occurring hyaluronic acid (hyaluronan (HA)) derivatives have been administered intra-articularly to humans with OA; preparations have varied widely in molecular weight (range from less than 100 000 to more than 1 000 000 daltons). HA has been reported to reduce joint pain and to improve mobility for prolonged periods in patients with OA[46–49]; the mechanism of action is unknown. However, there is evidence of an anti-inflammatory effect, particularly with high molecular weight preparations; of a short-term lubricant effect; of an analgesic effect, mediated perhaps by directly coating synovial nerve endings; and of an increase in the molecular weight of HA synthesized by the synovial lining cells following intra-articular injection[53,56].

Intra-articular injections of HA resulted in improvement in gait in the ovine medial meniscectomy model when given weekly for five weeks, beginning 16 weeks after the surgical procedure suggesting a reduction in lameness. A preparation with an average molecular weight of approximately 850 000 daltons was as effective as HA with an average molecular weight of approximately 2 000 000 daltons[50,51]. With both HA preparations, gross cartilage damage was less severe than in saline-treated controls, although osteophytosis was more marked. The authors suggested that the increase in osteophyte formation might have been associated with the improvement in gait and greater usage of the OA knee. In this ovine model, however, HA was not as effective as pentosan in reducing the severity of OA pathology[9].

In cruciate-deficient dogs, intra-articular injection of HA was reported to slow the development of pathologic changes and to improve the molecular characteristics of proteoglycans in the OA cartilage[52,53]. Recently, Dougados *et al*[54]. noted that intra-articular injection of HA in humans with knee OA slowed the progression of cartilage damage over a period of one year, as observed arthroscopically.

Recent short-term pain studies have shown that a chemically crosslinked hyaluronic acid preparation (Synvisc®) is equivalent in effectiveness to a non-steroidal anti-inflammatory drug[55]. However, no long-term studies have been performed to explore DMOAD properties of the crosslinked preparation.

Etidronate

Etidronate (ethane diphosphonate, Didronel®) belongs to the class of carbonyl phosphates, or bisphosphonates. Bisphosphonates, which have been extensively studied in treatment of Paget's disease of bone and osteoporosis, are adsorbed on to the surface of hydroxyapatite crystals, retarding flux of mineral ions and reducing bone loss[56,57].

Etidronate has been shown to suppress collagenase and prostaglandin E2 production in cultures of human articular chondrocytes[58], and to sharply reduce the collagenase content of growth plate cartilage[59]. Despite its suppressive effect on proteoglycan synthesis in sheep and rat cartilage culture systems, etidronate reduced the severity of joint pathology in the canine cruciate deficiency model of OA[60]. A series of 12, weekly, intra-articular injections, each containing 200 mg of etidronate, prevented osteophyte formation and reduced capillary invasion of the tidemark and cartilage collagenase levels. Whether other bisphosphonates have similar effects in OA is uncertain; no published studies exist of bisphosphonate treatment of OA in humans.

Calcitonin

Calcitonin, a peptide hormone, is synthesized by the C-cells of the thyroid gland as a high molecular weight precursor which undergoes modification before secretion. Calcitonin, particularly the salmon hormone, has been used extensively in treatment of osteoporosis, hypercalcemia, and Paget's disease of bone.

Salmon calcitonin inhibits osteoclast function and mildly stimulates osteoblast activity. Calcitonin appears to have a regulatory action on cartilage chondrocytes, mediated through specific receptors. Preliminary studies have indicated that calcitonin has anabolic effects on chondrocytes *in vitro*[61], for example, it stimulates incorporation of labeled glucose into glycosaminoglycans by chondrocytes from calf growth plate.

It has been suggested that calcitonin acts as a growth and maturation factor. For example, incubation of femoral cartilage from chick embryos with calcitonin stimulated cell growth and led to increases in the concentrations of hexosamine, hydroxyproline, DNA, and RNA in the cartilage matrix[62]: this action was synergistic with that of parathyroid hormone. In another study, a direct dose-response effect of human and salmon calcitonin was observed in embryonic chick pelvic cartilage, with increases in cartilage wet-weight and alkaline phosphatase activity, but no change in DNA concentration[63]. In studies of human articular chondrocytes in culture, calcitonin increased proteoglycan synthesis, incorporation of ^{3}H thymidine, and type II collagen synthesis in a concentration-dependent fashion (Manicourt, D., personal communication); no differences could be seen between the effects of the human and salmon hormone. In cultures of normal adult bovine chondrocytes, bovine calcitonin stimulated chondrocyte proliferation and increased GAG synthesis[61]. In cultures of articular cartilage from cruciate deficient dogs with OA, calcitonin stimulated proteoglycan and hyaluronan synthesis and led to increased retention of the newly synthesized proteoglycans within the matrix (Altman, R.D. — unpublished). In contrast, normal canine cartilage was essentially unaffected by calcitonin. Badursk, *et al.*[64] have reported that *in vivo* administration of calcitonin prevented the progression of OA in the rabbit partial meniscectomy model.

Doxycycline

In the early 1980s, Golub and Greenwald made the important observation that tetracyclines can inhibit the activity of mammalian collagenase, and that this was unrelated to the antimicrobial activity of these drugs[65]. Doxycycline, an analogue of tetracycline, when administered to patients with periodontitis, reduced the excessive collagenase levels in gingival crevicular

fluid[66]. Subsequently, Greenwald showed that doxycycline reduced collagenase in rat growth plate cartilages[67].

Doxycycline was tested as a potential DMOAD by Brandt and coworkers in the canine cruciate deficiency model of OA, in which joint breakdown was accelerated by L4–S1 dorsal root ganglionectomy[68]. Untreated OA controls developed extensive full-thickness ulceration of medial femoral condylar cartilage, whereas cartilage from dogs treated with doxycycline, 3–4 mg per kg per day, was grossly normal in some cases and showed only slight surface irregularity in others. Furthermore, matrix metalloproteinase activity (collagenase, gelatinase) was four- to five- fold higher in extracts of OA cartilage from the untreated controls than in those from the doxycycline treated animals. In addition, in the same canine model, oral administration of doxycycline reduced the severity of OA even when treatment was delayed until cartilage lesions had already developed[69]. These observations provide direct evidence for a strong DMOAD action of doxycycline under these specific conditions. Human trials on the potential DMOAD activity of doxycycline are under way.

Nonsteroidal anti-inflammatory drugs

Some NSAIDs have displayed DMOAD activity in animal models of OA; many NSAIDs exhibit a variety of biochemical and metabolic effects on cartilage[70–72]. Despite years of testing and experience, however, the DMOAD potential of this class of drugs, in humans, remains unclear. Examples of nonsteroidal anti-inflammatory drugs which have been reported to have activities consistent with a DMOAD effect are listed below.

Piroxicam

In vitro studies have suggested that piroxicam may have DMOAD activity[70]. Herman *et al.* found that when OA synovial membrane explants were cultured in the presence of clinically relevant concentrations of piroxicam, synthesis of factors which stimulated catabolism of cartilage was suppressed. Rainsford[71] has reported that other nonsteroidal anti-inflammatory drugs also reduce the *in vitro* production of cartilage catabolic factors by synovium. No *in vivo* studies testing the DMOAD effect of piroxicam are available.

Tenidap

In addition to its ability to inhibit the activities of cyclo-oxygenase and lipoxygenase, tenidap has been shown to reduce metalloproteinase synthesis, by down-regulation of IL-1 receptors, on chondrocytes in the canine cruciate deficiency model of OA[73]. Co-administration of the proton pump inhibitor, omeprazole, to cruciate-deficient dogs which were treated with tenidap, effectively protected against drug-induced gastroenteropathy[73]. Under these conditions, tenidap administration strikingly reduced the severity of OA pathology, in comparison with that in control dogs which did not receive the drug.

Tiaprofenic acid

Tiaprofenic acid, a propionic acid derivative, has been reported to have a number of actions which are not related to its action as a prostaglandin synthase inhibitor, but which might be potentially relevant to DMOAD activity. For example, because it inhibits plasminogen activator activity[74], and plasmin has been shown to be effective in converting the latent proenzyme forms of MMPs into active enzymes, tiaprofenic acid could theoretically inhibit cartilage breakdown. Indeed, proteoglycan catabolism has been shown to be reduced in cultures of human OA cartilage incubated with tiaprofenic acid[75]. Furthermore, oral administration of tiaprofenic acid improved the histological scores and preserved proteoglycan aggregate profiles in OA cartilage in the canine cruciate deficiency model of OA[76]. In a similar study using the cruciate-deficient model, tiaprofenic acid reduced the severity of OA lesions and levels of cartilage metalloproteases[74]. Vignon *et al.*[77] reported that treatment with oral tiaprofenic acid, for several days, was associated with a lower level of stromelysin in extracts of OA cartilage obtained from patients undergoing joint replacement surgery than that seen in extracts of OA cartilage from subjects treated with placebo.

Adrenal glucocorticoids

Oral corticosteroids are not indicated for treatment of human OA because of the limited level of inflammation in this disease and the variety of adverse reactions which may be caused by these agents. However, oral administration of steroids has been reported to reduce disease progression and joint erosion in some patients with rheumatoid arthritis[78], suggesting that steroids could reduce the frequency of secondary OA in patients with rheumatoid disease.

In vitro studies employing cartilage cells or explants, as well as *in vivo* studies in animal models, suggest that intra-articular injections of corticosteroids may have a DMOAD effect[79,80]. Theoretically, this could be explained by the observations that articular cartilage chondrocytes in OA exhibit reduced numbers of glucocorticoid receptors[81], and that collagenase activity is reduced and the level of the endogenous collagenase inhibitor, TIMP, increased by steroids[82]. However, for more than four decades concern has existed about potential corticosteroid-induced cartilage damage[83]. Previous studies indicate that corticosteroids suppress cartilage proteoglycan synthesis[84] and that intra-articular administration of corticosteroids can produce pathological lesions in normal cartilage and accelerate damage in OA joints. These results are difficult to interpret, however, insofar as the dosage of corticosteroids used in many of these studies was extremely high and doses were repeated at short intervals.

The role of corticosteroids as DMOADs must be evaluated in relation to the dose. The most recent information has been derived from studies in animal models. In cruciate-deficient dogs, an oral daily dose which, based on body weight, was equivalent to 5 mg per day for a 70 kg human, had no significant effect on cartilage[85]. However, in another study, protective effects were seen at a daily oral dose which was some three times larger[86].

In canine cruciate deficiency model of OA, two months after a single 20 mg intra-articular injection of methylprednisolone acetate, histologic changes of OA in articular cartilage of the unstable knee were less severe, and osteophytes on the tibial plateau and femoral condyles, smaller than in the controls[87]. A high percentage of the cells throughout the cartilage of the OA knee of the untreated dogs demonstrated immunohistochemical staining for stromelysin, while immunoreactive staining was less marked in the treated animals.

Anthraquinones

Diacerhein is a lipid-soluble acetylated form of the naturally occurring dihydroxyanthraquinone carboxylic acid, rhein. This agent has no effect on phospholipase A2, cyclo-oxygenase, or 5-lipoxygenase, but has been shown to stimulate synthesis of PGE_2 by chondrocytes in culture[88] and to inhibit expression of IL-1-induced collagenase[89,90]. It has been suggested that the latter effect is due to inhibition of the binding of activated c-fos and c-jun to the AP-1 site on the promoter region[91].

Absorption of diacerhein from the gastrointestinal tract is dependent on the formulation. With some preparations, loose bowel movements or diarrhea may occur in as many as 30 per cent of patients. The prominence of this adverse effect is related inversely to the efficiency of gastrointestinal absorption.

In animal models of OA, oral treatment with diacerhein has shown a tendency to protect against development of OA and to have an anti-inflammatory effect[92–94]. Clinical trials have demonstrated a modest reduction of joint pain in patients with OA; in a controlled trial in patients with hip OA, diacerhein and tenoxicam were both superior to placebo in relieving joint pain[95]. Further research is needed with respect to the DMOAD potential of this agent. Randomized placebo-controlled trials of the DMOAD effect of diacerhein in patients with hip OA and knee OA are currently in progress.

Lipids

Little information is available on the capacity of fatty acids, shark oil, and other similar natural products to serve as DMOADs. Recently, orally administered avocado / soy non-saponifiables (the components of oils which do not hydrolyze to form soap and glycerin) have been reported to modulate chondrocyte synthetic activity *in vitro*[96,97]. There have been some reports of decreases in joint pain and stiffness and reduction in the level of analgesic use by patients with OA taking such preparations[98]. No information is available with respect to a possible DMOAD effect of these agents.

Summary

Current therapy of OA is directed at symptomatic relief. However, agents are now being developed which have the capacity to modify basic pathologic processes and the progression of joint damage in this disease. Research into DMOADs is progressing swiftly. This is a field of rapid change; none of the agents discussed above may be the therapy of the future. However, they form the basis for research into agents that will serve as the DMOADs of the future and make it likely that the treatment of OA will change dramatically in the next several years.

References

1. Hutton, C.W. (1989). Osteoarthritis: the cause not result of joint failure? *Ann Rheum Dis*, **48**, 958–61.
2. Liang, M.H. and Fortin, P. (1991). Management of osteoarthritis of the hip and knee. (Editorial) *N Engl J Med*, **325:2**, 125–7.
3. Hicks, J.E. and Gerber, L.H. (1992). Rehabilitation in the management of patients with osteoarthritis. In *Osteoarthritis: diagnosis and medical/surgical management* (2nd edn) (ed. R.W. Moskowitz, D.S. Howell, V.M. Goldberg, *et al.*), pp. 427–64. W.B. Saunders, Philadelphia.
4. Lesquesne, M., Brandt, D., Bellamy, N., *et al.* (1994). Guidelines for testing slow acting drugs in osteoarthritis. *J Rheumatol*, **(suppl 41)21**, 65–73.
5. Moskowitz, R.W. (1992). Experimental models of osteoarthritis. In *Osteoarthritis: diagnosis and medical/surgical management* (2nd edn) (ed. R.W. Moskowitz, D.S. Howell, V.M. Goldberg, *et al.*), pp. 213–32. W.B. Saunders, Philadelphia.
6. Altman, R.D. and Dean, D.D. (1990) Osteoarthritis research: animal models. *Semin Arthritis Rheum*, **19(suppl 1)**, 21–5.
7. Ghosh, P., Armstrong, S., Read, R., *et al.* (1993). Animal models of early osteoarthritis: their use for the evaluation of potential chondroprotective agents. In *Joint destruction in arthritis and osteoarthritis* (ed. W.B. Vanden Berg, P.M. vander Kraan and P.L.E.M. Van Lent), pp. 195–206. Birkhauser Verlag, Basel.
8. O'Connor, B.L., Visco, D.M., Brandt, I.D., *et al.* (1992). Neurogenic acceleration of osteoarthrosis: the effects of previous neurectomy of the articular nerves on the development of osteoarthrosis after transection of the anterior cruciate ligament. *J Bone Joint Surg*, **74A**, 367–76.
9. Mitchell, N. and Shepherd, N. (1976). Resurfacing of adult rabbit articular cartilage by multiple perforations of the subchondral bone. *J Bone Joint Surg*, **58**, 230–3.
10. Altman, R.D., Kates, J., Chun, L.E., Dean, D.D., and Eyre, D.R. (1992). Preliminary observations of chondral abrasion in a canine model. *Ann Rheum Dis*, **51**, 1056–62.
11. Brittberg, M., Lindahl, A., Nilsson, A., *et al.* (1994). Treatment of deep cartilage defect in the knee with autologous chondrocyte transplantation. *N Engl J Med*, **331**, 889–95.
12. Rosenberg, L. and Hunzinker, E.B. (1995). Cartilage repair in osteoarthritis: the role of dermetan sulfate proteoglycans. In *Osteoarthritic disorders* (ed. K.E. Kuethner and V.E. Goldberg pp. 341–356). American Academy of Orthopedic Surgeons, Chicago.

13. Salter, R.B. (1989). The biologic concept of continuous passive motion of synovial joints: the first 18 years of basic research and its clinical application. *Clin Orthop*, **242**, 12–25.

14. Pelletier, J.P., Roughley, P.J., DiBattista, J.A., *et al.* (1991). Are cytokines involved in osteoarthritic pathophysiology? *Semin Arthritis Rheum*, **20**(**suppl 2**), 12–25.

15. Hunziker, E.B. and Rosenberg, L. (1994). Induction of repair in partial thickness articular cartilage lesions by timed release of TGF-beta. *Trans Orthop Res Soc*, **19**, 236.

16. Muller-Ladner, U., Roberts, C.R., Franklin, B.N., *et al.* (1995). Gene transfer of interleukin-1 receptor antagonist (IRAP) into human synovial fibroblasts and implantation into the SCID mouse. *Arthritis Rheum*, **38**, S398.

17. Wakitani, S., Goto, T., Pineda, S.J., *et al.* (1994). Mesenchymal cell-based repair of large, full-thickness defects of articular cartilage. *J Bone Joint Surg (Am)*, **76**, 579–92.

18. Hendrickson, D.A., Nixon, A.J., Grande, D.A., *et al.* (1994). Chondrocyte-fibrin matrix transplants for resurfacing extensive articular cartilage defects. *J Orthoped Res*, **12**, 485–97.

19. Cuevas, P., Burgos, J., and Baird, A. (1988). Basic fibroblast growth factor (FGF) promotes cartilage repair *in vivo*. *Biochem Biophys Res Comm*, **156**, 611–18.

20. Lippiello, L., Chakkalakai, D., and Connolly, J.F. (1990). Pulsing direct current induced repair of articular cartilage in rabbit osteochondral defects. *J Orthoped Res*, **8**, 266–75.

21. Bellamy, N. (1993). Osteoarthritis. In *Musculoskeletal clinical metrology* (ed. N. Bellamy), pp. 169–96. Kluwer Academic Publishers, Dordrecht.

22. Burkhardt, D. and Ghosh, P. (1987). Laboratory evaluation of antiarthritic drugs as potential chondroprotective agents. *Semin Arthritis Rheum*, **17**(**suppl 1**), 3–34.

23. DiPasquale, G. (1993). Pharmacological control of cartilage degradation in osteoarthritis. In Woessner JF, Howell DS (eds): *Joint cartilage degradation: basic and clinical aspects* (ed. J.F. Woessner and D.S. Howell), pp. 475–501. Marcel Dekker, New York.

24. Howell, D.S. and Altman, R.D. (1993). Cartilage repair and conservation in osteoarthritis: a brief review of some experimental approaches to chondroprotection. *Rheum Dis Clin North Am*, **19**, 713–24.

25. Dean, D.D., Muniz, O.E., Rodriguez, I., *et al.* (1991). Amelioration of lapine osteoarthritis by treatment with glycosaminoglycan-peptide association complex (Rumalon). *Arthritis Rheum*, **34**, 304–13.

26. Moskowitz, R.W., Reese, J.H., Young, R.G., *et al.* (1991). The effects of Rumalon, a glycosaminoglycan peptide complex, in a partial meniscectomy model of osteoarthritis in rabbits. *J Rheumatol*, **18**, 205–9.

27. Rejholec, V. (1987). Long-term studies of anti-osteoarthritic drugs: an assessment. *Semin Arthritis Rheum*, **17**(**suppl 1**), 35–53.

28. Muller, W., Panse, P., Brand, S., *et al.* (1983). *In vivo* study of the distribution, affinity for cartilage and metabolism of glycosaminoglycan polysulphate (GAGPS, Arteparon). *J Rheumatol*, **42**, 355–61.

29. Andrews, J.L., Sutherland, J., and Ghosh, P. (1985). Distribution and binding of glycosaminoglycan polysulfate to intervertebral disc, knee joint articular cartilage and meniscus. *Arzneimittel Forschung*, **35**, 144–8.

30. Altman, R.D., Dean, D.D., Muniz, O.E., and Howell, D.S. (1989). Prophylactic treatment of canine osteoarthritis with glycosaminoglycan polysulfuric acid ester. *Arthritis Rheum*, **32**, 759–66.

31. Altman, R.D., Dean, D.D., Muniz, O.E., *et al.* (1989). Therapeutic treatment of canine osteoarthritis with glycosaminoglycan polysulfuric acid ester. *Arthritis Rheum*, **32**, 1300–7.

32. Howell, D.S., Carreno, M.R., Pelletier, J-P., *et al.* (1986). Articular cartilage breakdown in a lapine model of osteoarthritis: action of glycosaminoglycan polysulfate ester (GAGPS) on proteoglycan degrading enzyme activity, hexuronate and cell counts. *Clin Orthop Rel Res*, **213**, 69–76.

33. Lust, G., Williams, A.J., Burton-Wurster, N., *et al.* (1992). Effects of intramuscular administration of glycosaminoglycan polysulfates on signs of incipient hip dysplasia in growing pups. *Am J Vet Res*, **53**, 1836–43.

34. Golding, J.C. and Ghosh, P. (1983). Drugs for osteoarthrosis. I: The loss of proteoglycans from articular cartilage in a model of osteoarthrosis induced in the rabbit knee joint by immobilization. *Curr Ther Res*, **32**, 173–84.

35. Smith, M.M., Ghosh, P., Numata, Y., *et al.* (1994). The effects of orally administered calcium pentosan polysulfate on inflammation and cartilage degradation produced in rabbit joints by intraarticular injection of a hyaluronate-polylysine complex. *Arthritis Rheum*, **37**; 125–36.

36. Cumming, G.J., Handley, C.J., and Preston, B.N. (1979). Permeability of composite chondrocyte- culture-Millipore membranes to solutes of varying size and shape. *Biochem J*, **181**, 257–66.

37. Burkhardt, D. and Ghosh, P. (1987). Laboratory evaluation of antiarthritic drugs as potential chondroprotective agents. *Semin Arthritis Rheum*, **17**(**suppl 20**), 3–34.

38. Busch, S.J., Martin, G.A., Barnhart, G.L., *et al.* (1992). Trans-repressor activity of nuclear glycosaminoglycans on fos and jun/AP-1 oncoprotein-mediated transcription. *J Cell Biol*, **116**, 31–42.

39. Howell, D.S., Kapila, P., Malinin, T., and Altman, R.D. (1987). Cartilage degradation and repair. In Huskisson EC, Shioda Y (eds). *New perspectives in rheumatological treatment. New trends in rheumatology 5* (ed. E.C. Huskisson and Y. Shioda), pp. 3–13. Exerpta Medica, Amsterdam.

40. Rogachefsky, R.A., Dean, D.D., Howell, D.S., *et al.* (1993). Treatment of canine osteoarthritis with insulin-like growth factor-1 (IGF-1) and sodium pentosan polysulfate. *Osteoarthritis Cartilage*, **1**, 105–14.

41. Klöcking, H-P., Hauptmann, J., and Richter, M. (1991). Profibrinolytic and anticoagulant properties of the pentosan polysulphate derivative bego 0391. *Pharmazie*, **46**, 543–4.

42. Smith, M.M., Ghosh, P., Numata, Y., and Bansal, M.K. (1994). The effects of orally administered calcium pentosan sulfate on inflammation and cartilage degradation produced in rabbit joints by intraarticular injection of a

hyaluronate-polylysine complex. *Arthritis Rheum*, **37**, 125–36.

43. Mazieres, B., Loyau, G., Menkes, C.J., *et al.* (1992). Chondroitin sulfate in the treatment of gonarthrosis and coxarthrosis. 5-month results of a multicenter double-blind controlled prospective study using placebo. *Revue du Rhumatisme*, **59**, 466–72.

44. Reichelt, A., Forster, K.K., Fischer, M., Rovati, L.C., and Setnikar, I. (1994). Efficacy and safety of intramuscular glucosamine sulfate in osteoarthritis of the knee. A randomised, placebo- controlled, double-blind study. *Arzneimittel Forschung — Drug Research*, **44**, 75–80.

45. Noack, W., Fisher, M., Forster, K.K., *et al.* (1994). Glucosamine sulfate in osteoarthritis of the knee. *Osteoarthritis Cartilage*, **2**, 51–60.

46. Balazs, E.A. and Denlinger, J.L. (1993). Viscosupplementation: a new concept in the treatment of osteoarthritis. *J Rheumatol*, **39(suppl)**, 3–9.

47. Peyron, J.G. (1993). Intraarticular hyaluronan injections in the treatment of osteoarthritis: state-of-the art review. *J Rheumatol*, **20(suppl 39)**, 10–15.

48. Dougados, M., Nguyen, M., Listrat, V., and Amor, B. (1993). High molecular weight sodium hyaluronate (hyalectin) in osteoarthritis of the knee: a 1 year placebo-controlled trial. *Osteoarthritis Cartilage*, **1**, 97–103.

49. Rydell, N. and Balazs, E.A. (1973). Effect of intra-articular injection of hyaluronic acid on the clinical symptoms of osteoarthritis and on granulation tissue formation. *Clin Orthop*, **80**, 25–32.

50. Ghosh, P., Read, R., Armastrong, S., *et al.* (1993). The effects of intraarticular administration of hyaluronan in a model of early osteoarthritis in sheep. I: gait analysis and radiological and morphological studies. *Semin Arthritis Rheum*, **22(suppl 1)**, 18–30.

51. Ghosh, P., Read, R., Numata, Y., *et al.* (1993). The effects of intraarticular administration of hyaluronan in a model of early osteoarthritis in sheep. II: cartilage composition and proteoglycan metabolism. *Semin Arthritis Rheum*, **22(suppl 1)**, 31–42.

52. Abatangelo, G., Botti, P., Del Bue M., *et al.* (1989). Intraarticular sodium hyaluronate injections in the Pond-Nuki experimental model of osteoarthritis in dogs. I: biochemical results. *Clin Orthop Rel Res*, **241A**, 278–85.

53. Schavinato, A., Lini, B.S., Guidolin, D., *et al.* (1989). Intraarticular sodium hyaluronate injections in the Pond-Nuki Experimental Model of osteoarthritis in dogs. II. morphological findings. *Clin Orthop Rel Res*, **241**, 286–99.

54. Dougados, M., Listrant, V., Ayral, X., *et al.* (1997). Arthroscopic evaluation of potential structure modifying activity of hyaluronan (Hyalgan) in osteoarthritis of the knee: a pilot, randomized controlled prospective study. *Osteoarthritis Cartilage*, **5**, 153–60.

55. Adams, M.E., Atkinson, M.H., Lussier, A., *et al.* (1995). The role of viscosupplementation with hylan G-F 20 (Synvisc) in the treatment of osteoarthritis of the knee: a Canadian multicenter trial comparing hylan G-F 20 with nonsteroidal anti-inflammatory drugs (NSAIDs) and NSAIDs alone. *Osteoarthritis Cartilage*, **3**, 213–25.

56. Jung, A., Bisaz, S., and Fleisch, H. (1973). The binding of pyrophosphate and two diphosphonates by hydroxyapatite crystals. *Calcif Tiss Res*, **11**, 269–80.

57. Russell, R.G. and Smith, R. (1973). Diphosphonates: experimental and clinical aspects. *J Bone Joint Surg*, **55B**, 66–86.

58. McGuire, M.K.B., Russell, R.G.G., Murphy, G., *et al.* (1981). Diphosphonates inhibit production of prostaglandin and collagenase by human cells *in vitro*. *Ann Rheum Dis*, **140**, 515.

59. Dean, D.D., Muniz, O.E., and Howell, D.S. (1989). Association of collagenase and tissue inhibitor of metalloproteinases (TIMP) with hypertrophic cell enlargement in the growth plate. *Matrix*, **9**, 366–75.

60. Howell, D.S., Altman, R.D., Pelletier, J-P., Martel-Pelletier, J., and Dean, D.D. (1995). Disease-modifying antirheumatic drugs: current status of their application in animal models of osteoarthritis. In *Osteoarthritic disorders* (ed. K.E. Kuettner and V.E. Goldberg), pp. 365–77. American Academy of Orthopedic Surgeons, Chicago.

61. Franchimont, P., Bassleer, C., Henrotin, Y., *et al.* (1989). Effects of human and salmon calcitonin on human articular chondrocytes cultivated in clusters. *J Clin Endocrinol Metab*, **69**, 259–66.

62. Kawashima, K., Iwata, S., and Endo, H. (1980). Growth stimulative effect of parathyroid hormone, calcitonin and N6,02′ -dibutyryl adenosine 3′,5′-cyclic monophosphoric acid on chick embryonic cartilage cultivated in a chemically defined medium. *Endocrinol Jpn*, **27**, 349–56.

63. Burch, W.M. (1984). Calcitonin stimulates growth and maturation of embryonic chick pelvic cartilage *in vitro*. *Endocrinol*, **114**, 1196–202.

64. Badurski, J.E., Schwamm, W., Popko, J., *et al.* (1991). Chondroprotective action of salmon calcitonin in experimental arthropathies. *Calcif Tiss Int*, **49**, 27–34.

65. Golub, L.M., Greenwald, R.A., Ramamurthy, N.S., *et al.* (1991). Tetracyclines inhibit connective tissue breakdown: new therapeutic implications for an old family of drugs. *CRC Crit Rev Oral Biol Med*, **2**, 297–321.

66. Golub, L.M., Ciancio, A., Ramamurthy, N.S., Leung, M., and McNamara, T.F. (1990). Low-dose doxy cycline therapy: effect on gingival and crevicular fluid collagenase activity in humans. *J Periodont Res*, **25**, 321–30.

67. Lovejoy, B., Cleasby, A., Hassel, A.M., *et al.* (1994). Structural analysis of inhibitor binding to the catalytic domain of human fibroblast collagenase. *Ann NY Acad Sci*, **732**, 378.

68. Yu, L.P. Jr, Smith, G.N. Jr, Brandt, K.D., *et al.* (1992). Reduction of the severity of canine osteoarthritis by prophylactic treatment with oral doxycycline. *Arthritis Rheum*, **35**, 1150–9.

69. Yu, L.P. Jr, Smith, G.N., Jr, Brandt, K.D., *et al.* (1993). Therapeutic administration of doxycycline slows the progression of cartilage destruction in canine osteoarthritis. *Trans Orthop Res Soc*, **18**, 724.

70. Herman, J.H., Appel, A.M., and Hess, E.V. (1987). Modulation of cartilage destruction by select nonsteroidal anti-inflammatory drugs: *in vitro* effect on the

synthesis and activity of catabolism-inducing cytokines produced by osteoarthritic and rheumatoid synovial tissue. *Arthritis Rheum*, 30, 257–65.

71. Rainsford, K.D. (1987). Effects of antiinflammatory drugs on the release from porcine synovial tissue *in vitro* of interleukin-1-like cartilage degrading activity. *Agents Actions*, 21, 337–40.

72. Pelletier, J-P., Haraoui, B., and Martel-Pelletier, J. (1993). Modulation of cartilage degradation in arthritic diseases by therapeutic agents. In *Joint cartilage degradation: basic and clinical aspects* (ed. J.F. Woessner and D.S. Howell), pp. 503–28. Marcel Dekker, New York.

73. Fernandes, J.C., Martel-Pelletier, J., Otterness, I.G., *et al.* (1995). Effects of tenidap on canine experimental osteoarthritis. I: morphologic and metalloprotease analysis. *Arthritis Rheum*, 38, 1290–303.

74. Fibbi, G., Serni, U., Pucci, M., *et al.* (1988). Plasminogen activators and tiaprofenic acid in inflammation: A preliminary study. *Drugs*, 35(suppl 1), 9–14.

75. Pelletier, J-P., Cloutier, J.M., and Martel-Pelletier, J. (1989). *In vitro* effects of tiaprofenic acid, sodium salicylate and hydrocortisone on the proteoglycan metabolism of human osteoarthritic cartilage. *J Rheumatol*, 16, 646–55.

76. Howell, D.S., Pita, J.C., Muller, F.J., *et al.* (1991). Treatment of osteoarthritis with tiaprofenic acid: biochemical and histological protection against cartilage breakdown in the Pond-Nuki canine model. *J Rheumatol*, 27(suppl 1), 138–42.

77. Vignon, E., Mathieu, P., Broquet, P., *et al.* (1990). Cartilage degradative enzymes in human osteoarthritis: effect of a nonsteroidal anti-inflammatory drug administration orally. *Semin Arthritis Rheum*, 19(suppl 1), 26–9.

78. Kirwan, J.R. and the Arthritis and Rheumatism Council Low-Dose Glucocorticoid Study Group. (1995). The effect of glucocorticoids on joint destruction in rheumatoid arthritis. *N Engl J Med*, 333, 142–6.

79. Neustadt, D.H. (1992). Intraarticular steroid therapy. In *Osteoarthritis: diagnosis and medical/surgical management* (2nd edn) (ed. R.W. Moskowitz, D.S. Howell, V.M. Goldberg, *et al.*), pp. 493–510. W.B. Saunders Philadelphia.

80. Gray, R.G., Tenenbaum, J., and Gottlieb, N.L. (1981). Local corticosteroid injection treatment in rheumatic disorders. *Semin Arthritis Rheum*, 10, 231–54.

81. DiBattista, J.A., Martel-Pelletier, J., Antakly, T., *et al.* (1993). Reduced expression of glucocorticoid receptor levels in human osteoarthritic chondrocytes: role in the suppression of metalloprotease synthesis. *J Clin Endocrinol Metab*, 76, 1128–34.

82. McGuire, M.B., Murphy, G., Reynolds, J.J., *et al.* (1981). Production of collagenase and inhibitor (TIMP) by normal, rheumatoid and osteoarthritic synovium *in vitro*: effects of hydrocortisone and indomethacin. *Clin Sci*, 61, 703–10.

83. Salter, R.B., Gross, A., and Hall, J.H. (1967). Hydrocortisone arthropathy: an experimental investigation. *Can Med Assoc J*, 97, 374–7.

84. Behrens, F., Shepard, N., and Mitchell, N. (1976). Metabolic recovery of articular cartilage after intra-articular injections of glucocorticoid. *J Bone Joint Surg*, 58A, 1157–60.

85. Myers, S., O'Connor, B., and Brandt, K. (1990). Low dose corticosteroid treatment after cruciate ligament transection in dogs fails to prevent osteoarthritis. *Arthritis Rheum*, 33, S117.

86. Pelletier, J-P. and Martel-Pelletier, J. (1989). Protective effects of corticosteroids on cartilage lesions and osteophyte formation in the Pond-Nuki dog model of osteoarthritis. *Arthritis Rheum*, 32, 181–93.

87. Pelletier, J-P., Mineau, F., Raynauld, J-P., *et al.* (1994). Intraarticular injections with methylprednisolone acetate reduce osteoarthritic lesions in parallel with chondrocyte stromelysin synthesis in experimental osteoarthritis. *Arthritis Rheum*, 37, 414–23.

88. Pomarelli, P., Perti, M., Gatti, M.T., and Mosconi, P. (1980). A non-steroidal anti-inflammatory drug that stimulates prostaglandin release. *Farmaco [Sci]*, 35, 836–42.

89. Pujol, J.P. (1993). Collagenolytic enzymes and interleukine I: their role in inflammation and cartilage degradation; the antagonistic effects of diacerhein on IL-1 action on cartilage matrix components (abstract). *Osteoarthritis Cartilage*, 1, 82.

90. Cruz, T., Tang, J., Pronost, S., and Pujol, J-P. (1996). Mécanismes moléculaires impliqués dans l'inhibition de l'espression de la collagénase par la diacerhéine. *La Revue du Praticien*, S6, 15–19.

91. Cruz, T. (1996). Effect of diacerhein on matrix metalloproteinases. *Abstracts of the Third International Congress (cannes), Research and Therapeutics in Osteoarthritis: interleukin-1 inhibitors*, p. 8. Negma-Stebu INT., The Netherlands.

92. Taccoen, A. and Berdah, L. (1993). Diacetylrhein, a new therapeutic approach of osteoarthritis. *Revue du Rhumatisme*, 60, 83s–86s.

93. Bendele, A-M., Bendele, R.A., Hulman, J.F., and Swann, B.P. (1996). Effects bénéfiques d'un traitement par la diacerhéine chez des cobayes atteints d'arthrose. *La Revue Du Praticein*, S6, 35–9.

94. Mazieres, B. and Berdah, L. (1993). Effect of diacerhein (ART50) on an experimental post-contusive model of osteoarthritis (abstract). *Osteoarthritis Cartilage*, 1, 47.

95. Nguyen, M., Dougados, M., Berdah, L., *et al.* (1994). Diacerhein in the treatment of osteoarthritis of the hip. *Arthritis Rheum*, 37, 529–37.

96. Harmand, J.F. (1985). Etude de l'action des insaponifiables d'avocat et de soja sur les cultures de chondrocytes articulaires. *Gazette Medicale de France*, 92, 29.

97. Loyau, G., Pujol, J.P., and Mauviel, A. (1991). Effect des insaponifiables d'avocat/soja aur l'activite collagenolytique de cultures de synoviocytes rhumatoides humains et de chondrocytes articularies de lapin traites par l'interleukine-1. *Revue du Rhumatisme*, 58, 241–5.

98. De Seze, S. (1984). Peut-on traiter l'arthrose? *Quotidien du Medecin*, No. 3254, pp. 1–14.

11.3 Advantages afforded by the use of animal models for evaluation of potential disease-modifying osteoarthritis drugs (DMOADs)

Michael E.J. Billingham

Introduction

The search for any therapy that will slow down or halt the progression of osteoarthritis (OA), like any chronic disease of man, relies on insight into the pathological process. This can come either from a clear understanding of the biochemical, biomechanical, and molecular mechanisms involved or from the understanding of the action of drugs that have been found, by chance, to influence disease progression. In the latter respect, OA has had very little success in comparison with rheumatoid arthritis, cancer, and atherosclerosis — but even Cinderella has her time. As the most common form of human disability, OA inevitably has become a major focus of medical research. Like so many chronic human diseases, OA research is hampered by a lack of information of the initiating events and mechanisms of progression. This can only be circumvented by the appropriate use of animal models, where time of onset is predictable and the outcome bears some resemblance to the human counterpart. Recent research into spontaneous OA in the knee of animals has addressed many of these issues.

Animal models of any human disease, however, only reach respectability when therapeutic agents which slow down or halt the progression of the animal model demonstrate similar disease-modifying activity in the human condition. There are presently no drugs which consistently moderate the progression of OA models or spontaneous OA disease in animals, and which have also proven useful in human OA. This is a pragmatic statement of the present situation; the reality is not quite so bleak. Our understanding of animal models, taken in context with the past and present search for agents which may influence disease progression — either discovered by serendipity, for example, diacetylrhein[1]; by design, for example, metalloproteinase inhibitors[2]; or by insight, for example, doxycycline[3] — have yielded some encouragement. It is now clear that

these agents slow the progression of spontaneous OA in the medial compartment of the knee in the guinea pig (a model system which is emerging as the prime vehicle for study of both the natural history of OA and the potential effectiveness of new therapies) or in the dog model involving cruciate ligament transection[3]. Clinical trials involving diacetylrhein are well under way in Europe, and it is likely that metalloproteinase inhibitors and bisphosphonates will enter trial in the near future.

Current concepts

Elsewhere in this book, detailed descriptions of the types, sites, prevalence, genetics, and predisposing factors of OA will be found, as will the tissues and matrix macromolecules involved. These will not be dealt with in any detail here. However, for an overview of OA which discusses the process of drug discovery, a few salient points need to be made. Some researchers refer to 'osteoarthritic diseases' to indicate that OA is not all the same problem[4], though the scientist with the responsibility for finding a disease-modifying drug for OA hopes for a single pathway leading to failure at all sites and in all circumstances. Also, the joint must be viewed as an organ with all the constituent tissues subserving the need for biomechanical stability[5]; change within one tissue, for example, ligament or bone, could alter the mechanical environment such that cartilage eventually fails, or vice versa. Adaptation and joint remodeling have been considered as the basis of OA[6] since 1962. Finally, the eminent dermatologist, Sam Schuster, pointed out to the Heberden Society in Newcastle, England in 1981, that for any medical scientific problem 'the facts will not be discovered until you first guess the answer'.

So, what is the answer? Probably stability, as mechanical stability requires that all the tissues involved in articulation should be in balance — in terms of tissue mass, composition, and strength — to resist the forces transmitted through them. An example of such a balance comes from elegant studies by Simon Rodbard, not in osteoarthrology, but from the control of vascular wall calibre and strength[7,8]: such principles apply equally to other connective tissues. Rodbard's thesis is that mesenchymal cells will respond to mechanical stress by producing materials (for example, elastin, collagen, proteoglycan) to counter such stress, or will remove these if the stress is diminished; this is under local control, but influenced by hormonal and other systemic factors. He noted that there is little elastin in arteries within bone fossae as there is no stretching at such sites with each pulse of blood and, therefore, no need for the recoil properties of elastin. Placement of a suture in the descending aorta of the dog increased pressure upstream and was associated with a loss of elastin upstream as the vessel wall increased in muscle and collagen to resist the pressure change, yet downstream the wall thinned as seen in post-stenotic dilatation. The suture involved an area of a few hundred microns, but the connective tissues were remodeled over several centimeters; this is relevant to the remodeling of the knee joint seen during the development of spontaneous OA in animals (p. 433). The most poignant observation of Rodbard in relation to OA, however, was the reaction to a steel wire placed through the intimal layers of the descending aorta[8]; here, the intimal mesenchymal cells were being compressed against a solid material, so they changed phenotype to chondrocytes and secreted cartilage around the wire to counter the compressive stress. This emphasizes the local nature of the control of tissue structure, and the facility to put down any component structure, anywhere in the body, depending on the mechanics.

Considering the joint as an organ, consisting of an outer capsule, a variety of stabilizing ligaments, subchondral bone, synovium, menisci, calcified and articular hyaline cartilage, all of which contribute to mechanical stability, any change within any component tissue will influence the synthetic and or degradative activity of cells in the other tissues as they strive to maintain mechanical stability. Surgical models of OA, or those involving intra-articular injection of degradative enzymes, destabilize the joint through the gross disruption of one or a number of tissues; these have been used in the search for drugs, but are more relevant to the sports injuries in man which lead to OA, for example, cruciate ligament rupture and meniscal tears. Recent descriptions of the development of spontaneous OA in the knees of mice[9,10], guinea pigs[11,12], and both

Rhesus and Cynomolgus macaques[13,14], present the drug hunter with potentially accurate model systems to determine if novel molecules can slow down the degenerative process of OA. No model can perfectly mimic the human situation, however, so the drug discovery process is essentially an expensive gamble that what can be achieved in animals will translate to the OA diseases of man. When the Battle of Britain was over during the Second World War, Winston Churchill commented, 'we are at the end of the beginning' — so it is with modeling of OA. A thorough understanding of the way spontaneous OA of animals initiates, of what the macromolecular changes comprise, and how the balance of synthetic and degradative processes influence disease progression will provide the strategies for discovery of therapeutic measures to control OA: this is the real advantage of using animal models, as it is difficult to obtain sequential human diseased tissue. What has been achieved, to date, with animal models of OA, in the search for DMOADs, will now be discussed.

Spontaneous OA in animals

Natural OA in animal species represents a model system for idiopathic human disease and should be considered separately from those induced models of arthritis involving surgical manipulation or enzymatic destruction of component structures. Comprehensive descriptions of medial compartment knee OA have been presented for mouse strains, the Dunkin Hartley guinea pig, and Rhesus and Cynomolgus macaque monkeys[9-14]. Recently, spontaneous OA in the knee of Wistar and Fischer 344 strains of rat has been described[15]. Apart from the mouse, very few reports of drug activity have been made, and the value of the larger species remains for the future — their importance lies in their similarities with idiopathic, human medial compartment knee OA, and the likelihood that mechanisms of initiation and progression will be discovered which are more relevant to human disease. This will enable drug discovery to proceed rationally and remove inaccurate guesswork from mechanistic approaches.

Spontaneous OA in mice

Nearly all inbred strains of mice develop some degree of OA, although the incidence, severity, and localization of the articular lesion varies between strains. The highest incidence and most severe form of the disease occurs in mice of the STR strains[16], STR / ORT and STR / IN. There have been several studies of these mice over the years but these have been mainly subjective and descriptive, and very few drug studies have been reported. It is generally agreed that the initial cartilage lesion is in the medial tibial plateau, but there is debate as to whether patella displacement precedes and, thus, causes cartilage degeneration. Radiographic assessment of the lesions in the knee[9] has demonstrated that male mice of the STR /ORT strain get more severe disease, and a higher incidence of it, than female mice. The conclusions reached by Evans *et al.*[9] and Collins *et al.*[10] were that patella displacement was not the predisposing factor, since by eleven months of age all mice had arthritis but not all had patella displacement.

Secondly, and particularly in male mice, they observed chondro-osseous metaplasia in the tendinous structures around the joint and the major ligament entheses, such as the patella ligament insertions. These had occurred by three months of age, preceding articular changes by at least a month, leading the authors to propose that this was the primary event in the development of OA in these strains of mice. Subsequently, as others had previously described[17,18], articular lesions appeared in the medial tibial plateau, initially as superficial fibrillation but eventually progressing to complete cartilage erosion with accompanying osteophyte formation. Interestingly, they noted that subchondral bone sclerosis was only seen in late disease and, in this respect, OA in mice differs from that seen in the knees of guinea pigs and macaques where subchondral bone changes, particularly sclerosis, precede the development of cartilage degeneration. Whether this disease can be considered a model of primary or idiopathic OA, since it is associated with early calcification of ligaments and tendons, was questioned by the authors[10]: nonetheless, it does have striking similarities with human knee OA. It also illustrates that change in one tissue or tissues, for example, calcification of ligaments and tendons, will lead to changes in others — in this case, the development of the cartilage degeneration and osteophyte formation typical of OA. Calcification of key ligaments will alter the mechanical stresses within the joint structures, and the ensuing tissue alterations can be viewed as an attempt, and failure, to maintain mechanical stability.

The advantage of mice for the search for DMOADs is their size, despite the fact that treatment will be needed for several months. For the medicinal chemist, this means less compound to prepare in comparison with that required for guinea pig and macaque models; but for the biochemist wishing to explore mechanisms, the small amount of cartilage available is a disadvantage. Radiographic analysis of disease development and progression has been used for drug evaluation[19] and has the advantage of being non-invasive, but the future may well lie with modern molecular biology techniques — such as differential display of genes that are activated or repressed during disease development — since these will enable objective assessment of disease inhibition over shorter time spans than are currently needed for the assessment of drug activity using histopathological evaluation. Of the drug studies reported to date, there are conflicting results with nonsteroidal antiinflammatory drugs (NSAIDS) and corticosteroids. Pataki *et al.*[20] found that the NSAIDS, indomethacin and diclofenac, were without effect in the OA that develops in C57BL mice. Previously, Maier and Wilhelmi had claimed that diclofenac had inhibited, and indomethacin exacerbated, mouse OA[21]. In relation to steroids, the experiments of Pataki *et al.*[20] showed a non-significant trend towards disease inhibition, whereas the earlier work of Silberberg and Silberberg[22] had demonstrated a protective effect of advenocorticotrophic hormone (ACTH). The problem with the interpretation of conflicting results is that differing dose levels and regimens, as well as differing strains of mice, are used by research groups. It has to be recognized that OA has not had as much attention as rheumatoid arthritis in terms of drug discovery, hence the reported drug studies are essentially anecdotal, and a consensus cannot be reached: this does not detract from the value of the model. It is quite simply 'early days' and we must await evaluation of agents such as diacetylrhein, bisphosphonates, matrixmetalloprotein (MMP) inhibitors, and others to determine whether this model will predict useful activity in the human disease.

Spontaneous OA in the guinea pig

The original observation of OA in the guinea pig was made by Silverstein and Sokoloff in 1958[23], but the model has come to prominence following the studies of Bendele *et al.*[11,12] and Meacock *et al.*[24] during the late 1980s. These fully described the natural history of the disease and male to female prevalence. Attention was focused initially on the cartilage changes, reflecting the general view that these are the initiating events. It is now apparent that all male guinea pigs of the Dunkin Hartley strain begin to show cartilage degeneration after three months of age[11,24]. The time that the lesion initiates is variable from animal to animal, but all will be involved by five months of age. Females show similar changes but these initiate around six months of age, essentially mirroring the development of OA seen in males, though the final outcome is not so severe as in the males. Initially, there is loss of proteoglycan and cell death in the center of the medial tibial plateau that is not covered by the meniscus. Loss of proteoglycan and cell death then progress to cover larger areas of the tibial plateau, fibrillation is significant by six months of

age, together with osteophyte formation, and the medial meniscus and femoral condyle are involved by nine months of age (Fig. 11.1). At one year of age, there can be complete loss of cartilage with exposure of bone in the medial femoral condyle and tibial plateau. Body weight can increase disease severity, and diet restriction, to keep the animals less than 900 gms, can essentially halve the rate of progression.

In studies involving magnetic resonance imaging (MRI) to follow progression non-invasively[25], it was observed that a change within the subchondral bone

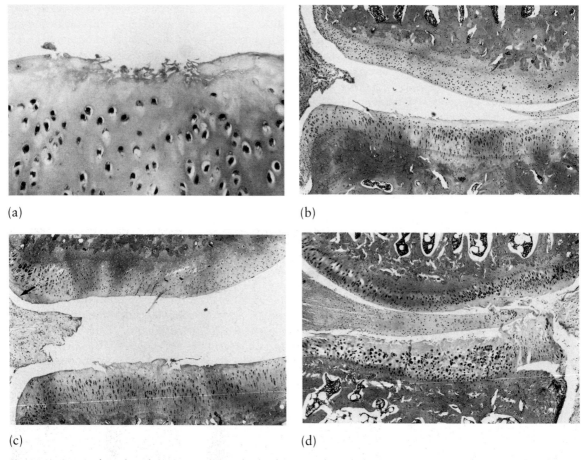

(a)   (b)

(c)   (d)

Fig. 11.1 Stages of cartilage degeneration during the development of OA in the guinea pig knee. (a) Twelve-week-old guinea pig. A minimal focal lesion on the surface of the medial tibial plateau. Note the loss of surface chondrocytes and cartilage matrix; this is the first sign of cartilage degeneration. (Hematoxylin and eosin (H & E) ×133.) (b) Twenty-one-week-old guinea pig. An extensive surface lesion on the medial tibial plateau with horizontal fibrillation, almost complete loss of surface chondrocytes, and increased hematoxylin staining of the lower cells. The femoral condyle is not involved at this stage. (H & E ×21.) (c) Thirty-week-old guinea pig. An extensive surface lesion on the medial tibial plateau with penetration to the middle zone of cells in the center. Note the early surface lesion on the medial femoral condyle near the cruciate junction (arrow). (H & E ×21.) (d) Thirty-seven-week-old guinea pig. Extensive lesions on the medial tibial plateau, on the medial femoral condyl, and on the tip of the intervening meniscus. Note the multiple clone formation and horizontal cleft at the tidemark in the medial tibial plateau, and the increased hematoxylin staining of the lower chondrocytes, adjacent to the lesions. (H & E ×17.)

was present at least as early as eight weeks of age, prior to any obvious change in the articular cartilage. X-radiography of thick, 1.5 mm slices of undecalcified knee in plastic revealed that, even prior to four weeks of age, considerable remodeling of the subchondral trabeculae in the tibial and femoral compartments was underway, particularly at the cruciate ligament insertion sites. These are illustrated in Fig. 11.2 where it can also be seen that the medial subchondral plate increases in thickness to compensate for the loss of trabeculae and to maintain mechanical stability. This loss of trabecular bone was associated with high levels of cathepsin B activity[26]. As with OA in mice, cartilage degeneration in the guinea pig is associated with, and preceded by, change in another tissue — in this case subchondral bone — though there may also be change within the cruciate ligaments that precipitates the bone remodeling. This provides a further illustration of Rodbard's thesis that a structure will alter if the mechanics change. Loss of trabecular bone initiates a series of structural changes that essentially place the cartilage between a 'rock and a hard place', leading to eventual failure. It is not possible, at present, to rule out that a change in articular cartilage precipitates the subchondral bone remodeling and that this model of OA is driven by such cartilage change. Osborne *et al.*[27]

have demonstrated that the ratio of 6-sulphated chondroitin to the 4-sulphated isomer on the glycosaminoglycan chains of cartilage proteoglycan is changing dramatically by eight weeks of age, but the appearance of the 3-B-3 minus mimitope, typical of the OA proteoglycan phenotype, is not present before nine weeks of age[28]. Debate on what changes first, hence initiating OA, may be considered academic but is, in fact, important when defining strategies for rational treatment of the disease. If bone change initiates and promulgates OA, then bone may be a worthwhile target for intervention. Progression to failure of the knee joint in human OA may be predicted by a positive scintigraph[29], using a technetium-labeled bone seeking bisphosphonate; remodeling of bone in late stage OA is a prerequisite for final failure.

Few drug studies have been reported in the literature on the model of OA in the guinea pig. Bendele *et al.* have presented results with diacetylrhein[1], an anthroquinone, demonstrating that this molecule can essentially reduce the rate of progression by at least 50 per cent when administered from three months of age to twelve or fifteen months. All aspects of the disease were inhibited — loss of cartilage from the tibial and femoral compartment, osteophyte formation, and the synovial hyperplasia which appears in the latter stages

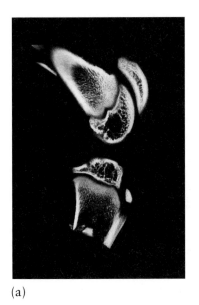
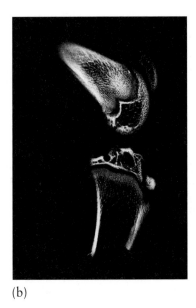
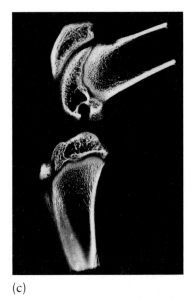

(a)   (b)   (c)

Fig. 11.2   X-radiography of 1 mm slices of the guinea pig knee, demonstrating bone remodeling prior to histological evidence of cartilage degeneration. Sagittal sections from the middle of the joint taken in the region of the cruciate ligament insertions (×1.9). (a), (b), and (c), respectively, demonstrate the loss of trabecular bone, cyst formation, and thickening of the subchondral plate at four, seven, and ten weeks of age. Remodeling of the subchondral bone occurs in both medial compartments of the knee and appears to initiate subjacent to the cruciate ligament insertion sites.

of the disease after nine months. Treatment from three months to seven months did not produce a significant reduction of disease progression, perhaps indicating that the drug is more effective against the final cartilage degeneration. This drug is currently in clinical trial in Europe and, if it is shown to influence human disease progression, it will validate the model in the guinea pig as a suitable vehicle for DMOAD discovery. Following from these studies on diacetylrhein, Carney *et al.*[30] investigated this drug and a series of analogues for an influence on cartilage proteoglycan metabolism. Sulphate incorporation into the 6 and 4 isomers of chondroitin sulphate was measured in both the tibial plateau and femoral condyle of young guinea pigs. Several of the compounds appeared to increase the half-life of the 4-sulphated isomer, with a lesser effect on the 6-isomer, and the effects were more marked with femoral proteoglycan. How this relates to the inhibition of OA seen with such compounds in the guinea pig is unclear, but this system may provide a more rapid screen for potential active compounds.

Initial reports are appearing on the effect of an MMP inhibitor, though a full paper is yet to appear. An orally active inhibitor of stromelysin, collagenase, and gelatinase from Ciba-Geigy (CGS 27023A) was fed in the diet, to guinea pigs, from six to twelve months of age; treatment was not commenced earlier so as not to interfere with bone remodeling during growth. Treatment with this MMP inhibitor produced a highly significant inhibition of the cartilage histopathology and loss of proteoglycan, and abolished the loss of chondrocytes seen as the disease progresses[31]. Similar effects of the compound were seen in the partial meniscectomy model in the rabbit[32]. Again, if the human disease can be similarly influenced by MMP inhibitors, the credentials of the model are established. Human trials of at least one such agent are about to commence. Another type of compound which deserves study in the model is the bisphosphonates, which can influence the resorption of bone by osteoclasts. Considering the involvement of bone in the pathogenesis of this model, the model in macaques, and the human counterpart, such agents are worthy of study. Experiments are in progress but have not been reported to date.

The guinea pig is proving to be a valuable model system for drug discovery and for seeking clues to the initiation and progression of human OA. Its disadvantage is the amount of compound necessary for long-term dosing — a daunting prospect for the medicinal chemist. It does, however, provide sufficient cartilage for detailed biochemical analysis and, as with the mouse, molecular biology technology may provide faster ways of discovering useful activity in compounds, as was attempted in a biochemical context by Carney *et al*[30].

Spontaneous OA in rhesus and cynomolgus macaques

OA in rhesus monkeys has been described by DeRousseau[33] and by Pritzker *et al.*[34]. However, the availability of this species for comprehensive study is limited, so the development of a similar disease pattern in the more prevalent cynomolgus species has enabled detailed study of a model of naturally occurring medial compartment knee OA in a primate species[14,35,36]. The value of this model is that it occurs in middle-aged to elderly animals which are bipedal, unlike mice and guinea pigs. Yet, there are considerable similarities between the OA initiation and progression in guinea pigs and monkeys, which resemble the human disease.

Carlson *et al.*[35] have pointed out the value of a model that develops insidiously and which simulates the human condition more closely than chemical, mechanical, and surgical manipulations, where extrapolation to the human condition should be done with caution. The earliest change they observed histologically was thickening of the subchondral plate, and this was followed by fibrillation and clefting of cartilage. This occurred initially in the medial plateau but, with severe disease, the lateral compartment became involved; a similar situation exists with involvement of the lateral compartment in guinea pig OA. The typical changes in histological appearance and X-radiography of 2 mm undecalcified sections of the joint are shown in Figs 11.3 and 11.4 respectively. The typical appearance of osteophytes is also clear from these figures. In their latest study[36], it was apparent that degeneration of cartilage did not occur until the subchondral bone had thickened to a significant degree. In fact, it had to reach 400 μm before the cartilage became involved. As with the guinea pig, the appearance of the 3-B-3 minus mimitope, seen on the OA phenotype of proteoglycans, occurred after the subchondral bone had increased in thickness[35]. It was also established that prevalence and severity of OA increased with age but these were not affected by gender or weight, providing some contrast with human OA of the knee. They concluded that thickening of the subchondral plate may be more important than the volume of epiphyseal/metaphyseal

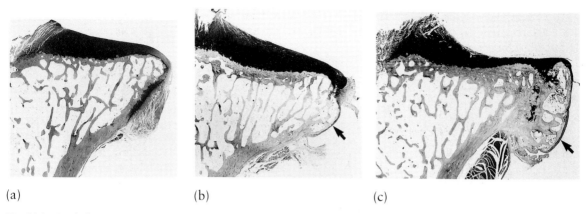

(a)   (b)   (c)

Fig. 11.3   Medial compartment OA in the knee of the Cynomolgus macaque. Low magnification photomicrographs (toluidine blue ×7) of sections of the medial tibial plateau of the same three joints as in Fig. 11.4: (a) normal, (b) moderately affected, and (c) severly affected. Thickening of the subchondral plate (arrowheads) and osteophytes (arrows) are evident in (b) and (c). There is slight fibrillation of cartilage in (b) and extensive loss of articular cartilage in (c). The average thickness of the subchondral plate in (a) is 272 μm; in (b), 750 μm; and in (c), 1120 μm.

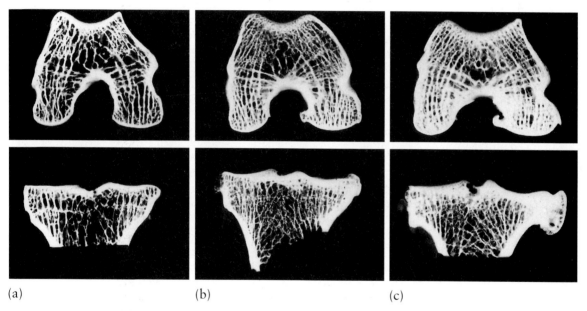

(a)   (b)   (c)

Fig. 11.4   Medial compartment OA in the knee of the Cynomolgus macaque. Microradiographs (×2.2) of one serial section of femur (top) and tibia (bottom) from a normal (a), moderately affected (b), and severely affected (c), knee joint. Note the extensive subchondral bone thickening and osteophyte formation as the disease progresses. In each joint, the medial aspect is to the right and the lateral, to the left.

bone in determining the mechanical stresses in the joint and in influencing the development of articular cartilage lesions.

Cynomolgus macaque OA provides another example of change in one tissue influencing change in other structures to maintain stability, yet, ultimately, failing to do so, thereby leading to OA and joint failure. Why the subchondral bone becomes thickened is unknown but perhaps ligament changes may be precipitative; this is a speculation, however, and needs to addressed. No drug studies have been performed, to date, to address an effect against OA progression, but since this species is closer to man than rodents it would appear an appropriate vehicle for drug studies, though expensive in terms of compound required and other factors. The Food and Drug Administration (FDA) requires a primary study for potential osteoporosis drugs, and the cynomolgus macaque is the species of choice. This may be a future requirement for OA.

Surgical and other models of OA which have been used for drug studies

As mentioned previously (p.00), surgical manipulations of the joint, causing an immediate joint laxity which clearly changes the mechanical influences on the joint, should be viewed as sports or traumatic injuries which may have a different pathway to joint failure than that occurring during spontaneous, primary, or idiopathic OA. The drug hunter will be hoping, however, that the mechanisms involved in cartilage degeneration will be the same, or similar to, those operating in other OA diseases. Surgery has been most frequently performed on rabbits and dogs, with the most studied being the section of the anterior cruciate ligament of the dog, originally described by Pond and Nuki[37]. A variety of ligament and meniscal manipulations have been described in the rabbit[38], including cruciate ligament section, with and without medial and collateral ligament section, total or partial meniscectomy, and meniscal tears (bucket-handle). Partial meniscectomy and cruciate or lateral ligament sectioning have also been reported in the guinea pig[24,39]; in this species, partial meniscectomy causes osteophyte formation within two weeks and major cartilage degeneration within six, greatly accelerating the underlying spontaneous disease.

In the dog, particularly, section of the cruciate ligament leads to cartilage hypertrophy with the chondrocytes responding vigorously to the change in mechanics. The cartilage thickens within a few weeks and osteophyte formation is marked by three months after surgery, though this process begins within days of ligament section[40]. General experience is that cartilage degeneration, seen as fibrillation, loss of surface tissue, and cloning of cells, is not markedly evident for many months after surgery, unless dorsal root ganglionectomy is also performed at the same time[3]; complete loss of cartilage to bone can then be observed within eight weeks. In the natural history of the model in the dog, failure of the joint, that is, loss of cartilage to bone, can take 3–5 years. The exception to these general findings are the studies of Fernandes *et al.*[41] where major loss of cartilage was reported within a few weeks of cruciate ligament section.

Despite the cost of using this model, several drug studies have been undertaken, the advantage being that there is ample cartilage for detailed biochemical studies. Tiaprofenic acid (an NSAID) has been claimed to reduce lesion severity and reduce protease levels within cartilage[42], though evidence for real efficacy in man with this or other NSAIDs is lacking or controversial. Tenidap, an agent with classical anti-inflammatory activity and cytokine inhibitory properties, has also been demonstrated to prevent cartilage damage by this same group of investigators[41]; the extent of cartilage damage was quite severe for this model at eight weeks and further confirmation of these fascinating results is required. Careful choice of dose with corticosteroids has demonstrated an inhibitory effect when given orally or intra-articularly, preventing osteophyte formation and reducing levels of the MMP stromelysin[43,44]. Both this model[45], and the medial meniscectomy model in the rabbit[46], have been used to demonstrate the efficacy of pentosan polysulphate, an agent considered to bind and present growth factors. In fact, when administered with IGF-1, this agent considerably protected against cartilage damage, and protease levels were reduced and TIMP increased within the cartilage[47]. The value of these heparinoid agents in OA models has recently been reviewed[48]. Finally, Brandt *et al.*[3] convincingly demonstrated that doxycycline could inhibit the accelerated model in the dog when ganglionectomy is performed. This agent prevented the major loss of cartilage seen in this model and reduced the levels of MMPs within the cartilage dramatically. Whether these varied agents will turn out to be DMOADs in man remains to be established. They influence cartilage metabolism certainly, but the definitive trials in man are not completed. As Howell states in his review[48], 'at the very least, they are agents with disease modifying properties under special experimental circumstances'.

Conclusion

Judging the value of the available models in the search for drugs for OA is at the stage of 'the jury is out'. Many agents have been identified with potentially useful properties against cartilage degradation, some of which have beneficial actions in various models of OA in animals. Until the feedback from clinical trials in man is available, however, the credentials of the models remain to be clarified. In this respect, OA lags a long way behind RA, where clinical feedback has established the value, or not, of the inflammatory arthritis models. To date, most attention has centered on surgically induced models of OA, with less on spontaneous disease. It is likely, however, that the latter will provide more relevant clues to the initiation and progression of idiopathic OA and lead to a more defined strategic approach to therapy. All this is in the future.

References

1. Bendele, A.M., Bendele, R.A., Hulman, J.F., and Swann, B.P. (1996). Effects benefiques d'un traitment la diacerheine chez des cobayes atteints d'arthrose. *Revue du Praticien*, **46**, 35–9.
2. O'Byrne, E.M., Blancuzzi, V., Singh, N.H., and Roberts, E.D., (1995). A matrix metalloproteinase inhibitor, CGS 27023A, in animal models of osteoarthritis. *Inflamm Res*, **44 (suppl 3)**, 255.
3. Yu, L.P. Jr, Smith, G.N. Jr, Brandt, K.D., Myers, S.L., O'Connor, B.L., and Brandt, D.A. (1992). Reduction of the severity of canine osteoarthritis by prophylactic treatment with oral doxycycline. *Arthritis Rheum*, **35**, 1150–9.
4. Dieppe, P.A. (1995). The classification and diagnosis of osteoarthritis. In *Osteoarthritic disorders* (ed. K.E. Kuettner and V.M. Goldberg), pp. 5–12. American Academy of Orthopedic Surgeons, Rosemont, IL.
5. Radin, E.L., Schaffler, M., Gibson, G., and Tashman, S.E. (1995). Osteoarthrosis as a result of repetitive trauma. In *Osteoarthritic disorders* (ed. K.E. Kuettner and V.M. Goldberg), pp. 197–203. American Academy of Orthopedic Surgeons, Rosemont, IL.
6. Johnson, L.C. (1962). Joint remodelling as a basis for osteoarthritis. *J Am Vet Med Assoc*, **141**, 1237–41.
7. Rodbard, S. (1970). Negative feedback mechanisms in the architecture and function of the connective and cardiovascular tissues. *Perspectives Biol Med*, **13**, 507–27.
8. Rodbard, S. (1974). Biophysical factors in vascular structure and caliber. In *Athersclerosis III* (ed. G. Schettlar and A. Weizel), pp. 46–63. Springer-Verlag, Berlin,
9. Evans, R.G., Collins, C., Miller, P., Ponsford, P.M., and Elson, C.J. (1994). Radiological scoring of osteoarthritis progression in STR/ORT mice. *Osteoarthritis Cart*, **2**, 103–9.
10. Collins, C., Evans, R.G., Ponsford, F., Miller, P., and Elson, C.J. (1994). Chondro-osseous metaplasia, bone density and patella cartilage proteoglycan content in the osteoarthritis of STR/ORT mice. *Osteoarthritis Cart*, **2**, 111–18.
11. Bendele, A.M. and Hulman, J.F. (1988). Spontaneous cartilage degeneration in guinea pigs. *Arthritis Rheum*, **31**, 561–5.

12. Bendele, A.M., White, S.L., and Hulman, J.F. (1989). Osteoarthritis in guinea pigs: histopathologic and scanning electron microscopic features. *Lab An Sci*, **39**, 115–21.
13. Pritzker, K.P.H., Chateauvert, J., Grynpas, M.D., Renlund, R.C., Turnquist, J., and Kessler, M.J. (1989). Rhesus macaques as an experimental model for degenerative arthritis. *P R Health Sci J*, **8**, 99–102.
14. Carlson, C.S., Loeser, R.F., Jayo, M.J., Weaver, D.S., Adams, M.R., and Jerome, C.P. (1994). Osteoarthritis in Cynomolgus macaques: a primate model on naturally occurring disease. *J Orth Res*, **12**, 331–9.
15. Smale, G., Bendele, A.M., and Horton, W.E. (1995). Comparison of age-associated degeneration of articular cartilage in Wistar and Fischer 344 rats. *Lab An Sci*, **45**, 191–4.
16. Sokoloff, L. (1956). Natural history of degenerative joint disease in small laboratory animals. 1. Pathological anatomy of degenerative joint disease in mice. *Arch Pathol*, **62**, 118–28.
17. Walton, M. (1977). Studies of degenerative joint disease in the mouse knee joint: histological observations. *J Pathol*, **123**, 109–22.
18. Schunke, M., Tillman, B., Bruck, M., and Muller-Ruchholtz, W. (1988). Morphologic characteristics of developing osteoarthrotic lesions in the knee cartilage of STR/IN mice. *Arthritis Rheum*, **31**, 898–905.
19. Pataki, A., Reife, R., Witzemann, E., Graf, H.P., and Schweizer, A. (1990). Quantitative radiographic diagnosis of osteoarthritis of the knee joint in the C57BL mouse. *Agents Actions*, **29**, 201–9.
20. Pataki, A., Graf, H.P., and Witzemann, E. (1990). Spontaneous osteoarthritis of the knee joint in C57BL mice receiving chronic oraltreatment with NSAIDs or prednisolone. *Agents Actions*, **29**, 210–17.
21. Maier, R. and Wilhelmi, G. (1987). Osteoarthrosis-like disease in mice: effects of anti-arthrotic and antirheumatic agents. In *Studies in osteoarthrosis, pathogenesis, intervention, assessment* (ed. D.J. Lott, M.K. Jasani, G.F.B. Birdwood), pp. 75–83. John Wiley and Sons, Chichester.
22. Silberberg, M. and Silberberg, R. (1955). Degenerative joint disease of mice as modified by adrenocorticotrophic hormone (ACTH). *Exp Med Surg*, **13**, 279–85.
23. Silverstein, E. and Sokoloff, L. (1958). Natural history of degenerative joint disease in small laboratory animals. 5. Osteoarthritis in guinea pigs. *Arthritis Rheum*, **1**, 82–6.
24. Meacock, S.C.R., Bodmer, J.L., and Billingham, M.E.J. (1990). Experimental osteoarthritis in guinea pigs. *J Exp Path*, **71**, 279–93.
25. Watson, P.J., Carpenter, T.A., Hall, L.D., and Tyler, J.A. (1994). Spontaneous joint degeneration in the guinea pig studied by magnetic resonance imaging. *Brit J Rheum*, **33 (suppl 1)**, 105.
26. Meijers, M.H.M., Bunning, R.A.D., Russell, R.G.G., and Billingham, M.E.J. (1994). Evidence for cathepsin B involvement in subchondral bone changes during early natural osteoarthritis in the guinea pig. *Brit J Rheum*, **33 (suppl 1)**, 90.

27. Osborne, D.J., Woodhouse, S., Meacock, S.C.R. (1994). Early changes in the sulfation of chondroitin in guinea-pig articular cartilage, a possible predictor of osteoarthritis. *Osteoarthritis Cart*, **2**, 215–23.

28. Caterson, B., Slater, R.R., Blankenship-Paris, T., Carney, S.L., Bendele, A.M., Chandrasekar, S. (1996). Natural osteoarthritis in guinea pigs. 1: expression of 3-B-3(–) mimotope in cartilage proteoglycans as a biochemical marker for the development of osteoarthritis. *Arthritis Rheum*, In revision.

29. Dieppe, P.A., Cushnaghan, J., Young, P., and Kirwan, J.R. (1993). Prediction of the progression of joint space narrowing in osteoarthritis of the knee by bone scintigraphy. *Ann Rheum Dis*, **52**, 557–63.

30. Carney, S.L., Hicks, C.A., Tree, B., Broadmore, R.J: (1995). An *in vivo* investigation of the effect of anthroquinones on the turnover of aggrecans in spontaneous osteoarthritis in the guinea pig. *Inflamm Res*, **44**, 182–6.

31. O'Byrne, E.M., Blancuzzi, V., Singh, N.H., and Roberts, E.D. (1996). Chondroprotective activity of a matrix metalloproteinase inhibitor in spontaneous osteoarthritis in guinea pigs. *Osteoarthritis Cart*, (submitted).

32. O'Byrne, E.M., Parker, D.T., Roberts, E.D., Goldberg, R.L., MacPherson, L.J., Blancuzzi, V., *et al.* (1995). Oral administration of a matrix metalloproteinase inhibitor, CGS 27023A, protects the cartilage proteoglycan matrix in a partial meniscectomy model of osteoarthritis in rabbits. *Inflamm Res*, **44 (suppl 2)**, S117–S118.

33. DeRousseau, C.J. (1985). Aging in the musculoskeletal system of rhesus monkeys. II. Degenerative joint disease. *Am J Phys Anthropol*, **67**, 177–84.

34. Kessler, M.J., Turnquist, J.E., Pritzker, K.P.H., and London, W.T. (1986). Reduction of passive extension and radiographic evidence of degenerative knee joint disease in cage-raised and free-ranging aged rhesus monkeys (Maccaca mulatta). *J Med Primatol*, **15**, 1–9.

35. Carlson, C.S., Loeser, R.F., Johnstone, B., Tulli, H.M., Dodson, D.B., and Caterson, B. (1995). Osteoarthritis in Cynomolgus macaques. II. Detection of modulated proteoglycan epitopes in cartilage and synovial fluid. *J Orth Res*, **13**, 399–409.

36. Carlson, C.S., Loeser, R.F., Purser, C.B., Gardin, J.F., and Jerome, C.P. (1996). Osteoarthritis in Cynomolgus macaques. III. Effects of age, gender, and subchondral bone thickness on the severity of disease. *J Bone Min Res*, **11**, 1209–17.

37. Pond, M.J. and Nuki, G. (1973). Experimentally-induced osteoarthritis in the dog. *Ann Rheum Dis*, **32**, 387–8.

38. Moskowitz, R.W. (1992). Experimental models of osteoarthritis. In *Osteoarthritis: diagnosis and medical/surgical management* (ed. R.W. Moskowitz, D.S. Howell and V.M. Goldberg) pp. 213–32. W.B. Saunders, Philadelphia, PA.

39. Bendele, A.M. and White, S.L. (1987). Early histopathologic and ultrastructural alterations in femorotibial joints of partial medial meniscectomised guinea pigs. *Vet Pathol*, **24**, 436–43.

40. Gilbertson, E.M.M. (1975). Development of periarticular osteophytes in experimentally induced osteoarthritis in the dog. *Ann Rheum Dis*, **34**, 12–25.

41. Fernandes, J.C., MartelPelletier, J., Otterness, I.G., Lopez Anaya, A., Mineau, F., Tardif, G., *et al.* (1995). Effects of Tenidap on canine experimental osteoarthritis. I. Morphologic and metalloprotease analysis. *Arthritis Rheum*, **38**, 1290–303.

42. Pelletier, J.P. and MartelPelletier, J. (1991). *In vivo* protective effects of prophylactic treatment with tiaprofenic acid or intraarticular corticosteroids on osteoarthritic lesions in the experimental dog model. *J Rheumatol*, **27 (suppl)**, 127–30.

43. Pelletier, J.P. and MartelPelletier, J. (1989). Protective effects of corticosteroids on cartilage lesions and osteophyte formation in the Pond-Nuki dog model of osteoarthritis. *Arthritis Rheum*, **32**, 181–93.

44. Pelletier, J.P., Mineau, F., and Raynauld, J.P. (1994). Intraarticular injections with methyl-prednisolone acetate reduce osteoarthritic lesions in parallel with chondrocyte stromelysin synthesis in experimental osteoarthritis. *Arthritis Rheum*, **37**, 414–23.

45. Altman, R.D., Dean, D.D., Muniz, O.E., and Howell, D.S. (1989). Therapeutic treatment of canine osteoarthritis with glycosaminoglycan polysulfuric acid ester. *Arthritis Rheum*, **32**, 1300–7.

46. Howell, D.S., Carreno, M.R., Pelletier, J.P., and Muniz, O.E. (1986). Articular cartilage breakdown in a lapine model of osteoarthritis: action of glycosaminoglycan polysulfate ester (GAGPS) on proteoglycan degrading enzyme activity, hexuronate and cell counts. *Clin Orthop*, **21**, 69–76.

47. Rogachevsky, R.A., Dean, D.D., Howell, D.S., and Altman, R.D. (1994). Treatment of canine osteoarthritis with insulin-like growth factor (IGF1) and sodium pentosan polysulfate. *Ann N Y Acad Sci*, **732**, 392–4.

48. Howell, D.S., Altman, R.D., Pelletier, J.P., MartelPelletier, J., and Dean, D.D. (1995). Disease modifying antirheumatic drugs: current status of their application in animal models of osteoarthritis. In *Osteoarthritic disorders* (ed. K.E. Kuettner and V.M. Goldberg), pp. 365–77. American Academy of Orthopedic Surgeons, Rosemont, IL.

11.4 The role of animal models in the discovery of novel disease-modifying osteoarthritis drugs (DMOADs)

Niall S. Doherty, R.J. Griffiths, and E.R. Pettipher

The currently available therapy for osteoarthritis (OA) is grossly inadequate. Palliative treatment with simple analgesics or nonsteroidal anti-inflammatory drugs (NSAIDs, prostaglandin synthesis inhibitors) provides some pain control, although NSAIDs may exacerbate joint damage and have significant gastrointestinal side effects (see Chapter 9.3). Disease-modifying osteoarthritis drugs for humans (DMOADs, as defined by Lequesne *et al.*) are, as yet, only a theoretical possibility rather than a proven reality[1] and the prospect facing the patient with OA is many years of pain and increasing disability. The scale of the problem in developed countries is growing as their population ages: an epidemic of OA can be anticipated as the 'baby boomers' reach their sixties, the age at which the disease incidence increases dramatically[2,3]. These factors have led, in recent years, to a great increase in research into OA and greater efforts to discover new therapeutic agents which will have significant disease-modifying activity and slow or stop the progressive damage to joint structures that leads to irreversible loss of function. Analgesics with greater efficacy and reduced adverse effects would also be of great benefit to patients with OA, but the present discussion will focus on disease-modifying drugs.

Animal models have long played an important role in the search for new therapeutic agents. The traditional mode in which they have been employed is to require that, before a compound is tested in man, it must exhibit 'therapeutic' activity in an animal model which resembles as closely as possible the targeted human disease. In this context, 'therapeutic efficacy' means that the compound shows efficacy against parameters similar to those that would be used in man, for example, joint swelling, radiographic changes, pain. In situations where activity in animal models of arthritis provides the sole justification for testing a compound in man (Fig. 11.5), it is essential that the models mimic the human disease as closely as possible because this

determines the ability of the model to predict therapeutic efficacy in humans. Over the years, this approach has led to the marketing of many drugs to treat arthritis (for example, NSAIDs) but, unfortunately, none of these agents has been proven to have a significant impact on the pathology of the disease in humans. This suggests that either the choice of animal models has been inappropriate or that fundamental differences exist between animals and humans which make true modeling of human arthritis impossible. Rather than initiate an endless search to find the perfect model of OA which faithfully predicts efficacy in human OA for all classes of compounds, we suggest that this paradigm of the drug discovery process be replaced by mechanism-based drug discovery. In this approach to drug discovery, *in vitro* screens are used to optimize the activity of compounds designed to interact with a molecular target believed to be important in the human disease (Fig. 11.5). This evolution in the drug discovery process requires reassessment of the role of animal models. The following discussion focuses on the issues concerning animal models of OA in this changing environment.

This chapter reviews the role of animal models in the discovery of DMOADs, highlights some of the limitations in the way they have been used in the past, and argues that the most effective method of selecting compounds for clinical development involves utilizing animal models to assess the pharmacodynamic properties of mechanism-based compounds. This paradigm of drug discovery has the potential to greatly enhance the value of clinical trials: in addition to assessing the clinical potential of the compound under investigation, the trial also offers the possibility of examining the underlying molecular mechanisms of OA. In this situation, even a negative result has considerable value. We also discuss a valuable role that animal models can play in the drug discovery process — identification of potential mechanisms of disease and potential sites of drug intervention. This application of animal models highlights

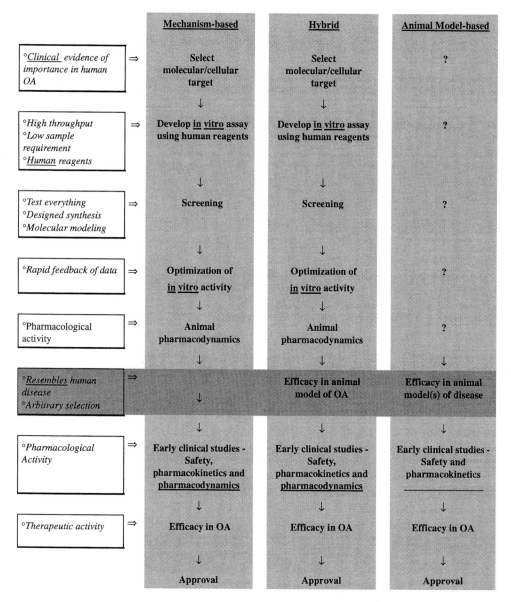

Fig. 11.5 Drug discovery paradigms. The mechanism-based paradigm for drug discovery involves: identification of a specific target believed to be important in the human disease; selection of compounds which have the appropriate *in vitro* properties against this target in assays utilizing the appropriate human reagents (e.g. enzymes, receptors, cells); ensuring that the compounds have the necessary pharmacodynamic properties (ability to deliver effective levels of drug to the target tissue / organ); and proceeding to evaluation of therapeutic efficacy in humans without requiring demonstration of 'therapeutic' efficacy in an animal model which is claimed to resemble the human disease. Animal model-based paradigms rely primarily on 'therapeutic' activity in an animal model of the human disease to justify evaluating compounds in man. The hybrid process resembles mechanism-based drug discovery but includes a requirement for demonstration of 'therapeutic' efficacy in animals, as a confidence-building measure, before proceeding to clinical trials in humans.

the need for close interaction between preclinical and clinical science to assess the relevance to human disease of studies of pathogenic mechanisms in experimental animals.

Animal models of human OA

A large number of animal models of OA have been described in the literature (Table 11.2), using different species, different mechanisms of induction of disease, and different end points; several comprehensive reviews have been published[4-10]. While we propose that inhibition of experimental pathology in animal models should not be a decision point for drug development, animal models can nonetheless supply important pharmacodynamic information for mechanism-based drugs. For example, an animal model in which the targeted enzyme or mediator is located at a site similar to that in the OA joint (for example, proteases secreted by chondrocytes in articular cartilage) may be useful in showing that a sufficient concentration of the drug has been achieved in the joint to penetrate cartilage and hit its target. When a model of OA is used in this way, inhibition of the targeted enzyme or mediator should be the experimental end point, not effects on experimental pathology. The following discussion, and Table 11.2, briefly survey some of the animal models of OA which may be used with pharmacodynamic end points but which have more frequently been used in attempts to demonstrate therapeutic efficacy.

The large number of models illustrates the fact that none of them is entirely satisfactory. The heterogeneity of the models does, however, reflect the heterogeneity of the disease in man. OA has been described as 'that ill-defined mass of joint damage which cannot be blamed on a specific disease such as gout or rheumatoid arthritis'[53]. Despite being lumped together under the heading OA, patients can be divided into different categories based on differences in etiology, pathology, and demographics[53]. Therefore, a given animal model may bear a closer resemblance to one particular subset of OA patients than to others. Animal models of OA can be produced by selecting animals in which the disease occurs spontaneously or by inducing the disease by some experimental manipulation of the animal. Since the initiating factors vary from model to model, it is likely that the underlying biochemical events also vary considerably. The so-called 'spontaneous models' may be more accurately described as models of unknown origin and there is no guarantee that the mechanisms involved are any more relevant to human OA than those in the various contrived models.

Models in which OA is deliberately induced are usually much more convenient operationally because the time of initiation is known, reproducibility is greater, and progression more rapid. However, these features can also make them very different from human OA and could potentially reduce their value in the evaluation of DMOADs. In a variety of models, OA is induced by physical methods. For example, knee instability induced by transection of the anterior cruciate ligament leads to altered load distribution, and the resulting unsuccessful biochemical attempts to compensate result in cartilage hypertrophy and osteophyte formation, followed by cartilage loss and a pattern of joint damage that is typical of OA[54]. Other methods of inducing instability which lead to, or exacerbate, joint damage include meniscectomy, myectomy, and denervation. Direct physical injury to cartilage, for example, contusion induced by blunt trauma, also induces a compensatory process which leads to an OA-like condition. Immobilization of joints perturbs physiological and biochemical processes and leads to loss of cartilage matrix.

OA-like conditions can also be induced by chemically perturbing the joint with intra-articular injections of degradative enzymes, metabolic poisons, growth factors, or proinflammatory stimuli. Even hypertonic saline can induce pathologic features of OA when injected into joints (Table 11.2).

Pitfalls associated with the use of animal models in the discovery of DMOADs

The etiology of OA is poorly understood, so it is not possible to measure how well any given model, although it may display some features of OA in humans, really mimics the human disease. This makes it impossible to determine how well therapeutic activity, in a particular animal model, predicts therapeutic activity in man. In particular, the importance of inflammation in OA is, at best, uncertain[55]. Therefore, use of models in which joint symptoms and damage are mediated by an inflammatory response in the joint could give false predictions of efficacy. Similarly, there is considerable ongoing debate concerning the importance of other etiologic factors (systemic increases in bone density, ligamentous laxity, inherited defects in collagen structure) which make it impossible to claim that any given animal model is a valid mimic of *all* aspects of human OA.

Major differences exist among species with respect to the relative contribution of different mediators, receptors, or enzymes to joint pathology. Such differences could lead to inappropriate extrapolation to humans of the therapeutic activity seen in animal models. One situation where species differences lead to an overestimation of human efficacy is the use of rodent models of arthritis in which NSAIDs have profound inhibitory activity on the disease process (including radiographic

Table 11.2   Examples of animals models of OA reported in the literature

Species/strain	Model	Inducing agent	Reference
Guinea pig, Hartley		Age obesity	11,12
Mouse, STR / ORT		Unidentified genetic predisposition	13–15
Mouse, C57 black	Spontaneous OA	Unidentified genetic predisposition	16–19
Mouse		Type II collagen mutation	20
Mouse		Type IX collagen mutation	21
Dog		Hip dysplasia	22
Primate		Unidentified genetic predisposition	23–25
Chicken		i.a. Iodoacetate	26
Rabbit		i.a. Papain	22
Guinea pig		i.a. Papain	27–29
Dog	Chemically induced	i.a. Papain	30
Guinea pig		i.a. Papain	31
Mouse		i.a. Papain	32
Mouse		i.a. Collagenase	32
Mouse		i.a. TGF-β	33
Rabbit		i.a. Hypertonic saline	34
Dog		Resection of ACL	35,36
Rabbit		Resection of ACL	37,38
Sheep		Meniscectomy	39
Rabbit		Meniscectomy	40–42
Guinea pig	Mechanically/Surgically	Meniscectomy	11
Guinea pig	induced	Myectomy	43–45
Rabbit		Patellar contusion	46,47
Rabbit		Immobilization	48,49
Dog		Immobilization	50,51
Dog		Denervation	52

i.a. = intra-articular; ACL = anterior cruciate ligament

changes) at doses which inhibit the formation of prostaglandins[56,57]. Unfortunately for RA and OA patients, however, prostaglandins do not play the same fundamental role in the disease pathology of human arthritis as they do in rodents, and the clinical use of NSAIDs is consequently limited to the partial relief of joint pain and swelling[58].

Underestimation of the therapeutic potential of novel agents on the basis of animal data could, on the other hand, lead researchers to abandon potentially useful agents. The slow-acting antirheumatic agents (gold, penicillamine, chloroquine, sulphasalazine) are effective in the treatment of RA, yet do not display efficacy in the animal models which have been routinely utilized in screening for antirheumatic drugs[59]. Because these drugs were discovered by serendipity, and their mechanisms of action are unknown, this salutary example clearly suggests that use of animal models of disease in drug screening could lead to the abandonment of novel mechanism-based agents with potential utility in the treatment of human arthritis.

One species difference is particularly appropriate in a discussion of OA: it has been assumed that interstitial collagenase (collagenase-1, MMP-1) is likely to make an important contribution to cartilage collagen damage in OA, and inhibitors of this enzyme are frequently evaluated in rodent models[60]. To date, however, a rodent homologue of collagenase-1 has not been identified and it seems likely that none exists[61]. Fortuitously, most matrix metalloprotease (MMP) inhibitors developed to date do not have great selectivity[62] and would be expected to inhibit the collagenase likely to be involved in cartilage collagen damage in rodents — now known to be collagenase-3 (MMP-13). Furthermore, a human form of collagenase-3 has been identified[63], occurs in human OA cartilage[64], and may play an important role in human OA[65]. The tissue distribution of collagenase-3 in rodents differs considerably from that in humans: human collagenase-3 is largely restricted to osteoarthritic cartilage, whereas in rodents collagenase-3 is widely expressed[64,65]. Therefore, inhibitors of collagenase-3 which do not inhibit collagenase-1 are particularly attractive as potential DMOADs: they should protect cartilage collagen but would not be expected to produce adverse effects in other connective tissues where only collagenase-1 is expressed. Given the broad tissue distribution of collagenase-3 in rodents, the use of rodent models to detect such an advantage could be very misleading.

Even assuming that a given mediator, receptor, or enzyme played a similar role in the pathogenesis of OA in humans and in a particular animal model, there is considerable precedent for the existence of differences in the ability of a given drug to interfere with the same molecular target in different species. For example, although leukotriene B_4 has similar chemotactic potency for human, mouse, and rabbit neutrophils, some antagonists show up to 1000-fold differences in potency in some of these species (Showell, personal communication; Sutherland *et al.*, presented at the Sixth International Conference of the Inflammation Research Association, White Haven, PA, 1992). With a mechanism-based agent, such species-specific differences in potency can be detected, and appropriate methods developed to make *in vivo* pharmacodynamic studies possible. One technique which has been used in this situation is the evaluation of compounds against an exogenously administered human enzyme or mediator. This technique has been used in the evaluation of MMP inhibitors by determining the ability of compounds to inhibit proteoglycan release from cartilage after injection of human stromelysin into the rabbit knee joint[66]. This method has advantages over traditional models in that the reagents are of human origin and the assay is rapid.

Use of animal models to identify potential cellular or molecular targets for development of DMOADs

As outlined above, there are many situations in which results obtained from animal models of OA could be misleading in the evaluation of potential DMOADs. Nonetheless, animal models of disease clearly do have an important role to play in basic research. By examining the mechanisms underlying the development of pathology in animal models, the *potential* for particular enzymes, mediators, or receptors to play a role in

human disease can be identified. However, merely because a particular molecular mechanism is important in an animal model does not guarantee that it is similarly important in man. One of the clearest proofs of the importance of a particular disease mechanism is the demonstration of a therapeutic effect following interference with that mechanism. Therefore, development of a mechanism-based drug frequently becomes an integral part of the analysis of the pathogenic mechanisms of human disease, and validation (or not) of the molecular target comes only after this long and costly experiment has reached Phase II clinical trials.

Initiation of clinical studies based on pharmacodynamic studies in animals

It is expected that, in the coming years, the majority of potential DMOADs will be mechanism-based drugs. Because no DMOAD has been validated in humans, for some time into the future all potential DMOADs will be prototypes. By definition, no validated animal model of OA can exist for prototypic compounds because demonstration of efficacy in man is required in order to validate the animal model. Therefore, the selection of compounds for evaluation in man should be based on pharmacodynamic demonstration in animals of their ability to affect a specific target which is implicated in human OA. The primary objective of early clinical studies is to define pharmacokinetics and toleration. However, in the case of mechanism-based drugs, it is important also to obtain pharmacodynamic data in these clinical studies. Only if a mechanism-based drug exerts the desired biochemical or pharmacological effect in the appropriate tissue, can lack of therapeutic efficacy can be interpreted as evidence that the molecular target is unimportant in the disease process. In the absence of such evidence of biochemical/pharmacological efficacy, lack of therapeutic activity could be due to failure of the agent to inhibit its target. Defining the plasma levels required to achieve the desired biochemical/pharmacological effect, also permits an estimate of the ratio of the pharmacologically effective dose to the maximum tolerated dose, greatly facilitating the design of studies to evaluate therapeutic efficacy.

It can be argued that the following hypothetical set of criteria provide a rationale for taking such a prototypic DMOAD into human trials without evidence of 'therapeutic' efficacy in an animal model of OA. The approach is outlined in Fig. 11.5, where it is compared with the empirical approach:

1. There is evidence from *in vitro* and *in vivo* studies of human tissues and cells that a particular molecular target (for example, mediator, receptor, enzyme, ion channel) is implicated in human OA, and it can be reasonably postulated that inhibition of its activity would produce a valuable therapeutic effect. For example, there is compelling evidence that MMPs play a key role in cartilage degradation in OA. This evidence is based on studies of the human enzymes which are capable of degrading cartilage matrix *in vitro*[64,65,67,68] and are expressed in OA synovium, cartilage, and synovial fluid[64,69–71]. In addition, *in vitro* degradation of human cartilage induced by IL-1 can be prevented by MMP inhibitors[72].

2. A specific inhibitor is identified using *in vitro* assays with purified, or recombinant, *human* MMPs.

3. *In vivo* animal studies demonstrate that systemic administration of the putative DMOAD leads to inhibition of human MMPs injected into an animal joint. These studies do not seek to demonstrate a therapeutic effect, but demonstrate that the compound hits its enzyme target in the joint *in vivo*. The plasma concentrations of the drug which are associated with biochemical efficacy are determined, and are used, to set the target plasma levels for human studies.

4. Pharmacokinetic projections from animals to man suggest that the plasma levels associated with biochemical efficacy in animals are achievable.

5. No undesirable pharmacological effects are observed *in vitro* or *in vivo* at relevant concentrations / doses.

6. The compound is found to have an acceptable profile in drug safety studies.

7. Clinical methods exist, which can be incorporated into early clinical studies, to determine whether the compound hits its target in humans. Sampling of joint tissues will not be possible in normal volunteers but there may be surrogate biochemical parameters (for example, MMP cleavage products of collagen[73,74]) that could be studied in blood or urine, and reflect overall matrix metalloproteinase activity under normal physiological conditions.

When studies progress to patients, biopsies of cartilage and synovium can be obtained for immunohistochemical studies of MMP cleavage products.

The amount of information obtained in the process outlined above should be sufficient to justify evaluating the human pharmacodynamics of a mechanism-based potential DMOAD in humans; therapeutic efficacy in an animal model of OA should not be needed.

Other advantages of mechanism-based drug discovery

An additional advantage of reducing the importance of animal disease models in the drug discovery process is that this could greatly reduce the number of experimental animals subject to pain and distress. It is obviously impossible to produce a model of arthritis devoid of pain and distress, but pharmacodynamic models can be relatively benign. Avoiding unnecessary use of animal models of OA, wherever possible, would certainly be in the spirit of Federal regulations on the use of animals in research and would show responsiveness to the widespread concern in the community on this subject.

Mechanism-based drug discovery can eliminate the need for testing of compounds in many animal disease models. If demonstration of therapeutic activity in an animal disease model were to be made a regulatory requirement, sponsors may be compelled to search through a wide range of animal species and models in order to identify the conditions in which therapeutic activity can be demonstrated: such an effort would generate a large amount of data of dubious relevance. All this would have to be reported and reviewed, adding to the already considerable burden on the sponsor, clinicians, and regulatory authorities. It would be to the benefit of all parties to reduce the size of regulatory documents and permit focus on the most relevant data. Proposals to regulatory authorities for the evaluation of mechanism-based compounds which contained little or no data from animal models of OA would achieve these objectives.

Although it seems reasonable to assume that the mechanism-based approach to discovery of DMOADs will be more successful over time than empirical methods, it certainly does not guarantee success for every project. For example, because compelling evidence from human clinical studies and *in vitro* studies with human tissues suggested that antagonists of platelet activating factor (PAF) would have significant therapeutic activity in asthmatic patients[75,76], several highly potent, selective, and bioavailable compounds were developed. However, rather than proving to be effective antiasthmatic agents, they have demonstrated that PAF is not an important mediator in human allergic asthma[77–79]. An explanation for why the early data implicating PAF proved to be misleading has yet to be found, but as a result of this failure the compounds which were developed are now available as tools to explore the role of PAF in other diseases. Completion of the necessary studies on safety, pharmacokinetic, and pharmacodynamic properties of several PAF antagonists has lowered the threshold for conducting more speculative clinical studies in other indications. It is exciting to speculate on the future availability of tools — such as specific inhibitors of MMPs, inhibitors of cytokine synthesis or action, growth factor agonists — arising out of the mechanism-based search for DMOADs and, regardless of their therapeutic efficacy in OA, being applied to the investigation of other diseases.

The 'warm feeling' factor

At present, the evidence needed to prove that a compound has DMOAD activity in humans is defined as reduction in the rate of joint damage as determined by imaging technologies[1]. With current technology and clinical trial design, these clinical properties will be extremely difficult and expensive to demonstrate, and require a lengthy period of observation. For example, it has been estimated[1] that 163 patients per treatment group would be required in a three-year placebo-controlled study to demonstrate a 0.5 mm difference in the loss of joint space in patients with hip OA, using conventional X-ray technology. The magnitude of these studies deters initiation of clinical trials of potential DMOADs and tends to induce a need for great reassurance from preclinical studies before proceeding.

In one arena, disease models of OA have an enormous advantage over pharmacodynamic models — they can be very effective in building confidence in the minds of the sponsor of the drug, the regulatory authorities, and the clinicians who will administer the new drug to volunteers and patients, that the compound will show therapeutic activity in humans. This 'warm feeling' does not have a strong scientific basis, as pointed out above, but it can be such a powerful factor

that proponents of a mechanism-based drug may find it necessary to find preclinical evidence for therapeutic efficacy, however, obscure the disease model, in order to build support for progressing the compound. This has resulted in the creation of a process for drug discovery in OA which is a hybrid between the traditional, animal model-based paradigm and the mechanism-based paradigm (Fig. 11.5). In the long term, however, use of disease models to select which mechanism-based drugs are advanced to clinical trials cannot be the most efficient way to discover DMOADs.

Reducing dependence on animal models of OA

The most effective means of reducing dependence on unreliable animal models of OA is to reduce the scale of the clinical studies required to demonstrate DMOAD activity. If the costs of a clinical DMOAD study could be greatly reduced, the confidence threshold for initiating a clinical trial would be reduced. Progress is being made in the development of more precise imaging technology to detect joint damage. Use of improved radioanatomic positioning of the patient for radiography of joints, microfocal X-ray generation, digital analysis of the image, magnetic resonance imaging, ultrasound, and arthroscopy, all show promise (see Chapters 11.5–11.9). Given the heterogeneity of OA, patient selection and trial design can also have an major impact. Defined subpopulations of patients with more rapidly progressive and/or more reproducible disease offer the possibility of much smaller studies with great statistical power[80].

The future role of animals in OA research — impact of new technologies

Genetic analysis of human disease is proceeding rapidly and future studies may identify the genes which predispose to OA. This information will effectively validate pathogenic processes in man, when the genes responsible for predisposition to OA are cloned and the biological functions of the expressed protein determined. With the advent of more powerful tools of molecular genetics, this process will be extended from the rare familial forms of OA, determined by a single dominant mutation[81], to the larger OA population in which the genetic component is much more complex[82–84]. It can be anticipated that information from this source will have greater and greater impact on the drug discovery process by validating the pathogenic mechanisms of human diseases without dependence on unreliable disease models in animals.

Transplantation of diseased human tissues into mice with severe-combined-immunodeficiency disease (SCID) has been investigated as a means of reproducing human disease in animals. Because these mice cannot reject the human tissues, long-term survival of such xenografts is achievable[85]. It is theoretically possible that these animals can be engineered to carry enough of the key components of a human disease to enable them to serve as valid disease models in drug discovery and investigation of disease mechanisms. For example, transplantation of human RA synovial tissue and cartilage[86], or RA synovial lymphocytes[87] into SCID mice, elicited a condition resembling RA. However, it is likely that murine cells will infiltrate the implanted human tissue and may participate in the disease process. A graft-versus-host reaction would also complicate interpretation of drug effects. Although this technology does not offer perfect disease models today, future developments may overcome many of the current limitations.

The number of biologicals (proteins) entering the pharmacopeia is growing rapidly. The data which justify testing a biological in humans are usually no different from those which would form the rationale for development of a low molecular weight drug. Biologicals, however, frequently move from basic research to clinical evaluation much faster than synthetic drugs, largely because they usually have inherent target specificity that eliminates the extensive search for specific analogues that is necessary with low molecular weight drugs. In addition, it has been argued that the biotechnology companies usually involved in developing biologicals can move more rapidly than the rest of the pharmaceutical industry because they have a greater willingness to take risks[88]. Whatever the explanation, conclusive proof of the importance of certain targets in human disease has been obtained by the use of biological reagents of high specificity. Anti-TNFα antibodies have demonstrated the importance of tumor necrosis factor-α (TNF-α) in RA[89] and have increased confidence in the potential value of low molecular weight drugs that will interfere with production or action of TNFα. In such circumstances, demonstration of therapeutic activity in an animal disease model becomes unnecessary. Biologicals may find a role in the therapy of OA, for example, growth factors, cytokine antagonists, antiproteases. It will be interesting to see whether the pharmaceutical industry can capitalize on such targets, validated in the human OA rather than animal models, by developing small molecules which are cheaper than biologicals, orally active, and non-immunogenic.

Summary

There is undoubtedly an important role for animal models of OA in exploring potential disease mechanisms and identifying targets to be investigated in man. However, animal disease models are being replaced by pharmacodynamic models in mechanism-based drug discovery strategies. Therefore, demonstration of the *in vivo* expression of a relevant mechanism in a pharmacodynamic model should be sufficient to justify initiating clinical trials. It is encouraging to note that the original recommendations for the testing of DMOADs, developed by a committee sponsored by the International League Against Rheumatism and the World Health Organization[1], have been refined to specifically support the mechanism-based drug discovery paradigm described in this chapter[90]. Because mechanism-based discovery efforts are becoming the norm, the impact of a decreased reliance on animal models of human OA could be:

(1)   a reduction in the size of the preclinical section of regulatory submissions;

(2)   considerably fewer animals subjected to pain and distress;

(3)   reduced risk of inappropriate rejection of mechanism-based agents;

(4)   increased rate of accumulation of valuable information about disease mechanisms.

This process will involve rheumatologists and other clinicians in studies which, at no increased risk to subjects, explore the underlying mechanisms of OA while they assess the clinical efficacy of a compound. However, the use of animal models of OA to justify the testing of compounds of unknown mechanism will continue and can be expected to generate some successes. However, the latter approach is not the most efficient process of drug discovery and it is likely that it will be gradually replaced by the evaluation of mechanism-based drugs in animal pharmacodynamic models.

References

1. Lequesne, M., Brandt, K., Bellamy, N., Moskowitz, R., Menkes, C.J., and Pelletiere, J-P. (1994). Guidelines for testing slow acting drugs in osteoarthritis. *J Rheumatol*, **21 (suppl 41)**, 65–71.

2. Badley, E.M. (1991). Population projections and the effects on rheumatology. *Ann Rheum Dis*, **50**, 3–6.

3. Hamerman, D: (1995). Clinical implications of osteoarthritis and ageing. *Ann Rheum Dis*, **54**, 82–5.

4. Warskyj, M. and Hukins, D.W. (1990). Animal models for osteoarthritis — ensuring experimental validity. *Br J Rheumatol*, **29**, 219–21.

5. Pritzker, K.P. (1994). Animal models for osteoarthritis: processes, problems and prospects. *Ann Rheum Dis*, **53**, 406–20.

6. Moskowitz, R.W. (1990). The relevance of animal models in osteoarthritis. *Scand J Rheumatol*, **81 (suppl)**, 21–3.

7. Jimenez, S.A. (1991). Molecular biological approaches to the study of heritable osteoarthritis. *J Rheumatol*, **27(suppl)**, 7–9.

8. Burton-Wurster, N., Todhunter, R.J., and Lust, G. (1993). Animal models of osteoarthritis. In *Inflammatory disease and therapy. Joint cartilage breakdown: basic and clinical* (ed. J.F. Woessner, Jr, D.S. Howell), pp. 347–84. Marcel Dekker Inc., New York.

9. Altman, R.D. and Dean, D.D. (1990). Osteoarthritis research: animal models. *Semin Arthritis Rheum*, **19**, 21–2.

10. Annefeld, M. (1992). Animal models in osteoarthritis research. In *Rheumatology, state of the art: XIIth European Congress of Rheumatology* (ed. G. Balint, B. Gomor and L. Hodinka), pp. 163–4. Excerpta Medica, Amsterdam.

11. Bendele, A.M. (1987). Progressive chronic osteoarthritis in femorotibial joints of partial medial meniscectomized guinea pigs. *Vet Pathol*, **24**, 444–8.

12. Bendele, A.M., Hulman, J.F., and Bean, J.S. (1989). Spontaneous osteoarthritis in Hartley Albino guinea pigs: effects of dietary and surgical manipulations. *Arthritis Rheum*, **32**, S106.

13. Das-Gupta, E.P., Lyons, T.J., Hoyland, J.A., Lawton, D.M., and Freemont, A.J. (1993). New histological observations in spontaneously developing osteoarthritis in the STR/ORT mouse questioning its acceptability as a model of human osteoarthritis. *Int J Exp Pathol*, **74**, 627–34.

14. Dunham, J., Chambers, M.G., Jasani, M.K., Bitensky, J., and Chayen, J. (1989). Quantitative criteria for evaluating the early development of osteoarthritis and the effect of diclofenac sodium. *Agents Actions*, **28**, 1–2.

15. Dunham, J., Chambers, M.G., Jasani, M.K., Bitensky, L., and Chayen, J. (1990). Changes in the orientation of proteoglycans during the early development of natural murine osteoarthritis. *J Orthop Res*, **8**, 101–4.

16. Okabe, T. (1989). Experimental studies on the spontaneous osteoarthritis in C57 black mice. *J Tokyo Med Coll*, **47**, 546–57.

17. Stanescu, R., Knyszynski, A., Muriel, M.P., and Stanescu, V. (1993). Early lesions of the articular surface in a strain of mice with very high incidence of spontaneous osteoarthritis-like lesions. *J Rheumatol*, **20**, 102–10.

18. Takahama, A. (1990). Histological study on spontaneous osteoarthritis of the knee in C57 black mouse. *J Jpn Orthop Assoc*, **64**, 271–81.

19. van der Kraan, P.M., Vitters, E.L., van Beuningen, H.M., van de Putte, L.B., and van den Berg, W.B. (1990). Degenerative knee joint lesions in mice after a single intra-articular collagenase injection. A new model of osteoarthritis. *J Exp Pathol*, **71**, 19–31.

20. Garofalo, S., Vuorio, E., Metsaranta, M., Rosati, R., Toman, D., Vaughan, J., *et al.* (1991). Reduced amounts of cartilage collagen fibrils and growth plate anomalies in transgenic mice harboring a glycine-to-cysteine mutation in the mouse type II procollagen α_1-chain gene. *Proc Natl Acad Sci (USA)*, **88**, 9648–52.

21. Nakata, K., Ono, K., Miyazaki, J-I., Olsen, B., Muragaki, Y., Adachi, E., *et al.* (1993). Osteoarthritis associated with mild chondrodysplasia in transgenic mice expressing α_1 (IX) collagen chains with a central deletion. *Proc Natl Acad Sci (USA)*, **90**, 2870–4.

22. Alexander, J.W. (1992). The pathogenesis of canine hip dysplasia. *Vet Clin North America: Small Animal Practice*, **22**, 503–11.

23. Alexander, C.J. (1994). Utilisation of joint movement range in arboreal primates compared with human subjects: an evolutionary frame for primary osteoarthritis. *Ann Rheum Dis*, **53**, 720–5.

24. Carlson, C.S., Loeser, R.F., Jayo, M.J., Weaver, D.S., Adams, M.R., and Jerome, C.P. (1994). Osteoarthritis in cynomolgus macaques: a primate model of naturally occurring disease. *J Orthop Res*, **12**, 331–9.

25. Chateauvert, J.M., Grynpas, M.D., Kessler, M.J., and Pritzker, K.P. (1990). Spontaneous osteoarthritis in rhesus macaques. II. Characterization of disease and morphometric studies (see comments). *J Rheumatol*, **17**, 73–83.

26. Kalbhen, D.A. (1987). Chemical model of osteoarthritis — a pharmacological evaluation. *J Rheumatol*, **130**, 130–1.

27. Marcelon, G., Cros, J., and Guiraud, R. (1976). Activity of anti-inflammatory drugs on an experimental model of osteoarthritis. *Agents Actions*, **6**, 191–4.

28. Coulais, Y., Marcelon, G., Cros, J., and Guiraud, R. (1984). An experimental model of osteoarthritis. II: biochemical study of collagen and proteoglycans. *Pathol Biol*, **32**, 23–8.

29. Coulais, Y., Marcelon, G., Cros, J., and Guiraud, R. (1983). Studies on an experimental model for osteoarthritis. I: induction and ultrastructural investigation. *Pathol Biol*, **31**, 577–82.

30. Leipold, H.R., Goldberg, R.L., and Lust, G. (1989). Canine serum keratan sulfate and hyaluronate concentrations. Relationship to age and osteoarthritis. *Arthritis Rheum*, **32**, 312–21.

31. Tanaka, H., Kitoh, Y., Katsuramaki, T., Tanaka, M., Kitabayashi, N., Fujimori, S., *et al.* (1992). Effects of

SL-1010 (sodium hyaluronate with high molecular weight) on experimental osteoarthritis induced by intra-articularly applied papain in guinea pigs. *Folia Pharmacol Jpn*, **100**, 77–86.

32. van der Kraan, P.M., Vitters, E.L., and van den Berg, W.B. (1989). Development of osteoarthritis models in mice by 'mechanical' and 'metabolical' alterations in the knee joints. *Arthritis Rheum*, **32**, S107.

33. van den Berg, W.B. (1995). Growth factors in experimental osteoarthritis: transforming growth factor beta pathogenic? *J Rheumatol*, (**Suppl 43**), 143–5.

34. Vasilev, V., Merker, H.J., and Vidinov, N. (1992). Ultrastructural changes in the synovial membrane in experimentally-induced osteoarthritis of rabbit knee joint. *Histol Histopathol*, **7**, 119–27.

35. Pond, M.J. and Nuki, G. (1973). Experimentally-induced osteoarthritis in the dog. *Ann Rheum Dis*, **32**, 387–8.

36. Brandt, K.D. (1994). Insights into the natural history of osteoarthritis provided by the cruciate-deficient dog: an animal model of osteoarthritis. *Ann NY Acad Sci*, **732**, 199–205.

37. Christensen, S.B. (1983). Localization of bone-seeking agents in developing experimentally induced osteoarthritis in the knee joint of the rabbit. *Scand J Rheumatol*, **12**, 343–9.

38. Vignon, E., Mathieu, P., Bejui, J., Descotes, J., Hartmann, D., Patricot, L.M., *et al.* (1991). Study of an inhibitor of plasminogen activator (tranexamic acid) in the treatment of experimental osteoarthritis. *J Rheumatol*, **27(suppl)**, 131–3.

39. Ghosh, P., Armstrong, S., Read, R., Numata, Y., Smith, S., McNair, P., *et al.* (1993). Animal models of early osteoarthritis: their use for the evaluation of potential chondroprotective agents. *Agents Actions*, **39(suppl)**, 195–206.

40. Fam, A.G., Morava-Protzner, I., Purcell, C., Young, B.D., Bunting, P.S., and Lewis, A.J. (1995). Acceleration of experimental lapine osteoarthritis by calcium pyrophosphate microcrystalline synovitis. *Arthritis Rheum*, **38**, 201–10.

41. Moskowitz, R.W. and Goldberg, V.M. (1987). Studies of osteophyte pathogenesis in experimentally induced osteoarthritis. *J Rheumatol*, **14**, 311–20.

42. Ehrlich, M.G., Mankin, H.J., Jones, H., Grossman, A., Crispen, C., and Ancona, D. (1975). Biochemical confirmation of an experimental osteoarthritis model. *J Bone Joint Surg (Am)*, **57**, 392–6.

43. Dedrick, D.K., Goulet, R., Huston, L., Goldstein, S.A., and Bole, G.G. (1991). Early bone changes in experimental osteoarthritis using microscopic computed tomography. *J Rheumatol*, **27(suppl)**, 44–5.

44. Layton, M.W., Arsever, C., and Bole, G.G. (1987). Use of the guinea pig myectomy osteoarthritis model in the examination of cartilage-synovium interactions. *J Rheumatol*, **125**, 125–6.

45. Arsever, C.L. and Bole, G.G. (1986). Experimental osteoarthritis induced by selective myectomy and tenotomy. *Arthritis Rheum*, **29**, 251–61.

46. Oegema, T.R.J., Lewis, J.L.J., and Thompson, R.C.J. (1993). Role of acute trauma in development of osteoarthritis. *Agents Actions*, **40**, 3–4.

47. Mazieres, B., Maheu, E., Thiechart, M., and Vallieres, G. (1990). Effects of N-acetyl hydroxyproline (oxaceprol (R)) on an experimental post-contusive model of osteoarthritis. A pathological study. *J Drug Dev*, **3**, 135–42.

48. Langenskiold, A., Michelsson, J.E., and Videman, T. (1979). Osteoarthritis of the knee in the rabbit produced by immobilization. Attempts to achieve a reproducible model for studies on pathogenesis and therapy. *Acta Orthop Scand*, **50**, 1–14.

49. Videman, T. (1982). Experimental osteoarthritis in the rabbit: comparison of different periods of repeated immobilization. *Acta Orthop Scand*, **53**, 339–47.

50. Howell, D.S., Muller, F., and Manicourt, D.H. (1992). A mini review: proteoglycan aggregate profiles in the Pond-Nuki dog model of osteoarthritis and in canine disuse atrophy. *Br J Rheumatol*, **31**, 7–11.

51. Ratcliffe, A., Beauvais, P.J., and Saed-Nejad, F. (1994). Differential levels of synovial fluid aggrecan aggregate components in experimental osteoarthritis and joint disuse. *J Orthop Res*, **12**, 464–73.

52. Vilensky, J.A., O'Connor, B.L., Brandt, K.D., Dunn, E.A., and Rogers, P.I. (1994). Serial kinematic analysis of the canine knee after L4-S1 dorsal root ganglionectomy: implications for the cruciate deficiency model of osteoarthritis. *J Rheumatol*, **21**, 2113–17.

53. Dieppe, P. (1991). Osteoarthritis: the scale and the scope of the clinical problem. In *Osteoarthritis: current research and prospects for pharmacological intervention* (ed. R.G.G. Russell and P. Dieppe), pp. 4–23. IBC Technical Services Ltd, London.

54. Brandt, K.D. (1991). Animal models: insights into osteoarthritis (OA) provided by the cruciate-deficient dog. *Br J Rheumatol*, **30**, 5–9.

55. Pinals, R.S. (1983). Approaches to rheumatoid arthritis and osteoarthritis: an overview. *Am J Med*, **75**, 2–9.

56. Blackham, A., Burns, J.W., Farmer, J.B., Radziowanic, H., and Westwick, J. (1977). An x-ray analysis of adjuvant arthritis in the rat. The effect of prednisolone and indomethacin. *Agents Actions*, **7**, 145–51.

57. Otterness, I.G., Larson, D., and Lombardino, J.G. (1982). An analysis of piroxicam in rodent models of arthritis. *Agents Actions*, **12**, 308–12.

58. Jobanputra, P. and Nuki, G. (1993). Nonsteroidal anti-inflammatory drugs in the treatment of osteoarthritis. *Curr Opin Rheumatol*, **6**, 433–9.

59. Zhang, J., Weichman, B.M., and Lewis, A.J. (1995). Role of animal models in the study of rheumatoid arthritis: an overview. In *Mechanisms and models in rheumatoid arthritis* (ed. B. Henderson, J.C.W. Edwards and E.R. Pettipher), pp. 363–72. Academic Press, New York.

60. Karran, E.H., Young, T.J., Markwell, R.E., and Harper, G.P. (1995). *In vivo* model of cartilage degradation — effects of a matrix metalloproteinase inhibitor. *Ann Rheum Dis*, **54**, 662–9.

61. Henriet, P., Rousseau, G.C., and Eekhout, Y. (1992). Cloning and sequencing of mouse collagenase cDNA. Divergence of mouse and rat collagenases from the other mammalian collagenases. *FEBS Lett*, **310**, 175–8.

62. Beeley, N.R.A., Ansell, P.R.J., and Docherty, A.J.P. (1994). Inhibitors of matrix metalloproteinases (MMP's). *Curr Opin Ther Patents*, **4**, 7–16.

63. Freije, J.M.P., Diez-Itza, I., Balbib, M., Snachez, L.M., Blasco, R., Tolivia, J., *et al.* (1994). Molecular cloning and expression of collagenase-3, a novel human matrix metalloproteinase produced by breast carcinomas. *J Biol Chem*, **269**, 16766–73.

64. Mitchell, P.G., Magna, H.A., Reeves, L.M., Lopresti-Morrow, L.L., Yocum, S.A., Rosner, P.J., *et al.* (1996). Cloning of matrix metalloproteinase-13 (MMP-13, collagenase-3) from human chondrocytes, expression of MMP-13 by osteoarthritic cartilage and activity of the enzyme on type II collagen. *J Clin Invest*, **97**, 761–8.

65. Billinghurst, R.C., Dahlberg, L., Ionescu, M., Reiner, A., Bourne, R., Rorabeck, C., Mitchell, P., Hambor, J., Diekmann, O., Tschesche, H., Chen, J., Vanwart, H. and Poole, A.R. (1997). Enhanced cleavage of type II collagen by collagenases in osteoarthritic articular cartilage . *J Clin Invest*, **99**, 1534–45.

66. Ganu, V., Parker, D., MacPherson, L., Hu, S-I., Goldberg, R., Raychaudhuri, A., *et al.* (1994). Biochemical and pharmacological profile of a non-peptidic orally active inhibitor of matrix metalloproteinases. *Osteoarthritis Cart*, **2 (suppl 1)**, 34.

67. Nguyen, Q., Murphy, G., Hughes, C.E., Mort, J.S., and Roughley, P.J. (1993). Matrix metalloproteinases cleave at two distinct sites on human cartilage link protein. *Biochem J*, **295**, 595–8.

68. Fosang, A.J., Last, K., Neame, P.J., Murphy, G., Knauper, V., Tschesche, H., *et al.* (1994). Neutrophil collagenase (MMP-8) cleaves at the aggrecanase site E373-A374 in the interglobular domain of cartilage aggrecan. *Biochem J*, **304**, 347–51.

69. Firestein, G.S., Paine, M.M., and Littman, B.L. (1991). Gene expression (collagenase, tissue inhibitor of metalloproteinases, complement and HLD-DR) in rheumatoid arthritis and osteoarthritis synovium. *Arthritis Rheum*, **34**, 1094–9.

70. Mohtai, M., Lane Smith, R., Schurman, D.J., Tsuji, Y., Torti, F.M., Hutchinson, N.I., *et al.* (1993). Expression of 92-kD collagenase/gelatinase (gelatinase B) in osteoarthritic cartilage and its induction in normal human articular cartilage by interleukin-1. *J Clin Invest*, **92**, 179–85.

71. Clark, I.M., Powell, I.K., Ramsey, S., Hazelman, B.L., and Cawston, T.E. (1993). The measurement of collagenase, tissue inhibitor of matalloproteinases (TIMP), and collagenase-TIMP complexes in synovial fluids from patients with osteoarthritis and rheumatoid arthritis. *Arthritis Rheum*, **36**, 372–8.

72. Mort, J.S., Dodge, G.R., Roughley, P.J., Liu, P., Finch, S.J., Dipasquale, G., *et al.* (1993). Direct evidence for active metalloproteinases mediating matrix degradation in interleukin-1 stimulated human articular cartilage. *Matrix*, **13**, 95–102.

73. Hassager, C., Risteli, J., Risteli, L., Jensen, S.B., and Christiansen, C. (1992). Diurnal variation in serum markers of type I collagen synthesis and degradation in healthy premenopausal women. *J Bone Miner Res*, **7**, 1307–11.

74. Bollen, A-M., Martin, M.D., Leroux, B.G., and Eyre, D.R. (1995). Circadian variation in urinary excretion of bone collagen cross-links. *J Bone Miner Res*, **10**, 1885–90.

75. Chung, K.F., Cuss, F.M., and Barnes, P.J. (1989). Platelet activating factor: effects on bronchomotor tone and bronchial responsiveness in human beings. *Allergy Proc*, **10**, 333–7.

76. Page, C.P. and Morley, J. (1986). Evidence favouring PAF rather than leukotrienes in the pathogenesis of asthma. *Pharmacol Res Commun*, **18(suppl)**, 217–37.

77. Spence, D.P.S., Johnston, S.L., Calverley, P.M., Dhillon, P., Higgins, C., Ramhamadany, E., *et al.* (1994). The effect of the orally active platelet-activating factor antagonist WEB 2086 in the treatment of asthma. *Am J Respir Crit Care Med*, **149**, 1142–8.

78. Benfield, T.L. and Lundgren, J.D. (1994). PAF receptor antagonists in the treatment of asthma. *Expert Opin Invest Drugs*, **3**, 733–42.

79. Koltai, M., Guinot, P., Hosford, D., and Braquet, P. (1994). Platelet-activating factor antagonists: scientific background and possible clinical applications. *Adv Pharmacol*, **28**, 81–167.

80. Spector, T.D., Hart, D.J., and Doyle, D.V. (1994). Incidence and progression of osteoarthritis in women with unilateral knee disease in the general population: the effects of obesity. *Ann Rheum Dis*, **53**, 565–8.

81. Jimenez, S.A. (1995). Genetic aspects of familial osteoarthritis. *Ann Rheum Dis*, **53**, 789–97.

82. Loughlin, J., Irven, C., Athanasou, N., Carr, A., and Sykes, B. (1995). Differential allelic expression of the type II collagen gene (COL2A1) in osteoarthritic cartilage. *Am J Hum Genet*, **56**, 1186–93.

83. Baldwin, C.T., Farrer, L.A., Adair, R., Dharmavaram, R., Jimenez, S., and Anderson, L. (1995). Linkage of early-onset osteoarthritis and chondrocalcinosis to human chromosome 8q. *Am J Hum Genet*, **56**, 692–7.

84. Loughlin, J., Irven, C., Fergusson, C., and Sykes, B. (1994). Sibling pair analysis shows no linkage of generalized osteoarthritis to the loci encoding type II collagen, cartilage link protein or cartilage matrix protein. *Br J Rheumatol*, **33**, 1103–6.

85. Bosma, G.C., Custer, R.P., and Bosma, M.J. (1983). A severe combined immunodeficiency mutation in the mouse. *Nature*, **310**, 527–30.

86. Geiler, T., Kriegsmann, J., Keyszer, G.M., Gay, R.E., and Gay, S. (1994). A new model for rheumatoid arthritis generated by engraftment of rheumatoid synovial tissues and normal human cartilage into SCID mice. *Arthritis Rheum*, **37**, 1664–71.

87. Tighe, H., Silverman, G.J., Kozin, F., Tucker, R., Gulizia, R., Peebles, C., *et al.* (1990). Autoantibody production by severe combined immunodifficient mice reconstituted with synovial cells from rheumatoid arthritis patients. *Eur J Immunol*, **20**, 1843–8.

88. Weisbach, J.A. and Moos, W.H. (1995). Diagnosing the decline of major pharmaceutical research laboratories: a prescription for drug companies. *Drug Dev Res*, **34**, 243–59.

89. Elliot, M.J., Maini, R.N., Feldmann, M., Kalden, J.R., Antoni, C., Smolen, J.S., *et al.* (1994). Randomized double-blind comparison of chimeric monoclonal antibody to tumor necrosis factor alpha (cA2) versus placebo in rheumatoid arthritis. *Lancet*, **344**, 1105–10.

90. Lequesne, M., Brandt, K., Bellamy, N., Moskowitz, R., Menkes, C.J., Pelletier, J-P., *et al.* (1995). Guidelines for testing slow acting drugs in arthritis — Addendum. *J Rheumatol*, **22**, 1442.

11.5 Assessment of changes in joint tissues in patients treated with a disease-modifying osteoarthritis drug (DMOAD): monitoring outcomes

11.5.1 Radiographic grading systems
Deborah J. Hart and Tim D. Spector

History of existing radiographic grading systems

In the past, attempts to classify osteoarthritis (OA) have set out to identify similar features of the disease and to apply changes in these features globally in all joints. It has now been shown that classification criteria cannot be developed to cover changes in this way, as OA manifests differently in each joint group it affects. The time sequence of exactly when articular cartilage is lost, subchondral bone alters, and new bone is formed is unclear. Choosing one as a marker for OA may lead to problems of misclassification should a different feature commonly appear first in a particular joint. For example, in the knee, osteophytes may be more prevalent and more closely associated with knee pain[1], whereas in the hip, joint space narrowing more strongly associates with pain and may be of more use in definition than osteophytes alone[2].

Radiographs are the most common method of classifying OA, particularly in epidemiological and clinical studies. Despite advantages of widespread availability, reproducibility, and good standardization, there are limitations: applying radiographic criteria to large populations may be expensive and ethically problematic; radiographs may show up to 40 per cent of the population have OA when they remain asymptomatic, and in contrast, others who have symptoms of arthritis show no radiographic signs[3]; classification of OA at some sites may be easier than at others; reproducibility of radiographic grading can be poor, and there are inconsistencies in interpreting existing criteria, thus affecting prevalence estimates in populations. For nearly 40 years, the radiological definitions of Kellgren and Lawrence[4], have been accepted as a 'gold standard', but there are many problems associated with this system[5]. In recent years, a number of developments have been made to classify OA using radiographs, which will be discussed here.

The method of grading radiographic change of OA was developed by Kellgren and Lawrence in 1957, and adopted by the World Health Organisation (WHO) in Rome, in 1961, as the accepted 'gold standard' for cross-sectional and longitudinal epidemiological studies. The original written definitions of the grading of radiographs were given in 1957 (Table 11.3), and it was intended that an atlas should accompany the definitions. However, the corresponding photographs used in a subsequent atlas[6], in some cases did not exactly match the written grades. For example, grade 2 was described as 'presence of definite osteophyte with minimal joint space narrowing', and later[7] as 'definite osteophyte but joint space unimpaired'. Definitions of the Kellgren and Lawrence grading system, as presented in 1963, are given in Table 11.3. These inconsistencies in interpretations of the system have led to problems of different classification in epidemiological studies by groups who believe that they have all applied the standard criteria. The Kellgren and Lawrence grading system has also been criticized for its reliance on the presence of the osteophyte for classification of disease[8]. The time sequence of when bony changes occur and articular cartilage is lost is still controversial. Thus, according to Kellgren and Lawrence, presence of a narrowed, sclerotic joint with deformity cannot be classified as osteoarthritic unless an osteophyte is also present. There also remains a problem of how to classify those individuals with a grade 1, doubtful osteophyte. Is it correct to classify these people as a normal group, or treat them as an affected group with early changes of OA? A recent review suggests that since no clear consensus exists as to whether grade 1 subjects are cases or controls, they should be treated as a separate grade[9]. This could be done by either excluding them from analysis or treating them as a separate subgroup.

Table 11.3 Description of the radiological features of the Kellgren and Lawrence grading system of OA[6]

The following radiological features were considered evidence of osteoarthrosis:

(1) formation of osteophytes on the joint margins or, in the case of the knee joint, on the tibial spines;

(2) periarticular ossicles — these are found chiefly in relation to the distal and proximal interphalangeal joints;

(3) narrowing of the joint cartilage associated with sclerosis of the subchondral bone;

(4) small pseudocystic areas with sclerotic walls, situated usually in the subchondral bone;

(5) alterted shape ends of bone ends, particularly in the head of the femur.

These changes have been graded numerically:

0	None	No features
1	Doubtful	Minute osteophyte, doubtful significance
2	Minimal	Definite osteophyte, unimpaired joint space
3	Moderate	Moderate diminution of joint space
4	Severe	Joint space greatly impaired, with sclerosis of subchondral bone

The imperfections of the Kellgren and Lawrence criteria were discussed at the 3rd International Symposium on Rheumatic Disease in New York, in 1966[10]. However, it was decided that in the absence of any improved, validated criteria, the Rome criteria should stand. There is an increasing acceptance that OA may not represent one disorder but that it is a disease spectrum with a series of subsets that lead to similar clinical and pathological alterations. In a recent editorial, the prevalent view that OA should no longer be thought of as a single disease, but as a group of 'osteoarthritic diseases' was emphasized[11]. The first step in classifying these diseases is to develop joint-specific definitions and criteria, and abandon trying to develop a single criteria that incorporates manifestations of the whole spectrum of the disease. A number of groups, aware of these existing problems, have developed new criteria for classifying OA radiographically, and have focused on improving radiographic criteria, particularly in solving the problems of emphasis on the osteophyte in the Kellgren and Lawrence atlas. These groups have selected particular joints and developed criteria relating to the differing pathological processes of OA that present as common individual features that accompany OA in that joint site.

Features of OA on radiographs and their utility

Radiographically, OA is characterized by joint space narrowing due to changes in articular cartilage, and by changes in the subchondral and marginal bone which manifest as osteophyte, cysts, and eburnation. It is not easy to detect these pathological joint changes on a plain radiograph. The following descriptions attempt to interpret these changes radiographically.

Osteophytes

An osteophyte is a fibrocartilage-capped bony growth. On a radiograph, marginal osteophytes appear as new spurs or lips of bone around the edges of a joint and are variable in size; they originate at tendon insertions and capsular attachments; they frequently predominate in one side of the joint and develop, initially, in areas of relatively normal joint space. Osteophytes can also occur in central areas of the joint in which remnants of articular cartilage still exist; these central osteophytes frequently lead to a bumpy contour on a radiograph. Osteophytes can be very large and can increase the size of a joint. They are almost always seen in association with some degree of cartilage loss, except in the interphalangeal joints of the hands. It has been proposed, by some authors, that the presence of osteophytes is attributed to age, rather than OA[12]. However, studies such as that by Brandt *et al.*, examining pathological correlates of OA by arthroscopy and radiography, found that patients with osteophytes and normal articular cartilage on arthroscopy were younger than the patient group as a whole, suggesting that osteophytes cannot be explained on the basis of age alone[13].

Joint space narrowing

Cartilage in a degenerating joint initially becomes thinned and roughened — 'fibrillation'. Later, larger areas of erosions begin, and this progressive cartilage loss leads to a common radiographic sign of OA narrowing and loss of joint space. In general, cartilage loss is most pronounced in areas of maximum weight-bearing, for example, the medial tibio-femoral compartment of the knee.

Sclerosis

Generally, after evidence of joint space loss, eburnation becomes apparent, followed by sclerosis — an increased localized area of density at the joint margin, seen as a dense white line extending vertically into deeper regions of the subchondral bone. Initially, the radiodense region may be uniform, leading to radiolucent lesions reflecting subchondral cyst formation. Reproducibility for grading sclerosis is often poor, as assessment is subjective and difficult to quantify.

Tibial spiking

A major radiological text states that 'spiking' (that is, an increase in height and reduction in angle) of the tubercles of the intercondylar eminence of the tibial plateau is an early sign of OA of the knee joint[14]. Most imaging centers uniformally report on spiking, without clear evidence of its significance. One study found spiking was more marked in OA patients, but did not look at other features of OA[15]. A recent, much larger population study found a modest association with degree of spike angle and presence of osteophyte and joint space narrowing. However, in patients with otherwise normal radiographs for OA, there was no association of spiking and pain, and isolated spiking was not a useful measure for knee OA[16].

Joint-specific radiographic features

The hand

OA of the distal and proximal interphalangeal joints (DIP/PIP) of the hand, and the trapeziometacarpal joint of the thumb base (1st CMC) are extremely common, especially in middle-aged, post-menopausal women. OA of the hand is characterized by the presence of multiple-affected joints and is usually symmetrical. OA of the DIP joints is more prevalent than OA of the PIPs and may be absent in the presence of DIP OA. A recent study examined inter-relationships of joint involvement and symmetry in the hand[17]. This study confirmed that clustering, commonly affecting the DIP and 1st CMC

joints, was greater than expected with increasing age. The most important determinants of pattern of involvement in the hand were, in order of importance, symmetry, clustering by row (DIP), then by ray (DIP followed by PIP).

Clinically, OA of the interphalangeal joint presents as bony enlargements around the joint, known as Heberden's and Bouchard's nodes respectively. These nodes may not always be seen as a radiographic bony deformity, and may also be undetectable in the presence of X-ray changes[18]. Malalignments and flexion deformity may also occur in severe cases of OA. X-ray of the hands reveal prominent osteophyte and joint space narrowing. In OA, the wavy contour of the distal phalanx resembles the wings of a bird (Seagull sign)[14]. There is sometimes mild to moderate subluxation at the distal or proximal joints, producing a zig-zag contour. Occasionally, at the joint margin, are what appears to be fractured osteophytes that have broken away from the articular surface.

OA of the wrist, in the absence of trauma, is rare, except at the trapeziometacarpal joint. Subluxation of the metacarpal base, with resulting joint space loss, is commonly seen, as well as osteophytosis and fragmentation of bone (Fig. 11.6).

The hip

In the hip joint, the most common feature of OA is joint space narrowing and the migration of the femoral head in either a superior, lateral, or medial direction. The most common loss of joint space on radiograph is superior-lateral. In later stages of OA, the femoral head may also appear flattened, with resulting proximal migration of the femur. Osteophytes appear most frequently on the superolateral acetabular surface, and less frequently on the femoral head and neck. In a

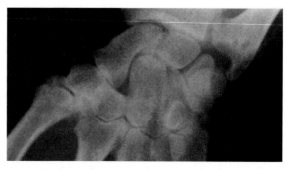

Fig. 11.6 Subluxation of the metacarpal base and osteophytosis.

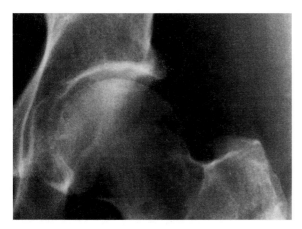

Fig. 11.7 Lateral acetabular margin showing mild osteo-phyte formation.

lateral acetabular osteophyte, the appearance is of a lip extending from the articular surface (Fig. 11.7). If the normal acetabular surface extends, this can often be misclassified as a mild osteophyte. Other features commonly seen at the hip are sclerosis and cysts.

The knee

The knee is made up of three compartments: medial and lateral tibiofemoral joint (TFJ) and the patellofemoral joint (PFJ). Common features of knee OA on radiographs are osteophyte, narrowed joint space, sclerosis, and cysts. Joint space narrowing is tra-

ditionally best seen on a weight-bearing film. Standard anterior-posterior views are useful for assessment of joint space in medial and lateral compartments. OA of the patellofemoral compartment is often seen in conjunction with the TFJ, and to a lesser extent on its own. The patellofemoral view is useful for assessing joint space narrowing and osteophyte on the patella side of the joint. Traditionally, two views of the PFJ have been used: the lateral, in approximately 30° of flexion, and the 'skyline' (30–60° flexion) or 'sunrise' view[19]. Recently, two studies have examined the relative merits of skyline versus lateral view for assessing the patello-femoral joint. In a small study of hospital cases, Jones *et al.* found grading of the skyline view was more reproducible than the lateral view, and allowed more precise localization of change[20]. This has been confirmed in a larger population-based study which also suggested that different osteophytes are detected by the two views, and may be complimentary[21].

Methods of grading features of OA

The hand

Kallman *et al.* were the first to produce an atlas of features of hand OA to include a graded scale of severity of osteophyte formation, narrowing of the joint space, subchondral sclerosis, subchondral cysts, lateral deformity, and cortical collapse[22]. Osteophyte and narrowing were to be graded using a 0–3 scale, and the other features scored present or absent (Table 11.4). In devel-

Table 11.4 Rating method used in scales for grading individual features of OA

Feature	Grade
Osteophytes	0 = None
	1 = Small (definite) osteophyte(s)
	2 = Moderate osteophyte(s)
	3 = Large osteophyte(s)
Joint space narrowing*	0 = None
	1 = Definitely narrowed
	2 = Severly narrowed
	3 = Joint fusion at at least one point
Subchondral sclerosis	0 = Absent
	1 = Present
Subchondral cysts	0 = Absent
	1 = Present
Lateral deformity⁺	0 = Absent
	1 = Present
Collapse of central joint cortical bone	0 = Absent
	1 = Present

*Narrowing between bone end plates, not osteophyte bridging
⁺ Malalignment of at least 15°
Modified from reference 22

oping the atlas, Kallman also graded all films using Kellgren and Lawrence for comparison: grade 1 Kallman was to correspond to Kellgren and Lawrence grade 2 (definite osteophyte), and grade 1 Kellgren and Lawrence (doubtful osteophyte) scored 0 on the Kallman scale. The grading scale appeared to be reliable when used cross-sectionally and in longitudinal data, and also compared well to the Kellgren and Lawrence scale. All features performed well for intraobserver reproducibility, but for interobserver reproducibility, osteophyte, narrowing, and Kellgren and Lawrence performed best, with cysts, deformity, and collapse performing less well. The interobserver agreement was best for dichotomous variables (96–99 per cent) and, for multiple categories, readers agreed most for osteophyte (86 per cent), followed by narrowing (79 per cent) and Kellgren and Lawrence (78 per cent). Reliability was good overall for osteophyte (interclass correlation (ICC) = 0.71), narrowing (ICC = 0.70), sclerosis (ICC = 0.60), and was best for Kellgren and Lawrence (ICC = 0.74): it was less good for cysts and deformity. Percentage agreement was higher within, than between, readers, and again, highest for dichotomous variables (98–99 per cent); osteophyte performed best (93 per cent), followed by narrowing (88 per cent) and Kellgren and Lawrence (85 per cent). Reliability within readers was better than between readers, for all measures. For the longitudinal data, readers also studied films 20–25 years apart. The authors suggested that one reader may be appropriate for longitudinal film data, as the different readers all determined progression similarly and intrareader reliability was almost perfect. Kallman *et al.* recommended different methods for reading X-rays for longitudinal studies. Firstly, paired films read side by side and assigned a progression score for time sequence and magnitude of change in the films — this carried the advantage of an increase in sensitivity, although films were subject to 'time sequence' bias. Secondly, read serial films one at a time, in random order, to eliminate 'time sequence' bias. The Kallman grading system is reproducible for both cross-sectional and longitudinal studies, and has been validated in other population studies[23], the only problem being the quality of the reproduced standard films which are difficult to read. The presence of the osteophyte remains the best way of defining OA of the hand.

The hip

Similar radiographic features have been tested to classify OA of the hip[2]. The features measured were:

(1) minimum joint space at four points around the joint arc, read by transparent ruler; (2) size of largest osteophyte; and (3) subchondral sclerosis. A composite score was also used. Joint space narrowing was more reproducible than osteophyte size; intraobserver kappas of 0.81 versus 0.44, and intraobserver, 0.70 versus 0.33. Narrowing of the joint space was more strongly associated with pain than osteophyte (56 per cent versus 34 per cent), suggesting that joint space narrowing may be of more importance in defining hip OA than the presence of osteophyte. Scott *et al.* studied 1363 women in the US and found that of the individual variables, joint space narrowing correlated best with pain, although a combination of osteophyte and joint space narrowing provided the best overall predictor of pain[24].

The knee

The earliest investigation into features of knee OA was performed by Ahlback in 1968[25]. This atlas made recommendations on views to be used, as well as gradings for measuring articular space, although these were crudely described and based on a subjective assessment likely to lead to variable interpretation. An atlas using individual features has been developed for the knee[26] and updated to include the skyline view[27] (the Spector atlas). Individual features of osteophyte and joint space narrowing were graded on a 0–3 scale, and sclerosis graded present or absent. This atlas also included a patellofemoral view, which was previously ignored in the Kellgren and Lawrence system. Reproducibility of reading lateral patellofemoral radiographs has, however, not been as good as tibiofemoral views[28,29]; recent data has shown that the skyline view is more reproducible for defining patellofemoral OA than the lateral view[20,21]. These knee criteria have been validated for observer reproducibility, and also compared to the Kellgren and Lawrence scale[26]. Features performed well within observers for both tibiofemoral and patellofemoral narrowing and osteophyte, and less well between observers; patellofemoral measurements between observers were poor. The individual features measured compared well to Kellgren and Lawrence grades.

These new criteria were compared to a number of other criteria for classifying knee OA, in a general population sample of 1954 knees[1]. The individual features, graded from the atlas, performed similarly well compared to Kellgren and Lawrence grades, precision ruler measurements, and automated digital analysis of joint space loss[30]. However, in analysis of predictors for knee pain in this group, using the Spector atlas, Kellgren and Lawrence grade 2 definite osteophytes (medial or lateral) were better predictors than narrowing. This suggests that, for reading conventional X-rays of the knee, the osteophyte may be the best predictor of clinical disease, and that joint space narrowing may be more useful for assessing disease severity or progression.

Another atlas for knee radiographs has been produced, assessing eight features of OA; both medial and lateral osteophytes, joint space narrowing and sclerosis; osteophytes of the tibial spines; and chondrocalcinosis. These signs were read in 30 films, by four readers, for reliability, who also read the films for a Kellgren and Lawrence grade. The results were good for all measures, with ICC ranging from 0.63–0.83 for inter-reader and 0.82–0.95 for intrareader: the poorest measures were sclerosis and tibial spiking. All measures were comparable to Kellgren and Lawrence grades, and narrowing performed as well as osteophytes grading[31].

Reproducibility of joint space measurement in conventional weight-bearing radiographs is a problem that must be addressed if this feature is to be useful for longitudinal studies. Problems may occur in two ways: positional problems (that is, variable knee flexion) which may result in large changes in joint space width; and precision of measurement. A coefficient of variation of 20–40 per cent has been estimated using conventional views and it is likely to be the major source of error[32]. One small study has examined the reproducibility of extended and semiflexed views of the medial compartment using computerized joint space measurement in optimal conditions[33]. The coefficient of variation (CV) was 9 per cent for the traditional method and 5 per cent for a standing semiflexed method, suggesting the latter may become more widely used.

In a preliminary study of radiographic progression of knee OA in 32 pairs of knees, it was found that joint space narrowing, followed by osteophyte, were the best variables in assessing progression[34]. We have recently assessed reproducibility of progression in 20 patients with knee OA, four years apart, and found changes in joint space narrowing, measured by atlas, to be internally more reproducible (k = 0.71) than changes in osteophyte (k = 0.50). Changes in joint space narrowing may be better for assessing progression, although these findings need to be confirmed. On current evidence, we believe that the osteophyte grade is the best way of defining OA of the knee in population studies, and that changes in knee joint space narrowing, with or without osteophyte, should be used for progression.

Other sites

Recent radiographic criteria have also been proposed for the thoracic and lumbar spine, as well as the hand and hip, using a similar scale of individual features[35]. These criteria have good reproducibility both between and within readers, but need to be validated in other populations.

A summary of the reproducibility for within and between observers for all radiographic grading systems is presented in Table 11.5.

Grading progression of radiographic changes

Relatively little is known of the determinants of the progression of OA. The disease is characterized by its slow evolution, and along with this, there are problems of lack of methods of assessment. A recent editorial urgently called for the development of standardized methods for detecting outcome of disease[36]. The authors believed that new methods of assessing progression are needed, in view of the advances being made in therapeutics to prevent and control the advancement of OA. In terms of standardizing radiographs, they stressed the importance of patient positioning, as small changes can affect the interbone distance in the knee. They also called for a consensus on which views of the knee and hip to use. In resolving these issues, it will be possible to develop consistency in data and permit direct comparison of radiographs between different studies.

In a recent workshop, convened in association with the World Health Organisation (WHO) and the American Academy of Orthopedic Surgeons (AAOS), guidelines were drawn up for methods to use in the assessment of progression of OA for clinical and intervention studies[37,38]. They aimed to set up a minimum set of standard methods that could be applied to all clinical studies of knee and hip OA. It was agreed that radiographs are currently the major outcome measure to assess development of OA over time, but were only of value if positioning of patients and assessment techniques were standardized. The committee recommended positioning of patients; the use of footmaps for reproducibility of knee radiographs; specific film cassette sizes and positions of X-ray beam; and, for the patellofemoral joint of the knee, the skyline view, with the knee in 45° of flexion. They did not recommend the lateral view, on the basis of current published data.

Table 11.5 A summary of interobserver and intraobserver reproducibility of radiographic grading scales

Joint	Feature	Kallman (1990) (P)		Hart (1993) (P)		Lane (1993) (P)		Croft (1990) (P)		Spector (1992) (P)		Cooper (1992) (H)		Scott (1993) (P)	
		Inter	Intra	Inter	Intra	Inter	Intra	Inter	Intra	Inter	Intra	Inter	Intra	Inter	Intra
DIP	OP	+++	+++	++	+++	+++	+++								
	N	+++	+++	+++	++	+++	+++								
	S	++	+++	+++		+	++								
PIP	OP	+++	++	+++	+++										
	N	+++	++	++	+++										
	S	++	+++	+++											
CMC	OP	+++	+++	++	+++										
	N	++	+++	+++	+++										
	S	+++	+++	+++											
Knee TFJ	OP									++	+++	++	+++	++	+++
	N									+	+++	++	+++	+++	+++
	S									++	++	+	++	+	+++
Knee PFJ	OP									++	+++	++	+++		
	N										+++	+	+++		
	S									+	++	+	++		
Hip	OP					+++	+++	+	+						
	N					+++	+++	+++	+++						
	S					+++	++	+	++						

H = Hospital based
P = Population based
DIP = Distal interphalangeal
PIP = Proximal interphalangeal
CMC = Carpometacarpal
TF = Tibiofemoral
PF = Patellofemoral
OP = Osteophyte
N = Joint space narrowing
S = Sclerosis
Inter = interobserver
Intra = intraobserver
+ = Poor
+ += Good
+ + + = Excellent

Table 11.6 Radiographic features to be recorded in cases of hip and knee OA*

Feature	Assessment of hip	Assessment of knee	
		TFJ	PFJ
Joint space narrowing	Graded 0–3 Millimeter measurement, (caliper optional)	Graded 0–3 Graded in 10ths of millimeters, perhaps with caliper	Graded 0–3
Osteophytes	Superior and inferior femoral graded 0–3, acetabular is difficult to judge and should be noted	Graded 0–3	Graded 0–3
Subchondral bony sclerosis	Femoral / acetabular sclerosis graded present / absent	Graded present / absent	Graded present absent
Attrition	Collapse of subchondral bony plate graded present / absent	Graded present / absent	
Subchondral bony cyst	Femoral / acetabular bony cyst graded 0–3		
Femoral migration	Superior and lateral migration should be noted present / absent		
Subluxation			Medial or lateral subluxation to be noted
Overall severity of OA	Kellgren & Lawrence or modified	Kellgren & Lawrence or modified	

*Modified from reference 38
TFJ = Tibiofemoral joint
PFJ = Patellofemoral joint

The recommended features to be recorded for the hip and knee are summarized in Table 11.6.

Summary

Current studies suggest that no single global system is suitable for the assessment of OA at all sites. They imply that different measures should be given different weight in different circumstances. At the hip, measurement of joint space is simple, reproducible, and might be preferred for the assignment of OA in epidemiologic studies. This may not be true at the knee, where precise location for joint space measurement, and tricompartmental structure of the joint, make assessment of this feature more difficult and assessment of the osteophyte, potentially, more useful.

This leaves the question of whether we should now abandon the system of Kellgren and Lawrence. It has been proposed that until consensus is reached on an improved method, we should not abandon it, but accept its deficiencies and use a standardized version. However, a recent consensus meeting also suggested that separate measurements of individual features are more likely to provide more information when used prospectively[5,38].

It can be seen that considerable advances have been made over the last thirty years in solving the problem of definition and criteria in OA, but we are still lacking a universal definition and classification of the disease. Radiological site, and perhaps compartment-specific definition of the disease, is now recognized as the major tool available in defining OA, and the way forward. There is general consensus that the grading of osteophytes and joint space narrowing at the major sites, using validated atlases, is an important advance, and a number of atlases with similar grading scales for most joints are available for general use[27,35,39].

References

1. Spector, T.D., Hart, D.J., Byrne, J., *et al.* (1993). Defining the presence of osteoarthritis of the knee in epidemiologic studies. *Ann Rheum Dis*, **52**, 790–794.
2. Croft, P., Cooper, C., Wickham, C., *et al.* (1990). Defining osteoarthritis of the hip for epidemiological studies. *Am J Epidemiol*, **132**, 514–22.
3. Lawrence, J.S., Bremner, J.M., and Bier, F. (1966). Osteoarthritis: prevalence in the population and relationship between symptoms and x-ray changes. *Ann Rheum Dis*, **25**, 1–23.
4. Kellgren, J.H. and Lawrence, J.S. (1957). Radiological assessment of osteoarthritis. *Ann Rheum Dis*, **16**, 494–501.

5. Spector, T.D. and Cooper, C. (1994). Radiological assessment of osteoarthritis in population studies: whither Kellgren and Lawrence? *Osteoarthritis Cart*, **1**, 203–6.

6. Kellgren, J.H., Jeffrey, M.R., and Ball, J. (1963). *The epidemiology of chronic rheumatism: atlas of standard radiographs, vol 2*. Blackwell Scientific, Oxford.

7. Lawrence, J.S. (1977). *Rheumatism in populations*, pp. 99–100. Heinemann, London.

8. Wood, P.H.N. (1976). Osteoarthritis in the community. *Clinics Rheum Dis*, **2**, 495–507.

9. Spector, T.D. and Hochberg, M.C. (1994). Methodological problems in the epidemiological study of osteoarthritis. *Ann Rheum Dis*, **53**, 143–6.

10. Bellamy, N., Bennett, P.H., and Burch, T.A. (1967). New York Symposium on Population Studies in Rheumatic Diseases: new diagnostic criteria. *Bulletin of the Rheumatic Disease*, **17**, 453–8.

11. Dieppe, P. and Kirwan, J. (1994). The localisation of osteoarthritis. *B J Rheum*, **33**, 201–4.

12. Hernborg, J. and Nilsson, B.E. (1973). The relationship between osteophytes in the knee joint, osteoarthritis and aging. *Acta Orthop Scan*, **44**, 69–74.

13. Brandt, K.D., Fife, R.S., Braunstein, E.M., and Katz, B. (1991). Radiographic grading of the severity of knee osteoarthritis: relation of the Kellgren and Lawrence grade to a grade based on joint space narrowing, and correlation with arthroscopic evidence of articular cartilage degeneration. *Arthritis Rheum*, **34**, 1381–6.

14. Resnick, D. and Niwayama, G. (1988). *Diagnosis of bone and joint disorders* (2nd edn), p. 1448. W.B. Saunders, Philadelphia.

15. Reiff, D.B., Heron, C.W., and Stoker, D.J. (1991). Spiking of the tubercles of the intercondylar eminence of the tibial plateau in osteoarthritis. *Br J Radiol*, **64**, 915–17.

16. Donelly, S., Hart, D.J., Doyle, D.V., and Spector, T.D. (1996). Spiking of the tibial tubercles — a radiological feature of osteoarthritis? *Ann Rheum Dis*, **55**, 105–8.

17. Egger, P., Cooper, C., Hart, D.J., Doyle, D.V., Coggon, D., and Spector, T.D. (1995). Patterns of joint involvement in osteoarthritis of the hand: the Chingford Study. *J Rheumatol*, **22**, 1509–13.

18. Hart, D.J., Spector, T.D., Egger, P., Coggon, D., and Cooper, C. (1994). Defining osteoarthritis of the hand for epidemiological studies: the Chingford Study. *Ann Rheum Dis*, **53**, 220–3.

19. Rosenberg, T.D., Paulos, L.E., Parker, R.D., Coward, D.B., and Scott, S.M. (1988). The 45 degree posterior-anterior flexion weightbearing radiographs of the knee. *J Bone Joint Surg*, **70A**, 1479–83.

20. Jones, A.C., Ledingham, J., McAlindon, T., *et al.* (1993). Radiographic assessment of patellofemoral osteoarthritis. *Ann Rheum Dis*, **52**, 655–8.

21. Ciccuttini, F.M., Baker, J., Hart, D.J., and Spector, T.D. (1996). Choosing the best method of radiological assessment of patello-femoral arthritis. *Ann Rheum Dis*, **55**, 134–6.

22. Kallman, D.A., Wigley, F.M., Scott, W.W., *et al.* (1989). New radiographic grading scales of osteoarthritis of the hand. *Arthritis Rheum*, **32**, 1584–91.

23. Hart, D.J., Harris, P.A., and Chamberlain, A. (1993). Reliability and reproducibility of grading radiographs for osteoarthritis of the hand. *B J Rheum*, **32 S1**, 137.

24. Scott, J.C., Nevitt, M.C., Lane, H.K., *et al.* (1992). Association of individual radiographic features of hip osteoarthritis with pain. *Arthritis Rheum*, **35** (**suppl**), s81.

25. Ahlback, S. (1968). Osteoarthritis of the knee: a radiographic investigation. *Acta Radiologica*, (suppl) **277**, 7–72.

26. Spector, T.D., Cooper, C., Cushnaghan, J., *et al.* (1992). A radiographic atlas of knee osteoarthritis. Springer Verlag, London.

27. Burnett, S.J., Hart, D.J., Cooper, C., and Spector, T.D. (1994). A radiographic atlas of osteoarthritis. Springer Verlag, London.

28. Cooper, C., Cushnaghan, J., Kirwan, J., *et al.* (1992). Radiological assessment of the knee joint in osteoarthritis. *Ann Rheum Dis*, **51**, 80–2.

29. Cooper, C., McAlindon, T., Snow, S., *et al.* (1994). Mechanical and constitutional risk factors for symptomatic knee osteoarthritis: differences between medial, tibio-femoral and patello-femoral disease. *J Rheumatol*, **21**, 307–13.

30. Dacre, J.E. and Huskisson, E.C. (1989). The automatic assessment of knee radiographs in osteoarthritis using digital image analysis. *B J Rheum*, **28**, 506–10.

31. Scott, W.W., Lethbridge-cejku, M., Reichle, R., Wigley, F.M., Tobin, J., and Hochberg, M.C. (1993). Reliability of grading scales for individual radiographic features of osteoarthritis of the knee. *Invest Radiol*, **28**, 497–501.

32. Spector, T.D. (1995). Measuring joint space in knee osteoarthritis: position or precision? *J Rheumatol*, **22**, 807–8.

33. Buckland-Wright, C., Macfarlane, D., Williams, S., and Ward, R. (1995). Joint space width measured more accurately and precisely in semi-flexed than extended view of OA Knees. *B J Rheum*, (**s1**)**34**, 121.

34. Altman, R.D., Fries, J.F., Bloch, D., *et al.* (1987). Radiographic assessment of progression in osteoarthritis. *Arthritis Rheum*, **30**, 1214–25.

35. Lane, N.E., Nevitt, M.C., Genant, H.K., *et al.* (1993). Reliability of new indicies of radiolographic OA of the hand and hip and lumbar disc degeneration. *J Rheumatol*, **20**, 1911–18.

36. Dieppe, P., Brandt, K.D., Lohmander, S., and Felson, D.T. (1995). Detecting and measuring disease modification in osteoarthritis. The need for standardized methodology. *J Rheumatol*, **22**, 201–3.

37. Dieppe, P.A. (1995). Recommended methodology for assessing the progression of osteoarthritis of the hip and knee joints. *Osteoarthritis Cart*, **3**, 73–7.

38. Kuettner, K.E. and Goldberg, V.M. (ed.) (1994). *Osteoarthritis disorders: workshop, Monterey, California*, pp. 481–96. American Academy of Orthopedic Surgeons.

39. Altman, R.D., Hochberg, M., Murphy, W.A. *et al.* (1995). Atlas of individual radiographic features in osteoarthritis. *Osteoarthritis and Cart*, **3** (**suppl A**), 3–70.

11.5.2 Quantitation of radiographic changes
J. Christopher Buckland-Wright

Radiography is the easiest way to identify the anatomical changes in joint structure that confirm the existence of osteoarthritis (OA). This characteristic, together with the ready availability and ease of interpretation of radiographs, has led to its use as the principal method for imaging OA joints. The features described in the pathology of the disease can be readily visualized, with joint space narrowing corresponding to cartilage loss[1,2] and subchondral sclerosis and osteophyte formation corresponding to the bone's response to the increased mechanical load consequent upon cartilage degeneration and loss[3]. Based upon pathological changes observed in OA joints, these radiographic features are considered specific to OA and have been used for diagnosis[4] and in clinical studies to classify the baseline status of the disease[5].

Results of standard radiography

Methods for assessing disease progression have been based upon scoring several radiographic features in parallel. Longitudinal studies[6,7] of the radiographic changes seen following the administration of non-steroidal anti-inflammatory drugs (NSAIDs) to patients with OA of the knee, showed no radiographic progression after two years and only minimal changes between treatment groups. The absence of significant changes in these investigations, and in other longitudinal studies of the knee[8,9], has led to the suggestion that radiographic features in OA joints remain relatively stable for long periods of time[6] and to the proposal that more sensitive techniques, such as microfocal radiography, should be evaluated[6,10].

Results of macroradiography

Microfocal radiography[11,12] utilizes a micron-sized X-ray source, permitting the object under examination to be placed close to the X-ray tube. The film is placed at 1–2 meters distance from the object, resulting in magnification (macroradiography) of the image with high spatial resolution. Such techniques have been used widely in both the United States[13] and Japan[14]. The work carried out by groups in those countries failed, however, largely due to limitations in the design of their X-ray machines, in which the minute size of the X-ray source could not be maintained. Furthermore, the macroradiographs which were obtained tended to be restricted both in their radiographic magnification (usually ×4, rarely ×6) and spatial resolution[11,12]. The design of the British tube[11,12] is based on a different approach, which ensures that the micron-sized X-ray source is retained throughout the life of the machine. These instruments are capable of producing radiographs of most parts of the human body at higher magnifications (from ×5 to ×20) and at a spatial resolution (25–50 μm) approximating that of histology[11,12]. The cost of the equipment, approximately £100 000 (including the patient table and fluoroscopic facility), is comparable to that of a good conventional X-ray unit.

Quantitative microfocal radiology[11,12] has been shown to be sufficiently sensitive to detect small changes in joint structure, so disease progression and drug effects can be recorded and accurately measured in a relatively short span of time[15-19]. This has been achieved through improvement in data quality, obtained by the use of high definition macroradiographs which record much finer structural detail[12] than standard radiographs and from the precision resulting from standardization of both radiographic and mensural procedures[20,21].

This chapter reviews the current procedures for standard radiography of OA joints (which make reliable measurements of radiographic features difficult) and the inconsistencies that are present in the methods for measuring radiographic features. Methods are described which standardize the radiographic and mensural procedures necessary to measure anatomical features recorded in standard radiographs of OA joints, to permit quantification of radiographic changes.

Problems in taking radiographic measurements

Several steps in the production of a standard radiograph make it difficult to ensure quality control:

1. The clinician making the request may not indicate precisely what is required (images of many OA knees are still obtained with the subject lying down).

2. The radiology technician performing the examination may have his or her own idiosyncratic methods of positioning patients, especially when faced with someone who has difficulty standing or walking.

3. The person making the measurements may be unaware of what has gone on beforehand.

   In addition to the variability due to the number of personnel involved, variability within the radiographic and mensural processes can lead to errors in assessment of the dimensions of features recorded in the radiographs.

Limitations in radiographic procedures

Radio-anatomical position

Without the use of special stereotaxic devices for examining leg alignment[22] or knee joint motion[23], there is no accepted method for positioning a joint for radiography which ensures that it is in precisely the same position for each patient and on successive occasions.

The present lack of protocols for radio-anatomical positioning of joints is evidenced by the variety of positions described for the anteroposterior view of the knee: this is most often taken in weight bearing, with the joint fully extended[24]. Although this view is occasionally specified[25], many studies fail to define the radiographic position of the joint[26-28]. Other views of the knee, in the standing-tunnel[29,30] or non-weight-bearing tunnel[31] position, have been recommended as providing more reliable assessment of joint space loss. This absence of a standard radio-anatomical position results in variable radiographic images of joints within and between patients (Fig. 11.8), compromising reliability

in assessments of the disease status of a joint, either for inclusion in a study or for quantifying the radiographic features of OA.

X-ray beam alignment

Another important variable is the position of the central ray of the X-ray beam relative to the center of the joint, that is, the joint space. Changes in the beam angle lead to partial overlapping of the anterior and posterior edges of a joint margin, obscuring the joint space and preventing accurate and reproducible serial measurements of bony features and joint space width (Fig. 11.8). Indeed, Fife *et al.*[25] found a marked decrease in joint space width in the knee when the X-ray beam was displaced by 1 cm from its original alignment centered at the mid-point of the patella.

Radiographic magnification

Radiographic magnification is not generally taken into account[32]. The distance between the center of a joint and the X-ray film will affect the degree of magnification which occurs in radiography. In an assessment of standard radiographs of the knee obtained in the standing extended view, the magnification was found to range from ×1.09 to ×1.35[33]. In knee or hip radiography, the distance between the center of the joint and the X-ray film can be large, and is influenced by factors such as obesity or restriction of joint movement from pain or osteophytosis. The common practice of assuming radiographic magnification in large joints to be ×1.0 leads to imprecise and inaccurate measurements of the joint space width — a surrogate for the thickness of articular cartilage[33].

Limitations in measurement procedures

Methods of measurement

Semiquantitative grading systems based on global scoring of the radiographic features[4] are still widely used to assess disease progression but suffer from two limitations, which are based on the following assumptions:

1. The change in any one radiographic feature is linear and constant during the course of disease progression.

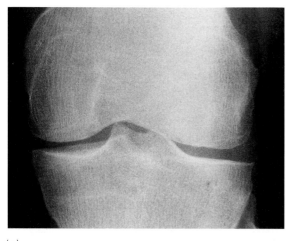

(a)

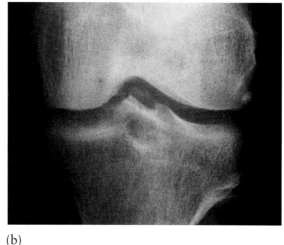

(b)

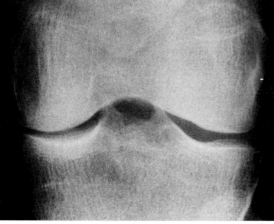

(c)

Fig. 11.8 Standard antero-posterior radiographs of different OA knee joints in the standing, fully extended view, illustrating the different radio-anatomical positions of the joint obtained in this position. Note that in each of the radiographs, the anterior and posterior margins of the tibial plateau in the medial compartment (left) are at different levels. Such variability makes it difficult to obtain accurate and precise measurements of either joint space width or other radiographic features.

2. The relationship between the different radiographic features is constant.

Therefore, these grading systems fail to take into account that different radiographic features may progress at different rates and at different times. As a consequence, recent workers[34–37] have turned to scoring individual radiographic features of OA, for example, joint space narrowing, osteophytes, subchondral sclerosis, and cyst formation. These methods remain susceptible, however, to fairly high levels of interobserver variation.

To determine the sensitivity of each of the radiographic features, far better knowledge is required of the natural history and outcome of the disease, of which little is known at present[38]. As already described,

measurement of radiographic features is dependent not only upon image quality but also upon the measurement procedure[32,39]. The latter varies among investigators; some do not describe their methods[6,27], others use a ruler[40] or calipers[1,41] and or a magnifying lens with a fitted graticule[42]. Measurement reproducibility is greatest with computerized techniques using digitally stored radiographic images[21,26], where inter- and intraobserver variability is virtually eliminated[21].

Landmarks for measurements

The selection of anatomical landmarks used to define the boundaries for measurements of radiographic features of OA can vary, and depend on the individual interpretation of the investigator. For example, measurements across the joint space may be taken either as a direct assessment of its width at (1) the mid-point; (2) the narrowest part of the joint space; (3) the sum of the distances measured in the medial and lateral tibiofemoral compartments within a knee[40]; or, as an assessment of the area between the bony margins, either as a 1 cm wide area[26], the mean joint space area within an anatomic compartment[43], or the sum of four equally spaced joint space width measurements in the hip[44]. Usually, the precise boundaries for this or other bony parameters have not been defined in published analyses.

Standardization of radiographic procedures

Protocols for OA joints

Protocols for precise radio-anatomical positioning of joints are essential if disease-related changes in joint anatomy are to be reliably assessed from sequential radiographic examinations. It cannot be emphasized strongly enough that their use is essential to maintain quality control in a procedure which involves several isolated steps with respect both to the number of personnel involved and the technical procedure. Indeed, worthwhile radiographic assessment for therapeutic trials require protocols defining the precise position of the joint, standard criteria for X-ray beam alignment, allowance for inherent radiographic magnification, and precise definition of anatomical boundaries for measurements of radiographic features. The following principles form the basis for such protocol:

1. The radio-anatomical position of a joint must occupy a plane in which the central ray of the X-ray beam will pass between the margins of the joint space, so that both margins and the space are optimally defined in a position consistent with the functional loading of that joint.

2. Standardization of the radio-anatomical position should ensure:
   (a) that the radiographic features to be evaluated can be assessed accurately and reproducibly in the same plane and on successive occasions;
   (b) that the dimensions obtained for the radiographic feature are accurately recorded in the

image, and are neither an underestimation nor overestimation of its actual size.

The rationale for the radio-anatomical position for the hand, knee, and hip is outlined in the following sections. Protocols for standard radiography of each joint are described in Appendix 5.

Dorsi-palmar radiography of the wrist and hand

In hand OA, joint space width is evaluated in joints from which cartilage loss may be uneven. Spreading the fingers will alter joint alignment, and can lead to an incorrect assessment of joint space narrowing. Fingers held together and in line with the axis of the wrist and forearm (Fig. 11.9) when laid flat on the X-ray film holder, will be under the combined action of both the flexor and extensor groups of the finger muscles. Thus, each joint will be under muscular load along its own axis, providing a reproducible method for evaluating the joint space.

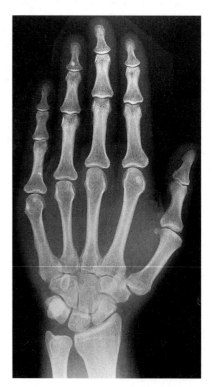

Fig. 11.9 Standard dorsi-palmar radiograph of a wrist and hand, with the fingers held in line with the axis of the wrist and forearm.

Knee radiography

The knee is one of the most difficult joints to examine well, radiographically, because of its structural complexity and wide range of movement. In addition, there is now an awareness that OA may affect different compartments of the joint and may be focally distributed even within compartments[18,45,46]. Recent epidemiological and clinical studies have highlighted the importance of examining the patellofemoral joint in evaluating OA of the knee[46–48]. Indeed, as these authors have shown, patellofemoral, or combined patellofemoral and medial tibiofemoral compartment disease is found in approximately 50 per cent of all patients with knee OA. Therefore, separate protocols describing the radio-anatomic positioning for the tibiofemoral and patellofemoral compartments are described.

Anteroposterior radiography of the tibiofemoral compartment

The standing, semiflexed anteroposterior view of the tibiofemoral compartment is the most reliable view for assessment of joint space width[18,21,33]. Each knee is flexed until the tibial plateau is horizontal, relative to the floor, parallel to the central X-ray beam and perpendicular to the X-ray film (Fig. 11.10). The degree of flexion ranges between 179° and 160°, depending on the angle of inclination of the tibial plateau, which varies from person to person. The center of the joint, defined by the joint space, is aligned with the center of the X-ray beam with the aid of the positioning light of the tube. The precise position of the knee is obtained visually with the aid of fluoroscopy. With the heel fixed, the foot is internally or externally rotated until the tibial spines appear centrally, placed relative to the femoral notch (Fig. 11.11). In this position, the joint is close to the normal anatomical standing position, the major contact stress points are opposed[49], and the surface of the tibial plateau is horizontal, parallel to the central ray of the X-ray beam and perpendicular to the X-ray film (Figs 11.10 and 11.11).

Axial radiography of the patellofemoral compartment

Examination of the patellofemoral joint in the axial or skyline view can be obtained using Ahlback's method[24], with the patient standing and the knee flexed to 30° from the vertical (Figs 11.12 and 11.13). In this

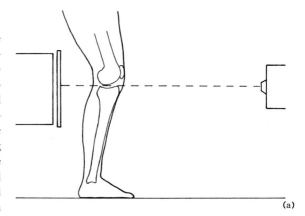

(a)

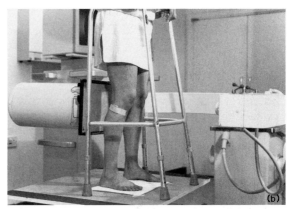

(b)

Fig. 11.10 (a) Diagram of the leg in the standing, semiflexed position, and its position relative to the X-ray tube on the right and the film cassette, placed in front of the image intensifier tube, to the left. In this position, the tibial plateau is horizontal, parallel to the central X-ray beam (broken line), and perpendicular to the X-ray film. (b) General view of the X-ray equipment for this view of the knee. The metal sphere is taped to the side of the knee. With this equipment, it has been necessary to use a table to raise the subject so that the knees were level with the horizontal X-ray beam.

position, the joint is under functional load, ensuring that the articular surfaces are in close apposition, providing a more reliable assessment of cartilage thickness than when the patient is radiographed in the supine position.

Anteroposterior radiography of the hip

Three factors affect the precision of joint space width assessment in the hip: patient position, limb rotation, and the direction of the center of the X-ray beam:

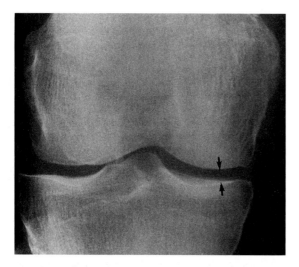

(a)

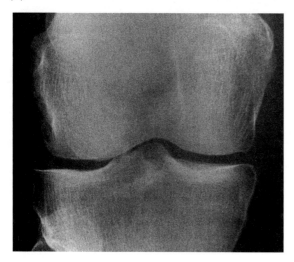

(b)

Fig. 11.11 Standard antero-posterior radiograph of an OA knee in the standing, semiflexed view, imaged on two separate occasions, with the X-ray beam centered on the joint space. The tibial spines are centrally located relative to the femoral notch, and the anterior and posterior margins of the medial compartment (right) are superimposed, illustrating the reproducibility of this view. The position of the minimum joint space width measurement is indicated by the arrows.

1. Recent radiographic studies[50,51], comparing OA hips of the same individuals after examination in both the supine and erect position, have shown that when the joint space is narrower than 2.5 mm, the measured interbone distance was significantly smaller (P < 0.03) when the patient was standing than it was when the subject was lying down.

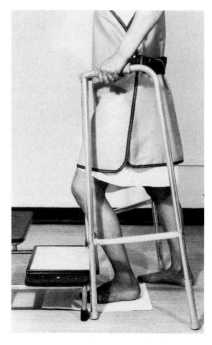

Fig. 11.12 General view showing the position of the patient and associated equipment for a skyline view of the patello-femoral compartment.

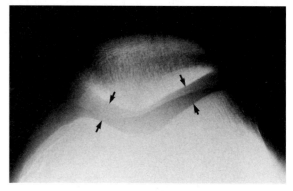

Fig. 11.13 Axial, or skyline, radiograph of a right patello-femoral compartment, with the knee in the standing, semiflexed view. The patello-femoral articular margins used in joint space width measurements are identified by the arrows.

2. Evaluation of the effect of limb rotation at the hip joint in nine cadavers in which radiographs were obtained in internal rotation, external rotation, and midway in a neutral position, showed that the joint space was narrower with the joint internally rotated than in the other positions. With the joint internally rotated, the minimum joint space (mean = 4.1 ± 0.6 mm) was smaller than in the

neutral position (mean = 4.6 ± 0.6 mm, P < 0.01, Wilcoxon signed rank test)[52]. The effect of internal rotation can be attributed to tightening of the powerful lateral rotator muscles of the hip joint, driving the femoral head medially into the acetabulum. Therefore, in those joints in which the status of the articular cartilage is to be assessed, the hip should be radiographed with the patient standing and the feet internally rotated to ensure the femoral head is closely applied to the articular surface of the acetabulum.

3. It has been established[21] that displacement of the X-ray tube away from the center of the joint can significantly alter the measurement of joint space width. It is recommended that the central ray of the X-ray beam be aligned with the center of the femoral head for accurate and precise measurements (Fig. 11.14).

Standardization of methods of measurement

Choosing the correct position for the radiographic examination and ensuring that the procedure used is reproducible, is, although fundamental, still only the starting point for quantifying outcome. The major radiographic features of OA are joint space narrowing,

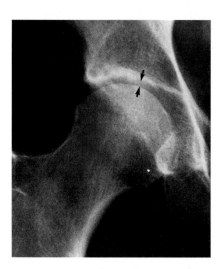

Fig. 11.14 Standard antero-posterior weight-bearing radiograph of an OA hip, taken with 10° of internal rotation of the foot. The position of the minimum joint space width measurement is indicated by the arrows.

osteophytes, subchondral sclerosis, and subchondral cysts. It is generally assumed that evidence of the slowing or of the progression of some, or all, of these features will occur with successful treatment. To detect such changes, measurements must be both accurate and precise.

Accuracy is defined as the agreement between the observed measurement and the true value of the measurement, and is dependent upon the spacial resolution of the radiographic image and the smallest change in the dimensions of a feature that can be measured.

Precision is defined as the reproducibility of a measurement (that is, how close the agreement is between repeat measurements of the same quantity) which is affected by any systematic errors and inter- and intraobserver variability.

Methods of measurement

Direct measurements are made of the area and distance of the radiographic features using either a ruler or magnifying lens fitted with a measuring graticule: these methods are susceptible to observer error and instrument reproducibility. It has been recommended by committees of the World Health Organization (WHO) and the International League of Associated Rheumatologists (ILAR) that manual measurement of joint space width should be performed using Lequesne's method[1,51] in which the points of a pair of dividers are used to measure the interbone distance on the radiograph[1]. The dividers are then used to prick a sheet of paper, and the distance between the center of each pin prick is measured using a x10 magnifying lens fitted with a 10 mm graticule with 0.1 mm divisions. Such assessments have been shown to have an intraobserver coefficient of variation for repeat measures of 3.8 per cent[33]. The development of microcomputers and image analysis techniques has provided a more accurate and reproducible method of measuring changes in joint anatomy than manual methods, and permits the handling of large amounts of numerical data. Measurements of bony changes may be obtained manually using a digitization tablet[20] linked to a microprocessor, but are not as precise as those obtained from digitally stored radiographic images in which the dimensions of specific features, such as joint space, are automatically measured by computer[21,26]. Observer error is virtually eliminated because the precision for repeat measurement is mainly determined by the system and is less than 1 per cent[21,26]. This method also saves a considerable amount of time, and readily lends itself to use in multicenter clinical trials.

Radiographic features to be measured

Should all features be measured in all joints and be given equal importance? The evidence to date suggests that this is not a useful approach because radiographic features of OA are variable, not only between joints (such as hip, hand, and knee[53]) but also within areas of a single joint (such as the tibiofemoral and patellofemoral compartments of the knee[46]). For each joint or compartment, a set of criteria needs to be developed for evaluating outcomes[46,53].

Landmarks for measurement

Joint space width, or interbone distance

Joint space narrowing has been shown to correlate with pathological change in OA cartilage[2] (Fig. 11.15). Because cartilage loss in OA is not uniform across the joint[54], minimum joint space width is the appropriate measurement, as recommended by WHO/ILAR[1]. The boundaries used for measuring this feature in concave-convex joints are:

(1) *for the convex surface*, the distal margin of the condylar cortex (Figs 11.11, 11.13, 11.14, and 11.18);

(2) *for the concave surface*, the margin of the bright radiodense band of the subchondral cortex in the floor of the articular fossa (Figs 11.11, 11.13, 11.14, and 11.18).

Osteophytes

The number of osteophytes can be counted, and their area measured, using either a planimeter or digitizing tablet[20] to trace around their perimeter. Alternatively, an estimate of their size can be obtained from the product of their width and height (Fig. 11.16). Change in osteophyte number and area are sensitive indicators of disease progression[15,16] and has been shown to be useful for assessing drug treatment[19] (Fig. 11.17).

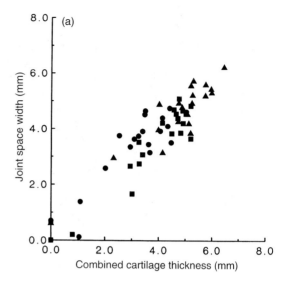

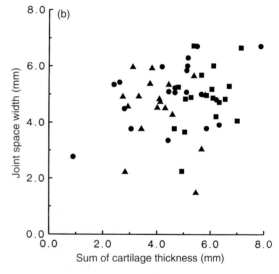

Fig. 11.15 Comparison of the joint space width (JSW) from plain film macroradiographs and the sum of femoral and tibial articular cartilages measured from the double contrast macroradiographs at the outer (●), middle (■), and inner (▲) sites in the (a) medial and (b) lateral tibiofemoral compartments. In the diseased medial compartment, JSW reliably measured cartilage thickness (correlation coefficient r > 0.91); the poor association between the two parameters in the lateral compartment is due to variability in the pattern of articular cartilage loss.

Subchondral sclerosis

Changes in the integrity of the articular cartilage, that precede physical loss of the cartilage (which is recognized radiographically as joint space narrowing), may result in thickening of both the cortical and trabecular

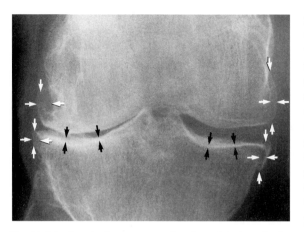

Fig. 11.16 Standard antero-posterior view of the knee in the standing, semiflexed position. The dimensions of the width and height of marginal osteophytes are indicated by the white arrows, and the thickness of the tibial subchondral cortex by the black arrows.

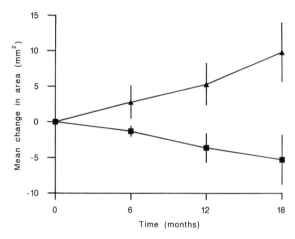

Fig. 11.17 Graph of the mean (SD) change in osteophyte area, at each 6-monthly visit, in knees with early OA (joint space width > 2 mm), of patients receiving either NSAID (■) or placebo (▲). Although the osteophyte size in the placebo group had increased significantly, by the end of 18 months, the treatment groups were not statistically significantly different, since their values lay within two standard deviations.

bone adjacent to the cartilage[17,18]. The thickness of the subchondral cortex at the convex and concave articular surfaces (Fig. 11.16 and 11.18) can be measured, for example, at three equidistant points along the joint margin, and the readings can then be averaged[15,17,18].

Juxta-articular radiolucencies

Although these features are referred to as 'erosions' by Altman *et al.*[53], the term 'juxta-articular radiolucencies'

is preferred, since the precise histopathologic characteristics of these radiographic features are, as yet, unknown. Although similar in distribution and appearance to the bony defects seen in rheumatoid arthritis[55], in patients with OA, these defects are smaller and the surrounding bone is not osteopenic (Fig. 11.18). These lucencies, which may be seen in the early stages of OA[15], appear to be associated with synovial inflammation[56], and have been described in OA of the hand[15,53] and larger joints[57]. Their number and size can be measured by using methods similar to those for osteophytes or by devising a transparent template with a spectrum of hole sizes, which can be placed over the radiograph.

Subchondral cysts

These lesions differ from the juxta-articular radiolucencies described above, insofar as they have a cavity with a clearly defined sclerotic margin. They tend to be located within bone of the load-bearing surface in joints with advanced disease and marked loss of joint space. Cysts appear to be more frequent in OA of the hip than in OA of other joints. Their number and size can be measured by using methods similar to those for juxta-articular radiolucencies.

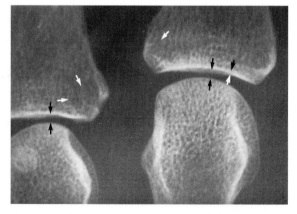

Fig. 11.18 Part of a macroradiograph of the metacarpophalangeal joints from a patient with hand OA, showing joint space narrowing, subchondral sclerosis, and large juxta-articular radiolucencies (white arrows). The position of the minimum joint space width measurement is indicated by the black arrows, and the thickness of the subchondral cortex by the black and white arrows on the right.

Effect of protocols upon measurement accuracy and precision

The effect of protocols for standardization of radiographic and mensural procedures upon the accuracy and precision of computerized measurement of minimum joint space width in the tibiofemoral compartment of the knee was assessed in the standing, semiflexed view for both standard and macroradiography of the knee. These findings were compared with the manual measurement of minimum joint space width in the standing, extended view of the knee, without correction for radiographic magnification. Twenty-five patients with knee OA and 10 subjects of similar age and sex, had standard and microfocal radiographs taken of the knee in both views, twice on the same day, and again, two weeks later. For each of the procedural comparisons listed in Table 11.7, reproducibility was calculated as the standard deviation in the four similar measurements for each knee, and accuracy as the mean absolute error with respect to the mean macroradiographic measurement. To assess improvement in reproducibility and accuracy of joint space width measurements between pairs of methods (Table 11.7), the respective difference between standard deviations and mean errors, obtained from those methods, were calculated.

The median differences are shown in Table 11.7. Although a more detailed explanation for the findings is presented elsewhere[33], the results show that for measurement of medial compartment joint space width, computerized was more accurate than manual; correction for radiographic magnification improved precision and accuracy; measurements in the semiflexed view were more precise and accurate than those in the standing position; and macroradiography increased measurement precision over that which could be achieved by standard radiography. In the lateral compartment, both the reproducibility and accuracy of measurements of joint space width were poor[33]. This is attributed to a variable pattern of joint space narrowing in this compartment, because cartilage loss can occur at either the inner or outer regions of the compartment[2].

Quantifying outcome

Sensitivity of radiographic features

Quantitative evaluation of the presence, extent, and progression of the different radiographic features have shown that in hand and knee OA[15-19], the most sensitive radiographic parameters for detecting the *presence* of OA disease are osteophytes, subchondral sclerosis, and juxta-articular radiolucencies. The only reliable and sensitive parameters for assessing disease *pro-*

Table 11.7 Pairwise comparisons showing the improvements in medial compartment joint space width measurement precision and accuracy for the four procedural modifications listed under the comparison.

Comparison	Knee group	No.	Precision of measurements; median improvement in SD[+] (95% confidence interval)		Accuracy of measurements; median improvement in mean error (95% confidence interval)	
Computerized over manual measurement	OA	25	−0.054 mm	(−0.169, 0.056)	0.436 mm[***]	(0.330, 0.874)
	Control	10	0.078 mm	(−0.116, 0.283)	0.034 mm	(−0.316, 0.880)
Magnification corrected over uncorrected	OA	25	0.067 mm[***]	(0.002, 0.125)	0.507 mm[***]	(0.275, 0.631)
	Control	10	0.046 mm	(−0.047, 0.304)	0.752 mm[***]	(0.566, 0.931)
Semiflexed over fully extended view	OA	25	0.079 mm[*]	(−0.023, 0.143)	0.123 mm[*]	(−0.072, 0.380)
	Control	10	0.102 mm[***]	(0.032, 0.354)	0.287 mm[***]	(−0.071, 0.681)
Microfocal over standard radiography	OA	25	0.072 mm[***]	(0.008, 0.173)	§	§
	Control	10	0.063 mm[**]	(−0.019, 0.154)	§	§

[*] $0.05 < P < 0.1$; [**] $0.01 < P << 0.05$; [***] $P < 0.01$ (Wilcoxon's matched pairs signed rank sum test).
[+]: standard deviation.
[§]: No comparison could be made between the accuracies of microfocal and conventional radiography protocols, since the results of the former protocol provided the standard for assessment of accuracy.

gression were changes in the number and size of osteophytes (Fig. 11.17) and joint space narrowing (Fig. 11.19). These observations indicate that in OA, bony changes appear to develop ahead of articular cartilage destruction, measured as joint space narrowing, and tend to support the hypothesis[15–18] that the bony features occur in association with the onset of biochemical and degenerative changes in articular cartilage[58]. In OA joints, different rates of joint space loss have been obtained by different investigators[1]. This variability may be attributed to the numbers of patients with either early or advanced disease in the study populations, insofar as it has been shown recently[19] that the rate of cartilage loss in knees with early disease is slower than in those with more advanced disease (Fig. 11.19).

Minimum interval change in joint space width measurement

Based on the results of the assessment of accuracy and reproducibility of joint space width measurements[33], it has been possible to calculate the minimum interval change in the medial compartment joint space width that can be measured with 95 per cent confidence in standard radiographs of the knee in the semiflexed position. In OA knees, over a broad range of disease severity (Kellgren and Lawrence grade 0–III)[4], this was found to be 9–15 per cent of the minimum joint space width. For macroradiography, the corresponding value was 4–9 per cent[33]. For both standard radiography and macroradiography, these figures are within the range of clinical usefulness for detecting cartilage loss over time in the medial tibiofemoral compartment of patients with OA.

Power calculations

The number of knees required for study of a DMOAD, in patients with early knee OA, that is, those most likely to respond to treatment[17,23], can be calculated from the standard deviation of the method used to measure joint space width[31] and the mean annual rate of joint space loss. These values were determined recently from macroradiographs of knees of subjects in the placebo group of an 18-month study of an NSAID[19]. For the analysis, 15 patients were selected who had early OA in the medial tibiofemoral compart-

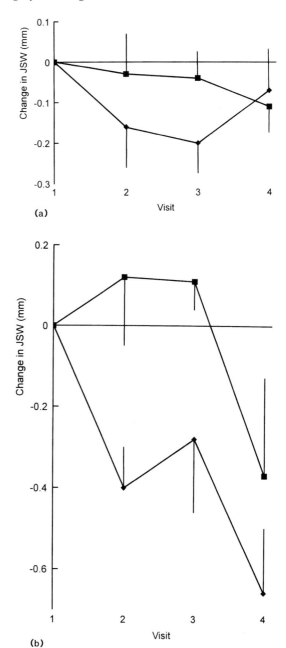

Fig. 11.19 Graphs of the mean (SD) change in joint space width (JSW) in the medial tibiofemoral compartment, at each 6-monthly visit, in knees with (a) early OA in the medial compartment (joint space width > 2 mm) and (b) late stage OA (joint space width < 2 mm), of patients receiving either a nonsteroidal anti-inflammatory drug (♦) or placebo (■)[17].

ment. All subjects had a history of pain in the target joint for at least 15 days of one month, radiographic evidence of osteophytosis and subchondral sclerosis, and a medial tibiofemoral compartment joint space width greater than 2 mm at the onset of the study. If the joint space width of both knees was greater than 2 mm, the knee with the smaller joint space was selected as the target joint, on the premise that it would be more likely to show progression of OA than a knee with greater cartilage thickness. The results of the analysis yielded a mean annual rate of joint space narrowing of 0.183 mm, with an associated standard deviation of 0.196 mm.

Using the above results, it is possible to estimate the total number of knees that would be needed to detect a significant difference in minimum medial compartment joint space width in a double-blind study of two years' duration which compared an active agent against placebo in treatment groups of equal size. Table 11.8 shows the results of such estimates. For example, for a DMOAD which resulted in a 50 per cent reduction in the rate of joint space loss, in comparison with the placebo, 40 knees per treatment group would be required to detect that drug effect with 90 per cent power at a significance level of p = 0.05, if computer measurements of joint space width were made on macrographs obtained with the patient in the standing, semiflexed position. In contrast, if standard radiographs were obtained (instead of macroradiographs), the required sample size would increase to 67 knees per treatment group.

It should be emphasized that the estimates of sample size required for a clinical trial of a DMOAD shown in Table 11.8 are based upon rates of joint space narrow-

ing and values for standard deviation of joint space width determined from analysis of a sample of only 15 knees; additional studies, employing larger numbers of subjects, are needed to determine the accuracy of these estimates. The numbers provided in Table 11.8, therefore, represent only a 'best guess' of required sample sizes. On the other hand, they provide an indication of the reduction in sample size that may be afforded by the use of macroradiography, in comparison with standard radiography.

In evaluating the different radiographic features of OA, the stage of the disease in the patients recruited and the duration of the study need to be controlled because they are variables which will influence the interpretation of the outcome measures. When the complexity of such an undertaking is considered in the light of what has been done to date, it becomes apparent that most imaging studies in OA have been technically flawed, so that even the simplest of clinical dogma, such as the statement, 'there is a poor correlation between symptoms and X-ray findings in OA'[38] must be re-evaluated. There may well be an excellent correlation if the correct views and appropriate measures are made at the correct time. Indeed, our preliminary findings indicate that growth of osteophytes correlates with joint pain[59]. In the future, real progress in the radiographic assessment of the efficacy of DMOADs will only be made by rigorous application of scientific methods of radioanatomic positioning of joints and of X-ray image analysis.

Table 11.8   Number of knees required for a 2-year clinical trial of a DMOAD in patients with early OA (JSW[‡] > 2 mm), using computerized measurement of minimum JSW from standard[*] radiographs and macroradiographs[**] of joints in the standing semiflexed position

X-ray technique	Power	Therapeutic effect[†]		
		30%	50%	80%
Standard radiography	95%	460	163	66
	90%	372	134	52
	80%	278	100	40
Macro-radiography	95%	274	100	40
	90%	222	80	32
	80%	166	60	24

† The therapeutic effect (the difference in joint space narrowing in the experimental group compared to that in the placebo group) is expressed as a % of joint space narrowing in the placebo group. For each effect size, the required number of knees has been determined[60] for each level of power shown, at a significance of P = 0.05.
‡JSW: joint space width
Mean annual rate of joint space narrowing (μ) = 0.183 mm/yr[19].
*with standard deviation for JSW measurement using standard radiography = 0.249 mm[33].
**with standard deviation for JSW measurement using macroradiography = 0.196 mm[19].

References

1. Lequesne, M., Brandt, K., Bellamy, R., Moskowitz, R., Menkes, C.J., and Pelletier, J-P. (1994). Guidelines for testing slow acting drugs in OA. Proceedings Vth joint WHO and ILAR task force meeting. *J Rheumatol*, **21 (suppl 41)**, 65–73.

2. Buckland-Wright, J.C., Macfarlane, D.G., Lynch, J.A., Jasani, M.K., and Bradshaw, C.R. (1995). Joint space width measures cartilage thickness in osteoarthritis of the knee: high resolution plain film and double contrast macroradiographic investigation. *Ann Rheum Dis*, **54**, 263–8.

3. Resnick, D. and Niwayama, G. (1995). *Degenerative disease of extraspinal locations; diagnosis of bone and joint disorders* (2nd edn) (ed. D. Resnick and G. Niwayama), pp. 1365–479. W.B. Saunders, Philadelphia.

4. Kellgren, J.H. and Lawrence, J.S. (1957). Radiological assessment of osteoarthrosis. *Ann Rheum Dis*, **16**, 494–501.

5. Larsen, A. (1982). Radiographic evaluation of osteoarthritis in therapeutic trials. In *Degenerative joints, test tubes, tissues, models, man* (ed. G. Verbruggen and E.M. Veys), pp. 179–82. Excerpta Medica, Amsterdam.

6. Dieppe, P., Cushnaghan, J., Jasani, M.K., McCrae, F., and Watt, I. (1993). A two-year, placebo-controlled trial of non-steroidal anti-inflammatory therapy in osteoarthritis of the knee joint. *Br J Rheumatol*, **32**, 595–600.

7. Williams, H.J., Ward, J.R., Egger, M.J., Neuner, R., Brooks, R.H., Clegg, D.O., *et al.* (1993). Comparison of naproxen and acetaminophen in a two-year study of treatment of osteoarthritis of the knee. *Arthritis Rheum*, **36**, 1196–206.

8. Massardo, L., Watt, I., Cushnaghan, J., and Dieppe, P. (1989). Osteoarthritis of the knee joint: an eight year prospective study. *Ann Rheum Dis*, **48**, 893–7.

9. Spector, T.D., Dacre, J.E., Harris, P.A., and Huskisson, E.C. (1992). Radiological progression of osteoarthritis: an 11-year follow up study of the knee. *Ann Rheum Dis*, **51**, 1107–10.

10. Peyron, J.G. (1991). Clinical features of osteoarthritis, diffuse idiopathic skeletal hyperostosis, and hypermobility syndromes. *Curr Opin Rheumatol*, **3**, 653–61.

11. Buckland-Wright, J.C. (1989). A new high definition microfocal X-ray unit. *Br J Radiol*, **62**, 201–8.

12. Buckland-Wright, J.C. and Bradshaw, C.R. (1989). Clinical applications of high definition microfocal radiography. *Br J Radiol*, **62**, 209–17.

13. Genant, H.K. and Resnick, D. (1995). Magnification radiography. In *Diagnosis of bone and joint disorders* (2nd edn) (ed. D. Resnick and G. Niwayama), pp. 84–107. WB Saunders, Philadelphia.

14. Takahashi, S. and Sakuma, S. (1975). *Magnification radiography*. Springer Verlag, Berlin.

15. Buckland-Wright, J.C., Macfarlane, D.G., Lynch, J.A., and Clark, B. (1990). Quantitative microfocal radiographic assessment of progression in osteoarthritis of the hand. *Arthritis Rheum*, **33**, 57–65.

16. Buckland-Wright, J.C., Macfarlane, D.G., and Lynch, J.A. (1991). Osteophytes in the arthritic hand: their incidence, size, distribution and progression. *Ann Rheum Dis*, **50**, 627–30.

17. Buckland-Wright, J.C., Macfarlane, D.G., and Lynch, J.A. (1992). Relationship between joint space width and subchondral sclerosis in the osteoarthritic hand: a quantitative microfocal study. *J Rheumatol*, **19**, 788–95.

18. Buckland-Wright, J.C., Macfarlane, D.G., Jasani, M.K., and Lynch, J.A. (1994). Quantitative microfocal radiographic assessment of osteoarthritis of the knee from weight bearing tunnel and semi-flexed standing views. *J Rheumatol*, **21**, 1734–41.

19. Buckland-Wright, J.C., Macfarlane, D.G., Lynch, J.A., and Jasani, M.K. (1995). Quantitative microfocal radiography detects changes in OA knee joint space width in patients in placebo-controlled trial of NSAID therapy. *J Rheumatol*, **22**, 937–43.

20. Buckland-Wright, J.C., Carmichael, I., and Walker, S.R. (1986). Quantitative microfocal radiography accurately detects joint changes in rheumatoid arthritis. *Ann Rheum Dis*, **45**, 463–7.

21. Lynch, J.A., Buckland-Wright, J.C., and Macfarlane, D.G. (1993). Precision of joint space width measurement in knee osteoarthritis from digital image analysis of high definition macroradiographs. *Osteoarthritis Cart*, **1**, 209–18.

22. Siu, D., Cooke, T.D.V., Broekhoven, L.D., Lam, M., Fisher, B., Saunders, G., *et al.* (1991). A standardized technique for lower limb radiography, practice, applications and error analysis. *Invest Radiol*, **26**, 71–7.

23. Jonson, H., Karholm, J., and Elmqvist, L-G. (1989). Kinematics of active knee extension after tear of the anterior cruciate ligament. *Am J Sports Med*, **17**, 796–802.

24. Ahlback, S. (1968). Osteoarthritis of the knee: a radiographic investigation. *Acta Radiol*, **277**(suppl), 7–72.

25. Fife, R.S., Brandt, K.D., Braunstein, E.M., Katz, B.P., Shelbourne, K.D., Kalasinski, L.A., *et al.* (1991). Relationship between arthroscopic evidence of cartilage damage and radiographic evidence of joint space narrowing in early osteoarthritis of the knee. *Arthritis Rheum*, **34**, 377–82.

26. Dacre, J.E., Coppock, J.S., Herbert, K.E., Perrett, D., and Huskisson, E.C. (1989). Development of a new radiographic scoring system using digital image analysis. *Ann Rheum Dis*, **48**, 194–200.

27. Dougados, M., Gueguen, A., Nguyen, M., Thiesce, A., Listrat, V., Jacob, L., *et al.* (1992). Longitudinal radiologic evaluation of osteoarthritis of the knee. *J Rheumatol*, **19**, 378–84.

28. Schouten, J.S.A.G., Ouweland, F.A., and van den Valkenburg, H.A. (1992). A 12 year follow up study in the general population on prognostic factors of cartilage loss in osteoarthritis of the knee. *Ann Rheum Dis*, **51**, 932–7.

29. Rosenberg, T.D., Paulos, L.E., Parker, R.D., Coward, D.B., and Scott, S.M. (1988). The forty-five-degree posteroanterior flexion weight-bearing radiograph of the knee. *J Bone Joint Surg*, **70-A**, 1479–83.

30. Messieh, S.S., Fowler, P.J., and Munro, T. (1990). Anteroposterior radiographs of the osteoarthritic knee. *J Bone Joint Surg*, **72-B**, 639–40.

31. Resnick, D. and Vint, V. (1980). The 'tunnel' view in assessment of cartilage loss in osteoarthritis of the knee. *Radiology*, **137**, 547–8.

32. Buckland-Wright, J.C. (1994). Quantitative radiography of osteoarthritis. *Ann Rheum Dis*, **53**, 268–75.

33. Buckland-Wright, J.C., Macfarlane, D.G., Williams, S.A., and Ward, R.J. (1995). Accuracy and precision of joint space width measurements in standard and macroradiographs of osteoarthritic knees. *Ann Rheum Dis*, **54**, 872–80.

34. Spector, T.D., Hart, D.J., Byrne, J., Harris, P.A., Dacre, J.E., and Doyle, D.V. (1993). Definition of osteoarthritis of the knee for epidemiological studies. *Ann Rheum Dis*, **52**, 790–4.

35. Croft, P., Cooper, C., Wickham, C., and Coggon, D. (1990). Defining osteoarthritis of the hip for epidemiological studies. *Am J Epidemiol*, **132**, 514–22.

36. Hart, D., Spector, T., Egger, P., Coggon, D., and Cooper, C. (1994). Defining osteoarthritis of the hand for epidemiological studies: the Chingford study. *Ann Rheum Dis*, **53**, 220–3.

37. Lane, N.E., Nevitt, M.C., Genant, H.K., and Hochberg, M.C. (1993). Reliability of new indices of radiographic osteoarthritis of the hand and hip and lumbar disc degeneration. *J Rheumatol*, **20**, 1911–18.

38. Dieppe, P., Cushnaghan, J., and McAlindon, T. (1992). Epidemiology, clinical course and outcome of knee osteoarthritis. In *Articular cartilage and osteoarthritis* (ed. K. Kuettner, R. Schleyerbach, J.G. Peyron and V.C. Hascall), pp. 617–27. Raven Press, New York.

39. Dieppe, P.A., Brandt, K., Lohmander, S., and Felson, D. (1995). Detecting and measuring modification in osteoarthritis: the need for standardized methodology. *J Rheumatol*, **22**, 201–3.

40. Jonsson, K., Buckwalter, K., Helvie, M., Niklason, L., and Martel, W. (1992). Precision of hyaline cartilage thickness measurements. *Acta Radiol*, **33**, 234–9.

41. Lequesne, M., Winkler, P., Rodriguez, P., and Rahlfs, V.W. (1992). Joint space narrowing in primary osteoarthritis of the hip. Results of a three year controlled trial. *Arthritis Rheum*, **35(suppl 9)**, S135.

42. Laoussadi, S. and Menkes, C.J. (1991). Amélioration de la précision de la mesure visuelle de la hauteur de l'interligne articulaire du genou et de la hanche à l'aide d'une loupe graduée. *Revue du Rhumatism et des Maladies Osteoarticulaires*, **58**, 678.

43. Byrne, J., Heald, G., James, M.F., Kay, M., Shorter, J.H., and Dacre, J.E. (1993). Digital image analysis, a rapid and reproducible method for joint space measurement. *Osteoarthritis Cart*, **1**, 60.

44. Rashad, S., Revell, P., Hemingway, A., Low, F., Rainsford, K., and Walker, F. (1989). Effect of non-steroidal anti-inflammatory drugs on the course of osteoarthritis. *Lancet*, **2**, 519–22.

45. Felson, D.T. and Radin, E.L. (1994). What causes knee osteoarthritis: are different compartments susceptible to different risk factors? *J Rheumatol*, **21**, 181–3.

46. Dieppe, P. and Kirwan, J. (1994). The localization of osteoarthritis. *Br J Rheumatol*, **33**, 201–3.

47. McAlindon, T.E., Snow, S., Cooper, C., and Dieppe, P.A. (1992). Radiographic patterns of the knee joint in the community: the importance of the patello-femoral joint. *Ann Rheum Dis*, **51**, 844–9.

48. McAlindon, T.E., Cooper, C., Kirwan, J., and Dieppe, P.A. (1992). Knee pain and disability in the community. *Br J of Rheumatol*, **31**, 189–92.

49. Maquet, P. (1976). Biomechanics of the knee. Springer-Verlag, Berlin.

50. Conrozier, T., Tron, A.M., Mathieu, P., Vignon, E., and Lequesne, M. (1993). Measurement of x-ray hip joint space in the weight bearing and non weight bearing position. *Revue du Rhumatisme et des Maladies Osteoarticulaires*, *(Engl. ed)*, **60**, 582.

51. Lequesne, M. (1995). Quantitative measurements of joint space during progression of osteoarthritis: chondrometry. *Osteoarthritic disorders*. (ed. K.E. Kuettner and V. Goldberg), pp. 427–44. American Academy of Orthopedic Surgeons, Rosemont.

52. Buckland-Wright, J.C. (1994). Unpublished results.

53. Altman, R., Fries, J.F., Block, D.A., Carstens, J., Cooke, T.D., Genant, H., *et al.* (1987). Radiological assessment of progression in osteoarthritis. *Arthritis Rheum*, **30**, 1214–25.

54. Thomas, R.H., Resnick, D., Alazraki, N.P., Daniel, D., and Greenfield, R. (1975). Compartmental evaluation of osteoarthritis of the knee. A comparative study of available diagnostic modalities. *Radiology*, **116**, 585–94.

55. Buckland-Wright, J.C. and Walker, S.R. (1987). Incidence and size of erosions in the wrist and hand of rheumatoid patients: a quantitative microfocal radiographic study. *Ann Rheum Dis*, **46**, 463–67.

56. Altman, R.D. and Gray, R. (1985). Inflammation in osteoarthritis. *Clin Rheum Dis*, **11**, 353–65.

57. Solomon, L. (1976). Patterns of osteoarthritis of the hip. *J Bone Joint Surg*, **58-B**, 176–83.

58. Mow, V.C., Setton, L.A., Ratcliffe, A., Howell, D.S., and Buckwalter, J. (1990). Structure-function relationships of articular cartilage and the effects of joint instability and trauma on cartilage function. In *Cartilage changes in osteoarthritis*, (ed. K.D. Brandt), pp. 22–42. Indiana University School of Medicine, Indianapolis.

59. Macfarlane, D.G., Buckland-Wright, J.C., Emery, P., Fogelman, I., Clark B., and Lynch, J.A. (1991). Comparison of clinical, radionuclide, and radiographic features of osteoarthritis of the hands. *Ann Rheum Dis*, **50**, 623–6.

60. Bourke, G.J., Daly, L.E., and McGilvray, J. (1985). *Interpretation and uses of medical statistics*. Blackwell, Oxford.

11.5.3 Magnetic resonance imaging
Charles G. Peterfy

Since its development approximately 15 years ago, magnetic resonance imaging (MRI) has become the imaging method of choice for evaluating internal derangements of the knee and other joints. Despite this, however, MRI has, until very recently, played only a minor role in the study of arthritis. This apparent paradox is in part because the MRI techniques originally developed for detecting abnormalities such as meniscal tear and cruciate ligament rupture offered relatively poor contrast among articular cartilage, synovium, and joint fluid, and only limited spatial resolution. Recent improvements in MRI hardware and the development of cartilage-selective techniques, such as fat-suppressed, T1-weighted three-dimensional (3D) gradient echo, and magnetization-transfer subtraction[1-3] (p. 484), have overcome these earlier difficulties and now offer an unprecedented opportunity to evaluate the arthritic joint in ways not imaginable in the past. The advantages of MRI for imaging arthritis include:

- multiplanar 2D and 3D image data

- high resolution capability

- unparalleled soft-tissue contrast allows direct examination of all components of joint

- potential for compositional analysis of tissues

- applicable to longitudinal evaluations

- non-invasive/high patient tolerance

- widely available.

In addition to delineating the anatomy, MRI is capable of quantifying a variety of compositional and functional parameters of articular tissues relevant to the degenerative process and osteoarthritis (OA). Moreover, since MRI is a non-destructive technique, multiple parameters can be analyzed in the same region of tissue and frequent serial examinations can be performed on even asymptomatic patients. These technical capabilities are, furthermore, widely available, and clinical MRI systems found at most major hospitals around the world can perform extremely sophisticated examinations making multi-institutional and even multinational investigations feasible[4]. Finally, as with other maturing technologies, the cost of MRI is rapidly decreasing (Table 11.9).

In addition to market forces, improvements in low-field MRI technology and the recent introduction of small-bore, dedicated extremity imaging systems (Fig. 11.20) have lowered the costs of clinical imaging in some institutions by as much as 50 per cent over the past five years. This trend in affordability will further facilitate the acceptance of MRI as a tool for evaluating arthritis. Therefore, although this particular application of MRI is still in its infancy, it deserves attention now, as it will undoubtedly play an increasingly important role in the development of our understanding of arthritis as well as in our efforts to combat the disease.

This chapter reviews the current status and future directions of MRI in the study of OA, with special emphasis on what is currently deliverable or imminently deliverable in terms of outcome measures for clinical studies.

Table 11.9 Relative costs of imaging the knee

Radiography[a]		$41
CT[b]		$290
Scintigraphy[c]	Conventional	$151
	Tomographic (SPECT)	$330
MRI		$566

Values are from 1995 Medicare fee schedule (technical and professional components) for California (area 5).
[a] Three views with weight-bearing or patellofemoral views.
[b] Knee imaging without contrast.
[c] Values are for imaging a single joint and include radiopharmaceutical administration.

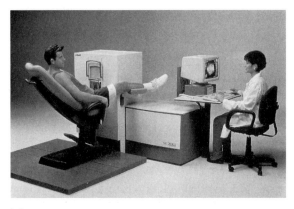

(a)

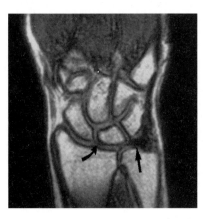

(b)

Fig. 11.20 Dedicated extremity MRI. Recently introduced dedicated extremity MRI systems reduce imaging cost and improve patient comfort and safety. In contrast to conventional whole-body MRI, only the limb is inserted into the dedicated extremity scanner — the remainder of the patient remains outside (a). This obviates problems associated with claustrophobia. The low magnetic field strength virtually eliminates any hazards associated with metallic objects near the magnet or in the patient. Also, dedicated systems cost only a fraction of the cost of whole-body scanners and, because of their small size and light weight, offer convenient and inexpensive siting. In addition to these practical and economic advantages, dedicated extremity MRI provides high quality images of articular anatomy (b). (b): coronal 3D gradient-echo image of a wrist acquired in less than 4 minutes using a dedicated extremity system (Artoscan: Lunar, Madison, WI). Small articular structures, such as the triangular fibrocartilage (*straight arrow*) and the scapholunate ligament (*curved arrow*) are seen well on this image.

MR imaging technique

The clarity and detail with which MRI depicts cross-sectional anatomy makes interpretation of the images

appear deceptively simple. In reality, MRI is a highly sophisticated technology, and while a detailed understanding of quantum physics may not be necessary to view the images, some background knowledge is essential to understand the findings, as well as to critically assess conclusions drawn from investigations that employ this technology. The following brief review of basic principles and terminology used in MRI is provided, therefore, to serve as an aid to understanding the remainder of the chapter. For the interested reader, there are several excellent books and articles that delve deeper into MRI physics and its applications in medicine[5-10].

Basic principles

MR imaging is based on the natural magnetic behavior of atomic nuclei as they spin about their axes (Fig. 11.21). Although a number of different nuclei (for example, sodium, phosphorus, hydrogen) could theoretically be used to generate MR images, only hydrogen is present in sufficient quantities within biological tissues to be feasible for clinical imaging. When the nuclei within a tissue are placed within the very high magnetic field in the bore of an MR imaging magnet, they show a net tendency to align their nuclear mag-

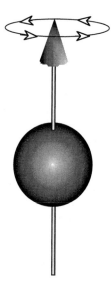

Fig. 11.21 The nuclear magnetic moment. Spinning (precessing) anatomic nuclei ('spins') generate small local magnetic fields analogous to the spinning planets. The magnitude of the magnetic moment depends on the rate of precession, or frequency, of the nucleus. The vector sum of individual magnetic moments for a pool of hydrogen nuclei ('protons') in fat or water is the essential parameter measured in clinical MRI.

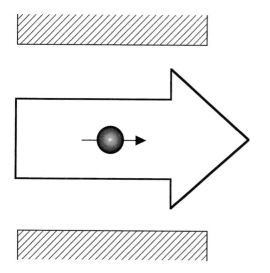

Fig. 11.22 Longitudinal magnetization. Protons placed within the strong magnetic field (*large open arrow*) in the bore of a MRI magnet tend to align their magnetic moments (*small arrow*) with this large magnetic field. The magnitude of this net longitudinal magnetic moment and, therefore, the maximal signal that could be generated during imaging varies directly with the field strength of the MRI magnet.

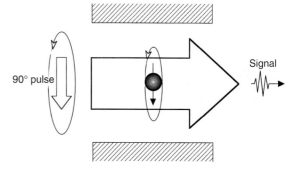

Fig. 11.23 Transverse magnetization. Protons that are longitudinally aligned with the high magnetic field (*large open arrow*) in the MRI magnet bore will realign (resonate) with a second, relatively smaller magnetic field (*small open arrow*) if this new field is tuned to the precessional frequency of these protons. Since this resonant frequency is in the same range as radiowaves, this second field is called a radio-frequency (rf) pulse. If the rf pulse is oriented transverse to the static magnetic field of the MRI magnet, it is said to have a 90° flip angle. If the rf pulse is also made to rotate in the transverse plane, the realigned (flipped) magnetic moment (*small solid arrow*) will also rotate transversely and induce an alternating current (by Faraday's Law) in receiver wires in an imaging coil placed near the patient. This induced current is the basis for the MR image.

netic moments along this static magnetic field (longitudinal magnetization) (Fig. 11.22). Exposure of these protons to a second field (rf pulse) that is rotating and perpendicular to the original static field of the magnet (90° rf pulse), realigns the protons transversely (transverse magnetization) (Fig. 11.23). This rotation of one magnetic field (the proton's) against another (the magnet's) induces an alternating electrical current in receiver coils, near the patient, in proportion to the magnitude of the net magnetic moment of these transversely aligned protons. This signal is then used to generate the MR images by computerized Fourier transformation.

Once the rf pulse is turned off, the protons relax to their original alignment with the static field of the magnet (Fig. 11.24). This process of recovering longitudinal magnetization is called T1 relaxation. T1 relaxation varies from tissue to tissue depending on the microenvironments of the different proton populations. In general, fat shows rapid T1 relaxation, while water shows slow T1 relaxation (Fig. 11.25). Under conditions of rapid rf pulsing (typically, a sequence of 192 to 512 rf pulses is used to generate an MR image), slow-T1 substances, such as water, are not given sufficient time to recover between the pulses and, therefore, exhibit low signal intensity, while fast-T1 substances,

such as fat, show high signal intensity (Fig. 11.25). Short-TR[1] sequences, therefore, generate contrast (relative signal intensity difference) among tissues on the basis of differences in T1, and are accordingly referred to as T1 weighted (Fig. 11.26).

Subtle T1 contrast (for example, between articular cartilage and synovial fluid) is usually overshadowed on T1-weighted images by the far greater difference in signal intensity that exists between fat and most other tissues (Fig. 11.26). However, by selectively suppressing the signal intensity of fat, it is possible to expand the scale of image intensities across smaller differences in T1 and, thus, to augment residual T1 contrast (Fig. 11.27). Another application of fat suppression is to increase contrast between fat and other substances, such as methemoglobin and gadolinium (Gd)-containing contrast material, which also show rapid T1 relaxation. The most widely used technique for fat suppression is based on the chemical-shift phenomenon: since the frequency of protons in fat differ from that of protons in water, the magnetization of fat (or water) can be selectively suppressed by a specifically tuned rf pulse at the beginning of the sequence (Fig. 11.28).

---

[1]The time between repeated 90° rf pulses in an MRI pulse sequence is called the repetition time (TR). The number and duration of the TR are the principal determinants of the imaging time.

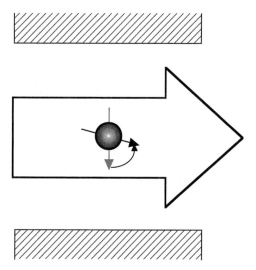

Fig. 11.24   T1 relaxation. When the rotating 90° rf pulse is turned off, the transversely oriented magnetic moment (*small solid arrow*) realigns with the static field of the magnet (*large open arrow*). This recovery of longitudinal magnetization is called T1 relaxation, and the parameter, T1, is a measure of the rate of this recovery. If the 90° rf pulse is repeated before longitudinal magnetization has fully recovered, only this smaller longitudinal component is flipped into the transverse plane and the image signal is correspondingly lower — these protons are said to be partially saturated.

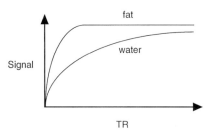

Fig. 11.25   Effect of TR on signal intensity. Repetition time (TR) is the time between successive rf pulses in an imaging sequence. Typically, 192 to 256 repetitions are necessary to generate an MR image. If the TR is less than five times the T1 of a substance, there is insufficient time for complete recovery of longitudinal magnetization and signal intensity is decreased. Therefore, as TR is shortened, substances with long T1 relaxation times (e.g. free water) begin to lose signal first, while substances with short T1 relaxation times (e.g. fat) retain signal until TR is very short. Short-TR sequences thus generate T1 contrast among tissues and are called T1-weighted.

A similar technique can also be used to suppress the signal of water indirectly through a mechanism called magnetization transfer. In this case, direct suppression of tightly constrained protons in macromolecules like collagen, which are thermodynamically coupled to freely mobile protons in bulk water, evokes a transfer of magnetization from the water proton pool to the macromolecular pool, to maintain equilibrium. This manifests as a loss of longitudinal magnetization and, therefore, signal intensity from water, in proportion to the relative concentrations of the two proton pools in the tissue and the specific rate constant for the equilibrium reaction. Since collagen (unlike fat) is strongly coupled to water, in this way, cartilage and muscle exhibit pronounced magnetization transfer effects[3,11-13] (Fig. 11.29). Magnetization-transfer techniques are, therefore, useful for imaging the articular cartilage, and could potentially be used to quantify the collagen content of this tissue.

Image contrast is also influenced by T2 relaxation. This phenomenon manifests as a loss of transverse magnetization and, therefore, signal over time as neighboring protons exposed to the transverse rf pulse gradually fall out of phase with each other. As for T1 relaxation, the rate of T2 relaxation or 'dephasing' of a group of protons, depends on their local microenvironment and, therefore, varies among different tissues. Freely mobile water protons (for example, in synovial fluid) show slow T2 relaxation and, therefore, retain signal over time, while constrained or 'bound' water protons (for example, by collagen or proteoglycan) show rapid T2 relaxation and signal decay (Figs 11.26 and 11.30).

In addition to the effects of neighboring protons on each other (T2 relaxation), fixed magnetic-field heterogeneities in a specimen also cause protons to dephase and lose transverse magnetization. The combined effects of these two causes of proton dephasing and signal loss is called T2* relaxation. Signal lost to fixed magnetic heterogeneity, but not that lost to T2 relaxation, can be recovered by rephasing the protons with a 180° rf pulse (spin echo) or, to a lesser extent, by rapidly reversing the magnetic gradient (gradient echo). Long echo time (TE) sequences thus generate contrast among tissues on the basis of T2 (Figs 11.26 and 11.30), and when combined with a long TR, to minimize the effects of T1 on contrast, are referred to as T2-weighted.

Local perturbations of the magnetic field typically arise at interfaces between substances that differ considerably in magnetic susceptibility (the degree to which a substance magnetizes in the presence of a magnetic field), such as between soft tissue and gas, metal or heavy calcification. Severe T2* at these sites is referred to as magnetic susceptibility effect. Spin-echo

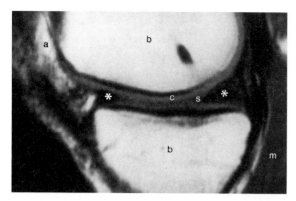

(a)

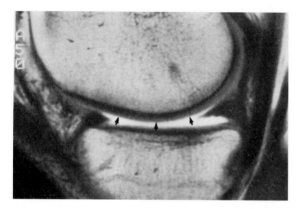

(b)

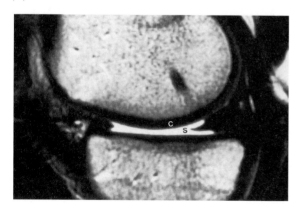

(c)

Fig. 11.26 T-weighted MRI. (a) Sagittal T1-weighted spin-echo image of a knee depicts structures that contain fat (*f*) (short T1) with high signal intensity, and structures that contain water (long T1) with low signal intensity. The small differences in T1 relaxation time among synovial fluid (*s*), articular cartilage (*c*), and muscle (*m*) are not sufficient to generate substantial contrast among these structures on this image. It is difficult, therefore, to delineate the articular cartilage surface. (b) Sagittal T1-weighted image of the same knee following intra-articular injection of Gd-containing contrast material that shortens the T1 of water, depicts the synovial fluid with high signal intensity, and clearly delineates the cartilage-fluid interface (*arrows*). (c) T2-weighted spin-echo image of the same knee before Gd-containing contrast injection depicts fat (relatively short T2) with intermediate signal intensity, and water in synovial fluid (long T2) with high signal intensity. Water in articular cartilage and muscle is relatively bound (short T2); these structures therefore show low signal intensity. High intrinsic contrast between cartilage (*c*) and synovial fluid (*s*) makes this technique useful for delineating the articular surface.

technique corrects for fixed magnetic heterogeneities and, therefore, can provide images with true T2 contrast. Gradient-echo technique is faster than spin echo, but does not correct for these effects and, therefore, provides only T2*-weighted images which are highly vulnerable to magnetic susceptibility effects, such as those caused by metallic prostheses. Magnetic susceptibility effects are more severe on high field strength magnets.

Finally, diffusion of protons (that is, water) within a specimen during the acquisition of an MR image will result in loss of phase coherence among the protons and, therefore, a loss in signal. This effect is usually insignificant in conventional MRI but can be augmented with the use of strong magnetic field gradients such as those employed in MR microimaging. Water diffusivity is, thus, an additional tissue parameter measurable with MRI[14,15] (p. 483).

Both T1-weighting (short TR) and T2-weighting (long TE) involve discarding MR signal. If these effects are eliminated, signal intensity reflects only the proton density. Accordingly, long-TR / short-TE images are often referred to as proton-density-weighted. However, even the shortest finite TE attainable is too long to completely escape T2 relaxation, and extremely long TRs (> 2500 msec) are not practical for imaging *in vivo*. Therefore, even so called proton-density-weighted images contain some T1 and T2 contrast. To generate true proton-density images (for example, for purposes of quantifying water content), multiple scans must be acquired, and TR and TE extrapolated to infinity and zero respectively (p. 483).

The spatial resolution of an MR image is defined by the dimensions of the individual volume elements, or

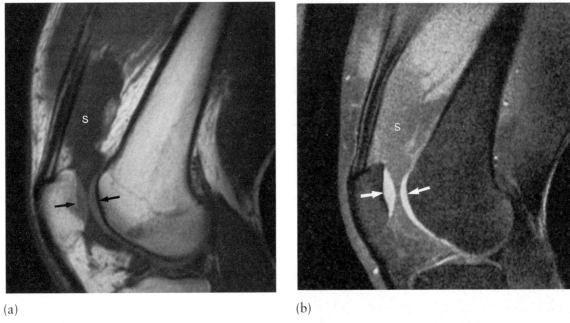

(a)   (b)

Fig. 11.27 Augmenting T1 contrast with fat suppression. (a) Sagittal, T1-weighted spin-echo image of a knee acquired with a somewhat shorter TR (300 msec) than usual (500–700 msec) depicts the articular cartilage (*arrows*) with a slightly higher signal intensity than the adjacent synovial fluid (*s*). Contrast between cartilage and water is greater on this shorter-TR image than on the conventional T1-weighted image shown in Fig. 11.26 (a) (TR = 600 msec), but is still overshadowed by the greater T1 contrast between fat and other tissues in the image. (b) The same sequence repeated with fat suppression generates greater contrast between articular cartilage (*arrows*) and synovial fluid (*s*) as their pixel intensities are rescaled across a broader range of greyscale values.

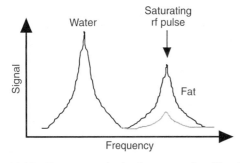

Fig. 11.28 Frequency-selective fat suppression. The chemical-shift phenomenon separates the resonant frequencies of water and fat (by 220 Hz at a magnetic field strength of 1.5 T). This allows the longitudinal magnetization of either of these proton pools to be selectively suppressed by an rf pulse tuned to the correct resonant frequency. Since the resonant frequency and the magnitude of the chemical shift both depend on magnetic field strength, this method of fat suppression is dependent on the homogeneity of the static magnetic field and is not feasible at very low field strengths.

voxels, comprising it. All signals within a single voxel are averaged. Therefore, if an interface with high signal

intensity on one side and low signal intensity on the other side passes through the middle of a voxel, the interface is depicted as an intermediate signal intensity band, the width of the voxel (Fig. 11.31). This effect is known as partial-volume averaging. Voxel size is determined by multiplying the slice thickness by the size of the in-plane subdivisions of the image, or pixels (picture elements). Pixel size, in turn, is determined by dividing the field of view by the image matrix, which most commonly ranges between 256 × 128 and 256 × 256. The smaller the voxel, the greater the spatial resolution. However, as voxel size decreases, so does signal-to-noise ratio (S/N). Accordingly, high-resolution imaging requires sufficient S/N to support the spatial resolution. S/N can be increased by shortening TE (less T2 decay), increasing TR (more T1 recovery), imaging at higher field strength (greater longitudinal magnetization), or utilizing specialized coils which reduce noise (small surface coil, quadrature coil, phased array of small coils)[16]. Specialized sequences, such as three-dimensional (3D) gradient echo, also provide greater S/N.

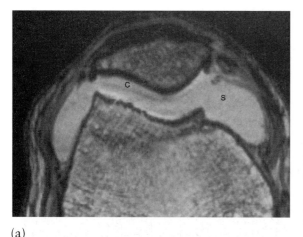

(a)

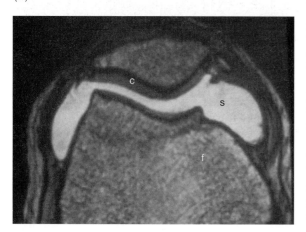

(b)

Fig. 11.29 Magnetization-transfer contrast. (a) Transverse (axial) $T2^*$ — weighted gradient-echo image of a knee shows poor contrast between articular cartilage (*c*) and adjacent synovial fluid (*s*). (b) Same image acquired with the addition of a magnetization-transfer pulse, which causes signal loss in collagen-containing tissues, such as articular cartilage (*c*) and muscle, but not synovial fluid (*s*) or fat (*f*).

Monitoring changes in articular cartilage

Normal cartilage

The MRI appearance of articular cartilage reflects its complex histological and biochemical composition[17–19]. The content and distribution of hydrophilic proteoglycan molecules, and the anisotropic organization of collagen (Fig. 11.32), influence the amount of water (that is, proton density) in cartilage as well as the relaxation

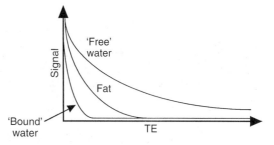

Fig. 11.30 Effect on TE on signal intensity. Echo time (TE) is the time between the initiating rf pulse and a subsequent 180° rephasing rf pulse (spin echo) or gradient reversal (gradient echo). The longer the TE, the greater the decay of transverse magnetization (and, therefore, signal intensity) by T2 or $T2^*$ relaxation. Substances with long T2 relaxation times (e.g. free water) retain the most signal intensity on long-TE (T2-weighted) sequences. Structures, such as tendons and menisci, that contain highly immobile water protons (bound water), show such rapid T2 relaxation that no attainable TE is short enough to recover any signal. These structures, therefore, appear dark on even the shortest-TE sequences.

properties (that is, T2) of this water, giving the tissue a characteristic 'zonal' appearance on MRI[20–23]. The T2 relaxation time of normal articular cartilage is between 10 msec and 20 msec. Therefore, on very short-TE (5–10 msec) images, cartilage, which is approximately 70 per cent water, exhibits a relatively high signal intensity, close to that of free water (that is, synovial fluid). However, immobilization of water protons in certain regions of the cartilage, such as the superficial tangential zone, where collagen fibrils form a dense tangentially oriented mat, or the upper radial zone, where the collagen fibrils are arranged in a tightly parallel array, dramatically shortens T2 at these sites, which accordingly appear as thin, low signal intensity bands at even the shortest TEs (Fig. 11.33).

Normal articular cartilage on short-TE images thus shows up to four lamina of alternating high and low signal intensity that correlate loosely with histological zones described in this tissue (Fig. 11.33): (1) a low-signal superficial lamina corresponding to the superficial tangential zone; (2) an intermediate-signal lamina incorporating the deep portion of the superficial tangential zone, the entire transitional zone, and the uppermost portion of the radial zone; (3) a low-signal stripe within the upper radial zone (this stripe is so thin that it may be obscured by partial-volume averaging on even mildly oblique imaging sections); and (4) an intermediate-signal lamina corresponding to the deep portion of the radial zone, and possibly the deep calcified layer.

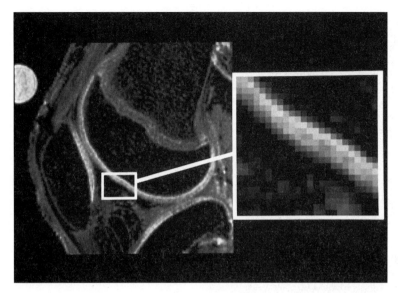

Fig. 11.31 Partial volume averaging. The smallest element of an MR image is the individual voxel (pixel size • slice thickness). Different signal intensities within a single voxel are averaged. This effect is most noticeable at high contrast interfaces as shown in the magnified view of the femoral cartilage on this sagittal, fat-suppressed, T1-weighted gradient-echo image of a knee.

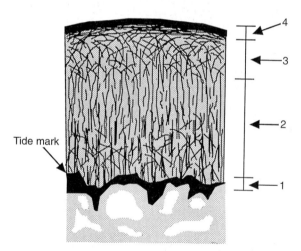

Fig. 11.32 Zonal organization of collagen in hyaline articular cartilage. Collagen forms a fibrous network that courses through the articular cartilage. The differing arrangement of collagen fibrils within the various cartilage zones results in heterogeneity of T2 relaxation and zonal signal behavior on MRI. The deepest layer of cartilage is calcified (1) and anchors a relatively parallel array of collagen fibrils that radiate through the radial zone (2). In the transitional zone (3), collagen fibrils adopt a more disorganized arrangement with a predilection for oblique orientation. The most superficial zone (4) is composed of a dense network of tangentially arranged collagen fibrils and is important to the load-bearing function of cartilage. (Modified from Peterfy, C., Linares, R., and Steinbach, L. (1994). Recent advances in magnetic resonance imaging of the musculoskeletal system. *Radiology Clinics of North America*, **32**,291–311; with permission.)

As TE is prolonged, signal decays from the deep radial lamina producing a trilaminar appearance in normal cartilage (Fig. 11.34): (1) a low-signal superficial lamina; (2) an intermediate-signal transitional and upper radial lamina; and (3) a low-signal deep lamina composed of the remainder of the upper radial, deep radial, and deep calcified zones. With very heavy T2-weighting, signal also drops out of the transitional lamina, and cartilage becomes homogeneously low in signal intensity (Fig. 11.34).

Abnormal cartilage

Superimposed upon this complex signal behavior are changes due to alterations of the normal structure of cartilage. Collagen loss from trauma, inflammation, or degeneration results in elevation of the water content of cartilage as resistance to the swelling pressure of hydrophilic proteoglycans is impaired[19,24–28]. Similarly, loss of proteoglycans, which usually accompanies collagen loss, tends to increase the volume occupied by water. This is intuitive, if one conceptualizes articular cartilage as being composed of two separate phases: a solid phase of proteoglycans and collagen, and a fluid phase of water and ions. In this biphasic model, loss of solid matrix, without an accompanying loss of thickness, would necessitate an increase in the water fraction. On MRI, damage to the cartilage matrix is associated with an increase in signal intensity both

Consistent with this, foci of high signal intensity are often seen in the cartilage of OA patients on T2-weighted images (Fig. 11.35), and have been shown

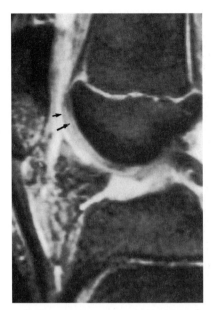

Fig. 11.33 Multilaminar appearance of articular cartilage on short- TE MRI. Sagittal short-TE gradient-echo image of the knee depicts the articular cartilage as a high signal intensity structure with a thin, low signal intensity lamina centrally (*long arrow*) and a narrow, low signal intensity lamina at the surface (*short arrow*). These low signal intensity lamina correspond to zones of dense and highly organized collagen, in which water protons are tightly constrained and, therefore, show rapid T2 relaxation and signal decay. Normal cartilage thus exhibits a maximum of four alternating lamina. However, either of the two low signal intensity lamina may be obscured by partial-volume averaging or by prolongation of T2 when the collagen fibrils in the lamina are oriented at 55° relative to the static magnetic field ('magic-angle phenomenon').

because the water content — and, therefore, the proton density — is increased, and because the intrinsic T2-shortening effects of the matrix on water are reduced. These are the earliest signs of cartilage injury and may be seen before any loss of thickness has occurred. There may, in fact, be mild swelling of the cartilage during this stage.

Fig. 11.34 Effect of TE on cartilage signal. (a) Short-TE (20 msec), proton-density-weighted spin-echo image of normal patellar cartilage shows diffuse intermediate signal intensity bounded superficially by a low signal intensity band (*arrow*). (b) As TE is doubled (40 msec), signal intensity decreases preferentially in the deep cartilage. Cartilage just beneath the low signal intensity superficial band remains intermediate in signal. (c) With further T2-weighting (TE = 80 msec), most of the cartilage becomes low in signal intensity and overall SN decreases. (Peterfy, C., Linares, R., and Steinbach, L. (1994). Recent advances in magnetic resonance imaging of the musculoskeletal system. *Radiology Clinics of North America* **32**, 291–311; with permission.)

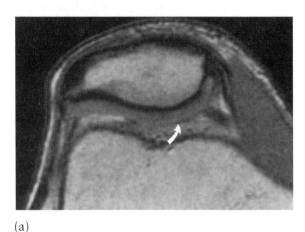

(a)

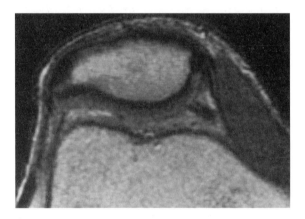

(b)

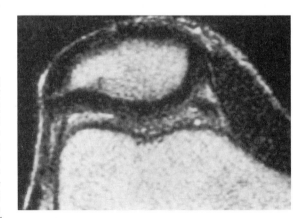

(c)

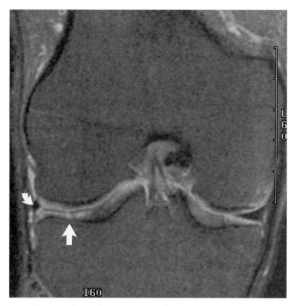

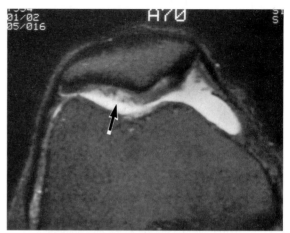

(a)

Fig. 11.35 Abnormal MRI signal in OA cartilage. Coronal, fat-suppressed, T2-weighted fast spin-echo image of the knee of a patient with remote lateral meniscectomy shows focal high signal intensity (*straight arrow*) in the cartilage over the lateral tibial plateau, indicative of chondromalacia. Signal intensity in the cartilage elsewhere in the knee is also mildly elevated, suggesting an element of diffuse chondromalacia in this patient. Note the small residual lateral meniscus (*curved arrow*).

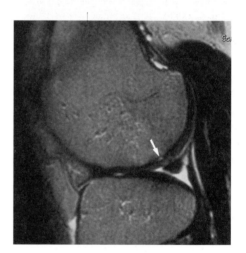

(b)

Fig. 11.36 Patterns of abnormal cartilage signal. (a) Transverse fat-suppressed, T2-weighted fast spin-echo image of a different patella shows transmural signal increase and surface fraying in the cartilage over the lateral facet (*arrow*). (b) Sagittal T2-weighted fast spin-echo image of an OA knee shows an isolated focus of increased signal intensity (*arrow*) in the deep cartilage of the weight-bearing region of the medial femoral condyle. The overlying cartilage shows a slightly increased signal intensity (compare with adjacent cartilage), but appears otherwise intact. This deep signal pattern may reflect early basal delamination of the cartilage resulting from mechanical failure, and may not be apparent on arthroscopy.

to correspond to arthroscopically demonstrable abnormalities[29,30]. Patterns of abnormal cartilage signal include superficial, transmural, and deep linear changes (Fig. 11.36). The latter may reflect deep degenerative changes initiated by basal delamination of the cartilage at the tide mark[31–33], and can be seen in young patients following trauma (Fig. 11.37) as well as in elderly patients with OA. Early changes such as these, confined to the deep layers of cartilage, may not be detectable by inspection of the articular surface alone during arthroscopy. We have frequently observed these MR signal abnormalities in cartilage adjacent to meniscal tears and in patients with established OA, in many cases before surface abnormalities were evident on MRI or arthroscopy. Others have also observed signal abnormalities in cartilage that were not apparent by arthroscopy[30,34–36]. This raises questions about the validity of arthroscopy as a 'gold standard' for assessing articular cartilage integrity — at least in very early disease. However, longitudinal data describing the natural history of these MRI findings, and their associ-

ation with subsequent cartilage loss and joint failure, are currently lacking.

Even more intriguing are applications of MRI that probe dynamic properties of tissues for which there are no direct histological correlates. For example, it is pos-

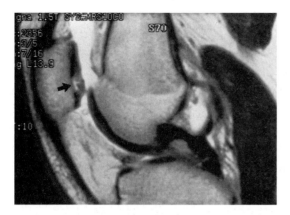

Fig. 11.37 Traumatic delamination of articular cartilage. Sagittal T2-weighted spin-echo image of a knee immediately following transient dislocation of the patella shows focal high signal intensity (*arrow*) in the patellar cartilage, extending from the surface to the subchondral cortex. In the deep calcified zone, this signal abnormality takes on a linear configuration and parallels the subchondral cortex. This pattern is consistent with traumatic delamination of the articular cartilage at the tide mark.

sible to quantify the diffusion coefficient for water in articular cartilage as well as to depict this parameter in image mode (diffusion-weighted image). With the aid of a high field strength (8.6 T) MR system and a highly specialized phase-sensitive MRI technique, Xia et al.[14] mapped true proton density and the diffusion coefficient of water in excised canine cartilage discs and cartilage-bone plugs at a resolution of 30 μm. The concentration of mobile protons (water content) in the cartilage specimens decreased slightly from the articular surface to the subchondral bone, consistent with the known gradient for water in this tissue[38]. Water diffusion also decreased towards the cartilage-bone interface, consistent with the normal distribution of proteoglycans which impart a high frictional drag to interstitial water movement in normal cartilage. Loss of proteoglycans from the articular cartilage is associated with decreased resistance to water movement and loss of compressive stiffness[19]. Using an 8.6 T spectrometer and a 4.7 T MRI system, Burstein et al.[15] showed a 20 per cent increase in the diffusion coefficient of water in bovine cartilage following the removal of proteoglycans by trypsin digestion. Although further development is necessary before this technique becomes applicable to *in vivo* imaging with conventional MR imaging hardware, water diffusion imaging may provide a sensitive way of monitoring early changes in degenerating articular cartilage.

The proteoglycan content in cartilage can be probed with the use of cationic MR contrast agents, such as manganese (Mn), which increase the signal intensity of cartilage on T1-weighted images in proportion to the fixed negative charge density (that is, glycosaminoglycan content) of the tissue. Fujioka et al.[39] have shown decreased Mn enhancement in OA cartilage. However, more work needs to be done before these agents become applicable for clinical use.

As discussed above, another MR relaxation mechanism in articular cartilage that can be harnessed to generate additional image contrast is magnetization transfer[3,11,40,41]. This phenomenon manifests as a loss of water signal in certain tissues due to equilibration of longitudinal magnetization between freely mobile water protons and tightly constrained protons associated with macromolecules within the same tissue. Collagen is a particularly good macromolecular substrate for this reaction, and cartilage, synovium, and muscle accordingly exhibit prominent magnetization-transfer effect. Fat and joint fluid, on the other hand, do not show any substantial magnetization transfer and, thus, do not lose signal intensity under conditions in which macromolecular protons are saturated. These tissue-dependent differences in magnetization transfer can be exploited to generate additional image contrast among articular structures[3,11,12]. (Figs 11.29 and 11.38). In addition, it may be possible to quantify specific macromolecular constituents, such as collagen, in different tissues by measuring the magnetization-transfer effect[41].

MRI thus shows considerable promise for detecting and monitoring very early compositional changes in degenerating articular cartilage. Delineation of subtle morphological changes, such as surface fraying and small focal defects, in later stages of degeneration, places additional demands on spatial resolution and contrast between cartilage and adjacent articular structures.

Fast spin-echo MRI provides high-resolution T2-weighted images in only a fraction of the time required for conventional T2-weighted spin-echo imaging[42], and is a superb technique for delineating articular surfaces of cartilage (Fig. 11.39). Higher spatial resolution can be achieved, however, with 3D gradient-echo techniques, both because thinner sections can be combined with large in-plane matrixes, and because S/N is inherently greater[43]. Additional contrast can be added to these sequences with magnetization-transfer subtraction[13] (Fig. 11.38), or fat-suppressed,

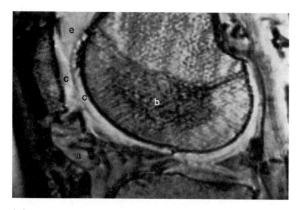

(a)

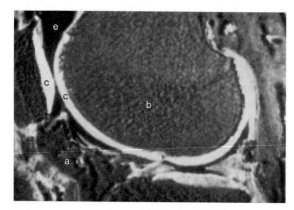

(b)

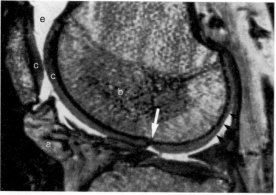

(c)

Fig. 11.38 Magnetization-transfer subtraction technique. Sagittal images of an amputated knee following intra-articular injection of 55 ml saline to simulate a joint effusion. (a) Conventional, T2*-weighted, thin-partitioned, sagittal 3D gradient echo shows poor contrast between cartilage (*c*) and joint fluid (*e*). (b) Addition of a magnetization-transfer pulse to the same imaging sequence markedly decreases signal intensity in cartilage (*c*) but not effusion (*e*), bone (*b*) or adipose tissue (*a*). This combines high cartilage-fluid contrast with sufficient spatial resolution to allow delineation of small surface defects in the cartilage (*long arrow*) in addition to more generalized areas of cartilage thinning (*arrowheads*). Contrast at the cartilage-bone interface, however, is decreased. (c) Magnetization-transfer subtraction image, generated by subtracting image (b) from image (a), maps the spatial distribution of magnetization transfer in the same knee. Hyaline articular cartilage (*c*) is depicted as a high signal-intensity structure, while effusion (*e*), bone (*b*), and adipose tissue (*a*) are low in signal intensity. Magnetization-transfer subtraction images thus provide high contrast at both the cartilage-effusion and cartilage-bone interfaces. Limitations of the subtraction technique include the extra imaging time necessary to acquire two sets of images (i.e. with and without magnetization transfer) and the risk of spatial misregistration (malalignment of the images) during subtraction. (Reproduced from reference 3; with permission.)

method, however, is twice as fast (since subtraction is not required), more widely available than magnetization-transfer subtraction, and offers greater contrast between cartilage and synovial tissue[3].

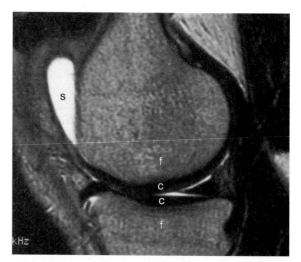

Fig. 11.39 Fast spin-echo imaging of cartilage. Sagittal T2-weighted fast spin-echo image of the knee shows high contrast between the low signal intensity articular cartilage (*c*) and adjacent high signal intensity synovial fluid (*s*), and intermediate signal intensity subchondral marrow fat (*f*).

T1-weighting[1,3,13] (Fig. 11.40). Both techniques depict the articular cartilage as an isolated band of high signal intensity, sharply contrasted against the adjacent low signal intensity joint fluid, intra-articular adipose tissue, and subchondral bone marrow[1,3,13]. The latter

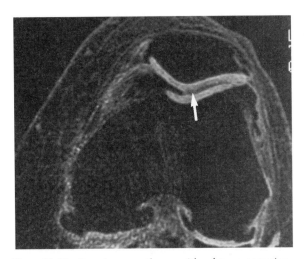

Fig. 11.40 Imaging cartilage with fat suppression. Transverse, thin-partitioned, fat-suppressed 3D gradient-echo image of a 62-year-old man with OA of the knee delineates cartilage with high resolution. Fibrillation of the surface of the patellar cartilage (*arrow*) is visible on this image. (Reproduced from reference 3; with permission.)

In a comparison of T1-weighted gradient echo (with and without fat suppression), T2*-weighted gradient echo, and conventional T1-weighted, proton-density-weighted, and T2-weighted spin-echo sequences in 10 elderly cadaver knees, Recht *et al.*[1] found fat-suppressed, T1-weighted gradient echo (flip angle = 60°, TE = 10 msec, voxel size = 469 μm × 938 μm × 1500 μm) to have the greatest sensitivity (96 per cent) and specificity (95 per cent) for demonstrating patellofemoral cartilage lesions visible on pathological sections. Disler *et al.*[36] similarly showed the same technique *in vivo* to have 93 per cent sensitivity and 94 per cent specificity for arthroscopically visible cartilage lesions. Fat-suppressed, T1-weighted gradient echo is, therefore, useful for detailed evaluation of the articular surfaces of diarthroidial joints; although, in small joints, such as the interphalangeal joints in the fingers, facet joints in the spine, or the temporomandibular joints, adequate S/N and spatial resolution may require specialized imaging sequences and coils (p. 490).

In addition to directly inspecting individual cross-sectional images for surface irregularities and focal defects of the articular cartilage, 3D image data can be analyzed in a variety of more sophisticated ways. For example, using established image processing techniques[12,13,44], shaded 3D renderings of individual cartilages can be produced, that visually depict the articular surface topography (Fig. 11.41). Such 3D renderings could be used to monitor the distribution and severity of cartilage surface irregularities in patients with arthritis, or to analyze contact areas between opposing articular surfaces in joint malalignment[45–47] (Fig. 11.42). This technique would be useful for exploring relationships between abnormal tracking and subsequent OA, as well as for directing and evaluating precise surgical correction of such disorders. Equivalent information cannot be derived from radiography since the surface topography of articular cartilage does not follow exactly the contour of the articular bone directly beneath it[48].

In addition to depicting the surface geometry of cartilage, 3D reconstructions of MRI data can be used to determine the exact volume of complex articular cartilages, such as that lining the femoral surface of the knee[13]. This is accomplished simply by summing the voxels contained within 3D reconstructions of this cartilage (Fig. 11.43). In a study using commercially available image processing software and only moderate-resolution (625 μm × 833 μm × 2000 μm) image data acquired with conventional clinical MRI equipment, this technique was found to provide greater than 95 per cent accuracy and 95 per cent reproducibility for measuring cartilage volume in the knee[13] and metacarpophalangeal joints[2]. Based on this performance, it should be possible to detect volume changes in the order of 10 per cent between serial examinations. Moreover, unlike cartilage thickness measurements made from individual sections, values for total cartilage volume are relatively unaffected by minor variations in the plane of section, and are less demanding in terms of spatial resolution. Total volume is, therefore, a more robust parameter for serial measurements in patients with arthritis.

One limitation of total volume measurements, however, is the lack of information about the distribution of cartilage changes in the joint. Total cartilage volume is accordingly insensitive to focal change. Theoretically, a loss of cartilage in one region could be balanced by an equivalent increase in volume elsewhere in the joint, and, thereby, elude detection by this method. By subdividing 3D reconstructions of the articular cartilage into several smaller regions[49], it is possible to evaluate the volume at specific sites, such as the weight-bearing surfaces of the femorotibial joints. However, the reproducibility of such measurements decreases as the subdivisions are made smaller. Ultimately, extremely high spatial resolution is necessary to maintain precision. If, however, sufficient resolution can be achieved within a reasonable imaging time, the prospect of mapping the cartilage thickness *in*

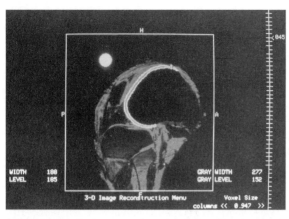

(a)

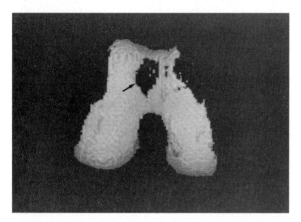

(b)

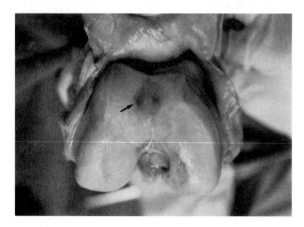

(c)

Fig. 11.41 Segmentation and 3D rendering of articular cartilage. (a) One slice of a T1-weighted, fat-suppressed 3D gradient-echo acquisition of the knee is shown with disarticulation
boundaries traced around the articular cartilage of the femur
during segmentation and 3D reconstruction of this cartilage.
(b) 3D surface rendering (viewed from an anterior vantage
point) of this femoral cartilage delineates a large focal
defect in the trochlear groove (*arrow*). (c) Gross anatomical
findings correlate well with the surface rendered 3D image.
(Reproduced from reference 13; with permission.)

Imaging other articular components in OA

In addition to evaluating the articular cartilage, MRI is
uniquely capable of imaging all of the other structures
that make up the joint, including the synovium and
joint fluid, articular bones, intra-articular menisci,
labra and discs, cruciate ligaments, collateral and other
capsular ligaments, and periarticular tendons and
muscles. Moreover, using the same voxel-counting
technique employed for quantifying articular cartilage
in 3D reconstructed images[2,13], it is possible to determine the volume of each of these components within
the same joint (Fig. 11.45).

Some degree of synovial thickening can be found in a
majority of OA joints[51]. Whether this synovitis contributes directly to articular cartilage loss in OA, or
simply arises in reaction to the breakdown of cartilage
by other causes, remains a controversy[52]. However,
synovitis may be important to the symptoms and disability of OA, and may pose different treatment
requirements than those directed only towards 'chondroprotection'. MRI is capable of imaging thickened or
inflamed synovium, but usually this requires the use of
special techniques, such as magnetization-transfer subtraction[3], fat-suppressed, T1-weighted imaging[3], or
intravenous injection of Gd-containing contrast material[3,53–55] (Fig. 11.46). By monitoring the rate of synovial enhancement with Gd-containing contrast over
time, using rapid, sequential MRI, it is, furthermore,
possible to grade the severity of the synovitis in these
patients. The majority of work in this area has,
however, focused on rheumatoid arthritis.

Osseous changes in OA are superbly depicted by
MRI. Both cortical and trabecular bone can be visualized with MRI (Fig. 11.47), and because of the tomographic nature of this modality, MRI is better at
delineating structures, such as central osteophytes and
subchondral cysts, that are often obscured by overlying
structures on conventional radiographs (Fig. 11.48).
Using high-resolution MRI techniques and sophisticated
texture analyses (for example, fractal dimension)[56,57], it

vivo becomes feasible [46,50] (Fig. 11.44). Cartilage thickness maps may render insight into the importance of
the location of cartilage lesions to the progression of
OA.

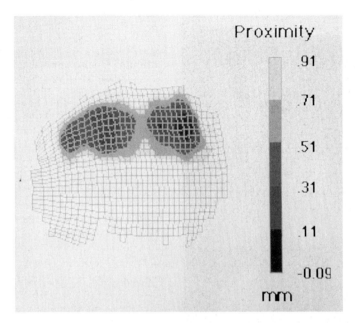

Fig. 11.42 Surface-contact mapping with MRI. Map of *in situ* contact areas for the patellar cartilage of the amputated knee shown in Fig. 11.38 by Ayeshian, G.A., Cohen, Z.A., Kwak, S.D., and Mow, V.C. (Columbia University, NY). MR images were segmented manually, and geometric models of the articular surfaces of the patellofemoral joint were generated from the contour curves, using parametric bicubic B-spline representations. Contact areas between the B-spline geometric models were determined by the proximity method[46] and depicted in intervals of 0.2 mm. In this example, the contact areas of the patellar cartilage on the femoral cartilage are shown in shades of orange.

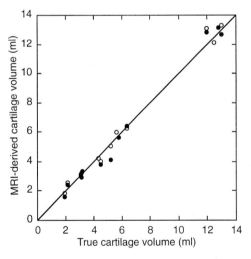

Fig. 11.43 Volumetric quantification of cartilage. The graph depicts cartilage volumes determined from fat-suppressed, T1-weighted 3D gradient-echo images (*open circles*) and magnetization transfer subtraction images (*closed circles*) plotted against volumes measured directly by water displacement. A total of 12 cartilage plates (six patellar, three tibial, three femoral) from six knees were included. Line represents theoretical 100% accuracy. (Modified from reference 13; with permission.)

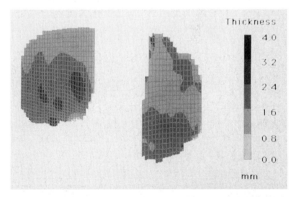

Fig. 11.44 Mapping cartilage thickness with MRI. B-spline geometric model of the tibial cartilage of the knee shown in Fig. 11.38 was generated by Ayeshian, G.A., Cohen, Z.A., Kwak, S.D., and Mow, V.C. (Columbia University, NY) using the same method as for *in situ* contact area mapping (Fig. 11.43). Regional cartilage thicknesses (perpendicular to the cartilage-bone interface) are depicted at intervals of 0.8 mm and shown in shades of orange.

may be possible to monitor trabecular changes in the subchondral bone, in order to determine their importance in the development and progression of OA.

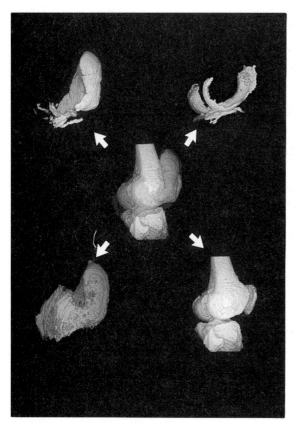

Fig. 11.45 'Exploded' 3D rendering of the knee shown in Fig. 11.38, showing individual components (clockwise from the top left: synovial fluid, cartilage, bone marrow, thickened synovium) surrounding a composite image viewed from a posterolateral vantage point.

In addition to delineating the calcified components of a bone, MRI is uniquely capable of imaging the marrow. Subchondral marrow edema is occasionally associated with not only acute trauma but also progressive OA[32] (Fig. 11.49). Focal bone marrow

edema in OA may be due to subchondral injuries caused by shifting articular contact points at sites of biomechanically failing cartilage, or pulsion of synovial fluid into uncovered subchondral bone. However, osteonecrosis, infection, and infiltrating neoplasms could theoretically produce a similar MRI appearance. Conventional radiographs are usually unremarkable in areas of bone marrow edema; although, bone scintigraphy may show increased uptake in these areas.

The menisci in the knee, and glenoid labrum in the shoulder, are important to the stability and functional integrity of these joints. Equally important are the cruciate ligaments and glenohumeral ligaments. The utility of MRI for evaluating these articular structures is already well established[58].

Tradeoffs in imaging specific joints

The knee

Each joint poses different challenges to proper imaging with MRI. Most work, thus far, has focused on the knee, not only because the knee is frequently affected by OA and because loss of knee function can be severely disabling, but also because the knee is a comparatively easy joint to image. Reasons for this include the relatively large size of this joint, which lowers demands on spatial resolution, and the relatively cylindrical structure of the knee, which minimizes perturbation of the static magnetic field — field homogeneity is critical to the performance of frequency-selective fat suppression techniques, and important in quantitative studies based on signal intensity measurements. The cylindrical shape also allows the use of circumferential imaging coils, which show greater homogeneity than surface coils[16]. In addition, since the knee is a relatively incongruent joint, contact areas between the hyaline

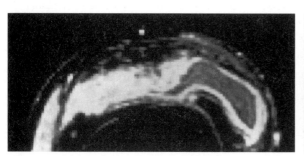
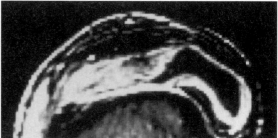

Fig. 11.46 Synovial imaging with MRI. Transverse images of the suprapatellar recess of the knee of a patient with rheumatoid arthritis, using magnetization-transfer subtraction (*left panel*) and fat-suppressed T1-weighted gradient echo (*right panel*). Both delineate the thickened synovial tissue with high contrast. (Reproduced from reference 13; with permission.)

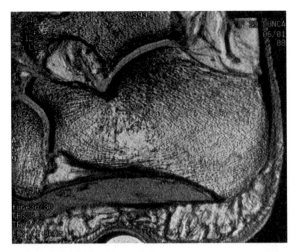

Fig. 11.47 High resolution MRI of cortical and trabecular bone. Sagittal high-resolution gradient-echo image of the calcaneus delineates both cortical and trabecular bone with high detail.

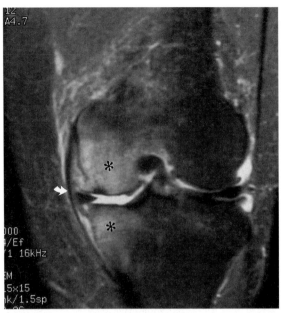

Fig. 11.49 Subchondral bone edema in OA. Coronal fat-suppressed T2-weighted fast spin-echo image of an OA knee shows areas of full-thickness cartilage loss in the medial femorotibial joint associated with local bone marrow edema (*asterisks*). The intact medial collateral ligament is also delineated on this image (*arrow*).

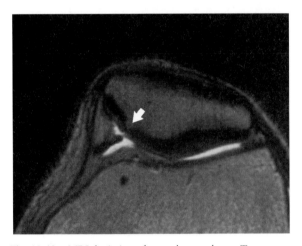

Fig. 11.48 MRI depiction of central osteophytes. Transverse T2- weighted fast spin-echo image shows focal cartilage loss with central osteophyte formation (*arrow*) over the medial facet of the patella.

cartilage plates, in all but the most severely degenerated joints, are small. Articular surfaces are, therefore, easy to separate from each other on MR images. Delineating the articular surfaces is facilitated by the relative abundance of synovial fluid in the knee, which provides high contrast at this interface on T2-weighted images and fat-suppressed, T1-weighted images. Since the articular surfaces are only gently curved, partial-volume averaging is not a major problem. Because of these forgiving imaging features, and the availability of effective surgical and arthroscopic therapies for many

of the internal derangements affecting the knee, MRI experience with knee is greater than for any other joint in the body.

These advantages, however, are offset to some extent by a number of inherent disadvantages. The knee is a highly complex joint composed of three articular compartments, one of which involves a sesmoid bone — the patella. The hyaline cartilage covering each of the articular surfaces accordingly shows somewhat different biomechanical properties and vulnerabilities. The joint contains two intra-articular ligaments, an intra-articular tendon, two menisci, intracapsular-extrasynovial fat pads, complex capsular ligaments (particularly laterally), and variable ontological remnants (plicas). Joint failure in the knee involves an equally complex interplay among these numerous articular constituents. Because the knee is a large joint, full coverage of the synovial cavity, including the suprapatellar recess, requires a relatively large field of view (12–18 cm). Since loose bodies tend to collect in the eddy pools within synovial recesses, incomplete coverage can result in important oversights. This can be particularly problematic in cases with large popliteal cysts dissecting down the calf. Larger fields of view, however, necessitate proportionately larger imaging matrices in order to maintain spatial resolution, and this increases the imaging time[3].

The hip

Next to the knee, the hip is the most important joint affected by OA from a disability stand point. Despite this, however, the hip has received only scant attention in terms of MRI evaluation for OA. This is at least, in part, because the hip poses significant challenges to proper imaging with MRI. It is a highly congruent joint, which makes separating the articular surfaces difficult. Delineation of the surfaces is further hampered by the relative lack of joint fluid in the tight synovial cavity of the hip. Moreover, the articular surfaces are highly curved, giving rise to severe partial-volume effects in all planes unless extremely high spatial resolution is employed. Accordingly, cartilage thickness measurements in the hip using MRI have been somewhat disappointing[59]. Achieving high spatial resolution in the hip is, itself, not an entirely straightforward matter. Since the hip is a relatively deep joint, signal drop off with small (less than 5 cm) surface coils is usually prohibitive. Larger surface coils could be employed, but these offer lower resolution and do not provide homogeneous signal for quantitative measurements. The anatomy of the hip prevents the use of small circumferential coils which could provide homogeneous images with high resolution. A large circumferential coil, such as the body coil, could be used in this way, but does not provide sufficient S/N to support the high spatial resolution needed. Multiple coils, configured in a phased array about the hip, offer high S/N, along with high spatial resolution (Fig. 11.50), and are probably the best alternative for this purpose.

The shoulder

Like the hip, the shoulder is a congruent, ball-in-socket joint with closely opposing articular surfaces[60] (Fig. 11.51). Because of the angular shape of the shoulder, magnetic field heterogeneities tend to develop laterally, near the greater tuberosity. While the field appears relatively undisturbed at the glenohumeral joint, lateral heterogeneities can limit the performance of fat suppression and complicate evaluation of the rotator cuff. Accurate assessment of the tendons of the

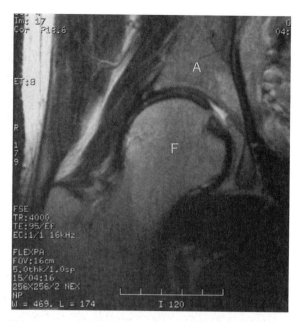

Fig. 11.50 MRI of the hip using phased array technique. Sagittal T2-weighted fast spin-echo image of a normal hip, acquired using two imaging coils arranged in a flexible phased array, shows high SN despite the relatively high-resolution employed. The articular cartilage is well delineated with this technique. F = femoral head, A = superior acetabulum.

rotator cuff is important, since the shoulder relies heavily on these structures for stability, and rotator cuff tear is an important risk factor for the development of OA in this joint. Shoulder stability is also dependent on the integrity of the glenoid labrum and the glenohumeral ligaments. However, reliable imaging of these labrocapsular structures can be extremely difficult, particularly in the absence of joint distention by significant synovial effusion. This can be improved by intra-articular injection of saline[61] or Gd-containing MRI contrast material (MR arthrography)[62,63].

Hand and finger joints

The joint most commonly affected by OA is the distal interphalangeal joint of the finger. The major challenge to imaging this small joint is the demand on spatial resolution. For this reason, small-bore, high-field magnets and small circumferential imaging coils are usually necessary[12]. The metacarpophalangeal joints are less frequently affected by OA, but are larger joints, and have been successfully imaged using conventional clinical MRI systems[2] (Fig. 11.52).

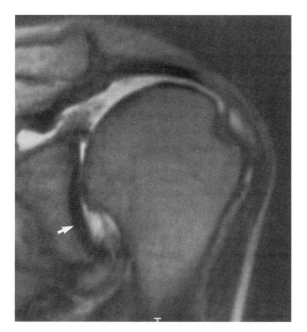

Fig. 11.51 MRI of OA shoulder. Oblique coronal (in plane with the long axis of the supraspinatus tendon), T2-weighted fast spin-echo image of an OA shoulder with a chronically torn and retracted rotator cuff, shows superior subluxation of the humerus and denuding of the cartilage over the humeral head. Relatively abundant articular cartilage is still present over the glenoid surface (*arrow*).

Conclusion

MRI is clearly a tool of unprecedented capabilities for evaluating joint disease and its potential treatments. The unparalleled tissue contrast of MRI allows it to directly examine all components of a joint simultaneously and, thus, evaluate the joint as a whole organ and OA as a disorder of organ failure, in which dysfunction may result from any one of a number of different causes. Especially intriguing is the unique potential of this technology for identifying very early changes associated with cartilage degeneration, and its ability to quantify subtle morphological and compositional variations in different articular tissues over time. Employing these techniques, MRI may provide more objective measures of disease progression and treatment response than are currently attainable by other methods. This will facilitate both the assessment of new therapies for OA and investigations of the pathophysiology in this disorder.

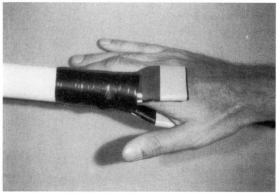

(a)

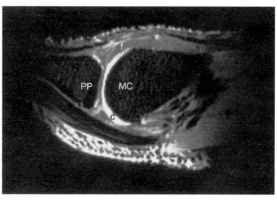

(b)

Fig. 11.52 MRI of the metacarpophalangeal joints. (A) Specialized imaging coil for finger joints is composed of two one-inch coils positioned on either side of the joint and housed in a plastic pipe. (B) Sagittal T1-weighted, fat-suppressed 3D gradient-echo image of a metacarpophalangeal joint acquired using the coil shown in (a) and conventional, clinical MRI hardware and software shows high contrast between articular cartilage (*c*) and adjacent effusion (*e*) and subchondral bone (*b*). (Reproduced from reference 2; with permission).

It is no exaggeration to say that only a minute fraction of the full potential of the capabilities of MRI has, thus far, been tapped. Investigators dealing with OA and other articular disorders should become more sophisticated in MRI, so that they can take full advantage of its unique capabilities and a more active hand in directing its development.

References

1. Recht, M.P., Kramer, J., Marcelis, S., Pathria, M., Trudell, D., Haghighi, P., *et al.* (1993). Abnormalities of articular cartilage in the knee: analysis of available MR techniques. *Radiology*, **187**, 473–78.

2. Peterfy, C.G., van Dijke, C.F., Lu, Y., Nguyen, A., Connick, T., Kneeland, B., *et al.* (1995). Quantification of articular cartilage in the metacarpophalangeal joints of the hand: accuracy and precision of 3D MR imaging. *AJR*, **165**, 371–5.

3. Peterfy, C.G., Majumdar, S., Lang, P., van Dijke, C.F., Sack, K., and Genant, H. (1994). MR imaging of the arthritic knee: improved discrimination of cartilage, synovium and effusion with pulsed saturation transfer and fat-suppressed T1-weighted sequences. *Radiology*, **191**, 413–19.

4. Dieppe, P., Altman, R.D., Buckwalter, J.A., Felson, D.T., Hascall, V., Lohmander, L.S., *et al.* (1995). Standardization of methods used to assess the progression of osteoarthritis of the hip or knee joints. In *Osteoarthritic disorders* (ed. K.E. Kuettner and V.M. Goldberg), pp. 481–96. American Academy of Orthopedic Surgons, Rosemont, IL.

5. Abragam, A. (1983). *The principles of nuclear magnetism.* Oxford University Press, Oxford.

6. Budinger, T. and Lauterbur, P. (1984). Nuclear magnetic resonance technology for medical studies. *Science*, **226**, 288–98.

7. Haacke, E. and Tkach, J. (1990). Fast MR imaging: techniques and clinical applications. *AJR*, **155**, 951–64.

8. Pykett, I. (1982). NMR imaging in medicine. *Sci Am*, **246**, 78–88.

9. Young, S. (1988). *Magnetic resonance imaging: basic principles.* Raven Press, New York.

10. König, S. and Brown, R. (1984). Determinants of proton relaxation in tissue. *Magn Reson Imag*, **1**, 437–49.

11. Woolf, S.D., Chesnick, S., Frank, J.A., Lim, K.O., and Balaban, R.S. (1991). Magnetization transfer contrast: MR imaging of the knee. *Radiology*, **179**, 623–8.

12. Hall, L.D. and Tyler, J.A. (1995). Can quantitative magnetic resonance imaging detect and monitor the progression of early osteoarthritis? In *Osteoarthritic disorders* (ed. K.E. Kuettner and V.M. Goldberg), pp. 67–84. American Academy of Orthopedic Surgeons, Rosemont, IL.

13. Peterfy, C.G., van Dijke, C.F., Janzen, D.L., Glüer, C., Namba, R., Majumdar, S., *et al.* (1994). Quantification of articular cartilage in the knee by pulsed saturation transfer and fat-suppressed MRI: optimization and validation. *Radiology*, **192**, 485–91.

14. Xia, Y., Farquhar, T., Burton-Wuster, N., Ray, E., and Jelinski, L.W. (1994). Diffusion and relaxation mapping of cartilage-bone plugs and excised disks using microscopic magnetic resonance imaging. *Magn Reson Med*, **31**, 273–82.

15. Burstein, D., Gray, M.L., Hartman, A.L., Gipe, R., and Foy, B.D. (1993). Diffusion of small solutes in cartilage as measured by nuclear magnetic resonance (NMR) spectroscopy and imaging. *J Orthop Res*, **11**, 465–78.

16. Kneeland, J.B. and Hyde, J.S. (1989). High-resolution MR imaging with local coils. *Radiology*, **171**, 1–7.

17. Hunziker, E. (1992). Articular cartilage structure in humans and experimental animals. In *Articular cartilage and osteoarthritis* (ed. K. Kuettner *et al.*), pp. 183–99. Raven Press, New York, NY.

18. Jeffery, A.K., Blunn, G.W., Archer, C.W., and Bentley, G. (1991). Three-dimensional collagen architecture in bovine articular cartilage. *J Bone Joint Surg (Br)*, **73-B**, 795–801.

19. Mow, V.C., Ratcliffe, A., and Poole, A.R. (1992). Cartilage and diarthroidial joints as paradigms for hierarchical materials and structures. *Biomaterials*, **13**, 67–97.

20. Modl, J.M., Sether, L.A., Haughton, V.M., and Kneeland, J.B. (1991). Articular cartilage: correlation of histologic zones with signal intensity at MR imaging. *Radiology*, **181**, 853–5.

21. Cole, P.R., Jasani, M.K., Wood, B., Freemont, A.J., and Morris, G.A. (1990). High resolution, high field magnetic resonance imaging of joints: unexpected features in proton images of cartilage. *Br J Radiol*, **63**, 907–9.

22. Fry, M.E., Jacoby, R.K., Hutton, C.W., Ellis, R.E., Pittard, S., and Vennart, W. (1991). High-resolution magnetic resonance imaging of the interphalangeal joints of the hand. *Skeletal Radiol*, **20**, 273–7.

23. Paul, P.K., Jasani, M.K., Sebok, D., Rakhit, A., Dunton, A.W., and Douglas, F.L. (1993). Variation in MR signal intensity across normal human knee cartilage. *JMRI*, **3**, 569–74.

24. Buckwalter, J., Rosenberg, L., and Hunziker, E. (1990). Articular cartilage: composition, structure, response to injury, and methods of facilitating repairs. In *Articular cartilage and knee joint function* (ed. J. Ewing), pp. 19–54. Raven Press, New York, NY.

25. Mow, V., Fithian, D., and Kelly, M. (1990). Fundamentals of articular cartilage and meniscus biomechanics. In *Articular cartilage and knee joint function* (ed. J. Ewing), pp. 1–18. Raven Press, New York, NY.

26. Mankin, H.J. and Thrasher, A.Z. (1975). Water content and binding in normal and osteoarthritic human cartilage. *J Bone Joint Surg*, **57A**, 76–9.

27. Armstrong, C.G. and Mow, V.C. (1982). Variations in the intrinsic mechanical properties of human cartilage with age, degeneration and water content. *J Bone Joint Surg*, **64A**, 88–94.

28. Maroudas, A. and Venn, M. (1977). Chemical composition and swelling of normal and osteoarthritic cartilage. II. Swelling. *Ann Rheum Dis*, **36**, 399–406.

29. Broderick, L.S., Turner, D.A., Renfrew, D.L., Schnitzer, T.J., Huff, J.P., and Harris, C. (1994). Severity of articular cartilage abnormality in patients with osteoarthritis: evaluation with fast spin-echo MR vs arthroscopy. *AJR*, **162**, 99–103.

30. Rose, P.M., Demlow, T.A., Szumowski, J., and Quinn, S.F. (1994). Chondromalacia patellae: fat-suppressed MR imaging. *Radiology*, **193**, 437–40.

31. Vener, M.J., Thompson, R.C.J., Lewis, J.L., and Oegema, T.R. (1992). Subchondral damage after acute transarticular loading: an *in vitro* model of joint injury. *J Orthop Res*, **10**, 759–69.

32. Vellet, A.D., Marks, P., Fowler, P., and Mururo, T. (1991). Occult posttraumatic lesions of the knee, prevalence, classification, and short-term sequelae evaluated with MR imaging. *Radiology*, **178**, 271–6.

33. Armstrong, C.G., Mow, V.C., and Wirth, C.R. (1985). Biomechanics of impact-induced microdamage to the articular cartilage: a possible genesis for chondromalacia. In *AAOS symposium on sports medicine: the knee* (ed. G. Finerman), pp. 70–84. W.B. Saunders, St. Louis.

34. Yulish, B.S., Montanez, J., Goodfellow, D.B., Bryan, P.J., Mulopulos, G.P., Modic, M.T. (1987) Chondromalacia patellae: assessment with MR imaging. *Radiology*, **164**,

35. Quinn, S.F., Rose, P.M., Brown, T.R., and Demlow, T.A. (1994). MR imaging of the patellofemoral compartment. *MRI Clin N Am*, **2**, 425–39.

36. Disler, D.G., McCauley, T.R., Wirth, C.R., and Fuchs, M.C. (1995). Detection of knee hyaline articular cartilage defects using fat-suppressed three-dimensional spoiled gradient-echo MR imaging: comparison with standard MR imaging and correlation with arthroscopy. *AJR*, **165**, 377–82.

37. Selby, K., Peterfy, C.G., Cohen, Z.A., Ateshian, G.A., Mow, V.C., Roos, M., *et al.* (1995). *In vivo* MR quantification of articular cartilage water content: a potential early indicator of osteoarthritis. *Book of abstracts: Society of Magnetic Resonance 1995* (p. 204). Society of Magnetic Resonance. Berkeley.

38. Volpi, M. and Katz, E.P. (1991). On the adaptive structures of the colagen fibrils of bone and cartilage. *J Biomechan*, **24**, 67–77.

39. Fujioka, M., Kusaka, Y., Morita, Y., Hirasawa, Y., and Gersonde, K. (1994). Contrast-enhanced MR imaging of articular cartilage: a new sensitive method for diagnosis of cartilage degeneration. *40th Annual Meeting, Orthopedic Research Society*. New Orleans.

40. Hajnal, J.V., Baudouin, C.J., Oatridge, A., Young, I.R., and Bydder, G.M. (1992). Design and implementation of magnetization transfer pulse sequences for clinical use. *J Comput Assist Tomogr*, **16**, 7–18.

41. Kim, D.K., Ceckler, T.L., Hascall, V.C., Calabro, A., and Balaban, R.S. (1993). Analysis of water-macromolecule proton magnetization transfer in articular cartilage. *Magn Reson Med*, **29**, 211–15.

42. Listerud, J., Einstein, S., Outwater, E., and Kressel, H.Y. (1992). First principles of fast spin echo. *Magn Reson Quarterly*, **8**, 199–244.

43. Tervonen, O., Dietz, M.J., Carmichael, S.W., and Ehman, R.L. (1993). MR imaging of knee hyaline cartilage: evaluation of two- and three-dimensional sequences. *JMRI*, **3**, 663–8.

44. Chan, W.P., Lang, P., Chieng, P.U., Davison, P.A., Huang, S.C., and Genant, H.K. (1991). Three-dimensional imaging of the musculoskeletal system: an overview. *J Formosan Med Assoc*, **90**, 713–22.

45. Ateshian, G.A., Soslowsky, L.J., and Mow, V.C. (1991). Quantification of articular surface topography and cartilage thickness in knee joints using stereophotogrammetry. *J Biomechan*, **24**, 761–76.

46. Ateshian, G.A., Kwak, S.D., Soslowsky, L.J., and Mow, V.C. (1994). A stereophotogrammetric method for determining *in situ* contact areas in diarthrodial joints, and a comparison with other methods. *J Biomechan*, **27**, 111–24.

47. Ateshian, G.A., Cohen, Z.A., Kwak, S.D., Wang, V., Kelkar, R., Raimondo, R., *et al.* (1995). *Determination of in situ contact areas in diarthrodial joints by MRI.* American Society of Mechanical Engineers, San Francisco CA,

48. Fulkerson, J.P. and Hungerford, D.S. (1990). *Disorders of the patello-femoral joint* (2nd edn) p. 294. Williams and Wilkins, Baltimore.

49. Pilch, L., Stewart, C., Gordon, D., Inman, R., Parsons, K., Pataki, I., *et al.* (1994). Assessment of cartilage volume in the femorotibial joint with magnetic resonance imaging and 3D computer reconstruction. *J Rheum*, **21**, 2307–21.

50. Eckstein, F., Sitteck, H., Gavazzenia, A., Milz, S., Putz, R., and Reiser, M. (1995). Assessment of articular cartilage volume and thickness with magnetic resonance imaging (MRI). *Trans Orthop Res Soc*, **20**, 194.

51. Fernandez-Madrid, F., Karvonen, R.L., Teitge, R.A., Miller, P.R., An, T., and Negendank, W.G. (1995). Synovial thickening detected by MR imaging in osteoarthritis of the knee confirmed by biopsy as synovitis. *Magn Reson Imag*, **13**, 177–83.

52. Brandt, K.D. (1995). Insights into the natural history of osteoarthritis and the potential for pharmacologic modification of the disease afforded by study of the cruciate-deficient dog. In *Osteoarthritic disorders* (ed. K.E. Kuettner and V.M. Goldberg), pp. 419–26. American Academy of Orthopedic Surgeons, Rosemont, IL.

53. Palmer, W.E., Rosenthal, D.I., Shoenberg, O.I., Fischman, A.J., Simon, L.S., Rubin, R.H., *et al.* (1995). Quantification of inflammation in the wrist with gadolinium-enhanced MR imaging and PET with 2-[F-18]-fluoro-2-deoxy- D-glucose. *Radiology*, **196**, 645–55.

54. König, H., Sieper, J., and Sorensen, M. K-J.W. (1991). Contrast-enhanced dynamic MR imaging in rheumatoid arthritis of the knee joint: follow-up study after cortisol drug therapy. *77th Scientific Assembly and Annual Meeting of the Radiological Society of North America.* Chicago, IL.

55. Yamato, M., Tamai, K., Yamaguchi, T., and Ohno, W. (1993). MRI of the knee in rheumatoid arthritis: Gd-DTPA perfusion dynamics. *J Comput Assist Tomogr*, **17**, 781–5.

56. Weinstein, R.S. and Majumdar, S. (1994). Fractal geometry and vertebral compression fractures. *J Bone Min Res*, **9**,

57. Majumdar, S., Genant, H.K., Grampp, S., Jergas, M.D., and Gies, A.A. (1994). Analysis of trabecular structure in the distal radius using high resolution magnetic resonance images. *Euro Radiol*, **4**, 517–24.

58. Resnick, D. (1995). Internal derangements of joints. In *Diagnosis of bone and joint disorders* (ed. D. Resnick), pp. 3063–9. W.B. Saunders, Philadelphia, PA.

59. Holder, J., Trudell, D., Pathria, M.N., and Resnick, D. (1992). Width of the articular cartilage of the hip: quantification by using fat-suppression spin-echo MR imaging in cadavers. *AJR*, **159**, 351–5.

60. Holder, J., Loredo, R., Longo, C., Trudell, D., Yu, J., and Resnick, D. (1995). Assessment of articular cartilage thickness of the humeral head: MR-anatomic correlation in cadavers. *AJR*, 165, 615–20.

61. Tirman, P.F.J., Stauffer, A.E., Crues, J.V., Turner, R.M., Nottage, W.M., Schobert, W.E., *et al.* (1993). Saline magnetic resonance arthrography in the evaluation of glenohumeral instability. *Arthroscopy*, 9, 550–9.

62. Palmer, W.E., Brown, J.H., and Rosenthal, D.I. (1994). Labral-ligamentous complex of the shoulder: evaluation with MR arthrography. *Radiology*, 190, 645–51.

63. Tirman, P.F.J., Bost, F.W., Garvin, G.J., Peterfy, C.G., Mall, J.C., Steinbach, L.S., *et al.* (1994). Postero-superior glenoid impingement: MRI and MR arthrographic findings with arthroscopic correlation. *Radiology*, 193, 431–6.

11.5.4 Arthroscopic evaluation of knee articular cartilage
Xavier Ayral and Roy D. Altman

To date, therapy for osteoarthritis (OA) has been directed at improving symptoms, primarily pain. Research is now exploring agents that may alter the course of OA. These potential disease-modifying drugs for OA (DMOADs) are being designed to prevent, delay, or even reverse OA changes in the joint. Research into DMOADS requires standardized and reproducible outcome measurements that evaluate changes in the joint. Since many of the potential DMOADS are directed at altering the breakdown of articular cartilage, a measurement of the quantity, integrity, and/or quality of articular cartilage would prove of value[1].

Arthroscopy provides a direct, inclusive, magnified view of the six articular surfaces of the knee. Direct visualization through the arthroscope is more sensitive than the plain radiograph or magnetic resonance imaging (MRI) in detecting cartilage lesions[2]. Indeed, arthroscopy is so sensitive and specific in the evaluation of cartilage, it has prompted some to view arthroscopy as the 'gold standard' for assessment of articular cartilage, whereby other methods will be judged[3]. Direct visualization permits evaluation of the synovium[4]. This is particularly significant in the anterior compartment of the knee where OA abnormalities are often patchy in distribution[5]. Direct visualization of the tissues by arthroscopy allows for guided biopsy of such focal abnormalities.

Over the last few decades, arthroscopy has been established to be of value for diagnosis and surgical intervention in numerous disorders of the knee. There is an evolving methodology that uses knee arthroscopy in clinical research, utilizing baseline and follow-up arthroscopy to monitor the course of knee OA. For this purpose, arthroscopy is used for diagnostic purposes,

and since it is mostly directed at evaluation of cartilage, it is often named 'chondroscopy'[6]. Sequential arthroscopies permit an evaluation of the natural history of OA. In clinical research, the natural history in one cohort of patients could easily be compared to an intervention in another cohort[6].

Issues that have interfered with the development of arthroscopy for clinical research include the following:

- the invasive nature of arthroscopy

- the lack of a validated, standardized scoring system of chondropathy

- the lack of standardized guidelines for video-recording the articular cartilage surfaces during arthroscopy.

Can arthroscopy be simplified?

Local anesthesia

Therapeutic arthroscopy is often performed under general or spinal anesthesia. The procedure requires a preoperative and operative anesthetist consultation, with as much as two days of hospitalization. Postoperative thigh rehabilitation is often necessary due to the potential deleterious effect of the tourniquet on nerve and muscle recovery[7]. Explorative arthroscopy conducted for research purposes can be simplified by the use of local anesthesia administered subcutaneously and intra-articularly. Lidocaine or marcaine can provide skin and synovial anesthesia. With the use of local anesthesia, the procedure is almost always performed on an outpatient basis in an ambulatory surgery center that may or may not be devoted to arthroscopy.

Arthroscopy under local anesthesia is safe, reliable, and relatively inexpensive, and is an alternative to arthroscopy under general or spinal anesthesia[8]. Eriksson *et al.* compared arthroscopy under local, spinal, and general anesthesia[8]. Patient satisfaction under local or spinal anesthesia was similar (77 per cent of satisfied patients), but not as good as general anesthesia (97 per cent of satisfied patients). Blackburn *et al.* compared arthroscopy under local anesthesia to magnetic resonance imaging (MRI) of the knee[2]: both were well tolerated by their 16 patients. When asked about which procedure they preferred, eight patients preferred arthroscopy, two preferred MRI, and six felt the two procedures were equally tolerable.

Ayral *et al.* evaluated local anesthesia in 84 patients undergoing chondroscopy[6]; tolerance was 'good' (62 per cent) or 'very good' (28 per cent) for 90 per cent of the patients[6]; there was no pain in 25 per cent, with some pain during or immediately following the procedure in 75 per cent. In relation to the ambulatory surgery, postarthroscopy daily activities were hampered in 79 per cent of the patients (for up to one day in 44 per cent, up to two days in 55 per cent, and up to one week in 79 per cent)[6]. One month after chondroscopy, 82 per cent of the patients felt improved.

As a guide to tolerability of anesthesia, in a clinical trial, 36 of 39 (95 per cent) patients accepted a second chondroscopy after one year of follow-up[9]. The lack of follow-up in the remaining three patients was not related to the technique[9].

McGinty and Matza compared the diagnostic accuracy of arthroscopy performed under local or general anesthesia with postarthroscopy visualization by arthrotomy[10]. Under this system, arthroscopy was slightly more accurate under local anesthesia (95 per cent) than general anesthesia (91 per cent). It appears that the benefits of local anesthesia are not outweighed by a loss in accuracy. Nevertheless, performance of arthroscopy under local anesthesia requires specific training, even for experienced arthroscopists.

Small glass lens arthroscope

Knee arthroscopy is often performed with a 4.0 mm glass lens arthroscope requiring a 5.5 mm trochar. Chondroscopy is intended to obtain information on the status of the articular surfaces. In some patients with contracted ligaments or residual muscle tension (because of local anesthesia), the posterior part of the femorotibial compartments may not be accessible with a standard 4.0 mm scope. The 2.7 mm arthroscope has a similar field of view as the 4.0 mm arthroscope and most often permits the inspection of all compartments. Continuous knee irrigation provided by the 2.7 mm arthroscope is adequate to clear the joint of blood and debris, allowing a clear field for visualization[6]. Technically, the 25 or 30 degree angle provides a wide field and a better view. Smaller diameter (1.8 mm about 16-gauge) fiberoptic arthroscopes (sometimes called 'needlescopes') can be inserted into the joint by needle puncture rather than stab incision but, among other disadvantages, they provide a smaller field of view, and a dimmer and grainier picture due to fiberoptic transmission and lower irrigation. They also tend to bend and fracture, and are often only straight viewing[11]. The images obtained by the needlescope appear to be insufficient for clinical research on cartilage and synovial lesions, as they tend to underestimate cartilage and synovial abnormalities. Compared to standard arthroscopy, the sensitivity for detecting abnormalities of needlescope arthroscopy is 89 per cent for cartilage and 71 per cent for synovial abnormalities[11].

Tourniquet

An inflated thigh tourniquet is routinely used under general or spinal anesthesia for therapeutic arthroscopy to minimize bleeding, but it cannot be tolerated under local anesthesia. Bleeding during chondroscopy is a potential problem for visualization rather than patient safety; chondroscopy includes enough joint irrigation so that bleeding is most often not of concern. However, some arthroscopists include epinephrine in the local anesthesia to reduce bleeding. Rapid absorption of the epinephrine could cause a transient adverse clinical event, but is avoided by verifying the absence of vascular puncture when performing local anesthesia.

Joint lavage

Ayral *et al.* found that one month after chondroscopy, 82 per cent of the patients felt improved[6]. It is believed the lavage performed during the procedure (usually one liter of normal saline) prompted clinical improvement of joint symptoms. This beneficial effect of joint lavage has been reported in controlled studies[12–14] and might partially counterbalance the invasive nature of the technic. This beneficial effect of arthroscopy needs to be considered when evaluating the benefits of any potential DMOAD.

How to score chondropathy?

Some degree of quantification of the severity of chondropathy is needed to monitor the lesions over time; this can provide the basis for comparing treatment in groups of patients. Articular cartilage lesions can be defined by three baseline parameters: depth, size, and location. Over the years, several arthroscopic classification systems have been devised in an attempt to describe and categorize the articular cartilage damage[15-20].

Previous classifications (Table 11.10)

Some systems only take into account the depth of the lesions (Beguin[15], Insall[16]) and give qualitative information on the surface appearance of articular cartilage. They do not provide a quantitative approach to cartilage lesions.

Some systems (Outerbridge[17], Hungerford and Ficat[18], Bentley[19], Casscels[20]) combine the depth and the size of the most severe chondropathy of the articular surface under a single descriptive category, but present obvious discrepancies.

The Outerbridge classification system[17] subdivides cartilage lesions: grade I — softening and swelling of the cartilage without fissuring (true chondromalacia); grade II — fragmentation and fissuring with a diameter of half an inch or less; grade III — fragmentation and fissuring with a diameter of greater than half an inch; grade IV — erosion of cartilage with exposure of subchondral bone. Grade II and III have identical depth and their size is estimated, while the size of grade I and IV is not described. This system has been used for classifying patients in a cross-sectional study[3] but appears inadequate for accurate outcome measurements of chondropathy in longitudinal studies as the size of grades I and IV is not evaluated, and the size of grades II and III is not a continuous variable.

Hungerford and Ficat subdivide cartilage lesions in closed and open chondromalacia[18]. Closed chondromalacia (grade I) represents true chondromalacia (softening-swelling), and open chondromalacia (grade II) represents open (fissurated) chondropathy. The size of a grade I lesion, according to Ficat and Hungerford, begins as 1 cm^2, in an area which extends progressively in all directions. This description leads to confusion as to the total extent of involvement of the surface area of any grade I lesion. Grade II includes three different depths of chondropathy: superficial and deep fissures, and exposure of subchondral bone, with no reference to the size. This system cannot lead to an accurate quantitative approach of articular cartilage breakdown.

In the classification proposed by Bentley and Dowd[19], grades I, II, and III have identical appearance (fibrillation or fissuring), and the distinction between the grades is based on the diameter of the involvement (Table 11.10). No mention is made of true chondromalacia. Grade IV describes two different depths of chondropathy: fibrillation with or without exposure of subchondral bone, with a fixed size of more than 2.0 cm. Which grade would be assigned to an exposure of subchondral bone less than 2.0 cm in size?

Casscels et al. assigned a specific size-range diameter, in centimeters, to a particular depth of lesion, with the prerequisite that the less the depth, the smaller the size[20] (Table 11.10). Which grade would be assigned to superficial lesions covering the entire articular surface?

The above systems lack consistency in providing information on depth, size, and location of cartilagenous lesions. Guidelines for a system suggest the following are needed:

1. All the different articular cartilage lesions of a given articular surface must be evaluated, and not only the most severe chondropathy, in order to score the overall articular cartilage breakdown.

2. Depth and size of each cartilage lesion must be rated separately.

3. The evaluation of depth must distinguish chondromalacia, superficial fissures, deep fissures, and exposure of subchondral bone.

4. The evaluation of size must be as accurate as possible to allow detection of change with time.

Location of chondropathy is a qualitative variable involving two types of information: (1) the articular surface of the knee that is affected by the chondral lesion; (2) the part of this articular surface that is affected by the chondral lesion. A system for scoring chondropathy can be applied globally to the joint or specifically to each of the three compartments of the knee, that is, patellofemoral, medial tibiofemoral, lateral tibiofemoral. Nevertheless, without quantitative joint mapping, the description of the location of chondropathy on a given articular surface remains qualitative.

Table 11.10 Review of previous classification symptoms of articular cartilage

Author	Surface description of articular cartilage	Diameter	Location
Outerbridge[*]	I — softening and swelling. II — fragmentation and fissuring. III — fragmentation and fissuring. IV — erosion of cartilage down to bone.	I — none II — < 1/2" III — > 1/2" IV — none	Starts most frequently on medial facet of patella; later extends to lateral facet 'mirror' lesion on intercondylar area of femoral condyles; upper border medial femoral condyle.
Hungerford and Ficat[*]	I — closed chondromalacia. Simple softening (small blister) macroscopically, surface is intact, varying degrees of severity from simple softening to 'pitting edema', loss of elasticity. II — open chondromalacia: (a) Fissures — single or multiple, relatively superficial or extending down to subchondral bone. (b)Ulceration — localized loss of cartilage substance, exposes dense subchondral bone. When extensive, bone has polished appearance (eburnated).	I — 1 cm² and then extends progressively in all directions. II — none.	Lateral facet — 2° excessive lateral pressure. Medial facet — 2° incongruence and combination of compression and shearing forces.
	Chondrosclerosis — abnormally hard, not depressible.	Not localized but involves entire contact zone.	
	Tuft formation — multiple deep fronds of cartilage separated from one another by deep clefts which extend to subchondral bone. Superficial surface changes — surface fibrillation; longitudinal striations present in the axis of movement of the joint.		Centered on crest separating medial and odd facets.
Bentley[*]	I — fibrillation or fissuring. II — fibrillation or fissuring. III — fibrillation or fissuring. IV — fibrillation with or without exposure of subchondral bone.	I — 0.5 cm II — 0.5–1.0 cm III — 1.0–2.0 cm IV — > 2.0 cm	Most common at junction of medial and odd facets of patella.
Casscels[*]	I — superficial area of erosion. II — deeper layers of cartilage involved. III — cartilage is completely eroded and bone is exposed. IV — articular cartilage completely destroyed.	I — < or = 1 cm II — 1–2 cm III — 2–4 cm IV — 'wide area'	Patella and anterior femoral surfaces.
Insall[*]	I — swelling and softening of cartilage (closed chondromalacia). II — deep fissures extending to subchondral bone. III — fibrillation. IV — erosive changes and exposures of subchondral bone (osteoarthrosis).	None	I–IV: midpoint of patellar crest with extension equally onto medial and lateral patellar facets. IV: also involves opposite or mirror surface of femur. Upper and lower 1/3 nearly always spared (patella); femur never severe.
Beguin/ Locker	I — softening — swelling. II — superficial fissures. III — deep fissures, down to bone. IV — exposure of subchondral bone.	None	None

[*] Reproduced from reference 21, with the kind permission of the publishers, the American Journal of Sports Medicine.

Newer classifications

Noyes and Stabler

In 1989, Noyes and Stabler proposed a system for grading articular cartilage lesions at arthroscopy.[21] They separate the description of the surface appearance, the depth of involvement, and the diameter and location of the lesions (Table 11.11). They distinguish three surface grades: articular surface intact (grade 1), articular surface damaged, open lesion (grade 2), and bone exposed (grade 3). Each grade is divided into subtypes A or B, depending upon the depth of involvement. Grade 1 implies chondromalacia. Type 1A corresponds to a moderate degree of softening of the articular cartilage; type 1B corresponds to an extensive softening resulting in swelling of the articular surface. A grade 2 lesion is characterized by any disruption of the articular surface without visualized exposure of bone. A type 2A lesion is less than one-half thickness (superficial fissures); type 2B is more than one-half thickness (deep fissures, down to bone). Grade 3 indicates any surface with exposed bone. Type 3A indicates that the normal bony contour remains; type 3B indi-

cates cavitation or erosion of bone surface. Lesions are reported on a knee diagram, and the diameter of each lesion is estimated by the examiner in millimeters using a graduated probing hook. Depending on the diameter and depth of the lesion, a point scaling system is used to calculate the score of chondropathy for each compartment and, finally, to calculate an overall joint score.

This system is the first attempt to score chondropathy; we offer this critique:

1. In this system, all the chondral lesions are represented on the knee diagram as a full circle with a unique diameter defined by the graduated hook. This is a semiobjective estimate of size because most cartilage lesions are not circular, but rather oval or irregularly shaped. Moreover, degenerative cartilage lesions often have the appearance of escharotic skin lesions, with the deepest breakdown located at the middle central point, surrounded by more superficial cartilage lesions. A diameter cannot be attributed to this 'surrounding lesion' which is crown-shaped.

Table 11.11 Classification of articular cartilage lesions[*]

Surface description	Extent of involvement	Diameter (mm)	Location	Degree of knee flexion
1 Cartilage surface intact	(a) Definite softening with some resilience remaining	< 10 ≤ 15 ≤ 20 ≤ 25 > 25	Patella (a) Proximal 1/3 Middle 1/3 Distal 1/3 (b) Odd facet Middle facet Lateral facet Trochlea Medial femoral condyle	Degree of knee flexion where the lesion is in weight-bearing contact (e.g. 20–45 degrees)
	(b) Extensive softening with loss of resilience (deformation)			
2 Cartilage surface damaged: cracks, fissures, fibrillation, or fragmentation	(a) < 1/2 thickness (b) ≥ 1/2 thickness		(a) Anterior 1/3 (b) Middle 1/3 (c) Posterior 1/3 Lateral femoral condyle	
3 Bone exposed	(a) Bone surface intact (b) Bone surface cavitation		(a) Anterior 1/3 (b) Middle 1/3 (c) Posterior 1/3 Medial tibial condyle (a) Anterior 1/3 (b) Middle 1/3 (c) Posterior 1/3 Lateral tibial condyle (a) Anterior 1/3 (b) Middle 1/3 (c) Posterior 1/3	

[*] Reproduced from reference 21, with the kind permission of the publishers, The American Journal of Sports Medicine.

2. In this system, any lesion less than 10 mm in diameter is not considered clinically significant and, therefore, no points are subtracted: this induces a lack of sensitivity. In monitoring the outcome of DMOAD, all lesions, even the smallest, must be described.

3. The point scaling system proposed to score, simultaneously, depth and diameter of chondral lesions, is arbitrary. It is not based on statistical methodology, nor on clinical assessment of the severity of the lesions.

4. This system has not been validated.

Ayral et al.

In 1993, Ayral *et al.*[6] proposed two methods for scoring chondropathy. The first method is a subjective approach based on the overall assessment by the investigator of chondropathy, reported on a set of 100 mm visual analogue scales (VAS) in which '0' indicates the absence of chondropathy and '100', the most severe chondropathy. One VAS is used for each articular surface of the knee: patella, trochlea, medial femoral condyle, lateral femoral condyle, medial tibial plateau, and lateral tibial plateau. A VAS score is calculated for each of the three compartments of the knee and is obtained by averaging the VAS scores from the two corresponding articular surfaces of the compartment.

The second method is a more objective and analytic approach which includes an articular diagram of the knee with grading for location, depth, and size of all the different cartilagenous lesions (Fig. 11.53 and Table 11.12).

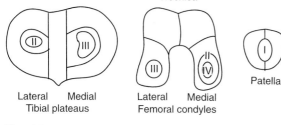

Fig. 11.53 An example of articular cartilage lesions visualized by arthroscopy and recorded on a knee diagram (right-knee) with grades according to Beguin and Locker classification[15].

Location
Areas defined included the patella, trochlea, medial femoral condyle, medial tibial plateau, lateral femoral condyle, and the lateral tibial plateau.

Depth
The system is based on the classification of chondropathy proposed by French arthroscopists Beguin and Locker[15] (Fig. 11.54):

1. Grade 0: normal cartilage.

2. Grade I: chondromalacia, including softening with or without swelling. It can be assimilated to grade 1, type A and B, of Noyes and Stabler[21].

3. Grade II: cartilage demonstrates superficial fissures, either single or multiple, giving a 'velvet-like' appearance to the surface; grade II also includes superficial erosion. Fissures and erosions do not reach subchondral bone and can be assimilated to the grade 2A of Noyes and Stabler in which lesions are less than one-half thickness.

4. Grade III: there are deep fissures of the cartilage surface, down to subchondral bone, which is not directly visualized but may be touched with an arthroscopy probe. Grade III lesions may take different aspects: a 'shark's mouth-like' aspect, or a detached chondral flap, due to a single deep fissure; a 'crab meat-like' aspect due to multiple deep tears. Grade III also includes deep ulceration of the cartilage creating a crater which remains covered by a thin layer of cartilage. Grade III can be assimilated to the grade 2B of Noyes and Stabler in which lesions are more than one-half thickness.

5. Grade IV: there is exposure of subchondral bone with intact bone surface or with cavitation. It can be assimilated to grade 3, type A and B, of Noyes and Stabler.

The different grades are summarized in Fig. 11.54. In knee OA, cartilage breakdown often shows a combination of different grades, the most severe grade being surrounded by milder lesions (Fig. 11.53 and Table 11.12).

Size
The size and shape of each grade of chondropathy is recorded on a knee diagram (Fig. 11.53) by the arthroscopist: this step is crucial for evaluation. Then, the size is evaluated as a percentage of the articular surface.

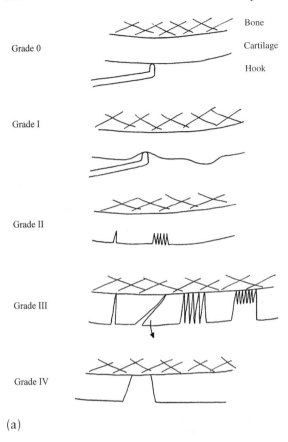

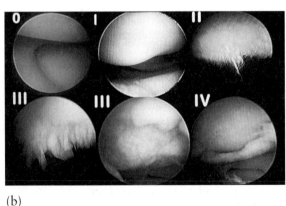

Fig. 11.54 (a) Depth of articular cartilage lesions according to the classification proposed by Beguin and Locker[15]. (b) Examples: chondroscopy; 2.7 mm arthroscope; local anesthesia. Reading from left to right: grade 0 = normal medial femorotibial compartment; grade I = swelling of the lateral femoral condyle; grade II = 'velvet-like' aspect of the patella; grade III = 'crab-meat-like' aspect of the patella; grade III = deep ulceration of the medial femoral condyle; grade IV = exposure of subchondral bone of the medial femoral condyle.

The percentage can be calculated by computer using numerization of the drawing on the knee diagram, or calculated directly from the diagram by a trained investigator. Unless fully trained, the investigator has a tendency to overestimate the size of the lesions. A practical way to calculate the size of each chondropathy covering a given articular surface is to determine the number of times this area could be traced within the whole (100 per cent) articular surface on the diagram. Dividing 100 per cent by the resulting number indicates the size of chondropathy as a percentage. As an example, if tracing a given chondropathy four times on the diagram of the femoral condyle fills the diagram, the size of this given chondropathy is 25 per cent of the femoral condyle, (obtained by dividing 100 per cent, the whole articular surface of the femoral condyle, by four). Examples of different sizes of chondropathy of varying severity are shown in Fig. 11.55.

Location, depth and size of the different chondropathies are reported on a special form[6] (Table 11.12). This form lists ten different quantitative variables, that is, sizes of chondropathy from grade 0 to grade IV for each compartment. The comparison of chondropathy severity between patients and/or between arthroscopies performed at different times in the same patient, required the integration of these different quantitative variables in a single score of chondropathy. For this purpose, the French Society of Arthroscopy carried out a prospective, multicenter study with 14 arthroscopists, selected on the basis of their experience in arthroscopy and considered in this study as 'standard of reference'. Seven hundred and fifty-five subjects who had undergone arthroscopy of the knee were enrolled in this study. Criteria for assessment of severity of chondropathy were as follows: (1) overall assessment by the investigator, using a 100-mm-long visual analogue scale (VAS); and (2) depth, size, and location of cartilage lesions recorded on a diagram. For the establishment of chondropathy scoring, multivariate analyses were carried out using logistic multiple regression in which overall assessment of chondropathy by the investigator using the VAS comprised the dependent variable, and the depth and size of the lesion were the independent variables. Multivariate parametric and non-parametric analyses were performed on two-thirds of the patients and resulted in two systems of assessing chondropathy: the SFA scoring system[22,23] and the SFA grading system[22]. After the SFA systems were established, their validity was evaluated and confirmed on the remaining one-third of the patients by correlating the SFA score

Table 11.12 Calculation of SFA score [†] and SFA grade [‡] from one example of articular cartilage lesions visualized by arthroscopy and recorded on case record form (see Figure 11.53)

Grade[*]	Location								
	Medial compartment			Lateral compartment			Femoropatellar compartment		
	Femur	Tibia	Mean value	Femur	Tibia	Mean value	Patella	Trochlea	Mean value
0	60[**]	65	62.5	80	75	77.5	80	100	90
I	0	0	0.0	0	0	0.0	20	0	10
II	30	0	15.0	0	25	12.5	0	0	0
III	0	35	17.5	20	0	10.0	0	0	0
IV	10	0	5.0	0	0	0.0	0	0	0

[*]0, normal; I, softening–swelling; II, superficial fissures; III, deep fissures; IV, exposure of subchondral bone (Beguin and Locker classification[15])
[**]example: the number represents the size of the corresponding grade expressed in percentage of the corresponding whole articular surface. Each column totals 100%.
[†] SFA score = size (%) of grade I lesions × 0.14 + size (%) of grade II lesions × 0.34 + size (%) of grade III lesions × 0.65 + size (%) of grade IV lesions × 1.00
• Medial score: (15 × 0.34) + (17.5 × 0.65) + (5 × 1.00) = 21.475
• Lateral score: (12.5 × 0.34) + (10 × 0.65) = 10.75
• Femoropatellar score: 10 × 0.14 = 1.4
[‡] SFA grade (definition: see Table 11.13)
• Medial grade = IV
• Lateral grade = III
• Femoropatellar grade = I

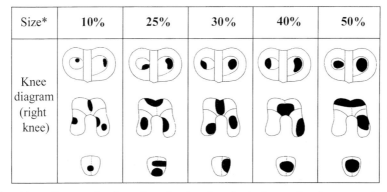

Fig. 11.55 Examples of knee diagrams, by the author, showing size of articular cartilage lesions. Each solid black area represents the % of cartilage damage of each articular surface.

and SFA grade with overall assessment by the investigator using the VAS.

The SFA score is a continuous variable graded between '0' and '100'. The score is obtained for each compartment as follows:

SFA score = A + B + C + D; where

  A = size (per cent) of grade I lesions x 0.14
  B = size (per cent) of grade II lesions x 0.34
  C = size (per cent) of grade III lesions x 0.65
  D = size (per cent) of grade IV lesions x 1.00

Size (per cent) = average per cent of surface for the medial femoral condyle and medial tibial plateau (medial tibiofemoral compartment), lateral femoral condyle and lateral tibial plateau (lateral tibiofemoral compartment), or trochlea and patella (patellofemoral compartment).

The coefficients of severity of chondropathy (0.14, 0.34, 0.65, 1.00) were obtained by parametric multivariate analysis[23].

The SFA grade is a semiquantitative variable. The above numbers [size (per cent) of grade 0 to IV lesions] are placed in a formula to provide a summary grade (or category of chondropathy severity of the compartment) for each of the knee compartments (Table 11.13). The formula for each compartment was obtained by non-parametric multivariate analysis, using a tree-structured regression[22]. There are six categories for the patellofemoral compartment (0 to V) and five categories for the medial and lateral tibiofemoral compartments (0 to IV). One example of the SFA score and the SFA grade is calculated in Table 11.12

Klashman et al.

In 1995, a committee of the American College of Rheumatology (ACR) proposed a scoring system for cartilage[24]. This system takes into account depth, size, and location of chondral lesions, recorded on a knee diagram. Depth of each lesion is assessed by the grades proposed by Noyes and Stabler; the size of each lesion is evaluated as a percentage. An arbitrary point scaling system is applied to obtain an overall score, called damage score; the reliability of the damage score has been evaluated[24]. Videotapes of 10 arthroscopies were each viewed on two separate occasions by three rheumatologist–arthroscopists, in blinded fashion.

Damage score demonstrated significant intraobserver reliability (r = 0.90, 0.90, 0.80; p < 0.01 for each) and interobserver reliability (r = 0.82, 0.80, 0.70; p < 0.05 for each).

The validation of arthroscopic quantification of chondropathy by using VAS score and SFA scoring and grading systems

Ayral *et al.* investigated their system for practicality of chondroscopy in terms of simplicity, reliability, validity, clinical relevance, sensitivity to change, and discriminant capacity.

Simplicity

Arthroscopy will always be an invasive procedure because of stab the incision required, but can be rendered less complex by the use of local anesthesia, performance on an outpatient basis, elimination of the tourniquet, and use of a small-bore glass lens arthroscope[6] (see p. 494–495).

Table 11.13 French Society of Arthroscopy (SFA) system for grading chondropathy during knee arthroscopy

Category	Grade* 0 (%**)		Grade III (%)	Grade IV (%)
Medial tibiofemoral compartment				
0	100			
I	≥80	<100		0
II	<80		<15	0
III	<80		≥15	0
	or ≥65			≥1
IV	<65			≥1
Lateral tibiofemoral compartment				
0	100			
I	≥85	<100	<10	<10
II	<85		<10	<10
III			≥10	<10
IV				≥10
Patellofemoral compartment				
0	100			
I	≥85	<100	<10	<2.5
II	<85		<10	<2.5
III			≥10	<2.5
IV				≥2.5 <25
V				≥25

*Grade derived from cartilage surface changes (Beguin and Locker classification[15]), see p. 6 and Table 11.12
**% derived from extent of surface involved with the grade changes, see p. 6,7 and Table 11.12
Adapted from reference 22.

Reliability

Intraobserver reliability of chondropathy measurement using either VAS score of chondropathy, or SFA score and SFA grade is good[6,25], and better than interobserver reliability[6] (reliability coefficient, 0.928 and 0.989 for intraobserver reliability of the arthroscopic quantification of chondropathy by using SFA score and VAS score, respectively; reliability coefficient, 0.529 and 0.936 for interobserver reliability by using SFA score and VAS score, respectively[25]). Thus, it appears that arthroscopy videotapes from a clinical study should be reviewed by a single trained investigator. For multicenter studies, training sessions will be needed to improve interobserver evaluations of depth and size of the cartilage lesions.

Validity

Intrinsic validity was evaluated by calculating the correlations between the different arthroscopy scales (VAS score and SFA systems). A strong correlation was found between these different systems, as the evaluation of cartilage status by the SFA scoring system accounts for 84, 81, and 83 per cent of the variability of the overall assessment (VAS score) of the medial, lateral, and femoropatellar compartment ($r = 0.92$, 0.90, 0.91, respectively), and the evaluation by the SFA grading system accounts for 75, 77 and 78 per cent of the variability of the overall assessment for these compartments ($r = 0.87$, 0.88, 0.88, respectively)[25]. Nevertheless, the three methods of quantifying chondropathy (VAS score, SFA score, and SFA grade) appear to be of complementary interest and are used together, at this time, in clinical trials in OA. The VAS score and the SFA score are more appropriate to detect minimal changes in severity of chondropathy over time, as they represent a continous variable. SFA grade permits classification of a population of OA patients into homogenous categories of chondropathy severity and investigation of specific subgroups of OA patients. Although a highly significant correlation exists between the VAS and the SFA score, there are some discrepancies between these two technics; the SFA score usually shows a lower value than the VAS score[25]. This is likely due to the fact that evaluating, objectively, the extent of chondropathy as a percentage, lowers the final SFA score; a single deep fissure represents impressive chondropathy (high subjective VAS score) but a very small surface (low objective SFA score). Moreover, the investigator might be influenced by the location of chondropathy on the articular surface (weight-bearing areas or not) when recording his subjective overall assessment of the severity of chondropathy on the 100 mm visual analogue scale.

Extrinsic validity was evaluated by calculating the correlations between the arthroscopic quantification of chondropathy and radiological joint space narrowing on weight-bearing X-rays[6,25]. Arthroscopic and roentgenographic evaluations of chondropathy are closely correlated. There was a strong correlation between: (1) the overall assessment of chondropathy (VAS) and radiological medial joint space narrowing evaluated in percentage ($r = 0.646$, $p < 0.0001$)[6]; (2) the SFA score and joint space narrowing of the medial and lateral femorotibial compartments evaluated in millimeters ($r = -0.59$, $p < 0.01$; and $r = -0.39$, $p < 0.01$, respectively)[25]; (3) the SFA grade and joint space narrowing of the medial and lateral femorotibial compartments evaluated in millimeters ($r = -0.48$, $p < 0.01$; and $r = -0.31$, $p < 0.01$, respectively)[25]. Nevertheless, arthroscopy appears to be more sensitive than plain radiographs. Mild cartilage lesions, but also severe and deep cartilage erosions, may remain undetected, even on weight-bearing radiographs[3,6,25]. In 33 patients fulfilling ACR criteria for OA[6] with joint space narrowing of the medial compartment of less than 25 per cent on weight-bearing X-rays, chondropathy was found at arthroscopy in 30 patients, with a mean VAS score of 21 mm, ranging from 2 to 82 mm, and above 10 mm in 24 patients[6].

Clinical relevance

Ayral *et al.* evaluated clinical relevance in a cross-sectional study of the severity of chondropathy at arthroscopy[25]. This was correlated with the clinical characteristics of the patients, including demographic data, baseline characteristics, and clinical activity of OA. They found a statistically significant correlation ($p < 0.05$) between articular cartilage damage: (1) of the three compartments (medial, lateral, femoropatellar) of the knee and patient age; and (2) of the medial compartment and the body mass index. At variance, no statistically significant correlation was found between articular cartilage damage of the knee and clinical activity (pain, Lequesne's index[27], Arthritis Impact Measurement Scale (AIMS2)[28]. Conversely, a longitudinal study performed with a one-year arthroscopy follow-up in 41 patients showed that changes in the severity of cartilage lesions correlated with changes in functional disability (Lequesne's index: $r = 0.34$, p = 0.03) and quality of life (AIMS2: r = 0.35, p = 0.04)[25].

Sensitivity to change

Chondroscopy demonstrated statistically significant worsening in knee OA cartilage lesions between two arthroscopic evaluations performed one year apart in 41 patients[25]. The mean VAS score of the medial compartment moved from 45 ± 28 at entry to 55 ± 31 after one year (p = 0.0002) and the SFA score from 31 ± 21 to 37 ± 24 (p = 0.0003). Significant worsening was also reported in a one-year trial of 26 patients with post-traumatic patella chondromalacia[29]. Sensitivity to change might be explained by the precision of the technique and enrollment of patients with active OA of the knee. These patients had prior failure of analgesics, NSAIDs, physical exercises, and intra-articular glucocorticoid injection leading to joint lavage. It should be noted that several longitudinal arthroscopic studies that demonstrated cartilage abnormalities noted reversible changes in occasional patients[25,29,30].

Discriminant capacity

A preliminary study of repeated hyaluronic acid injections suggested that chondroscopy may be capable of identifying chondromodulating agents[9].

Guidelines for videorecording articular cartilage surfaces at knee arthroscopy

Arthroscopies conducted for clinical or research purposes are most often recorded on videotape. The arthroscopist needs to prepare for the videorecording by making sure the appropriate equipment is available and functional. For clinical trials, centralized reading and grading of arthroscopies may be needed.

Clarity of the image

Clarity of the videorecording can be improved by:

(1) Using a local intra-articular anesthesia with epinephrine to reduce bleeding;

(2) Performing abundant articular lavage before starting to record, in order to remove debris and cellular material;

(3) continuously focusing the camera;

(4) maximizing light intensity by providing enough light for visualization but avoiding overexposure ('flash') of the articular cartilage;

(5) removing any condensation on the camera or scope.

Complete exploration

The aim of arthroscopy is to explore the entire six articular surfaces of the knee joint. Areas of normal cartilage should receive as much attention as areas of damage, in order that the reader can assess what percentage of the total cartilage is damaged. The arthroscopist can briefly assess any cartilage lesion, but should not focus on specific lesions before making a general examination by sweeping along the whole articular surface from medial to lateral edge, and inversely, and from back to front, in order to allow the reader to assess the size of any lesion. The exploration of each articular surface should be performed twice, and slowly, to ensure that no area is missed. The femoral condyles should be explored from 20° to 90° of knee flexion, whilst maintaining valgus or varus pressure, to allow the inspection of their posterior surfaces.

Conclusion

Arthroscopy, performed under local anesthesia, is a relevant outcome measure of OA in clinical research. Arthroscopy could potentially lead to reducing the duration and number of patients in clinical trials on DMOADs in OA.

References

1. Lequesne, M., Brandt, K., Bellamy N., Moskowitz, R., Menkes, C.J., Pelletier, T.P., *et al.* (1994). Guidelines for testing slow acting drugs in OA. *Journal of Rheumatology*, **21** (4 suppl), 65–71.
2. Blackburn, P.M., Kramer, J., Marcelis, S., Pathria, M.N., Trudell, D., Haghighi, P., *et al.* (1994). Arthroscopic evaluation of knee articular cartilage: a comparison with plain radiographs and magnetic resonance imaging. *Journal of Rheumatology*, **21**, 675–9.
3. Fife, R.S., Brandt, K.D., Braunstein, E.M., Katz, B.P., Shelbourne, K.D., Kalinski, L.A., *et al.* (1991). Relationship between arthroscopic evidence of cartilage damage and radiographic evaluation of joint space narrowing in early OA of the knee. *Arthritis and Rheumatism*, **34**, 377–82.

4. Kurosaka, M., Ohno, O., and Hirohata, K. (1991). Arthroscopy evaluation of synovitis in the knee joints. *Arthroscopy*, 7, 162–70.

5. Lindblad, S. and Hedfors, E. (1987). Arthroscopic and immunohistologic characterization of knee joint synovitis in OA. *Arthritis and Rheumatism*, 30, 1081–8.

6. Ayral, X., Dougados, M., Listrat, V., Bonvarlet, J.P., Simonnet, J., Poiraudeau, S., *et al.* (1993). Chondroscopy: a new method for scoring chondropathy. *Seminars in Arthritis and Rheumatism*, 22, 289–97.

7. Dobner, J. and Nitz, A. (1982). Postmeniscectomy tourniquet palsy and functional sequelae. *American Journal of Sports Medicine*, 10, 211–14.

8. Eriksson, E., Haggmark, T., Saartok, T., Sebik, A., and Ortengren, B. (1986). Knee arthroscopy with local anesthesia in ambulatory patients. *Orthopedics*, 9, 186–8.

9. Listrat, V., Ayral, X., Patarnello, F., Bonvarlet, J.P., Simonnet, J., Amor, B. *et al.* (1997). Arthroscopic evaluation of potential structure modifying activity of hyaluronan (Hyalgan®) in osteoarthritis of the knee. *Osteoarthritis and cartilage*, 5, 153–60.

10. Mc Ginty, J.B. and Matza, R.A. (1978). Arthroscopy of the knee. *Journal of Bone and Joint Surgery*, 60-A, 787–9.

11. Ike, R.W. and Rourke, K.S. (1993). Detection of intra-articular abnormalities in OA of the knee. A pilot study comparing needle arthroscopy with standard arthroscopy. *Arthritis and Rheumatism*, 36, 1353–63.

12. Livesley, P.J., Doherty, M., Needhoff, M., and Moulton, A. (1991). Arthroscopic lavage of osteoarthritic knees. *Journal of Bone and joint Surgery*, 73-B, 922–6.

13. Ike, R.W., Arnold, W.J., Rothschild, E., and Shaw, H.L. (1992). The Tidal Irrigation Cooperating Group. Tidal irrigation versus conservative medical management in patients with OA of the knee: a prospective randomized study. *Journal of Rheumatology*, 19, 772–9.

14. Chang, R.W., Falconer, J., Stulberg, S.D., Arnold, W.J., Manheim, L.M., and Dyer, A.R. (1993). A randomized, controlled trial of arthroscopic surgery versus closed-needle joint lavage for patients with OA of the knee. *Arthritis and Rheumatism*, 36, 289–96.

15. Beguin, J. and Locker, B. (1983). Chondropathie rotulienne. In *2ème journée d'arthroscopie du genou*, No. 1, pp. 89–90. Lyon.

16. Insall, J.N. (1984). Disorders of the patellae. In *Surgery of the knee*, pp. 191–260. Churchill Livingstone, New York.

17. Outerbridge, R.E. (1961). The etiology of chondromalacia patellae. *Journal of Bone and Joint Surgery*, 43-B, 752–7.

18. Ficat, R.P. Philippe, J., and Hungerford, D.S. (1979). Chondromalacia patellae: a system of classification. *Clinical Orthopaedics and Related Research*, 144, 55–62.

19. Bentley, G. and Dowd, G. (1984). Current concepts of etiology and treatment of chondromalacia patellae. *Clinical Orthopaedics and Related Research*, 189, 209–28.

20. Casscels, S.W. (1978). Gross pathological changes in the knee joint of the aged individual: a study of 300 cases. *Clinical Orthopaedics and Related Research*, 132, 225–35.

21. Noyes, F.R. and Stabler, C.L. (1989). A system for grading articular cartilage lesions at arthroscopy. *American Journal of Sports Medicine*, 17, 505–13.

22. Dougados, M., Ayral, X., Listrat, V., Gueguen, A., Bahuaud, J., Beaufils, P., *et al.* (1994). The SFA system for assessing articular cartilage lesions at arthroscopy of the knee. *Arthroscopy*, 10, 69–77.

23. Ayral, X., Listrat, V., Gueguen, A., Bahuaud, J., Beaufils, P., Beguin, J., *et al.* (1994). Simplified arthroscopy scoring system for chondropathy of the knee (revised SFA score). *Revue du Rhumatisme (English Edition)*, 31, 89–90.

24. Klashman, D., Ike, R., Moreland, L., Skovron M.L., and Kalunian, K. (1995). Validation of an OA data report form for knee arthroscopy. *Arthritis and Rheumatism*, 38 (9 suppl), S 178, Abstract 154.

25. Ayral, X., Dougados, M., Listrat, V., Bonvarlet, J.P., Simonnet, J., Amor, B. (1996). Arthroscopic evaluation of chondropathy in osteoarthritis of the knee. *Journal of Rheumatology*, 23, 698–706.

26. Altman, R., Asch, E., Bloch, D., Bole, G., Borenstein, D., Brandt, K., *et al.* (1986). Development of criteria for the classification and reporting of osteoarthritis. Classification of osteoarthritis of the knee. *Arthritis and Rheumatism*, 29, 1039–49.

27. Lequesne, M., Mery, C., Samson, M., Gerard, P. (1987). Indexes of severity for osteoarthritis of the hip and knee. Validation — value in comparison with other assessment test. *Scandinavian Journal of Rheumatology*, 85 (65 suppl), 85–9.

28. Poiraudeau, S., Dougados, M., Ait-Hadad, H., Pion-Graff, J., Ayral, X., Listrat, V., *et al.* (1993). Evaluation of the French version of a quality of life scale (AIMS2) in rheumatology patients. *Revue du Rhumatisme (English Edition)*, 60, 466–72.

29. Raatikainen, T., Vaananen, K., and Tamelander, G. (1990). Effect of glycosaminoglycan polysulfate on chondromalacia patella. A placebo controlled 1 year study. *Acta Orthopaedica Scandinavica*, 61, 443–8.

30. Fujisawa, Y., Masuhara, K., and Shiomi, S. (1979). The effects of high tibial osteotomy on OA of the knee. An arthroscopic study of 54 knee joints. *Orthopedic Clinics of North America*, 10, 585–608.

11.5.5 Bone scintigraphy
Donald S. Schauwecker

Radiographic techniques, such as microfocal spot radiography magnification and computed tomography, provide exquisite anatomic details of the joint in osteoarthritis (OA). Joint narrowing, subchondral cysts, subchondral sclerosis, the size and number of osteophytes, and so on — all can be evaluated. Unfortunately, these anatomic changes are a historic record of the response to past insults: they are of no use in assessing physiologic changes or disease 'activity' at the time of the radiographic examination.

Scintigraphy provides information about alterations in physiology that are occurring at the time of the study — it has two drawbacks, however. First, the image resolution is much poorer than radiography. Second, because bone cells respond to many insults, such as trauma, infection, and tumor invasion by increasing bone turnover, scintigraphy has high sensitivity but poor specificity. The physiologic information from scintigraphy complements the anatomic information of the radiologic examination.

From the point of view of the patient, a nuclear medicine bone scan is a relatively innocuous procedure. The patient lies on a table and receives an intravenous injection of the radiopharmaceutical through a small gauge needle while the nuclear angiogram or perfusion study is obtained. The patient then is free to spend about three hours as he or she wishes while the radiopharmaceutical localizes to the bone. The delayed imaging of the bone then takes 30 to 60 minutes.

At least three different scintigraphic approaches have been taken for the evaluation of OA. These have been directed toward the articular cartilage, joint perfusion, and the bone, respectively.

Because many of the early changes of OA occur in the cartilage, a cartilage imaging agent might theoretically provide the best approach. Several preliminary attempts have been made to develop a cartilage imaging agent; however, these have met with only limited success[1,2]. Therefore, it is necessary today to use more indirect approaches for the scintigraphic evaluation of OA.

Two approaches have been used to study perfusion of the joint, which is increased when inflammation is present. The more elegant is the injection of Xe-133

into the joint, which is then washed out at a rate proportional to the perfusion. Phelps *et al.* found a biexponential washout curve following intra-articular injection of Xe-133[3]. They hypothesized that the faster component related to perfusion of the synovial membrane, while the slower component represented washout from the articular fat. Six rabbits with surgically induced OA of the knee were compared with controls: the OA knee showed significantly greater synovial perfusion than the control knee.

A less elegant, but more readily available indication of perfusion is the nuclear angiogram performed in conjunction with the bone scan. Serial 2–4-second images of the desired joints are obtained following the injection of the bone scanning agent: sites of OA exhibit increased perfusion compared to control joints. Interpretation is only qualitative, and is based upon direct comparison of the OA joint to the normal control. In general, this approach has proved less accurate in the evaluation of OA joints than the evaluation of increased bone turnover[4,5].

The most common scintigraphic approach to the study of OA is the use of delayed bone scan images obtained three to four hours after the injection of the radiopharmaceutical. Historically, many agents have been used which are incorporated into calcium hydroxyapatite crystals as the bone remodels. The current agents of choice are biphosphonates, which are chemisorbed on to the surface of microcrystals of calcium hydroxyapatite in the bone[6]. The more rapid the rate of bone turnover, the greater the localization of the radiopharmaceutical, given an adequate blood supply. Most of the bone scintigraphy discussed in the remainder of this chapter was obtained using this approach.

The bone scan images are obtained using a gamma camera, a sophisticated instrument that detects gamma rays and locates the source of the ray in a two-dimensional plane. Because the injected radiopharmaceutical produces far fewer gamma rays than the number of X-rays produced by the cathode ray tubes used in radiography, the resolution of the image is much poorer. The bone scan images resemble low resolution radiographs. (For example, see Fig. 11.56) When

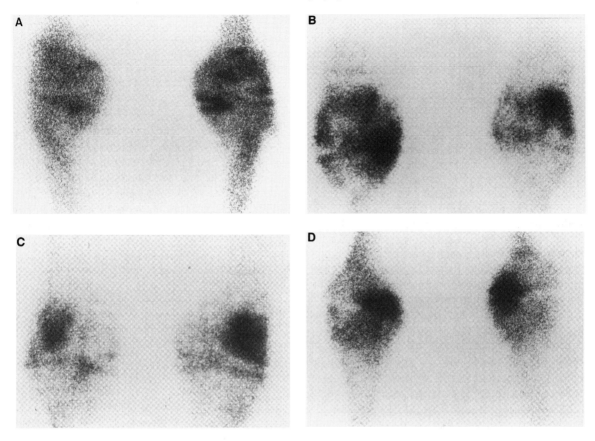

Fig. 11.56 Four patterns of OA are seen on the delayed (4-hour) bone scan image, as described by McCrae *et al.*[4]. In the tramline pattern (a), increased retention is seen along the joint line. This corresponded to the presence of joint pain and to subchondral sclerosis on the plain radiograph. In the extended pattern (b), uptake is seen in the subchondral bone. This was associated with more severely damaged knees, with joint space narrowing, and subchondral sclerosis. The 'hot patella' sign (c) is associated with patellofemoral OA change (note that a tramline pattern is also present in (c)). The generalized pattern (d) shows a diffuse increase in uptake around the joint. This was associated with pain and radiographic evidence of osteophytosis. (Adapted and modified from McCrae *et al.*[4], with permission.)

the gamma camera is rotated around the patient, it is possible to produce cross-sectional images in any plane, such as those obtained with magnetic resonance imaging. This technique is called single photon emission computed tomography (SPECT).

The resolution of bone scintigraphy is approximately 1 cm. Scintigraphic evaluation of OA in large joints, such as the hip and knee, will be considered separately, therefore, from that of OA of smaller joints, such as those in the fingers and toes. In large joints, semiquantitative measurements can be made by comparing pixel counts at various sites within the joint with those at a control site, such as the midshaft of the adjacent long bone. The limited resolution of the gamma camera prevents such comparisons for the smaller joints.

It has been known for years that bone-seeking isotopes are rapidly taken up by OA joints. In 1963, Danielsson *et al.* found a relationship between isotope uptake and the radiographic severity and rate of progression of OA of the hip[7]. While the technique is non-specific, it may be highly sensitive and may reveal more extensive and severe changes of OA than other imaging modalities[8].

Christensen found that the distribution of ^{99m}Tc-methylene diphosphonate uptake was similar to that of the histochemical localization of bone acid and alkaline phosphatase activity in the OA joint[9]. The most intense uptake was seen in subchondral bone, at the osteochondral junction of osteophytes, and in the walls of bone cysts.

Sharif *et al.* compared the bone scan results with synovial fluid markers of bone and cartilage turnover in 35 patients with OA of the knee[10]. They found a statistically significant correlation between the intensity of the bone scan and the level of osteocalcin, a biochemical marker of bone turnover. A weaker association was present between the synovial fluid concentrations of keratan sulfate and chondroitin sulfate epitopes and bone scan intensity, suggesting a poorer correlation with cartilage turnover. These observations reinforced the suggestion that scintigraphy provided an index of bone remodeling in OA.

Using an experimental model of secondary OA in the rabbit, Christensen showed that uptake of ^{99m}Tc-methylene diphosphonate was increased in the unstable knee within one week following surgical destabilization. Uptake was confined to sites of developing osteophytes[11]. Later, however, the same sites did not exhibit increased localization of the radiopharmaceutical, although increased localization was then seen in the subchondral bone beneath areas of cartilage damage. These studies in experimentally induced OA suggested that scintigraphy might *predict* the subsequent development of pathologic changes in OA.

Scintigraphic studies of hand OA in humans

Hutton *et al.* utilized the above information to examine the ability of scintigraphy to predict radiographic changes in hand joints of subjects with OA, taking advantage of the fact that many joints within the hand are susceptible to OA and that progression of changes within and between hand joints is often rapid[12]. In a cross-sectional survey of 33 patients with hand OA, in whom bone scans and plain radiographs were performed, the bone scans showed abnormalities in a number of joints that were normal on the plain radiograph. In several other cases, the radiograph showed evidence of OA but the bone scan was normal (Table 11.14).

In a subsequent study, 14 of the above patients were followed for three to five years to relate the initial scintigraphic findings to subsequent development of osteoarthritis[13]. The results indicated that positive scans were associated with a greater likelihood of subsequent radiographic evidence of OA progression than negative scans (Table 11.15). In several instances, initial scan abnormalities preceded radiographic changes of OA in the same joint by months or years. In some cases, scan positivity subsided as abnormalities in the involved joint became stable on plain radiography (Table 11.15).

These results were corroborated by Buckland-Wright *et al.*, who studied 35 patients with OA of the hand and wrist using serial magnification radiographs and four-hour bone scan images[14]. They found that the intensity on the bone scan correlated well with the size and number of osteophytes, but not with joint space width, subchondral sclerosis, or juxta-articular radiolucencies. During the one-year follow-up, joints with increased activity on the bone scan exhibited growth in the size or remodeling of the osteophytes, but no significant change in the number of osteophytes. In contrast, in those joints in which the bone scan was essentially normal, little change was detected in the size and number of osteophytes.

These data suggest that the onset of disease activity in the OA joint is marked by increased localization of the radiopharmaceutical, which is followed eventually by radiographic changes of OA. As disease activity stabilizes, the bone scan subsequently returns to normal.

Table 11.14   Cross-sectional data from scintigraphic studies in OA of the hand[*]

Site	X-ray + Normal	X-ray + Scan +	X-ray – Scan –	Scan +
DIP	37	32	25	6
PIP	57	24	11	9
MCP	91	2	1	7
TB	17	55	12	17

[*]Numbers indicate the percentage of joints with each feature, based on analysis of all joints in the hand in 33 patients with OA.

DIP = distal interphalangeal joints; PIP = proximal interphalangeal joints; MCP = metacarpophalangeal joints; TB = thumb base.

+ = positive, – = normal

From reference 12.

Table 11.15 Longitudinal data from scintigraphic studies in OA of the hand[*]

	Total	No change	Progression	Regression	Ankylosis
Normal	288	262 (91)	26 (9)	0	0
X+, S–	59	43 (73)	8 (14)	6 (10)	2 (3)
X+, S+	81	46 (57)	30 (37)	3 (4)	2 (2)
X–, S+	20	6 (30)	14 (70)	0	0

[*] Numbers indicate the total number and, in parentheses, the percentage of joints showing change in 14 patients with OA of the hand.
X = radiograph, S = scintigraph, + = positive, –= normal
From reference 13.

In individual patients, different stages in the evolution of OA may exist concurrently within joints of the same hand.

Not all authors agree fully with the results of Hutton et al.[13] and Buckland-Wright et al.[14]; Balblanc et al.[15] studied hand radiographs and bone scans of 15 patients with symptomatic hand OA at baseline and four years later. Correlation was noted between the radiographic score and the scintigraphic score assessed either at entry or at follow-up. An attempt was made to quantitate bone uptake in the scintigram by expressing the data as a joint-to-bone reference area ratio. Joints in which an initially normal bone scan had become positive four years later, or in which both bone scans were abnormal, were more likely to show worsening of the radiographic score than those in which both bone scans were normal. However, in contrast to the results of the studies noted above[13,14], quantification of initial isotope retention and changes in the scintigraphy score had *no* predictive value for progression of the score for radiographic severity of OA.

Scintigraphic studies of knee OA in humans

Joints of the hand are too small to permit ready analysis of uptake within different areas of the joint. Hutton et al.[12] dealt with the limited resolution of bone scintigraphy by combining the first carpometacarpal joint and scaphotrapezoid joint, and calling this 'thumb base'. The images of the remainder of the carpal bones were combined and called 'the wrist'. However, the knee is a much larger structure than the hand or wrist, and analysis of uptake in different areas of that joint is possible. A recent scintigraphic assessment of OA of the knee revealed four different image patterns on the delayed (four-hour) bone scan (Fig. 11.56)[4]. Generalized retention of isotope around the joint, in either the early (flow) or late (bone) phase of the bone scan, was less common than focal areas of uptake around the margin of the patella or in the subchondral bone, which were observed only in the late phase scans. As noted in the above studies of hand OA, some knees with abnormal scans were radiographically normal, while others that exhibited evidence of OA on the radiograph were normal on the scintigraphic study. Retention of isotope along the joint line correlated with joint pain clinically and subchondral sclerosis on the radiograph, while a generalized pattern of uptake was associated with the presence of osteophytes[4].

In the knee, planar scintigraphy often superimposes activity in the patellofemoral space upon that in the medial and lateral tibiofemoral compartments. Theoretically, a lateral view of the knee could separate activity in the patellofemoral compartment from that in the tibiofemoral compartment. However, no large series has used this approach to date. Thomas et al. found that planar bone scintigraphy was no more sensitive than clinical evaluation or conventional radiography when used to identify patellofemoral OA[8]. Collier et al., using single photon emission computed tomography[5], studied 27 patients with chronic knee pain. With arthroscopy used as the 'gold standard', they found that the sensitivity for cartilage damage and synovitis of single photon emission computed tomography (SPECT) was 91 per cent, while that of planar bone scintigraphy was 57 per cent, radionuclide angiography (the perfusion study obtained at the time of the radiopharmaceutical injection), 39 per cent, conventional radiography, 22 per cent, and clinical examination, 17 per cent.

Dieppe et al. suggested that bone scintigraphy could predict progression of knee OA in patients who already exhibited clinical and radiographic evidence of the disease[16]. In this study, patients who had knee radiographs and bone scans in 1986 underwent repeat radiography in 1991. Criteria for progression of knee OA were: (1) joint surgery; or (2) a decrease in the tibiofemoral joint space of more than 2 mm. Of the 94 patients enrolled in this study, ten died, nine were lost to follow-up over the five-year interval, and 15 underwent knee surgery (22 knees). Eighty-seven knees had bone scan abnormalities at the initial evaluation, and 52 (60 per cent) had progression of radiographic abnormalities or surgery during the five-year period. Notably, of the 32 knees that exhibited severe radiographic abnormalities at the outset of the study, 28 (88 per cent) showed progression. On the other hand, *none* of the 55 knees in which knee scintigraphy was normal at entry into the study showed progression of OA.

Three caveats should be raised, however, with regard to this study. First, the criteria for joint surgery were not defined. This is important because the basis for the decision to proceed with arthroplasty varies markedly among clinicians. It is often related to joint pain and function, and may have had nothing to do with progression of joint pathology in the involved knee [17]. Second, the sequential knee films were plain radiographs, that is, an anteroposterior standing view in full extension and a lateral taken in 30° of flexion. Because no particular effort was made to standardize radioanatomic positioning for the serial radiographs, changes in joint space width due to errors in beam alignment or increased knee flexion (that is, due to joint pain) may have resulted in artifactual narrowing of the joint space in the standing anteroposterior view (see Chapter 11.5.1). Third, the bone scan results were interpreted as 'normal' or 'abnormal'; criteria for scoring were not defined, nor was any attempt made to quantify radionuclide uptake.

Currently, scintigraphy is not part of the routine clinical evaluation of a patient with OA. The above data suggest that bone scintigraphy may prove useful in diagnosing *preclinical* OA, for example, in identifying involved joints before the appearance of clinical or radiographic evidence of the disease. In addition, scintigraphy may predict future radiographic changes of OA.

If the strong negative predictive value of bone scintigraphy reported by Dieppe *et al.*[16] is confirmed, the procedure would be very useful in screening patients for enrollment in controlled clinical trials of disease-modifying drugs for OA. Indeed, use of a nega-

tive baseline bone scan as an exclusion criterion could sharply decrease the number of subjects required to demonstrate a statistically significant effect of the drug under study and, therefore, significantly reduce the cost of the study.

In conclusion, although the data relating to scintigraphic evaluation of OA are less extensive than those for some other diseases, from the perspective of scintigraphy, the overall pattern of disease progression in OA is similar to that in many diseases of bone, such as osteomyelitis [18], stress fracture [19], and Paget's disease[20]. Initially, the bone suffers some insult or injury and responds with accelerated bone turnover. At that stage, the bone scan will be positive but the radiograph will still be normal. With the passage of time, increased bone remodeling may result in anatomic changes. At this stage, both the bone scan and the radiograph will be abnormal. Later, if the insult has stabilized or healed, bone turnover returns to normal. At this stage, the bone scan will be normal, although residual anatomic changes may be present on the radiograph.

The major limitations of bone scintigraphy are its low spatial resolution, in comparison with plain radiography and computed tomography, and, because bone responds to most insults with increased turnover, its poor specificity for OA.

The chief advantage of scintigraphy is its extreme sensitivity for activity of the disease at the time the scan is obtained: this may permit scintigraphy to predict future anatomic changes. Conversely, if, as suggested, the technique proves to have a strong negative predictive value, it may be very helpful in predicting joints which will not be affected by OA.

Bone scintigraphy is rarely used to make the diagnosis of OA, but the localization of disease activity seen on the bone scan could prove to be helpful in planning treatment. For example, relative disease activity in the knee can be determined separately for the patellofemoral and the medial and lateral tibiofemoral compartments. If, as Dieppe *et al.*[16] have shown, a normal bone scan tends to remain normal in patients with OA, it might be possible to use scintigraphy to help identify subjects who are candidates for an osteotomy or unicompartmental arthroplasty, rather than total joint replacement. Finally, scintigraphy may have potential in clinical trials which require monitoring of the effects of disease-modifying drugs for OA.

References

1. Cassiede, P., Amedee, J., Vuillemin, L. *et al.* (1993). Radioimmunodetection of rat and rabbit cartilage using a monoclonal antibody specific to link proteins. *Nucl Med Biol*, **20**, 849–55.

2. Yu, W.K.S., Shaw, S.M., Bartlett, J.M., *et al.* (1989). The biodistribution of [^{75}Se]bis-[b-(N,N,N-Trimethylamino)ethyl]selenide diiodide in adult guinea pigs. *Nucl Med Biol*, **16**, 255–9.

3. Phelps, P., Steele, A.D., and McCarty, D.J. (1972). Significance of Xenon-133 clearance rate from canine and human joints. *Arthritis Rheum*, **15**, 360–70.

4. McCrae, F., Shouls, J., Dieppe, P., *et al.* (1992). Scintigraphic assessment of osteoarthritis of the knee joint. *Ann Rheum Dis*, **51**, 938–42.

5. Collier, B.D., Johnson, R.P., Carrera, G.F., *et al.* (1985). Chronic knee pain assessed by SPECT: comparison with other modalities. *Radiology*, **157**, 795–802.

6. Francis, M.D. (1969). The inhibition of calcium hydroxyapatite crystal growth by polyphosphonates and polyphosphates. *Calc Tiss Res*, **3**, 151–62.

7. Danielsson, L.G., Dymling, J.F., and Heripret, G. (1963). Coxarthrosis in man studied with external counting of ^{85}Sr and ^{47}Ca. *Clin Orthop*, **31**, 184–99.

8. Thomas, R.H., Resnick, D., Alazraki, N.P., *et al.* (1975). Compartmental evaluation of osteoarthritis of the knee: a comparative study of available diagnostic modalities. *Radiology*, **116**, 585–94.

9. Christensen, S.B. (1985). Osteoarthrosis: changes of bone, cartilage and synovial membrane in relation to bone scintigraphy. *Acta Orthop Scan*, **56**(suppl 214), 1–43.

10. Sharif, M., George, E., and Dieppe, P.A. (1995). Correlation between synovial fluid markers of cartilage and bone turnover and scintigraphic scan abnormalities in osteoarthritis of the knee. *Arthritis Rheum*, **38**, 78–81.

11. Christensen, S.B. (1983). Localization of bone-seeking agents in developing experimentally induced osteoarthritis in the knee joint of the rabbit. *Scand J Rheumatol*, **12**, 343–9.

12. Hutton, C.W., Higgs, E.R., Jackson, P.C., *et al.* (1986). ^{99m}TcHMDP bone scanning in generalized nodal osteoarthritis. I. Comparison of the standard radiograph and four hour bone scan image of the hand. *Ann Rheum Dis*, **45**, 617–21.

13. Hutton, C.W., Higgs, E.R., Jackson, P.C., *et al.* (1986). ^{99m}TcHMDP bone scanning in generalized nodal osteoarthritis. II. The four hour bone scan image predicts radiographic change. *Ann Rheum Dis*, **45**, 622–6.

14. Buckland-Wright, J.C., Macfarlane, D.G., and Lynch, J.A. (1995). Sensitivity of radiographic features and specificity of scintigraphic imaging in hand osteoarthritis. *Rev Rhum (English Ed)*, **62**, 14S–26S.

15. Balblanc, J.C., Mathieu, P., Mathieu, L., *et al.* (1994). Second scintigraphy and radiographic progression of digital osteoarthritis. *Osteoarthritis and Cartilage*, **2**, 38.

16. Dieppe, P., Cushanghan, J., Young, P., *et al.* (1993). Prediction of the progression of joint space narrowing in osteoarthritis of the knee by bone scintigraphy. *Ann Rheum Dis*, **52**, 557–63.

17. Wright, J.G., Coyte, P., Hawker, G., *et al.* (1995). Variation in orthopedic surgeons' perceptions of the indications for and outcomes of knee replacement. *Can Med Assoc J*, **152**, 687–97.

18. Howie, D.W., Savage, J.P., Wilson, T.G., *et al.* (1983). The technetium phosphate bone scan in the diagnosis of osteomyelitis in childhood. *J Bone Joint Surg*, **65-A**, 431–7.

19. Zwas, S.T., Elkanovitch, R., and Frank, G. (1987). Interpretation and classification of bone scintigraphic findings in stress fractures. *J Nucl Med*, **28**, 452–7.

20. Wellman, H.N., Schauwecker, D.S., Robb, J.A., *et al.* (1977). Skeletal scintimaging and radiography in the diagnosis and management of Paget's disease. *Clin Orthop*, **127**, 55–62.

11.5.6 Ultrasonography
Stephen Myers

Pharmacologic agents are now available which, in experimental models of Osteoarthritis (OA), favorably influence the progression of the disease[1]. This raises the possibility that such agents, which can alter pathogenic mechanisms within the joint and are termed 'disease-modifying OA drugs' (DMOADs)[2], may have utility in the prevention or treatment of OA in humans. The exciting prospect of evaluating these drugs has prompted considerable interest in identification of sensitive and reliable methods to measure the progression of this disease[3]. As discussed in previous chapters, modifications of standard radiographic and MR imaging techniques have been devised to improve their performance as measures of OA severity and progression, but none of these methods are entirely satisfactory, or readily available to the clinician[3]. Other approaches, such as measurement of the concentration of cartilage-derived 'marker' molecules in serum or synovial fluid, have also been proposed for monitoring disease progression, but some investigators have expressed reservation that measurement of the body fluid concentration of *any* cartilage-derived molecule will be useful in monitoring changes in an index joint, evidence of which is likely to be required in a clinical trial of a DMOAD[4].

Clearly, better ways to evaluate the OA joint are needed. This chapter reviews diagnostic ultrasonic imaging, or sonography, a rapidly evolving imaging technique whose clinical value in the evaluation of some musculoskeletal problems has been established, and which may prove to be a powerful tool for the assessment of OA cartilage. Sonography is a safe, non-invasive, and relatively inexpensive technique that can readily distinguish synovial fluid from tendon, cartilage, and bone, and can provide a real-time visual display of the anatomical relationships of articular and periarticular tissue in a two-dimensional imaging plane. It represents a powerful technology that, with appropriate instrumentation, may be useful in obtaining serial measurements of the thickness and surface characteristics of articular cartilage in clinical trials of DMOADs.

Production of the sonographic image

The objective of diagnostic sonography is to obtain and interpret images of living tissue by probing it with very high frequency (ultrasonic) sound waves. Although the features and complexity of the electronic equipment used to acquire, process, and display such images depend on the tissue to be evaluated, the equipment that is used to image the extremities typically employs pulse-echo ultrasound technology to produce a grey-scale image[5-8]. A basic understanding of this technology can help us understand the image it produces and some of its limitations.

An electrical ultrasound generator, or transducer, that emits acoustic energy at a characteristic sonic frequency, is the primary element in any sonographic imaging system[7]. Several identical transducers can be aligned to enlarge the area which is imaged. In most applications, the transducer serves also as a microphone, or receiver, for high frequency sound energy reflected from the target tissue. The transducer-receiver used clinically for diagnostic external sonography is pressed against the skin of the patient by the examiner, and beams short bursts of ultrasound signal through the skin. As the signal pulse encounters each successive layer of tissue or body fluid, part of its energy is reflected, part is transmitted, and a small fraction is absorbed.

The acoustic energy reflected from the tissues under the transducer-receiver is detected as a spectrum of ultrasonic echoes. This 'A-mode' signal is amplified, processed, and then temporarily stored as an acoustic characterization of that site. To obtain a two-dimensional 'B-mode' image that can be more readily interpreted, multiple A-mode signals are displayed in a linear array. These signals can be obtained one at a time, by moving the transducer laterally to a series of adjacent locations, or from a device that contains an aligned array of multiple transducers that work in concert. In either case, the lateral distance between the location of the first and last signal corresponds to the x-axis of the B-mode sonographic image (Fig. 11.57). The y-axis of this image represents the time required for the ultrasound pulse to travel from the transducer to an organ or subcutaneous tissue, for example, tendon, and to be reflected from this point back to the surface as an echo; the position of the echo on the y-axis indicates its distance from the transducer. In 'grey-scale' sonography, the acoustic intensity of the echo corresponds to the brightness of the displayed image. Accordingly, tissues that reflect very little acoustic energy, such as synovial fluid, appear nearly black, while those such as tendon or bone, which are highly reflective (echogenic), appear very bright (Fig. 11.58). The high-speed image acquisition and

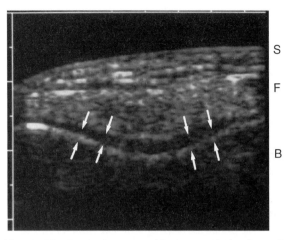

Fig. 11.58 External sonographic image of the femoral trochlea in a patient with OA. Transverse view, B-mode scan obtained with a diagnostic (7.5 MHz) transducer positioned above the superior pole of the patella, with the knee in 90° of flexion. Note skin (S); suprapatellar fat pad (F); nearly anechoic band of articular cartilage (between arrows); and subchondral bone (B). The cartilage on the lateral trochlear ridge (on left) is 30–40% thinner than that in the midline, or on the medial trochlear ridge.

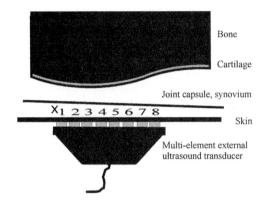

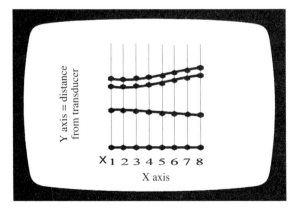

Fig. 11.57 Display format of a B-mode ultrasound image acquired with a multi-element external transducer. Pulse-echo data representing the tissues under each element of the transducer are displayed along the x-axis of the video screen to create a two-dimensional image. The position of each echo signal on the y-axis of the image corresponds to the distance between the transducer and the tissue that produced the echo.

display capabilities of the sonography equipment available today yield a real-time image and, when necessary, the operator can redirect the transducer to optimize image quality. Observations made during voluntary movements, such as contraction of the quadriceps muscle, can help identify anatomical landmarks and improve visualization of structures such as tendons and bursae[8].

Acoustic properties of connective tissue

The usefulness of diagnostic sonography, and how far it can 'see' into the body, depend on the characteristics of the transducer, its placement, and the acoustic properties of the target tissues. The absorption, reflection, and transmission of incident sound energy by tissue are related to the frequency of the ultrasound waves emitted by the transducer, and these parameters determine the sonographic appearance of each tissue or organ, and the resolution and accuracy of the imaging system[7–12].

Body fluids, including blood and hyaluronan-rich fluids, such as synovial fluid and aqueous humor,

Table 11.16   Velocity and absorption of ultrasound in connective tissues

Tissue	Sonic velocity (meters/second)	Sonic attenuation coefficient @ 1 MHz (decibels/meter)
Blood	1540	9
Aqueous humor	1500	7
Muscle	1630	350
Fat	1430	60
Tibial bone	2888	1900*
Skull bone	3050	870
Articular cartilage (human)	1658	na
Articular cartilage (bovine)	1700	na

na = not available
* = measured at 5 MHz

transmit sound efficiently. This can be expressed in terms of tissue sonic impedance, which relates the pressure in a sound wave to the size and velocity of the wave in the tissue; the impedance of blood (1.5×10^6 kg per m²) is similar to that of skeletal muscle and fat [7,9,13]. The velocity of sound in blood (1540 m per sec, Table 11.16) is nearly five times faster than that of sound traveling through air. Although sound travels at approximately the same velocity (1430–1630 m per sec, Table 11.16) through blood, fat, and muscle, more acoustic energy is absorbed and scattered by musculoskeletal tissue than by body fluids. This difference in sonic absorption, or attenuation, among tissues is frequency-dependent, and is expressed as an attenuation coefficient that ranges from 9 dB per m in blood to 1900 dB per m in bone (Table 11.16). The speed of sound in cortical bone is much faster (2888–3406 m per sec) than that in blood or other tissues but, because bone has a very high acoustic impedance (5×10^6 kg per m²) and reflects and absorbs incident sonic energy, rather than transmitting it [6,11,12], external sonography reveals only the surface of bone. Like bone, calcifications in tendon or other soft tissue, and most foreign bodies, are highly echogenic [6].

The acoustic velocity and impedance of non-calcified articular and periarticular tissues, including cartilage, tendon, muscle, and fat, resemble those of blood more than of bone [9,12,13] (Table 11.16). It is important to point out that adjacent tissues cannot be distinguished with sonography unless their acoustic impedances differ, because this difference determines how much incident acoustic energy each will reflect [7]. When the velocity of sound in adjacent tissues differs, the direction of travel of an ultrasound wave passing from one to the other is altered, or refracted, at the interface.

The complex interactions of the ultrasound signal and target tissue yield scattered echo patterns (speckle) that produce the characteristic sonographic appearance of each tissue or organ [10].

The diagnostic sonography system typically used to evaluate the extremities has an operational sonic frequency of 3–10 MHz [6]. The spatial resolving power of the system is proportional to its operating frequency, and the theoretical maximum resolving power that can be achieved at an imaging frequency of 7.5 MHz is approximately 0.2 mm [10]. Soft tissue structures several inches below the skin can routinely be imaged with such equipment, and diagnostic sonography is often used to localize structures, for example, tumors or foreign bodies, no more than a few millimeters in diameter.

Precise measurements of skin thickness (± 0.05 mm) have been obtained with a 20 MHz transducer array designed specifically for this application [14]. This high-resolution instrument can resolve adjacent structures separated by less than 0.3 mm. However, because the effective imaging range of external ultrasound is inversely proportional to the operating frequency, it does not achieve sufficient tissue penetration to permit study of even a superficial joint, or of deeper structures, such as the knee. Recently, inflammatory pannus, tenosynovitis, tendon rupture, and joint effusions in the hands and wrists of patients with rheumatoid arthritis have been identified with a 13 MHz imaging system [15,16]. Although it is possible that good visualization of marginal osteophytes and synovial cysts in the interphalangeal joints and first carpometacarpal joint in patients with OA could be obtained with this technique, the feasibility, sensitivity, and precision of such imaging has not been evaluated.

External sonography of the knee and hip

Images of the articular surface of portions of the human femoral condyle can be obtained with external sonography[6,16–25]. Optimal, full-thickness images of the cartilage are obtained, however, only when the transducer-receiver can be positioned perpendicular to the articular surface. A gel, or liquid-filled pad, is often interposed between the transducer and the skin to improve the quality of the image[6]. The patient must be able to maintain the knee in a flexed position for several minutes, and careful positioning of the joint and transducer are required because of the contours of the femoral condyles and the acoustic barrier created by the patella[20]. Extraneous echoes from the intervening skin and subcutaneous fat, muscle, tendon, joint capsule, and synovium tend to reduce the quality of the cartilage image.

Because of its higher fat content, synovium is less echogenic than the fibrous joint capsule. In some knees, synovium can be identified as a distinct echo band between the capsule and the anechoic synovial fluid[16,17]. Synovitis and hypertrophic synovial villi are often present in OA, but there is insufficient evidence, even in rheumatoid arthritis, that sonography can provide a reliable estimate of the severity of synovial proliferation[16]. External sonography readily detects synovial effusions in the knee and other joints because the joint fluid is readily distinguished as a black, anechoic area in the image[26]. Although a sonographic method that estimated synovial fluid volume accurately would be useful in studies that determine the concentration of a cartilage-derived 'OA marker' in the synovial fluid, and then relate the quantity of the molecule in the joint to cartilage catabolism and repair[27], this approach has not been tested.

The characteristic appearance of normal articular cartilage in images obtained with external sonography is a uniformly hypoechoic band with a smooth surface which follows the contour of the subchondral bone (Fig. 11.58). The interface between the synovial fluid and the articular surface produces a thin line of echoes at the surface of this band[23], while the deep chondral margin is defined by echoes from the highly echogenic interface between the cartilage and subchondral bone. In such images, the width of the hypoechoic band provides an estimate of cartilage thickness[16]. The fibrocartilaginous menisci yield a more intense, relatively homogeneous pattern of echoes which distinguish them from articular cartilage. Meniscal defects have been detected with external sonography[24,28], but the technique is considered unreliable[8].

The anatomy of the knee imposes strict limits on the chondral surfaces that can be evaluated with external ultrasound. A transverse view of the trochlea (Fig. 11.58) can be obtained with a 5–7.5 MHz linear array transducer, when the joint is positioned in 80–120° of flexion[16,23]. Even though this degree of flexion cannot always be achieved in the OA knee, the possibility that this view might be used to evaluate the severity of OA has been explored because it depicts the thickness and contour of that portion of the trochlear cartilage which is loaded by contact with the patella[23]. Longitudinal views, obtained 1–2 cm medial or lateral to the midline of this portion of the trochlea, and aligned with the femoral shaft, have been used to complement these transverse images[22]. The cartilage on small areas of the posterior portion of the medial and lateral condyles has also been imaged with a transducer centered over the anterior, lateral, or posterolateral aspect of the condyle, just proximal to the joint line[19,21]. Notably, neither patellar nor tibial cartilage, nor the central, habitually loaded regions of the femoral condyles that are typically the site of fibrillation in early OA, can be adequately evaluated with external sonography.

In sonograms of the OA knee, the normal, well-defined boundary between articular cartilage and soft tissue often appears blurred. Some investigators have concluded that subjective estimates of the severity of OA, based on the degree of blurring and thinning of the cartilage, may be more useful than efforts to measure cartilage thickness from these images[20]. In one series, measurements of cartilage thickness were least reliable when areas of eburnated bone were present, but good correlation was reported between the severity of chondral ulceration in gross specimens obtained at the time of knee arthroplasty and grades of OA severity assigned by evaluation of preoperative sonograms[20].

The average thickness of the cartilage on the normal femoral trochlea, as determined by external sonography, is 2.1–2.3 mm[16,20–22]. A strong correlation ($r = 0.86$) has been shown between such measurements and those of cartilage thickness obtained with gadolinium-DTPA- enhanced magnetic resonance imaging[16], although the precision of values obtained with ultrasound cannot exceed the 0.2 mm limit imposed by the operating frequency of the transducer[23]. In cartilage obtained from patients at the time of knee arthroplasty, histologic measurements of the thickness of trochlear cartilage did not differ significantly from the values obtained by preoperative sonography[22]. In another series[21], sonograms from both knees of 60 patients with symptomatic and radiographic evidence of OA showed the articular cartilage on the medial, lateral, and central aspect of the trochlea, proximal to the intercondylar notch, was significantly thinner (mean thickness = 0.94, 0.99, 1.35 mm, respectively) than that in a group of 30 knees of age-matched controls (mean thickness 1.77 mm, 1.87 mm, 2.20 mm, respectively; p < 0.01). It should be noted that even though most of the subjects with OA in these series[20-22] had advanced disease, the mean thickness of the trochlear cartilage (1.4 mm) was only 36 per cent less than that in normal knees. This suggests that measurement of cartilage thickness at the trochlea, by any method, is unlikely to be a sensitive indicator of disease progression. While the clinical role of external sonography of the OA knee has not been fully evaluated, the technique does not appear well suited to studies designed to serially monitor therapeutic response or disease progression.

External sonograms obtained with a hand-held, 5 MHz linear array transducer have been used experimentally to determine the apparent thickness of the articular cartilage of the femoral head in adults with no radiographic evidence of OA[28]. These images showed the cartilage as a relatively sonolucent band, immediately adjacent to an echogenic, curvilinear band (Fig. 11.59) that represented the subchondral bone of the anterior femoral head. Measurements of joint space obtained from these sonograms had a coefficient of variation of 19 per cent and more reproducible measurements of the joint space in the same subjects were obtained from either plain radiographs or MR images of the hip. At present, sonography has no role in the assessment of hip OA.

Investigational sonography of OA cartilage

Of the methods now available for evaluation of the articular cartilage in OA, only direct, arthroscopic inspection of the joint can quantitate roughening of the articular surface, detect swelling or changes in turgor of the cartilage, or map the extent of chondral ulceration[29]. Arthroscopy, however, reveals little about

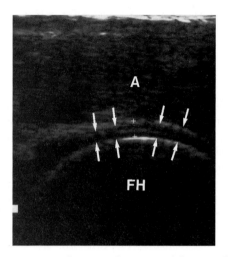

Fig. 11.59 External sonographic image of the normal hip. Longitudinal scan obtained with a 5 MHz transducer. Note the acetabulum (A) and the nearly anechoic band (between the arrows) representing the articular cartilage, immediately adjacent to the echogenic band representing the subchondral bone of the femoral head (FH). A measurement of cartilage thickness (2.5 mm) was obtained with the cursors (+) superimposed on the image.

the thickness of the cartilage, which varies with location on the femoral condyle. Cartilage thickness can be increased in early OA[30], but diminishes with progression of the disease. Interest has arisen, therefore, in the possibility that *intra-articular* sonography can be used to complement and enhance radiographic and orthoscopic assessment of the knee in subjects with OA.

The feasibility of mapping the thickness of the articular cartilage with high-frequency, 20 MHz ultrasound was established in *ex vivo* studies of the human acetabulum[31]. These pioneering studies showed that echoes from the smooth articular surface of normal cartilage could be distinguished from the hypoechoic cartilage matrix and from deeper echoes produced by the osteochondral junction. The accuracy of thickness measurements in this series was approximately 0.08 mm, or about the same as that reported for 20 MHz measurements of skin thickness[14]. Sonographic analysis of the acetabulum revealed that, while this surface was nearly spherical, the contour of the calcified osteochondral interface was far more variable.

Recently, a pulse-echo technique, similar to that used to evaluate the acetabulum, and a focused 25 MHz transducer were used *in vitro* to determine the velocity of sound in normal and OA human articular cartilage, and the thickness of articular cartilage on canine and human femoral condyles[32,33]. The speed of sound in normal human articular cartilage averaged 1658 ± 185 m per s; a slightly lower value, 1581 ± 148 m per s, was obtained for OA cartilage. Although the water, proteoglycan, and collagen content of OA cartilage differ from those of normal cartilage, no significant correlation was found between the speed of sound in OA cartilage and any of these variables. These data allay concern[31] that changes in the biochemical composition of the cartilage matrix in OA could affect the precision of sonographic measurements of cartilage thickness.

Investigators in several laboratories have used ultrasound to obtain B-mode cross-sectional images of canine, bovine, porcine, and human articular cartilage specimens immersed in degassed saline[23,32,33–36]. Typically, after the specimen has been excised, a high-frequency transducer (18–50 MHz) has been moved over the articular surface in order to image the cartilage and, in some cases, the attached subchondral bone. In images of normal cartilage, the interface between the saline bath and articular surface is seen as a smooth, echogenic band (Fig. 11.60), while the cartilage matrix yields almost no echoes. The interface between the cartilage and calcified cartilage/subchondral bone produces a second, distinct band of strong echoes. No important species-specific differences in the sonographic appearance of normal cartilage have been described.

B-mode images of OA cartilage reflect the severity of fibrillation and ulceration of the articular surface. The surface of severely fibrillated cartilage completely disrupts the salinecartilage interface, so that the fibrillated matrix is seen as a band of chaotic internal echoes that extends from the cartilage surface into the matrix (Fig. 11.61). In contrast, mechanical abrasion of the surface of normal cartilage with fine sandpaper, so as to produce a minor degree of fibrillation, significantly increases the number and intensity of the surface echoes that represent the saline-cartilage interface, but leaves the deeper matrix echo free.

In specimens of OA cartilage in which fibrillation extended only 0.1–1.2 mm beneath the articular surface, the width of the surface echo band in B-mode scans, obtained with a 25 MHz transducer, was proportional to the depth of fibrillation (r = 0.78)[33]. Other work suggests that a modified ultrasonic technique, which measures either the scattering of 10–30 MHz ultrasonic waves from the cartilage surface[34] or the frequency-dependent intensity of this acoustic backscatter[36,37], could provide a quantitative measure of the degree of cartilage fibrillation without the need for the controlled movement of the transducer across the joint surface that is needed to acquire a B-mode image.

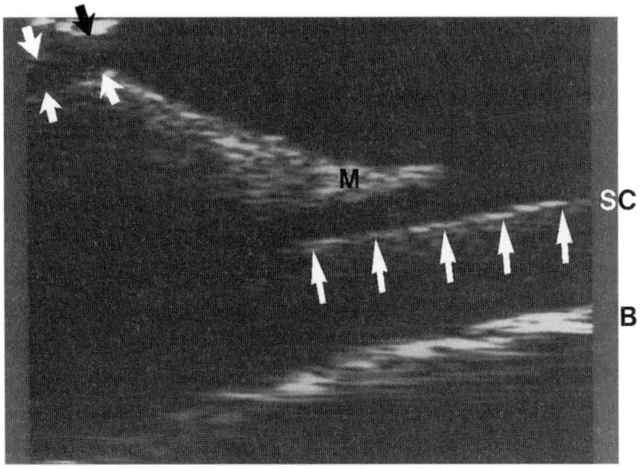

Fig. 11.60 Sonographic image of human tibial plateau obtained *ex vivo* with high frequency (25 MHz) B-mode scanner. Note the wedge-shaped medial meniscus (M) and the echogenic band representing the subchondral bone (B). Echoes from the saline-cartilage interface (SC) delineate the smooth surface of the hypoechoic articular cartilage (arrows), except where the cartilage is eclipsed by the overlying meniscus. An artifactual defect produced with a scalpel in the relatively echogenic meniscus is represented by an area of diminished echogenicity (open triangles) in the upper left corner of the figure.

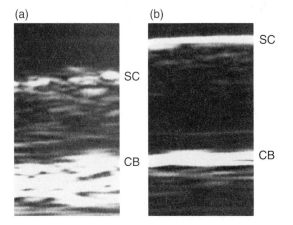

Fig. 11.61 High frequency (25 MHz) B-mode sonographic images, obtained *ex vivo*, of a specimen of cartilage and subchondral bone from a patient with OA (a) and from an individual with normal joints (b). Note the saline-cartilage (SC) and cartilage-bone (CB) echo bands. In the specimen from the patient with OA, the normally smooth SC interface is disrupted by superficial fibrillation of the articular surface and the cartilage is thinned.

The distance between the echo bands produced by the saline-cartilage and cartilage-bone interfaces in the B-mode image of a full-thickness specimen of normal articular cartilage is proportional to the thickness of the cartilage[31,33]. Measurements of this distance permit estimations of cartilage thickness with a precision of approximately 0.1 mm and a mean coefficient of variation of less than 2 per cent[33]. The thickness of OA cartilage determined from scans obtained with a 25 MHz transducer showed a high degree of correlation (r = 0.87) with measurements of the cartilage thickness, from the surface to the zone of calcified cartilage, in histologic sections of the cartilage cut in the plane of the scan[33].

These results establish the feasibility of using high-frequency (for example, 20–30 MHz) sonography for evaluation of articular cartilage changes in OA. Because ultrasound, as it passes though connective tissue, is attenuated to a far greater extent at these frequencies than at 5–7 MHz, this technique is likely to be practical only when the transducer can be placed within the joint[38]. It may be feasible to design an instrument that could be used during arthroscopy, to supplement visual inspection of the knee with measurements of cartilage thickness and surface roughening. A practical scanning device is likely to contain one or more small transducers, such as those developed for intravascular sonography[39], and a mechanism to permit alignment of the instrument with the articular surface.

References

1. Brandt, K.D. (1995). Toward pharmacologic modification of joint damage in osteoarthritis. *Ann Intern Med*, **122**, 874–5.
2. Lequesne, M., Brandt, K., Bellamy, N., Moskowitz, R., Menkes, C.J., Pelletier, J.P., *et al.* (1994). Guidelines for testing slow-acting and disease-modifying drugs in osteoarthritis. *J Rheumatol*, **suppl 41** 41, 65–71.
3. Adams, M.E. and Wallace, C.J. (1991). Quantitative imaging of osteoarthritis. *Semin Arthritis Rheum*, **20**, 26–39.
4. Myers, S.L., Brandt, K.D., and Eilam, O. (1995). Even low-grade synovitis significantly accelerates the clearance of protein from the canine knee. Implications for measurement of synovial fluid 'markers' of osteoarthritis. *Arthritis Rheum*, **38**, 1085–91.
5. Harcke, H.T., Grissom, L.E., and Finkelstein, M.S. (1988). Evaluation of the musculoskeletal system with sonography. *Amer J Roentgenology*, **150**, 1253–61.
6. Kaplan, P.A., Matamoros, A. Jr, and Anderson, J.C. (1990). Sonography of the musculoskeletal system. *Amer J Roentgenology*, **155**, 237–45.

7. Hussey, M. (1985). *Basic physics and technology of medical diagnostic ultrasound*, pp. 12–119. Elsevier, NY.
8. Fornage, B.D. (1992). Musculoskeletal and soft tissue. In *General ultrasound* (ed. C.A. Mittelstaedt), pp. 1–58. Churchhill Livingstone, NY.
9. Wells, P.N. (1993). Physics of ultrasound. In *Ultrasonic exposimetry* (ed. P.A. Lewin and M.C. Ziskin), pp. 9–45. CRC Press, Boca Raton.
10. Harris, R.A., Follett, D.H., Halliwell, M., and Wells, P.N.T. (1991). Ultimate limits in ultrasonic imaging resolution. *Ultrasound Med Biol*, **17**, 547–58.
11. Newman, J.S., Adler, R.S., Bude, R.O., and Rubin, J. (1991). Detection of soft-tissue hyperemia: value of power Doppler sonography. *Amer J Roentgenology*, **163**, 385–9.
12. Kratochwil, A. (1978). Ultrasonic diagnosis in orthopaedic surgery. In *Handbook of clinical ultrasound*, (ed. M.de Vlieger, J.H. Holmes, A. Kratochvil, E. Kagner, R. Kraus, G. Kossoff, *et al.*), pp. 945–53. J. Wiley and Sons, New York, USA.
13. Sanders, R.C. (1984). Sonography of fat. In *Ultrasound annual 1984*, (ed. R.C. Vaunder and M. Hill) pp. 71–94. Raven Press, NY.
14. Turnbull, D.H., Starkoski, B.G., Harasiewicz, K.A., and Semple, J.L. (1995). A 40–100 MHZ B-scan ultrasound backscatter microscope for skin imaging. *Ultrasound Med Biol*, **21**, 79–88.
15. Grassi, W., Tittarelli, E., Blasetti, P., Pirani, O., and Cervini, C. (1995). Finger tendon involvement in rheumatoid arthritis. Evaluation with high-frequency sonography. *Arthritis Rheum*, **38**, 786–94.
16. Ostergaard, M., Court-Payen, M., Gideon, P., Wieslander, S., Cortsen, M., Lorenzen, I., *et al.* (1995). Ultrasonography in arthritis of the knee. A comparison with MR imaging. *Acta Radiologica*, **36**, 19–26.
17. Cooperberg, P.L., Tsang, I., Truelove, L., and Knickerbocker, W.J. (1978). Gray scale ultrasound in the evaluation of rheumatoid arthritis of the knee. *Radiology*, **126**, 759.
18. Derks, W.H.J., De Hooge, P., and Van Linge, B. (1986). Ultrasonographic detection of the patellar plica in the knee. *J Clin Ultrasound*, **14**, 355–62.
19. Richardson, M.L., Selby, B., Montana, M.A., and Mack, L.A. (1988). Ultrasonography of the knee. *Radiol Clin North Am*, **26**, 63–75.
20. McCune, W.J., Dedrick, D.K., Aisen, A.M., and MacGuire, A. (1990). Sonographic evaluation of osteoarthritic femoral condylar cartilage. Correlation with operative findings. *Clin Orthop*, **254**, 230–5.
21. Iagnocco, A., Coari, G., and Zappini, A. (1992). Sonographic evaluation of femoral condylar cartilage in osteoarthritis and rheumatoid arthritis. *Scand J Rheumatol*, **21**, 201–3.
22. Martino, F., Ettorre, G.C., Angelelli, G., Macarini, L., Patella, V., Moretti, B., *et al.* (1993). Validity of echographic evaluation of cartilage in gonarthrosis. *Clin Rheumatol*, **12**, 178–83.
23. Aisen, A., McCune, W.J., MacGuire, A., Carson, P.L., Silver, T.M., Jafri, S.Z., *et al.* (1984). Sonographic evaluation of the cartilage of the knee. *Radiology*, **153**, 781–4.

24. Gerngross, H. and Sohn, C. (1992). Ultrasound scanning for the diagnosis of meniscal lesions of the knee joint. *Arthroscopy*, **8**, 105–10.

25. Pathria, M.N., Zlatkin, M., Sartoris, D.J., Scheible, W., and Resnick, D. (1988). Ultrasonography of the popliteal fossa and lower extremities. *Radiol Clin North Am*, **26**, 77–85.

26. Koski, J.M. (1992). Ultrasongraphy in detection of effusion in the radio carpal and midcarpal joints. *Scand J Rheumatol*, **21**, 79–81.

27. Lohmander, L.S. (1994). Articular cartilage and osteoarthritis. The role of molecular markers to monitor breakdown, repair and disease. *J Anat*, **184**, 477–92.

28. Jonsson, K., Buckwalter, K., Helvie, M., Niklason, L., and Martel, W. (1992). Precision of hyaline cartilage thickness measurements. *Acta Radiologica*, **33**, 234–9.

29. Ike, R.W. (1993). The role of arthroscopy in the differential diagnosis of osteoarthritis of the knee. *Rheum Dis Clin North Am*, **19**, 673–96.

30. Adams, M.E. and Brandt, K.D. (1991). Hypertrophic repair of canine articular cartilage in osteoarthritis after anterior cruciate ligament transection. *J Rheumatol*, **18**, 428–35.

31. Rushfeldt, P.D. and Mann, R.W. (1981). Improved techniques for measuring *in vitro* the geometry and pressure distribution in the human acetabulum — Ultrasonic measurement of acetabular surfaces, sphericity and cartilage thickness. *J Biomech*, **14**, 253–60.

32. Sanghvi, N.T., Snoddy, A.M., Myers, S.L., Brandt, K.D., Reilly, C.R. Franklin, T.D. Jr. (1990). Characterization of normal and osteoarthritic cartilage using 25 MHZ ultrasound. Ultrasonics, Ferroelectrics and Frequency Control Society 1990 Ultrasonics Symposium Proceedings, *Institute of Electronic and Electromechanical Engineering*, **3**, 1413–16.

33. Myers, S.L., Dines, K., Brandt, K.D., and Albrecht, M.E. (1993). Experimental assessment by high frequency ultrasound of articular cartilage thickness and osteoarthritic changes. *J Rheumatol*, **22**, 109–16.

34. Kim, H.K.W., Babyn, P.S., Harasiewicz, L., and Foster, F.S. (1993). Ultrasound backscatter microscopy of porcine articular cartilage (abstr.). *Trans Orthop Res Soc*, **18**, 187.

35. Senzig, D.A. and Forster, F.K. (1992). Ultrasonic attenuation in articular cartilage. *J Acoust Soc Am*, **92**, 676–80.

36. Adler, R.S., Dedrick, D.K., Laing, T.J., Chiang, E.H., Meyer, C.R., Bland, P.H., *et al.* (1992). Quantitive assessment of cartilage surface roughness in osteoarthritis using high frequency ultrasound. *Ultrasound Med Biol*, **18**, 51–8.

37. Chiang, E.H., Adler, R.S., Meyer, C.R., Rubin, J.M., Dedrick, D.K., and Laing, T.J. (1994). Quantitative assessment of surface roughness using backscattered ultrasound: the effects of finite surface curvature. *Ultrasound Med Biol*, **20**, 123–35.

38. Chivers, R.C. and Hill, C.R. (1975). Ultrasonic attention in human tissue. *Ultrasound Med Biol*, **2**, 25–9.

39. Barry, B., Golberg and Ji-Bin, Liu. (1992). Endoluminal ultrasound: vascular and nonvascular. *Ultrasound Quart*, **9**, 245–70.

11.5.7 Defining and validating the clinical role of molecular markers in osteoarthritis

L. Stefan Lohmander and David T. Felson

Osteoarthritis (OA) is associated with a loss of the normal balance between synthesis and degradation of the macromolecules that are necessary to provide articular cartilage with its biomechanical and functional properties. Concomitantly, changes occur in the structure and metabolism of the synovium and subchondral bone of the joint. These processes result in the destruction of joint cartilage and changes in the function of the affected joints, which cause pain and physical disability.

Current therapy of OA is largely symptomatic, and is focused on decreasing pain and improving function with analgesics, nonsteroidal anti-inflammatory drugs, or arthroplasty. However, new interventions are being proposed for treatment of joint disease[1-2] which may have the ability to decrease the rate of joint destruction

in OA. The ability to reproducibly and sensitively monitor disease progression and outcome for both joint and patient in intervention trials is critical to the development of new disease-modifying treatment strategies in OA. There are three general means by which OA can be assessed:

(1) *patient-related measures of joint pain and disability* (algofunctional scores such as WOMAC[3], index of severity of knee or hip disease[4]);

(2) *measurements of the structural (anatomical) changes in the affected joints* (plain radiographs[5], magnetic resonance imaging[6], arthroscopy[7], high frequency ultrasound[8]);

(3) *measurements of the disease process exemplified by changes in metabolism or functional properties of the articular cartilage, subchondral bone, or other joint tissues* (body fluid markers of cartilage and bone metabolism[9], bone scintigraphy[10], measurement of cartilage compression resistance by indentation or streaming potentials[11]).

Algofunctional scores, plain radiographs, and arthroscopy are in use to assess OA trials. Of these methods, only the algofunctional scores have yet been fully validated as outcome instruments.

Standardized imaging of joints by plain X-ray examination is proposed as the current 'gold standard' to detect changes in joint structure in clinical trials of disease-modifying drugs in OA[12]. Even with improved techniques for patient positioning and image measurements, and a future validation, plain X-ray examination remains, at best, an indirect measure of cartilage destruction — a 'surrogate marker' — not a direct measure of the disease process in OA. Magnetic resonance imaging will not doubt find increasing use as a measure of joint changes in OA. Until methods to monitor joint cartilage quality or composition by MRI appear, the technique suffers from the same weakness as X-ray examination: it provides only an indirect measure of the current disease process, but documents the consequences of it.

Methods which could provide rapid information on the function, composition, and metabolic processes in arthritic joint cartilage would, thus, be of considerable value in evaluating the role of new and old interventions in OA[13].

The destruction of joint cartilage in OA involves the degradation of matrix molecules, which are released as fragments to joint fluid, blood, and urine, where they may be detected. Such molecular 'markers' of cartilage matrix metabolism could be used to diagnose, prognosticate, and monitor joint diseases such as rheumatoid arthritis and OA, and to identify disease mechanisms on the molecular level. For overviews and further references, several recent reviews and books are available[9,14–17]. Although many publications have described the increased release of markers of cartilage, bone, or synovial metabolism into joint fluid, serum, and urine in OA (Table 11.17), the goal of using these markers to assess the disease process in OA remains elusive[18].

The word 'marker' has been used in many different contexts. Cytokines, enzymes and their inhibitors, cartilage matrix components and their fragments, antibodies to cartilage collagen and membrane proteins of chondrocytes, and even growth factors, have been suggested to be markers for OA. We will, in this chapter, focus on markers which are directly associated with turnover of joint tissue matrix molecules, such as matrix molecule fragments and proteases potentially associated with their generation. We will briefly summarize the current status of research on these molecular markers of OA, and discuss requirements for them to fulfill their promises.

The relationship between marker concentration and joint cartilage metabolism

Specific issues need to be considered with regard to a putative molecular marker of OA:

(1) is the relationship known between the marker concentration and the metabolic rate in joint cartilage of the molecule in question? This relationship, in turn, is dependent on:

(2) the relationship between concentrations of a marker in different body fluid compartments such as joint fluid, blood, or urine;

(3) the influence of changes in synovial inflammation, liver, and kidney function on marker concentrations in these compartments;

(4) the specificity of the marker molecule for cartilage, in general, and joint cartilage, in particular.

Our understanding of the relationship between changes in marker concentrations in a body fluid compartment and changes in cartilage matrix metabolism is limited. For example, the concentration of a marker of cartilage matrix degradation in joint fluid may depend not only on the rate of degradation of cartilage matrix, but also on other factors such as the rate of elimination, (clearance) of the molecular fragment in question from the joint fluid compartment[19–21] and the amount of cartilage matrix remaining in the joint[22] (Fig. 11.62). Since the clearance of macromolecules from the joint fluid compartment is increased by inflammation,[20,23] differences in the rates of release of markers from joint cartilage into joint fluid, between control joints and diseased joints with inflammation, may actually be underestimated. An estimate of the degradation rate of a cartilage matrix molecule in arthritis, based on the

Table 11.17 Molecular markers in synovial fluid or serum of joint tissue metabolism in human OA

Marker[a]	Process[b]	OA markers in synovial fluid[c,d] (references)	OA markers in serum[c,d] (references)
Cartilage			
Aggrecan			
Core protein epitopes	Degradation of aggrecan	⇑ (24,66)	
Core protein epitopes (cleavage site specific neoepitopes)	Degradation of aggrecan	⇑[e] (54–56)	
Keratan sulfate epitopes	Degradation of aggrecan	⇑ (58,67)	⇑ ⇔ ⇓ (32, 42–44, 47, 67, 68)
Chondroitin sulfate epitopes (846, 3B3, 7D4, etc.)	Synthesis/degradation of aggrecan	⇑ (32,69–71)	⇑ (32)
Chondroitin sulfate ratio 6S/4S	Synthesis/degradation of aggrecan	⇓ (72)	
Small proteoglycans	Degradation of small proteoglycans	⇑[e] (73)	
Cartilage matrix proteins			
Cartilage oligomeric matrix protein	Degradation of COMP	⇑ (25,74)	⇑ (52)
Cartilage collagens			
Type II collagen C-propeptide	Synthesis of type II collagen	⇑ (26,75)	
Type II collagen α chain fragments	Degradation of type II collagen	⇑[e] (76)	
Matrix metalloproteinases and inhibitors	Synthesis and secretion	⇑ From synovium or joint cartilage?	⇑ ⇔ Tissue source? (see below)
Meniscus			
Cartilage oligomeric matrix protein	Degradation of COMP	⇑ From joint cartilage, meniscus or synovium?	
Small proteoglycans	Degradation of small proteoglycans		
Synovium			
Hyaluronan	Synthesis of hyaluronan	⇑ (51, 77,78)	
Matrix metalloproteinases and inhibitors			
Stromelysin (MMP-3)	Synthesis and secretion of MMP-3	⇑ (24)	⇑ ⇔ (79–81)
Interstitial collagenase (MMP-1)	Synthesis and secretion of MMP-1	⇑ (24,82)	⇔ (81)
Tissue inhibitors of metalloproteinases	Synthesis and secretion of TIMPs	⇑ (24, 81)	⇔ (79)
Type III collagen N-propeptide	Synthesis/degradation of type III collagen	⇑ (83)	⇑ (83)
Bone			
Bone sialoprotein	Synthesis/degradation of BSP	⇑ ⇔ (84)	⇑[f] (84)
Osteocalcin	Synthesis of osteocalcin	⇑ ⇔ (85)	⇔ (67)
3-hydroxypyridinium crosslinks[g]	Degradation of bone collagens		

⇑ ⇔ ⇓: Increased, unchanged, or decreased concentrations, respectively, compared with healthy controls

a Markers have been assigned a predominant tissue source with regard to marker occurrence in joint fluid and serum.
b As discussed in this chapter (see e.g. Figs 11.62 and 11.63) some individual marker levels may change both as a result of changes in synthesis and in degradation.
c A predominant increase or decrease, respectively, is assigned on the basis of representative publications on 'active', not end-stage OA.
d Some recent and representative literature references are given: this is not intended to be a comprehensive review of the literature.
e In human OA cartilage.
f After acute knee injury.
g Results published only for urine, and show increased excretion[86,87].

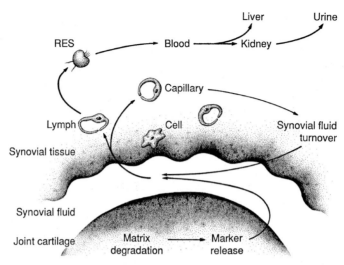

Fig. 11.62   Molecular fragments generated by degradation of cartilage matrix, or released from synovial tissue or bone into the joint fluid compartment, are cleared by bulk flow through the synovial tissue matrix into the lymphatic vessels.[21] Some fragments are eliminated or further degraded in the regional lymph nodes. Many, and possibly most, products of cartilage matrix metabolism are taken up and degraded in the liver. Some specific types of fragments, such as collagen cross-links, are not metabolized, but are found in urine. (From reference 14, with permission.)

joint fluid concentration of its fragments, may, thus, actually lead to an underestimation of its metabolic rate.

In spite of these confounding factors, marker concentrations in joint fluid, in general, seem to correlate with the expected metabolic rate of joint cartilage matrix molecules[9]. For example, the temporal changes in joint fluid concentrations of fragments of aggrecan, cartilage oligomeric matrix protein (COMP), and of collagen II C-propeptide, after joint injury and in developing OA[24-26], are consistent with the changes in metabolic rate observed for these molecules in animal models *in vivo* and in human OA cartilage *in vitro*[27-30].

The identification of the specific source of the molecular fragment can be a problem with regard to both process and tissue. An increased rate of release of molecular fragments may be present both as a result of a net increase in degradation (resulting in net loss), or as a result of an increased rate of degradation in the presence of an increased rate of new synthesis and replenishment (resulting in a steady state with regard to tissue concentration of the critical molecule). We, therefore, need markers specific for both degradative and synthetic events. An example of the former is aggrecan fragments, of the latter, collagen II C-propeptide.

Even with a molecular marker being unequivocally associated with degradative events, the specific process source may need to be further considered. For example, the fragments identified could result from the degrada-

tion of a newly synthesized matrix molecule which has not yet been incorporated into a functional matrix, a molecule recently incorporated into cell-associated matrix, or a resident matrix molecule which is a critical functional part of the mature matrix (Fig. 11.63). The ensuing consequences on cartilage matrix function may

Cartilage matrix turnover

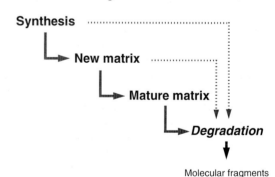

Fig. 11.63   Fragments of cartilage matrix molecules may be generated by degradation of newly synthesized molecules which are never incorporated into the functional matrix, molecules which have recently been incorporated into a functional matrix, and molecules which have been long-time members of the 'resident' functional matrix. At present, it is not always possible to distinguish these different sources of fragments. Another source of heterogeneity is the origin of fragments from pericellular, territorial, and interterritorial matrix, as well as from superficial and deep layers of the joint cartilage.

well be different. In general, markers are not specific to these processes. This issue is also related to the largely unresolved question of the specific cartilage matrix compartment source (pericellular, territorial matrix, or interterritorial matrix) of a molecular marker present in joint fluid, blood, or urine. *In vitro* experimentation suggests that the metabolic rates of these cartilage matrix compartments may differ significantly[31]. Assay of some low-abundance epitopes associated with chondroitin sulfate sulfation patterns may help identify populations of newly synthesized aggrecan molecules[15,32–34].

It may be suggested that fragments, in joint fluid, of matrix molecules normally resident in cartilage, are generated by metabolism of cartilage matrix. This assumption may or may not be true. It relies, in turn, on the assumption that the molecule in question is significantly more abundant in cartilage than in any other joint tissue, or that its metabolic rate in cartilage is higher than other joint tissues. While it may be true that cartilage contains the far greater total mass of joint aggrecan compared to, for example, the meniscus,[22] the total mass of COMP in the menisci of the knee may approach that in the joint cartilage of the knee[35]. Both chondrocytes and synovial cells produce stromelysin-1,[36,37] but the cell number in synovial tissue may be higher than in cartilage, suggesting that a significant proportion of the stromelysin-1 detected in joint fluid originates in the synovium. The specific source of the molecule or molecular fragment identified in joint fluid may, thus, not always be entirely evident, and is likely to be often more complex than originally proposed.

The question of the tissue source of markers of cartilage metabolism is even more relevant for markers assayed in serum or urine samples. Joint cartilage represents only a minority of body hyaline cartilage, probably less than 10 per cent. Sources of the marker other than cartilage will also have to be considered. Moreover, in monoarticular disease, any markers released from the single affected joint are mixed with markers released from normal joints. It would, thus, seem reasonable to suggest that determinations of cartilage markers in serum or urine may be of use in polyarticular or systemic disease, but are less likely to be useful in monoarticular disease.

As discussed above for joint fluid markers, extra-articular factors which affect the clearance of the marker from the serum or urine compartment have to be considered. Physical activity may change the concentrations of some markers in both synovial fluid and serum[38]. Circadian variations occur in urinary excre-

tion of collagen crosslinks[39]. The lymph nodes and the liver are responsible for the elimination of a great part of the molecular fragments released from cartilage and other connective tissues. Any change in the function of these organ systems will, thus, affect the clearance of cartilage markers from serum (Fig. 11.62). For example, the serum concentration of hyaluronan is greatly affected by changes in liver function[40].

Potential uses of markers

The demands on a marker may differ, depending on if it is to be used as a diagnostic test, a prognostic test, or an evaluative test[41]. For example, the diagnostic test focuses on the ability to detect differences between affected and non-affected individuals, often expressed in terms of sensitivity and specificity of the test. The evaluative test, on the other hand, focuses on the ability of the marker to monitor change over time in the individual patient, often expressed as sensitivity to change or effect size.

Markers could serve as *diagnostic tests*, helping to distinguish joints with OA from unaffected joints or other joint diseases. Examples of frequently used serological diagnostic tests in rheumatoid arthritis include rheumatoid factor and antinuclear antibody (ANA). The concentration of keratan sulfate in serum was originally suggested to serve as a diagnostic test for generalized OA[42,43]. Subsequent experience has, however, not fulfilled this promise[32,44], although this serum marker may yet serve to reflect cartilage proteoglycan degradation in specific situations[45,46]. A considerable overlap exists between affected and non-affected individuals, and serum concentrations are influenced by age and gender[47]. Other studies have shown differences in knee joint fluid concentrations of aggrecan fragments, COMP fragments, and matrix metalloproteinases and their inhibitors between knee-healthy reference groups, rheumatoid arthritis, reactive arthritis, and OA[18,24,25,48,49]. While these investigations show significant differences of mean values between the study groups, with only moderate overlap, interpretation is confounded by the fact that comparisons between groups are cross-sectional and retrospective[18,41]. These studies should, therefore, be regarded only as hypothesis-generating and will require confirmation in prospective studies.

The term 'marker' might also be used for a test evaluating *disease severity*, rather than its presence or absence classifications Tumor Node Metastasis (TNM) for cancers are measures of disease severity or stage, rather than diagnostic markers. Some biochemical tests, like that for thyroid stimulating hormone (TSH), serve both as diagnostic tests (for example, for hypothyroidism) and as measures of disease severity. In OA, disease severity (or stage) is measured by, for example, Kellgren and Lawrence grade of radiological changes, by the amount of cartilage loss on arthroscopy, or by the degree of functional impairment of the patient. Several reports have suggested that assay of molecular markers of cartilage metabolism may provide complementary information on joint disease stage[22,50]. While further experience in this area is needed, molecular markers clearly have the potential to provide unique information on joint cartilage quality not currently available by other modalities of staging.

Biochemical assays of molecular markers developed to evaluate OA have also been promoted as *prognostic markers* and tested to see whether they predict the later occurrence or worsening of the disease. For example, it was shown that levels of serum hyaluronan (but not keratan sulfate), in patients with diagnosed knee OA at study entry, predicted subsequent progression of knee OA at the five-year follow-up[51]. In the same study population, an increase in serum COMP during the first year after study entry was associated with radiographic progression of OA at five-year follow-up[52]. Studies on rheumatoid patient groups have indicated that serum levels of COMP and the chondroitin sulfate epitope 846 are associated with rapid disease progression in that condition[53]. These reports describe results obtained on patient groups of limited size, and often do not specify the strength of the relationship between marker levels and disease progression. However, they suggest that further progress in the area of prognostic markers is very likely with prospective, longitudinal studies on larger patient cohorts.

Measures of disease dynamics evaluate the ongoing repair and degradative processes occurring within a joint, and might be classified as prognostic measures. As discussed, concentrations in joint fluid of molecular markers, for both degradation and synthesis, are consistent with the changes in metabolic rate observed for these molecules in animal models *in vivo* and in human OA cartilage *in vitro*.

Markers may also be used to *predict response to therapy* — such as estrogen receptors for breast cancer treatment. Structure analysis of the fragments released from or remaining in the cartilage matrix may yield important information on the character of the meta-

bolic process or protease responsible. Results obtained on aggrecan fragments may here serve as an example. The structures of the fragments released into joint fluid, and of those remaining in the matrix, are consistent with two different proteolytic activities in cartilage matrix in OA[54–56]. One of these proteases generates fragments consistent with the action of a 'classic' matrix metalloprotease such as stromelysin; while the other, as yet unidentified protease, generates fragments consistent with the action of an unidentified protease, 'aggrecanase'. Similar and ongoing structure analysis of fragments of cartilage collagens and matrix proteins may yield information on the role of different proteases in different phases of disease development — critical for our understanding of cartilage metabolism. This information may, in turn, be used to predict responsiveness to treatment specific for proteolytic activity such as a collagenase or 'aggrecanase'. The usefulness of this concept relies on the demonstration of disease mechanisms with at least a relative specificity for a condition or disease stage, and on the availability of agents specific for these processes.

Molecular markers have also been suggested as being useful to *monitor response to therapy* in OA; to be used as sensitive surrogate outcome measures in clinical trials of new disease-modifying treatments. Here, advances in our understanding of disease mechanisms, assisted by structure analysis of molecular fragments released from human joint cartilage, as outlined in the preceding paragraph, will be critical. Obviously, with the current absence of disease-modifying treatments in OA, the role of molecular markers in this area remains speculative. Experience from the treatment of rheumatoid patients is also limited, but suggests that cartilage molecular markers are responsive to treatment[49,57,58]. Randomized, controlled clinical trials of new disease-modifying treatments of OA will represent a precious opportunity to validate OA markers as outcome measures.

Different aspects of validity

Given that markers reflect the dynamic state of cartilage metabolism, it is likely that markers will be used clinically to evaluate the dynamic changes in disease: as prognostic tools to identify those at high risk of rapid progression, or as measures of response to treatment, to identify the responders and assess the degree of response. Other potential uses of markers (for example,

Table 11.18   Relevant types of validity and their interpretation in the context of marker studies

Type of validity	Meaning	Marker studies
Face validity	Is it credible?	Strong biologic rationale (a molecule found in cartilage or joint whose genesis or role is understood).
Construct validity	Are results in same direction as other similar measures?	Many possibilities. Examples: do other markers of degradation correlate with measures? Do markers reflecting synthesis increase after known stimulus for synthesis?
Content validity	Is it relevant across multiple domains of disease?	Is marker relevant across multiple different joints, and at multiple stages of disease (n.b. some markers may be valid only for severe or end-stage OA, others for early OA).
Criterion validity	Does it predict or correlate with gold standard?	Does marker level predict change in disease status using an accepted gold standard such as X-ray, arthroscopy, or algofunctional index?

as diagnostic tests) will possibly be less attractive. Assuming that clinical utility will fall into the realm of prognostic or evaluative tools, we outline different aspects of the validity of these measures (Table 11.18)[59,60]. Validity is defined as 'the extent to which any instrument measures what it is intended to measure'[61]. Using validity as a goal, we further suggest criteria that should be met before these markers can be widely used as clinical tools. These criteria can serve as specific goals for marker studies.

A starting point in evaluating the validity of a molecular marker for OA is asking whether it is credible or has *face validity*. Markers are likely to be credible if they are molecules present in the joint fluid or in cartilage, and where the metabolic process that generates them in cartilage is understood. Several markers under study, such as aggrecan and collagen fragments, can be said to aspire to these features.

In testing any marker, a *construct validity* will necessarily be an important component of validation studies. Construct validity is complex, but essentially focuses on whether results of marker studies show the direction that might be expected. If, for example, the marker were a measure of cartilage matrix synthesis, an increase would be expected in concentration in synovial fluid if the patient or joint were treated with factors that induced increased synthesis of cartilage matrix; the collagen type II C-propeptide may be a relevant example. Also, construct validity would be satisfied, in part, if concentrations of other measures of cartilage synthesis correlated with the putative marker. Other measures might include radiolabel incorporation studies or the simultaneous measurement of other molecular factors known to be reflective of cartilage matrix synthesis. Similar arguments could be made for markers of cartilage degradation. Studies that confirm the construct validity of a marker provide a rich foundation of corroborative evidence that suggest that a marker is valid. Testing whether marker concentrations are different in those with OA, versus those without disease, is also an example of construct validity.

Content validity may or may not be important in the validation of a molecular marker for OA. If the marker is reported to reflect the dynamic metabolism of cartilage in OA at all stages of disease and in all joints, the content validity is high. On the other hand, it is possible that some markers may be present only at certain stages of disease (or even in certain joints), in which case content validity or validity across the spectrum of disease range and joints would be less evident.

Perhaps the most critical element in validating a marker is whether it has *criterion validity*. For dynamic measures of disease activity such as molecular markers, criterion validity speaks as to whether marker concentration predicts changes in disease status over time. With the slow progression characteristic of OA, the longitudinal, prospective studies necessary to show criterion validity will need to use follow-up times of several years. Moreover, an appropriate 'gold standard' must be available for comparison, such as data collected using a validated algofunctional index or radiographs obtained under standardized conditions.

For evaluative tests, *discriminant validity* is critical. This dimension of validity concerns the sensitivity of the marker to a clinically relevant change in disease status. The *effect size* is dependent on the amount of change for the test, divided by the baseline variation in the test. Knowledge of longitudinal, within-patient variability and correlations with other measures of disease activity is, thus, important[41].

It is quite possible that using a combination of several markers, or their ratios, will prove to be more useful than focusing on a single marker[12], preliminary data to this effect have been presented[18].

Markers in osteoporosis — a model for OA

Biochemical markers of bone formation and bone resorption, that utilize commercially available assays based on serum and urine, have become accepted. They are primarily indices of bone turnover — the dynamic balance between resorption and formation of bone matrix. As will likely be the case for OA, comparisons of different assays that presumably measure the same type of bone activity, such as resorption, are not necessarily consistent in their sensitivity to change or discriminant validity. Some markers are measured with more precision than others; others may be more specific for bone; and, yet others, may have variable rates of metabolism by liver and other organs, and may, therefore, not always accurately reflect bone turnover[62,63]. Despite these limitations, bone marker studies have been used to identify women with high bone turnover states, and to follow treatment, especially with therapy aimed at diminishing bone turnover[64].

In transferring the concepts of osteoporosis to OA, several caveats are in order:

1. Bone turnover, while not necessarily systemic, can be measured readily in the serum. Cartilage turnover in a single joint may not be so easily detected in serum and may require synovial fluid sampling.

2. Variations in clearance from synovial fluid, with the degree of inflammation, is a concern unique to arthritis.

3. A number of practical barriers will make it harder to validate the clinical usefulness of markers in OA, compared to osteoporosis: obtaining synovial fluid is more difficult, and determining expected levels of markers in synovial fluid in non-diseased joints is especially challenging. Serum levels would be easier to determine in normals, but may not be as relevant.

4. Precise and accurate bone mineral density assessments in osteoporosis have provided a consensus 'gold standard' and simplified prognostic studies of bone markers. Similar quantitative measures of disease status in an OA joint are more difficult, so that detecting change over time is not easily feasible. Markers may, therefore, be more difficult to validate and use clinically in OA than they have been in osteoporosis.

Validating markers

As an example, we suggest criteria to validate a prognostic marker:

1. Strong biological rationale (*face validity*); marker identifiable in cartilage or periarticular bone; marker's role in pathogenesis of OA is at least partly understood.

2. Marker measured at baseline, in a body fluid, predicts the course of OA (*predictive validity*). Course of OA at baseline and follow-up is determined independently of marker measurement using conventional clinical means.

3. Marker present in high concentrations in appropriate tissue or fluid from patients with OA and concentration; correlates with other measures of disease dynamics (*construct validity*).

4. Marker validated in patients with spectrum of mild/severe disease and OA of different etiologies (for example, post-traumatic versus primary) (*content validity*).

5. Marker measurement is reliable (*repeatable*) and described in sufficient detail so as to be replicable by others.

Each of the criteria is necessary, but not sufficient, for validation. First, a prognostic marker should have a strong biological rationale. The marker should be identifiable in cartilage or periarticular bone. A prognostic marker should correlate strongly with the course of OA in an individual. If the level of a marker is abnormal at baseline, then the risk of subsequent joint deterioration should be magnified. The evaluation of the course of OA should be made by means that are conventionally accepted and are independent of the marker. The marker should be found in high concentrations in most, if not all, OA patients or their joints, and should correlate with other appropriate measures of disease dynamics. If joint biology suggests that a marker is relevant at all disease stages, the marker should be found in high concentrations in those with different stages of disease and disease of different etiologies.

Markers might also serve as predictors of responsiveness to treatment. Such a putative marker should be assayed at baseline in a longitudinal treatment study, and those who respond to treatment, defined independently of the marker, should have a different marker level at baseline than those who did not respond to treatment. For a marker of treatment response, measures at baseline and after treatment should be obtained. Normalization or improvement in the level of marker should occur in those who respond to treatment.

For all suggested uses of markers, but perhaps, in particular, for markers used to monitor treatment response, we shall require knowledge of the variability over time both in the individual and between individuals in representative and stable cohorts of appropriate size. Such data can be used to calculate the necessary number of patients and the required response to treatment in a clinical trial setting. Only few such data have yet been presented[65]. Similarly, we will need marker data for age- and gender-matched groups of joint-healthy and arthritic individuals at different stages of disease development. On the basis of such data, sensitivity and specificity for diagnostic tests may be calculated. Again, only few such calculations have been presented[18]. The future use of markers for any of the uses proposed here will, finally, require the general availability of both reproducible assays and standards.

Conclusion

In conclusion, molecular markers for OA could serve different purposes. Since markers reflect ongoing dynamic changes in joints, they are likely to serve as measures of prognosis and of response to treatment. Obviously, some markers may serve multiple functions. To operate as adequate tests, they should meet a set of standards. It is only when these markers have met such criteria that they will be generally accepted in the research and clinical community, and will become widely used.

References

1. Vincenti, M.P., Clark, I.M., and Brinckerhoff, C.E. (1994). Using inhibitors of metalloproteinases to treat arthritis. Easier said than done? *Arthritis and Rheumatism*, 37, 1115–26.
2. Campion, G. (1994). The prospect for cytokine-based therapeutic strategies in rheumatoid arthritis. *Annals of the Rheumatic Diseases*, 53, 485–7.
3. Bellamy, N., Buchanan, W.W., Goldsmith, C.H., Campbell, J., and Stitt, L.W. (1988). Validation study of WOMAC: A health status instrument for measuring clinically important patient relevant outcomes to antirheumatic drug therapy in patients with osteoarthritis of the hip or knee. *Journal of Rheumatology*, 15, 1833–40.
4. Lequesne, M.G., Mery, C., Samson, M., and Gerard, P. (1987). Indexes of severity for osteoarthritis of the hip and knee. Validation — value in comparison with other assessment tests. *Scandinavian Journal of Rheumatology*, suppl 65, 85–9.
5. Spector, T.D. and Cooper, C. (1993). Radiographic assessment of osteoarthritis in population studies: whither Kellgren and Lawrence? *Osteoarthritis and Cartilage*, 1, 203–6.
6. Chan, W.P., Lang, P., Stevens, M.P., Sack, K., Majumdar, S., Stoller, D.W., et al. (1991). Osteoarthritis of the knee: comparison of radiography, CT, and MR imaging to assess extent and severity. *American Journal of Roentgenology*, 157, 799–806.
7. Dougados, M., Ayral, X., Listrat, V., Guegen, A., Bahaud, J., Beaufils, P., et al. (1994). The SFA system for assessing articular cartilage lesions at arthroscopy of the knee. *Arthroscopy*, 10, 69–77.
8. Myers, S., Dine, K., Albrecht, M., Brandt, D., Wu, D., and Brandt, K. (1994). Assessment by high frequency ultrasound (HFU) of the thickness and subsurface characteristics of normal and osteoarthritic human cartilage. *Transactions of the Orthopaedic Research Society*, 19, 215.
9. Lohmander, L.S. (1994). Articular cartilage and osteoarthrosis — the role of molecular markers to monitor breakdown, repair and disease. *Journal of Anatomy*, 184, 477–92.
10. Dieppe, P., Cushnagan, J., Young, P., and Kirwan, J. (1993). Prediction of the progression of joint space narrowing in osteoarthritis of the knee by bone scintigraphy. *Annals of the Rheumatic Diseases*, 52, 557–63.
11. Bonassar, L.J., Frank, E.H., Murray, J.C., Paguio, C.B., Moore, V.L., Lark, M.W., et al. (1995). Changes in cartilage composition and physical properties due to stromelysin degradation. *Arthritis and Rheumatism*, 38, 173–83.
12. Dieppe, P. (1995). Recommended methodology for assessing the progression of osteoarthritis of the hip and the knee. *Osteoarthritis and Cartilage*, 3, 73–7.
13. Dieppe, P., Brandt, K.D., Lohmander, L.S., and Felson, D. (1995). Detecting and measuring disease modification in osteoarthritis — the need for standardised methodology. *Journal of Rheumatology*, 22, 201–3.
14. Lohmander, L.S. (1991). Markers of cartilage metabolism in arthrosis. a review. *Acta Orthopaedica Scandinavica*, 62, 623–32.
15. Poole, A.R. (1994). Immunochemical markers of joint inflammation, skeletal damage and repair; where are we now? *Annals of the Rheumatic Diseases*, 53, 3–5.
16. Saxne, T. and Heinegård, D. (1995). Matrix proteins: potentials as body fluid markers of changes in the metabolism of cartilage and bone in arthritis. *Journal of Rheumatology*, 22 (suppl 43), 71.
17. Ed. Lohmander, L.S., Saxne, T., and Heinegård, D. (1995). Molecular markers of joint and skeletal diseases. *Acta Orthopaedica Scandinavica*, 66 (suppl 266), 1–212.
18. Lohmander, L.S., Roos, H., Dahlberg, L., and Lark, M. W. (1995). The role of molecular markers to monitor disease, intervention and cartilage breakdown in

osteoarthritis. *Acta Orthopaedica Scandinavica*, **66** (suppl 266), 84–7.

19. Wallis, W.J., Simkin, P.A., Nelp, W.B., and Foster, D.M. (1985). Intraarticular volume and clearance in human synovial effusions. *Arthritis and Rheumatism*, **28**, 441–9.

20. Wallis, W.J., Simkin, P.A., and Nelp, W.B. (1987). Protein traffic in human synovial effusions. *Arthritis and Rheumatism*, **30**, 57–63.

21. Levick, J.R. (1992). Synovial fluid. Determinants of volume turnover and material concentration. In *Articular cartilage and osteoarthritis*. (ed. K.E. Kuettner, R. Schleyerbach, J.G. Peyron and V.C. Hascall), pp. 529–41. Raven Press, New York.

22. Dahlberg, L., Ryd, L., Heinegård, D., and Lohmander, L.S. (1992). Proteoglycan fragments in joint fluid — influence of arthrosis and inflammation. *Acta Orthopaedica Scandinavica*, **63**, 417–23.

23. Pejovic, M., Stankovic, A., and Mitrovic, D.R. (1995). Determination of the apparent synovial permeability in the knee joints of patients suffering from osteoarthritis and rheumatoid arthritis. *British Journal of Rheumatology*, **34**, 520–4.

24. Lohmander, L.S., Hoerrner, L.A., and Lark, M.W. (1993). Metalloproteinases, tissue inhibitor and proteoglycan fragments in knee synovial fluid in human osteoarthritis. *Arthritis and Rheumatism*, **36**, 181–9.

25. Lohmander, L.S., Saxne, T., and Heinegård, D. (1994). Release of cartilage oligomeric matrix protein (COMP) into joint fluid after injury and in osteoarthrosis. *Annals of the Rheumatic Diseases*, **53**, 8–13.

26. Lohmander, L.S., Yoshihara, Y., Roos, H., Kobayashi, T., Yamada, H., and Shinmei, M. (1996). Procollagen II C-propeptide in joint fluid. Changes in concentrations with age, time after joint injury and osteoarthritis. *Journal of Rheumatology*, **23**, 1765–9.

27. Eyre, D.R., McDevitt, C.A., Billingham, M.E., and Muir, H. (1980). Biosynthesis of collagen and other matrix proteins by articular cartilage in experimental osteoarthritis. *Biochemical Journal*, **188**, 823–37.

28. Aigner, T., Stöss, H., Weseloh, G., Zeiler, G., and von der Mark, K. (1992). Activation of collagen type II expression in osteoarthritic and rheumatoid cartilage. *Virchows Archiv B Cell Pathology*, **62**, 337–45.

29. Carney, S.L., Billingham, M.E.J., Muir, H., and Sandy, J.D. (1984). Demonstration of increased proteoglycan turnover in cartilage explants from dogs with experimental osteoarthritis. *Journal of Orthopaedic Research*, **2**, 201–6.

30. Sandy, J.D., Adams, M.E., Billingham, M.E., Plass, A., and Muir, H. (1984). *In vivo* and *in vitro* stimulation of chondrocyte biosynthetic activity in early experimental osteoarthritis. *Arthritis and Rheumatism*, **27**, 388–97.

31. Mok, S.S., Masuda, K., Häuselmann, H.J., Aydelotte, M.B., and Thonar, E.J. (1994). Aggrecan synthesized by mature bovine chondrocytes suspended in alginate. Identification of two distinct metabolic matrix pools. *Journal of Biological Chemistry*, **269**, 33021–7.

32. Poole, A.R., Ionescu, M., Swan, A., and Dieppe, P.A. (1994). Changes in cartilage metabolism in arthritis are reflected by altered serum and synovial fluid levels of the cartilage proteoglycan aggrecan — implications for pathogenesis. *Journal of Clinical Investigation*, **94**, 25–33.

33. Caterson, B., Griffin, J., Mahmoodian, F., and Sorrell, J.M. (1990). Monoclonal antibodies against chondroitin sulphate isomers: their use as probes for investigating proteoglycan metabolism. *Biochemical Society Transactions*, **18**, 820–3.

34. Visco, D.M., Johnstone, B., Hill, M.A., Jolly, G.A., and Caterson, B. (1993). Immunohistochemical analysis of 3-B-3(–) and 7-D-4 epitope expression in canine osteoarthritis. *Arthritis and Rheumatism*, **36**, 1718–25.

35. Hauser, N., Geiss, J., Neidhart, M., Paulsson, M., and Häuselmann, H.J. (1995). Distribution of CMP and COMP in human cartilage. *Acta Orthopaedica Scandinavica*, **66** (suppl 266), 72–3.

36. Hutchinson, N.I., Lark, M.W., MacNaul, K.L., Harper, C., Hoerrner, L.A., McDonnell, J., *et al.* (1992). *In vivo* expression of stromelysin in synovium and cartilage of rabbits injected intraarticularly with interleukin-1 beta. *Arthritis and Rheumatism*, **35**, 1227–33.

37. Wolfe, G.C., MacNaul, K.L., Buechel, F.F., McDonnell, J., Hoerner, L.A., Lark, M.W., *et al.* (1993). Differential *in vivo* expression of collagenase messenger RNA in synovium and cartilage. Quantitative comparison with stromelysin messenger RNA levels in human rheumatoid arthritis and osteoarthritis patients and in two animal models of acute inflammatory arthritis. *Arthritis and Rheumatism*, **36**, 1540–7.

38. Roos, H., Dahlberg, L., Hoerrner, L.A., Lark, M.W., Thonar, E.J -M.A., Shinmei, M., *et al.* (1995). Markers of cartilage matrix metabolism in human joint fluid and serum — the effect of exercise. *Osteoarthritis and Cartilage*, **3**, 7–14.

39. Bollen, A.M., Martin, M.D., Leroux, B.G., and Eyre, D.R. (1995). Circadian variation in urinary excretion of bone collagen cross-links. *Journal of Bone and Mineral Research*, **10**, 1885–90.

40. Laurent, T.C. and Fraser, R.E. (1992). Hyaluronan. *FASEB Journal*, **6**, 2397–404.

41. Ward, M.M. (1995). Evaluative laboratory testing. *Arthritis and Rheumatism*, **38**, 1555–63.

42. Thonar, E.J-M.A., Lenz, M.E., Klintworth, G.K., Caterson, B., Pachman, L.M., Glickman, P., *et al.* (1985). Quantification of keratan sulfate in blood as a marker of cartilage catabolism. *Arthritis and Rheumatism*, **28**, 1367–76.

43. Sweet, M.B., Coelho, A., Schnitzler, C.M., Schnitzer, T.J., Lenz, M.E., Jakim, I., *et al.* (1988). Serum keratan sulfate levels in osteoarthritis patients. *Arthritis and Rheumatism*, **31**, 648–52.

44. Spector, T.D., Woodward, L., Hall, G.M., Hammond, A., Williams, A., Butler, M.G., *et al.* (1992). Keratan sulphate in rheumatoid arthritis, osteoarthritis, and inflammatory diseases. *Annals of the Rheumatic Diseases*, **51**, 1134–7.

45. Thonar, E.J-M.A., Shinmei, M., and Lohmander, L.S. (1993). Body fluid markers of cartilage changes in osteoarthritis. *Rheumatic Diseases Clinics of North America*, **19**, 635–57.

46. Thonar, E.J-M.A., Masuda, K., Häuselmann, H.J., Uebelhart, D., Lenz, M.E., and Manicourt, D.H. (1995). Keratan Sulfate in body fluids in joint disease.

Acta Orthopaedica Scandinavica, **66** (**suppl 266**), 103–6.

47. Lohmander, L.S. and Thonar, E.J-M.A. (1994). Serum keratan sulfate concentrations are different in primary and posttraumatic osteoarthrosis of the knee. *Transactions of the Orthopaedic Research Society*, **19**, 459.

48. Saxne, T., Heinegård, D., Wollheim, F.A., and Pettersson, H. (1985). Difference in cartilage proteoglycan level in synovial fluid in early rheumatoid arthritis and reactive arthritis. *Lancet*, **8447**, 127–8.

49. Saxne, T., Heinegåd, D., and Wollheim, F.A. (1987). Cartilage proteoglycans in synovial fluid and serum in patients with inflammatory joint disease. *Arthritis and Rheumatism*, **30**, 972–9.

50. Saxne, T. and Heinegård, D. (1992). Synovial fluid analysis of two groups of proteoglycan epitopes distinguishes early and late cartilage lesions. *Arthritis and Rheumatism*, **35**, 385–90.

51. Sharif, M., George, E., Shepstone, L., Knudson, W., Thonar, E.J.M.A., Cushnaghan, J., et al. (1995). Serum hyaluronic acid level as a predictor of disease progression in osteoarthritis of the knee. *Arthritis and Rheumatism*, **38**, 760–7.

52. Sharif, M., Saxne, T., Shepstone, L., Kirwan, J.R., Elson, C.J., Heinegård, D., et al. (1995). Relationship between serum cartilage oligomeric matrix protein levels and disease progression in osteoarthritis of the knee joint. *British Journal of Rheumatology*, **34**, 306–10.

53. Månsson, B., Carey, D., Alini, M., Ionescu, M., Rosenberg, L.C., Poole, A.R., et al. (1995). Cartilage and bone metabolism in rheumatoid arthritis. Differences between rapid and slow progression of disease identified by serum markers of cartilage metabolism. *Journal of Clinical Investigation*, **95**, 1071–7.

54. Sandy, J.D., Flannery, C.R., Neame, P.J., and Lohmander, L.S. (1992). The structure of aggrecan fragments in human synovial fluid: evidence for the involvement in osteoarthritis of a novel proteinase which cleaves the glu 373-ala 374 bond of the interglobular domain. *Journal of Clinical Investigation*, **89**, 1512–16.

55. Lohmander, L.S., Neame, P., and Sandy, J.D. (1993). The structure of aggrecan fragments in human synovial fluid: evidence that aggrecanase mediates cartilage degradation in inflammatory joint disease, joint injury and osteoarthritis. *Arthritis and Rheumatism*, **36**, 1214–22.

56. Lark, M.W., Bayne, E.K., and Lohmander, L.S. (1995). Aggrecan degradation in osteoarthritis and rheumatoid arthritis. *Acta Orthopaedica Scandinavica*, **66** (**suppl 266**), 92–7.

57. Saxne, T., Heinegård, D., and Wollheim, F.A. (1986). Therapeutic effects on cartilage metabolism in arthritis as measured by release of proteoglycan structures into the synovial fluid. *Annals of the Rheumatic Diseases*, **45**, 491–7.

58. Carroll, G.J., Bell, M.C., Laing, B.A., McCappin, S., Blumer, C., and Leslie, A. (1992). Reduction of the concentration and total amount of keratan sulphate in synovial fluid from patients with osteoarthritis during treatment with piroxicam. *Annals of the Rheumatic Diseases*, **51**, 850–4.

59. Tugwell, P. and Bombardier, C. (1982). A methodologic framework for developing and selecting endpoints in clinical trials. *Journal of Rheumatology*, **9**, 758–62.

60. Felson, D. (1995). Validating markers on osteoarthritis. *Acta Orthopaedica Scandinavica*, **66** (**suppl 266**), 205–7.

61. Carmines, E.G. and Zeller, R.A. (1979). *Reliability and validity measurements*. Sage Publications Inc., Beverly Hills.

62. Delmas, P.D. (1995). Biochemical markers of bone turnover. *Acta Orthopaedica Scandinavica*, **66** (**suppl 266**), 176–82.

63. Baron, R. (1995). Molecular mechanisms of bone resorption. *Acta Orthopaedica Scandinavica*, **66** (**suppl 266**), 66–70.

64. Riggs, B.L. and Khosla, S. (1995). Role of biochemical markers in assessment of osteoporosis. *Acta Orthopaedica Scandinavica*, **66** (**suppl 266**), 14–18.

65. Lohmander, L.S. (1995). Molecular markers to monitor outcome and intervention in osteoarthritis (promises, promises …). *British Journal of Rheumatology*, **34**, 599–601.

66. Lohmander, L.S., Dahlberg, L., Ryd, L., and Heinegård, D. (1989). Increased levels of proteoglycan fragments in knee joint fluid after injury. *Arthritis and Rheumatism*, **32**, 1434–42.

67. Campion, G.V., Delmas, P.D., and Dieppe, P.A. (1989). Serum and synovial osteocalcin (bone Gla protein) levels in joint disease. *British Journal of Rheumatology*, **28**, 393–8.

68. Mehraban, F., Finegan, C.K., and Moskowitz, R.W. (1991). Serum keratan sulfate — quantitative and qualitative comparisons in inflammatory versus noninflammatory arthritides. *Arthritis and Rheumatism*, **34**, 383–92.

69. Hazell, P.K., Dent, C., Fairclough, J.A., Bayliss, M.T., and Hardingham, T.E. (1995). Changes in glycosaminoglycan epitope levels in knee joint fluid following injury. *Arthritis and Rheumatism*, **38**, 953–9.

70. Slater Jr, R.R., Bayliss, M.T., Lachiewicz, P.F., Visco, D.M., and Caterson, B. (1995). Monoclonal antibodies that detect biochemical markers of arthritis in human. *Arthritis and Rheumatism*, **38**, 655–9.

71. Lohmander, L.S., Ionescu, M., and Poole, A.R. (1995). Changes in aggrecan structure and metabolism after knee injury and in osteoarthritis. *Transactions of the Orthopaedic Research Society*, **20**, 412.

72. Shinmei, M., Miyauchi, S., Machida, A., and Miyazaki, K. (1992). Quantitation of chondroitin 4-sulfate and chondroitin 6-sulfate in pathologic joint fluid. *Arthritis and Rheumatism*, **35**, 1304–8.

73. Witsch-Prehm, P., Miehlke, R., and Kresse, H. (1992). Presence of small proteoglycan fragments in normal and arthritic human cartilage. *Arthritis and Rheumatism*, **35**, 1042–52.

74. Saxne, T. and Heinegård, D. (1992). Cartilage oligomeric matrix protein: a novel marker of cartilage turnover detectable in synovial fluid and blood. *British Journal of Rheumatology*, **31**, 583–91.

75. Shinmei, M., Ito, K., Matsuyama, S., Yoshihara, Y., and Matsuzawa, K. (1993). Joint fluid carboxy-terminal type II procollagen peptide as a marker of cartilage collagen biosynthesis. *Osteoarthritis and Cartilage*, **1**, 121–8.

76. Hollander, A.P., Heathfield, T.F., Webber, C., Iwata, Y., Bourne, R., Rorabeck, C., *et al.* (1994). Increased damage to type II collagen in osteoarthritic cartilage detected by a new immunoassay. *Journal of Clinical Investigation*, **93**, 1722–32.

77. Goldberg, R.L., Lenz, M.E., Huff, J., Glickman, P., Katz, R., and Thonar, E.J.-M.A. (1991). Elevated plasma levels of hyaluronate in patients with osteoarthritis and rheumatoid arthritis. *Arthritis and Rheumatism*, **34**, 799–807.

78. Hedin, P-J., Weitoft, T., Hedin, H., Engström-Laurent, A., and Saxne, T. (1991). Serum concentrations of hyaluronan and proteoglycan in joint disease. Lack of association. *Journal of Rheumatology*, **18**, 1601–5.

79. Yoshihara, Y., Obata, K.I., Fujimoto, N., Yamashita, K., Hayakawa, T., and Shimmei, M. (1995). Increased levels of stromelysin-1 and tissue inhibitor of metalloproteinases-1 in sera from patients with rheumatoid arthritis. *Arthritis and Rheumatism*, **38**, 969–75.

80. Zucker, S., Lysik, R.M., Zarrabi, M.H., Greenwald, R.A., Gruber, B., Tickle, S.P., *et al.* (1994). Elevated plasma stromelysin levels in arthritis. *Journal of Rheumatology*, **21**, 2329–33.

81. Manicourt, D.H., Fujimoto, N., Obata, K., and Thonar, E.J. (1994). Serum levels of collagenase, stromelysin-1, and TIMP-1. Age- and sex-related differences in normal subjects and relationship to the extent of joint involve-ment and serum levels of antigenic keratan sulfate in patients with osteoarthritis. *Arthritis and Rheumatism*, **37**, 1774–83.

82. Clark, I.M., Powell, L.K., Ramsey, S., Hazleman, B.L., and Cawston, T.E. (1993). The measurement of collagenase, tissue inhibitor of metalloproteinases (TIMP), and collagenase-TIMP complex in synovial fluids from patients with osteoarthritis and rheumatoid arthritis. *Arthritis and Rheumatism*, **36**, 372–9.

83. Sharif, M., George, E., and Dieppe, P.A. (1996). Synovial fluid and serum concentrations of amino-terminal propeptide of type III procollagen in healthy volunteers and patients with joint disease. *Annals of the Rheumatic Diseases*, **55**, 47–51.

84. Lohmander, L.S., Saxne, T., and Heinegård, D. (1996). Increased concentrations of bone sialoprotein in joint fluid after knee injury. *Annals of the Rheumatic Diseases*, **55**, 622–6.

85. Sharif, M., George, E., and Dieppe, P.A. (1995). Correlation between synovial fluid markers of cartilage and bone turnover and scintigraphic scan abnormalities in osteoarthritis of the knee. *Arthritis and Rheumatism*, **38**, 78–81.

86. Astbury, C., Bird, H.A., McLaren, A.M., and Robins, S.P. (1994). Urinary excretion of pyridinium crosslinks of collagen correlated with joint damage in arthritis. *British Journal of Rheumatology*, **33**, 11–15.

87. Thompson, P.W., Spector, T.D., James, I.T., Henderson, E., and Hart, D.J. (1992). Urinary collagen crosslinks reflect the radiographic severity of knee osteoarthritis. *British Journal of Rheumatology*, **31**, 759–61.

12 | Design of clinical trials for evaluation of DMOADs and of new agents for symptomatic treatment of osteoarthritis

Nicholas Bellamy

Regardless of the musculoskeletal condition, assessing the clinical response to treatment necessitates the use of valid, reliable, and responsive measurement techniques. (See pp. 535–536 for definition). Such techniques are numerous and include questionnaires, clinical examination techniques, and mechanical or electromechanical devices[1]. Thus, decisions regarding what to measure, and how to conduct measurement are fundamental methodologic questions.

Decisions regarding what to measure can be based on conceptual principals or by reference to techniques used in prior studies, or by adhering to existing outcome measurement guidelines. It should not be assumed that because osteoarthritis (OA) is generally a more indolent, slowly progressive disorder than the inflammatory arthropathies, outcome assessment is simpler. To the contrary, measurement options are more complex because of a tendency for the condition to either be confined to a single joint, or to show different patterns of multi-joint involvement in different patients. Furthermore, the volume of accumulated data referring to the clinical metrology of OA is much

smaller than that concerning conditions such as rheumatoid arthritis or ankylosing spondylitis.

Decisions regarding how to measure the response require a thorough knowledge of the characteristics and metrologic properties of different measuring instruments: these have been summarized recently in a textbook of metrology[1]. It is reasonable to question whether theoretical concerns regarding measurement issues have practical consequence — two examples serve to illustrate the point. In a comparative study of naproxen-CR versus regular naproxen, two different measures were used to assess physical function[2] (Table 12.1). Based on the Steinbrocker classification[3], no change in physical function was noted in the majority of subjects on either formulation. In contrast, a more responsive activities of daily living (ADL) scale was able to detect degrees of both improvement and deterioration missed by the Steinbrocker index. This example illustrates the importance of selecting the correct instrument, and the importance of understanding the properties of different forms of scaling.

Table 12.1 Relative responsiveness of two measures of physical function: comparison from a double-blind randomized controlled trial of naproxen (CR) versus standard naproxen (SN)

	Better (%)	Same (%)	Worse (%)
Steinbrocker			
Naproxen (CR) (n = 102)	5	95	0
Naproxen (SN) (n = 103)	7	91	2
Ability to work, play, exercise			
Naproxen (CR) (n = 102)	30	53	17
Naproxen (SN) (n = 105)	3	54	11

Andersson *et al.*[4], have studied the effects of different indices for categorizing the outcome of orthopedic surgery (Table 12.2). Using the Judet and Judet scale[5], it would be concluded that 97.5 per cent of outcomes were good. However, a completely different conclusion would be reached using the Harris scale[6]. This second example illustrates the complexities of placing more importance on some aspect of the disease than on others (weighting), combining information (aggregation), and categorizing the final score (transformation). It also indicates that data from composite indices require cautious interpretation.

Experience with measuring outcomes in OA trials encompasses the orthopedic surgery, physiotherapy, and pharmacology (drugs and devices) literature. Progress in the development of pharmacologic agents has been such that a new phase of drug evaluation has been reached, and it will be necessary to assess the potential of some new compounds to modify the disease process in OA. Such drugs might affect joint pathology but not have any effect on symptoms, while others may influence joint pathology *and* reduce symptoms. It is usually expected that drugs in the NSAID class will have a beneficial effect on pain, stiffness, and physical disability in OA (that is, symptom modifying osteoarthritis drugs — SMOAD), but will not have any effect on joint pathology. Thus, the dimensionality of the response between agents in the DMOAD class and those in the SMOAD class may differ. Furthermore, disease modification, itself, may result in more favorable long-term outcomes, as measured in terms of dependency, employability, or necessity for orthopedic intervention. Thus, the instrumentation required to assess the extent of the dimensionality of the response to DMOADs may need to be greater than that previously used to assess the dimensionality of the response to SMOAD-class drugs.

Design options

In general, the double-blind randomized controlled parallel trial is the most appropriate design for large scale comparative studies of SMOADs and DMOADs. Although sample size requirements may be greater than for a comparable crossover study, the design offers simplicity without any danger of carryover effects[7]. Furthermore, crossover designs are only appropriate where the intervention has a relatively fast onset and offset of action. Thus, while crossover designs may be suitable, in some instances, for studying the effect of fast-acting SMOADs (FASMOADs), they cannot be used to assess slow-acting SMOAD (SASMOAD) or DMOAD effects. An interesting variation of the crossover design, applicable to assessing individual response to FASMOADs, is the N-of-1 trial design in which patients undergo repeated crossovers to determine whether any statistically significant and/or clinically important difference exists between competing alternative treatments administered in a double-blind fashion[8].

In general, non-randomized comparative group designs and one-group non-comparative open designs lack the necessary rigor essential for assessing the relative and absolute efficacy and tolerability of antirheumatic compounds. The importance of double-blinding in SMOAD trials is unchallenged. Its value in DMOAD trials, where the principal outcome is radiographic, is less obvious. In such studies, radiographs may be read blind by a third party. However, DMOAD trials are likely to be of several years' duration, and the lack of blinding of patients and assessors may cause an expectation bias, one result of which may be that patients on traditional therapy will terminate prematurely because of therapeutic nihilism on the part of the patient, or the assessor, or both. Therefore, it is prefer-

Table 12.2 Comparative results (as %) of categorizing the outcomes of orthopedic surgery using seven different rating scales on the same group of 27 patients.

	Judet & Judet	Stinchfield *et al.*	Merle d'Aubigne	Shepherd	Larson	Harris	Andersson & Möller-Nielsen
Good	97.5	62.5	35	49	49	36	36
Fair	2.5	28.5	17	33	13	24	38
Bad	0.0	9.0	48	18	38	40	26

Courtesy of the Editor of the *Journal of Bone and Joint Surgery*. Adapted from reference 4 and published

able to use blinding procedures in both SMOAD and DMOAD trials.

What constitutes an adequate trial duration is contentious. However, the following *minimum* durations are commonly used or have been recommended[9].

- FASMOAD: 6–12 weeks

- SASMOAD: 4–6 months

- DMOAD: 2–3 years

In early trials of new SMOADs, where efficacy has not been proven, a placebo comparison group should be chosen or, alternatively, an NSAID group should be employed. Where feasible, both could be used in initial studies of these agents. In DMOAD trials, the comparison group will depend on the level of symptoms. In trials of asymptomatic individuals, a placebo group could be employed, while studies of mildly symptomatic subjects could employ an analgesic group. However, in trials of more symptomatic subjects, the comparison group should include subjects taking an NSAID that is not known to have an effect on joint pathology.

Patient selection

In selecting patients for SMOAD or DMOAD trials, a decision must be made whether to study localized or generalized OA and, in the case of the latter, whether the focus will be on a single joint or all affected joints. In SMOAD studies, patients are often selected on the basis of having demonstrated their potential responsiveness to an anti-inflammatory drug during a washout period. In DMOAD studies, a number of patient groups might be selected[9].

(1) subjects at risk of developing OA (for example, prior injury known to be associated with the development of OA) in studies assessing the ability of a drug to prevent OA;

(2) patients with established OA (with or without symptoms) in studies assessing the ability of a drug to retard disease progression;

(3) patients with established OA (with or without symptoms) in studies assessing the ability of a drug to repair damaged cartilage.

In general, selection criteria (at least in early studies of new compounds) attempt to exclude patients in whom the probability of response is decreased, and the probability of an adverse reaction increased. The statistical efficiency of studying a relatively homogeneous group of compliant patients with potentially responsive disease, needs to be weighed against the more limited generalizability of the study result.

Randomization and stratification

In a comparative trial, the relative effectiveness of two anti-rheumatic drugs can be demonstrated only if the two treatment groups are known to be prognostically similar. However, there is considerable variability in the response to anti-inflammatory drugs, and the key determinants of this variability have proven extremely difficult to define. As a result, randomization has generally been used to increase the probability that treatment groups are comparable[10]. It should be noted, however, that randomization does not guarantee group comparability, it only increases the probability that prognostically important factors have been evenly distributed.

In contrast, stratification is a process in which patients are categorized into two or more groups with respect to certain defined variables of potential prognostic importance, such that their distribution is guaranteed[10]. Randomization is then performed separately within each of the resulting strata. Identification of stratification variables has proven difficult. The initial pain level might be used as a stratification variable in SMOAD studies, although it has not been employed or proved to be necessary in previous NSAID studies. Given the possible association between obesity and disease progression in middle-aged females, the body mass index (BMI) might be used as a stratification variable in DMOAD studies. It should be noted that while there may be current enthusiasm for selecting or stratifying patients at increased risk of progressive OA, there is no evidence whether the disease process in this group is more or less amenable to disease modification than that in the bulk of subjects with OA.

Intervention, cointervention, contamination, and compliance

The term, intervention, is applied to the use of a specific treatment in a study. The agent tested may be given in a fixed dose, or may be titrated according to a predetermined schedule or to the requirements of the patient. Although clinical practice is best simulated by the titration strategy — because it commits patients to neither excessive nor inadequate therapy and, thereby, minimizes response failures because of either inefficacy or adverse reactions — it renders dose-based comparative analyses difficult because of the small residual sample size at each dose level[11]. In contrast, a fixed dose strategy permits conclusions to be drawn about the efficacy and tolerability of a single specified dose, but fails to address the issue of optimal therapy in routine clinical practice.

For SMOAD studies, drug administration may be preceded, punctuated, or followed by a 'washout' period — such periods may be NSAID-free or totally drug-free. Studies may be single-blinded, double-blinded, triple-blinded, or unblinded. For practical and ethical reasons, 'rescue' analgesia with acetaminophen is usually allowed during the washout period. Because withdrawal may be poorly tolerated by some patients, a provision is usually made to advance such patients, prematurely ('trap door' provision), to the active treatment phase after 3–7 days. In spite of these problems, washout periods are advantageous in that they allow assessment of the baseline status of study patients and amplify any subsequent response to active SMOAD therapy, thereby minimizing sample size requirements for detecting statistically significant improvements. Also, they facilitate assessment of patient responsiveness and absolute magnitude of the change, minimize carryover effects from prior treatments, allow clinical baselines to be re-established in crossover studies and, when performed at the end of a trial, serve to redefine group comparability and the persistence of patient responsiveness.

Cointervention

Cointervention refers to the administration of another potentially efficacious treatment at the same time as the intervention treatment[12]. It can take many forms, including concomitant use of analgesic drugs, hospitalization, physiotherapy, and surgery. Because these often have a major biasing effect and confound interpretation of trial results, cointervention should be minimized, monitored, and taken into account in for-

mulating any conclusions. Because pain relief is the principal outcome measure in most SMOAD trials, such caution is particularly relevant for concomitant analgesics because their use is ubiquitous, whether they are officially permitted or not. Unrecognized differential analgesic consumption rates can minimize between-group differences in pain control and lead incorrectly to the assumption that no difference exists. Analgesic consumption is a surrogate measure of pain control and, therefore, is itself an important end-point.

Contamination

Contamination is rarely a problem in well-structured clinical trials of anti-rheumatic drugs. It occurs when an individual, instead of receiving the intended medication, receives a drug specifically designated for individuals in one of the other treatment groups. Its biasing effects are obvious, and if the effects are unrecognized, patients will be analyzed according to the drug that they were scheduled to receive, rather than that which they truly received.

Compliance

Compliance is a measure of the extent to which a patient adheres to the protocol, in general, and to drug ingestion, in particular[13]. It can be measured in four ways: by direct observation, patient report (verbal or diary), pill counting, and plasma drug level monitoring. Each method has its limitations, so that non-compliant patients can appear compliant, and vice versa. Even when the monitoring procedure is satisfactory, there is no standard definition for any level of compliance below which the therapeutic response is significantly compromised. In clinical trials, a level of compliance greater than 80 per cent is often considered acceptable. Furthermore, because enrollment is entirely voluntary, and because patients are in pain and under close supervision, compliance levels are generally high, and patient report (by diary) and pill counting are probably adequate[14] in short-term studies. However, in studies of DMOADs, in which the treatment period must be several years in length, compliance may be a problem. Whether a strategy such as the use of computerized medicine caps offers any real advantage in compliance monitoring has yet to be established.

Outcome assessment

The timing and nature of outcome assessment should respect both the potential adverse and beneficial effects of test compounds. Thus, although adverse reactions to SMOADs and DMOADs can occur at any time after administration, the induction-response (efficacy) interval for FASMOADs will be shorter than for SASMOADs and both, in turn, will be much shorter than that for DMOADs. The experience with disease-modifying antirheumatic drug therapy in rheumatoid arthritis is that certain toxic effects (for example, thrombocytopenia) occur more rapidly than others (for example anemia) because of physiologic variability in the half-life of the target cells. For both safety and scientific rigor, patients should be appropriately monitored for both clinical and laboratory tolerance to a drug, in accordance with its known pharmacokinetics and pharmacodynamics. Some assessment points may assess toxicity, others efficacy, and still others, both.

Clinical tolerance can be monitored by spontaneous patient report or open-ended or close-ended questioning. In general, the more rigorous the probe, the greater the incidence of 'intolerance' and the more difficult the task of attributing it to the studied drug. Even in a healthy population there is a background level of transient symptoms, such as headache, diarrhoea, and dyspepsia. For this reason, the term 'adverse event' is often used in preference to the term 'drug side effect'.

Outcome measures used to assess drug efficacy should be able to detect the smallest clinically important change and, at the same time, should be both reliable and valid with respect to capturing the dimensionality of clinical and pathophysiologic responses. To avoid bias, both patients and assessors should not know who is receiving what treatment (double-blinded study). Usually, the test treatments are given in an identical format, either as indistinguishable compounds or using the 'double-dummy' technique. When only a single-blinded technique is used, either the patient, or, more usually, the assessor can be compromised by an expectation bias that may either enhance or abrogate the clinical result. In a triple-blinded format, not only the patient and assessor are blind, but also a third party, who has responsibility for administering certain aspects of the trial — for example, termination of the study on ethical grounds if adverse reactions or response failure are unexpectedly frequent or severe in one or other treatment group. In a triple-blinded scheme, such decisions can be made without prejudice.

Irrespective of the specific protocol, ten criteria, important for selecting evaluative indices for clinical trials (Fig. 12.1), should be considered[15]:

1. The measurement process must be ethical. Measurement procedures that are painful, embar-

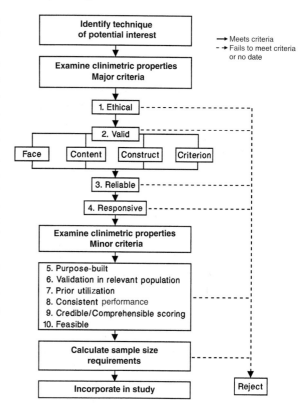

Fig. 12.1 Conceptual framework for selecting efficacy outcome measures from amongst existing techniques (Courtesy of Kluwer Academic Publishers. From Bellamy, N. (1993). *Musculoskeletal clinical metrology*.)

rassing, or hazardous to study subjects raise ethical issues. Such issues must be fully disclosed to participants and, if possible, less invasive procedures sought. The necessity for data collection must be carefully weighed against the risks, and the final procedures reviewed by an independent committee versed in judging ethical issues in biomedical research.

2. Validity should be adequate for achieving measurement objectives[16]. There are four types of validity: face, content, criterion, and construct.

(a) Face validity
A measure has face validity if informed individuals (investigators and clinicians) judge that it measures part or all of the defined phenomenon.

(b) Content validity
An instrument can have face validity but fail to capture the dimension of interest in its entirety. A measure, therefore, has content validity if it is comprehensive;

that is, it encompassees all relevant aspects of the defined attributes (for example, the Health Assessment Questionnaire (HAQ) contains not only questions on walking but also questions on dressing, grooming, arising, eating, hygiene, reaching, and gripping). Like face validity, content validity is subjective, but can be conferred either by a single individual or by a group of individuals using one of several consensus-development techniques.

In general, evaluative instruments for clinical trials should include some measures that comprehensively probe symptoms that occur frequently and are clinically important to patients. The definition of importance can be decided by groups of patients polled to assess the dimensions of their symptoms or by clinical investigators whose decision is based on their perception of the symptoms of the patient.

(c) Criterion validity

Criterion validity is assessed statistically by comparing the new instrument against a concurrent independent criterion or standard (concurrent criterion validity), or against a future standard (predictive criterion validity). It is, therefore, an estimate of the extent to which a measure (for example, the perceived difficulty of the patient in walking) agrees with the true value of an independent measure of health status (for example, the actual observed performance of the patient in walking a set distance or for a defined period of time), either present or future. The attainment of concurrent criterion validity is usually frustrated by the lack of any available standard, whereas predictive criterion validity is not immediately relevant to evaluative objectives.

(d) Construct validity

Construct validity is of two types: convergent and discriminant. Both represent statistical attempts to demonstrate adherence between instrument values and a theoretical manifestation (construct) or consequence of the attribute. Convergent construct validity testing assesses the correlation between scores on a single health component, as measured by two different instruments. If the coefficient is positive and appreciably above zero, the new measure is said to have *convergent* construct validity. In contrast, *discriminant* construct validity testing compares the correlation between scores on the same health component, as measured by two different instruments (for example, two different measures of physical function), and between scores on that health component and each of several other health components (for example, separate measures of social

and emotional function). A measure has discriminant construct validity if the proposed measure correlates better with a second measure, accepted as more closely related to the construct, than it does with a third, more distantly related measure. Validity, like reliability, has no absolute level, and its adequacy depends on the measurement objective.

3. Reliability should be adequate for achieving measurement objectives[16]. Reliability is a synonym for consistency, or agreement, and is the extent to which a measurement procedure yields the same result on repeated applications[37], when the underlying phenomenon has not changed. Because repeated measures rarely equal one another exactly, some degree of inconsistency is common. This form of measurement error is referred to as noise or random error. Low levels of reliability are reflected in the magnitude of the standard deviation and result in increased sample size requirements for clinical trials using such instruments. In contrast to systematic error, that is, bias, random error can be minimized by increasing sample size. Although there is no absolute level of acceptable reliability, in general, reliability coefficients should exceed 0.80.

4. An evaluative index must be responsive to change, that is, be capable of detecting differential change in health status occurring in two or more groups of individuals exposed to competing interventions[17]. This is an absolute prerequisite for an evaluative instrument and requires careful documentation. Not only should the instrument be responsive in general, but it should also be specifically responsive in the clinical setting in which it is to be applied.

5. The index should be designed for a specific purpose. Thus, instruments developed for one form of arthritis may not be applicable to, or as efficient in, the measurement of other forms of arthritis. The Ritchie index[18], for example, which was developed for rheumatoid arthritis, has been modified by Doyle *et al.* for application in OA subjects, principally by including the distal interphalangeal joints and lumbar spine in the count[19]. The WOMAC OA index[20–36] focuses on lower extremity involvement in OA and does not include upper extremity items contained in other indices, such as the HAQ[37] and AIMS[38] instruments. Furthermore, although some indices may

be applicable to the study of pathologic aspects of disease or to the radiographic appearance of the articulations, other equally specific and sophisticated instruments may be needed to assess the clinical progress of patients with chronic arthritis. Finally, the different research objectives of description, prediction, and evaluation should be kept clearly separate because each requires a different type of instrumentation.

6. The index should have been validated on individuals or groups of patients having characteristics similar to those of the proposed study population. Validation studies were reported infrequently for earlier indices, but are now a requirement for new measuring instruments. In particular, while an index may be responsive in one setting (for example, joint replacement surgery), it may be too insensitive to detect smaller responses, accompanied by greater variability, in another setting (for example, NSAID therapy). The instruments selected for a clinical trial, therefore, should be of demonstrated reliability, validity, and responsiveness in the relevant clinical setting.

7. Use of the index should have been adopted by other clinical investigators. This is a retrospective judgment and a relative one, because poor indices may be repeatedly used, possibly because they are familiar, whereas high-performance indices may be neglected because they are either novel or use innovative, but incomprehensible, statistical techniques.

8. Index performance should have been maintained in subsequent applications under similar study conditions. The repeated observation of expected relationships between intergroup differences and differential index scores, when the instrument has been used under similar study conditions, provides evidence for consistent performance. Such consistency has been observed, for example, in the measurement of pain in OA by visual analogue and categorical Likert-type scales.

9. The method of deriving index scores, particularly in composite indices, should be credible and comprehensible[39,40]. Although clinical investigators and the biostatisticians, with whom they associate, may understand the construction of index scores, the methods may not be readily appreciated by physicians, in general, who will be the appliers of any new knowledge. The responsibility of the investigators to convey the methods used in score derivation cannot be overemphasized. This is particularly true of composite indices for which analytic techniques integrate the magnitude and variability of any change occurring on each of several different dimensions, but may disregard the relative clinical importance of the contribution of each of the components.

10. The feasibility of data collection should not be constrained by time or cost. Measurement procedures that are complex and excessively lengthy run the risk of patient and assessor fatigue, with a resultant decline in data quality. Similarly, measurement methods that are prohibitively expensive lack general applicability, although for certain projects, cost may not be an overriding consideration.

Structuring efficacy outcome assessment

A conceptual approach to efficacy assessment is currently lacking. Although linkages between the different consequences of disease may be rather loose, it is, pragmatically speaking, reasonable to consider a series of consequences arising from the cellular pathology. In particular, we can recognize the development of clinical pathology which leads to clinical manifestations and, thereafter, to a series of clinical outcomes (impairment → disability → handicap or even death)[15]. The terms 'impairment,' 'disability', and 'handicap' have been given definition by the World Health Organization (WHO)[41]. Impairment is defined as any loss or abnormality of psychologic, physiologic, or anatomic structure or function. Disability includes any restriction or lack of ability to perform an activity in the manner considered normal. A handicap is manifest as a disadvantage experienced by an individual as a result of an impairment or disability, such that it limits or prevents the fulfillment of a role considered normal for that individual. In essence, therefore, impairment occurs at the organ level (intellectual, sensory, visceral, musculoskeletal), disability at the personal level (behavior, self-care, locomotion, dexterity), and handicap at the social level (independence, geographic mobility, employability, social integration). Having identified the consequences of disease, even though they may not exist in a strict hierarchy, one can develop measurement strata corresponding to each. Depending on the dimension of interest, one could use (or develop) one or more appropriate instruments to probe each of the strata, or as many as are relevant given the research question and the known or predicted pharmacodynamic properties of the SMOAD or DMOAD under study (Fig. 12.2).

The measurement challenge is different for studying regional OA (ROA) versus generalized OA (GOA), and different for ROA depending on whether the hips, knees, hands, or other joints are the focus of study. For this reason, the measurement process requires greater consideration than apparently more complex problems of assessing changing health status in patients with rheumatoid arthritis or ankylosing spondylitis. Existing

guidelines, whether they be from the FDA[42], EULAR[43], or WHO/ILAR[9] focus principally on the hip and knee. This is best exemplified by considering the current lack of a valid, reliable, and responsive internationally accepted functional index for specifically assessing OA of hand joints. This stands in stark contrast to the WOMAC[20-36] and Lequesne indices[44], which have been developed specifically to assess patients with hip and knee OA.

Two statistical problems arise in measuring multiple outcomes. First, the sample size may be quite different for different measures and, second, where multiple variables are being assessed, the issue of multiple comparisons arises. Furthermore, while we have reasonable

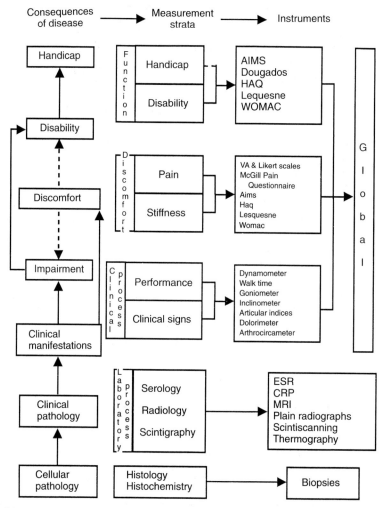

Fig. 12.2 Conceptual framework for outcome measurement in musculoskeletal clinical trials. (Courtesy of Kluwer Academic Publishers. From Bellamy, N. (1993). *Musculoskeletal clinical metrology*.)

estimates of the sample size requirements for certain variables, and a familiarity with the magnitude of the response which may occur, we have relatively little knowledge of these same issues with respect to so-called generic health status or quality-of-life measures.

Selecting specific measures for efficacy outcome assessment

The four key anatomic areas for research into the treatment of peripheral joint OA with SMOAD and DMOAD agents are: generalized OA (GOA), hip OA, knee OA, and hand OA (Table 12.3). The principal manifestations of these conditions are pain, stiffness, and physical dysfunction and, if they are sufficiently severe, compromise the quality of life of the patient. While stiffness may be of short duration, it is a common problem in hip and knee OA, and one to which patients attach importance[22]. Indeed, in a recent study of this problem, the percentage importance attached to being free of pain versus free of stiffness versus free of physical disability was 42 per cent, 21 per cent and 37 per cent, respectively[33].

It is difficult, at the present time, to recommend a particular quality-of-life instrument for OA studies, as there is relatively little experience in the clinical trials literature with these instruments. However, the SF-36 is popular and has been shown by Bombardier *et al.* to provide complementary data to the WOMAC OA index[45]. Both are high performance indices, one probing overall health, and the other, disease-specific aspects of lower extremity OA. Our own experience, to date, in comparing the WOMAC with the Lequesne, HAQ, AIMS, and FSI indices is that overall, the WOMAC may be a more sensitive measure, not only in lower extremity OA[23,24,34], but also in lower extremity rheumatoid arthritis[46]. As a result, my preference is to

recommend the WOMAC index, SF-36, and separate global assessments by patient and physician as core clinical measures for OA hip and knee studies[47].

There is no entirely satisfactory OA hand index, as yet, but we are encouraged by our recent experience with a new hand index (Auscan hand OA index), and also the work of Dreiser *et al.*[48]. In OA hand studies, I would recommend a similar strategy (that is, SF-36, patient and physician global assessments) and a regional index probing pain, stiffness, and function (i.e. Auscan). For studies of generalized OA, the regional indices are not satisfactory, unless used in combination, and only then in patients whose disease is confined to the hips, knees, and hands. For GOA studies, I prefer to use either the HAQ or AIMS indices, the SF-36, and patient and physician global assessments.

Some of the measures of physical performance (for example, 50-foot walk time, grip strength, range of motion) require observer training procedures[49–52]. Changes recorded on these measures often lack any individual definition of their clinical importance, and in the case of the 50-foot walk time, there is some suggestion that the measure is poorly responsive[21]. For these reasons, while such measures were recommended in previous guidelines, we now place little importance on them, compared to other measures, in current studies of FASMOADS. Whether they prove to be more useful in the study of SASMOADs or DMOADs is debatable.

Details of individual clinical measures are discussed in Chapter 10, while radiographic and biologic measures are discussed in Chapters 10,11. The careful selection of an imaging technique for a DMOAD study is paramount. In contrast, the validity, reliability, and responsiveness of biologic markers of OA progression have yet to be established. Additional measures are required to assess tolerability and to examine pharmacoeconomic issues. Finally, it should be noted that four other basic types of OA exist, each of which requires a different approach to efficacy measurement: (1) erosive

Table 12.3 Clinical outcome measurement batteries for OA trials

Measure	Generalized OA	Hip OA	Knee OA	Hand OA
Pain	VA or Likert	VA or Likert	VA or Likert	VA or Likert
Stiffness	VA or Likert	VA or Likert	VA or Likert	VA or Likert
Physical function (indices)[*]	HAQ or AIMS(2)	WOMAC or Lequesne	WOMAC or Lequesne	Auscan or Dreiser
Global assessment	MD/patient	MD/patient	MD/patient	MD/patient
Generic health status/QOL[**]	SF-36	SF-36	SF-36	SF-36

[*] Many of these indices contain their own subscales
[**] While the SF-36 is popular, there may be alternatives, e.g. EuroQol, Nottingham Health Profile, Health Utilities Index

OA; (2) axial degeneration involving the facet joints and/or intervertebral discs; (3) axial degeneration associated with enthesopathy, that is, Forrestier's disease; and (4) atypical OA, in which there is unusual joint involvement or episodes of inflammation, for example, in calcium pyrophosphate deposition disease.

Statistical issues

Statistical issues can be subdivided into those relating to sample size calculation and those relevant to statistical analysis of the resulting data. Both are quite complex, and those readers less experienced in this area of clinical research may find it advantageous to recruit a biostatistician to the research team. Sample size requirements may be calculated from several standard formulas which differ, depending on the trial design and whether the analysis compares means or proportions[53,54]. In addition to setting the Type I (α) and Type II (β) error rate, the calculation requires definition of the minimum clinically important difference (Δ) to be detected and the variance (SD) or, in the case of proportions, the differential event rates of interest. (The Type I error is the risk that the investigator takes of erroneously concluding that a difference between treatments exists, and the Type II error is the risk of erroneously concluding that no difference exists, when the converse is true.) The key difficulty, currently, is in obtaining estimates of the Δ and SD for comparisons of mean values. However, for knee OA studies, this has been made easier by the recent publication of statistical tables for sample size calculation[55].

The results should be analyzed and presented in a way that demonstrates both their clinical importance and their statistical significance. Two types of analytic philosophy are commonly used: explicative, or per protocol; and management, or intention to treat[56]. In the explicative approach, all patients failing to complete the study exactly according to protocol are excluded from analysis. In contrast, in a management trial, all patients entered into the trial are included in the analysis. Although the former strategy is operationally simple, it runs the risk of producing a biased result, usually by eroding any true differences in drug efficacy or tolerability. In the management strategy, patient drop outs, who often represent important drug-dependent events, are included in the analysis. For this reason, the management approach is currently the preferred method for analysis in most studies. We recommend that if an explicative strategy is used, the analysis be duplicated using a management approach, to establish the stability of the result and the integrity of the conclusions.

In addition to these basic approaches, which often employ statistical methods appropriate to the analysis of repeated measurements of continuous variables, it may be important to examine the time-dependent rate at which patients withdraw from treatment due to inefficacy, intolerance, or both. Methods applicable to the comparison of multiple proportions may be required for these analyses, as well as for other efficacy comparisons and most tolerability comparisons.

Interpretation

Caution is necessary in extrapolating results of a study and in generalizing them to other patient groups (for example, the elderly) that may differ in their response, be they beneficial or adverse. The results of a trial should be reviewed, therefore, in the appropriate clinical context[57]. Furthermore, they should be interpreted with respect to other relevant data from trials of similar or different design, and knowledge gained from case reports and case series. Finally, it is important to be aware of the possible existence of unpublished studies, some of which may contain negative results. With respect to published trials, the Cochrane Collaborative Project[58] should greatly facilitate the identification and evaluation of clinical trials data. This tremendously important initiative has attracted considerable interest and international collaboration. One of the primary goals of the Cochrane Project in OA is to identify, appraise, and collate clinical trials data in order to subject such data to meta-analysis. This endeavor should contribute significantly to the practice of evidence-based medicine.

References

1. Bellamy, N. (1993). The evolution of assessment techniques. In *Musculoskeletal clinical metrology*, pp. 5–9. Kluwer Academic Publishers, Dordrecht.

2. Canadian Multi-center OA/RA Study Group. (1988). Clinical evaluation of a new controlled-release formulation of naproxen in osteoarthritis and rheumatoid arthritis. *Current Medical Research and Opinion*, **11**(1), 16–27.

3. Steinbrocker, O., Tragus, C.H., and Batterman, R.C. (1949). Therapeutic criteria in rheumatoid arthritis. *Journal of the American Medical Association*, **140**, 659–62.

4. Andersson, G. (1972). Hip assessment: a comparison of nine different methods. *Journal of Bone and Joint Surgery (Br)*, **54-B**, 621–5.

5. Judet, R. and Judet, J. (1952). Technique and results with the acrylic femoral head prosthesis. *Journal of Bone and Joint Surgery (Br)*, **34-B**, 173–80.

6. Harris, W.H. (1969). Traumatic arthritis of the hip after dislocation and acetabular fractures: treatment by mold arthroplasty — an end-result study using a new method of result evaluation. *Journal of Bone and Joint Surgery(Am)*, **51-A**, 737–55.

7. Lequesne, M. and Wilhelm, F. (1989). *Methodology for the clinician. Compendium and glossary*, pp. 9–152. Eular Publishers, Basel.

8. Guyatt, G.H., Heyting, A., Jaeschke, R., Keller, J., Adachi, J.A., and Roberts, R.S. (1991). N of 1 randomized trials for investigating new drugs. *Controlled Clinical Trials*, **11**, 88–100.

9. Lequesne, M., Brandt, K., Bellamy, N., Moskowitz, R., Menkes, C.J., Pelletier, J-P., *et al.*, (1994). Guidelines for testing slow acting drugs in osteoarthritis. *Journal of Rheumatology* (**suppl 41**)21, 65–73.

10. Feinstein, A.R. (1985). Implementation of the outline: manoeuvres. In *Clinical epidemiology — the architecture of clinical research*, pp. 291–9. W.B. Saunders Company, Philadelphia.

11. Bellamy, N., Buchanan, W.W., and Grace, E.G. (1986). Double-blind randomised controlled trial of isoxicam vs piroxicam in elderly patients with osteoarthritis of the hip and knee. *British Journal of Clinical Pharamcology*, **22**, 149S–155S.

12. Feinstein, A.R. (1985). Randomised clinical trials. In *Clinical epidemiology — the architecture of clinical research*, pp. 683–717. W.B. Saunders Company, Philadelphia.

13. Gordis, L. (1979). Conceptual and methodologic problems in measuring patient compliance. In *Compliance in health care* (ed. R.B. Haynes, D.W. Taylor and D.L. Sackett), pp. 23–45. Johns Hopkins University Press, Baltimore.

14. Deyo, R.A., Inui, T.S., and Sullivan, B. (1981). Noncompliance with arthritis drugs: magnitude, correlates and clinical implications. *Journal of Rheumatology*, **8**, 931–6.

15. Bellamy, N. (1993). Future perspective. In *Musculoskeletal clinical metrology*, pp. 253–68. Kluwer Academic Publishers, Dordrecht.

16. Bellamy, N. (1993). Reliability and validity. In *Musculoskeletal clinical metrology*, pp. 11–29. Kluwer Academic Publishers, Dordrecht.

17. Bellamy, N. (1993). Responsiveness. In *Musculoskeletal clinical metrology*, pp. 31–5. Kluwer Academic Publishers, Dordrecht.

18. Ritchie, D.M., Boyle, J.A., McInnes, J.M., Jasani, M.L., Dalakos, T.G., Grieveson, P., and Buchanan, W.W. (1968). Clinical studies with an articular index for the assessment of joint tenderness in patients with rheumatoid arthritis. *Quarterly Journal of Medicine (New Series XXXVII)*, **37**, 393–406.

19. Doyle, D.V., Dieppe, P.A., Scott, J., and Huskisson, E.C. (1981). An articular index for the assessment of osteoarthritis. *Annals of the Rheumatic Diseases*, **40**, 75–8.

20. Bellamy, N. (1982). Osteoarthritis — an evaluative index for clinical trials. MSc Thesis. McMaster University, Hamilton, Canada.

21. Bellamy, N. and Buchanan, W.W. (1984). Outcome measurement in osteoarthritis clinical trials: the case for standardisation. *Clinical Rheumatology*, **3**(3), 293–303.

22. Bellamy, N. and Buchanan, W.W. (1986). A preliminary evaluation of the dimensionality and clinical importance of pain and disability in osteoarthritis of the hip and knee. *Clinical Rheumatology*, **5**(2), 231–41.

23. Bellamy, N., Buchanan, W.W., Goldsmith, C.H., Campbell, J., and Stitt, L. (1988). Validation study of WOMAC: a health status instrument for measuring clinically-important patient-relevant outcomes following total hip or knee arthroplasty in osteoarthritis. *Journal of Orthopaedic Rheumatology*, **1**, 95–108.

24. Bellamy, N., Buchanan, W.W., Goldsmith, C.H., Campbell, J., and Stitt, L.W. (1988). Validation study of WOMAC: a health status instrument for measuring clinically important patient relevant outcomes to antirheumatic drug therapy in patients with osteoarthritis of the hip or knee. *Journal of Rheumatology*, **15**, 1833–40.

25. Bellamy, N., Buchanan, W.W., Goldsmith, C.H., Campbell, J., and Duku, E. (1990). Signal measurement strategies: are they feasible and do they offer any advantage in outcome measurement in osteoarthritis? *Arthritis and Rheumatism*, **33**(5), 739–45.

26. Bellamy, N., Goldsmith, C.H., Buchanan, W.W., Campbell, J., and Duku, E. (1991). Prior score availability: observations using the WOMAC Osteoarthritis Index. *British Journal of Rheumatology*, **30**, 150–1.

27. Bellamy, N., Wells, G., and Campbell, J. (1991). Relationship between severity and clinical importance of symptoms in osteoarthritis. *Clinical Rheumatology*, **10**(2), 138–43.

28. Bellamy, N., Kean, W.F., Buchanan, W.W., Gerecz-Simon, E., and Campbell, J. (1992). Double blind randomized controlled trial of sodium meclofenamate (Meclomen) and diclofenac sodium (Voltaren): Post validation reapplication of the WOMAC Osteoarthritis Index. *Journal of Rheumatology*, **19**, 153–9.

29. Bellamy, N., Buchanan, W.W., Chalmers, A., Ford, P.M., Kean, W.F., Kraag, G.R., *et al.*, (1993). A multicenter study of tenoxicam and diclofenac in patients with osteoarthritis of the knee. *Journal of Rheumatology*, **20**, 999–1004.

30. Griffiths, G., Bellamy, N., Kean, W.F., Campbell, J., and Gerecz-Simon, E. (1993). A study of the time frame dependency of responses to the WOMAC Osteoarthritis Index. *Inflammopharmacology*, **2**, 85–7.

31. Barr, S., Bellamy, N., Buchanan, W.W., Chalmers, A., Ford, P.M., Kean, W.F., *et al.* (1994). A comparative study of signal versus aggregate methods of outcome measurement based on the WOMAC Osteoarthritis Index. *Journal of Rheumatology*, **21**, 2106–12.

32. Bellamy, N., Campbell, J., Stevens, J., Pilch, L., Stewart, C., and Mahmood, Z. (1994). Validation study of a computerized version of the WOMAC VA 3.0 Osteoarthritis Index. Australian Rheumatology Association 38th Annual Scientific Conference, May 22–24, 1994, Melbourne, Australia. *Scientific Program*, p. 102.

33. Bellamy, N., Wells, G.A., and Campbell, J. (1994). PARIS sectogram: a method for weighting and aggregating the WOMAC Osteoarthritis Index. Second International Congress of the Osteoarthritis Research Society, December 9–11, 1994, Orlando, Florida. *Osteoarthritis and Cartilage,* **2** (suppl 1), 37.

34. Griffiths, G., Bellamy, N., Bailey, W.H., Bailey, S.I., McLaren, A.C., and Campbell, J. (1995). A comparative study of the relative efficiency of the WOMAC, AIMS and HAQ instruments in evaluating the outcome of total knee arthroplasty. *Inflammopharmacology,* **3,** 1–6.

35. Choquette, D., Bellamy, N., and Raynauld, J.P. (1994). A French–Canadian version of the WOMAC Osteoarthritis Index. 58th National Scientific Meeting of the American College of Rheumatology, October 23–27, 1994, Minneapolis, Minnesota. *Arthritis and Rheumatism,* **37, No. 9 (suppl),** Abstract No. 400, S226.

36. Bellamy, N. (1995). *WOMAC Osteoarthritis Index. A user's guide.* London, Ontario.

37. Fries, J.F., Spitz, P., Kraines, R.G., and Holman, H.R. (1980). Measurement of patient outcome in arthritis. *Arthritis and Rheumatism,* **23,** 137–45.

38. Meenan, R.F., Gertman, P.M., and Mason, J.H. (1980). Measuring health status in arthritis: the arthritis impact measurement scales. *Arthritis and Rheumatism,* **23,** 146–52.

39. Bellamy, N. (1993). Weighting and aggregation. In *Musculoskeletal clinical metrology,* pp. 45–52. Kluwer Academic Publishers, Dordrecht.

40. Bellamy, N. (1993). Composite indices. In *Musculoskeletal clinical metrology,* pp. 135–46. Kluwer Academic Publishers, Dordrecht.

41. Wood, P.N.H. (1980). Appreciating the consequences of disease: the international classification of impairments, disabilities and handicaps. *WHO Chronicle,* **34,** 376–80.

42. US Department of Health and Human Services, Public Health Service, Food and Drug Administration. (1988). *Guidelines for the clinical evaluation of anti-inflammatory and anti-rheumatic drugs (adults and children),* pp. 12–15.

43. World Health Organization, Regional Office for Europe, Copenhagen, European League Against Rheumatism. (1985). *Guidelines for the clinical investigation of drugs used in rheumatic diseases, European drug guidelines series 5,* pp. 21–4.

44. Lequesne, M.G., Mery, C., Samson, M., and Gerard, P. (1987). Indexes of severity for osteoarthritis of the hip and knee. Validation-value of comparison with other assessment tests. *Scandinavian Journal of Rheumatology,* **65**(suppl), 85–9.

45. Bombardier, C., Melfi, C.A., Paul, J., Green, R., Hawker, G., Wright, J., *et al.* (1994). Comparison of a generic and a disease-specific measure of pain and physical function after knee replacement surgery. *Medical Care,* **33, No. 4, suppl,** AS131–44.

46. Hobby, K.J. (1994). The effects of aerobic walk-based exercise on women with rheumatoid arthritis. MSc. Thesis, The University of Western Ontario, London, Ontario, Canada.

47. Bellamy, N. (1995). Outcome measurement in osteoarthritis clinical trials. *Journal of Rheumatology* **(suppl 43)22,** 49–51.

48. Dreiser, R.L., Maheu, E., Guillou, G.B., Caspard, H., and Grouin, J.M. (1995). Validation of an algo-functional index for osteoarthritis of the hand. *Revue du rhumatisme — (English edn)* **No.6(suppl. 1),** 43S–53S.

49. Bellamy, N., Carette, S., Ford, P.M., Kean, W.F., le Riche, N.G.H., Lussier, A., *et al.* (1992). Osteoarthritis antirheumatic drug trials. I. Effects of standardization procedures on observer dependent outcome measures. *Journal of Rheumatology* **19,** 436–43.

50. Bellamy, N., Carette, S., Ford, P.M., Kean, W.F., le Riche, N.G.H., Lussier, A., *et al.* (1992). Osteoarthritis antirheumatic drug trials. II. Tables for calculating sample size for clinical trials. *Journal of Rheumatology,* **19,** 444–50.

51. Bellamy, N., Carette, S., Ford, P.M., Kean, W.F., le Riche, N.G.H., Lussier, A., *et al.* (1992). Osteoarthritis antirheumatic drug trials. III. Setting the delta for clinical trials — results of a consensus development (Delphi) exercise. *Journal of Rheumatology,* **19,** 451–7.

52. Bellamy, N. (1993). Standardised procedures for outcome measurement and parameters for calculating sample size for antirheumatic drug studies. In *Musculoskeletal clinical metrology,* pp. 193–251. Kluwer Academic Publishers, Dordrecht.

53. Colton, T. (1974). Inference on means. In *Statistics in medicine,* pp. 99–150. Little, Brown, Boston. 99–150.

54. Colton, T. (1974). Inference on proportions. In *Statistics in medicine,* pp. 151–88. Little, Brown, Boston.

55. Bellamy, N. (1993). Standard deviation tables for sample size calculation in rheumatoid arthritis, osteoarthritis, ankylosing spondylitis and fibromyalgia clinical trials. In *Musculoskeletal clinical metrology,* pp. 337–57. Kluwer Academic Publishers, Dordrecht.

56. Sackett, D.L. and Gent, M. (1979). Controversy in counting and attributing events in clinical trials. *New England Journal of Medicine,* **301,** 1410–12.

57. Bellamy, N. and Buchanan, W.W. (1993). Clinical evaluation in rheumatic diseases. In *Arthritis and allied conditions,* (ed. D.J. McCarty and W.J. Koopman), pp. 151–78. Lea and Febiger, Philadelphia.

58. Cochrane, A.L. (1972). *Effectiveness and efficiency. Random reflections on health services.* Nuffield Provincial Hospitals Trust, London.

Appendix 1

The American College of Rheumatology (ACR) criteria for the classification and reporting of osteoarthritis

Table A1.1 ACR criteria for the classification and reporting of OA of the hip*

Hip pain and at least 2 of the following 3 features:

    ESR < 20 mm/hour
    Radiographic femoral or acetabular osteophytes
    Radiographic joint space narrowing (superior, axial, and/or medial).

* This classification method yields a sensitivity of 89% and a specificity of 91%.

ESR = erythrocyte sedimentation rate (Westergren)

From Altman, R., Alarcón, G., Appelrouth, D., *et al.* (1991). The American College of Rheumatology criteria for the classification and reporting of osteoarthritis of the hip. *Arthritis and Rheumatism*, **34**, 505–14.

Table A1.2 ACR criteria for the classification and reporting of osteoarthritis of the knee

Clinical and laboratory	Clinical and radiographic	Clinical[†]
Knee pain + at least 5 of 9:	Knee pain + at least 1 of 3:	Knee pain + at least 3 of 6:
Age > 50 years Stiffness < 30 minutes Crepitus Bony tenderness Bony enlargement No palpable warmth ESR < 40 mm/hour RF < 1:40 SF OA	Age > 50 years Stiffness < 30 minutes Crepitus + osteophytes	Age > 50 years Stiffness < 30 minutes Crepitus Bony tenderness Bony enlargement No palpable warmth
92% sensitive 75% specific	91% sensitive 86% specific	95% sensitive 69% specific

ESR = erythrocyte sedimentation rate (Westergren); RF = rheumatoid factor; SF OA = synovial fluid signs of OA (clear, viscous, or white blood cell count < 2000/mm^3).

† Alternative for the Clinical category would be 4 of 6, which is 84% sensitive and 89% specific.

From Altman, R., Asch, E., Bloch, G., *et al.* (1986). Development of criteria for the classification and reporting of osteoarthritis: classification of osteoarthritis of the knee. *Arthritis and Rheumatism*, **29**, 1039–49.

Table A1.3   ACR criteria for the classification and reporting of osteoarthritis of the hand

Hand pain, aching, or stiffness, and 3 or 4 of the following features:

   Hard tissue enlargement of 2 or more of 10 selected joints[*]
   Hard tissue enlargement of 2 or more DIP joints
   Fewer than 3 swollen MCP joints
   Deformity of at least 1 of 10 selected joints

[*] The 10 selected joints are the second and third distal interphalangeal (DIP), the second and third proximal interphalangeal, and the first carpometacarpal joints of both hands. This classification method yields a sensitivity of 94% and a specificity of 87%.

MCP = metacarpophalangeal

From Altman, R., Alarcón, G., Appelrouth, D., *et al.* (1990). The American College of Rheumatology criteria for the classification and reporting of osteoarthritis of the hand. *Arthritis and Rheumatism*, 33, 1601–10.

Appendix 2

Lequesne's Algofunctional Lower Limb Indices

Table A2.1 Algofunctional Index for hip OA

Pain or discomfort	
During nocturnal bedrest	
None or insignificant	0
Only on movement or in certain positions	1
With no movement	2
Morning stiffness or regressive pain after rising	
1 minute or less	0
More than 1 but less than 15 minutes	1
15 minutes or more	2
After standing for 30 minutes	0 to 1
While ambulating	
None	0
Only after ambulating some distance	1
After initial ambulation and increasingly	
with continued ambulation	2
After initial ambulation, not increasingly	1
With prolonged sitting (2 hours)	0 to 1
Maximum distance walked (may walk with pain)	
Unlimited	0
More than 1 km, but limited	1
About 1 km (0.6 mi), (in about 15 min)	2
From 500 to 900 m (1.640–2.952 ft or	
0.31–0.56 mi) (in about 8–15 min)	3
From 300 to 500 m (984–1.640 ft)	4
From 100 to 300 m (328–984 ft)	5
Less than 100 m (328 ft)	6
With one walking stick or crutch	1
With two walking sticks or crutches	2
Activities of daily living[*]	
Put on socks by bending forward	0 to 2
Pick up an object from the floor	0 to 2
Climb up and down a standard flight of stairs	0 to 2
Can get into and out of a car	0 to 2

[*]: without difficulty: 0; with small difficulty: 0.5; moderate: 1; important difficulty: 1.5; unable: 2

Reproduced with the kind permission of the author, Dr Michel Lequesne.

Table A2.2   Algofunctional Index for knee OA

Pain or discomfort

During nocturnal bedrest	
None or insignificant	0
Only on movement or in certain positions	1
With no movement	2
Morning stiffness or regressive pain after rising	
1 minute or less	0
More than 1 but less than 15 minutes	1
15 minutes or more	2
After standing for 30 minutes	0 to 1
While ambulating	
None	0
Only after ambulating some distance	1
After initial ambulation and increasingly	
with continued ambulation	2
After initial ambulation, not increasingly	1
While getting up from sitting without the help	
of arms	0 to 1
Maximum distance walked (may walk with pain)	
Unlimited	0
More than 1 km, but limited	1
About a km (0.6 mi), (in about 15 min)	2
From 500 to 900 m (1.640–2.952 ft or 0.31–0.56 mi) (in about 8–15 min)	3
From 300 to 500 m (984–1.640 ft)	4
From 100 to 300 m (328–984 ft)	5
Less than 100 m (328 ft)	6
With one walking stick or crutch	1
With two walking sticks or crutches	2
Activities of daily living[*]	
Able to climb up a standard flight of stairs	0 to 2
Able to climb down a standard flight of stairs	0 to 2
Able to squat or bend on the knees	0 to 2
Able to walk on uneven ground	0 to 2

[*]: without difficulty: 0; with small difficulty: 0.5; moderate: 1; important difficulty: 1.5; unable: 2

Reproduced with the kind permission of the author, Dr Michel Lequesne.

Appendix 3

WOMAC Osteoarthritis Index Version LK3.0

Instructions to patients

In Sections A, B, and C, questions will be asked in the following format and you should give your answers by putting an 'X' in one of the boxes.

Note:

1. If you put your 'X' in the left-hand box, that is

None	Mild	Moderate	Severe	Extreme
☒	☐	☐	☐	☐

then you are indicating that you have no pain.

2. If you put your 'X' in the right-hand box, that is

None	Mild	Moderate	Severe	Extreme
☐	☐	☐	☐	☒

then you are indicating that your pain is extreme.

3. Please note:

   (a) that the further to the right you place your 'X', the more pain you are experiencing;
   (b) that the further to the left you place your 'X', the less pain you are experiencing;
   (c) please do not place your 'X' outside the box.

You will be asked to indicate on this type of scale the amount of pain, stiffness, or disability you have experienced in the last 48 hours.

Remember, the further you place your 'X' to the right, the more pain, stiffness, or disability you are indicating that you experienced. Finally, please note that you are to complete the questionnaire with respect to your study joint(s). You should think about your study joint(s) when answering the questionnaire, that is, you should indicate the severity of your pain, stiffness, and physical disability that you feel is caused by arthritis in your study joint(s). Your study joint(s) has been identified for you by your health care professional. If you are unsure which joint(s) is your study joint, please ask before completing the questionnaire.

Section A

Instructions to patients

The following questions concern the amount of pain you have experienced due to arthritis in your study joint(s). For each situation please enter the amount of pain experienced in the last 48 hours. (Please mark your answers with an 'X').

Question: How much pain do you have?

1. Walking on a flat surface.

None	Mild	Moderate	Severe	Extreme
☐	☐	☐	☐	☐

PAIN1   _____

2. Going up or down stairs.

None	Mild	Moderate	Severe	Extreme
☐	☐	☐	☐	☐

PAIN2   _____

3. At night while in bed.

None	Mild	Moderate	Severe	Extreme
☐	☐	☐	☐	☐

PAIN3   _____

4. Sitting or lying.

None	Mild	Moderate	Severe	Extreme
☐	☐	☐	☐	☐

PAIN4   _____

5. Standing upright.

None	Mild	Moderate	Severe	Extreme
☐	☐	☐	☐	☐

PAIN5   _____

Section B

Instructions to patients

The following questions concern the amount of joint stiffness (not pain) you have experienced in the last 48 hours in your study joint(s). Stiffness is a sensation of restriction or slowness in the ease with which you move your joints. (Please mark your answers with an 'X'.)

6. How severe is your stiffness after first wakening in the morning?

None	Mild	Moderate	Severe	Extreme
☐	☐	☐	☐	☐

STIFF1   _____

7. How severe is your stiffness after sitting, lying or resting later in the day?

None	Mild	Moderate	Severe	Extreme
☐	☐	☐	☐	☐

STIFF2   _____

Section C

Instructions to patients

The following questions concern your physical function. By this we mean your ability to move around and to look after yourself. For each of the following activities, please indicate the degree of difficulty you have experienced in the last 48 hours due to arthritis in your study joint(s). (Please mark your answers with an 'X'.)

Question: What degree of difficulty do you have?

8. Descending stairs.

None	Mild	Moderate	Severe	Extreme		PFTN8	_____
☐	☐	☐	☐	☐			

9. Ascending stairs.

None	Mild	Moderate	Severe	Extreme		PFTN9	_____
☐	☐	☐	☐	☐			

10. Rising from sitting.

None	Mild	Moderate	Severe	Extreme		PFTN10	_____
☐	☐	☐	☐	☐			

11. Standing.

None	Mild	Moderate	Severe	Extreme		PFTN11	_____
☐	☐	☐	☐	☐			

12. Bending to floor.

None	Mild	Moderate	Severe	Extreme		PFTN12	_____
☐	☐	☐	☐	☐			

13. Walking on flat.

None	Mild	Moderate	Severe	Extreme		PFTN13	_____
☐	☐	☐	☐	☐			

14. Getting in/out of car.

None	Mild	Moderate	Severe	Extreme		PFTN14	_____
☐	☐	☐	☐	☐			

15. Going shopping.

None	Mild	Moderate	Severe	Extreme		PFTN15	_____
☐	☐	☐	☐	☐			

16. Putting on socks/stockings.

None	Mild	Moderate	Severe	Extreme		PFTN16	_____
☐	☐	☐	☐	☐			

17. Rising from bed.

None	Mild	Moderate	Severe	Extreme		PFTN17	_____
☐	☐	☐	☐	☐			

18. Taking off socks/stockings.
    None   Mild   Moderate   Severe   Extreme   PFTN18   _____
     ☐   ☐   ☐   ☐   ☐

19. Lying in bed.
    None   Mild   Moderate   Severe   Extreme   PFTN19   _____
     ☐   ☐   ☐   ☐   ☐

20. Getting in/out of bath.
    None   Mild   Moderate   Severe   Extreme   PFTN20   _____
     ☐   ☐   ☐   ☐   ☐

21. Sitting.
    None   Mild   Moderate   Severe   Extreme   PFTN21   _____
     ☐   ☐   ☐   ☐   ☐

22. Getting on/off toilet.
    None   Mild   Moderate   Severe   Extreme   PFTN22   _____
     ☐   ☐   ☐   ☐   ☐

23. Heavy domestic duties.
    None   Mild   Moderate   Severe   Extreme   PFTN23   _____
     ☐   ☐   ☐   ☐   ☐

24. Light domestic duties.
    None   Mild   Moderate   Severe   Extreme   PFTN24   _____
     ☐   ☐   ☐   ☐   ☐

THANK YOU FOR COMPLETING THE QUESTIONNAIRE

Appendix 4

Design and conduct of clinical trials in patients with osteoarthritis*

Recommendations from a task force of the Osteoarthritis Research Society

Results from a workshop

Steering Committee:
ROY ALTMAN, MIAMI, FL, U.S.A.
KENNETH BRANDT, INDIANAPOLIS, IN, U.S.A.
MARC HOCHBERG, BALTIMORE, MD, U.S.A.
ROLAND MOSKOWITZ, CLEVELAND, OH, U.S.A.

Committee members:
NICHOLAS BELLAMY, CANADA
DANIEL A. BLOCH, STANFORD, CA., U.S.A.
JOSEPH BUCKWALTER, IOWA CITY, IO, U.S.A.
MAXIME DOUGADOS, PARIS, FRANCE
GEORGE EHRLICH, PHILADELPHIA, PA, U.S.A.
MICHEL LEQUESNE, PARIS, FRANCE
STEFAN LOHMANDER, LUND, SWEDEN
WILLIAM A. MURPHY, JR. HOUSTON, TX, U.S.A.
THERESA ROSARIO-JANSEN, CINCINNATI, OH, U.S.A.
BENJAMIN SCHWARTZ, ST. LOUIS, MO, U.S.A.
STEPHEN TRIPPEL, BOSTON, MA, U.S.A.

CONTENTS

*Reproduced in its entirety from *Osteoarthritis and Cartilage* 4, 217–43. Reproduced with the kind assistance of the Osteoarthritis Research Society.

A. Introduction

There have been many recent advances in understanding the pathophysiology and evolution of osteoarthritis (OA). These advances have led to improvement in diagnosis and therapy, and have prompted a re-evaluation of the methodology and metrology involved in the performance of clinical trials in OA. Recently, a combined committee of the World Health Organization (WHO) and International League of Associations for Rheumatologists (ILAR) has defined two classes of symptomatic therapy based on the onset and duration of the response to treatment[1], and has proposed a third classification for agents that may alter the disease process. In addition, a workshop sponsored by the WHO and the American Academy of Orthopedic

Surgeons (AAOS) has reviewed methods to assess progression of OA of the hip and knee[2]. At the request of the U.S. Food and Drug Administration, an independent committee has developed a set of guiding principles for the development of a new drug for OA[3]. Subsequently, the European Group for the Respect of Ethics and Excellence in Science (GREES), through a subcommittee, has made recommendations regarding the methods to be used for registration of drugs for OA[4]. Most recently, the Outcome Measures in Arthritis Clinical Trials (OMERACT) group has recommended a core set of measures to be used in OA clinical trials[5].

The Osteoarthritis Research Society also established a Task Force to address the issue of clinical trial guidelines for OA. Through a series of meetings, a draft manuscript was developed. The intent of the Task Force was to bring together the ideas on the conduct of clinical trials generated by the relevant active working groups, and to add sufficient detail to be of help to any party involved in the design of clinical trials. The Task Force was composed of academic and clinical physicians, researchers in the pharmaceutical industry and members of GREES. Representatives of regulatory agencies were invited to attend all meetings.

On May 26 and 27, 1996, a Workshop attended by representatives of the basic and clinical sciences, the pharmaceutical industry, GREES, and regulatory agencies was held in Washington, D.C. to discuss the working document of the Task Force. The present document resulted from the Workshop and reflects a consensus of the participants (See Appendix I).

It can be expected that the metrology and methodology of clinical trials of drugs for OA will change in the future, as they have in the past[6,7]. The following recommendations for the design of clinical trials in patients with OA are made with the understanding that they will require modification as new information becomes available. Investigators, regulatory and sponsoring agencies should be aware of the likelihood of such changes. Investigators and sponsors will need to incorporate new methodologies into their protocol design, and regulatory agencies will require flexibility to adapt to the newer technologies and methodologies. Indeed, as part of the advancement of science, it is expected that OA protocols will contain both validated measures and investigational outcome measures still requiring validation. The following are recommendations, or guidelines, not rigid rules for the conduct of clinical trials in OA. Many of the recommendations are supported by published clinical research. However, some recommendations have yet to be validated and are based on the best judgment of the Task Force and the participants of the Workshop.

B. *Objectives for treatment of OA*

Medications for OA may affect symptoms and/or modify structure (joint pathology). Demonstration of these benefits will depend upon the trial design and outcome parameters selected. Trial design will depend on the mechanism of action of the drug and the expected response.

For trials related to symptoms, some measure of joint pain will usually be the primary outcome variable. Factors that are considered in trial design include, but are not limited to, the pharmacodynamics of the drug, time to clinical response, duration of benefit after discontinuation of treatment, route of administration, frequency and severity of adverse events, effects on pain, effects on inflammation and effects on other symptoms and signs of the disease. In contrast to a prior consensus publication[1], the majority of the members of the Task Force and participants in the Workshop felt that there is no advantage in creating a separate class for those agents that produce a rapid symptom response from those with a slower onset of benefit. Medications used to treat symptoms have generally included analgesics and nonsteroidal anti-inflammatory drugs (NSAIDs). Examples of agents that may prove to be of benefit with a particularly prolonged onset to pain relief include intra-articular (IA) hyaluronic acid, glucosamine, chondroitin sulfate and diacerrhein. For the purpose of this report, the term symptom modifying drugs for OA will be used for both rapid and slow onset agents.

A drug may have effects on joint structure/function independent of its effects on symptoms. Studies of drugs that are expected to modify the pathologic process of OA should measure outcome parameters that reflect an alteration of joint structure. Such drugs may (1) prevent the development of OA, and/or (2) prevent, retard, reverse, or stabilize the progression of established OA by altering the underlying pathologic process(es). A drug that affects the pathology of OA may have no effect on joint symptoms. Symptomatic improvement may occur only after a prolonged period of administration. Demonstration of symptomatic improvement is not required if no claim is made for this outcome. Indeed, the GREES group have clearly separated those drugs that may alter the structure

without an affect on symptoms from those that modify structure and do effect symptoms[4]. Whether related to symptoms, function or some other variable, the primary outcome measure should be clinically relevant.

Drugs with a potential for structure modification have been labeled as 'chondroprotective,' 'disease modifying drugs for OA' (DMOADs), 'anatomy modifying agents,' 'modifiers for morphology,' etc. There is no uniformity of opinion concerning the term that best reflects the action of these agents. For the purposes of this report, and to provide consistency in the literature[4], the term structure modifying drugs will be used. To date, no agent has been proved to have structure modifying properties in humans. It should be pointed out that a symptom modifying drug may prove to have structure modifying properties (favorable or deleterious), just as a structure modifying drug may have symptom modifying properties.

C. *Levels of clinical trials for OA*

Preclinical studies are helpful in assessing potential modes of action and the dose range for benefit/toxicity, and may shorten the duration of clinical testing of a potential structure modifying drug. Although they are not essential, studies that demonstrate efficacy in animal models of OA will strengthen the rationale for clinical trials of structure modifying drugs in humans.

Medications undergoing clinical investigation are allocated to different levels of development as described below[8].

C.1. Phase 1 trials

Phase 1 trials are directed principally at demonstrating pharmacokinetics and safety. They may also contain a dose-finding component. Escalating dose trials are desirable for initial evaluation of drug safety. Mechanism based pharmacological evaluations, including those at the site of action (i.e., in joint tissues), are common. Initially, the presence of comorbid conditions should be minimized: later studies may target special populations, such as individuals taking concomitant medication. Phase 1 trials may be performed in normal volunteers or in a patient population appropriate for the target indication. Double-blind, placebo-controlled, single and multiple dose Phase 1 trials are desirable for the initial evaluation of drug safety. Evaluation of efficacy is not the primary purpose of Phase 1 trials. A

Phase 1 trial cannot adequately address the benefits of structure modifying the drugs.

C.2. Phase 2 trials

The goals of Phase 2 trials are to define an ideal effective dose range and regimen (Phase 2 trials must take into account both drug activity and toxicity) and to provide sufficient patient exposure to demonstrate safety in order to justify progression to Phase 3 trials (See Below). The duration of the study and number of patients studied should be based on the mechanism of action of the drug, duration of action of the drug, outcome variable being assessed, variability of the outcome parameters, and the intended patient population. Dose ranging in these and subsequent studies should identify the minimal effective does and dose-response profile, and may define the maximum tolerated dose of the drug in patients with OA.

C.2.1. Symptom modifying drugs

Phase 2 studies of symptom modifying drugs for OA should be placebo controlled, randomized and double-blind. Efficacy can often be demonstrated within days. Longer studies (weeks) are needed to demonstrate slow onset or persistent benefit. Even longer studies are required for safety. In studies of long duration, rescue analgesia may be necessary. A short-acting analgesic is suggested with a suitable washout employed prior to efficacy assessment.

C.2.2. Structure modifying drugs

As an alternative to demonstrating effects on joint structure, dose-ranging studies in Phase 2 trials of a structure modifying drug may utilize other measures of mechanism-based drug activity. Because these are measures of physiology and not efficacy endpoints, multiple dose regimens may be needed in late Phase 2 (2b) or 3 trials. The duration of Phase 2 studies for a structure modifying drug will also depend on its mode of action.

C.3. Phase 3 trials

Phase 3 trials are intended to convincingly demonstrate efficacy and safety of the optimal regimen and dose(s) of the test agent. Replication of pivotal studies (studies of primary importance for registration of drugs) for demonstration of efficacy is recommended. There

should be only one target joint in a single trial. These studies are designed to clearly define the dose/regimen of the test drug to be recommended for clinical use, further define toxicity, and compare the test drug with a reference drug and/or placebo. Sample size and study duration should be calculated to assure that subjects will be followed for a sufficient time period to detect a clinically relevant, as well as a statistically significant, difference between treatment and control groups with respect to efficacy — outcome parameters (see Statistical Methods). Sufficient data must be supplied to the appropriate regulatory agency(ies) to satisfy safety concerns. The number of patients and length of time to assess safety should follow the recommendation for chronic diseases of the *Guidelines for Industry*[9].

C.3.1. Symptom modifying drugs

Phase 3 trials of drugs with a rapid onset of effect can be as short as 4 weeks. At times, shorter trials are appropriate. Longer trials may be needed to evaluate efficacy for drugs with a slower onset of action. In studies of long duration, rescue analgesia may be necessary. A short-acting analgesic is suggested with a suitable washout prior to assessment of efficacy. A Phase 3 double blind study may be followed by a long-term double-blind study or open-label extension to evaluate safety.

C.3.2. Structure modifying drugs

There are no proven structure modifying drugs. Hence, the extent of testing needed to demonstrate this effect is not established. The duration of the trial should be pre-determined, and it is recommended that it be at least 1 year. The duration will depend on the mode of action of the drug, the anticipated response rate, the primary outcome variable and the length of time needed to show a difference in comparison with a control (i.e., placebo) group. Structural changes are required as primary endpoints. The size of the study population should be ideally calculated on the basis of preliminary data from Phase 2 trials in the particular population to be studied (see Statistical Section).

C.4. Phase 4 trials

Phase 4 studies are performed after the agent has been approved for clinical use by the regulatory agency. These studies may be used to support clinical observations leading to expanded indications. They also permit exploration of uncommon adverse events that can be discovered only in studies with a large sample size. It also provides supportive evidence of long-term benefit. Some Phase 4 trials may be open label. To date, Phase 4 trials have been published only for symptom modifying drugs.

C.5. Regulatory issues

When evaluating OA medications, it is advisable (when applicable) for the sponsor to schedule a pre-investigational new-drug meeting with the appropriate regulatory agency to define the preclinical and clinical requirements prior to initiation of Phase 1 trials. The sponsor should maintain communication with the regulatory agency as the drug progresses through Phase 2 and Phase 3 studies.

D. Entering patients in OA trials

This section addresses several aspects of the study design, including the protocol, admission criteria, selection of the study population and the definition of what is to be studied. Baseline assessment should provide information on joint localization (site), etiology (primary, secondary), severity of symptoms, structural abnormality in the joint, concomitant therapy and comorbidity[4].

D.1. Overview of the protocol

The study protocol should be divided into sections that encompass background information, rationale for the study, the question(s) being asked, size and site(s) of the study, method of patient selection (including inclusion and exclusion criteria), the method of procedure, clearly defined primary and secondary outcome variables, specific measures to be performed at each visit, drug dispensing format, method of reporting adverse events, statistical analysis and regulatory issues (including drug accountability, Institutional requirements, etc.).

It is desirable to include a table (or flow sheet) that outlines the method of procedure, information from selected references (e.g., disease classification, radiographic criteria), the informed consent statement, protocol worksheets, drug accountability forms, the data collection forms, etc.

The protocol should carefully define the investigators, their study sites, the method of randomization,

patient monitoring procedures, technical aspects of imaging techniques, laboratory tests, methods of documenting adverse events, methods of blinding and method of documenting medication intake for each patient (active drug, placebo, rescue analgesia), and the method of maintaining the medication log for each participating center.

D.2. Demographics

Demographics recorded in the protocol should include identifying information, such as the patient's name, address and telephone number, which should be kept confidential. The patients name should be coded by letters/numbers for data processing and future reference.

As a minimum, sociodemographic and clinical data collected at the time of enrollment into the study should include age (date of birth), sex, race, height, weight, marital status and years of formal education.

D.3. Diagnosis

Criteria for diagnosis of OA should be clearly stated. Patients should fulfill validated criteria for the classification of OA, such as those published by the American College of Rheumatology (ACR)[10,11,12]. The disease should be classified as primary or secondary. Study populations should be as homogenous as possible with regard to the presence of idiopathic (primary) or secondary OA[10]. If patients with secondary OA are studied, the underlying condition should be specified and should be the same in all patients (e.g., post-traumatic arthritis, mechanical derangement of the knee). It is suggested that in studies of patients with idiopathic OA, exclusions for secondary OA of the study joint include septic arthritis, inflammatory joint disease, gout, Pagets disease of bone, recurrent pseudogout, articular fracture, major dysplasias or congenital abnormality, ochronosis, acromegaly, hemachromatosis, Wilsons disease and primary osteochondromatosis[4].

D.4. Radiographs

The radiographic severity of OA in each patient should be quantified and documented using either aggregate radiographic criteria (e.g., Kellgren and Lawrence scale[13,14]) or grading of specific radiographic features[15,16,17]. This estimate of anatomic alteration on images should be acquired no longer than 3 months prior to entry. The range of grades used for entry criteria, as well as variations in grade among treatment and placebo (or control) groups should be comparable and similar. These radiographic entry criteria should also be appropriate for the specific study design. For example, a cohort that included advanced severity might be appropriate in studies of a symptom modifying drug while a cohort limited to minimal severity would be more appropriate for studies of a structure modifying drug intended to retard progression.

D.5. Study population

The source of the patient population (e.g., clinic-based, community-based, hospital-based) should be defined in the protocol. Considerable controversy exists regarding the use of broad vs narrow patient eligibility criterion. Broad patient eligibility allows for generalizable application of positive results; however, because of the larger amount of variation, broad patient eligibility increases the sample size of the study population required to demonstrate clinical and statistically significant differences, and may mask the presence of subsets receiving benefit (unless extensive stratification is performed). At the Workshop, the consensus was that patient eligibility should define specific populations and that, where appropriate, stratification of subgroups should be employed within studies of secondary endpoints of interest.

Examples of high-risk groups that might be considered for inclusion in studies of structure modifying drugs include obese women with unilateral radiographic knee OA[18], men or women who have undergone meniscectomy[19,20]. Examples of variables to be considered for stratification of the source population might include prior surgical intervention of the index joint, and high- vs low-risk groups. Examples of subjects who might be considered for exclusion might be either low- or high-risk populations, such as young age (< 45 years old) and those with protrusio acetabuli, concentric femoral head migration, extensive surgery of the reference joint, excessive varus/valgus deformity, and those involved with litigation/compensation related to the reference joint.

D.5.1. Symptom modifying drugs

For studies of symptomatic response, the level of symptoms at baseline should be of sufficient severity to permit detection of change, i.e., not too mild. After washout (see Section E.5.), inclusion criteria for symptomatic response should include the following:

- Pain of at least mild intensity: e.g., 100 mm visual analog scale (VAS) recording of ≥ 25 mm; or 5 point categorical (Likert) scale grade ≥ 1 (where 0 is no pain and 4 is extreme pain);
- Definite radiographic changes of OA, using an established scale and atlas, e.g., Kellgren and Lawrence radiographic grade ≥ 2 for tibiofemoral OA (i.e., presence of a definite osteophyte); modified Croft scale ≥ 2 for hip OA[13,14,21,22].

D.5.2. Structure modifying drugs

For studies of structure modifying drugs, as discussed above, special subpopulations of subjects who are at high risk for development of OA or rapidly progressive OA may be advantageous (as above). In addition, the following should be considered:

- Kellgren and Lawrence radiographic entry criteria: Prevention studies: grades 0 or 1 (i.e., absence of a definite osteophyte); disease retardation/reversal studies: grades 2 or 3 (i.e., sufficient remaining interbone distance to permit detection of worsening/progression);
- Current or previous pain in the index joint is not essential. However, changes in pain may be examined as a secondary outcome measure.

Preliminary data suggest that some molecular markers in serum may predict radiographic progression of established OA[23,24]. Analysis of molecular markers may select subpopulations who are most likely to show progression in OA.

D.6. Inclusions/exclusions

Inclusion criteria should be clearly defined and should specify the population to be studied by age, sex, diagnostic criteria, joint with OA, degree of symptoms, and radiographic grade.

Exclusion criteria should similarly be clearly defined with regard to degree of symptoms, radiographic grade, concomitant disease, prior peptic ulcer disease (if a drug is perceived to have gastrointestinal effects), concomitant medications, pregnancy/contraception, IA depocorticosteroid or hyaluronic acid injection, tidal lavage, and secondary OA (listed above).

Opinion varies concerning the proximity to the beginning of a study for administering IA medication into the reference joint. All agreed that there should be a sufficient interval between the time of the injection and the beginning of the study to eliminate the confounding effects of the injection on joint pain. The consensus of the participants at the Workshop was that a minimum of 3 months should elapse between the time of the IA injection and the trial (e.g., IA corticosteroids). This interval may be longer for specific types of IA therapy (e.g., IA hyaluronan), but sufficient evidence is not available to provide more definitive guidance at this time. The investigator should consider stratification of patients receiving prior IA therapy, administered within a year of the study.

Additional exclusions are significant injury to the affected joint within 6 months of trial start; arthroscopy of the affected joint within 1 year; disease of spine or other lower extremity joints of sufficient degree to affect assessment of the target joint, use of assistive devices other than a cane (walking stick) or knee brace, concomitant rheumatic disease (e.g., fibromyalgia), or poor general health interfering with compliance or assessment.

As with any investigational drug, women of childbearing potential should be screened for pregnancy, and if pregnant, shall be excluded from the trial.

D.7. OA history

The OA history is used to characterize the study population and should include the location and number of symptomatic OA joints; presence of hand OA (e.g., Heberden's nodes in patients with hip or knee OA); duration of symptoms; duration of the diagnosis of OA; history of prior medications for OA; surgical procedures performed on the study joint (including arthroscopy), with the date of the most recent procedure; use of assistive devices, such as canes, crutches, knee braces (in studies of lower extremity OA); history of prior IA injection (e.g. depocorticosteroid or hyaluronate injection), with date of most recent injection (see above).

D.8. History (other)

Other baseline history that may be of value includes smoking history, hormonal status in postmenopausal women, concomitant chronic disease, and concomitant medications, e.g., estrogens, anti-inflammatory drugs.

D.9. Study joint

Protocols should be limited to the evaluation of a single joint site (e.g., knee, hip) or in the case of hand OA,

either both hands or the symptomatic hand (preferably the dominant hand).

D.9.1. Symptom modifying drugs

Although data may be collected for both right and left joints (e.g. knee, hip), for symptom studies only one should be the primary joint evaluated (except for hands as above). This is most often the signal (more symptomatic) side. Changes in the contralateral joint should be considered as a secondary outcome variable.

D.9.2. Structure modifying drugs

For studies of a structure modifying drug, the more involved side of a single joint site (e.g., hip, knee) should be studied as the primary outcome variable. In these cases, changes in the contralateral joint can serve as a secondary outcome variable. However, changes in the contralateral joint, which may not yet be symptomatic or have definite OA, may be selected as the primary outcome variable (e.g. Chingford data).

For studies of both symptom and structure modifying drugs, additional joint sites may be evaluated as secondary outcome variables.

D.10. Physical examination of the index joint

Baseline information about the index joint helps characterize the study population and provides reference data for assessing how variables of interest have changed during the course of treatment. Evidence of inflammation (e.g., joint effusion), joint deformity, and joint contractures should be noted. For large joints, loss of range of motion and presence of severe valgus/varus deformity may be useful as exclusion criteria. Although it is important to record the presence of clinical signs of inflammation, including synovial effusion, these should not be used as a primary outcome measure in trials of structure modifying drugs.

D.11. Function

Measuring the degree of functional impairment can identify the severity of disease in the study population. Functional impairment should be defined using a segregated, validated multidimensional index (SMI) such as the Western Ontario and McMasters Universities (WOMAC)[25] OA index for hip and knee OA, or an aggregated multidimensional index (AMI) such as the Algo-functional Index (AFI) for hip or knee[26]. At this time, although the AFI has been validated, separate pain, stiffness and physical function subsections have not been validated for independent application.

D.12. General physical examination

A general physical examination should be performed at the onset of the study and again at the end of the study.

D.13. Informed consent

Guidelines for information to be contained in the Informed Consent statement should be in accordance with the Declaration of Helsinki[27]. Patient participation requires understanding, and completion of an informed consent document that has been approved by the appropriate institutional review board.

E. Conduct of the study

This section deals with the procedures used during the study, exclusive of individual outcome variables.

E.1. Study design

Studies should generally be single joint, controlled, randomized, double-blind; and parallel in design. Occasionally, crossover studies or other designs may be appropriate.

The study should include a screening and baseline visit. The two visits allow the collection of more reliable baseline data, assure that the patients fulfill entry criteria and may be used to help reduce noncompliance ('faintness-of-heart test'[28]), collect biological specimens, etc. For treatment group assignment, patients should be randomized in the order in which they are enrolled into the study, to receive treatment according to a randomization schedule specifically designed to meet study objectives.

At each visit, vital signs (blood pressure, pulse, and weight) should be recorded and a report of adverse experiences (see below) obtained.

In order to minimize unwanted sources of variation in patient assessment, to the extent possible, the same examiner should examine the same patient at each visit, at the same time of day (and preferably also on the same day of the week) throughout the duration of the trial.

E.2. Primary study outcome

Efficacy studies of OA drugs should preferably identify a single clearly defined primary outcome variable. The choice of this variable will depend upon the nature of the desired drug effect and the objective of the study.

An alternative approach might involve the use of several outcome variables. With this latter approach, adjustments to the significance level are required for multiple analyses performed. (See Outcome Measures below.)

E.3. Secondary study outcomes

The inclusion of one or more secondary outcome variables will strengthen the study design. Collection of information for the secondary outcome variables should not interfere with collection of data for the primary outcome variable.

E.4. Examiner

The method used for training and masking of the examiner and masking of the patient must be specified. Both a blinded investigator (to assess the patient for efficacy and adverse events) and an unblinded investigator may be needed to administer the test medication and monitor toxicity in some studies.

E.5. Washout requirements
E.5.1. Symptom modifying drugs

All symptom-oriented studies require discontinuation of prior analgesic and anti-inflammatory medications, including topical agents, prior to initiating treatment with the test drug in order to permit an evaluation of unmodified pain severity. The time of withdrawal should be the time required for the clinical effect to disappear (e.g., 5 half-lives of the drug). During the washout period, subjects may use acetaminophen (or paracetamol) as rescue analgesia (up to 4 g/day in the U.S. and up to 3 g/day in Europe). This must be discontinued in sufficient time for the clinical effects of the rescue drug to disappear.

Worsening of symptoms during the washout period — although not necessarily a requisite for subject inclusion into the trial — should be documented.

E.5.2. *Structure modifying drugs*

A washout period is not required in trials of a structure modifying drug. If however, the effect of the drug on symptoms is to be tested, then the use of a washout period should be considered.

E.6. Administration of study medication

Control agents may include placebo or active (e.g., analgesic or NSAID) agents. Use of placebo may be influenced by ethical and regulatory agency considerations. Active control agents offer the advantage of demonstrating improved efficacy over existing therapies, but may require large numbers of subjects.

E.6.1. *Topical*

Topical test medications should be dispensed in containers which are identical in appearance to those containing the comparison agent (drug or placebo). The comparison agent should mimic the test medication in appearance, odor and local effects on the skin. Clear instructions regarding use must be provided to the patient both orally and in written form and must be contained in the Informed Consent. Compliance should be monitored by weighing the returned tubes or measuring the returned liquid. Placebo responses are particularly frequent with this technique of drug delivery, so placebo controlled trials are particularly important, as are to be carefully defined, homogeneous study populations.

E.6.2. *Oral*

Oral test medications should be formulated to provide an appearance identical to that of the comparison drug (placebo or other). If this is not feasible, a 'double dummy' technique (two non-identical active agents, each with an identical matching placebo) should be used.

Preferably, medication should be dispensed in blister packs with the label clearly stating the day and time of administration. Compliance should be monitored by counting returned unused medications or by use of medication vials with computerized caps.

Concomitant medication (e.g., rescue analgesia and NSAIDs in studies of structure modifying drugs) may be dispensed in bottles. The pills should be counted at each visit. Analgesic drugs with a short half-life should not be taken from the evening prior to the day of the evaluation if pain is to be evaluated.

E.6.3. *Parenteral medication*

Parenteral medication should be formulated to provide an appearance identical to that of the comparison drug. If this is not possible, the parental medication should be dispensed by a person other than the blinded investigator (e.g., by an unblinded investigator) and the injectable agent should be concealed from both the patient and the blinded evaluator.

E.6.4. *IA medication*

IA study medication should be formulated to provide an appearance identical to that of the comparison drug. If this is not possible, the medication should be injected by a physician other than the blinded investigator (e.g., unblinded investigator). The volume of control (carrier) injected should equal the volume of the test agent. The joint should be aspirated to remove any existing effusion as completely as possible prior to instillation of the drug, and the volume of fluid removed should be recorded. The injectable should be concealed from both the patient and the blinded evaluator. Placebo responses are particularly frequent with this technique of drug delivery, so placebo controlled trials are particularly important, as is the use of carefully defined homogeneous study populations.

E.7. Compliance and subject retention

It is essential for studies of structure modifying drugs, that strategies be employed to maximize and document patient compliance. For example, contact might be maintained with patients at 4–8 week intervals by telephone. The method of communication and time spent with patients should be standardized as much as possible without jeopardizing the relationship with the patient.

E.8. Socioeconomic measures

Sponsors should consider performing pharmaco-economic analyses in all OA clinical trials[29,30].

E.9. Use of concomitant medications
E.9.1. *Symptom modifying drugs*

It is impractical to expect patients to participate in a long-term trial without some potential for use of rescue medications for pain. For long-term trials, use of concomitant medication should be permitted on a limited basis. An example may be the use of acetaminophen (or paracetamol) for escape analgesia (up to 4 gm/day in the U.S. and up to 3 gm/day in Europe). Any escape medication must be discontinued in sufficient time for the clinical effects of the agent to disappear prior to the assessment. Protocol design should include a record of the consumption of analgesics, NSAIDs, and IA injections. However, the use of such information as an outcome in clinical trials has not been validated.

IA depocorticosteroids should not be permitted in studies of symptom modifying drugs, except as part of the protocol design.

E.9.2. *Structure modifying drugs*

Concomitant therapy may interfere with the evaluation of outcome measures and should ideally be excluded. However, in long-term studies, it is neither ethical nor practical to exclude all concomitant treatments. In all trials, concomitant therapies (drugs or other interventions) that are likely to affect joint structure should be excluded, and rescue therapy should be standardized, carefully recorded and monitored. As noted above, participants may use acetaminophen (or paracetamol) for escape analgesia (up to 4 g/day in the U.S. and up to 3 g/day in Europe). Analgesics and NSAIDs must be discontinued prior to the assessment in sufficient time for the clinical effects of the rescue medication to disappear.

The consumption of analgesics, NSAIDs, and IA injections should be documented at each visit. However, methods need to be developed to effectively control for these confounding variables in the analysis and the use of this information has not been validated as an outcome variable.

E.10. Concomitant non-medicinal therapy

Concomitant treatment with physical and/or occupational therapy should be either standardized or adjusted for in the analysis to ensure that the effects of exercise programs on disease progression do not bias the outcome of the study. Information on weight change (reduction or gain), changes in use of ambulatory support (cane, crutches, walker), and introduction of, or changes in, physical or occupational therapy during the study should be incorporated into the study design.

E.11. Laboratory tests

For most multicenter studies, routine laboratory tests (complete blood count, urinalysis, serum chemistry determinations) should be performed in a central laboratory.

Routine synovial fluid analyses should be performed at each site, and should include an examination for cells and crystals.

For studies routinely performing arthrocentesis with injection of an IA agent, culture of the synovial fluid should be performed as clinically indicated.

E.12. Adverse events

Adverse events should be ascertained in an open-ended manner, rather than by checklist. They should be recorded at each visit and between visits, as appropriate. The date of onset, severity, a judgment with respect to the relationship between the adverse event and the test agent, treatment and the duration and resolution of the adverse event should all be recorded.

Serious adverse events should be reported to regulatory authorities immediately.

E.13. Protocol violation

Reasons for termination of a subject from the study due to protocol violation must be specified in the protocol. Intake of rescue medications (other than those specifically prescribed), use of oral or topical agents, or devices targeted towards pain relief during the course of the study should be prohibited. Information on the use of such agents should be obtained at each visit and recorded, and the patient should be warned about such co-interventions. Patients in repeated violation of the protocol may need to be dropped from the study.

Screening for protocol violations by performing blood or urine analyses for blood for salicylates or related agents is not considered useful.

E.14. Case report forms and supplies

Investigators must maintain adequate records showing the receipt, dispensing, return, or other disposition of the investigational drug, including the date, quantity, batch or code number, and identification of subjects who received the study drug. Investigators must maintain completed case report forms and informative source documents. Case report forms must be kept in locked cabinets to maintain security. There are no special requirements for OA trials.

F. Outcome measures of OA

Instruments used to measure outcome in clinical trials of OA should be valid, reliable and responsive to change, when such measures exist. Clinical trials in OA should use published instruments that have been used in other studies, thus permitting comparison of results across trials of different therapeutic interventions. Clinical trials in OA should include a core set of validated measures[5] (Appendix II):

- Pain
- Physical function
- Patient global
- Imaging (for studies ≥ 1 year in duration)

Additional measures that are recommended include the following:

- Quality of life/utility (strongly recommended)
- Physician global

Optional measures for trials in OA include the following:

- Signs of inflammation
- Biologic markers
- Stiffness
- Performance based measures of function
- Presence of 'flares'
- Time to surgery
- Analgesic consumption

The items listed below pertain mostly to phase 3 trials. These measures should be recorded at baseline and serially at appropriate intervals.

F.1. Symptom modifying drugs

For studies of drugs designed to affect symptoms, the primary outcome variable should usually be joint pain reported by the patient. Measurement should be serially recorded at appropriate intervals, at least monthly. However, this is dependent upon the target joint and study design.

F.1.1. Pain

The degree of joint pain in the index joint(s) should be graded. Pain should be recorded on a five-point Likert scale (e.g., none, mild, moderate, severe, very severe) or on a 100 mm VAS. Single questions about pain can be used but the activity causing pain should be specified: e.g., weight bearing, resting, nocturnal, post exercise, stair climbing. Alternatively, a validated pain instrument can be used (e.g., WOMAC pain subscale[24]). Other pain indices include the Health Assessment Questionnaire (HAQ)[31] and Arthritis Impact Measurement Scale (AIMS)[32].

F.1.2. Function

The AFI[25] and the function subscale of the WOMAC[24] have been validated and are recommended for studies of OA of the hip and knee. Other indices which have been used include the HAQ disability index[28], and AIMS[33]. Disability indices specifically designed to measure hand function are under development[34,35].

F.1.3. Global status

F.1.3.a. Patient assessment of global status. The patient's assessment of his/her global status should be measured using a Likert or VAS scale. The optimal method by which this should be measured is not well established. However, a standard question should be asked, e.g., 'Considering all the ways your OA (joint site) affects you, how are you doing (time frame)?'

F.1.3.b. Physician assessment of global status. A measure of the physician assessment of global status may be required by some regulatory agencies. There is no generally accepted method for measurement of this variable. A question such as 'Considering all information, how is the patients OA [joint site] today?' should be used with a VAS or Likert scale.

F.1.4. Quality of life scales

Measurement of health-related quality of life and utility based measures at appropriate intervals is strongly recommended; although, these are not a part of the core set of measures. Examples of health related quality of life instruments include the Medical Outcomes Study, 36 question short form (SF-36)[36], Sickness Impact Profile (SIP)[37]. Nottingham Health

Profile (NHP)[38], and EuroQol[39]. Examples of utility instruments include the Time Trade Off, the Standard Gamble and Techniques and Feeling Thermometer and the Health Utilities Index (HUI)[40,41].

F.1.5. *Joint examination*

Measures of range of motion, intermalleolear distance, knee interbone distance, heel to buttock measurements, knee circumference, etc. have been validated to a variable degree[42]. The usefulness of these measures in clinical trials remains unclear and their inclusion is optional.

F.1.6. *Performance-based measures*

Performance-based measures which include such items as grip strength, time to walk a specified distance (e.g., 6 or 15 m, 50 ft), distance walked in a specified time (e.g., 6 min)., have been studied to a variable degree. Some composite measure exist[43]. The usefulness of these measures in clinical trials remains unclear and their inclusion is optional.

F.1.7. *Inflammation*

Clinimetric properties of methods designed to measure inflammation have not been well elucidated. The usefulness of these measures in clinical trials remains uncertain.

F.1.8. *Response criteria*

There is no definition of a minimum clinically important response for the above measures. Available information does not allow setting of predetermined limits for improvement. This is particularly true for the composite indices. At this time, the Task Force recommends that each protocol predefine a significant response, based upon statistically significant improvement in a carefully defined primary efficacy variable (see the Statistical section below). The Task Force does not recommend using an individual response criterion such as has been recommended in rheumatoid arthritis[44].

F.2. Structure modifying drugs

For studies of potential structure modifying drugs, the primary outcome variable should be a measure of joint morphology; e.g., imaging (see below) or direct visualization, i.e. arthroscopy. As stated above, time to joint replacement surgery is not recommended as a primary outcome variable due to its dependence on factors unrelated to disease progression. Clinical followup of patients participating in trials of structure modifying drugs should be at intervals of 3 months or less.

F.2.1. *Radiography*

The primary radiograhic evaluation should be of a single joint (knee, hip, hand). Outcome should assess the effect of the drug on joint structure. Although assessment should include both cartilage and bone, the primary radiographic outcome variable for studies of progression of the hip and knee should be minimum joint space width (JSW) since this measure is more sensitive than global scoring[45–49]. Osteophytes and other bone changes should be assessed as secondary outcome variables either by measurement or by grading, using published atlases[13–17]. In contrast, for studies of prevention, the primary radiographic outcome variables should include osteophytes, since this feature is most strongly associated with knee pain, is a basic component of the ACR classification criteria, and is the hallmark of the Kellgren-Lawrence scale of the knee. Outcome variables for hand OA should be based on published atlases agreed upon by the study group in advance.

Obtaining reproducible X-rays on successive visits is a prerequisite for reliable assessment of progression of OA. The sources of variability in joint space width measurement are numerous (patient positioning, radiographic procedure, measurement process, etc.). Protocols have been proposed for hip and knee joints[50–52]. It is essential to standardize radiographic technique based on published, validated data (Appendix III). The method should define the radioanatomic position of the joint, beam alignment, and, the anatomic landmarks for measurements. Positioning of the patient should also be based on validated published methods, but in all cases, weight bearing (standing) anteroposterior views should be used in studies involving the hip or knee. Repositioning of the joint can be facilitated by use of foot maps drawn at the time of the initial examination. Correction for radiographic magnification has been shown to improve accuracy and precision of measurements[53]. Techniques that improve the precision of measurements might lead to studies requiring smaller sample sizes.

Quality assurance should include: training sessions for technologists at the onset of the study as well as for any technologists recruited during the study. Radiographic quality, including patient positioning, exposure, labeling, etc., should be monitored throughout the study. Even minor changes in technique may significantly alter the precision of measures of joint anatomy and hence conclusions about treatment response. It is, therefore, critical that the technique be identical at all centers involved in a multi-institutional study and remain consistent throughout the study.

The number of readers, method of blinding and the method of manual measurement should be agreed upon in advance by the study group. Quality control of the readings should include an initial training session and periodic assessments of performance. Validated methods of computerized reading of digitized radiographs can decrease observer-based error. Enhanced anatomical detail provided by microfocal magnification radiography can further improve precision and accuracy of measurements[54].

F.2.2. Magnetic resonance imaging (MRI)

MRI is uniquely capable of visualizing all components of the joint simultaneously, and therefore offers an opportunity to assess the joint as an organ. MRI is capable of quantifying a number of morphological and compositional parameters of articular tissues relevant to OA. Recently developed techniques for non-invasively quantifying cartilage volume, thickness and water content, particularly in early disease, show promise as potential outcome measures for future therapeutic studies (Appendix IV). While some cross sectional measures have been validated, their performance in longitudinal studies has yet to be determined.

F.2.3. Other imaging modalities

Computed tomography, ultrasonography and scintigraphy have not been adequately validated and cannot be recommended for use in long-term studies.

F.2.4. Arthroscopy

Arthroscopy can directly visualize cartilage and other intraarticular structures, including fibrocartilagenous menisci, synovium, ligaments and chondrophytes. Attempts to quantify this information have followed two strategies. The first transforms information from each cartilage lesion into a numeric score, weighted mainly by depth and size of the lesion. When several lesions are found, as occurs frequently in OA, a composite score is derived from the scores of individual lesions. The second approach calls for the arthroscopist to globally assess cartilage degeneration in a compartment-by-compartment fashion, recording each impression on a VAS. Both strategies are being employed in the two systems currently under evaluation, with intra- and inter-observer reliability determined for both[55,56], and sensitivity to change (utilizing videotaped records from two points in time) has been shown for the French system[51].

Other systems yet to be devised may prove superior for assessment of particular aspects of OA, examining biomechanical characteristics of cartilage (which might be shown better by a probe) or features of the accompanying synovitis. The precision and sensitivity to change of any system employed in an OA outcomes trial should be determined by a study group before the system is implemented. Management of arthroscopic data by videotaping each procedure provides an immutable record that can be reviewed by a blinded evaluator. However, video records do not convey certain impressions obtained in real time, such as three-dimensional perception and tactile feedback from probing the cartilage. Regardless of the recording technique, a systematic uniform method of collecting arthroscopic data is essential, and should be specifically delineated in any protocol. Discussion of the technical aspects of the arthroscopic procedure is beyond the purview of this statement. However, the size and type of instrument used and conditions under which the procedure is performed should be uniform for all investigators in any particular study.

F.2.5. Molecular markers

Molecular markers have not been validated as outcome measures in clinical trials of OA (Appendix V). However, molecular markers have the potential of offering a unique way of assessing drug effects on specific disease mechanisms, and modes of action of drugs in phase 1 clinical trials[57–59]. The field is developing rapidly. For these reasons, trials should include collections of body fluid samples. Standardization of methods for collection and storage is important.

G. Statistical methods

There are specific statistical tasks in the design, implementation and analysis components of a clinical trial.

General textbooks cover a broad range of topics regarding clinical trial research[60,61].

G.1. Design

The predominant activity of the statistician is working with the researcher in developing the protocol. The protocol must clearly list the primary and secondary study objectives. Where appropriate, these objectives should be rephrased as null versus alternative hypothesis to be tested.

All protocols should specify the outcome measure(s) to be used for evaluating the study treatments and should contain sample size calculations for all primary outcomes, indicating the required number of patients to achieve prestated power and significance levels, or a calculation of the power provided with a prestated sample size. Sample size calculations are based on the choice of experimental design (e.g. parallel groups, factorial design, more than one treatment group vs control) and require that explicit assumptions be made regarding the variance(s) in outcomes among study subjects and the desired magnitude of change(s) in the outcome variable(s) during the study period; these assumptions should be stated explicitly in the protocol. Phase 3 studies should require a 5% or lesser level of significance and 80% or greater power to detect a protocol defined minimal clinically meaningful difference in the expected outcome between the treatment and control groups. These assumptions should, when possible, be based on available clinical/epidemiological data.

Randomization is a method for assigning patients to a test or control treatment that is free of selection bias. The method of randomization should be specified in the protocol. Two general designs exist for randomization of patients to treatments: fixed randomization and adaptive randomization. Fixed randomization schemes may be completely random or may be constrained so as to ensure balance in the number allocated to various treatment groups (randomization in blocks of fixed size, stratified random sampling). Randomization in blocks should be considered if patient enrollment is likely to continue over an extended period of time, or if the study population can be expected to change over the course of treatment. Stratification should be considered when patients are recruited from many sites. Adaptive randomization schemes should be considered when investigators require that balance be achieved on multiple factors.

G.2. Implementation

Statistical quality control procedures are essential to ensure the validity of the data collection and computer entry methods. Key data variables should be run through checking programs to ensure, at a minimum, that the data are within the permissible range of possible values, that missing data are flagged, that patients meet inclusion and exclusion criteria, and that patients data forms are obtained in a timely fashion, as per protocol. Double entry of all keyed data is preferred. A random sample of data coded on data entry forms should be checked against original sources (e.g. forms from laboratories and/or the medical record).

Once study eligibility is validated, subjects are enrolled (and possibly stratified on baseline factors), assigned a study identification and thereby randomized to treatment following the predetermined randomization plan.

G.3. Analysis

Generally, comparisons among treatment groups should be made as an 'intent-to-treat' analysis; that is, (1) patients should be counted in the treatment group to which they were randomly assigned, (2) the denominator for a treatment should be all patients assigned to that treatment, and (3) all events (whether believed to be related to the disease process under treatment or not) should be counted in the comparison(s) of primary interest.

An intent-to-treat analysis can lead to an underestimate of the true treatment effect, especially if compliance is low, there are many treatment crossovers, or the denominator includes many patients who could not be followed for the outcome of interest. Secondary analyses might then be carried out on completers (those staying on the program to study end), controlling for compliance levels. In general, analyses focused on an individual patient's longitudinal response, using composite (multidimensional) outcomes, should be encouraged. The outcome dimensions could include symptoms and/or structural measurements.

Some analytic methods used to compare treatments in trials are as follows:

G.3.1. Comparison of proportions

This method is valid provided that patients are subject to the same length of follow-up and the loss of follow-up is low, and occurs for the same reasons, across treatment groups. Statistical evaluation of the difference in proportions can be performed using Fishers' exact tests or chi-square test for larger samples. Examples include: proportion who are 'pain free', proportions experiencing serious adverse medical events. An example with respect to structure modifying drugs, might include proportions developing joint space narrowing.

G.3.2. *Lifetable analysis*

This approach provides a means of dealing with varying duration of follow-up to achieve the primary endpoint and for dealing with cases where the primary endpoint does not occur by the end of the study ('censored data'). Statistical comparisons of lifetable rates are often performed using a 'log rank' test. Examples include: time until pain resolves, time until normalization of a laboratory parameter.

G.3.3. *Comparison of means*

This method is valid subject to the same conditions required for comparing proportions (see above). Statistical evaluation of the difference in means can be performed using a two-sample *t*-test or the standard normal distribution for larger samples. Example: comparing average change in pain over the study period.

G.3.4. *Descriptive methods*

These are useful for assessing the baseline comparability of the treatment groups, and for secondary analyses assessing compliance issues. Descriptive statistics often include means, standard deviations, and percent of subjects in different strata (e.g. gender).

G.4. Adjustment procedures

To be valid, evaluation of treatment effects must be performed on treatment groups that are comparable with respect to their baseline characteristics. Statistical adjustment for one or more sources of variation is often performed by using regression models. Multiple linear regression models are used for quantitative outcomes, multiple logistic regression models are used for binary outcomes, and Cox proportional hazards models are used to adjust rates calculated from lifetables. These methods are especially useful if the randomization scheme failed or if randomization was not used in allocating patients to treatment groups.

G.5. Interim analysis

The concept of interim analysis is that patients assigned to the inferior treatment should be removed from it as soon as the choice is clear. These methods provide statistically valid *P*-values by accounting for the multiple looks at the outcome data during the study period. The scheme for interim analyses should suit the particular trial. The procedure of O'Brien and Fleming is one statistically valid method for adjusting the *P*-value.

G.6. Repeated measures analyses

These methods are useful for quantifying the trend and tempo of outcomes repeatedly assessed during the course of a trial and during the extended follow-up period. Statistical evaluation of the difference in summary statistics (e.g. trend, or slope) can be performed using the analysis of variance for repeated measures. Comparisons across treatment groups are valid provided that patients are followed for the same length of time and there is no differential loss to follow-up.

H. *Summary*

H.1. Symptom modifying drugs

The primary outcome variable is a specific aspect of joint pain, although a 'signal' symptom or some measure of function may also be studied. Trials of drugs with a rapid onset of effect can be as short as 1–4 weeks but may be as long as 12 weeks, with evaluations performed weekly. Longer trials (up to 2 years) may be needed to evaluate longer-term toxicity, determine optimal long term dosing regimes, or establish long-term benefit. Supplemental escape analgesia should be minimized, monitored and discontinued prior to evaluation of efficacy.

Some agents that provide symptom relief may not provide benefits until weeks after initiation of therapy. Under these circumstances, trials will vary from 3–12 months in length. If the agent is administered in courses, episodic readministration of the drug may be needed in long-term trials. Longer trials (up to 2 years) may be required to exclude toxicity or establish long-term benefit.

H.2. Structure modifying drugs

These drugs are intended to prevent, retard, stabilize or reverse development of the morphologic changes of OA. Although this has been called 'chondroprotection,' the term is misleading and should be avoided because all structures of the joint are involved in OA, not articular cartilage alone. The benefits of disease modifying therapy may not be apparent until years after the onset of treatment. The selection of high-risk groups may shorten the time of investigation. Improvement in symptoms (i.e., joint pain) is not a requisite for the efficacy of a drug in this category. In these studies, it may be necessary to permit concomitant use of drugs for relief of symptoms (NSAIDs, analgesics). The confounding effects of glucocorticoids and NSAIDs in these trials is not yet understood and very restricted use of IA steroids is recommended.

Demonstrations of structure modification will require the use of direct measures of joint anatomy, such as radiography, particularly measurement of the radiographic joint space. As stated above, the plain radiograph is presently the most reproducible and readily available method for assessment of disease modification. Studies are needed to validate surrogate markers of disease activity, since they may help shorten phase 2 structure modifying drug trials. As an alternative to radiography, some trials may utilize arthroscopy.

As we approach the beginning of the twenty first century, concepts of clinical trials of OA drugs is changing. Methodology and techniques for the evaluation of new agents for OA have been refined dramatically over the last decade. We look forward to the future with excitement as we anticipate the development of new agents that may alter the symptoms and course of OA. The above recommendations are intended to help us ascertain which of these new agents are effective.

Acknowledgements

The Osteoarthritis Research Society would like to acknowledge the tireless and efficient work of our Executive Secretary, Evie Altman Orbach, in organizing the Task Force meetings and the Workshop. We wish to recognize the cooperation and participation of the International League Of Associations For Rheumatologists (ILAR) and the American College Rheumatology. We wish to also recognize the participation and support of the European Group for the Respect of Ethics and Excellence in Science (GREES) and our industrial partners.

References

1. Lequesne M., Brandt K., Bellamy N., *et al.* Guidelines for testing slow acting drugs in osteoarthritis: J Rheumatol 1994;21Suppl 41:65–71.
2. Kuettner K., Goldberg V., editors. Osteoarthritic Disorders. Rosemont: American Academy of Orthopedic Surgeons, 1995.
3. Furst D. Guiding Principles for the development of drugs for osteoarthritis, 1995.
4. Group for the Respect of Ethics and Excellence in Science (GREES: osteoarthritis Section). Recommendations for the registration of drugs used in the treatment of osteoarthritis. Ann Rheum Dis 1996;55:552–7.
5. Bellamy N., Kirwan, J., Boers M., Brooks P., Strand V., Tugwell P., *et al.* Recommendations for a core set of outcome measures for future phase III clinical trials in knee, hip, and hand osteoarthritis: consensus development at OMERACT III. J Rheumatol 1996.
6. Altman R.D., Hochberg M.C.: Degenerative joint disease, Clin Rheum Dis 1983;9:681–93.
7. Rataiu J.S., Hochberg M.C. Clinical trials: a guide to understanding methodology and interpreting results. Arthritis Rheum 1990;33:131–9.
8. FDA Document #77-3040. General considerations for the clinical evaluation of drugs. CDER Executive secretarial staff, HFD-8, FDA (Center for Drug Evaluation and Research, 5400 Fisher's lane, Rockville, MD 20857.
9. FDA Document: Guidelines for industry. The extent of population exposure to assess clinical safety: for drugs intended for long term treatment of non-life-threatening conditions, ICH-EIA, March 1995; Federal Register March 1, 1995 (60FR11270).
10. Altman R.D., Asch E., Bloch D., Bole G., Borenstein D., *et al.* Development of Criteria for the Classification and Reporting of Osteoarthritis: Classification of Osteoarthritis of the Knee. Arthritis Rheum 1986;29:1039–49.
11. ACR Subcommittee on Classification Criteria of Osteoarthritis — Altman R.D., Chairman: The American College of Rheumatology Criteria for the Classification and Reporting of Osteoarthritis of the Hand. Arthritis Rheum 33:1990;1601–10.
12. ACR Subcommittee on Classification Criteria of Osteoarthritis — Altman R.D., Chairman: The American College of Rheumatology Criteria for the Classification and Reporting of Osteoarthritis of the Hip. Arthritis Rheum 1991;34:505–14.
13. Kellgren J.H., Lawrence J.S. Radiological assessment of osteoarthritis. Ann Rheum Dis 1957;16:494–501.
14. Kellgren J.H. The Epidemiology of chronic rheumatism. Atlas of standard radiographs of arthritis, 2nd edn. Philadelphia. F.A. Davis Co. 1963:1–13.

15. Burnett S., Hart D.J., Cooper C., and Spector T.D. A radiographic atlas of osteoarthritis. London. Springer Verlag 1994.

16. Kalman D.A., Wigley F.M., Scott W.W., *et al.* New radiographic grading scales of osteoarthritis of the hand. Arthritis Rheum 1989;32:1584–91.

17. Altman R.D., Hochberg M., Murphy W.A., *et al.* Atlas of individual radiographic features in osteoarthritis. Osteoarthritis Cart 1995;3:3–70.

18. Spector T.D., Hart D.J., Doyle D.V. Incidence and progression of osteoarthritis in women with unilateral knee disease in the general population: the effect of obesity. Ann Rheum Dis 1994;53:565–8.

19. Neyret P., Donell S.T., DeJour D., De Jour H. Partial miniscectomy and anterior cruciate ligament rupture in soccer players: a study with a minimum 20-yr followup. Am J Sports Med 1993;21:455–60.

20. Roos H., Lindberg H., Gardsell P., Lohmander L.S., Wingstrand H. The prevalence of gonarthrosis and its relation to meniscectomy in former soccer players. Am J Sports Med. 1994;22:219–22.

21. Croft P., Cooper C., Wickham C., Coggon D. Defining osteoarthritis of the hip for epidemiologic studies. Am J Epidemiol 1990;132:514.

22. Hochberg M.C., Lane N.E., Pressman A.R., Genant H.K., Scott J.C., Nevitt M.C. The association of radiographic changes of osteoarthritis of the hand and hip in elderly women. J. Rheumatol 1995;22:2291–4.

23. Sharif M., George E., Shepstone, L., *et al.* Serum hyaluronic acid level as a predictor of disease progression in osteoarthritis of the knee. Arthritis Rheum 1995;38:760–7.

24. Sharif M., Saxne T., Shepstone L., *et al.* Relationship between serum cartilage oligomeric matrix protein level and disease progression in osteoarthritis of the knee joint. Br J Rheumatol 1995;34:306–10.

25. Bellamy N., Buchanan W.W., Goldsmith C.H., Campbell, Stitt L.W. Validation of WOMAC: a health status instrument for measuring clinically important patient relevant outcomes to antirheumatic drug therapy in patients with osteoarthritis of the hip or knee. J Rheumatol 1988;15:1833–40.

26. Lequesne M., Meezy C., Samson M., *et al.* Indices of severity for osteoarthritis of the hip and knee. Scand J Rheumatol 1987; Suppl 65:85–9.

27. U.S. Food and Drug Administration Regulations 21 CFR Parts 50.20–50.27.

28. Haynes R.B., Dantes R. Patient compliance and the conduct and interpretation of therapeutic trials. Controlled Clin Trials 1987;8:12–29.

29. Drummond M.F. Principles of economic appraisal in health care. Oxford: Oxford University Press, 1980.

30. Ehrlich G.E. Treatment decisions, side-effect liability and cost-effectiveness in osteoarthritis. Inflammopharmacology 1996;4:137–40.

31. Fries J.F., Spitz P., Kraines R.G., Holman J.H. Measurement of patient outcome in arthritis. Arthritis Rheum 1980;23:137–45.

32. Meenan R.F., Gurtman P.M., Mason J.H. Measuring health status in arthritis: the Arthritis Impact Measurement Scales. Arthritis Rheum 1980;23:146–54.

33. Mason J.H., Anderson J.J., Meenan R.F. Application of a health status model to osteoarthritis. Arthritis Care Res 1989;2:89–93.

34. Treves R., Maheu E., and Dreiser R-L. Therapeutic trials in digital osteoarthritis. A critical review. Revue Rheumatisme Engl edition 1994;626 Suppl 1:33S–41S.

35. Bellamy N., Haraoui B., Buckbinder R., *et al.* Development of a disease-specific health status measure for hand osteoarthritis clinical trials. 1. Assessment of the symptom dimensionality. Scand J Rheumatol 1996;Suppl 106:5.

36. Ware J.E. Jr., Sherborune C.D. The MOS 36-item short-form health survey (SF36): I. Conceptual framework and item selection. Med Care 1992;30:473–83.

37. Bergner M., Bobbitt R.A., Carter W.B., Gilson B.S. The Sickness Impact Profile: development and final revision of a health status measure. Med Care 1981;19:778–805.

38. Hunt S., McEwan P. The development of a subjective health indicator. Social Health Illness 1980;2:231–46.

39. Euroqol Group: Euroqol: A new facility for the measurement of health related quality of life. Health Policy 1990;16:199–208.

40. Torrance G.W. Social preferences for health status. An empirical evaluation of the measurement techniques. Socio-economic Planning Sciences 1976;10:128–36.

41. Feeny D., Furlong W., Barr R.D., *et al.* A comprehensive multiattribute system for classifying the health status of survivors of childhood cancer. J Clin Oncol 1992;10:923–8.

42. Theiler R., Stucki G., Schutz R., Hofer H., Seifert B., Tyndall A., Michel B.A. Parametric and non-parametric measures in the assessment of knee and hip osteoarthritis: interobserver reliability and correlation with radiology. Osteoarthritis Cart 1994;2:1–24.

43. Rejeski W.J., Ettinger W.H. Jr., Schumacker S., *et al.* Assessing performance related disability in patients with knee osteoarthritis. Osteoarthritis Cart 1995;3:157–68.

44. Felson D.T., Anderson J.J., Boers M., Bombardier C., Furst D., Goldsmith C., *et al.* American College of Rheumatology Preliminary definition of improvement in rheumatoid arthritis. Arthritis Rheum 1995;38:727–35.

45. Hochberg M.C. Quantitative radiography: osteoarthritis — analysis. Bailliere's Clin Rheum 1996;10:In Press.

46. Dougados M., Villers C., Amor B. Sensitivity to change of various roentgenological severity scoring systems for osteoarthritis of the hip. Rev Rhum 1995;[Engl Ed]62:169–84.

47. Lequesne M. Chondrometry quantitative evaluation of joint space width and rate of joint space loss in osteoarthritis of the hip. Rev Rhum 1995;[Engl Ed]62:155–8.

48. Buckland-Wright J.C., Macfarlane D.G., Williams S.A., Ward R.J. Accuracy and precision of joint space width measurements in standard and macroradiographs of osteoarthritic knees. Ann Rheum Dis 1995;54:872–80.

49. Ravaud P., Giraudeau B., Auleley G.R., *et al.* Radiographic assessment of knee osteoarthritis: reproducibility and sensitivity to change. J Rheumatol 1996;35:761–6.

50. Dieppe P., Altman R., Buckwalter J., *et al.* Standardization of methods used to assess the progres-

sion of osteoarthritis of hip and knee. In: New Horizons in Osteoarthritis, Kuettner K. and Goldberg V., eds. Rosemont: American Academy of Orthopedic Surgeons 1995;481–96.

51. Buckland-Wright C. Protocols for precise radio-anatomical positioning of the tibiofemoral and patellofemoral compartments of the knee. Osteoarthritis Cart 1995;3(Suppl A):71–80.

52. Ravaud P., Auleley G.R., Chastang C., *et al.* An experimental study of the influence of radiographic procedure and joint positioning on knee joint space width measurement. Br J Rheumatol 1996;35:761–766.

53. Mazzuca S., Brandt K.D., Katz B. Is conventional radiography suitable for evaluation of a disease-modifying drug in patients with knee osteoarthritis. Osteoarthritis Cart 1997;5,217–226.

54. Buckland-Wright J.C., Macfarlane D.G. Radio-anatomic assessment of therapeutic outcome in osteoarthritis. In: Kuettner K.E., Goldberg V.M., eds. Osteoarthritic Disorders, Rosement: American Academy of Orthopedic Surgeons, 1995, pp. 51–65.

55. Klashman D., Ike R., Moreland L., Skovron M.L., Kalunian K. Validation of an osteoarthritis data report form for knee arthroscopy. Arthritis Rheum 1995;38(suppl 9):S178.

56. Ayral X., Dougados M., Listrat, Bonvarlet J-P, Simonnet J., Amor B. Arthroscopic evaluation of chondropathy in osteoarthritis of the knee. J Rheumatol 1996;23:698–706.

57. Poole A.R. Immunochemical markers of joint inflammation, skeletal damage and repair; where are we now? Ann Rheum Dis 1994;53:3–5.

58. Lohmander L.S. Articular cartilage and osteoarthrosis — the role of molecular markers to monitor breakdown, repair and disease. J Anat 1994;184:477–92.

59. Lark M.W., Bayne E.K., Lohmander L.S. Aggrecan degradation in osteoarthritis and rheumatoid arthritis. Acta Orthop Scand 1995;66 Suppl 266:92–7.

60. Hully S.B., Cummings S.R. Designing Clinical Research Baltimore, Williams and Wilkins, 1988.

61. Meinert C.L. Clinical Trials, New York: Oxford University Press, 1986.

Appendix I

Workshop participants

Code

[1] Organizing chairperson
[2] Plenary session chairperson
[3] Speaker
[4] Chairperson — Breakout Session
[5] Co-chairperson — Breakout Session
[6] Scribe — Breakout Session

Roy Altman, Miami, FL, U.S.A. [2, 3]
Marliese Annefeld, Monza, Italy

Roberto Arinoviche, Santiago, Chile
Bernard Avouac, Creteil, France
Xavier Ayral, Paris, France [3, 5]
Nicholas Bellamy, London, ON, Canada [3, 4]
Daniel Bloch, Palo Alto, CA, U.S.A. [4]
Kenneth Brandt, Indianapolis, IN, U.S.A. [5]
Peter Brooks, Sydney, Australia [3]
J.C. Buckland-Wright, London, U.K. [3, 4]
Roland Chang, Chicago, IL, U.S.A.
Xavier Chevalier, Creteil, France
Cyrus Cooper, Southampton, U.K. [6]
Philipe Coste. Cpurbevoie, France
L. Crasborn., Brussels, Belgium
J.P. Devogelaer, Brussels, Belgium
Paul Dieppe, Bristol, U.K. [5]
Maxime Dougados, Paris, France [3]
Elliot Ehrich, Chatham, NJ, U.S.A.
George Ehrlich, Philadelphia, PA, U.S.A. [6]
Dominique Ethgen, Staines, U.K.
Walter Ettinger, Winston-Salem, NC, U.S.A. [6]
Yoshimasa Fujita, Tokyo, Japan
Daniel Furst, Seattle, WA, U.S.A. [3]
Peter Ghosh, Sydney, Australia
Klaus Peter Guenther, Ulm, Germany
George Bernard Guillou, Courbevoie, France
Laurie Hall, Cambridge, U.K.
Paul Haraoui, Monteal, PQ, Canada
Yves Henrotin, Liege, Belgium
Rosemarie Hirsch, Bethesda, MD, U.S.A.
March Hochberg, Baltimore, MD, U.S.A. [1, 2, 5]
Zeb Horowitz, Cincinnati, OH, U.S.A. [5]
Robert Ike, Ann Arbor, MI, U.S.A. [4]
T. Ishihara, Tokyo, Japan
Sergio Jimenez, Philadelphia, PA, U.S.A.
Kent Johnson, Bethesda, MD, U.S.A.
E.A. Jones, Amsterdam-Zuidoost, Netherlands
Joanne Jordan, Chapel Hill, NC, U.S.A.
Ken Kalunian, Los Angeles, CA, U.S.A.
Linda Katz, Rockville, MD, U.S.A. [4]
Seiichi Kobayashi, Ibaraki, Japan
Nancy Lane, San Francisco, CA, U.S.A.
Michael R.G. Leeming, Sandwich, U.K.
Richard Leff, West Haven, CT, U.S.A.
Arleette Lepot, Boulogne, France
Michel Lequesne, Paris, France [3]
Bruce Littman, Groton, CT, U.S.A.
Stefan Lohmander, Lund, Sweden [2, 4]
Leland Loose, Groton, CT, U.S.A.
Carlos Lozada, Miami, FL, U.S.A.
Ron Magolda, Wilmington, DE, U.S.A.
Emmanuel Maheu, Paris, France
Henry Mankin, Boston, MA, U.S.A.

Joe Markenson, New York, NY, U.S.A.
Joel Menkes, Paris, France [4]
Joan Meyer, Cincinnati, OH, U.S.A.
Christopher Mojcik, West Haven, CT, U.S.A.
Roland Moskowitz, Cleveland, OH, U.S.A.
Richard Newmark, Summit, NJ, U.S.A.
Pat O'Brien, Woburn, MA, U.S.A.
Michael O'Regan, Brindisi, Italy
Laurence Paolozzi, Paris, France
J.P. Pelletier, Montreal, PQ, Canada [2, 4]
Charles Peterfy, San Francisco, CA, U.S.A. [6]
Stanley Pillemer, Bethesda, MD, U.S.A.
Bernard Prigent, Kirkland, PQ, Canada
Ruth Raiss, Wiesbaden, Germany
Philippe Ravaud, Paris, France
J.Y. Reginster, Liege, Belgium [2]
Charles Rivest, Montreal, PQ, Canada
Harald Roos, Helsingborg, Sweden [6]
Teresa Rosario-Jansen, Cincinnati, OH, U.S.A. [5]
Lucio Rovati, Monza, Italy
Alan Rubinow, Jerusalem, Israel
Eric Sauvage, Courbevoie, France
Thomas Schnitzer, Chicago, IL, U.S.A. [5]
Benjamin Schwartz, St. Louis, MO, U.S.A. [6]
William Scott, Baltimore, MD, U.S.A. [5]
Umberto Serni, Florence, Italy
Vibeke Strand, San Francisco, CA, U.S.A.
Takashi Sugiyama, Tokyo, Japan
Eugene Thonar, Chicago, IL, U.S.A. [6]
J. Carter Thorne, Newmarket, OH, Canada
Stephen Trippel, Boston, MA, U.S.A. [6]
Y. Tsouderos, Courbevoie, France
Peter Tugwell, Ottowa, ON, Canada
Jenny Tyler, Cambridge, U.K.
Robert Vender, Wilmington, DE, U.S.A.
Gust Verbruggen, Ghent, Belgium [5]
Koju Watanabe, Tokyo, Japan
Michael Weisman, San Diego, CA, U.S.A.
Fred Wolfe, Wichita, KS, U.S.A.

Appendix II

Clinical assessment techniques

Nicholas Bellamy

Core set measures

The core set of outcome measures for OA clinical trials developed at OMERACT III, contain three clinical measures: pain, physical function and patient global assessment with imaging for studies of 1 year or longer[1].

Pain

Pain is usually measured on a rating scale (Likert or VAS) which grades perceived pain severity in one or several situations (e.g., nocturnal, stair climbing, walking, rest, global)[2]. The pain subscale of the WOMAC OA Index has been validated for use in patients with hip and/or knee OA[3–6]. WOMAC is available in both Likert and 10 cm VA scaled formats and in a large number of alternate language translations. Although not recommended for use as a distinct pain scale, the AFI have been validated for use in hip and knee studies where the goal is to provide a weighted clinical severity score in which scores for pain/discomfort, stiffness, maximum distance walked and activities of daily living are summated into a single value[7,8]. A similar approach can be used with the WOMAC in situations where a composite score (based on pain, stiffness and physical function) is required, using weights derived from the Patient Assessment of the Relative Importance of Symptoms (PARIS) Sectogram[6]. The Health Assessment Questionnaire (HAQ)[9] pain scale or the AMIS[10!] or AIMS2[11] may be of limited value for studies focusing on a single joint, because they are appropriated for studies measuring pain severity in both the upper and lower extremities. Options for OA hand studies are limited but early experience with the pain subscale of an instrument termed the Australian/Canadian (AUSCAN) Osteoarthritis Hand Index has been favorable[12].

Physical function

Physical function/disability is usually measured on a rating scale (Likert, VA) which grades the perceived severity or degree of disability in one or more activities of daily living (e.g., stair climbing, walking, etc)[13]. The physical function subscale of the WOMAC index has been validated for use in patients with hip and/or knee OA[3]. The index is available in both Likert and 10 cm VA scaled formats and in a large number of alternate language translations. Although not recommended as a distinct physical function scale, the Algofunctional indices have been validated for use in hip and knee studies, where the goal is to provide a weighted clinical severity score in which scores for pain/discomfort, stiffness, maximum distance walked and activities of daily living are summated into a single score[7,8]. A similar approach can be used with the WOMAC by weighting and aggregating the pain, stiffness and physical function subscale using PARIS Sectogram weights[6]. An AFI developed by Dreiser and colleagues contains 10 questions directed at functional disability in the hand[14]. Early experience with the function subscale of the AUSCAN Osteoarthritis Hand Index has been favorable[12]. In studies and measuring physical disability in both the upper and lower extremities, the physical function subscale of the HAQ[9] or AIMS[10] (or AIMS2)[11] instruments is appropriate.

Patient global assessment

The patient's perception of the clinical severity of their OA is usually assessed by a direct question, e.g., 'Considering all the ways your OA affects you, how would you rate your condition today?' Suitable response scales could include the following: Likert — very poor, poor, fair, good, very good; or 10 cm horizontal VAS anchored to very poor (left hand end) and very good (right hand end). Alternatively, or in addition, at the end of the study a change in score could be derived using a similar question, e.g., 'Considering all the ways your OA has affected you, how do you feel now compared with the beginning of the study?' Responses could be made on Likert scale, e.g., 'much better', 'better', 'no change', 'worse', 'much worse'. There is currently no standard question and no standard response format[15]. It should be noted that depending on the research hypothesis, there are several ways of phrasing the global question, e.g., musculoskeletal condition, OA in the study knee, overall health, etc. Investigators should be guided by questions and response formats that have been used successfully in past studies or should develop and validate new standardized questions.

Non-core set measures

Health related quality of life (HRQOL) and utility (UT) measures

HRQOL and/or UT measures are increasingly being considered as very important components of the measurement battery for studies of 6 months or longer. They not only allow measurement of the patient's quality of life or the utility of their health state, but also facilitate pharmacoeconomic and cross-disease comparisons of outcome. There is relatively little experience to date with these instruments (e.g., SF-36[16], EuroQol[17], Nottingham Health Profile[18], Health Utilities Index[19], Standard Gamble[20], Time Trade Off[21], Category Scaling[22] in OA trials. However, because of their potential importance, use of HRQOL and/or UT measures is highly recommended in Phase 3 trials of six months or longer. It is expected that there will be improvement in our knowledge of the performance of one or more of these instruments, their role in Phase 3 clinical trials and the relative impact that interventions have on different measures will evolve over the next few years. Comparing different measures in the same trial would be particularly useful.

Physician global assessment

The physician's perception of his or her patient's OA can be based on a number of different variables, e.g., symptoms, signs, imaging, and, possibly, in the future, biologic markers. It is important to specify in the question or in accompanying instructions which variables should be considered in making the assessment. Usually, this will be based on symptoms, and since the clinical encounter will likely be quite brief, the question should be phrased with respect to the day of assessment, e.g., 'Considering all the ways OA affects your patient, how would you rate his or her condition today?' Suitable response scales could include the following: Likert — very poor, poor, fair, good, very good; or 10 cm horizontal VAS anchored to very poor (left hand end) and very good (right hand end). Alternatively, or, in addition, at end of study a change score can be derived using a similar question, e.g., 'Considering all the ways OA has affected your patient, how do you rate their condition now compared with the beginning of the study?' Responses could be made on a Likert scale, e.g., much better, better no change, worse, much worse. There is currently no standard question and no standard response format[15]. Investigators should be guided by questions and response formats that have been used successfully in past studies or should develop and validate new standardized questions. It should be noted that depending on the research hypothesis, there are several ways of phrasing the global question, e.g., musculoskeletal condition, OA in study knee, overall health, etc.

Performance-based measures

Many performance based measures are available, some of which are of demonstrated reliability, validity and responsiveness[15,23]. Although providing numerical estimates of performance, the clinical consequence to individual patients of any change for the better or worse on such measures lacks clarity. As a consequence, while sometimes useful in certain types of studies, they are not included in the core set. Measures that have been employed include: walking distance, walk time, grip strength[23]. It is important with these measures to use standard techniques and to train assessors to acceptable levels of inter-observer reliability[15].

Examination based measures

The clinical examination provides an opportunity to detect swelling (bony, soft tissue, effusion), crepitus, heat, range of movement, deformity, ligamentous laxity, range of movement (goniometer, plurimeter, intermalleolar straddle, intercondylar distance, heel to buttock test)[15,23]. These assessments require standard methods applied by trained assessors[15]. In general, as with performance-based measures, changes for the better or worse occurring on these examination-based measures lack defined levels of clinical importance to individual patients. They may be useful in some types of study but are not in the core set.

Miscellaneous

'Stiffness' is a sense of resistance or decreased ease during active movement of the joint. Some, but not all, patients have difficulty differentiating between pain and stiffness. When stiffness is measured in clinical trials, it is preferable to use the WOMAC[3-6] or AFI[7,8] (depending on whether a segregated or aggregated stiffness score is required) for hip and knee studies. The assessment of stiffness may be useful in some types of studies but has not been validated as an outcome in OA and is not in the core set.

'Inflammation' has not been extensively studied in OA clinical trials. As a result, the validity, reliability and responsiveness of inflammatory-based measures remain in doubt. They may be useful in some types of study but are not validated in OA and are not in the core set.

'Number of "Flares"' and the occurrence of disease 'flares' in OA lacks precise definition and as a result is difficult to reliably identify. This variable has not been included in the core set.

'Time to surgery' is influenced by a large number of factors, independent of the study intervention, e.g., the dynamics of scheduling operating time. Although this variable may be useful in some studies it has not been validated as an outcome in OA and is not included in the core set.

'Analgesic consumption' is an important source of cointervention; however, the precision with which analgesic consumption can be monitored, particularly in long-term studies, is suboptimal.

Response criteria

Response criteria may apply to groups of patients or individuals. The definition of a minimum clinically important difference between two groups of patients exposed to different interventions, depends on a number of factors relating to patient characteristics, disease features, the nature of the interventions, and the primary outcome measures selected. It is difficult to determine estimates of minimum clinically important differences for OA clinical studies[15]. At the present time there are no standard criteria for defining the success, or failure, of treatment in individual OA patients in a clinical trial.

Summary

The core set of outcome measures for OA clinical trials requires measurement of pain, physical function, patient global assessment, and imaging procedures for studies of one year or longer. Depending on the research hypothesis, one of several existing validated measures can be selected for evaluating change in each of the four domains.

References

1. Bellamy N., Kirwan J., Bores M. *et al.* Recommendations for a core set of outcome measures for future phase III clinical trials in knee, hip and hand, osteoarthritis. Consensus development at OMERACT III. J Rheumatol 1996;24:799–802.
2. Bellamy N. Pain measurement. In: Musculoskeletal Clinical Metrology. Dordrecht: Kluwer Academic Publishers, 1993:65–76.
3. Bellamy, N. Osteoarthritis — An evaluation index for clinical trials. MSc Thesis, McMaster University, Hamilton, Canada. 1982.
4. Bellamy N., Buchanan W.W., Goldsmith C.H., Campbell J., Stitt L.W. Validation study of WOMAC: a health status instrument for measuring clinically important patient-relevant outcomes to antirheumatic drug therapy in patients with osteoarthritis of the hip or knee. J Rheumatol 1988;15:1833–40.
5. Bellamy N., Campbell J., Buchanan W.W., Goldsmith C.H., Stitt L.W. Validation study of WOMAC: a health status instrument for measuring clinically-important patient-relevant outcomes following total or knee

arthroplasty in osteoarthritis. J Orthopaed Rheumatol 1988;1:95–108.

6. Bellamy N. WOMAC Osteoarthritis Index — A User's Guide. London: London Health Science Centre, 1996.

7. Lequesne M., Mery C., Samson M., Gerard P. Indexes of severity for osteoarthritis of the hip and knee: validation-value in comparison with other assessment tests. Scandinavian J Rheumatol 1987;Suppl 65:85–9.

8. Lequesne M. Indices of severity and disease activity for osteoarthritis. Semin Arthritis Rheum 1991;20:48–54.

9. Fries J.F., Spitz P., Kraines R.G., Holman H.R. Measurement of patient outcome in arthritis. Arthritis Rheum 1980;23:137–45.

10. Meenan R.F., Gurtman P.M., Mason J.H. Measuring health status in arthritis: the Arthritis Impact Measurement Scales. Arthritis Rheum 1980;23:146–52.

11. Meenan R.F., Mason J.H., Anderson J.J., Guccione A.A., Kazis L.E. AIMS2. The content and properties of a revised and expanded Arthritis Impact Measurement Scales Health Status Questionnaire. Arthritis Rheum 1992;35:1–10.

12. Bellamy N., Haraoui B., Buchbinder R., *et al.* Development of a disease-specific health status measure for hand osteoarthritis clinical trials. I. Assessment of symptom dimensionality. [Abstract] Scand J Rheumatol 1996;Suppl 106:5.

13. Bellamy N. Health status instruments and functional indices. Musculoskeletal Clinical Metrology. Dordrecht: Kluwer Academic Publishers, 1993:77–101.

14. Dreiser R.L., Maheu E., Guillou G.B., Caspard J., Grouin J.M. Validation of an algofunctional index for osteoarthritis of the hand. Revue du rhumatisme 1995;(English edn)Suppl 1:43S 53S.

15. Bellamy N. Standardized procedures for outcome measurement and parameters for calculating sample size for antirheumatic-drug studies. In Musculoskeletal Clinical Metrology. Dordrecht: Kluwer Academic Publishers, 1993:193–251.

16. Ware J.E., Sherborune C.D. The MOS 36-item Short-Form Health Status Survey (SF-36): I. Conceptual framework and item selection. Medical Care 1992;30:473–83.

17. Economic and Health Outcome Research Group: Jobanputra P., Hunter M., *et al.* Validity of Euroqol — a generic health status instrument in patients with rheumatoid arthritis. Br J Rheumatol 1994;33:655–62.

18. The European Group for Quality of Life and Health Measurement. European Guide to the Nottingham Health Profile, 1992.

19. Feeny D., Furlong W., Barr R.D., *et al.* A comprehensive multiattribute system for classifying the health status of survivors of childhood cancer. J Clin Oncol 1992;10:923–8.

20. Von Neumann J., Morgenstern O. Theory of games and economic behaviour. Princeton NJ: Princeton University Press; 1953.

21. Torrance G.W., Thomas W.H., Sackett D.L. A utility maximization model for evaluation of health care programs. Health Services Research. 1972;7:118–33.

22. Torrance G.W. Social preferences for health states: an empirical evaluation of three measurement techniques. Socioeconomic Planning Sciences. 1976:10(3):128–36.

23. Bellamy N. Mechanical and electromechanical devices. In Musculoskeletal Clinical Metrology. Dordrecht: Kluwer Academic Publishers, 1993:117–34.

Appendix III

Radiographic imaging techniques

J. Christopher Buckland-Wright, William W. Scott Jr, Charles Peterfy

The reproducibility of the radiographic technique is dependent on control of a number of technical issues. The discussion below presents a few methods that attempt to standardize many of the relevant techniques. Such standardization is essential in order to reliably assess sequential changes in joint anatomy. The most consistent results will be obtained by carefully adhering to standardized radiographic procedures, based on published, validated data. Quality control of personnel and procedures is essential for multicenter or comparative studies. The methods described below require no special facilities other than fluoroscopy.

Hip joint

Patient position

Anteroposterior radiographs are obtained with the patient standing. Weight bearing compresses the joint space to its most narrow configuration[1,2]. The feet are positioned in internal rotation with the toes subtending an angle of $15 \pm 5°$[3]. A foot map, used to facilitate repositioning at successive visits may improve measurement reproducibility. However, a foot map alone does not assure identical repositioning as the body can torque about the knee. Reproducibility requires multipoint control.

X-ray beam alignment

With a focus to film distance of 100 cm, the X-ray beam must be horizontal and perpendicular to the film. When the X-ray beam is centered on the superior aspect of the symphysis pubis to radiograph both hips together. There is less accuracy and precision in the joint space width measurement than when the central ray of the x-ray beam is aligned with the center of each femoral head[3,4,5].

Radiographic magnification

In view of the variable distance between hip joint and film among individuals, variable radiographic magnification can occur. A metal sphere of known size (5 mm), mounted in a semi-radiolucent material and taped to the skin over the greater trochanter can be used to correct for radiographic magnification at the joint. This is needed only if significant weight change has occurred between visits to alter this distance. An increase in the number of study patients may be needed without correction for radiographic magnification.

Knee joint: tibio-femoral compartment

Standing fully extended view[6-9]

Patient position

Separate antero-posterior radiographs of each knee are obtained with the patient standing and the weight equally distributed to both feet. The knee must be in full extension, with the back of the knee as near as possible to the vertical cassette. With the aid of fluoroscopy, the lower limb is rotated so that the tibial spines appear centrally placed relative to the femoral notch. A foot map may be used to facilitate repositioning at successive visits.

X-ray beam alignment

The central ray of the X-ray beam is centered on the joint space and inclined downward to ensure that the medial tibial plateau is parallel to the X-ray beam.

Correction for radiographic magnification

It is only necessary to correct for radiographic magnification if the distance between the back of the knee and the vertical cassette is altered in subsequent examinations (see above).

Standing partially flexed view[3,10,11]

Patient position

Separate antero-posterior radiographs of each knee are obtained with the patient standing. Each knee is flexed until the tibial plateau is horizontal relative to the

floor, and therefore parallel to the central X-ray beam which is oriented perpendicular to the X-ray film. The degree of flexion varies among individuals due to differences in the angle of inclination of the tibial plateau. The precise inclination is obtained with the aid of fluoroscopy. With the heel fixed, the foot is internally or externally rotated until the tibial spines appear centrally placed relative to the femoral notch. A foot map may be used to facilitate joint repositioning at successive visits. Patients are provided with hand supports to ensure their stability.

X-ray beam alignment

With a focus to film distance of 100 cm, the X-ray beam, must be horizontal to the floor, perpendicular to the film, and aligned with the center of the joint.

Radiographic magnification

Correction for the effect of radiographic magnification is essential. A metal sphere of known size (5 mm) is taped above the head of the fibula. The dimension of this ball is used to determine the degree of radiographic magnification at the joint. This is only needed if there is variation in knee to film distance between visits.

Published studies may guide the calculation of numbers needed for a structure modifying drug trial[3,12].

Wrist and hand joints

Patient position

Dorsopalmar radiographs of the wrist and hand are obtained with the fingers held together and in line with the axis of the wrist and forearm, since spreading the fingers may alter joint alignment and lead to an incorrect assessment of joint space loss. A hand map may be used to facilitate precise repositioning at successive visits.

X-ray beam alignment

The tube is positioned at a focus to film distance of 100 cm. The central ray of the X-ray beam is centered vertically at the head of the third metacarpal bone.

Landmarks for measurement

Joint space width, or interbone distance

Joint space narrowing correlates with cartilage thickness in OA[13]. Because cartilage loss in OA is not uniform across the joint[14], minimum joint space width is the appropriate measurement[15].

References

1. Lequesne M. Quantitative measurement of joint space during progression of osteoarthritis: 'chondrometry'. In: Kuettner K.E., Goldberg V., Eds. Osteoarthritic disorders. Rosemont: American Academy of Orthopedic Surgeons 1995;427–444.
2. Conrozier T., Tron A.M., Mathieu P., Vignon E. Quantitative assessment of rarliographic normal and osteoarthritic hip joint space. Osteoarthritis Cart 1995;3Suppl A:81–7.
3. Buckland-Wright J.C. Quantitation of radiographic change. In: Brandt K.D., Lohmander S., Doherty M., Eds Textbook of Osteoarthritis. Oxford: University Press 1997: in press.
4. Fife R., Brandt K., Braunstein E., *et al.* Relationship between arthroscopic evidence of cartilage damage and radiographic evidence of joint space narrowing in early osteoarthritis of the knee. Arthritis Rheum 1991;34:377–82.
5. Lynch J.A., Buckland-Wright J.C., Macfarlane D.G. Precision of joint space width measurement in knee ostcoanhritis from digital Image analysis of high definition macroradiographs. Osteoarthritis Cart 1993;1:209–18.
6. Dieppe P.A. Recommended methodology for assessing the progression of osteoarthritis of the hip and knee joint. Osteoarthritis Cart 1995;3:73–77.
7. Ravaud P., Auleley G., Chastang C., *et al.* Knee joint space width measurement: an experimental study of the influence of radiographic procedure and Joint positioning. Br J Rheumatol 1996;35:761–6.
8. Ravaud P., Graudeau B., Aulelcy G., *et al.* Radiographic assessment of knee osteoarthritis: reproducibility and sensitivity to change. J Rheumatol 1996;23:1756–64.
9. Ravaud P., Chastang C., Auleley G., *et al.* Assessment of joint space width in patients with osteoarthritis of the knee: a comparison of four measuring instruments. J Rheumatol 1996;23:1–15.
10. Buckland-Wright J.C. Protocols for precise radio-anatomical position of the tibiofemoral and patcllofemoral compartment of the knee. Osteoarthritis Cart 1995;3Suppl A:71–80.
11. Buckland-Wright J.C., Macfarlane D.O., Williams S.A., Ward R.J. Accuracy and precision of joint space width measurement in standard and macroradiographs of osteoarthritis knees. Ann Rheum Dis 1995;54:872–880.
12. Mazzuca S., Brandt K.D., Katz B. Is conventional radiography suitable for evaluation of a disease-modifying drug in patients with knee osteoarthritis. Osteoarthritis Cart 1997;5,217–226.
13. Bourke G.J., Daly L.E. McGilvray J. Interpretation and uses of medical statistics. Oxford, Blackwell, 1985;312–4.
14. Buckland-Wright J.C., Macfarlane D.G., Lynch J.A., Jasani M.K., Bradshaw C.R. Joint space width measures cartilage thickness in osteoarthritis of the knee: high resolution plain film and double contrast macroradiographic investigation. Ann Rheum Dis 1995;54:263–268.
15. Thomas R.M., Resnick D., Alazraki N.P., D. Eel D., Greenffeld R. Compartmental evaluation of osteoarthritis of the knee. A comparative study of available diagnostic modalities. Radiology 1975;116:585–594.
16. Lequesne M., Brandt K., Bellamy N., Moskowitz R., Menkes C.J., Pelletier J-P. Guidelines for testing slow acting drugs In OA. Proceedings Vth Joint WHO and ILAR Task Force Meeting. J Rheumatol 1994;21Suppl 41:65–7.

Appendix IV

Magnetic resonance imaging

Charles Peterfy

MRI is a relatively new imaging technique, but its utility for evaluating structural derangements of diarthrodial joints, such as meniscal tears, cruciate ligament ruptures and bone injuries is already well-established in clinical practice. Recent techniques show promise for serial quantification of the volume, thickness, geometry and composition of articular cartilage[1]. These techniques are so new, however, that only a few have been validated cross-sectionally and none has been assessed longitudinally.

Possible uses of MRI

MRI is uniquely suited for monitoring structural changes in OA, for its is capable of directly examining all components of the joint simultaneously. In addition to delineating anatomy, however, MRI shows promise for quantification of compositional and functional parameters of articular tissues.

Measuring cartilage morphology

Fat-suppressed, T-weighted three-dimensional (3D) gradient echo imaging can delineate articular cartilage morphology in the knee[2–6] and fingers[7,8]. In a recent study of 48 knees[4,5], this technique demonstrated a sensitivity of 86% and specificity of 97% for identifying cartilage defects which were visible on arthroscopy. The surface topography of individual cartilage plates as well as contact-areas between opposing articular surfaces can be mapped[9]. Accurate measurement of cartilage thickness requires a spatial resolution better than 10% of that thickness (e.g., 200 μmg in-plane resolution for a 2-mm thick cartilage). This is possible with conventional MRI, but generally beyond what is performed during routine clinical imaging. Considerably less resolution is required to quantify cartilage volume in the knee[3] or the metacarpophalangeal[7]. Validation of the longitudinal reproducibility of cartilage volume measurement and its sensitivity to volume changes will not be available for several years.

Measuring cartilage quality

MRI may be able to probe the composition of articular cartilage. Areas of matrix loss and increased water content in the cartilage may cause focal signal intensity alterations and it may be possible to map the fractional water content of normal and abnormal cartilage[10]. This technique, however, must await further optimization and validation. Other parameters of articular cartilage integrity, such as water diffusivity[11,12], proteoglycan content[11,14], collagen content and organization[14,15] and compressive stiffness, may be measurable in the future. Should these advancements occur, MRI may replace radiography as the standard imaging method.

Evaluating other articular tissues in OA

MRI also provides information about the severity of synovial inflammation, the integrity of intra-articular ligaments and menisci, the status of periarticular muscles and tendons, the presence of subarticular bone marrow edema, and the morphology of the articular bones (including the size, number and location of osteophytes and subchondral cysts)[16,17].

References

1. Peterfy C.G., Genant H.K. Emerging applications of magnetic resonance imaging for evaluating the articular cartilage. Radiol Clin N Am 1996;34:195–213.
2. Peterfy C.G., Majumdar S., Lang P., van Dijke C.F., Sack K., Genant H. MR imaging of the arthritic knee: improved discrimination of cartilage, synovium and effusion with pulsed saturation transfer and fat-suppressed T1-weighted sequences. Radiology 1994;191:413–9.
3. Peterfy C.G., van Dijke C.F., Janzen D.L., Gluer C., Namba R. Majumdar S., Lang P., Genant H.K. Quantification of articular cartilage in the knee by pulsed saturation transfer and fat-suppressed MRI: optimization and validation. Radiology 1994;192:485–91.
4. Recht M.P., Pirraino D.W., Paletta G.A., Schils J.P., Belhobek G.H. Accuracy of fat-suppressed three-dimension! spoiled gradient-echo FLASH MR imaging in the detection of patellofemoral articular cartilage abnormalities. Radiology 1996;198:209–12.
5. Disler D.G., McCauley T.R., Kelman C.G., Fuchs M.C., Ratner L.M., Wirth C.R., Hospodar P.P. Fat-suppressed three-dimensional spoiled gradient-echo MR imaging of hyaline cartilage defects in the knee: comparison with standard MR imaging and arthroscopy. AJR 1996;167:127–32.
6. Recht M.P., Kramer J., Marcelis S., Pathria M., Trudell D., Haghighi P. ,Sartoris D.J., Resnick D. Abnormalities of articular cartilage in the knee: analysis of available MR techniques. Radiology 1993;187:473–8.
7. Peterfy C.G., van Dijke C.F., Lu Y. Nguyen A., Connick T, Kneeland B., Tirman P.F.J., Lang P., Dent S., Genant H.K. Quantification of articular cartilage in the metacarpophalangeal joints of the hand: accuracy and precision of 3D MR imaging. AJR 1995;165:371–5.
8. Robson M., Hodgson R., Herrod N., Tyler J., Hall L. A combined analysis and magnetic resonance imaging technique for computerized automatic measurement of cartilage thickness in the distal interphalangeal joint. Magnetic Resonance Imag 1995;13:709–18.
9. Ateshian G.A., Cohen Z.A., Kwak S.D., Wang V., Kelkar R., Raimondo R., Feldman F., Miller T.R., Mun I.K., Bigliani L.U., Mow V.C., Peterfy C.G. Determination of an in situ contact areas in diarthroidial joints by MRI. International Mechanical Engineering Congress and Exposition. San Francisco, CA, November: 1995.
10. Selby K., Peterfy C.G., Cohen Z.A., Ateshian G.A., Mow V.C., Roos M., Wong S., Newitt D.C., van Dijke C.F., Wendland M., Genant H.K. *In vivo* MR quantification of articular cartilage water content: a potential early indicator of osteoarthritis. Book of Abstracts: Society of Magnetic Resonance 1995. Berkeley: Society of Magnetic Resonance, 1995:204.
11. Burstein D., Gray M.L., Hartman A.L., Gipe R., Foy B.D. Diffusion of small solutes in cartilage as measured by nuclear magnetic resonance (NMR) spectroscopy and imaging. J Orthop Res 1993;11:465–78.
12. Xia Y., Farquhar T., Burton-Wuster N., Ray E., Jelinski L.W. Diffusion and relaxation mapping of cartilage-bone plugs and excised disks using microscopic magnetic resonance imaging. Magn Reson Med 1994;31:273–82.
13. Kusaka Y., Grunder W., Rumpel H., Dannhauer K-H., Gersone K. MR microimaging of articular cartilage and contrast enhancement by manganese ions. Magn Reson Med 1992;24:137–48.
14. Eng J., Ceckler T., Balaban R.S. Quantitative 1 H magnetization transfer imaging *in vivo*. Magn Reson Med 1991;17:304–14.
15. Rubenstein J.D., Kim J.K., Morava-Protzner I., Stanchev P.L., Henkelamn R.M. Effects of collagen

Orientation on MR imaging characteristics of bovine cartilage. Radiology 1993;188:219–26.

16. Peterfy C.G., Genant H.K. Applications of magnetic resonance imaging in arthritis. In W. Koopman, J., ed. Arthritis and Allied Conditions. A Textbook of Rheumatology. Lea and Sebiger, 1996.

17. Resnick D. Internal derangements of joints. In: D. Resnick, ed. Diagnosis of Bone and Joint Disorders. Philadelphia: W.B. Saunders, 1995:3063–3069.

18. Bell R.A. Economics of MRI technology. JMRI 1996;6:10-2519. Peterfy C.G., Roberts T., Genant H.K. Dedicated extremity MRI: an emerging technology. In J.B. Kneeland, ed. Radiol Olin N Am. Philadelphia: W.B. Saunders, 1996.

Appendix V

Methods for collection and storage of body fluid samples

Stefan Lohmander

Most of the published studies on markers have focused on analyzing cartilage-derived products; however, markers of the metabolism of other joint tissues, such as meniscus, synovium and bone should also be considered. In addition, markers of genetic susceptibility, and cellular activity or other processes that might be relevant to the pathogenesis of osteoarthritis should also be given consideration. The following represents an update and summary of the previously published guidelines for sample collection and storage[1].

Sample collection

Three biological fluids are potential sources for markers in OA studies: urine, blood and synovial fluid. Guidelines for collecting these samples should minimize manipulations at the site of collection. While this probably does not present difficulties with urine and blood, some special problems are noted below for synovial fluids. In general, samples should be processed so that they may be frozen at the collection site in small screw-cap tubes designed for storage. Additional manipulations, involving dilution, aliquoting, storage and shipping of collected specimens to laboratories performing the marker assays would be best accomplished by a referral center with appropriate facilities and trained personnel. Due to the possibility of circadian variations in marker levels, care should be taken to collect samples at the same time of the day in longitudinal studies.

Urine

Specimens should be obtained as the second void in the morning; spot sampling would be acceptable; however, time of collection must be recorded. Specimens should be chilled at 4 °C and clarified in a clinical centrifuge within 4 h. Approximately 25 ml should be aliquoted into a 50 ml polypropylene tube and screw cap. The specimen should be clearly labeled and stored frozen (see below).

Blood

Approximately 25 ml of blood should be taken from the antecubital vein after fasting, and collected in either plain, heparin or EDTA tubes. The choice of tubes is dictated by the effect either may have on the marker assays eventually chosen. For example, some heparin samples may contain interfering substances in assays for carbohydrate epitopes on chondroitin sulfate or keratan sulfate. The samples should be kept at 4 °C until plasma (or serum) can be prepared by centrifugation in a clinical centrifuge, preferably within 4 h. The clarified plasma (or serum) should be aliquoted into 'Eppendorf type' tubes (1 ml per tube). The tubes should be clearly labeled and stored frozen (see below). Although the collection of serum may be simpler, it was argued that plasma samples could be preferred for some marker assays, and may also be a source of DNA for analysis of genetic susceptibility. If analysis of genetic material is planned as a specific target, preparation and frozen storage of buffy coat is recommended.

Synovial fluid

Synovial fluid should, if at all possible, be collected undiluted, i.e. without lavage. In cases without joint swelling and exudate, synovial fluid volumes will be small. Up to 10 aliquots of 1 ml should be distributed into 1.5–2.0 ml 'Eppendorf type' tubes. Any remaining larger volumes can be stored in larger size aliquots. The tubes should contain EDTA in appropriate amounts to prevent fibrin clot formation. The tubes should be suitable for centrifugation in a higher speed centrifuge, such as a microfuge. The higher speeds are required to remove cells and debris from the samples which are frequently very viscous. Samples should be kept at 4 °C and centrifuged within 4 h. Clarified supernatants should be transferred into appropriate sized (2 or 20 ml) polypropylene tubes with screw caps. The specimens should be clearly labeled and stored frozen, preferably at −70 °C, prior to shipment to a referral center. A recommendation for sample centered information that should always be available, to complement the core clinical data, is included (Table I).

Table I.
Sample centered data to be collected with all specimens

Urine
    First or subsequent a.m. void, or other time of 'spot' sample

Serum
    Site of venepuncture
        (if not antecubital vein, where)

Synovial fluid
    Total volume withdrawn
    Lavage used (yes/no) — if yes, volume

For all
    Date and time sample was taken
    Have guidelines for handling the storage been adhered to
        (if no, provide details)
    At what temperature have samples been stored

Referral collection centers

The collection center should have defined protocols for thawing, diluting, aliquoting, coding (consider bar coding), freezing and storing the specimens received. Accompanying clinical and chemical data, required by the clinical protocol and any accessory information, would be encoded into a data bank system. This center would also distribute appropriate sample sets to laboratories conducting the marker assays. Results of the assays would be sent to this center and entered into the data bank. For synovial fluid samples, volumes will often be small, and a minimum set of aliquots could be prepared based upon a 1 ml volume. A measured volume, e.g. 1 ml, should be diluted with 4 volumes of physiological saline supplemented with either EDTA or heparin depending upon the original choice. Aliquots of 250 μl should then be distributed into small volume, coded polypropylene tubes with O-rings and screw caps. This dilution and sampling protocol will yield around 20 identical samples for each original synovial fluid sample. For synovial fluid samples with larger volumes, we recommend preparing at least one such set of 20 identical standards, and then storing the remainder of the 1:4 diluted samples in larger aliquots (5 or 10 ml) in appropriate tubes for long term storage. All storage should be −70 °C.

Freezing and shipping

Freezing and thawing of samples should be minimized, as some markers may loose antigenicity in the process. Storage at −70 °C is preferable if such freezer capabilities are available at the site of sample collection. In this case, the samples can be stored for long periods of time. If this option is not available, samples can be stored at −20 °C in a freezer which does not have an automatic defrost cycle. Samples collected during a week should then be sent on dry ice to a referral collection center.

References

1. Dieppe P., Altman R., Buckwalter J., Felson D., Hascall V., Kuettner K., Lohmander L.S., Peterfy C., Roos H. Standardization of methods used to assess the progression of osteoarthritis of hip and knee. In: Kuettner K., Goldberg V. Eds. Osteoarthritis Disorders. Rosemont: American Academy of Orthopedic Surgeons 1995;481–96.

Appendix 5

Protocols for radiography[*]

J. Christopher Buckland-Wright

Protocol for dorsipalmar radiography of the hand and wrist

Preparation for radiography

1. The X-ray tube is positioned so that the central ray of the X-ray beam is vertical and perpendicular to the film, with a film-to-focus distance of 1 m.

2. A sheet of paper the size of the X-ray film is placed over the film holder.

Radiography

1. Each hand is X-rayed separately.

2. The hand is laid flat on the X-ray film holder with the thumb slightly extended. The fingers are held together and in line with the axis of the wrist and forearm.

3. The center of the wrist and hand is aligned with the center of the X-ray beam, by placing the positioning light of the tube directly over the head of the third metacarpal bone.

4. The radiograph is taken immediately this position is obtained (Fig. 11.9).

5. Following the exposure, the outline of the wrist and hand is drawn on the paper, to facilitate joint repositioning at subsequent visits.

6. The other extremity is X-rayed, following the procedure described above.

[*] This appendix relates to Chapter 11.5.2 ('Quantitation of radiographic change') by J. Christopher Buckland-Wright.

No correction for radiographic magnification is required since the extremities are in almost direct contact with the film.

Protocol for anteroposterior radiography of the tibiofemoral compartment

Preparation for radiography

1. The X-ray tube is positioned so that the central ray of the X-ray beam is horizontal and parallel to the floor, and with a film-to-focus distance set to 1 m.

2. A large sheet of paper, or the back of the patient's X-ray envelope, is placed immediately in front of the film holder and fixed to the floor with adhesive tape.

3. The floor is marked so that the sheet of paper can be repositioned in exactly the same place, relative to the film holder and X-ray tube, for each patient and at each subsequent visit.

4. A metal sphere (5 mm), mounted in a semiradiolucent material (to improve the definition of the margin of the ball), is placed on the head of the fibula of each knee.

Radiography

1. Each knee is X-rayed separately.

2. The center of the joint, defined by the joint space, is aligned with the center of the X-ray beam with the aid of the positioning light of the tube.

3. With the patient standing straight, the back of the heel is placed on the back edge of the sheet of paper, the knee is flexed until the tibial plateau is horizontal and perpendicular to the X-ray film (Fig. 11.10).

4. The precise position of the knee is confirmed visually with the aid of fluoroscopy. The tibial plateau is horizontal when the anterior and posterior margins of the medial compartment are superimposed (Fig. 11.11).

5. With the heel fixed, the foot is internally or externally rotated until the tibial spines appear centrally, placed relative to the femoral notch.

6. The radiograph is taken immediately this position is obtained (Fig. 11.11).

7. Following the exposure, the outline of the foot is drawn on the paper, to facilitate joint repositioning at subsequent visits.

Protocol for axial radiography of the patellofemoral compartment

Preparation for radiography

1. The X-ray tube is positioned so that the X-ray beam is directed vertically downwards and the film-to-focus distance is set to 1.5 m.

2. A large sheet of paper is placed partly under the step and at the front of the patient support (Fig. 11.12), and fixed to the floor with adhesive tape using pre-existing marks. Marks on the floor are used to reposition the sheet of paper, the step, and patient support in exactly the same place, for each patient and at each subsequent visit.

3. For computing radiographic magnification, a metal sphere (5 mm), as described above, is placed on the anterior surface of the knee.

Radiography

1. Each knee is radiographed separately.

2. With the patient standing, the foot of the knee under examination is placed on the sheet of paper, with the front part of the foot under the step. The knee is flexed to 30° from the vertical, and the leg is positioned so that it is aligned in the vertical plane. In this position, the anterior surface of the patella is positioned above and, a little in front of, the toes. The patient's stability is maintained by a support frame (Zimmer or 'walker' frame) and, in this instance, by resting the front of the tibia against the cross-bar of the frame (Fig. 11.12).

3. The radiographic plate is placed on the box or step, positioned below the knee.

4. The tube is positioned vertically above the patellofemoral joint. This may require the tube to be moved to a position above the head of the patient.

5. With the aid of the positioning light of the tube the central ray of the X-ray beam is directed so as to project through the patellofemoral joint space.

6. The radiograph is taken immediately this position is obtained (Fig. 11.13).

7. The outline of the foot is drawn on the paper, to facilitate joint repositioning at subsequent visits.

Protocol for anteroposterior radiography of the hip

Preparation

1. The X-ray tube is positioned so that the central ray of the X-ray beam is horizontal and parallel to the floor, and with a film-to-focus distance set to 1 m.

2. A large sheet of paper, or the back of the patient's X-ray envelope, is placed immediately in front of the film holder and fixed to the floor with adhesive tape using pre-existing marks, for the reasons given above.

3. To identify the position of the femoral head, the skin overlying the femoral pulse (or at a point 2.5 cm distally along the perpendicular bisector of the line joining the pubic symphysis and the anterior superior iliac spine) should be marked. Should this surface mark be located with the patient supine, it will need to be reconfirmed when the patient stands, since the skin often moves between the two positions.

4. A metal sphere (10 mm), as described above, is placed on the skin overlying the greater trochanter.

Radiography

1. Each hip is X-rayed separately.

2. With the patient standing straight, the back of the heels are placed on the back edge of the sheet of paper. The center of the joint under examination, defined by the skin mark over the femoral head, is aligned with the center of the X-ray beam.

3. The feet are internally rotated to between 5° to 10°, so that the inside edge of the big toes touch. The angle subtended between the long axes of the feet should be approximately 15–20 degrees.

4. Care should be taken to ensure that the pelvis is neither rotated nor tilted, and that the anterior superior iliac spines are equidistant from the film placed behind the patient.

5. The radiograph is taken immediately this position is obtained (Fig. 11.14).

6. Following the exposure, the outline of the foot is drawn on the paper, to facilitate joint repositioning at subsequent visits.

Index

Page numbers in *italics* indicate tables or figures.

Abbreviations used in sub-headings: ACR, American College of Rheumatology; CPPD, calcium pyrophosphate dihydrate; DMOAD, disease-modifying osteoarthritis drug; MMP, matrix metalloproteinase; MRI, magnetic resonance imaging; NSAID, nonsteroidal anti-inflammatory drug; TGF-β, transforming growth factor β.